eLearning

Self-directed learning activities that foster independence in nursing practice, collaboration in caring for the public's health, and opportunities for advanced learning. You are limited only by your curiosity.

Web Links provide direct access to relevant web sites, including professional organizations, the government, and health care organizations.

Case Studies allow you to turn theory into practice, on-line, with "no harm done" to you or the patient.

Community Health Nursing eLearning

Karen Saucier Lundy and Sharyn Janes

CHAPTER 1

Web Links

Case Studies

Critical Thinking Activities

Stories from the Field

Back to Chapters

Quick Jump to Chapter:

Select

Community Health Nursing Home

These activities foster the critical thinking that is necessary in the home situation and in thinking "globally."

communitynursing.jbpub.com

Copyright 2000-2001 Jones and Bartlett Publishers
Contact webmaster@jbpub.com

Stories from the Field are anecdotal inspirations, quotes, and humorous and unusual nursing situations that offer insights into community health nursing.

Access to the **eLearning** tools is restricted to students who have purchased this textbook. A unique, one-time-use passcode is included with all new books. If you did not receive a passcode with this book, you may purchase one online at **http://communitynursing.jbpub.com**

COMMUNITY HEALTH NURSING
Caring for the Public's Health

Karen Saucier Lundy, Ph.D., R.N.

ASSOCIATE PROFESSOR
COLLEGE OF NURSING
UNIVERSITY OF SOUTHERN MISSISSIPPI
HATTIESBURG, MISSISSIPPI

Sharyn Janes, Ph.D., R.N., A.C.R.N.

PROFESSOR
COLLEGE OF NURSING
UNIVERSITY OF SOUTHERN MISSISSIPPI
HATTIESBURG, MISSISSIPPI

JONES AND BARTLETT PUBLISHERS
Sudbury, Massachusetts
BOSTON   TORONTO   LONDON   SINGAPORE

World Headquarters
Jones and Bartlett Publishers
40 Tall Pine Drive
Sudbury, MA 01776
978.443.5000
www.jbpub.com
info@jbpub.com

Jones and Bartlett Publishers Canada
2406 Nikanna Road
Mississauga, ON L5C 2W6
CANADA

Jones and Bartlett Publishers International
Barb House, Barb Mews
London W6 7PA
UK

Library of Congress Cataloging-in-Publication Data not available at time of printing
ISBN: 0-7637-0706-6

Production Credits
Chief Executive Officer: Clayton Jones
Chief Operating Officer: Don W. Jones, Jr.
Executive Vice President and Publisher: Tom Manning
V.P., Managing Editor: Judith H. Hauck
V.P., Design and Production: Anne Spencer
V.P., National Sales Manager: Paul Shepardson
V.P., Manufacturing and Inventory Control: Therese Bräuer
Acquisitions Editor: Penny Glynn
Production Editor: Rebecca S. Marks

Associate Editor: Christine Tridente
Editorial Assistant: Thomas Prindle
Developmental Editor: Tom Lochhaas
Marketing Director: Kimberly Brophy
Interior Design: PageMasters and Company
Composition: Graphic World Inc.
Cover Design: Stephanie Torta
Cover Illustrator: Anne Whittenbarger
Printing and Binding: DB Hess
Cover Printing: DB Hess

Photo Credits: Backgrounds: Digital Imagery® copyright 1999 PhotoDisc, Inc.; Page 15: Used with Permission, American Nurses Association Standards of Public Health Nursing Practice, American Nurses Association; Page 15: Used with Permission, Minnesota Department of Health, Division of Community Health Services, Section of Public Health Nursing; Page 54: Courtesy of Caroline Cremo; Page 70: Courtesy of The Mississippi State Department of Health; Page 83: Courtesy of the Visiting Nurse Service of New York; Page 88: Courtesy of the Frontier Nursing Service of Wendover, Kentucky; Pages 87, 91, 406, 408, 414, 551, 866, 882: Courtesy of The Mississippi State Department of Health; Pages 100, 396, 406, 408, 414, 882: Courtesy, Mississippi State Department of Health; Page 150: Courtesy, *The Hattiesburg American,* Hattiesburg Mississippi; Page 350: Used with permission, University of Michigan Press; Page 352: Used with permission of the American Holistic Nurses Association; Page 478: Used with permission of the University of Colorado, Boulder, Department of Journalism; Page 546: Courtesy of American Red Cross; Page 610: Courtesy of National Broadcasting Network; Pages 686, 982, 985, 986: Courtesy of Ruth Berry; Page 694: Used with permission of Blackwell Scientific Publications; Page 756: Courtesy of Dr. B.Y. "Jay" Lee; Page 829: Used with permission American Nurses Association Standards of Gerontological Nursing Practice Health Nursing; Page 836: Courtesy of North Mississippi Medical Center, Tupelo, Mississippi; Page 884: Courtesy of North Mississippi Medical Center, Tupelo, Mississippi; Page 886: Used with permission of the National League for Nursing; Page 911: Used with permission of Mosby Publishing Company; Page 932: Courtesy of Dan Fairchild; Page 953: Used with permission, American Nurses Association Standards of Occupational Health Nursing; Pages 968, 977: Courtesy of University of Southern Mississippi Public Relations Department; Page 988: Courtesy of Second Presbyterian Church, Lexington, Kentucky.

Printed in the United States of America
05 04 03 02 01   10 9 8 7 6 5 4 3 2 1

Dedication

I am honored to dedicate this book to my family and friends who make up my life community and who provided me with the love and commitment needed to see this book come to life. To bring a text of this size and breadth to print consumes time, energy, and focus from many. Special recognition to my husband, Dr. Chris Lundy, who acted as gentle critic and editor and gave me the time and space when I needed it. Thank you for staying the distance with me and making my dream, your dream. For my son, Parker Lundy, who still believes that anything is possible; you are the joy of my existence and my connection to the faculty of wonder. For my father, Marshall Saucier, from whom I learned the value of intellectual curiosity and the importance of the circle of community that gives life meaning. You have always been my inspiration. I am eternally grateful for your love and intellectual presence in my life. And I am most grateful to Marcelle Saucier Stinson, Wayne Saucier, and John Lundy for the encouragement needed to see this to the end. And for being a part of this book in so many ways, I thank Judy Barton and Ann Lanier for their belief in me and being with me through the years, sharing your hearts and your wisdom. A special thanks to Tom Lochhaas, for giving me my first publishing opportunity when I had little to say or to offer in publishing: I am grateful that you had faith in me and that I benefited from your extraordinary editing talents on this text as well. It was a fitting completion of our publishing journey together over the past decade. I am thankful for the good fortune, in the face of extraordinary personal challenges, to benefit from the healing gifts of Nagan Bellare, MD. You helped me find my way back to health, which made it possible for me to complete this text. For the healing environment created by Charlotte McDonnell, RN, BSN, OCN, and your nursing staff and to Dolly Mathis, RN, BSN, and Brad Archer, RN, BSN, you all have been critical to my healing and embody the essence of good nursing care. And to my friend and co-author, Dr. Sharyn Janes, without whom this book would not have happened. Thank you for helping me to believe that anything was possible, even when the rest of the world seemed to suggest otherwise. For your friendship and shared vision of this text, I remain eternally grateful.

Karen Saucier Lundy

This dedication is for all of my family and friends who have encouraged and supported me along the way and who gave me the strength to complete the journey that was the creation of this book. A very special thanks to you my mother, Joan Janes, for always believing in me and helping me to believe in myself and to my daughter, Heather Rakauskas Sherry, for always making me proud of you in every way and for your special contributions to this book. To my son-in-law Cliff Sherry, my sisters Diane Janes and Joan Kilvitis, and my brother and sister-in-law Harry and Lana Janes—thank you for being an endless source of love and encouragement. My siblings are nurses who have provided constant "feedback" and support for this project. Special thanks to Justin, Holly, and Oscee just for being you and loving me. There are three very special friends deserving of mention: First, Dr. Gale Spencer, professor and director of my master's program at SUNY Binghamton, who introduced me to the world of public health. Your friendship and guidance helped shape the early stages of my career. For Evelyn Jenkins, who has been a nurse for more than 50 years and is truly a role model for professional nursing. You taught me that to be a "good" nurse you must care about your clients, your profession, and yourself. Finally Dr. Kay Lundy, my friend and colleague, who has given me both professional and personal opportunities that I could only have imagined in my dreams. We have shared laughter, tears, and most of all the belief in a common dream. You are much more than a friend. You are family.

Sharyn Janes

About the Authors

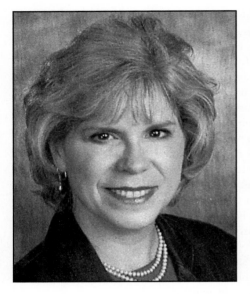

Karen Saucier Lundy, PhD, RN, is currently an Associate Professor at the University of Southern Mississippi College of Nursing in Hattiesburg, Mississippi. She has practiced in community and public health in diverse settings, such as state health departments, migrant health programs, the U.S. Public Health Service, school health, and high-risk maternity and child health. She has also functioned in neonatal intensive care as a staff nurse, clinical instructor, and transport nurse in regional referral medical centers. Dr. Lundy has taught community health at the baccalaureate and master's levels. In addition, Dr. Lundy has taught holistic health, research, maternal child health, and philosophy of science in the doctoral program. She has been responsible for undergraduate and graduate courses in community health nursing and doctoral courses in philosophy of science and qualitative research. Dr. Lundy served as Dean at Delta State University School of Nursing in Cleveland, Mississippi, and was on faculty at the University of Mississippi, Loretta Heights College in Denver, Colorado, and the University of Colorado School of Nursing in Denver. Dr. Lundy has also taught sociology at the University of Colorado in Boulder, including courses in family, gender roles, deviance, and social theory. Her scholarly presentations and publications have been in the areas of community health, philosophy of science, gender role and the family, media, and international health and education in Great Britain, Germany, Jamaica, and Cuba. She holds a BS in nursing from the University of Southern Mississippi College of Nursing, an MS in community health nursing from the University of Colorado School of Nursing in Denver and an MA and PhD in sociology from the University of Colorado in Boulder. Dr. Lundy is the author of *Perspectives in Family and Community Health,* which was named an American Journal of Nursing Book of the Year in 1990.

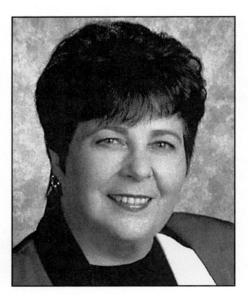

Sharyn Janes, PhD, RN, ACRN, is currently a professor in the University of Southern Mississippi College of Nursing in Hattiesburg, Mississippi, where she teaches community health nursing at the baccalaureate and master's levels. She also teaches health care policy at the doctoral level, international health courses in Cuba and Jamaica, and graduate and undergraduate courses in transcultural nursing. Dr. Janes is the Director of the Cuba Studies Program in the University of Southern Mississippi College of International and Continuing Education. Prior to her tenure at the University of Southern Mississippi, Dr. Janes was an associate professor in the School of Nursing at Florida Agricultural and Mechanical University in Tallahassee, Florida. She earned her BSN at Marywood College, Scranton, Pennsylvania; her MS in community health nursing at the State University of New York at Binghamton; and her PhD in Higher Education at Florida State University, Tallahassee. Dr. Janes has practiced nursing in a variety of community settings, including home health, hospice, and school health and in several acute care settings, including medical-surgical units and emergency departments. She holds certification in HIV/AIDS nursing. Her scholarly presentations and publications are predominantly in the areas of HIV/AIDS education and prevention; cultural issues in nursing education, practice, and research; and international health and education.

Contributors

Barbara Aranda-Naranjo, PhD, RN, ACRN, FAAN
Branch Chief
SPNS/HIV/AIDS Branch
Health Resources and Services Administration
U.S. Department of Health and Human Services
Rockville, Maryland

A. Serdar Atav, PhD
Assistant Professor
Decker School of Nursing
Binghamton University
Binghamton, New York

Susan Scoville Baker, PhD, RN, CS
Associate Professor and Director
Canseco School of Nursing
Texas A&M International University
Loredo, Texas

Joan H. Baldwin, DNSc, RN
Professor
College of Nursing
Brigham Young University
Provo, Utah

Judith A. Barton, PhD, RN
Associate Professor
School of Nursing
University of Colorado Health Sciences Center
Denver, Colorado

Kaye W. Bender, MS, RN, PhD(c), FAAN
Deputy State Health Officer
Mississippi State Department of Health
Jackson, Mississippi

Ruth D. Berry, RN, MSN
Associate Professor
Community Health Nursing/Administration
College of Nursing
University of Kentucky
Parish Nurse, Second Presbyterian Church
Lexington, Kentucky

Lucy Bradley-Springer, PhD, RN, ACRN
Associate Professor and Director
Mountain Plains AIDS Education and Training Center
School of Medicine
University of Colorado Health Sciences Center
Denver, Colorado

Ann Elizabeth Kaiser Brown, MSN, RN
School Nurse Consultant
Natchez, Mississippi

Margaret A. Burkhardt, PhD, RN, CS, HNC
Director
Healing Matters
Beckley, West Virginia

Ronald L. Burr, PhD
Associate Professor
Department of Philosophy and Religion
The University of Southern Mississippi
Hattiesburg, Mississippi

Angeline Bushy, PhD, RN, CS
Bert Fish Endowed Chair
Professor
School of Nursing
University of Central Florida–Daytona Beach
Daytona Beach, Florida

Patricia Butterfield, PhD, RN
Associate Professor
College of Nursing
Montana State University–Bozeman
Bozeman, Montana

Janie B. Butts, DSN, RN
Assistant Professor
College of Nursing
The University of Southern Mississippi
Hattiesburg, Mississippi

Venus Callahan, RNC, MSN, FNP, WHNP
Family Nurse Practitioner
Mississippi State Department of Health
Mississippi Family Health Care Center
Pascagoula, Mississippi

Ann H. Cary, RN, MPH, PhD, A-CCC, FAAN
Professor and Coordinator of Doctoral Program
College of Nursing and Health Science
George Mason University
Fairfax Station, Virginia

Emily Chandler, MS, MDiv, PhD, RN
Coordinator of Psychiatric/Mental Health Nursing Track
Graduate Program in Nursing
MGH Institute of Health Progressions
Boston, Massachusetts

Cynthia O'Neill Conger, PhD, RN
Assistant Clinical Professor
School of Nursing
University of Texas at Austin
Austin, Texas

Virginia Lee Cora, DSN, RN, CS
Adult/Geriatric Nurse Practitioner
Assistant Professor
Division of Geriatrics
School of Medicine
University of Mississippi Medical Center
Jackson, Mississippi

Norma G. Cuellar, DSN, RN
Assistant Dean
College of Nursing
The University of Southern Mississippi
Hattiesburg, Mississippi

Debrynda B. Davey, EdD, RN
Associate Professor
School of Nursing
University of Mississippi Medical Center
Jackson, Mississippi

Valerie M. DeCoux, PhD, RN
Coordinator
Office for Disability Accommodations
The University of Southern Mississippi
Hattiesburg, Mississippi

Susan Oliver Dodds, MSN, RN, CRNP
Family Nurse Practitioner
Private Practice
Marlton, New Jersey

Joseph E. Farmer, RN, MSN
Instructor
College of Nursing
The University of Southern Mississippi–Gulf Park
Long Beach, Mississippi

Janet Gottschalk, DrPH, RN, FAAN
Visiting Professor
Canseco School of Nursing
Texas A&M International University
Laredo, Texas

Gail A. Harkness, DrPH, RN, FAAN
Professor and Chair
Department of Nursing
School of Health and Human Services
University of New Hampshire
Durham, New Hampshire

Sherry Hartman, DrPH, RN
Associate Professor
College of Nursing
The University of Southern Mississippi
Hattiesburg, Mississippi

Jean Haspeslagh, DNS, RN
Associate Professor
The University of Southern Mississippi
Hattiesburg, Mississippi

Peggy "Margaret" Hickman, EdD, RN
Associate Professor
College of Nursing
University of Kentucky
Lexington, Kentucky

Edith L. Hilton, MS, CS, ANP, DSN, CRRN
Assistant Professor
College of Nursing
University of Southern Mississippi
Hattiesburg, Mississippi

Mary H. Huch, PhD, RN, ANP
Professor of Nursing
College of Nursing
The University of Southern Mississippi
Hattiesburg Clinic, P.A.
Hattiesburg, Mississippi

Loretta Sweet Jermott, PhD, RN, FAAN
Associate Professor and Director, Center for Urban
    Health Research
School of Nursing
University of Pennsylvania
Philadelphia, Pennsylvania

Marilyn Givens King, DNSc, RN
Associate Professor
College of Nursing
Medical University of South Carolina
Charleston, South Carolina

Harriet J. Kitzman, PhD, RN
Loretta C. Ford Professor of Nursing
School of Nursing
University of Rochester
Rochester, New York

Anne C. Klijanowicz, MS, PNP, CS
Senior Advanced Practice Nurse, Pediatrics
University of Rochester Medical Center
Rochester, New York

Pat Kurtz, PhD, RN
Assistant Dean
College of Nursing
University of Southern Mississippi
Hattiesburg, Mississippi

Debra K. Lance, RN, MSN
Branch Office Manager
South Mississippi Home Health, Inc.
Hattiesburg, Mississippi

Sarah Steen Lauterbach, MSPH, EdD, RN
Associate Professor
College of Nursing
University of Southern Mississippi
Hattiesburg, Mississippi

**Madeleine Leininger, PhD, RN, LHD, DS,
    CTN, FAAN, FRCNA, LL**
Founder of Transcultural Nursing
Leader of Human Care Research
Adjunct Professor, University of Nebraska Medical Center
    (Omaha) College of Nursing
Professor Emerita, Wayne State University–Detroit
Omaha, Nebraska

Frances R. Martin, PhD, CFNP
Family Nurse Practitioner and Associate Director
Student Health Services
Hattiesburg, Mississippi

Linda G. McDowell, PhD
Director of Grant Projects
Department of Special Education
The University of Southern Mississippi
Hattiesburg, Mississippi

Russell C. McGuire, RN, MSN
Director
Clinical Services
Appalachian Regional Healthcare, Inc.
Hazard, Kentucky

Nancy Milio, PhD, MA, RN, FAPHA, FAAN
Professor of Nursing and Health Policy and Administration
School of Public Health, Nursing
University of North Carolina at Chapel Hill
Chapel Hill, North Carolina

Lindsay Lake Morgan, PhD, RN, GNP
Assistant Professor and Director
O'Connor Office of Rural Health Studies
Decker School of Nursing
Binghamton University
Binghamton, New York

Michelle Cousins Mott, RN, MSN, CRNP
Family Nurse Practitioner
Penn Nursing Network Practices
School of Nursing Center for Urban Health Research
University of Pennsylvania
Philadelphia, Pennsylvania

Carol J. Nyman, CRN, FNP, MPH
Family Nurse Practitioner
U.S. Public Health Service
White Earth Indian Reservation
White Earth, Minnesota

Ruth A. O'Brien, PhD, RN
Associate Professor
School of Nursing
University of Colorado Health Sciences Center
Denver, Colorado

Bonita R. Reinert, PhD, RN
Professor
College of Nursing
University of Southern Mississippi
Hattiesburg, Mississippi

Bonnie Rogers, DrPH, COHN-S, RN, FAAN
Associate Professor and Director
Occupational Health Nursing Program
School of Public Health
University of North Carolina at Chapel Hill
Chapel Hill, North Carolina

Julia B. St. Lawrence, MSN, RN, CNM
Certified Nurse Midwife
Maternal Health Center
Bettendorf, Iowa

Janet St. Lawrence, PhD
Chief of Behavioral Interventions and Research Branch
Division of STD Prevention
National Center for HIV, STD, TB Prevention
Centers for Disease Control and Prevention
Atlanta, Georgia

Marla E. Salmon, ScD, RN, FAAN
Associate Vice President for Nursing Science
Woodruff Health Sciences Center
Dean and Professor
Nell Hodgson Woodruff School of Nursing
Emory University
Atlanta, Georgia

Heather Rakauskas Sherry, MS, PhD(c)
Student Services Policy Specialist
Florida State Board of Community Colleges
Former Legislative Assistant
Florida House of Representatives
Tallahassee, Florida

Jean Shreffler, PhD, RN
Assistant Professor
College of Nursing
Montana State University–Bozeman
Missoula, Montana

Gale A. Spencer, PhD, RN
Associate Professor and Director
Kresge Center for Nursing Research
Decker School of Nursing
Binghamton University
Binghamton, New York

Mary E. Stainton, MS, RN-C, FAAN
Retired President
South Mississippi Home Health, Inc.
Hattiesburg, Mississippi

Linda Beth Tiedje, PhD, RN, MA, FAAN
Adjunct Associate Professor
College of Human Medicine
Department of Epidemiology
Michigan State University
East Lansing, Michigan

Karen B. Utterback, RN, MSN
Vice President of Operations
South Mississippi Home Health, Inc.
Hattiesburg, Mississippi

H. Lorrie Yoos, PhD, CPNP
Associate Professor of Clinical Nursing
School of Nursing
University of Rochester Medical Center
Rochester, New York

Contributors to Chapter Special Features

Margaret M. Aiken, PhD, RN
Sexual Assault Nurse Examiner (SANE)
Memphis Sexual Assault Resource Center
Memphis, Tennessee

Ilene Purvis Bloxsom, BSN, RN
Director
Dale Medical Center Home Health
Ozark, Alabama

Miriam Cabana, MSN, RN
Coordinator of Learning Center
College of Nursing
The University of Southern Mississippi
Hattiesburg, Mississippi
Former Nursing Supervisor
Mississippi State Penitentiary
Parchman, Mississippi

Lynne Cameron, ANP
Skagway Medical Center
Skagway, Alaska

Alvara Leonard Castillo
Assistant Professor of Nursing
Instituto Superior De Ciencias Medicas
President of Havana Chapter of Cuban Nurses Society
Havana, Cuba

Pamela N. Clarke, PhD, MPH, RN
Past President, Association of Community Health Nursing
Educators (ACHNE)
Chair and Professor
Department of Nursing
Idaho State University
Pocatello, Idaho

Betty Dickson
Executive Director and Lobbyist
Mississippi Nurses Association
Jackson, Mississippi

Mary Fisher
Author and AIDS Activist
Washington, DC

Marjaneh Fooladi, PhD, RN
Assistant Professor
College of Nursing
The University of Southern Mississippi
Hattiesburg, Mississippi

Betty Ford
Former First Lady
Founder of the Betty Ford Center
Rancho Mirage, California

Loretta C. Ford, EdD, RN, FAAN
Cofounder, First Nurse Practitioner Program
University of Colorado School of Nursing
Dean and Professor Emerita
Wildwood, Florida

Toni D. Frioux, MS, CNS, ARNP
Chief, Nursing Service
Oklahoma State Department of Health
Oklahoma City, Oklahoma

Sherry Hartman, DrPH, RN
Associate Professor
College of Nursing
The University of Southern Mississippi
Hattiesburg, Mississippi

Jim Jones, BEd, RN
Case Manager and Home Health Nurse
South Mississippi Home Health
Hattiesburg, Mississippi

Carolyn Keil, PhD, RN
Associate Professor
School of Nursing
University of Alaska
Anchorage, Alaska

Felton Keyes, BSN, RN
Staff Nurse
Forrest General Hospital
Hattiesburg, Mississippi

Deborah Konkle-Parker, MSN, RN, FNP, ACRN
Family Nurse Practitioner
Department of Medicine
Division of Infectious Diseases
The University of Mississippi Medical Center
Jackson, Mississippi

Ann Thedford Lanier, PhD
National Science Foundation
Washington, DC

Jerri Laube, PhD, RN, CS, FAAN
Director, Personal Growth Center
Professor Emerita and former Dean
The University of Southern Mississippi
College of Nursing
Hattiesburg, Mississippi

Judith K. Leavitt, MEd, RN, FAAN
Professor of Nursing
School of Nursing
The University of Mississippi Medical Center
Jackson, Mississippi

James A. Lopresti, PhD
Poet
Denver, Colorado

Debendra Manandhar, MPA
Community Development Consultant with NGOs
Kathmandu, Nepal

Lic. Juana Daisy Berdayes Martinez
Associate Dean for Graduate Studies and Research
Julio Trigo School of Nursing
Instituto Superior de Ciencias Medicas
Havana, Cuba

Arlene McFarland, DNS, RN
Family Therapist and Author
Fort Payne, Alabama

Anayda Fernandez Naranjo, MD
Dean
Julio Trigo School of Medical Sciences
Instituto Superior de Ciencias Medicas
Havana, Cuba

Sharon L. Oswald, PhD
Associate Professor of Management
Director of Graduate Management Programs
College of Business
Auburn University
Auburn, Alabama

Regina Hood Posey, MSN, RN
Instructor
The University of Southern Mississippi
College of Nursing
Hattiesburg, Mississippi

Johnny R. Purvis, EdD
Professor and Director of Education Service Center
College of Education and Psychology
The University of Southern Mississippi
Hattiesburg, Mississippi

James Ryan, MSN, RN
Memorial Hospital at Gulfport
Gulfport, Mississippi

Elizabeth A. Simnons
Graduate Student
Auburn University
Auburn, Alabama

Connie Thompson, BSN, RN, ACRN
HIV Case Manager
Delta Region AIDS Education and Training Center
The University of Mississippi Medical Center
Department of Medicine
Division of Infectious Diseases
Jackson, Mississippi

Ntombodidi Muzzen-Sherra (Zodidi) Tshotsho, MCur, DCur
Deputy Director
Child Youth, Women and Mental Health in the National
Directorate: Mental Health and Substance Abuse
Pretoria, South Africa

Jean Watson, PhD, RN, FAAN, HNC
Distinguished Professor of Nursing
Endowed Chair in Caring Science
University of Colorado Health Sciences Center
Denver, Colorado

Anna Frances Z. Wenger, PhD, RN, FAAN
Affiliate Faculty, Neil Hodgson Woodruff School of Nursing
Faith and Health Consortium Coordinator
Interfaith Health Program
Rollins School of Public Health
Emory University
Atlanta, Georgia

Reviewers

Patricia L. Ackerman, RN, PhD
California State University
Division of Nursing
Sacramento, California

Joan H. Baldwin, DNSc, RN
Professor
Brigham Young University
College of Nursing
Provo, Utah

Kaye W. Bender, MS, RN
Deputy Health Officer
Mississippi State Department of Health
Jackson, Mississippi

Ilene Purvis Bloxsom, BSN, RN
Director
Dale Medical Center Home Health
Ozark, Alabama

Sue Boos, RN, MS, CS, ARNP
Fort Hays University
Department of Nursing
Hays, Kansas

Laura Elliott Brower, MS, RN
Vice President of Administration
North Mississippi Medical Center
Tupelo, Mississippi

Donna Darity, MSN, RN
Assistant Professor
Florida Agriculture and Mechanical University
Tallahassee, Florida

Sandra DeBella, RN, EdD
Sonoma State
Division of Nursing
Rohnert Park, California

Ann Dollins, RN, PhD, CNM
Northern Kentucky University
Department of Nursing
Highland Heights, Kentucky

Charlene Douglas, PhD, MPH
George Mason University
College of Nursing and Health Science
Fairfax, Virginia

Donna Gates, EdD, MSN, MSPH, RN
University of Cincinnati
College of Nursing
Cincinnati, Ohio

Ruth Seris Gresley, RN, PhD, MSN
Concordia University
Graduate Program in Nursing
St. Paul, Minnesota

Joan L. Klein, RN, MS
St. Xavier University
Department of Nursing
Chicago, Illinois

Ann Thedford Lanier, PhD
University of Texas at San Antonio
Department of Sociology
San Antonio, Texas

Marilyn Lauria, RN, EdD
Monmouth University
Marjorie K. Unterberg School of Nursing
West Long Branch, New Jersey

Debbie Lindell, RN, CS, MSN
Case Western Reserve University
Francis Payne Bolton School of Nursing
Cleveland, Ohio

Joel Christopher Lundy, EdD
Academic Counselor
Pearl River Community College
Poplarville, Mississippi

Shirley Mason, RN, EdD
University of North Carolina at Chapel Hill
School of Nursing
Chapel Hill, North Carolina

Kathleen Masters, DNS, RN
Instructor
The University of Southern Mississippi
College of Nursing
Hattiesburg, Mississippi

Janette S. McCrory, MSN, RN
Instructor
Delta State University
School of Nursing
Cleveland, Mississippi

Marjorie McCullagh, RN, PhD
North Dakota State University
Department of Nursing
Fargo, North Dakota

Carol O'Neil, RN, PhD
University of Maryland-Baltimore
School of Nursing
Baltimore, Maryland

Lisa Paine, CNM, DrPH, FAAN, FACNM
Boston University
School of Public Health
Boston, Massachusetts

Heather R. Sherry, BA, MS, PhD(c)
Student Services Specialist
Florida State Board of Community Colleges
Former Legislative Analyst
Florida House of Representatives
Tallahassee, Florida

Nancy A. Sowan, RN, PhD
University of Vermont
School of Nursing
Burlington, Vermont

Mary Stewart, MSN, RN, PhD(c)
Assistant Professor
William Carey College
Hattiesburg, Mississippi

Pat Torsella, RN, DNSc
Bloomsburg University
Department of Nursing
Bloomsburg, Pennsylvania

Contents

PART ONE   Community-Focused Nursing Care

PART TWO   Community-Based Nursing Care

PART THREE   Diversity in Community Health Nursing Roles

Foreword

The health of people is a reflection of the communities in which they live, play, work, and learn. Communities shape the lifestyles that people adopt and their likelihood of living safe, fulfilling, and productive lives. For those who seek to understand human health, the community is an important force to understand. For those who wish to improve the health of others, the community is an essential factor in the equation of people's health and well-being.

The relationship between the health of people and their communities lies at the core of nursing's work. As a profession whose hallmark is concern for human health, nursing has had a long history of engagement in the community. Nurses have practiced in this context, have exercised social activism and advocacy for community causes, and are themselves active members of their communities. Many of nursing's greatest leaders have come from the ranks of nurses working in community and public health.

Despite the close relationship between nurses and the community, the advancement of medical technology, the rise of institutions in which people receive care, and the financial systems supporting services have overshadowed the roles that nurses play in the community context. The public perception of nurses is frequently one in which the nurse is seen as a provider of services to people in hospitals. This view, coupled with the fact that the majority of nurses do work in institutional settings, has had a negative impact on the development of specialties within the community—and the education that prepares them for these roles. One indication of this is the relatively small number of outstanding texts available for teaching community health nursing.

Fortunately, community health nursing is now moving into its renaissance. The fastest growing context for nursing services is now the community. And, there is widespread recognition that the challenges facing health care today can only be addressed if early interventions to populations at risk are delivered in the community context. In short, the day of community health nursing has arrived.

This text heralds the arrival of this new era for community health nursing. It does so in a manner that sets it apart from previous works of this type. It is an exciting and innovative collection of important information, ideas, and perspectives that promise to meet the challenge of educating nurses for effective, population-based, community health nursing practice. It is also a text that makes significant connections between theory, practice, and learning, in ways that are grounded in the emerging reality of community health nursing.

There are many important and useful features to this text. First, it has value as a text specifically designed for undergraduate BSN nursing programs. Second, the text is designed to support education that integrates community health nursing across content and specialty practice areas. It can also support individual specialty course work in community health nursing. This is a text that has widespread applicability across types of education and curricular designs.

The contributors to this book are also noteworthy in that they represent some of the very best thinkers in the field. They are practitioners, researchers, educators, policy makers, and innovators in the field. They bring important viewpoints, challenging readers to think beyond conventional views of community health.

Perhaps most important is that this book is a significant and timely contribution to the advancement of the public's health. The theme that ties this work together is one that focuses on the real goal of nursing education and practice: meeting the health needs of people everywhere. This theme is one that recurs throughout the text with great clarity.

The editors of this book are really its architects—they have conceptualized and brought to fruition a wonderfully designed project that serves its mission very well. They had the foresight to see the movement of community health nursing into new importance in the health of people and to help move the field forward through enhancing the education of those practicing in its specialties.

Marla E. Salmon, ScD, RN, FAAN
Associate Vice President for Nursing Science
Woodruff Health Sciences Center
Dean and Professor
Nell Hodgson Woodruff School of Nursing
Emory University
Former Director, The Division of Nursing
U.S. Department of Health and
    Human Services

Preface

Community health nursing has historically responded to changes in health care needs of the population and met those needs in a variety of diverse roles and settings. As we enter the 21st century, the health care needs of the public can seem overwhelming to the beginning nurse. The health care system in the United States has produced technological advancements never thought possible at the beginning of the last century. Public health, along with scientific and technological progress, has resulted in an ever-increasing average life span for Americans while other parts of the world struggle to meet basic health care needs. Greater life expectancy of individuals with chronic and acute conditions has continued to challenge the health care system's ability to provide efficient and quality care for its population. As the population of the United States has become increasingly more diverse, the need for change in community health nursing is imperative; practice must now reflect an awareness of these diverse values and beliefs of populations from the homeless to children with AIDS. Morbidity and mortality statistics reveal significant disparities among population groups, while socioeconomic and cultural factors have led to increased violence and substance abuse. Health care must be provided within the client population's cultural context, whether influenced by age, gender, race, or ethnicity. In this text, we have attempted to represent diversity among our authors, in the selection of chapter content, and in the general visual presentation of the text. By doing so, we hope to have produced a textbook that is more representative of what communities are in the United States—a unified society made up of many different populations and unique health perspectives.

This text is intended to serve as a primary text for undergraduate BSN nursing students throughout the curriculum with an ***emphasis on population-based nursing*** directed toward health promotion and primary prevention in the community. It is both community-based and community-focused, reflecting the current dynamics of the health care system. The Association of Community Health Nursing Educators *Essentials of Baccalaureate Nursing Education for Entry Level Practice in Community/Public Health Nursing (C/PHN)* (2000) guided the conceptual development of chapter selection, structure, and content of the book.

Rising costs and an aging population have both contributed to the shift to a population-based health care system. As Baby Boomers move into their aging years, their rising expectations for a healthy life span have resulted in a shift from episodic, acute care management to a more chronic focus.

Such a change has contributed to population-based outcomes. The community has largely become the setting for chronic disease management and prevention. BSN nurses, to provide care for defined populations in all settings, must have the additional skills and knowledge in such areas as epidemiology and environmental sciences. Nurses will need to demonstrate skills in managed care at both the individual and group level, keeping an ever-vigilant eye on population influenced variables, such as age, gender, and cultural factors.

During the last 30 years of the 20th century, the cost of health care in the United States approached 15% of the gross national product (GNP). No longer just the interests of economists and policy makers, everyone has joined the debate about how to pay for the public's increasing expectations of quality health care at every life stage. More than 40 million U.S. citizens lack adequate health insurance while certain health indicators lag behind those of other comparable advanced countries who are spending far less for health care. The growing economic and health disparity between competing segments of the population has taken on national political significance, as all political parties struggle to find acceptable solutions. Health policy is no longer confined to nurses in leadership or government positions. Although nurses have historically remained uninvolved in the policy arena, this too is changing. The impact of federal and state policy on the delivery of community health services cannot be ignored if nurses in the community expect to influence the delivery of appropriate services to the population. This text provides chapters on economics, managed care, and health policy by prominent nurse scholars who help beginning nurses understand how the knowledge of these often abstract forces can be used in everyday clinical practice.

With the *technological explosion* of the past decade, advances in digital technology have increased applications in telehealth, bringing together health providers and clients without regard to geographical proximity. The community health nurse of the 21st century must use computer technology as the public health nurse of the 18th century used quill and ink. With faster and more current data access in community and acute care settings, new dimensions are emerging in client assessment and intervention. This text is the first community health nursing text to include a chapter on nursing informatics in the community.

With advances in information technology and global travel, global health issues create challenges for all nurses, not just those who work in international settings. With the global community becoming smaller with every passing day, the spread of disease as well as health information occurs in *hours* rather than the *years* of the past. These dramatic risks have created the need for different approaches for the community health nurse. Opportunities are vast for nurses in global health, and inaccessible populations throughout the world can now be reached through the advent of telehealth and telecommunications.

The passive health consumer of yesterday has given way to the well-informed, fully participating client of today. With almost total access to information, which until recently has been available only to health professionals and scientists, individuals can participate as full partners in their care decisions and in the management of their health, which has raised expectations of care outcomes for clients and nurses. Through the almost phenomenal proliferation of the World Wide Web, most individuals can access unlimited information about health and health choices. This has greatly increased the power of consumer groups in health and has resulted in greater demands for services and access. The nurse in the community setting will have even greater responsibilities in the educator role as community populations demand the most current information and become more assertive about securing services.

The increased interest in the use of complementary and alternative, non-Western health practices among Americans to enhance health, healing, and a more holistic sense of well-being continues to influence the health care system. Nurses in the community are often confronted with unfamiliar health practices that may or may not have a research basis for use. Attempts to legitimatize many unconventional approaches are occurring at research medical centers and through the federal government. A greater interest in the spiritual aspects of health is part of the movement among health care consumers for more emphasis on the subjective experience of health. With greater awareness of health information and greater participation in alternative health practices, community health nurses must be more prepared to understand these revolutionary changes. Nurses in the community are in an ideal position to help families and populations navigate through these uncharted and unfamiliar areas, making ethically sound and informed decisions. This text includes a chapter on complementary holistic health to prepare the nurse for these challenges, *breaking new ground for community health nursing textbooks.*

With the extension of life through technology and improved living conditions, *end-of-life issues have changed dramatically as well.* The traditional approaches to caring for the dying are no longer as acceptable to clients accustomed to having more control in health care decisions. More clients and families are electing to die at home with hospice services and nurses as part of this team approach to a more dignified and humane end of life. In recognition of these needs, this text includes an *extended section on hospice* in the chapter on home visiting and home health nursing.

This text features a unique collaborative model of chapter authorship. Nursing education is moving to integrate a more collaborative and interdisciplinary practice in the curriculum at the undergraduate level. The BSN nurse will take the leadership role in such coordinated care in an increasingly complex health care system. Although most of our authors are community health nurse specialists, we also use other specialists in chapters that benefit from diverse perspectives. We believe that by securing well-known authors from nursing and other community health–related fields, we present a strong text and support our ideology of a more integrated approach to community health nursing. The inclusion of clinical practitioners as authors further provides a clinical authenticity that is often missing from nursing textbooks. A further strength of this text was in our review process. In addition to the traditional review process by community health nurse authors and faculty, we included nurses in other specialties; student nurses at all levels, including RN to BSN students; and beginning practicing nurses and experienced nurses in community health practice. These reviews were extremely enlightening, and we believe that through such an extensive and diverse group of reviewers, the text is more accessible for a broader section of nursing students and the final version of the text is more grounded in current practice.

Change has always been a certainty in the U.S. health care system. These changes present community health nurses with unlimited opportunities to influence the public's health. It is up to the student nurses of today to fully realize such possibilities. Nurses of the future must be in partnership with the health care system, which requires a broad understanding of community structure and process. The need for a commitment to lifelong learning and critical thinking skills emerges as critical for the nurse who will be successful in the challenging nursing roles of the future. We challenge faculty and students to use this text as the basis for their future professional practice, whatever the setting or role.

Organization

The book is organized into 3 parts with 8 units and 42 chapters and is designed to be used throughout the undergraduate nursing curricula, as well as in the traditional community health nursing theory and clinical courses. The central focus of the 5 units and 29 chapters in **Part I** is community-/population-focused health care. **Unit I** provides an overview of community and public health, which includes the history of public and community health nursing, the Lundy-Barton Model for community and population health assessment and intervention, the science of epidemiology, and an examination of the current U.S. health care system.

Unit II addresses the major influences on the health of a community. Health care and nursing are viewed through the lenses of economics, ethics, and culture. Environmental influences on community health are explored and discussed. The influence of politics and the law on health care delivery is described and examined, along with the role of the community/public health nurse in the formation of health policy.

Unit III presents the nursing care of communities and populations. The increasing use of complementary therapies as well as innovative health-promotion and health education concepts and models are discussed within the context of public health nursing. Nursing informatics, along with the use of technology in the practice of community and public health nursing, is introduced and examined. A definition of groups and an explanation of group process assists the new community health nurse in working with groups in the local community. World health issues are examined, and the global initiative of primary care as delineated by the Declaration of Alma Ata is explored. A unique and interesting feature of this chapter includes essays on the health care systems of five developing nations: Cuba, the Czech Republic, Iran, Nepal, and South Africa.

Common community health problems provide the focus for **Unit IV.** Communicable diseases, including sexually transmitted diseases and HIV/AIDS, are examined from a global public health perspective. Both violence, as the number one public health problem in the United States, and substance abuse are addressed within both family and community nursing frameworks. Chronic health problems in the community are examined, and examples of population-focused nursing interventions are provided. Disaster preparedness and population-focused interventions are addressed as essential components of public health nursing practice.

Unit V presents an overview of vulnerability, including social, economic, cultural, and political factors. Specific needs of homeless and migrant populations, pregnant teens, and people living with disabilities are addressed in both rural and urban settings.

Part II contains two units and eight chapters with a focus on community-based nursing care. This part of the book can be used to supplement learning throughout nursing curricula. The emphasis is on the health care of families and individuals as they move between acute care and community settings. **Unit VI** is focused on the foundations of family care and nursing interventions for both healthy and unhealthy families, whereas the chapters in **Unit VII** address the health issues specific to women, men, children, and elders, as well as mental health issues in the community.

Part III provides a view of the diversity in community health nursing roles and functions. The six chapters in this unit describe the rapidly changing and constantly evolving functions of nurses in many community settings, including public health departments, homes, schools, and workplaces. Advanced practice roles for nurses working with populations are explored. Health ministries have appeared in recent years as a method of delivering health care to faith communities using a spiritual framework. The successful role of nurses within this framework is examined.

Pedagogy

The chapters are organized to facilitate faculty use and enhance student learning. Most chapters contain the following:

- *An outline of chapter content and a list of questions to be considered in the chapter*

- *Key terms*
- *Research briefs*
- *Case studies*
- *Short original essays, interviews, or quotes from well-known persons representing diverse views relevant to the chapter focus*
- *Poems, quotes, and other featured boxed material which enhance learning of chapter content*
- Healthy People 2010 *Objectives*
- *FYI boxes containing interesting facts*
- *A web icon at the end of every chapter, directing the reader to the accompanying web site (http://communitynursing.jbpub.com) for more information about topics covered in the chapter*
- *Critical thinking activities*
- *Carefully selected photographs and graphics to enhance reading and understanding of chapter content*
- *A reference list*

Teaching Support

An Instructor's Manual is available to supplement the teaching aids already provided by the chapter features in the text. The Instructor's Manual is an integrated package of teaching and learning tools that enhances teaching effectiveness. The Instructor's Manual also provides non–community health instructors with specific directions and ample clinical examples of how to make the community-based portion of the text in Unit II relevant to their content areas in the curriculum. In addition, there is a web site that provides regular updates, student and faculty resources, web links, in-depth and current material for further inquiry for each chapter, a sample course syllabus, a testbank, and PowerPoint presentation outlines for each chapter and communication with text authors.

Available to accompany this text is *Hospital to Home: A Pocket Guide*. The pocket guide serves as a convenient reference for nurses assisting clients with the transition from hospital to home.

Acknowledgments

Many people have contributed to the development and completion of this book. The contributing chapter authors have honored us with their contributions to this text and have enriched our lives through our interactions with them. We thank them for making this book come to life. The ideas and eventual structure of this text have evolved over many conversations and interactions with faculty, colleagues, and students over many years. We thank those who have inspired us and given us the hope and confidence that the time was right for such a text. We remain in debt to the following people for their encouragement and belief in seeing us through this project with their professional support: Lenell Ford,

Dr. Gerry Cadenhead, and the University of Southern Mississippi College of Nursing faculty and students. And for Jones and Bartlett Publishers who believed in the importance of this project, especially Tom Lochhaas, for his insights, which go far beyond the critical eye of a manuscript editor—you saved us in so many ways, our debt is immeasurable; Amy Austin and John Danielowich, for their early work on the book; Christine Tridente, for contributions during the last critical stages of manuscript completion; Dr. Penny Glynn, for her insights and valuable critical evaluation of the entire manuscript; and Rebecca Marks for her determination and production expertise. For those who participated in the critical review of this text, we thank them for their interest, enthusiasm, and courage to produce candid, detailed evaluations of this text throughout the many stages of development: Kaye Bender; Dr. Joan Baldwin; Brigham Young University faculty and students; University of Southern Mississippi undergraduate and graduate students in community health nursing; Juanita Mikell and John Hodnett, for their extraordinary reviews and constructive suggestions; Dr. Judith A. Barton; Dr. Chris Lundy; Dr. Arlene McFarland; and Dr. Jerri Laube for the extra attention to context and detail.

We honor and acknowledge the work of our colleague and friend, Dr. Sherry Hartman, who contributed her energy and passion during the early stages of this text.

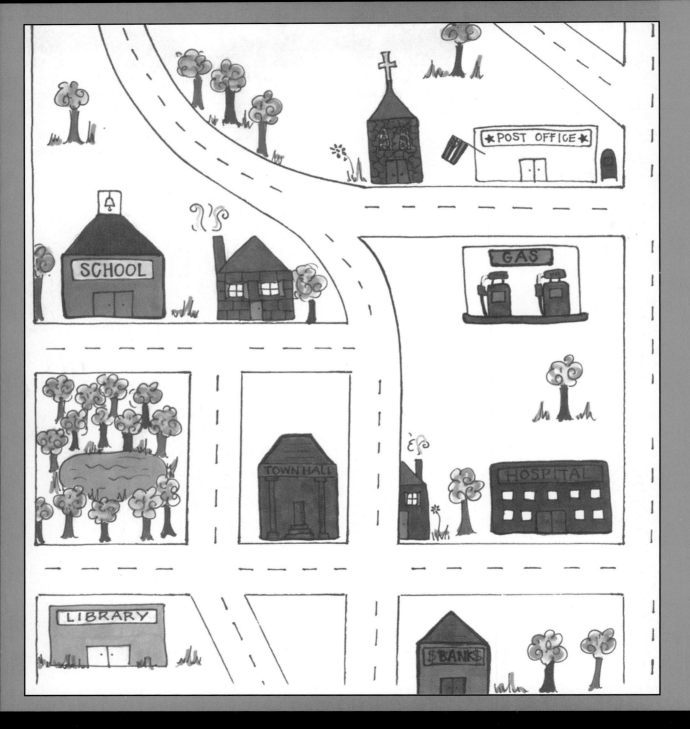

PART ONE

Community-Focused Nursing Care

What does it mean to take care of a community? Community-focused nursing care is often difficult to define and even more difficult to practice. Baccalaureate nurses are educated to practice nursing in all health care settings. Community health nurses care for populations. Since the late 1800s, professional public health nurses have cared for communities. Those communities have changed over time, and the practice of community health nursing has changed as well. Community health nursing has evolved into a complex, multifaceted nursing specialty that is constantly challenged by rapidly changing delivery systems. While reading about the history of community and public health nursing, both similarities and differences in today's community health nursing practice will emerge. Community health nursing, which evolved from public health nursing and is accountable to the public for meeting the population's health care needs, has responded to changes in society to include the care of such diverse populations as school children, women with HIV/AIDS (human immunodeficiency virus/acquired immunodeficiency syndrome), and the homeless. Part One introduces the student to the world of the community health nurse: the focus, the settings, and the historical issues relevant to today's community health practice. As a broadly based specialty, community health nursing practice is more affected by structural changes in society than are other nursing specialties. The community health nurse must be aware of the health care system, social trends, economics, and culture to deliver effective care to the public. Part One assists the student in understanding the uniqueness of community health nursing and the structural influences that must be considered when delivering effective care for an entire community.

Unit I
The Context

Chapter 1
Opening the Door to Health Care in the Community

Karen Saucier Lundy, Sharyn Janes, and Sherry Hartman

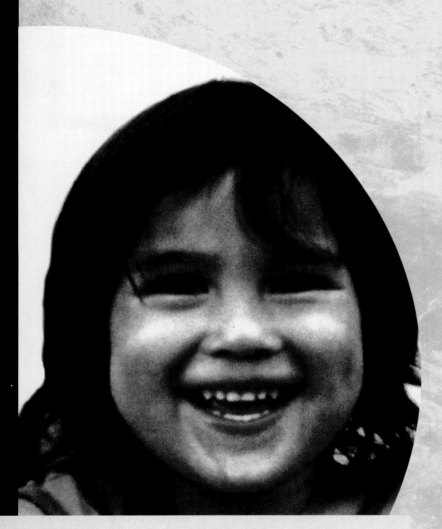

Money would be better spent in maintaining health in infancy and childhood than in building hospitals to cure diseases.

Florence Nightingale, 1894

CHAPTER FOCUS

A Closer Look at Health
- Historical Insights

Nursing in the New Millennium
- Educating Nurses for Community Health Nursing Practice

Community-Based, Population-Focused, and Community-Focused Care
- Communities and Populations
- Acute Care Versus Community-Based Nursing
- Public Health Nursing

Reform and Reinvention of Systems of Care
- Nursing's Agenda for Health Care Reform
- Managed Care and the Future of Nursing

Back to the Future: From Hospital to Community, from Cure to Prevention
- Home Health Care
- Cure and Prevention: Can We Really Do It All?
- Benefits Versus Costs
- Health People 2010: Goals for the Nation
- Core Functions of Public Health
- Influences on a Community's Health: Culture, Environment, and Ethics

Epidemiology: The Science of Public Health

Measuring a Community's Health: How Do We Know When We Get There?

Healthy People 2010: Priority Areas

QUESTIONS TO CONSIDER

After reading this chapter, answer the following questions:

1. How does the definition of health affect the way we care for populations?
2. How have settings for health care changed in recent decades?
3. What implications does managed care have for nurses?
4. What is health care reform and prevention and how has it influenced the U.S. health care system?
5. What is the significance of Nursing's Agenda for Health Care Reform?
6. What is the role of the Association of Community Health Nursing Educators in shaping baccalaureate community health nursing content?
7. What is Healthy People 2010 and how does it influence the health care system related to a policy of prevention?
8. What are the distinctions of the concepts of community health, population-focused care, and acute care?
9. What is a community and a population?
10. What are the Core Functions of Public Health?
11. What are the three major influences on community health?
12. What is epidemiology?
13. What is the relationship between the natural history of disease and the three levels of prevention?
14. How is a population's health measured?

KEY TERMS

Association of Community Health Nursing Educators (ACHNE)
Care management
Community
Community assessment
Community partnerships
Community-based nursing
Core Functions of Public Health
Culture

Environment
Epidemiology
Essentials of Baccalaureate Nursing Education for Entry Level Community/Public Health Nursing Practice
Ethics
Florence Nightingale
Future of Public Health
Health

Health care policy
Health care reform
Healthy People 2010
Home health care
Managed care
National League for Nursing (NLN)
Natural history of disease
Nursing's Agenda for Health Care Reform
Population

Population-focused nursing
Primary prevention
Public health nursing
Secondary prevention
Tertiary prevention
World Health Organization (WHO)

It is cheaper to promote health than to maintain people in sickness.

Florence Nightingale, 1894

At a recent nursing conference, participants were asked to close their eyes and visualize "a nurse in action." After a few minutes, they were told to open their eyes and asked how many saw a nurse at a client's hospital bedside. The overwhelming majority raised their hands in the affirmative. The speaker was quick to use this exercise to illustrate the need for nurses to change their "vision" of nursing. For many nurses the rapid changes in health care have bypassed how they view nursing. The speaker suggested that in the future, the nurse's place was at the client's side in any setting, not only at the bedside in the hospital. Wherever individuals live, work, play, learn, worship, shop, surf on the Web, or call a hot line, the professional nurse has an opportunity to promote health care for people in communities.

The world of nursing and the nurse's role are always changing, but it is probably safe to say that those who choose nursing at the new millennium are caught in unprecedented currents of change: change in health care and change in nursing. These forces for change have been developing for some time now, engulfing all health care professionals in "shifting sands" in their practice. In response to new demands, new opportunities, new

A CONVERSATION WITH...

Nursing's story is a magnificent epic of service to mankind. It is about people: how they are born, and live and die; in health and in sickness; in joy and in sorrow. Its mission is the translation of knowledge into human service.

Nursing is compassionate concern for human beings. It is the heart that understands and the hand that soothes. It is the intellect that synthesizes many learnings into meaningful administrations.

For students of nursing the future is a rich repository of far-flung opportunities around this planet and toward the further reaches of man's explorations of new worlds and new ideas. Theirs is the promise of deep satisfaction in a field long dedicated to serving the health needs of people.

—Professor Martha Rogers, PhD
The Education Violet, June 1966,
New York University.

possibilities, and a complex health care environment, current nursing students are in a curriculum that their predecessors might not recognize. The **National League for Nursing (NLN),** which nationally accredits nursing programs that meet the highest standards of excellence, has developed its "Vision for Nursing Education" (Box 1-1) based on these dramatic changes to a community-based environment. Even if the world around us appears to remain chaotic and complex, as some suggest, the nursing ideals and commitments will fulfill the promise of the dreams that bring most nurses to the profession. The American

BOX 1-1 A VISION FOR NURSING EDUCATION

Nursing's vision for a health care system that ensures access, quality, and cost containment through a new approach to the delivery of care is within reach. The nursing education system required by that new approach must move quickly to provide adequate numbers of appropriately prepared nurses.

Successful implementation of nursing's approach to health care delivery requires the following:

- Significant increases in the numbers of advanced nurse practitioners prepared to provide primary health care to communities and primary care services in group and interdisciplinary practice

- A shift in emphasis for all nursing education programs to ensure that all nurses—whatever their basic and graduate education and wherever their basic and graduate education and wherever they choose to practice—are prepared to function in a community-based, community-focused health care system

- An increase in the numbers of community health nursing centers and their increased utilization as model clinical sites for nursing students

- A shift in emphasis for nursing research and an increase in the numbers of studies concerned with health promotion and disease prevention at the aggregate and community levels

- Targeted national initiatives to recruit and retain nurse providers, faculty, administrators, and researchers from diverse racial, cultural, and ethnic backgrounds

Source: A vision for nursing eduction. New York: National League for Nursing, 1993.

Association of Colleges of Nursing (AACN), which sets standards for and promotes bachelor of science in nursing (BSN) and higher degree education, sets forth a position that "preparation for the entry level professional nurse now requires a greater orientation to community-based primary health care, and emphasis on health promotion, maintenance and cost-effective coordinated care that responds to the needs of increasing culturally diverse groups and underserved populations in all settings" (AACN, 1993, p. 1).

With the headlines often heralding hospital closures, mergers, and downsizing, where does that leave the nurse? What is the story behind where we are today? What kind of job will there be for you after graduation? When you graduate from nursing school, you will join more than 2.2 million registered nurses (RNs) in the United States. The good news is that the federal government predicts that RN will be one of the top 10 careers, with the most job openings in the year 2006 (Bureau of Labor Statistics, 1998).

The Division of Nursing of the Bureau of Health Professions in the Health Resources and Services Administration (HRSA), a division of the Department of Health and Human Services, released its national survey of registered nurses in the United States in 1997. Although nearly 60% of RNs still work in hospitals, that percentage has dropped more than 6 points since 1992. The greatest changes have been an increase in the percentage of nurses who work in community-ambulatory care, home health, public health, and other community-based settings (National Sample Survey of Registered Nurses, 1997). McKinnon (1997) predicts that by the year 2002, fewer than half of all nurses will work in hospitals. Dramatic changes in the way health care is delivered have led to the discharge of sicker clients to their homes. As managed care continues to result in fewer hospitalizations, nurses in acute care settings are facing assignments on a daily basis to different units and in diverse settings, including outpatient, home health, and other community-based agencies housed in or associated with their own facility. As the client census (the number of occupied beds in a hospital on a daily basis) fluctuates, nurses must be flexible, willing, and competent in multiple settings. So no matter where you ultimately choose to work as a nurse, community health will be an influence on you and on your clients' lives.

According to Gebbie (1997), the U.S. vision of public health is that of healthy people *in healthy communities* because individual health can be fully realized only if the community itself is in good shape as well. For a closer look at how much our health is influenced by public health measures, see "A Personal Look at Public Health."

In this chapter the history, context, and setting for nursing practice are discussed, as well as some of the current controversies and confusions specific to the "new" move to "the client's side" in the community. So many things influence health: In this century we continue to find out through research how much in the environment, in our own behavior, and in the kind of health care we deliver affects whether we are healthy or ill. Why some people get sick and some people don't has intrigued health care providers for centuries. This chapter introduces health as a concept, presents the historical insights we have learned, and reveals what we can expect nursing and health care to look like in the new millennium. Sometimes, the ways in which we use terms can confuse and obscure the focus of community and public health nursing. In this chapter the terms related to community, population, and nursing roles are discussed in the context of health care delivery. The ways in which a population's health is determined are introduced as well as concepts related to disease and illness prevention and health promotion.

A Closer Look at Health

• •

We hear much of "contagion and infection" in disease. May we not also come to make health contagious and infectious?
Florence Nightingale, 1890

• •

Before we can talk in more detail about the U.S. health care system and nursing roles in today's health care arena, we need an understanding of what "health" is. That seems simple; after all, everyone knows what health is. However, there are many definitions and descriptions of health depending on one's perspective and purpose. The most well-known and widely cited description of health is the **World Health Organization's (WHO)** definition of **health** as "a state of complete physical, mental, and social well-being and not merely the absence of disease or infirmity" (WHO, 1958). When this definition was drafted in 1948, it began a trend that has persisted for more than 50 years to define health more broadly, including social terms in addition to medical terms. In 1986, the WHO definition of health was expanded to include a community concept of health. WHO now defines health as "the extent to which an individual or group is able, on the one hand, to realize aspirations and satisfy needs; and on the other hand, to change or cope with the environment. Health is, therefore, seen as a resource for everyday life, not the objective of living; it is a positive concept emphasizing social and personal resources, as well as physical capacities" (WHO, 1986). An individual or community then must be able to attain and use resources effectively and exhibit a resilience when facing change.

Although WHO's definition of health is the most common, many other definitions also imply a social or community focus. Health has been defined as "a purposeful and integrated method of functioning within an environment" (Hall & Weaver, 1977, p. 7), and "the common attainment of the highest level of physical, mental, and social well-being consistent with available knowledge and resources at a given time and place" (Hanlon & Pickett, 1984). Even Florence Nightingale's definition of health as "not only to be well, but to use well every power that we have"

FYI

A Personal Look at Public Health

The first rays of sunlight peek through your bedroom curtains, accompanied by the fresh air of a new day. You breathe deeply and enjoy the clean air that public health protects by monitoring radiation levels and developing strategies to keep them low.

Rousing the children, you usher them into the bathroom for their showers. You brush your teeth, knowing the water won't make you sick because safe drinking water is the responsibility of public health.

You check your smile in the mirror. You can't remember your last cavity, thanks in part to the fluoride public health helps add to the water. Through similar programs, public health has always sought to promote good health by preventing disease altogether.

The family clambers to the table just as you finish pouring the milk, which is safe to drink because the State Department of Health checks and monitors it from the dairy to the grocery store.

After breakfast, you call your sister—who is pregnant with her first child—and find out her routine doctor's visit went perfectly. Even in the small town where she lives, your sister can visit a local doctor. Public health recognized the need for doctors in rural areas and helped place one there.

Your sister tells you her doctor suggested she visit the county health department and enroll in the Women, Infants, and Children Program, another public health service that ensures children get the proper nutrition to prevent sickness later in life.

You walk outside and guide the children into the car. You buckle their seatbelts without realizing it. Seatbelts have become a habit now, because public health has explained how proper seatbelt use has greatly reduced automobile-related deaths nationwide.

Playmates greet your children at the child care center with yelps of youthful joy. As you watch the children run inside to play, you know they'll stay safe while you're away at work. Public health has licensed the center and made certain the staff knows the proper ways to avoid infectious disease outbreaks that can occur among young children.

And thanks to the immunizations your children have gotten, you know they'll be safe from life-threatening diseases like polio and whooping cough.

In fact, public health has eliminated the deadly smallpox virus worldwide, so your children will never catch it. Maybe your children's children won't have to worry about polio or whooping cough.

You arrive at work and find a flyer for a new exercise program tacked to the bulletin board. You decide to sign up, remembering the public health studies that show you can reduce the risks of chronic disease by staying physically active.

The morning goes well, and you feel good because your company became a smoke-free work place this month. Science shows that tobacco can cause cancer and other ailments in those who use tobacco and among those who breathe second-hand smoke. Public health encourages people and organizations to quit smoking so that all people can live more healthful lives.

Walking to a nearby fast food restaurant for lunch, you pass a bike rider with a sleek, colorful helmet, another example a public health message that can influence healthy behaviors. Inside, you order a hamburger and fries.

You notice the food service license signed by the State Health Officer on the wall, and you know the food is sanitary and free of disease-causing organisms. Still, a State Department of Health public service announcement from TV rings in your head, and you make a mental note to order something with a little less cholesterol next time.

You finish your day at work, pick up the kids, and head to the community park to let the children play. You watch the neighborhood children launch a toy sailboat into the park pond, knowing public health protects lakes and streams from dangerous sewage runoff.

At home, your spouse greets you at the door. You sort the mail and discover a letter from your uncle. He's doing fine after his surgery in the hospital and will head back to the nursing home in 2 days. You know he's getting quality care at both facilities because public health monitors and licenses them to ensure a commitment to quality standards.

Even the ambulance that transported him to the hospital met public health standards for emergency medical services.

After dinner, you put the children to bed and sit to watch the evening news. The anchor details a new coalition dedicated to preventing breast and cervical cancer. A representative of the State Department of Health issues an open invitation for members from all walks of life. You jot down the telephone number and promise yourself you'll call first thing tomorrow.

As you settle into bed, you decide that public health is more than a point-in-time recognition. Without even realizing it, you'll rely on public health every day for an entire lifetime.

Source: Mississippi State Department of Health Annual Report (1997), pp. 2–3.

can be used to describe health for both individuals and communities (Nightingale, 1860).

Many social issues surround the concept of health, making it difficult to limit it to only one definition and perspective. Health is defined by the society and culture in which we live. How individuals, families, and communities perceive what health means is often determined by social, cultural, and economic conditions that limit health choices (Kuss, Proulx-Girouard, Lovitt, Katz, & Kennelly, 1997). To put this another way: Health is highly dependent on where and how we live. A 20-year-old man may consider himself healthy only if he can run up the stairs at work. For an 80-year-old woman, retrieving her own mail at the mailbox may be her idea of health.

• •

[Health is] a way of life, an attitude, an outlook, a history, a context with socio-cultural norms, a belief, and a tradition. Being healthy is managing, negotiating, achieving, growing, becoming, and helping others grow and become. Being and becoming healthy may be parts of a whole perception of health. Becoming healthy is hopefulness, transcending worries, realizing options, advocating, and accessing resources.

A. L. Meleis, 1996

• •

• •

Health [is rather] a modus vivendi enabling imperfect men to achieve a rewarding and not too painful existence while they cope with an imperfect world.

Rene Dubos, 1968

• •

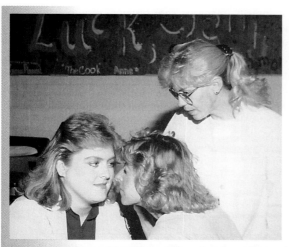

Chapter author, Dr. Karen Saucier Lundy, assists nursing students learning individual assessment skills. Community health nursing skills often involve additional data collection, such as morbidity and mortality statistics.

Nurses differ in their perception of health and are influenced by their own background, age, and experiences. In a study that explored the perceptions of community health nurses about health, the nurses interviewed described health as an "interactive vision" between nurses and client (Leipert, 1996). This vision of health varies with each nurse-client relationship, depending on the values and characteristics of the nurse, the client, and the setting where the interaction occurs. Some of the characteristics that can greatly affect the vision of health are age, culture, social environment, and economic status. Clients in this context include individuals, families, groups, and communities.

Historical Insights

Sickness and suffering have always been a part of human existence. As a result, from the beginning there have been men and women who served as caregivers to the sick and injured. Early on, most care was provided by family members. As human society evolved, moral consciousness became formalized into religious codes, and religious groups assumed more responsibility for the ill. Although efforts were commendable, they were limited because so little was known about disease management or prevention. In chapter 2 the historical dimensions of community health will be explored more fully.

Florence Nightingale is recognized as the founder of modern professional nursing, as well as for developing the first school of nursing at London's St. Thomas' Hospital in 1860. Although her initial efforts focused on preparing nurses to care for the sick in hospitals and infirmaries, she continued throughout her life to promote "well" nursing in the community. Nightingale's directive was to manipulate the patient's environment to allow "nature" to take its course in the healing process.

Through scientific inquiry during the 19th century, causes of the devastating communicable diseases of these earlier centuries began to emerge and professional intervention became possible. During the mid to late 1800s, public health measures were established as the process of contagion between human hosts and their environment became better understood.

Throughout the 20th century medical science grew in leaps and bounds, and the manipulation of "nature" became the drive that resulted in significant medical discoveries and inventions. The United States experienced unprecedented growth in technology and medical science in the 20th century. We learned more about the causes of diseases and generated a broad knowledge base about disease and injury detection, treatment, and prevention. The resulting health care system, which early on was divided into public and private sectors, focused on the diagnosis and treatment of disease in the highly specialized and centralized setting of the hospital. For most individuals, health care was synonymous with the local hospital. During the 20th century, most nurses were employed in hospital settings as skilled caregivers for the acutely ill; nursing education was mostly focused on care of the sick. Nursing students gained experience almost exclusively in hospitals. But even as we were credited worldwide with having the most advanced health technology for treating disease, and while health care spending vastly increased during the 1960s and 1970s, health professionals expressed a growing concern that the health care needs of all citizens were not being met.

In the 1990s, we came to realize that as a society our obligation is to provide an environment in which achievement of good health for all is not only possible but expected. Yet there are population groups, such as the homeless, the elderly, and the poor, whose illnesses and death rates exceed those of the general population and may require additional resources to achieve good health. Health care costs in the United States already amount to more than 14% of the gross domestic product (GDP), more than twice that of other countries that can boast better health statistics.

Americans would probably be willing to live with the high price tag of health care if it made us all healthier than people in other countries (*Consumer Reports,* 1990). However, that is not the case. In the United States, where the health care system is heralded as the most sophisticated in the world, when compared with similar countries such as Great Britain, Germany, or France, we are lagging behind:

- *We have high infant mortality rates relative to other highly developed industrialized nations.*
- *We rank 12th in the world in life expectancy, behind Japan, Italy, France, and the Scandinavian countries.*
- *At least one third of our population has limited access to basic health services and one third of the uninsured are children.*
- *We are the only industrialized nation in the world without guaranteed access to basic health care services.*

Much must be done in this country for many to achieve levels of health that are acceptable and equitable. Many deaths and disabilities could be reduced by environmental improvements and lifestyle changes. A hundred years ago, most deaths were caused by infectious diseases; today the leading causes of death are related to societal influences, lifestyle, and behavioral choices. Progress in technology has created environmental threats to our air, water, and food. Health problems such as addiction and violence have emerged as serious threats to our well-being. "Good

health cannot be achieved without a social concern for ethical, humane decision-making . . . a just and caring society does not withhold health care from its citizens; sickness after all is never something people deserve" (Keck, 1994, pp. 4–5).

Beyond looking at our own country's struggle with internal decisions about health care delivery and connecting it with the broader determinants of health, there has been a concurrent recognition of the global connectedness and importance of concerns for health. As the millennium dawns, the achievement of world health has increasingly become a global expectation. Although nurses are still needed as skilled caregivers who improve the health of the individual, a broader perspective has evolved as population health interventions are realized to be at least equally if not more significant in the attainment of health for all. Solutions to the health problems of populations worldwide now exceed the resources and control of any one individual (McKenzie & Pinger, 1997).

Nursing in the New Millennium

Trossman (1998, p. 1), in *American Nurse,* stated that "in the early part of the next century, hospitals will still be a major place of employment for nurses. The type of work will slowly change, though, as these hospitals become the care zones for the nation's oldest and sickest individuals. At the same time, other settings, such as home health and community based care, will provide increased opportunities for R.N.s." Hospitals are relinquishing their role as the recognized hub of care delivery while health care services continue to increase at home, at work, at play, in schools and churches, online with the World Wide Web through the Internet, and on the telephone. *Who* delivers health care, *what* is provided, and *when* and *where* clients are seen have changed. Cost containment, managed care systems, technology, societal expectations, and politics have all influenced these changes. Clients stay less often in the hospital, and when they do, they stay fewer days. Clients are generally sicker when they are admitted and when they are discharged than they have been in the past. There has not been a significant decrease in client numbers, but rather the settings for care have changed; with this shift, pop-

FYI

Health Care Spending Projected to Double in Decade

Spending for health care in the United States will double over the next decade, reaching $2.1 trillion by the year 2007, according to U.S. government projections. Spending per person will jump from $3,759 in 1996 to $7,100 in 2007. Hospitals will account for only 30% of all health care expenditures by 2007, compared with 35% in 1996, as the trend continues toward more community-based care.

Source: The Wall Street Journal, *September 14, 1998.*

ulation health issues have become more of a focus. There are greater demands on the health care system than ever before, and nurses are needed more than ever. Nurses, as always, continue to meet the needs of clients; we move to care for populations in whatever setting they are found.

In a study conducted by the American Nurses Associations' (ANA) Department of Labor Relations and Workplace Advocacy, nurse executives from acute, home health, extended, and managed care settings reported on the skills seen as most important for the next generation of nurses. Nurses should possess skills of self-reliance, independence, flexibility, and decision making, as well as a "systems-thinking" approach to health care, client education and critical thinking skills, and computer skills. The conclusion of the study was that nurses need to be prepared to provide the four rights of nursing practice: give the right care, in the right setting, at the right time, and at the right cost (Canavan, 1996).

Educating Nurses for Community Health Nursing Practice

The *Essentials of Baccalaureate Nursing Education for Entry Level Community/Public Health Nursing Practice,* a document endorsed by the **Association of Community Health Nursing Educators (ACHNE)** in 2000, provides recommendations regarding the baccalaureate educational content essential for entry level in community health nursing practice. ACHNE is the only organization that represents community health nurse educators throughout the United States and many other parts of the world. To survive as a profession, ACHNE recognizes that nursing

must evolve along with the health care system. Nurses of the future will practice in a more complex health care system that involves both care of individuals outside of hospital settings (community-based care) and care of whole populations (community-focused care). This book uses the ACHNE document as the basis for its content and organization (ACHNE, 2000).

One of the most intriguing and challenging aspects of the health problems that we face in the new millennium is that we already know effective interventions for many diseases and conditions in our society. According to Salmon and Vanderbush (1990), "Never before have we known as much about health as we do now; what we don't know is how to put this knowledge into action" (p. 192). Chapter 3 discusses how early nursing leaders like Florence Nightingale and Lillian Wald discovered that to truly make a difference in people's lives, more—much more—was needed than just their tireless and dedicated individual efforts at the bedside. These women recognized that health policies, and those who make these policies, make health care accessible, available, and appropriate to the needs of the population, thus making the most difference for the largest number of persons in a society.

Community–Based, Population–Focused, and Community–Focused Care

How can a nurse care for an entire community? Don't we have enough to do taking care of the individual client? *Community-*

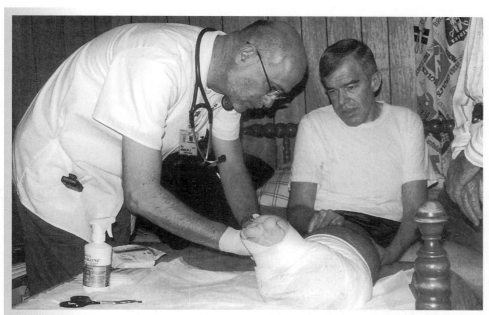

Home health nursing practice is the fastest growing community health nursing role.

based, population- and community-focused, and *personal client care*—what do these phrases actually mean? What does it mean that health care is "moving out" to the community? **Community-based nursing** refers to both the *setting* and the *practice* of the nursing role. The *setting* usually means any kind of health care *other than acute care settings.* The nurse who practices community-based nursing is referred to as a *community health nurse* (CHN). To further complicate our use of terms, a hospital may have both acute care (labor and delivery, coronary care units, emergency care) and community-based health care (outpatient

BOX 1-2 TERMS TO KNOW . . .

A community *is a group of people who share something in common and interact with one another, who may exhibit a commitment with one another and may share a geographic boundary.*

A population *is a group of people who have at least one thing in common and who may or may not interact with each other.*

surgery, day care for children and elders in home health) within its scope.

Communities and Populations

When we think of the word *community,* we may have many pictures in our mind, because the word has a variety of meanings. Andy Griffith lived in the community of Mayberry, and Mr. Rogers' neighborhood is also a community. Most television situation comedies revolve around a community, such as the shows *Seinfeld* or *Friends.* In this text the word **community** is defined as *a group of people who share something in common and interact with one another, who may exhibit a commitment with one another and may share a geographic boundary.* A **population** is defined as *a group of people who have at least one thing in common and who may or may not interact with each other.*

Examples of communities include the following:

- *Lesbians in a communal living setting*
- *The town of Nederland, Colorado*
- *The nursing faculty at the University of West Virginia*
- *The "Devil's Own" neighborhood urban gang*

Examples of populations include the following:

- *People who drink alcohol and drive*
- *Parents with preterm infants*
- *Sexually active teenagers*
- *Nurses who work the night shift*
- *Professional athletes*
- *Foreign-educated RNs*
- *Teenagers with diabetes*

According to Schultz (1994), interaction is essential in a community, whereas members of a population may or may not interact with one another. To put it another way, communities are usually aware of their "communityness," which binds them into a collective entity and "to which they give a name" (Cottrell, 1976, pp. 114–115). Some populations evolve into communities over time; elderly persons who participate in a water aerobics class, for example, may develop into a cohesive community of older women who share other common activities and interests.

The move toward *population-focused health care* is rooted in the realization that the health of individuals and families is closely connected to the health of the communities in which they live (Gebbie, 1997; Hall & Stevens, 1995). Notably, in population-focused health care the environment of the target population (social, cultural, biological) must be considered in the promotion of health (Baldwin, Conger, Abegglen, & Hill, 1998). Population-focused health care is defined as "interventions aimed at disease prevention and health promotion that shape a community's overall profile" (U.S. Department of Health and Human Services/Public Health Service, 1994, p. 27). An example of population-focused health care is a media campaign directed toward the prevention of smoking in teens. The average life span of Americans

RESEARCH BRIEF

Seldes, R., Grisso, J., Pavell, J., Berlin, J., Tan, V., Bowman, B., Kinman, J., Fitzgerald, R. (1999). Predictors of injury among adult recreational in-line skaters: A multicity study. American Journal of Public Health, 89(2), 238–242.

The rising number of injuries caused by in-line skating has resulted from the increased popularity of this sport. An estimated 105,000 in-line skating injuries occurred in 1996, representing a 191% increase from 1993. This research study focused on the population of adults who participate in recreational skating. The researchers interviewed 964 skaters and administered a questionnaire about skating activities, use of safety equipment, procedures, and frequency of skating. In addition, interviewers made observations about the presence of safety equipment. Use of safety gear was generally low. Helmets and elbow, wrist, and knee guards were reportedly used sometimes or nearly never by 96% of those sampled. Eleven percent of those sampled reported injuries, including injuries to the wrist and knee, fractures, and contusions; 65% of the injuries required medical treatment. Only 7% of the injured skaters reported wearing safety gear at the time of the accident. The study concluded that safe skating education programs should recognize this at-risk population and consider specifically targeting more advanced skaters in their campaigns.

increased from 45 years to 75 years during the 20th century, but it is interesting to note that only five of those years are attributable to individual preventive or curative interventions such as cardiac surgery. Twenty-five of the additional years of life have resulted from public health efforts to provide for safe water, effective waste disposal, adequate housing, and other improvements in the overall health of communities (Bunker, Frazier, & Mosteller, 1994).

There are many ways in which nurses are moving into new settings and expanding their application of population-focused skills. Although these nurses are bringing expertise on acute care and technology to community settings, they are often lacking in their knowledge of community dynamics and public health concepts (Gebbie, 1996). If nurses are to continue to be a dynamic part of health care in the future, we must be able to understand the complex and community-based nature of health promotion, illness prevention, recovery from illness and injury, and health restoration (Kurtzman et al., 1980). We need to expand our knowledge and expertise in the care of individuals and our skills in hospital-based clinical management of illness and injury to include care of populations and groups in community settings (Hall & Stevens, 1995). By using our knowledge and experience in medical-surgical, maternal-child, and psychiatric nursing, we can assist individuals, families, and groups to make choices that promote health and wellness (Smith, 1995).

Practicing **population-focused nursing** is obviously not just for community health or public health nurses. All BSN nurses will have the ability to use population-focused skills in any clinical practice, including hospitals, just as community and public health nurses can apply individual client skills in the home or community setting. However, *how those skills are used* will be different. In the acute care setting, where caring for the individual client takes priority, population skills are secondary. In turn, a nurse employed in a school or business setting will use a *population perspective* as the basis of care, which will improve the health of individuals and families (Baldwin, Conger, Abegglen, & Hill, 1998). According to Schultz (1987), in the evolution of nursing concepts, nursing must now extend the definition of client/person to "pluralities of persons" such as families, groups, organizations, and communities.

Acute Care Versus Community-Based Nursing

Let's compare acute care and community-based nursing to more fully understand how these nursing roles differ both in setting and practice focus. In the acute care setting, there is the issue of provider control. Clients are well aware of who is in

FYI

Common Definitions in Community Health Nursing

Community-based nursing refers to both the setting and the practice of the nursing role. Nursing care that occurs in a setting other than acute care; also referred to as *community health nursing* (CHN).

Population- and community-focused care refers to interventions aimed at health promotion and disease prevention that shape a community's overall health status.

Public health nursing is population-focused, community-oriented nursing practice and the dominant responsibility is to the care of the larger community.

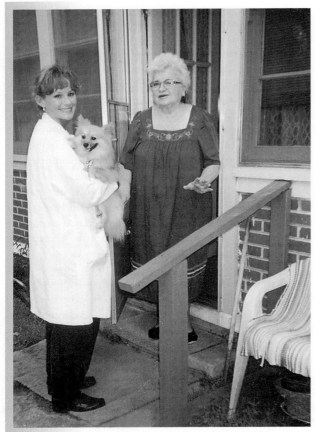

Community nurses work with clients in their homes to improve health. For many elders, pets are considered "family."

tified by their "condition" (e.g., the gallbladder in room 214), are isolated from friends, family, and pets, who are excluded from the "health" care setting. Little individualized care that takes into consideration the client's lifestyle and preferences is given. When the client changes into a hospital gown, the role of client is assumed. Personal items such as medications, glasses, and false teeth are often relinquished, and self-care is limited, with permission often required from nurses for activities taken for granted at home. Many questions are asked, sometimes over and over by different health professionals, and most often these questions are of a very personal and intimate nature. Rarely does the client receive any explanation for why information is needed, for to question is to risk being labeled a "difficult" client—and we know what that means (Armentrout, 1998)! (Refer to Table 1-1 for differences in nursing interventions by setting.) The controlled environment of the acute care setting, however, has many benefits for the nurse:

- *Predictable routine*
- *Maintenance of hospital policy*
- *Predictability of nursing and medical goals*
- *Resource availability, both human and material*
- *Collegial collaboration and consultation*
- *Controlled client compliance with plan of care: the client takes correct medicine and treatment on time*
- *Standardization of care*

The community-based setting is completely different from acute care, especially in home care. Nurses tend to be dependent on clients' willingness to adhere to the plan of care, and clients on their own "turf" act very differently than in the acute care setting. A significant advantage is that the nurse is able to assess environmental conditions, food and other critical resources, lifestyle influences, and social support system, such as friends, family, and pets. Transportation issues, which impact the ability to adhere to medical and nursing goals, often become overriding concerns that are not even considered in the hospital setting. The lack of colleagues to consult about problems and challenges encountered in community settings is a cause of stress among new graduates and nurses who have never worked outside the con-

control in the hospital setting—the health care professional. The client is in a subordinate position to the nurse, who remains the ultimate authority regarding when to go to sleep, what to wear, when and how much to urinate, what kind of diet to eat and when, and whether visitors are allowed. Treatments and interventions are done "to" the client and scheduled at staff and hospital convenience. Clients, who are often iden-

TABLE 1-1	DIFFERENCES IN NURSING INTERVENTIONS BY SETTING	
HEALTH PROBLEM	ACUTE CARE SETTING: HOSPITAL	COMMUNITY-BASED SETTING: HOME HEALTH
Osteoporosis resulting in degenerative hip disease	Treatment Surgery and recovery (total hip replacement)	Teach client how to walk after surgery. Involve family with encouraging activity and flexibility exercises.

trolled environment of the hospital (Armentrout, 1998). Benefits for the community client include the following:

- *Familiar and comfortable environment*
- *Routine that is less determined by the nurse or health professional*
- *Diverse resources, including friends, family, pets, available for support and comfort*
- *Autonomy and choice in health decisions*

Public Health Nursing

The role of the public health nurse is population focused, which means that the dominant responsibility is to the care of the larger community. **Public health nursing** is a nursing specialty that synthesizes public health sciences and nursing theory. You will learn in this text about the public health sciences of epidemiology, ecology, biostatistics, and other subjects that affect *groups* of people, populations, and communities. Early public health nurses often gave direct, hands-on care to clients afflicted with communicable diseases, but their nursing interventions focused on education, mass immunizations, and isolation techniques to control the spread of these diseases in the target population. As the control of these communicable diseases became possible, public health nurses focused on other types of care, such as prenatal education, substance abuse, accident prevention, school health, and workplace health (Buhler-Wilkerson, 1985). *"Public health" in this text refers to the health of the people as a whole* (Neufeldt & Guralnik, 1994, p. 1087). Public health as a specialty in community health nursing still has disease prevention and health promotion as its primary focus (see appendix A and p. 1000). Although all BSN nurses are prepared to deliver population-focused care, for the public health nurse, such care becomes the primary focus of the role. Public health nursing applies nursing theory in a broader context; people are viewed as part of the larger social system. The central mission of public health is to improve the health of *population groups in communities*. Population-based care can be further understood by the identification of *where the point of nursing intervention occurs:* individual-focused, community-focused, or systems-focused (Keller, Strohschein, Lia-Hoagberg, & Schaffer, 1998). Table 1-2 illustrates these interventions and provides examples from practice.

The role of the public health nurse is determined by focus of *practice* rather than *setting*. In a 1996 report titled "Preparing Currently Employed Public Health Nurses for Changes in the Health Care System," Gebbie describes the *context* of public health nursing practice to be influenced by the following, among others:

- *Social forces (e.g., increased number of elders)*
- *Economic changes (e.g., the demand for lower taxes and increased access to health services)*
- *Government changes (e.g., the lack of a coherent health policy at the national level)*
- *Changes in technology and science, health and illness forces (expansion of definition of health, such as teen violence)*
- *Care system changes (increased numbers of uninsured citizens)*

TABLE 1-2	EXAMPLES OF POPULATION-BASED CARE INTERVENTIONS BY LEVEL
Individual focused	Conduct home safety assessment on home visits to families with young children.
Community focused	Provide childhood injury prevention tips to parents of children enrolled in a local day-care center.
System focused	Plan and implement "Safety First" media campaign focusing on childhood safety measures.

Source: Adapted from Minnesota Department of Health, Division of Community Health Services, Section of Public Health Nursing. (1997, October). Public health interventions: Examples from public health nursing. Used with permission.

TABLE 1-3   COMPARISON OF THE COMMUNITY HEALTH NURSE, THE PUBLIC
HEALTH NURSE, AND THE HOME HEALTH NURSE AND FOCUS OF CARE

Caregiver	Home health nurse	Community health nurse	Public health nurse
Primary focus	Individuals and families in the home setting	Individuals and families in community-based setting, such as schools and industry	Communities and populations
Secondary focus	Community	Community	Individuals, families
Intervention	Assess client. Manage treatment plan for client and family: drugs, diet, therapeutics.	Identify community priorities. Mobilize resources. Organize groups. Manage care. Provide primary care.	Provide empowerment, partnerships, and policy strategies. Link with government resources. Use population care management.
Evaluation	Identified individual health indicators; adherence to the plan of care.	Outcomes, statistics Critical path outcomes Outcome studies of care	Statistical indicators Epidemiological descriptive and analytical study outcomes

From this lengthy list one can surmise that public health nursing practice is intrinsically related to social justice philosophy, which refers to the concept of how each member of a given society is allocated his or her fair share of collective burdens and benefits (Turnock, 1997). Entry level for the practice of public health nursing, or population-focused nursing, begins with a baccalaureate degree, with advanced practice specialization at the masters and doctoral levels. Table 1-3 provides a comparison of the focus of care for the community health (community-based) nurse, the public health nurse, and the home health nurse.

Reform and the Reinvention of Systems of Care

Our health care system is but one of the many overlapping and interacting systems created by society. Societies create systems that reflect the commonly held values of that society. This is the realm of policy, politics, and power. **Health care reform** initiatives arise in this realm of competing and conflicting values. Groups who advocate values related to well-being, sustenance, quality of life, equity, fairness, and justice often compete with other values related to economic self-interest. Even when values do not seem to be in conflict, the methods recommended to act on those values often cannot be agreed upon. The capitalistic values of the health care delivery system in the United States have been questioned by health care leaders and policy makers in other countries (Moon, 1993). They often do not understand how we can consider ourselves a highly industrialized and civilized country and not provide basic, essential health care for all. A caring society would not allow individuals (especially children) to be deprived of health care. Many find our "nonsystems" approach to health care confusing.

Indeed, among Americans as well, there are few who would not argue that, although the health-illness system has changed, it still needs improvement. Many of the authors throughout this text make reference to health care reform. Enacted reforms, proposed reforms, and preferred reforms all have actual and possible effects on the populations for which nurses provide care and the conditions under which they provide it. Reform is not new, nor is it controlled; rather it is *episodic,* responding to multiple forces for change. *Reform* implies some major change in the process of the delivery of health care. We often refer to reform as change that originates at the national level but is implemented by the states, by payers, or by provider systems. When change is not a "broad" and "sweeping" reform, it is considered an "incremental change," meaning smaller adjustments occur over time. This is the type of health care reform that occurred during the 1990s.

Historically, there have been numerous reform proposals. Major health care reform was attempted following World War II, in 1948, when President Harry Truman proposed national health insurance. What many thought were the beginnings of broad health coverage were introduced in the 1960s as Medicaid and Medicare. In the 1970s, Senator Edward Kennedy (D-Massachusetts) was one of the major supporters of nationwide reform. Most recently, the presidential campaigns of the early 1990s were marked by health reform issues. Despite various proposals from both political parties, no reform initiatives were passed. Even though there was initial support from diverse stakeholders, many of these stakeholders, such as businesses, physicians, and insurance companies, eventually opposed the reform approaches. In addition, the public was confused and did not recognize the cost and choice consequences to individuals (Starr, 1993).

Nursing's Agenda for Health Care Reform

The failed effort of the 1990s to redesign the American health care system had at least one positive consequence for nursing. In an unprecedented collaboration, more than 75 nursing associations endorsed the document jointly developed by the ANA and the NLN, *Nursing's Agenda for Health Care Reform*. This document was significant in terms of its expression of nursing's values and in furthering an understanding of the profession itself. Values such as health services for all, illness prevention, and wellness were prominent. Many nurses played influential and visible roles during the health care reform attempts. Nursing supported the need for cost containment but wanted assurance of quality of care, reduced barriers to advanced practice nursing, and promotion of nursing care as the link between consumers and the health care system. According to the document, "the cornerstone of nursing's plan for reform is the delivery of primary health care services to households and individuals in convenient, familiar places" (ANA, 1991, p. 9).

Managed Care and the Future of Nursing

Although major health care reform proposals are still debated, significant change at the national level is unlikely in the near future. The controversial issues most debated are expanding federal coverage (access) and controlling costs. Many policy and regulation changes, however, have had significant impact on health care delivery systems and providers. **"Managed care"** and a market approach based on "managed competition" have emerged as our major strategies to control costs. These connected strategies have together transformed the organization and methods of care delivery. **Care management** is a growing practice arena for nurses. Within the managed care environment, there is a focus on care management, which is the attempt to provide more timely and coordinated care for individuals. Individuals move among the following possible states: being well and promoting that state, having acute care needs, needing outpatient surgery, needing follow-up home care, and so on (ANA, 1994).

Health care organizations now see the economic and quality outcome benefits of caring for clients and managing client care over a continuum of possible settings and needs. Traditional health care was episodic, with individuals moving with little connection from one episode of need to the next (often waiting until the need for care was acute) and one facility to another. When care is managed, the term *discharge planning* is now more accurately referred to as *transition planning*. The client does not "leave" the system but merely requires another type of care, including wellness care or health promotion. Clients are followed much more closely both during illness care and with follow-up when well. Care managers can practice from a base in many settings, including the offices of a payer. To more clearly conceptualize this change in thinking, instead of a client being "discharged" from the hospital, more importantly, he or she is being "admitted" back to the community.

When the health care providers in a system have the responsibility for all types of care for the plan's "enrolled population," they have an incentive to coordinate or "manage" that care efficiently. The goal is to provide the best value in the most efficient way to be competitive in the health care market. A market economy for health care delivery dramatically changes health care services and incentives. For nurses who are historically committed to "doing whatever it takes" for their clients, cost consciousness is an unfamiliar and often resisted viewpoint. Nurses in today's health care system must remain informed about the complexities of managed care to sustain professional identity and to assist clients in the navigation through the market systems. The continued growth of managed care as a system for health financing and delivery provides unique challenges and opportunities for nurses, especially those prepared in community health. Nurses remain the only health care professionals who are specifically educated to assess health status and risks, unhealthful lifestyles, and health education needs for clients and families; who provide support and reassurance while caring for present and potential health problems; and who act as advocates for primary and preventive care services. Managed care organizations, as well as all agencies that provide health care services in a managed care environment, have come to value quality and recognize the importance of prevention, wellness, and early intervention. The community health nurse is especially well prepared to provide managed care with the direction needed to focus on providing a full range of quality, cost-effective services in the promotion of a population's health (ANA, 1994). Health care delivery in the context of managed care will be discussed in chapter 6.

. . . .

Money would be better spent in maintaining health in infancy and childhood than in building hospitals to cure diseases.
Florence Nightingale, 1894

. . . .

Back to the Future: From Hospital to Community, from Cure to Prevention

As we have learned from the history of health care, early attempts to improve health, treat disease, and prevent disability occurred primarily in the home. The primary characteristic of the emerging system has been the move back to the community practice setting. Perhaps the major force behind much of the change has been economic, with efforts to contain what many see as the exploding costs of our health care system. One cost-related factor encouraging a population focus has been the movement of clients out of expensive acute care facilities into community settings, where many of their illness needs can be adequately met at a much lower cost. This movement has encouraged the growth of home care, hospice care, outpatient clinics, and outpatient

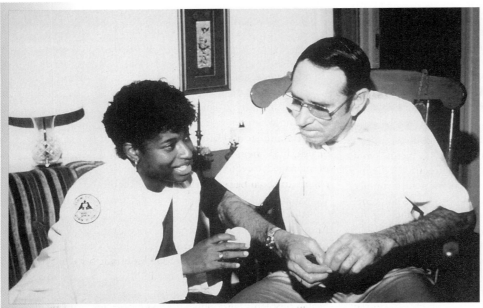

Home health nurses deliver care in the client's home. A goal of home care is to teach clients and their families self-care.

surgeries. Another among the many results of cost-containment efforts has been the recognition of the connection between prevention and keeping populations healthy. Healthy populations have lower morbidity (disease rates) and mortality (death rates) statistics.

· ·

My view, you know, is that the ultimate destination of all nursing is the nursing of the sick in their own homes. . . . I look to the abolition of all hospitals and workhouse infirmaries. But no use to talk about the year 2000.
Florence Nightingale, 1867

· ·

Home Health Care

Home health care is the fastest growing community-based nursing role outside of the acute care setting. This is just one of many roles available in community health and is covered in various chapters in the text. Home health nursing is discussed briefly here as an example of an emerging role that has resulted from changes in the way health care is delivered and paid for. One attempt at major health care cost containment in the early 1980s was the shift from cost reimbursement to prospective payment for hospital care, which means that payment was based on standard disease categories. Because of this change, hospitals could make money if they were efficient in taking care of the clients' problems and could discharge them quicker. Home

health boomed as clients were discharged while still needing nursing care in their homes. Even with recent government attempts to regulate the growth of home health by changing reimbursement patterns, home health continues to grow and present new and challenging opportunities for nursing. In addition to offering community-based practice with individuals and families in the home, some see the role expanding to include practice that addresses the needs of populations of home care clients (Trossman, 1998).

Cure and Prevention: Can We Really Do It All?

Most people spend little time thinking about or planning for their own good health or the community's health. Research tells us that our health is influenced more by our social and biological environment, lifestyle choices, and self-care initiatives than by our inherited traits, yet we continue to pour money into newer and better treatments rather than into learning about what we can do to promote health and prevent illness from the beginning. We are discovering that we have overemphasized cure with a disease-based medical model for health care. As early as 1977, the Centers for Disease Control and Prevention (CDC) reported an analysis of the proportional contributions to mortality in the United States of four "health field elements": lifestyle, human biology, environment, and health care. Their conclusions were that approximately 50% of premature mortality in the United States is due to lifestyle, 20% to human biology, 20% to environment, and only 10% to inadequacies in health care. Seventy percent of the potential for reducing premature mortality lies in the areas of health promotion and disease prevention, but only about 3.5% of the health care dollar is spent in those areas. Therefore, although the health status of a population is related more to the determinants of health than it is to the causes of disease, we have developed a system that pays for illness care rather than a system designed to create the healthiest population possible.

Certainly, people having access to competent and skilled health practitioners and technologies related to the diagnosis and treatment of disease is important, but no more so than having clean water to drink, safe food to eat, meaningful employment with an adequate wage, adequate housing and childcare, a good education, a life free of discrimination, and a safe environment. Such insights are leading to a "reinvention" of health services organizations at all levels—from single facilities organized to serve sick clients to complex networks organized to serve populations of mostly well people (Shortell & Gilles 1995).

Prevention activities and population-focused care are often contrasted with the more immediately "gratifying" and "exciting" acute care. Population-focused care is long term, often behind the scenes, taken for granted, and largely unseen unless something goes amiss. Nurses have always promoted the welfare and health of those in their care. Wolf (1989) contends that nursing has difficulty being visible because much of the work of nursing goes unnoticed. Health care reform and the move to health promotion and illness prevention may provide the opportunity for nursing to shine as a profession.

Despite the "excitement" of acute care, there are many economic, social, and political factors that suggest that the future focus of health care should be on health promotion and disease prevention in a health-based model with a "community orientation" (Proenca, 1998). These areas and such networking have traditionally been the domain of the less visible and less financially supported practice of public health. Mechanic (1998) has pointed out that an alignment of public health with the growing managed care health plans would be a logical and potential benefit to the mission of our public health system. The vision of public health for more than a century has been one of health promotion and disease prevention that depends on a population perspective to activate identification of risks and protective and restorative interventions.

Health care providers in managed care plans are increasingly subject to competition and are evaluated on their successes in improving outcomes for their plan's enrollees. They have become more interested in the population activities and methods long carried out by public health. Acknowledging the economic value of population health promotion and disease prevention activities within the health care marketplace encourages the adoption of these approaches. Thus the focus on community health nursing roles is twofold: a transition in practice setting to the community for many nurses caring for individuals and a renewed and enlarged scope of practice for nurses whose expertise includes population-focused practice.

Nurses have been optimistic about the trends in health care practice and reform. With the increasing impetus for health promotion, nurses seem well poised as a result of their longstanding commitment to and expertise in keeping people healthy. In the past, when nurses have made claims about the benefits of health promotion and disease prevention strategies, the thoughts have been on benefits to the individual, not on any financial benefit or loss. Now we as nurses are beginning to embrace the possibilities of teaming up with a market-driven business world to also realize financial benefits and improved health for populations.

Benefits Versus Costs

Anderson (1997) cautions against a naive understanding of what we take for granted. Indeed, she describes the case of smoking cessation programs, proven to have economic benefits. However, a potential financial loss scenario is possible for preventing cardiopulmonary diseases in middle-aged clients. Prevention may actually increase managed care costs by prolonging a person's life and thus incurring greater costs for the complex medical problems of old age. Similarly, early detection of HIV in at-risk populations should permit early drug treatment to prevent costly AIDS-related illnesses. For a managed care organization, early detection would imply costly antiviral treatment at thousands of

A CONVERSATION WITH...

I am more convinced than ever that the major health problems in this and future decades— chronicity, aging, the personal and public health problems generated by social and economic dislocations, the prevention of illness, and the promotion of healthy communities—are all within the nursing genius to address and ameliorate. These are the very things that we are known for. They are the things we do best and we are the best to do them. . . . I truly believe that we are at a place in nursing that we will never see again. This is our big chance. . . . We cannot wait for anybody to let us do anything . . . . We have more capacity to play in the health care game, we have the obligation to take charge, to endorse professional values and improve health outcomes.

—Melanie C. Dreher, PhD, RN, FAAN
Past President of Sigma Theta Tau International. December 6, 1997, Indianapolis, Indiana, cited in *Reflections* (1998), first quarter, pp. 36–37.

dollars yearly. Nondetection and an early death would actually save money for a private health care provider and increase its profits. Nurses are socialized to value life. Health care companies are in business to make a profit first.

With those warnings, nurses must realize the competing values often at work in the health care arena. Population-focused health promotion strategies also can face ideological, political, and religious differences that cause conflict. Needed sex education to prevent teenage pregnancy has long met with resistance from some groups. Strategies must be developed at the individual and societal levels to bring about change that aligns with all interested parties' goals and needs. In the case of smoking cessation, other community groups could be approached to encourage health promotion interventions and policies. Employers could be motivated to realize the financial gain of less employee illness and fewer work days lost. They would then negotiate for managed care plans that cover health promotion activities.

Healthy People 2010: Goals for the Nation

Even before the more recent reform efforts and regulations encouraged increased use of prevention practices, it became obvious in the 1970s, based on the CDC's study of premature deaths, that health promotion and disease prevention could save lives and perhaps reduce health care costs. In 1980, the federal government issued a set of national health objectives that were evaluated to measure progress in the nation's health goals and health care services. The process proved valuable and was repeated with the issuing of a new set of objectives to guide the 1990s. That plan was titled Healthy People 2000: National Health Promotion and Disease Prevention Objectives.

The process was again repeated, culminating in the release of a *Healthy People 2010* document in October 2000. Two overarching goals, "increase years of healthy life" and "eliminate health disparities," are proposed. Four enabling goals provide support. They are concerned with promoting healthful behav-

HEALTHY PEOPLE 2010

PRIORITY AREAS

Promote Healthy Behaviors
1. Physical activity and fitness
2. Nutrition
3. Tobacco use

Promote Healthy and Safe Communities
4. Educational and community-based programs
5. Environmental health
6. Food safety
7. Injury/violence prevention
8. Occupational safety and health
9. Oral health

Improve Systems for Personal and Public Health
10. Access to quality health care services
    1. Preventive care
    2. Primary care
    3. Emergency services
    4. Long-term care and rehabilitative services

11. Family planning
12. Maternal, infant, and child health
13. Medical product safety
14. Public health infrastructure
15. Health communication

Prevent and Reduce Diseases and Disorders
16. Arthritis, osteoporosis, and chronic back conditions
17. Cancer
18. Diabetes
19. Disability and secondary conditions
20. Heart disease and stroke
21. HIV
22. Immunization and infectious diseases
23. Mental health and mental disorders
24. Respiratory diseases
25. Sexually transmitted diseases
26. Substance abuse

Source: DHHS, 2000.

iors, protecting health, achieving access to quality health care, and strengthening community prevention. These objectives provide a tool that the creators envision for public health policy makers and all policy makers at both state and local levels as well. Meeting these objectives requires that all health care providers move toward a community-based practice or focus. They must move from illness and cure to health promotion and illness prevention.

. . . .

Of all the forms of inequality, injustice in health care is the most shocking and inhumane.

Martin Luther King

. . . .

Core Functions of Public Health

The **Core Functions of Public Health,** as identified in the Institute of Medicine report on *The Future of Public Health* (1988), are assessment, policy development, and assurance. These functions involve assessing the health care needs of the community, supporting the development of comprehensive **health care policy,** and assuring access to and availability of health care services in the community. See appendix A for the detailed Core Functions of Public Health.

The roles for nurses in the delivery of community-based and population-focused health care are reflective of the changing systems and are rooted in the core public health functions. The starting point for determining what nursing interventions are needed to ensure that the core public health functions are carried out and the *Healthy People 2010* objectives are met is the formation of partnerships between nurses and the communities being served. When community members are involved as partners in determining the services needed, planning and implementing interventions, and evaluating outcomes, health care services are seen as more responsive to the needs of the community and are better utilized and supported (Flynn, 1997). **Community partnerships** provide community members with the skills and resources needed to make healthy choices based on community needs. Partnerships also provide a sense of "ownership" to the community members, which then puts the power back into the hands of the people (Kuss et al., 1997). If the community members have an investment in the health services and feel empowered, they will continue working to keep their communities "healthy."

Community assessment is the first of the core public health functions. It involves monitoring the health status of a community to identify existing or potential health problems. Nurses, in partnership with community members and other health care professionals, diagnose and investigate health problems in the community. Through education and empowerment, community partnerships serve to mobilize communities to identify and solve health problems (Gebbie, 1997). For example, a

nurse may conduct an assessment of a neighborhood community and, with community residents, develop strategies to create a more healthful environment for children.

Another essential public health role for nurses is support for the *development of health care policy.* Nurses work at the local, state, national, and international levels to develop and support legislation that promotes the health and well-being of the population. Nurses' roles in policy development can range from something as complex as serving on a committee to draft legislation addressing a specific community health issue to something as simple as voting in a public election.

Assuring access to health care is probably the most complex task of all. The United States spends billions of dollars each year on a health care system that is the most technologically advanced in the world, yet many Americans, including the poor and vulnerable, do not receive the health care services needed to meet their basic needs (Whelan, 1995). Hall and Stevens (1995) describe access to health care as "not only access to professional services but also access to the knowledge, skills, support, safety, and resources that people need to be healthy." Barriers to access to care can be physical, financial, political, social, cultural, educational, or environmental. All nurses educated at the baccalaureate level must have the skills needed to apply the Core Functions of Public Health in any setting that serves the public (Baldwin et al., 1998).

. . . .

Preventable disease should be looked on as a social crime.

Florence Nightingale, 1894

. . . .

Influences on a Community's Health: Culture, Environment, and Ethics

There are so many different things that influence health care that it is difficult to decide which are the most important. For the nurse to isolate any one factor for assessment and intervention with both individuals and communities is like the captain of a ship seeing only the tip of the iceberg and not looking for the real threat to the ship's safety that lies underneath. However, there are three major components of health care that are addressed in this first chapter because they have a profound affect on all aspects of client care. The influence of **culture, environment,** and **ethics** are discussed in greater detail in later chapters.

Culture

The numerous global, social, demographic, economic, and political changes in recent years have alerted health care professionals to the need to provide attention to increasing diversity in our society and the affect of that diversity on people's health (Meleis, 1996). International travel and advances in communication through the Internet and satellite television make it essential for today's nurses to have the skills needed to provide care that recognizes complexities and differences among clients (Janes & Hobson, 1998).

The United States is the most culturally diverse nation in the world. In fact, in 1994, *Time Magazine* designated the United States "the first universal nation" (Grossman, 1994). The 1990 census reported that almost 25% of Americans were members of ethnic minority groups, including 12% African Americans, 9% Hispanics, and 2.9% Asian Americans. It is predicted that by the year 2050, the African American population will increase to 16%, Hispanics to 21%, and Asian Americans to 11% (Norbeck, 1995).

So what exactly do we mean by the term *culture*? According to Madeleine Leininger (1995), culture refers to the "learned and shared beliefs, values, and life ways, of a designated or particular group which are generally transmitted intergenerationally and influence one's thinking and action modes." Giger and Davidhizar (1995) say the culture is "a patterned behavioral response that develops over time as a result of imprinting the mind through social and religious structures and intellectual and artistic manifestations." Purnell and Paulanka (1998) define culture as "the totality of socially transmitted behavioral patterns, art, beliefs, values, customs, life ways, and all other products of human work and thought characteristics of a population of people that guide their world view and decision making." Obviously, culture is more than just ethnicity. Culture is language, religion, food, traditions, customs, clothing, and everything that makes one group of people unique from another. Cultural values, beliefs, and behaviors can also be related to age, gender, sexual orientation, socioeconomic status, and profession. There is a "culture of nursing" that all nurses belong to, with its own language, values, and traditions, that often clashes with clients whose cultural beliefs about health care differ from those of their nurses.

When considering cultural issues, we need to look beyond the borders of our own country. Those who hold privileged and recognized positions in societies by virtue of specialized expertise, such as nursing, have an obligation to give back to those societies. To make such contributions, nurses should become "global citizens" holding a broad vision of international health. In today's connected world, no profession can be truly effective without interactions and viewpoints that include international perspectives. Community health nurses especially, who by definition practice within a broad systems perspective, must incorporate understandings from international health efforts in their own interventions. Comparing and drawing insights from methods and successes of nurses delivering care in other countries holds the promise of improving the care to U.S. populations. In addition, there is a need to understand and support collaborating agencies at the international level. Principles of pluralism, consultation, coherence, consensus, compassion, partnership, and cooperation are the hallmarks of nurses who practice and embrace global citizenship (Neufield, 1992). For example, control measures for effectively reducing AIDS infections have involved the active cooperation of most countries worldwide.

Environment

The environment has been a concern for nursing since the days of Florence Nightingale. In *Notes on Nursing* (1860), Nightingale emphasizes the fact that recovery from illness can occur only in a bright, clean, well-ventilated environment. She states:

> The very first canon of nursing, the first and the last thing upon which a nurse's attention must be fixed, the first essential to a client, without which all the rest you can do for him is nothing, with which I had almost said you may leave all the rest alone, is this: TO KEEP THE AIR HE BREATHES AS PURE AS THE EXTERNAL AIR, WITHOUT CHILLING HIM.

When Nightingale spoke of the patient's environment, she meant the room in the hospital or home in which the patient stayed during the course of his or her illness. In more recent years, the public health definition of environment has come to mean all the surroundings and conditions that affect the health of individuals, families, and communities. The environment has many different components, including social, cultural, political, economic, and ecological factors.

. . . .

The work we are speaking of has nothing to do with nursing disease, but with maintaining health by removing the things which disturb it . . . dirt, drink, diet, damp, draughts, and drains.

Florence Nightingale, 1860

. . . .

Environmental issues have been in the forefront of many political campaigns during the last few years and seem to be gaining momentum, with many governmental and private community groups supporting legislation to protect the environment. Most of this activity has been focused on the ecological component of environmental health—primarily clean air and water and a safe food supply.

Nurses are beginning to take a more active role in promoting environmental health, reducing environmental health risks, and protecting the earth's resources. In fact, several nursing organizations, such as the American Holistic Nurses Association and the International Council of Nurses, have developed position statements to delineate the nurse's role in promoting environmental health. A specialty organization called Nurses for Environmental and Social Responsibility has been formed specifically to educate nurses and the public about environmental health hazards.

Ethics

Since the time of Florence Nightingale, the nursing profession has been addressing ethical concerns related to patient care issues. The ANA's *Code for Nurses with Interpretive Statements* (1985) provides guidance for ethical decisions made by nurses in the clinical setting. The ANA *Code for Nurses* is being updated to address current practice issues and is expected to be approved in the year 2000 (Savage & Bosek, 1998).

Ethical dilemmas have traditionally included such things as informed consent and individual freedom of choice, autonomy, truth telling, protection of privacy and confidentiality, and discrimination. In addition, public health nurses have also had to make ethical decisions related to the dual obligation to protect the public's welfare while respecting the rights of individual clients (Folmar, Coughlin, Bessinger, & Sacknoff, 1997). However, today's changing health care delivery system brings with it additional ethical dilemmas for nurses. We are now concerned with problems related to equity in health care delivery, environmental safety, politicization of health care interventions, euthanasia, elder abuse in nursing homes, provider-client relationships, and community partnerships (Graham, 1997). Recent advancements in science and technology are presenting ethical dilemmas that Florence Nightingale could not have envisioned in even her wildest fantasies. These include such issues as physician-assisted suicide, living wills, gene therapy, in vitro fertilization, and human cloning. All nurses would do well to follow Spicer's advice to nursing students in an editorial in *Imprint* (1998). She says, "As you prepare for your careers, remember your professional commitment to place your patient first in all decisions. Take time to establish your ethical boundaries. . . . Base your decisions from your head and your heart."

Epidemiology: The Science of Public Health

Whether a person is healthy or ill results from numerous constantly changing interacting forces. The actual occurrence of disease results from a triad of factors, referred to as the *epidemiological model* or *triangle.* The triad is composed of the host, the agent, and the environment. The host is the human body influenced by such variables as gender, age, race, and behavior. The agent is a physical, chemical, or biological element that can cause illness or injury. Examples might include a tuberculosis bacilli or nicotine. The environment is perhaps the most complex component. As we learn more about health and its determinants, the environment holds more and more keys to explaining health risks to our human hosts. The environment not only includes the physical environment, such as climate and terrain, but also the sociocultural-political environment, such as poverty, racism, and other stressors that influence health.

Prevention strategies are made up of measures that protect people from disease and take the form of efforts that we use to protect ourselves and others from specific diseases and conditions and their resulting consequences. There are three levels of prevention: primary, secondary, and tertiary. Nurses in all settings use all three levels of prevention as a basis for practice. The nurse caring for clients in an acute care setting may primarily use secondary and tertiary interventions, and the occupational health nurse may use primary and secondary interventions in his or her role. These levels of prevention were originally conceptualized by Leavell and Clark in 1953 and were tied to what these authors described as the **natural history of disease.** Their assumption is that disease in humans is a process: The conditions that promote either health or disease are present in the human's biological, physical, emotional, and social environments as well as in the human host itself.

The relationship between levels of prevention and the natural history of any given disease condition or health state is the basis for community health interventions. Disease occurs in two stages: prepathogenesis and pathogenesis. The intervention strategies or levels of prevention must coincide with predictable events within the stages of prepathogenesis (predisease) and pathogenesis (disease, condition, or injury). One can readily see that applying the levels of prevention requires that the nurse know the natural history of a given disease or condition. The less known about the disease or condition, the greater the likelihood of interventions occurring in secondary or tertiary prevention levels. In other words, the more we learn about disease, disability, and injury, the earlier we can intervene to prevent the illness from occurring. The goal of preventive health then is to intervene at the earliest possible stage in the natural history of disease in order to prevent complications, limit disability, and halt irreversible changes in health status (Leavell & Clark, 1979).

Primary prevention refers to those measures that focus on prevention of health problems *before* they occur. Primary prevention is *not* therapeutic, which means that it does *not* consist of symptom identification and use of the typical therapeutic skills of the nurse (Shamansky & Clausen, 1980). This level includes both generalized health promotion and specific protection against certain identified diseases or conditions. The purpose is to reduce the person's vulnerability to the illness by strengthening the human host's capacity to withstand physical, emotional, and environmental stressors. An example would be teaching a person about adequate nutrition, exercise, and hygiene. Specific protection includes numerous interventions associated with public health nursing: immunizations, bicycle helmets, auto seatbelts, safety caps on electrical outlets, handrails on bathtubs, and drug education for children.

Secondary prevention begins when pathology is involved and is aimed at early detection through diagnosis and prompt treatment. This level of prevention is aimed at halting the pathological process, thus shortening its duration and severity and getting the client back to a normal state of functioning. All screening tests, such as breast self-examinations, hypertensive assessments, and Pap smears, are included in this level of prevention. The goal of this level is to identify groups of individuals who have early symptoms of disease so that they may be treated as soon as possible in the natural history of the disease, condition, or injury. If the disease, condition, or injury cannot be cured, further complications and disability move the level of prevention to that of tertiary prevention.

Tertiary prevention consists of activities designed around rehabilitation of a person with a permanent, irreversible condition. The goal of tertiary prevention goes beyond halting the disease process to restoring the client to an optimal level of functioning *within the constraints of the disability*. Nursing strategies at this level might include teaching a stroke patient how to ambulate with assistance or assisting a child with cystic fibrosis to reduce risks of respiratory infection while maintaining an active lifestyle.

The boundaries between secondary and tertiary prevention are often fuzzy and more difficult to identify as either one or the other. One feature that helps in this identification is that tertiary intervention takes place *only if the condition results in a permanent disability* (Shamansky & Clausen, 1980). This may be influenced by the age or development of the patient rather than by the condition itself. For example, if a 15-year-old high school athlete suffers a simple broken femur during a soccer game, intervention would occur at the secondary prevention level. Although the athlete may require extensive physical rehabilitation after the cast is removed, unless there are serious complications, she should eventually be able to return to her normal state of health. Compare this with a 75-year-old man who falls from a roof and suffers the identical injury. Most likely, this client would need both secondary and tertiary intervention strategies because of the aging process, recovery, and the likelihood of permanent disability resulting from this fall.

Shamansky and Clausen (1980) use the following example to illustrate how all levels of prevention are often used with the same client and family:

> A nurse is conducting a group session with young parents and uses values clarification as a method to discuss issues of parental responsibility for providing a safe yet stimulating environment for the young, curious child. This is primary prevention; health promotion occurs, since the discussion is general and directed toward nonspecific efforts to ensure the well-being of the young child. Later, on a home visit, the nurse encourages a mother to use screens on a second story window, since she perceives the window is dangerously accessible to the active three year old. This, too, is primary prevention, an example of specific protection, because one is attempting to remove a risk factor from the environment of a vulnerable child. If the screen is not used and the child falls out of the window onto a cement driveway below, the mother's and emergency personnel's use of appropriate emergency first aid would be secondary prevention through the use of prompt treatment. If the child sustained a severe head injury, was hospitalized (and secondary measures were used in the hospital), and later released to home care, teaching the mother to turn, feed, and give range of motion exercises would represent the disability limitation aspect of secondary prevention. Several months later if the child is found to have some permanent brain damage, tertiary prevention would take the form of referrals to special education classes, or physical or speech therapy to increase the child's maximum potential level of functioning, although the damage itself is irreversible. (pp. 106–107)

Measuring a Community's Health: How Do We Know When We Get There?

Outcomes and measurements of population and community health interventions take the form of health statistics such as birth rates, infant mortality rates, and incidence and prevalence rates for various diseases and age groups. Most threats to health do not occur at random (i.e., by chance). Natural forces influence health threats, but by no means do they dictate the outcome. In this century we have learned through epidemiological research that most threats or risks to our health and well-being are associated with *patterns* of human activity and behavior. It is those patterns that we use to evaluate health interventions and the multitude of influences on people's health (Cohen, 1989). For example, breast cancer rates in the United States are high compared with other countries such as Japan and China. In other words, breast cancer is not universal among all females, nor is it randomly distributed in the female population (Cohen, 1989).

We can see from epidemiological research that individual behavior has a significant effect on a person's "chance" of developing breast cancer. Breast cancer may be associated with a high-fat, high-protein, high-calorie diet, and with high levels of estrogen (either produced by the woman's own body or ingested in diet and medication). Women who do not have or nurse children or have them later in life have higher rates of breast cancer. These lifestyle factors clearly influence the chances of a woman's contracting breast cancer in her lifetime. The availability of cutting edge technology and diagnostic interventions cannot prevent women from contracting breast cancer; they can improve chances of survival only once cancer is detected (Kolata, 1987; Marx, 1986; Winick, 1980). In another example, maternal death risk in childbirth plummeted during the 20th century in developed countries as a result of research application of prenatal care, use of antibiotics, and infectious disease control. In the United States, a woman has only a 1 in 3,700 chance of dying in childbirth, yet in Latin Amer-

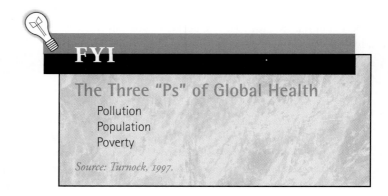

FYI

The Three "Ps" of Global Health
Pollution
Population
Poverty

Source: Turnock, 1997.

TABLE 1-4   A COMPARISON OF INDIVIDUAL, FAMILY, COMMUNITY, AND GLOBAL POPULATION-FOCUSED CARE

INDIVIDUAL CARE	FAMILY	COMMUNITY	GLOBAL
Injuries suffered by woman in violent spousal domestic relationship	Family dysfunctions, such as inability to provide appropriate behavioral roles for conflict resolution Children exhibiting early and inappropriate use of firearms	Child unable to function in school setting because of disruptive behavior in classroom Gang violence resulting in neighborhood isolation, decreased population, diminished economic base because of business closure and decreased funds available for education and family assistance	Woman and child refugees in war-torn Bosnia, injuries and from acts of violence war abuse during acts of resulting in U.N. intervention

ica, a woman's mortality risk is 1 in 130 and women in parts of Africa have an alarming *1 in 16 chance* of dying as a result of childbearing (Whaley & Hashim, 1995). Table 1-4 provides an illustration of the links among all levels of care. You will learn in this text how these group rates of disease, health, injury, and disability reflect more accurately the values of a society and how health professionals measure not only their interventions but the influences of many variables on health.

CASE STUDY

Community-Focused and Community-Based Care: An Example from Practice

A 3-year-old child is brought to a public health department for her first set of immunizations. As the nurse assesses the child, she finds that the child has a generalized red rash all over her body. The mother complains that the child scratches and cries about the rash and that she has been using a cortisone skin cream for three days. The nurse attends to the immediate concerns of the mother about home care comfort measures and possible causes. The nurse then delivers direct client care to the child and to her family, while considering the following community implications:

- Does anyone else in the family exhibit those symptoms?
- Does the child go to day care?
- Have there been any other children in the clinic recently with similar symptoms? If so, how does this case compare with cases in recent months?
- What is the likely pathogen that is causing the rash?
- Are there any pregnant women in the clinic or in the home setting?

1. What are possible conclusions that the nurse can make that have individual implications?
2. Are there community and public health issues that may be present that the nurse must address?

CONCLUSION

In community-focused care, the community is the primary client. Although a nurse in a community-focused setting may care for individuals and families and groups, the community health nurse must consider the impact, implications, and consequences of that care on the health of a community. To treat the community, the nurse considers the community assessment data, resources in the community, and interventions at the population level, such as isolation, education of others, and community reaction, including political and policy implications. Although the *focus* of the nurses' practice may be on the individual client initially, the ultimate *target focus* is the population at large. In this chapter you have learned about the various influences on a community's health and how the health care system has organized services around societal needs and expectations. Nurses will play a critical role in the future of managed care, which is organized around prevention and a healthy population. **Epidemiology** is the science that provides community and public health with a framework for addressing the primary, secondary, and tertiary health needs for a population and directs community health nursing practice. The health of populations and the personal well-being of individuals are more than an individual matter. Humankind does not live in isolation, unaffected by others. Community health is a dynamic of the community and is influenced by the context of where and how the population lives, works, and addresses health care needs.

CRITICAL THINKING ACTIVITIES

1. After reading "A Personal Look at Public Health" on p. 8, respond to the following questions:
   - What three risks described in the essay were unknown a century ago?
   - What is the responsibility of the individual in creating a safe environment?
   - What three public safety measures mentioned in the essay do not exist in underdeveloped countries?

2. How can heart disease be both a personal health problem and a community health problem?

3. For several decades now, nurses have worked primarily in hospitals using a medical model approach to health and illness. Does nursing have a vision of the profession with community at the center or has nursing become so institutionalized into hospital-based practice over the past decades that we will resist the tremendous opportunities to care for people in a myriad of settings and situations?

4. After reading this chapter, watch an episode of *ER, Chicago Hope,* or any program on television that features a trauma setting. Identify the kinds of problems that are presented on the program. Which ones could have been prevented? How?

5. Identify public health prevention strategies that could have prevented the problems encountered at the trauma center.

6. Could a community health nurse work in such an environment? If so, what would the role be?

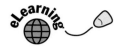

Explore Community Health Nursing on the web! To learn more about the topics in this chapter, use the passcode provided to access your exclusive web site: http://communitynursing.jbpub.com
If you do not have a passcode, you can obtain one at this site.

REFERENCES

American Association of Colleges of Nursing (AACN). (1993). *Nursing education's agenda for the 21st century.* Washington, DC: Author.

American Nurses Association (ANA). (1980). *ANA social policy statement.* Kansas City, MO: Author.

American Nurses Association. (1985). *Code for nurses with interpretive statements.* Kansas City: Author.

American Nurses Association. (1986). *Standards of community health nursing practice.* Kansas City: Author.

American Nurses Association. (1991). *Nursing's agenda for health care reform: Executive summary.* Washington, DC: Author.

American Nurses Association. (1994). *Managed care: challenges and opportunities for nursing.* Washington, DC: Author.

American Public Health Association. (March, 1996). *The definition and role of public health nursing.* A statement of the Public Health Nursing Section. Washington, DC.

Anderson, C. (1997). The economics of health promotion. *Nursing Outlook, 45*(3), 105–106.

Armentrout, G. (1998). *Community-based nursing. Foundation for practice.* Stamford, CT: Appleton & Lange.

Association of Community Health Nursing Educators. (2000). *Essentials of baccalaureate education for community health nursing.* Louisville, KY: University of Kentucky.

Baldwin, J. H., Conger, C. O., Abegglen, J. C., & Hill, E. M. (1998). Population-focused and community-based nursing: Moving toward clarification of concepts. *Public Health Nursing, 15*(1), 12–18.

Buhler-Wilkerson, K. (1985). Public health nursing: In sickness and in health? *American Journal of Public Health, 75,* 1155.

Bunker, J. P., Frazier, H. S., & Mosteller, F. (1994). Improving health: Measuring effects of medical care. *Milbank Quarterly, 72,* 225–258.

Bureau of Labor Statistics. (1998). *Statistics of employment 1996–2006: A summary of BLS projection* (Bulletin No. 2502). Washington, DC: U.S. Government Printing Office.

Canavan, K. (1996). Nursing education on cusp of shift in focus: Faculty grapple with preparing students for changing health care delivery. *American Nurse, 28*(6), 1, 11.

Cohen, M. (1989). *Health and the rise of civilization.* New Haven, CT: Yale University Press.

Consumer Reports. (1992, July). Wasted health care dollars, 435–448.

Consumer Reports. (1990, September). The crisis in health insurance part 2, 608–617.

Cottrell, K. (1976). The competent community. In B. H. Kaplan, R. N. Wilson, & A. H. Leighton (Eds.), *Further explorations in social psychology.* New York: Basic Books.

Dubos, R. (1968). *Man, medicine and environment.* New York: Mentor.

Flynn, B. C. (1997). Are we ready to collaborate for community-based health services? *Public Health Nursing, 14*(3), 135–136.

Folmar, J., Coughlin, S. S., Bessinger, R., & Sacknoff, D. (1997). Ethics in public health practice: A survey of public health nurses in southern Louisiana. *Public Health Nursing, 14*(3), 156–160.

Gebbie, K. M. (1996, November 18). *Preparing currently employed public health nurses for changes in the health care system: Meeting report and suggested action steps.* New York: Columbia University School of Nursing Center for Health Policy and Health Sciences Research. (Report based on meeting in Atlanta, GA, July 11, 1996.)

Gebbie, K. M. (1997). Using the vision of Healthy People to build healthier communities. *Nursing Administration Quarterly, 21*(4), 83–90.

Giger, J. N., & Davidhizar, R. E. (1995). *Transcultural nursing. Assessment and intervention* (2nd ed.). St. Louis: Mosby.

Graham, K. Y. (1997). Ethics: Do we really care? *Public Health Nursing, 14*(1), 1–2.

Grossman, D. (1994). Enhancing your cultural competence. *American Journal of Nursing, 94*(7), 58–62.

Hall, J. M., & Stevens, P. E. (1995). The future of graduate education in nursing: Scholarship, the health communities, and health care reform. *Journal of Professional Nursing, 11*(6), 332–338.

Hall, J. E., & Weaver, B. R. (1977). *Distributive nursing practice: A systems approach to community health.* Philadelphia: Lippincott.

Hanlon, J. J., & Pickett, G. E. (1984). *Public health: Administration and practice* (8th ed.). St. Louis: Mosby.

Heinrich, J. (1983). Historical perspectives on public health nursing. *Nursing Outlook, 32*(6), 317–320.

http://odphp.osophs.dhhs.gov/pubs/hp2000/newsbit.html.

Institute of Medicine. (1988). *The future of public health*. Washington, DC: National Academy Press.

Keck, E. W. (1994). Community health: Our common challenge. *Family and Community Health, 17*(2), 1–9.

Keller, L. O., Strohschein, S., Lia-Hoagberg, B., & Schaffer, M. (1998). Population-based public health nursing interventions: a model from practice. *Public Health Nursing, 15*(3), 207–215.

Kolata, G. B. (1987). !Kung hunter-gatherers: Feminism, diet, and birth control. *Science, 185,* 932–934.

Kurtzman, C., Ibgui, D., Pogrund, R., & Monin, S. (1980, December). Nursing process at the aggregate level. *Nursing Outlook, 28*(12), 737–739.

Kuss, T., Proulx-Girouard, L., Lovitt, S., Katz, C. B., & Kennelly, P. (1997). A public health nursing model. *Public Health Nursing, 14*(2), 81–91.

Lancaster, J. (1984). History of community health and community health nursing. In M. Stanhope & J. Lancaster (Eds.), *Community health nursing. Process and practice for promoting health* (pp. 3–31). St. Louis: Mosby.

Leininger, M. (1995). *Transcultural nursing. Concepts, theories, research, & practices* (2nd ed.). New York: McGraw-Hill.

Leipert, B. D. (1996). The value of community health nursing: A phenomenological study of the perceptions of community health nurses. *Public Health Nursing, 13*(1), 50–57.

Janes, S., & Hobson, K. (1998). An innovative approach for affirming cultural diversity among baccalaureate nursing students and faculty. *Journal of Cultural Diversity,* Winter Issue.

Leavell, H. R., Clark, E. G. (1953). *Preventive medicine for the doctor in his community.* New York: McGraw-Hill.

Leavell, H. R., Clark, E. G. (1979). *Preventive medicine for the doctor in his community: An epidemiological approach* (3rd ed.). Huntington, NY: RE Dreges.

Marx, J. (1986). Viruses and cancer briefing. *Science, 241,* 1039–1040.

McKenzie, J. F., & Pinger, R. R. (1997). *An introduction to community health.* Boston: Jones and Bartlett.

McKinnon, R. H. (1997). *Community health nursing: A case study approach.* New York: Lippincott-Raven.

Mechanic, D. (1998). Topics of our times: Managed care and public health. *American Journal of Public Health, 88*(6), 84–85.

Meleis, A. I. (1990). Being and becoming healthy: The core of nursing knowledge. *Nursing Science Quarterly, 3,* 107–114.

Meleis, A. L. (1996). Culturally competent scholarship: Substance and rigor. *Advances in Nursing Science, 19*(2), 1–16.

Moon, M. (1993). Health care reform. *The Future of Children, 3*(2), 21–36.

Division of Nursing, Bureau of Health Professions, Health Resources and Services Administration, Health and Human Services. (1997). *National Sample Survey of Registered Nurses.*, Washington, DC: U.S. Government Printing Office.

Neufield, V. (1992). Training: a Canadian perspective. In Pan American Health Organization (Ed.), *International health: North south debate.* (Human Resource Development Series, pp. 95, 193–203). Washington, DC: Pan American Health Organization.

Neufeldt, V., & Guralnik, D. B. (Eds.). (1994). *Webster's new world dictionary* (3rd college ed.). New York: Prentice Hall.

Nightingale, F. (1860). *Notes on nursing: What it is and what it is not.* London: Harrison.

Norbeck, J. S. (1995). Who is our consumer? Shaping nursing programs to meet consumer needs. *Journal of Professional Nursing, 11*(6), 325–331.

Proenca, E. J. (1998). Community orientation in health services organizations: the concept and its implementation. *Health Care Management Review, 23*(2), 28–38 (51 ref.).

Purnell, L. D., & Paulanka, B. J. (1998). *Transcultural health care. A culturally competent approach.* Philadelphia: F. A. Davis.

Salmon, M., & Vanderbush, P. (1990). Leadership and change in public and community health nursing today: The essential intervention. In J. C. McCloskey, & H. K. Grace (Eds.), *Current issues in nursing* (3rd ed., pp. 187–193). St. Louis: Mosby.

Savage, T. A., & Bosek, M. S. D. (1998). Moments of courage: Reconciling the real and ideal in the clinical practicum. *Imprint, 45*(3), 31–34.

Schultz, P. R. (1987). When client means more than one: extending the foundational concept of person. *Advances in Nursing Science, 10*(1), 71–86.

Schultz, P. R. (1994). *On the matter of populations, aggregates, and communities.* Unpublished manuscript, University of Washington, Seattle.

Shamansky, S. L., & Clausen, C. L. (1980, February). Levels of prevention: Examination of the concept. *Nursing Outlook, 28*(2), 104–108.

Shortell, S. M., & Gilles, R. R. (1995). Reinventing the American hospital. *Milbank Quarterly, 73*(2), 131.

Smith, C. M. (1995). Responsibilities for care in community health nursing. In C. M. Smith, & F. A. Maurer (Eds.), *Community health nursing. Principles and practice* (pp. 3–29). Philadelphia: Saunders.

Spicer, G. (1998). Learning right from wrong. *Imprint, 45*(3), 4.

Starr, P. (1993). The framework of health care reform. *New England Journal of Medicine, 329,* 1666–1672.

Trossman, S. (1998, March/April). Self-determination: The name of the game in the next century. *The American Nurse,* 1.

Turnock, B. (1997). *Public health: What it is and how it works.* Baltimore: Aspen.

U.S. Department of Health and Human Services. (1994). *Consensus conference on the essentials of public health nursing practice and education: Report of the conference.* Rockville, MD: Author.

Whaley, R. F., & Hashim, T. J. (1995). *A textbook of world health.* New York: Parthenon.

Whelan, E. M. (1995). The health corner: A community-based nursing model to maximize access to primary care. *Public Health Reports, 110*(2), 184–188.

Winick, M. (1980). *Nutrition in health and disease.* New York: John Wiley.

Wolf, Z. R. (1989, October). Uncovering the hidden work of nursing. *Nursing and Health Care, 10*(8), 462–467.

World Health Organization. (1958). *The first ten years of the World Health Organization.* New York: Author.

World Health Organization. (1986). Health promotion. A discussion document on the concept and principles. *Public Health Reviews, 14*(3–4), 245–254.

APPENDIX A

Scope and Standards of Public Health Nursing Practice
Author: Quad Council of Public Health Nursing
   Organizations
American Nurses Association
Washington, DC
1999

STANDARDS OF CARE

Standard I. Assessment

The public health nurse assesses the health status of populations using data, community resources identification, input from the population, and professional judgment.

Standard II. Diagnosis

The public health nurse analyzes collected assessment data and partners with the people to attach meaning to those data and determine opportunities and needs.

Standard III. Outcomes Identification

The public health nurse participates with other community partners to identify expected outcomes in the populations and their health status.

Standard IV. Planning

The public health nurse promotes and supports the development of programs, policies, and services that provide interventions that improve the health status of populations.

Standard V. Assurance: Action component of the nursing process for public health nursing

The public health nurse assures access and availability of programs, policies, resources, and services to the population.

Standard VI. Evaluation

The public health nurse evaluates the health status of the population.

Chapter 2
Community and Population Health: Assessment and Intervention

Karen Saucier Lundy and Judith A. Barton

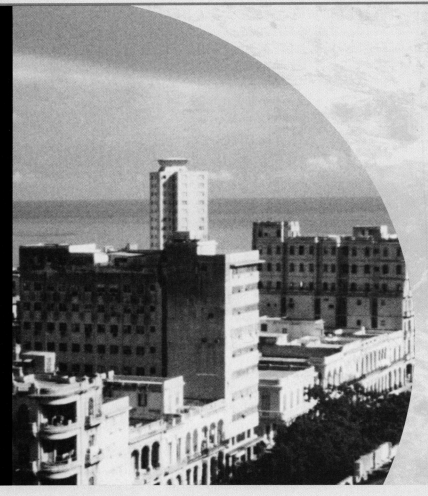

We are all longing to go home to some place we have never been—a place, half-remembered, and half-envisioned we can only catch glimpses of from time to time. Community: Somewhere, there are people to whom we can speak with passion without having the words catch in our throats. Somewhere a circle of hands will open to receive us, eyes will light up as we enter, voices will celebrate with us whenever we come into our own power. Community means strength that joins our strength to do the work that needs to be done. Arms to hold us when we falter. A circle of healing. A circle of friends: Someplace where we can be free.

Starhawk from *Dreaming in the Dark*

QUESTIONS TO CONSIDER

After reading this chapter, answer the following questions:

1. What is a population-focused approach to health care?
2. How does the baccalaureate-prepared nurse use population assessment in health care settings?
3. What is "the community as client"?
4. What is the difference between a community and a population?
5. What do the terms *status*, *structure*, and *process* refer to?
6. What is the Healthy Cities initiative?
7. How are community assessment frameworks or models used in the assessment process?
8. What are examples of community assessment frameworks or models?
9. How does a community health nurse gain entry into the community?
10. What are the five methods of collecting community data?
11. What is a community diagnosis, and what is an example of one?
12. What occurs in the planning and prioritization phase of the community assessment process?
13. What occurs in the implementation phase of the community assessment process?
14. What are examples of strategies that the community health nurse can use to assist communities in healthy change?
15. What is media advocacy?

KEY TERMS

Collaborative arrangement
Community
Community- and
  population–focused
  care
Community as client
Community assess-
  ment frameworks
  and models
Community assessments

Community
  competency
Community
  empowerment
Community-focused
  intervention
Community forums
Community health
  diagnoses
Constructed surveys

Focus groups
Healthy change
Healthy communities
Informant interviews
Key informant
Media advocacy
Observation
Planning phase
Population
Population assessment

Population level
  interventions
Primary informant
Process
Secondary analysis of
  existing data
Secondary data
Status
Structure
Windshield surveys

Community nurses have traditionally conducted nursing assessments of entire geopolitical communities and of vulnerable populations within communities. The focus of the nursing assessment is on the community or population's health status rather than the individual's health status, and consequently the assessment takes on a different form and process.

Today more than ever the community health nurse has the unique responsibility of defining problems and proposing solutions at the community/population level (Baldwin, Conger, Abegglen, & Hill, 1998; Gebbie, 1996; Keck, 1994; Williams & Highriter, 1978). Furthermore, baccalaureate-prepared nurses will be expected to practice population-based nursing in all settings as managed care of populations becomes the basis of organizational survival.

The U.S. health care system's trend toward community- and population-focused care was well documented in the previous chapter. The shift from location-based care (e.g., hospital, outpatient clinic care) to community-based care will demand a greater emphasis on nursing assessments of both geopolitical communities and high-risk populations. In other words, to plan care, carry out interventions, and evaluate care outcomes when the client is either a geopolitical community or population at risk, there is a need for all nurses to have skills in community and population assessment. Although community and population assessment, planning, intervention, and evaluation are receiving greater attention in today's health care system, these skills have always been associated with community health nursing role expectations (Hegyvary, 1990).

Historically, community/population assessment, the initial step in community-/population-focused care, was first seen as a nursing practice role by Florence Nightingale. Nightingale was concerned with assessing the physical and social environment as a possible cause of illness. Nightingale's own community assessments included an analysis of the 1861 census data of England, which served as the foundation of England's sanitary reform acts (Kopf, 1986). She also included community assessment as a nursing role for district nurses. These nurses were to assess both the physical and social environments of the community to determine what health teaching and social reform programs were needed by the community (Montero, 1985). From its earliest history, the nursing profession has viewed community and population assessment as an important role directed toward improving the health of entire communities.

Today, recommitment toward community and population assessment is a vital nursing practice role, as identified by all organizations that set standards for community health nursing (AACN, 1986; ACHNE, 1990, 1993; ANA, 1986; APHA, 1981). This recommitment to seeing the community as client has emerged as a critical function of the community health nurse as more and more research connects the important role that physical and social environments play in health and disease (Cassel, 1976; Gordon, 1990, 1993; Lalonde, 1974; Rodgers, 1984). Such findings also influence health policy

formation, the establishment of priorities when financing health care, and the potential of the nursing community to establish itself as a leader in health care reform. Knowledge of community and population assessment is now considered essential for the baccalaureate nurse (Ruth, Eliason, & Schultz, 1992). The diagnoses and interventions that result from the community and population assessment process are population-based, community-focused interventions. Such interventions are directed at groups of persons within a community; activities are geared toward changes in community norms, greater consciousness about health issues and solutions, and healthy practices and behaviors, to name a few (Keller, Strohschein, Lia-Hoagberg, & Schaffer, 1998).

•••••••••••••••••••••••••••••••••••

Health [is rather] a modus vivendi enabling imperfect men to achieve a rewarding and not too painful existence while they cope with an imperfect world.

Rene Dubos, 1968

•••••••••••••••••••••••••••••••••••

This chapter introduces the **community as client,** how to get to know the community patient, and how to practice skills of community and population assessment in actual community assessment examples. The future of nursing depends to a large degree on our understanding of the "big picture" of health care delivery (Aiken & Salmon, 1994). As we become more and more dependent on outcome measures, such as evaluation of morbidity and mortality statistics, this chapter will help the beginning nurse use the community/population assessment process in all practice settings (Reinhart, 1984) (Box 2-1).

This chapter also discusses how to interpret community and population level data and plan interventions more appropriately and efficiently as we work within the limited resources of the present health care environment. Our health care system can no longer rely on quick fixes. For example, in developed countries the nature of fatal diseases has changed. In the course of recent human history, when people were fighting diseases such as smallpox, diphtheria, or polio, immunizations were an easy, quick, and sure prevention. As we learned more about infectious disease and the contribution of human factors, such as lifestyle, heredity, and behavior, solutions became more complex. Chronic disease and disabling conditions are continuing to grow as we extend the life span through technology and advancement of diagnosis and treatment. Today many diseases and conditions require that we are much more attentive to the totality of variables that influence health and illness (Gebbie, 1996). Achieving prevention and control requires much more effort on the part of communities and changes in thinking about the impact of the structure of society (e.g., economics, culture, and politics) on the health of community (*Community Facilitator Implementation Manual,* 1996).

- Applying for grants to provide health care for specific populations, such as pregnant adolescents
- Conducting a "mini" assessment during orientation to a new position in any setting to be better prepared for serving the agencies' target population
- Avoiding burnout by going beyond personal care of clients, identifying better ways of delivering care, and using staff and material resources
- Justifying new projects by establishing the needs of a selected population
- Joining a community group such as the Parent Teacher Organization or American Cancer Society, volunteering to do an assessment and follow-through program planning
- Conducting an assessment of unfamiliar locales, both national and international, to determine possible relocation possibilities

Communities and Populations

The significance of the community/population nursing process becomes evident only when community health nurses define the community as client. A nurse would not even consider omitting individual client assessment and basing interventions only on intuition or a standard formula, but this is what happens when community health nurses fail to do a focused community/population assessment when planning and implementing health care for clients. For example, we would not even consider examining just the arm of a client and totally ignoring the other systems of the body when we plan our nursing care. And yet by looking at only a few aspects of a selected community or population, such as the number and availability of hospitals, we are examining just the "arm" and ignoring the rest of the "body" of the community or population.

The first step in delivering **community- and population-focused care** is to define the boundaries of the group to be assessed. We often use the term **community** in various ways, as was discussed in chapter 1, so defining the boundaries of a community or population becomes critical in the early stages of **community-focused intervention**. Community is defined in this text as *a group of people who share something in common, who interact with one another, and who may exhibit a commitment to one another.* A population is defined as *a group of people who have at least one thing in common and who may or may not interact with each other.* From these definitions one can see that *interaction* is essential in

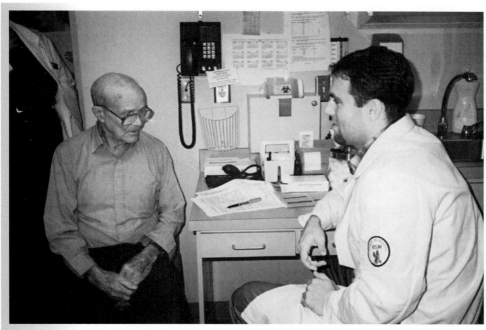

Nurse providing individual care.

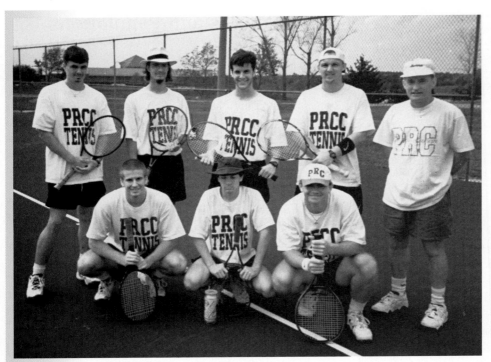

This college tennis team has formed a community after 1 year of common and meaningful interactions.

a *community*, whereas members of a *population* may or may not interact with one another. To put it another way, community members are usually aware that they are part of a community and most often have an identified name (Box 2-2). **Populations** may or may not have such self-awareness (Box 2-3). Some populations do evolve into communities. For example, adults who

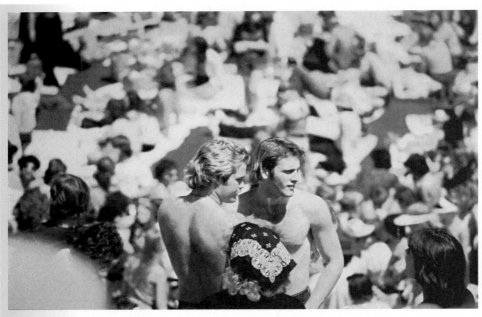

An example of a noninteracting population of young concertgoers.

> **BOX 2-2 EXAMPLES OF COMMUNITIES**
>
> - Retirement apartment community
> - Corvette Club of San Francisco
> - Town of Blackhawk, Colorado

> **BOX 2-3 EXAMPLES OF POPULATIONS**
>
> - Cross-country truck drivers
> - Elders with chronic asthma
> - College soccer players
> - Street musicians
> - Ice skaters

> **BOX 2-4 BASIC COMPONENTS OF COMMUNITY AND POPULATION HEALTH WITH EXAMPLE INDICATORS**
>
> *DIMENSIONS*
>
> *Status*
> - Vital statistics
> - Leading causes of death
> - Mental health statistics
> - Crime rates
>
> *Structure*
> - Hospitals, community health clinics
> - Health professionals, government structures, etc.
> - Statistics related to use of health resources
> - Population characteristics (e.g., gender, age, socioeconomic status)
>
> *Process*
> - Commitment of members
> - Self and other awareness
> - Articulateness
> - Effective communication
> - Conflict resolution
> - Active participation by members
> - Management of social interactions with larger society/environment
> - Machinery for effective resource procurement and utilization
>
> *Source: Schuster, G. F., & Goeppinger, J. (1996). Community as client: Using the nursing process to promote health. In M. Stanhope, & J. Lancaster (Eds.), Community health nursing: Promoting health of aggregates, families, and individuals (pp. 289–314). St. Louis: Mosby.*

have disabilities and attend a day program in a certain community may develop into a cohesive, interactive group over time. Whether or not the population being assessed has self-awareness, the environment (e.g., the social, cultural, ecological environment of a particular community or the greater society) of the target population must be considered in order for effective health interventions to occur (Baldwin et al., 1998).

The Health of Communities and Populations

Public health professionals often describe **healthy communities** and populations in three different ways: status, structure, and process. See Box 2-4 for a summary of these components.

Status is what we most commonly use to describe communities and populations and is the component you are most familiar with. When we talk about life expectancy rates and the morbidity (or illness) rates of a community or population, these are the "outcome" measures of *physical* or *biological* determinants of health. The *emotional aspects* of a community's or population's health status are often measured by such indices as specific mental health rates (e.g., suicide or drug addiction). The *social* determinants are reflected by such indices as crime rates and juvenile delinquency. As we have learned more about the health and the "ills" of modern society, we have discovered that most status outcome measures reflect the influences of all three status components. For example, teen drug use is associated with risky behavior such as unprotected sex, which may result in high rates of teen pregnancy, sexually transmitted diseases, and associated higher infant mortality rates.

Structure refers to aspects of a community's or population's health such as health organizations, health professionals, utilization rates of health services and facilities, and characteristics of the community structure itself. How the community or population is structured is reflected in such measures as socioeconomic and educational levels; demographics of race, age, and gender; and how the members of a community access and use resources related to health. Research has linked education, socioeconomic status, and health outcomes, so these components are aspects that reflect the health status of a group to that end (Shuster & Goeppinger, 1996).

Process is a measure of community or population health that reflects how well a community/population functions to keep healthy. Just as the care of the individual client commonly includes an assessment of personal competence to maintain health, a community or population can be described in relation to **community competency**. This notion of community competency has been around for some time. George Herbert Mead (1934), the noted sociologist, linked our individual behaviors to what eventually emerges as collective behavior. These collective behaviors ultimately take the form of social institutions, such as a church, the Microsoft Corporation, or the American Red Cross. Mead contends that it is only this "organized self" and the resulting group response that makes communities possible and survival likely. For example, people exhibit varying degrees of competency at meeting social needs. Each individual who is intrinsically tied to the group through social interaction is changed by the interaction—each participant then not only becomes a part of the "other" but learns his or her part, as well as the part of the other (Mead, 1934). Cottrell (1976) defines community competence as a process in which the components of a community—families, organizations, and populations—"are able to collaborate effectively in identifying the problems and needs of the community; can achieve a working consensus on goals and priorities, can agree on ways and means to implement the agreed-on goals; and can collaborate effectively in the required action" (p. 197).

An important distinction must be made between individual competence and community competence: Although we often assume that a community made up of competent citizens and health professionals results in a competent community, these are not sufficient conditions. The complexity of community requires that we look not only beyond the individual parts of a community but also to the "whole" and the interactions between and among community constituents (Goeppinger, Lassiter, & Wilcox, 1982). Goeppinger, Lassiter, and Wilcox (1982) developed a nursing process–related model for community assessment designed to address the importance of community processes and community competence. To assess community competencies, the nurse examines the health capabilities and potential health actions of the community. The basic assumption of the community competency model is that health assessments need to include the community's strengths and abilities to improve their own health status. The model is based on research conducted by Goeppinger and Baglioni (1986) that was designed to discover indices of community competence. These competencies are not considered mutually exclusive, but are interrelated. Table 2-1 summarizes essentials for community competency and includes examples from Goeppinger and Baglioni's research on indices of community competency (1986).

Healthy Cities

The World Health Organization (WHO) developed the Healthy Cities initiative as a global approach to community-focused health promotion and preventive health. The Healthy Cities movement began in 1984 in Canada, and in 1986, WHO initiated the project in Europe. The largest Healthy City in Europe in the WHO project is St. Petersburg, Russia, while Indiana and California have the longest history with Healthy Cities in the United States. Approximately half the world's population lives in urban areas, where health problems are the most complex. As an international movement, Healthy Cities (Box 2-5) now involves

TABLE 2-1	ESSENTIAL CONDITIONS FOR COMMUNITY COMPETENCE
Commitment	Evidence that community members are attached to their community—people within the community demonstrate loyalty and pride.
Self-other awareness	Evidence that community members are aware of how they fit into their community—as outsiders or insiders, as having power or not having power.
Articulateness	Evidence that the community is able to clearly express its own issues, needs, and strengths as compared with other similar communities in order to effectively secure resources to meet needs.
Effective communication	Evidence of good communication within a community—the people say that they feel they are always well informed about issues ahead of time so that good decisions can be made.
Conflict containment and accommodation	Evidence that the community has been able to deal effectively with conflicts within the community such as growth policies or taxes for local school districts.
Participation	Evidence that all populations (different age groups, ethnic groups, etc.) participate in community organizations and governmental decisions.
Management of relations with larger society	Evidence that the community is able to secure resources from county, state, or federal governments as needed.
Machinery for facilitating participant interaction and decision making	Evidence that a community's governmental structure has built-in processes that encourage participation by the members of the community for good decision making.

Source: Adapted from Goeppinger, J., Lassiter, P. G., & Wilcox, B. (1982). Nursing Outlook, 30(8), 464–467.

more than 1,000 cities throughout the world where public, private, and not-for-profit partnerships work together to address the complex health and environmental problems in urban areas (Flynn, Ray, & Rider, 1994). Based on the belief that the health of a community is largely influenced by the social and physical environments in which people live and work, Healthy Cities projects promote change in the complex web of city life (Flynn & Dennis, 1996). Community assessment is a critical and early step in the process of identifying the health needs of cities and working with residents to develop realistic and community-identified solutions (Hancock, 1993). The underlying philosophy of such an approach is based on the belief that when residents work out their own locally defined health issues, they will find sustainable solutions to those problems (Flynn, 1994).

Difference and Similarities Among Communities and Populations

Chapter 1 introduced the idea that baccalaureate nurses are prepared to deliver population-focused care. The Association of Community Health Nursing Educators (ACHNE) has identified in its *Essentials of Baccalaureate Nursing Education for Entry Level Practice in Community/Public Health Nursing* (2000) community assessment, diagnosis, and community planning as essential skills for the BSN nurse.

For advanced-degree nurses specializing in community-based public health nursing, population-focused care becomes the primary focus of the role. For baccalaureate-prepared nurses not specializing in public health nursing, such care may be a secondary focus. However, baccalaureate-prepared nurses practicing in all settings (hospital settings as well as community settings) will need to have skills in population-focused care. Baccalaureate-prepared nurses will be expected to move beyond being able to just provide care for individual patients. They will be expected to move beyond incorporating only pathophysiological, psychological, pharmacological, and family factor knowledge into their nursing assessments of individual patients. They will need to incorporate population knowledge—population knowledge that includes an understanding of the common needs of all clients who share one or more characteristics (Salmon, 1993).

These characteristics may include, for example, a common disease, gender, occupation, or age range. For example, an emergency room nurse noted that most of the patients she was caring for had some condition related to substance abuse. Perhaps they had been involved in an automobile accident caused by drunk driving, or perhaps they suffered a gunshot wound that occurred during a drug deal. Conducting a **population assessment** to better understand the demographic, political, economic, and health system factors affecting this population will eventually lead to **population level interventions** such as an initiative to coordinate care of substance abusing clients with mental health professionals. Such efforts may improve not only the health of the individuals within this population, but also the efficiency of the health care system.

Nurses also participate as team members in communitywide health assessments. **Community assessments** differ from population assessments only in that they are not focused on a specific group of individuals who share one or more common characteristics. City municipalities are an example of a community. The individuals in a city municipality interact to achieve goals of employment, the exchange of goods and services, law and order, and so on. A hospital is an example of a community. The individuals within the hospital environment interact to achieve the goals of the organization. You could think of community assessment as more expansive, more complex than a population assessment. In addition, the process of community assessment usually requires a team of researchers to complete a comprehensive analysis of the health of a community. In the following section, four models for community assessment are presented. Please note that although these models use the language of community assessment and were developed for community assessment, they can be and are adapted for use in population assessments.

Community Assessment Frameworks

Just as there are models, theories, and organizing frameworks that guide nursing practice for individual and family care, there are theoretical perspectives for understanding community dynamics and assessing the needs and strengths or assets of communities. In addition to providing guidance on the criteria or systems to be assessed when the client is a community, these theoretical perspectives also provide guidance for the development of community diagnoses, program planning, and the process for data collection, analysis, and dissemination of the findings. All **community assessment frameworks and models** presented in this chapter are based on the underlying assumption that successful health programs are those that emerge from empowered communities that participate in all phases of program planning, implementation, and evaluation, with community assessment being the first phase of the empowerment process (Eisen, 1994).

Community Empowerment

The WHO has provided leadership in the use of **community empowerment** as a means toward health for all. WHO's International Conference on Primary Health Care, held in 1978 at Alma-Ata, U.S.S.R., concluded that people throughout the world have little control over their own health care and that more positive health outcomes would occur if people had a greater sense of power over programs that address their needs (Glick, Hale, Kulbok, & Shettig, 1996). The term *community empowerment* means "a social-action process in which individuals and groups act to gain mastery over their lives in the context of changing their social and political environment" (Wallerstein & Bernstein, 1994). Based on the work of Brazilian educator Paulo Freire, community empowerment involves a participatory educational process in which people are not just the recipients of political, educational, or health care projects, but become active participants in naming their problems and proposing solutions. For example, empowerment projects should not begin with a nurse-conducted assessment of an at-risk population. Instead, participants from the identified population at risk are recruited by nurses to co-conduct the assessment. Of course, this recruitment process involves a level of trust that has developed between the nurses and the identified population at risk. For more information on building trust when the client is a community, see "Gaining Entry into the Community" later in this chapter.

Community empowerment is also considered the prerequisite to health promotion. Indeed, the World Health Assembly observes that "the effective participation of the community is indispensable to guarantee the development of health activities and the prevention and control of disease" (*Handbook of Resolutions and Decisions of the World Health Assembly and the Executive Board*, 1984, p. 75). Just as individual clients cannot participate in health promotion until their basic needs are met and they feel some control over their lives, populations and communities must also feel empowered in order to participate in prevention and health promoting projects.

Community assessment, viewed within the context of community empowerment, is just one part of the methodology that hopefully will lead to health for all. It is an essential component leading to effective, acceptable, affordable health care for our so-

ciety and all other societies. It is one of the core competencies for nursing practice directed toward communities.

Keck (1994) believes that for community health to become a reality, all health care professionals will need to learn how to empower citizens to take responsibility for decision making related to the community's health, as well as their own. Empowering our clients requires that health professionals give up some of their power and rely on true partnership and collaboration for the community good. Such thinking brings resistance because to promote "power sharing" means to rely on community involvement, not just "lip service," for the advancement in a community's health status. An example of giving up power to the community is when the nurse facilitates the establishment of a board of directors for a community health center made up entirely of community members as the voting members with health care professionals as ad hoc members. Keck (1994, p. 8) contends that "our common challenge [in community health] is the facilitation of that [empowering] process."

Four Community Assessment Frameworks/Models

Many community assessment frameworks and models have been designed to guide the process of community assessment. The four theoretical perspectives described here have either been developed by public health nurses or are often used by public health nurses when conducting a community assessment. Two other important approaches to community assessment not included in this chapter are *Community Competence: A Positive Approach to Needs Assessment* by Goeppinger and Baglioni (1986) and *The Sunrise Model* by Leininger, which will be addressed in chapter 10. Use of a framework or model to help guide a community assessment project is an essential step in the process. A framework/model provides a frame of reference for data collection. Concepts or elements within a theoretical framework or model can be transposed into categories for data collection, diagnosis, and planning. Example concepts or elements that can be transposed into categories for data collection include safety, community boundaries, lines of resistance, and government systems. The following sections of this chapter give examples of how theoretical concepts can be used as criteria for assessment, community diagnoses, and planning.

General Ethnographic and Nursing Evaluation Studies in the State (GENESIS) Framework

GENESIS is a community assessment framework developed in 1979 by nurse anthropologist Jodi Glittenberg (1981). The primary method for conducting community assessments before the time Glittenberg developed the model was to dissect or "segregate the health system into neat little piles and pieces of roles, functions, needs, resources and by so doing take the problem out of its social context" (Glittenberg, 1981, p. 143). Furthermore, the health and health care system within communities was typically defined exclusively by "encultured health professionals"

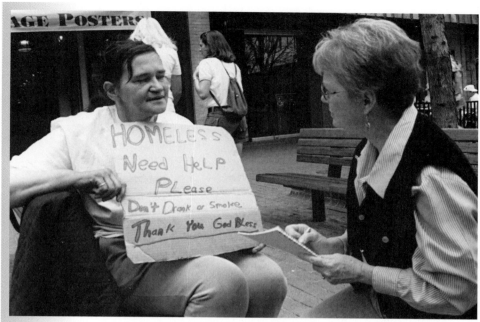

Chapter author, Dr. Judith Barton, conducting an ethnographic interview using the GENESIS framework as a theoretical guide for the conduct of a community health assessment, with a community member who is homeless.

(Glittenberg, 1981, p. 143) without including community members' perspectives on their state of health and health care system. Glittenberg asserted that if nursing professed to view clients holistically, community health assessment must include community member perspectives, and the health needs of a community must be viewed as interrelated with the environmental, economic, social, educational, and cultural needs of the community (Magilvy, McMahon, Bachman, & Evenson, 1986; Schultz & Magilvy, 1988; Stoner, Magilvy, & Schultz, 1992).

Project GENESIS was developed in Colorado when the state was on the verge of rapid growth. Then, as now, there was tremendous pressure to do a fast, simple community health assessment. In other words, just gather health statistics and demographic data on the population and develop health programs based on that data alone. But each community has its own uniqueness and means of problem solving, and these strengths are lost when health programs are not community based. What the GENESIS framework does is to combine the use of demographic statistics (i.e., census data) and epidemiology (i.e., health and vital statistics) with ethnographic field methods developed in the disciplines of anthropology and sociology. The goal is to generate a comprehensive and holistic portrait of a community through both a secondary analysis of existing quantitative data (e.g., census and health statistics data) and qualitative methods (Stoner, Magilvy, & Schultz, 1992).

There are five steps involved in using GENESIS as a guide for conducting a community assessment:

1. Collect and analyze **secondary data**, including, at a minimum, census data, health statistic data, historical documents, and community resources.

2. Identify and interview **key informants** (formal and informal leaders in the community representing a cross section of all age groups—a variety of town officials, school personnel, student leaders, community service leaders, etc.) using an ethnographic approach (i.e., open-ended questions related to community life).

3. Interview **primary informants** selected randomly throughout the community under study representing different community roles and population segments in the community (e.g., shoppers, post office foot traffic, laundromat users).

4. Analyze secondary data (i.e., existing data on the community such as census data and health statistics) and primary data (i.e., data from the ethnographic interviews) and compare and contrast these analyses. Do the quantitative data support, partially support, or contradict the qualitative data gathered in the interviews? Develop a list of strengths, weaknesses, and net health values, resulting in recommendations to improve the health status of the community. (See Table 2-2 for a sample GENESIS community

TABLE 2-2	SUMMARY OF *SOCIAL/CULTURAL ISSUES CATEGORY* DERIVED FROM AN ANALYSIS OF ETHNOGRAPHIC IN-TERVIEW DATA AND SECONDARY DATA USING THE GENESIS FRAMEWORK FOR COMMUNITY ASSESSMENT

STRENGTHS	WEAKNESSES	NET VALUE
People, primarily young people, move to beautiful mountain area by choice A high emotional bonding to the community as described by many residents High level of education	A labile transient population with perceived unmet needs by social services Limited community participation by commuting residents Limited cultural diversity	A young, educated population who have chosen and bonded to the community with unique needs regarding transients and cultural homogeneity

Recommendations:
Continue development of programs that sensitize and inform the residents about different cultural values and practices.
Investigate ways to promote increased involvement of the commuter population.
Address transient population situation with county government.

assessment outcome or community issue presented in a format listing strengths, weaknesses, and net value with recommendations.)

5. *Present a written and verbal report to the community asking for feedback before finalizing the written report in case community members find errors in the interpretation (Barton, Smith, Brown, & Supples, 1993; Smith & Barton, 1992).*

Community-as-Partner Model

The *community-as-partner model* includes community assessment as the first phase of the nursing process to be used when the client is a community. The model is based on nursing theorist Betty Neuman's (1989) total-person model for viewing individual patient problems. Nurse authors Anderson and McFarlane (1996) developed the model to help guide public health nurses in their practice with communities. The authors explain that the title of the model is purposeful in that the underlying philosophy of the model is primary health care with an emphasis on community empowerment. The model is also intended to be a synthesis of public health and nursing.

The community-as-partner model is a systems perspective that gives direction to types of community systems (e.g., educational system and transportation system) that need to be assessed when conducting a community assessment. It also provides direction for the analysis of the data collected to illuminate community dynamics related to health. Concepts in the model include the *community core*, eight interacting community *subsystems*, community *stressors*, and boundaries titled *normal level of defense*, *flexible line of defense*, and *lines of resistance*.

The *core* of any community is its people. Included in the core are the demographics of the population and their values,

beliefs, and history. The core in turn affects and is affected by eight interacting subsystems. Those subsystems are physical environment, education, safety and transportation, politics and government, health and social services, communication, economics, and recreation. In addition to assessing the core people within a community and the eight interacting subsystems, the community-as-partner model directs the nurse to assess current stressors that are producing tension within the community, the normal level of defense or current level of health within the community, the flexible line of defense representing current temporary responses to stressors or threats to health within the community, and lines of resistance or established community strengths that weave through all the interacting subsystems. Table 2-3 is a summary of all concepts or elements included in the community-as-partner model and their definitions.

After assessing *all* elements in the model, the researchers are directed to develop community diagnoses that include community responses to stressors (i.e., problem identification), causative factors leading to each problem, and a list of supporting data to validate each community diagnoses. In other words, the outcome of the community assessment using the community-as-partner model is a set of community diagnoses developed in the same format as nursing diagnoses. In turn, these community diagnoses lay the groundwork for health planning. For an example community diagnoses and plan see Table 2-4.

Although the community-as-partner model does not specifically direct the nurses to develop an interview guide based on the model's elements, an interview guide using an ethnographic open-ended approach has been developed and can be found in Box 2-6.

TABLE 2-3   **COMMUNITY-AS-PARTNER MODEL: CONCEPTS FOR ASSESSMENT**

Community core	The people who reside in a geopolitical community or the population of a community. Criteria to evaluate when assessing the core include the community's history, current demographics, and the values and beliefs of community residents.
Interrelated subsystems:	
Physical environment	Observations of the climate, terrain, natural boundaries, commercial systems, neighborhoods, religious symbols, planning studies, etc.
Health and social services	Hospitals and clinics, home health care, extended care facilities, public health services, counseling and support services, clothing, food, shelter, and special needs services
Economics	Household median income, percentage of persons living in poverty, employment status, occupational categories, and union activity
Safety and transportation	Information about protection services (fire, police, water treatment, solid waste) and air quality. Information on public transportation
Politics and government	Type of city government, political action groups, and political party affiliation
Communication	Formal communication sources (e.g., newspapers) and informal communication sources (e.g., bulletin boards, posters)
Education	Educational status of community members and educational sources
Recreation	Recreational facilities
Stressors	Tension-producing situations within the community such as an increase in substance abuse among teens within the community
Normal level of defense	Health statistics for the community (e.g., mortality and morbidity)
Flexible line of defense	Community responses to current stressors
Lines of resistance	Established strengths within the community (e.g., shelters, food banks)

Source: Anderson, E. T., & McFarlane, J. (1996). Community as partner: Theory and practice in nursing. *Philadelphia: Lippincott.*

TABLE 2-4   **COMMUNITY DIAGNOSIS FOR HEALTH PLANNING USING THE COMMUNITY-AS-PARTNER MODEL**

RESPONSE (PROBLEM)	RELATED TO (CAUSES)	AS MANIFESTED BY (DATA)
Community disorganization and medical/social services economic crisis	Increase in illegal immigrant workers from Mexico not eligible for government benefits Noncoordinated efforts between agencies within one community and among neighboring communities	Increase in nonreimbursed emergency room care at community hospital Increase in free school lunches at local schools Increase in delayed prenatal care and lower-birth-weight infants

GOAL	OBJECTIVE(S)	EVALUATIVE INDICATORS
Regional coordination of efforts to meet the needs of medical and social underserved populations	Establish a task force made up of service providers and community leaders representing the medically and socially underserved populations to design appropriate and feasible solutions/programs to deal with current community disorganization and medical/social services economic crisis	Reduced nonreimbursed emergency room costs, free school lunches, and low birth weight rates Increase in first trimester prenatal care

BOX 2-6 EXAMPLE KEY INFORMANT ETHNOGRAPHIC INTERVIEW GUIDE BASED ON COMMUNITY-AS-PARTNER MODEL

INTRODUCTION BY INTERVIEWER

Explain the purpose of the interview (i.e., to better understand the culture and the customs of your community). In addition, confirm that you will be taping the interview so that you do not have to take notes the whole time. Tell the informant that he or she may ask you to stop the taping at any time. Finally, assure the informant that his or her identity will remain confidential in all reports.

Grand Tour Question: What is it like to live in your community?

Mini-Tour Questions (some of the following questions, which target community subsystems, may have been thoroughly covered in response to grand tour question):

- What do you do for fun?
- What would you tell someone new to your community about the natural resources (environment) in your community?
- What are the schools like? Where do people go if they want to further their education?
- How safe do you feel in your community? How do you get around (transportation) in your community?
- Who has the political power in the community (i.e., who is the most powerful figure[s] in your community)? Discuss your rationale (reasons).
- Describe your perceptions of the health of your community. Where do you personally go for your health care needs? How adequate are the services available to you?
- Please describe the formal and informal types of communication in your community.
- How would you describe the economic trends/future for your community? If I moved here, how easy would it be to make a living, buy groceries and clothes, and have a place to live?
- Can you tell me something about the cultural and spiritual/religious aspects of your community (e.g., family life, philosophy of community)?
- Is there anything else you would like to tell me about your community?

Source: University of Colorado Health Sciences Center School of Nursing, master course materials for Community Analysis Project, *1996.*

General Systems Model for Community Assessment

Lundy and Barton's (1995) *General Systems Model for Community and Population Assessment and Intervention* is based on general systems theory as originally conceived by Von Bertalanffy (1968). A general systems approach is the basis for many nursing theories and has widespread usage in most all scientific disciplines. This approach to community assessment directs the research team to focus on the whole community, not on the parts of a community. Two broad concepts for assessment using this model include community *structure* and *process*.

The **structure** of any system can be defined as an arrangement of *interacting subsystems* or parts at a given point in time. The system as a whole has specified boundaries that determine what is inside the system and what is outside the system. In turn, each subsystem has boundaries that specify what is inside the subsystem and what is outside. Similar to the community-as-partner assessment model, subsystems within the community system include schools, churches, self-help groups, health systems, and so on. Systems also have a *suprasystem,* the larger construct of which the system is a part. For example, if the community system is identified as a municipality or a city, the county and state where the municipality is situated become suprasystems to the community system and have great relevance to the community system and the community assessment process.

Community health nurses using the general systems assessment approach to community assessment begin by identifying the target system and its boundaries. For example, if the assessment is to be carried out on a geopolitical community named Jonestown, the researchers must ask the following questions:

1. *Do the boundaries for Jonestown stop at the city's geopolitical limits or does the community consider a neighboring smaller crossroads community as within its boundaries?*
2. *What are the critical subsystems within the target community system?*
3. *What are the critical suprasystems impacting the community?*
4. *What types of relationships exist among the subsystems and between the target community and its suprasystems?*
5. *Are the boundaries between subsystems, the system, and its suprasystems open and cooperative, or is there a lack of cooperation and support between these systems?*
6. *Does the target community system and its subsystems have a sense of integrity or are the boundaries too open?*

In assessing *community process,* nurses need to determine how the community system works to meet its needs or goals. Questions to be asked include the following: How is the community system responding (termed *throughput*) to internal and external stimuli or *inputs*? What are the results or *outputs* of the community system's response? (An example of a result or output to a stressor such as air pollution might be stricter auto emission policies.) Is the output successful (negative feedback) or does the Environmental Protection Agency fine the community for having too many poor air quality days per year (positive feedback)? In other words, does the community return to a *steady state* or does it continue to experience *disequilibrium*? and How can the community continue to grow from the ongoing processes of *input, response, output,* and *feedback*?

The Lundy-Barton Model also includes a process for the nurse to use as a follow-through to the community assessment. This process is a familiar one to both nursing and medicine. One assesses the client (i.e., the community), arrives at several diagnoses, develops a plan of action, evaluates the outcomes, and revises the plan as needed. Table 2-5 is a summary of all concepts found in the Lundy-Barton Model, their definitions, and examples of types of data to collect. A community assessment guide based on the Lundy-Barton Model can be found in appendix A.

Planned Appr

The Planned App conceptual guide for the mid-1980s by the tion (CDC). PATCH w theory, which specifies hea people to increase control o health. It is a comprehensive g collecting, organizing, and an health-related data; choosing healt prehensive intervention plan; and key strategy in PATCH is to encoura munity and among the community an ment, universities, and other regional and national organizations that can provide data, resources, and consultation. Any interested group within a community can request a PATCH concept guidebook from the CDC, and most state health departments

---

TABLE 2-5   **LUNDY-BARTON MODEL: CONCEPTS FOR ASSESSMENT WITH EXAMPLE QUESTIONS**

COMMUNITY STRUCTURE

Target system	*Observations:* Are the boundaries for the target community geopolitical or geographic? How would you describe the natural environment? Describe cultural symbols noted.
	Measurements: Demographics, health and social service statistics.
	Interactions: History of community, values and beliefs.
Subsystems	*Observations:* Windshield survey of public institutions such as schools, churches, businesses, recreational facilities, etc.
	Measurements: Literature on various subsystems within community.
	Interactions: Interview key community leaders to find out how the community subsystems interact.
Suprasystems	*Observations:* Compare and contrast target community environment with suprasystems (e.g., in comparison to other cities within county).
	Measurements: Demographic and health statistic data for most relevant suprasystem (e.g., state statistics) to compare target system with suprasystem.
	Interactions: Interview key community leaders to find out how the target community interacts with state or county agencies.

COMMUNITY PROCESS

Goals	*Observations:* Windshield survey may reveal new construction sites indicating growth direction.
	Measurements: Seek community planning documents, interview key community leaders concerning goals of community.
	Interactions: Does there seem to be agreement among key community leaders about community goals?
Inputs	*Observations:* Attendance at community meetings to gain information about particular community stressors (inputs). Windshield survey to observe for environmental hazards.
Responses/ throughputs	*Measurements:* Review of literature obtained from various community agencies to determine ongoing community initiatives (responses or throughputs). Interviews with key community
Results/outputs	members to learn more about final outcomes of initiatives and if the initiatives met their
Feedback	objectives (results or outputs and feedback).
	Interactions: Is the community experiencing a steady state or is it experiencing disequilibrium?

Source: Lundy, K. S., & Barton, J. A. (1995). Assessment: Data collection of the community client. In P. J. Christensen & J. W. Kenney (Eds.), Nursing process: Application of conceptual models (4th ed., pp. 102–119). St. Louis: Mosby.

ATCH and a state coordinator who serves
act for PATCH. The CDC promotes the use of
helping achieve the year 2010 national health objec-
Fundamental to PATCH is active participation by a wide
range of community members. The community health team provides leadership and guidance, but community members actively
participate in collecting community health data, analyzing the
data, setting priorities, and planning intervention activities.

Similar to the GENESIS framework, PATCH promotes the
collection of both *quantitative* and *qualitative data* during the

community health assessment phase of the process. Box 2-7 includes recommended quantitative data to be collected according
to PATCH. These include demographics, health statistics, and
behavioral risk factor data. PATCH directs the assessment team
to collect these data on both the local community level and the
state level to compare the local community with some standard.

Qualitative information to be collected using the PATCH
process is opinion data from community leaders. According to
PATCH, community leaders are people in positions of power
who have the reputation for getting things done, who made key
decisions on previous community issues, who actively volunteer
their time to help the community, or who are formal or informal
neighborhood or community leaders. PATCH emphasizes that
the opinions of the community must be heard and respected if
there is to be community ownership of community health planning. Opinion information provides viewpoints from the community about health awareness, needs, and perceived health
problems. A comparison of quantitative information with the
opinion data will either substantiate or disprove the opinions of
the community. For example, community opinion might perceive that the cancer rate in the community is high and that it is
connected to their "smelly water." However, the mortality and
morbidity data collected on the community showed lung cancer
as the prominent type of cancer, whereas digestive cancers were
extremely rare. Thus, the community designed an intervention
program to target lung cancer by reducing tobacco use. Box 2-8
includes the recommended community leader opinion survey as
designed by PATCH.

**BOX 2-7 ESSENTIAL QUANTITATIVE DATA
TO COLLECT AND ANALYZE USING THE
PATCH PROCESS FOR COMMUNITY
HEALTH PLANNING**

- Community profile data
- Unemployment rate
- Per capita income
- Families below poverty level (%)
- Age distribution in years
- Number of households, by household size
- Annual household income
- Marital status
- Racial/ethnic composition
- Number of people enrolled in educational programs
- Educational achievement levels
- Mortality and morbidity data
- Unique health events (e.g., health legislation, special health promotion activities)
- Number of deaths and years of potential life lost by major disease categories
- Five leading causes of death by age groups
- Comparison of mortality rates for leading causes of death by race, sex, and age groups
- Behavioral data
- State-collected Behavioral Risk Factor Surveil-lance System (BRFSS) extrapolated to commu-nity subgroups; BRFSS data includes items on seatbelt use, obesity, current smoking, drink-ing, sedentary lifestyle, leisure-time activities, hypertension, exercise, and cholesterol screen-ing levels

Source: Planned approach to community health: Guide for the local coordinator. (1992). Atlanta: U.S. Department of Health and Human Services, Centers for Disease Control and Prevention, NCFCDP & HP.

**BOX 2-8 COMMUNITY LEADER OPINION
SURVEY AS DESIGNED BY PATCH**

1. What do you think the main health problems are in our community?
2. What do you think are the causes of these health problems?
3. How can these problems be reduced or elimi-nated in our community?
4. Which one of these problems do you con-sider to be the most important one in our community?
5. Can you suggest three other people with whom I might talk about the health problems in our community?

   Thank you for your help. Right now I do not have any more questions, but may I contact you in the future if other issues come up?

Source: Planned approach to community health: Guide for the local coordinator. (1992). Atlanta: U.S. Department of Health and Human Services, Centers for Disease Control and Prevention, NCFCDP & HP.

A Comparison of the Four Community Assessment Frameworks/Models

More often than not a community assessment project is guided by a blend of two or more perspectives to meet the objectives of the assessment. For example, the PATCH model provides specific directions for involving the target community not only in planning and participating in the assessment, but also in diagnosing assets and needs as well as program planning to build on assets and address needs. Although project GENESIS does not provide specific directions for involving the target community in the assessment process, GENESIS may be the theoretical framework of choice if the research team needs to develop a trusting relationship with the community while simultaneously collecting data. The process is similar to that of the cultural anthropologist who lives in the study community while "talking" (i.e., conducting ethnographic interviews) with community members to learn about the cultural ways of the community. When conducting ethnographic interviews, the community member is the expert and the nurse is the learner. This philosophical stance helps build a trusting relationship between the community and the nurse. Finally, the PATCH and GENESIS frameworks guide the team to specifically include both quantitative and qualitative data.

Both the community-as-partner model and the Lundy-Barton Model use a systems approach to community assessment. The goal of both perspectives is to arrive at an integrated or holistic view of the target community. Both perspectives also include a four-step process for nurses to follow. That process includes assessment as phase one, diagnosis as phase two, action plans as phase three, and evaluation as phase four.

Although the authors of the community-as-partner model discuss the concept of community empowerment and explain that the title of the model is purposeful, there are no specific directions in the model for including the community in the assessment process. The same is true of the Lundy-Barton Model and the GENESIS framework, although the GENESIS framework specifically includes the ethnographic interview as integral; that process in and of itself can be empowering for community members, and in particular, community leaders. See Table 2-6 for a comparison of the four community assessment frameworks/models discussed in this chapter.

Using the Nursing Process for the Community
Conducting a Community Assessment

More often than not a community assessment project will be guided by a blend of two or more theoretical perspectives. In addition, a community assessment model or blended model can be used to conduct a population assessment *in any practice setting*. For example, a nurse in a postpartum unit of a regional medical center noted that there had been an influx of Mexican immigrants. These immigrants were Spanish-speaking only, and no staff spoke Spanish, nor was patient education literature available in Spanish. The nurse in this case realized that she needed to provide the leadership role in conducting a population assessment. Her population assessment included an examination of population demographics in both the hospital and the general community. She then examined the hospital's human resources for language translation and available Spanish-language educational materials. She also inter-

---

TABLE 2-6   A COMPARISON OF THE FOUR COMMUNITY ASSESSMENT FRAMEWORKS/MODEL

GUIDELINES	FRAMEWORKS/MODELS			
	GENESIS	COMMUNITY AS PARTNER	GENERAL SYSTEMS ASSESSMENT	PATCH
Directs researchers in collection of quantitative data (e.g., health statistics)	Yes	Yes	Yes	Yes
Directs researchers in collection of qualitative data (e.g., interviews)	Yes	No	No	Yes
Directs researchers to use a systems approach	No	Yes	Yes	No
Directs researchers to include community members as experts or as assessment team members	Yes	No	No	Yes
Directs researchers to use a four-step process from data collection to diagnosis to planning to evaluation	No	Yes	Yes	Yes

viewed personnel (key informants familiar with the population) on the unit and some of the inpatients as well (primary informants). The nurse, with the support of the nurse manager of the unit, raised the consciousness of the hospital administration that patient educational materials and translators should be available for Spanish-speaking patients. The nurse then developed a culturally sensitive child education program including written materials in Spanish. The program was implemented by nurses on the postpartum unit and was well accepted by the immigrant patients and nurses on the unit. Recommendations were made to administration for the program's continuation with support from the Hispanic community. The nurse in this example adapted the GENESIS model as her conceptual guide for the population assessment. She conducted key and primary informant interviews,

she gathered some secondary data (e.g., community resources for the population and some census data on the population), and she analyzed both sources of data to define the strengths and limitations of the population and recommendations for interventions at the population level. Clearly this nurse used her understanding of the connection between population health and individual care regardless of setting (Baldwin et al., 1998).

Once a theoretical perspective or a combination of theoretical perspectives has been chosen to guide the community assessment process, general tenets from the nursing process (i.e., assessment techniques, planning based on the assessment, interventions implemented at the community or population level, and evaluation) will apply. Box 2-9 summarizes steps in the process of a community health assessment.

BOX 2-9   STEPS IN COMMUNITY-FOCUSED INTERVENTION

Community defined; partnership established
Identification of the community
Promotion of the partnership of the community

ASSESSMENT

What are the characteristics of the population (age, gender, race)?

What changes are occurring in the characteristics of the people in the community (births, deaths, migrations)?

What health problems exists in the community (morbidity rates)?

What health problems are causing deaths in the population (mortality rates)?

How do these health problems compare with other populations? Are they increasing or decreasing?

NURSING DIAGNOSES

Name the:

Risk of (a specific problem or health risk in the community)

Among (the specific group or population affected by the problem/risk)

Related to (strength and weaknesses in the community that influence the specific health risk in the community)

PLANNING

What factors that are changeable (environmental, behavioral) increase the risk of the health problem?

What can most effectively reduce risk among the population?

What can be done in the community to reduce risk?

How much change in the health problem is desired over what period of time in the population (goals and objectives)?

Who can most effectively affect the outcome of the plan?

IMPLEMENTATION

What is the role of the community health nurse in the action phase?

What strategies can facilitate healthy change in the community?

EVALUATION

Was the plan carried out?

Was it acceptable to the community or population?

Was the health problem changed as planned?

Was the program effective?

What would be done differently?

What are recommendations for future community health promotion?

Source: Watson, N. M. (1984). Community as client. In J. A. Sullivan (Ed.), Community health nursing. Boston: Blackwell.

Gaining Entry into the Community

The collection of meaningful data about a community depends on the nurse's successfully gaining entry into the community. According to Goeppinger and Schuster (1988, p. 262), "gaining entry or acceptance into the community is perhaps the biggest challenge in assessment."

Just as you would never just enter a client's room in a hospital or knock on the door of a home health client and say, "Turn over in bed, I am here to give you a 'shot,'" the population-focused nurse should not expect to just walk into a community and plan to conduct a community-focused intervention without going through some stages of getting to know the community as client. As Kauffman (1994) explains in her study of the experience of white nurse researchers who conducted an ethnography of a senior citizen center in a poor, inner-city black ghetto, "getting in" a community is "a process of gaining, building, and maintaining trust with the group under study" (p. 179). Differences in characteristics such as social status, ethnicity, age, and class between the researchers, who are the *outsiders,* and the community being studied, the *insiders,* may create an environment of prejudicial and discriminatory responses that impede *getting in.* In other words, would the community be willing to share their issues with a community assessment team that just barged in and said they were here to study their health and health care needs? Would the results of an assessment set up in this manner produce valid results? Is it not possible that the outsiders could commit flagrant errors in their interpretations that might even promote prejudice and discrimination toward the very community that they intended to assist?

Another strategy found to be helpful is to use a variety of communication channels to "reach" the target population. Using existing personal networks (e.g., clubs, social groups) and social institutions (e.g., voluntary health organizations, churches, schools) that the target population depends on for support and information can both yield positive access results. If the target group has an established health network (e.g., a group of diabetic elders), contacting those medical/health societies to seek support and approval can provide valuable entry. The nurse must be aware, however, that all members of a subgroup may not be reached through any one organization, thus necessitating the use of diverse means in attempts to initially establish contact with the target population. With the Internet, many new opportunities for developing contact and securing information about target groups are possible and hold great promise in this stage of community assessment. Another way to demonstrate the community team's commitment to reach the community is to participate in community activities. Community team members may stay in local motels, rather than chains, and patronize local eateries.

If the community assessment team is very different in social characteristics from the community under study, it would be easy for the outsiders to err by underestimating the effects of ethnicity, age, and class on insiders' responses. They may use inappropriate data collection tools, or they may assume the insiders are just not knowledgeable enough or educated enough to be able to articulate their health beliefs and health issues. If the assessment team believes the community is not knowledgeable, they may patronize the group (i.e., treat the community with unseemly deference rather than as equals). Locals and important leaders in communities and target populations can function as valuable "cultural brokers," controlling entry into the group, especially to underserved populations. These brokers are often laypersons who might be called "natural helpers," people to whom the community turns for help in times of health concerns and other crises. Identifying these significant persons takes time because they may not be the formal leaders of a group. These brokers can impede "outside" projects or provide invaluable assistance in accessing the group. By serving as local "interpreters," these brokers can translate culture for both the health team and residents and promote collaboration for assessment activities.

Note that it is not detrimental to be an outsider when studying a community. The sociological concept of the "professional stranger" has taught us that being an outsider studying the group allows the researcher to not be caught up in the commitments of the group and therefore to be able to raise questions unlikely to be raised by insiders.

Kauffman (1994) proposes five phases of "getting in" to a community to build trust that will lead to a valid study of the community. These five phases are impressing, behaving, swapping, belonging, and "chillin' out." Kauffman points out that several phases may sometimes occur simultaneously. However, at all times the processes are mutual, interactive, and context specific.

Impressing is the initial and sometimes lengthy process of outsiders and insiders evaluating one another. Social myths are explored; stereotypes and traits of the other (e.g., skin color, clothes, social courtesies) are observed. Rejection is possible by either side. Strategies for the community assessment team to maintain include (1) maintaining political, institutional, and personal neutrality; (2) avoiding obligations to any sponsor or patron of the assessment project; (3) following the rules or customs of all the insiders, not just the leaders; (4) continuing to return to the community and clarifying the assessment process; (5) keeping abreast of local events; and (6) identifying key informants who represent all different groups within the community. An important aspect of a cultural system is its members' valued ideas—those notions about how things should be done. As is so often the case, community members and the community assessment team have different "valued ideas," and cultural clashes occur.

Behaving occurs when actions and interactions between outsiders and insiders begin to erode myths about each other, and each sees the other as fellow human beings, although each side may still guard against rejection. Strategies for continuing the trust-building process in this phase include (1) demonstrating nonjudgmental and unconditional regard, (2) being genuine and avoiding trying too hard to be accepted, (3) learning the language of the group (e.g., the meaning of cultural slang words, perhaps phrases of a foreign language), and (4) placing the insider as the esteemed teacher of community life and health. The gender and age of team members and community members can also play an important part in this phase. For example, using a very young community interviewer in an elderly population may be less effective than using a middle-aged person. Wax (1986) found that middle-aged or older women are more able than any other age or gender to collect data across ages and gender categories. Of course, generalizations must be avoided in any context; however, ignoring age and gender influences can often impede or distort data collection.

Swapping involves reciprocal giving and sharing between the outsiders and insiders. Giving and sharing helps break down the remaining barriers to mutual acceptance and trust between the outsiders and insiders. Strategies used in the swapping process include telling insiders more about the roles of the outsiders (e.g., health programs involved in, outcomes of previous community assessments). Going to community events is an important swapping activity that often allows for informal interviews.

Belonging is the culmination of the process. During this phase, outsiders and insiders are able to talk about issues that heretofore provoked discomfort. Issues such as racism, prejudice, and discrimination are open to discussion. Insider language no longer seems foreign to the outsider, who understands the meaning of the language. Greetings and good-byes include physical displays of affection such as hugging. Socially deviant acts such as drug use may no longer be hidden from the outsider.

Chillin' out begins as the outsiders near the end of their community assessment phase and begin (hopefully) a long-term partnership with the community for the improvement and maintenance of community health. Outsiders should give insiders an idea of what to expect in the future, such as the amount of help that will always be available from health care experts.

Collecting Data

What kinds of data do nurses look for when conducting a community assessment, and where do they find it? The primary goal of data collection is to acquire meaningful and useful information about the community and its health. A systematic and informed nursing assessment in partnership with the community involves a variety of techniques and resources. The scope of a community or population assessment is determined by the purpose of the assessment and the complexity and nature of the identified community or population. For community assessments of large geopolitical communities, the process may take several months to a year or more and may require an interdisciplinary team.

Confidentiality regarding sensitive or controversial data is a critical issue for nurses conducting a community assessment (Goeppinger & Schuster, 1988). Just as a nurse must safeguard information obtained from the individual client as an ethical and legal responsibility, the information derived from the community may involve a more concerted effort. Because there are often many team members collecting information from a variety of sources, it may be necessary to assign anonymous names to com-

munity members and even to other organizations within the community.

There are seven methods of collecting community data: **informant interviews, observation, secondary analysis of existing data, constructed surveys, focus groups, community forums,** and **windshield surveys.** The community health nurse should attempt to collect data using several different methods because no method is without bias. The process of using multiple complementary methods is termed *triangulation.*

Informant interviews involve directly questioning community residents. The nurse uses appropriate communication techniques in directed conversations with selected members of a community. These interviews can be structured, with planned questions, or unstructured, in which the informants guide the interviews. Data gathered through informant interviews are considered subjective and can yield valuable information about the residents' perspectives on health values and health care; for example, how do the residents perceive their community health care services? Such data are recorded in the resident's own words and noted as direct quotations in the interaction column of the assessment tool. Both formal and informal leaders of groups and communities will yield important information about the community.

The nurse uses *observation* by purposefully looking and listening for significant events that are taking place in the community. Examples include city council meetings, high school basketball games, county fairs, barber shop conversations, and other similar social events. The nurse systematically records these observations. Relevant conversations of community residents are recorded in the interaction column of the assessment tool.

Secondary analysis is analysis of records, documents, and other previously collected data. The nurse may not have to collect new data when conducting the community assessment. Such data may already exist in the form of census data, historical accounts, diaries, previous studies of the community or aggregate, court records, minutes from community meetings, and research studies on population risks. The following research brief describes risks for cross-country truck drivers. The results of this research can be incorporated in a population assessment of cross-country truck drivers and is an example of the use of secondary data in a population health assessment. These are invaluable sources of information that can reveal the characteristics of the community as well as the attitudes of people in the community and how they cope with their lives on a daily basis.

Voluntary agencies, such as the American Heart Association, can provide aggregated data on specific health issues. These data are often organized in a more useful and focused format than official agencies. *Healthy People 2010* can be an excellent resource for specific health issues, including baselines and progress in preventive health. State health departments, the U.S. Public Health Service, the National Center for Health Statistics, and the U.S. Census provide a wide array of mortality and morbidity statistics and demographic profiles of populations. The CDC is an excel-

RESEARCH BRIEF

Renner, D. A. (1998). Cross country truck drivers: A vulnerable population. Nursing Outlook, 46(4), 164–168.

Cross-country truck drivers were identified as a vulnerable population and studies were analyzed that explored the risks of this occupational group. There are more than 2.9 million commercial truck drivers in the United States who generate more than $362 billion in annual gross revenue (1994). As the author points out, "anything that touches your life was brought to you by a truck and a truck driver." The article identifies health risks for drivers that are related to the stress, monotony, and transient nature of the work: 50% of drivers admitted to smoking one to two packs of cigarettes a day, and 25% revealed that they had concerns about their alcohol drinking pattern. Almost 90% of the drivers cited exercise as a rare or infrequent health practice and complained of stress related to the hypervigilant state of driving long distances. Other risks included cardiovascular disease, back disorders, muscle and joint disorders, decreased circulation of the lower extremities, kidney disease, and herniated lumbar intervertebral disks caused by the prolonged stationary seated position. Combined with the vibration of the truck, the increased intraluminal pressure contributed to their high incidence of hemorrhoids and disorders such as appendicitis. Social risks are related to disenfranchisement from family, friends, and coworkers as a result of long days on the road and the isolation of the work. Most truckers do not have adequate health insurance, especially those who are self-employed, and they rarely seek health care unless in a state of emergency. The author suggests that interventions for truckers need to occur both at the policy level (by changing standards of work conditions) and in delivery by ensuring access to preventive health care. Other suggestions include the need for focused research on the health beliefs of truckers and working with truckers and trucker unions to create appropriate, accessible health resources.

lent source for information about national illness and health patterns as well as aggregated state health information.

In **constructed surveys,** community or aggregate members in a random sample of the population provide answers to written or oral questions. This technique is costly and time-consuming and is used only when other resources have been exhausted. For example, if a nurse is interested in abortion attitudes and if very little information is available through other techniques, a survey of

community members may provide useful information about this issue.

A **focus group** can be used very effectively to derive information about health needs of specific groups in the community or population. The focus group is a qualitative approach to learning about subgroups within the population regarding sociocultural and other specific characteristics. Members of a focus group differ from other small groups in that the members are usually chosen to be fairly homogenous in regard to specific characteristics, such as gender, age, or other social variables. By being highly selective about the membership of a focus group, the nurse can learn a great deal about that particular subpopulation's needs and perceptions about viable, acceptable solutions to health problems. The average group meeting lasts 2 to 3 hours and can be a very efficient way to determine group perceptions (Basch, 1987).

A **community forum,** which involves having an open meeting for all members of a community or population, can also be used to obtain information concerning the needs and perceptions of community members. In contrast to the focus group, a community forum is open to all; no attempt is made to structure a homogenous group. A town hall meeting is a variation of the community forum and was used by President Bill Clinton to bring his health care reform package to the grass roots level. Even though community forums are not necessarily representative of the entire target population, they can be used effectively in a short period of time, with little cost, as one strategy for community members to voice their views.

The nurse can conduct a **windshield survey** of the geopolitical community as a technique for data collection. These observations through the window of an automobile are a way of collecting information about a community's environment. As an initial data collection technique, a windshield survey often reveals common characteristics about the way people live (e.g., transportation primarily by automobile, little pedestrian traffic), where they live, and the type of housing they live in.

Community Diagnosis

Conclusions about data collected on the community client is a natural outcome of the assessment process. Eventually, these stated analyzed conclusions identify "labels" or names for the health problems in the community; these are called **community health diagnoses** (Higgs & Gustafson, 1985). The gathered data and generated data form a composite database. At this phase of the nursing process, as raw data are analyzed, themes begin to emerge and needs are noted, as are problems, strengths, and community resources. Community members continue to be involved in this process as both subjective and objective data are compiled.

Written community health diagnoses differ significantly from those written for the individual client. Most systems of classification developed for nursing diagnoses have focused on the individual. Hamilton (1983) analyzed various theories and diagnostic classification schemata and concluded that research is needed in both the application of individual models of diagnoses and the clarification of the *target* of care, whether that be the community, individuals in the community, or individuals influenced by the community. Viewing the community as a client who has varying degrees of ability to meet its own needs extends the focus to include response to illness and change, social problems, or any areas in which the community client needs assistance in order to function optimally (Higgs & Gustafson, 1985). Data from the target community or population are compared with similar populations in other settings. Comparing data such as infant mortality rates or accident rates can reveal significant differences and point to specific disparate health risks in the target population. During this phase, the community health nurse compares conclusions about the community's health status with accepted standards of health and judgments are made as to strengths and concerns of a community's functioning (Lundy & Barton, 1995).

Identified problems are now stated in the form of a community health diagnosis. Each diagnosis is documented, the recipient of care is identified (the community as opposed to the individual), and factors contributing to the problem are explicated.

A common nursing diagnosis format that has been modified for community use has been developed by Schuster and Goeppinger (1996) and Muecke (1984). Here the **diagnosis** takes the following form:

1. *Risk of (a specific problem or health risk in the community)*
2. *Among (the specific group or population that is affected by the problem/risk)*
3. *Related to (strengths and weaknesses in the community that influence the specific problem or health risk in the community)*

The following are some sample community/population diagnoses using the aforementioned format:

- *Risk of hearing loss among studio musicians related to constancy of loud music in occupational settings and nonuse of hearing protection*
- *Risk for increased incidence of pregnancy among teens at Rydell High School related to increased sexual activity and nonuse of contraceptive services or methods*
- *Risk for lung damage among migrant farm workers in the Mississippi delta related to presence of pesticide pulmonary irritants in the occupational environment*
- *Risk of eating disorders among professional ballet dancers related to occupational pressure to stay underweight for professional advancement*
- *Risk of sleep deprivation among nurses who are permanent night shift workers at Bayview Medical Center related to erratic and interrupted day sleep*
- *Build on community strength of coordination among community agencies to address all risks or identified community health issues*

- *Support beginning efforts by faith communities within community to address family solidarity through church-sponsored day-care facilities*

Planning and Prioritization Phase

During the **planning phase**, priorities are established, goals and objectives are identified based on those priorities, and community-focused interventions are developed. Unlike a clinical individual diagnosis, a community diagnosis requires more than simple establishment of the presence of a health problem. More than one health problem is always present in a community or population; consequently, diagnoses require prioritizing problems for community action. Criteria must be established to determine how resources and energies will be allocated toward addressing the identified needs (Watson, 1984).

The WHO has published criteria that may be used to prioritize health problems identified in communities. These criteria are listed in Box 2-10.

Goeppinger (1984) has also developed a set of criteria to guide the prioritization of community health problems. Those criteria are as follows:

- *Community awareness of the problem*
- *Community motivation*
- *Nurse's or team's ability to influence problem solution*
- *Availability of expertise*
- *Severity of consequences to society if problems left unresolved*
- *Quickness with which the problem can be resolved*

Reviewing the identified health problems using a set of criteria is a critical step in the process to address complex community health problems. In addition, community members repre-

---

BOX 2-10   CRITERIA FOR SELECTING A HEALTH PROBLEM FOR COMMUNITY INTERVENTION

- Significance of the problem (in terms of numbers affected or consequences)
- Level of community awareness and priority
- Ability to reduce risk
- Cost of reducing risk (economic, social, ethical)
- Ability to identify the target population
- Availability of resources to intervene in the reduction of risk

Source: Adapted from World Health Organization (WHO). (1976, October 11–15). Criteria to be considered in selecting a preventive health action. In Report of the first interdisciplinary workshop on psychosocial factors and health. Stockholm: Author.

senting multiple subpopulations within the community (e.g., different age groups, ethnic groups), community leaders, and assessment team members should be involved at this stage.

Once the prioritized problem list emerges, goals, objectives, strategies, and plans are developed. *Goals* are broad and general statements of concern that are usually considered long range. *Objectives* are specific, measurable statements of desired outcomes and are often viewed as short term. An example of the planning phase of the community health process is shown in the figure on pp. 52–53.

All planning group members, community representatives, and other experts within the appropriate areas are involved in this process, especially those who will be most affected and who are in a position to influence the implementation of solutions. The importance of this involvement cannot be overemphasized. Many community interventions have failed and undermined future professional assistance because community teams excluded community members from participating in this process. We know from research that when communities and populations develop a vested interest in the identification of health needs and proposed solutions, there is a greater likelihood of sustaining these intervention strategies over time. In other words, the community must be willing to "pay the price" of whatever objectives and goals are proposed (Watson, 1984).

Community health nurses are often members of teams who are conducting community or population level assessments, and as such the identified health problems and concerns are rarely limited to the use of nursing interventions. The complexity of group-identified health concerns requires an interdisciplinary approach, and planning and intervention strategies usually reflect the involvement of other professionals (e.g., social workers, audiologists, physicians, and psychologists) and community resources' utilization.

Implementation Phase

The implementation phase is the action phase. It translates the objectives and strategies into reality. Strategies should be selected based on not only currently available resources in the community but also the likelihood that the means will have some long-term availability. During implementation, lay leaders in the communities, professionals, and organizations must be included and their support acquired. In the long run, it is always better to educate others on how to implement these strategies than for the nurse and other team members to control the implementation. The tendency toward paternalism is strong among health professionals and for many has been reinforced through acute care organizational structures and roles; one must safeguard against the problems of paternalism. In the implementation phase, those community leaders who have greatest probability of achieving success—those whom the community respects and looks to for guidance—are identified. In general, a pilot test should be planned if possible as a trial run of the implementation. In this way, using a few individuals from target groups for feedback, delivery and design issues may be dis-

FYI

New Orleans Musicians as a Population: A Community-Focused Intervention Implemented Through a Collaborative Arrangement Between Health Professionals and Community Leaders

After noticing that musicians from the New Orleans entertainment district, the French Quarter, often sought medical attention late in an illness, nurses and MDs at Louisiana State University Medical Center conducted a population assessment of the target group. They found that musicians rarely had any health insurance and only sought health care when desperate. After seeking collaboration with musicians in the New Orleans area, the LSU Medical Center Musicians Clinic opened as an affordable, focused primary health clinic. A musician's union card is all that is needed to qualify for the clinic services. The clinic is managed with a board of musicians, business owners, and community health professionals. The MDs and nurse practitioners donated their time and musicians pay minimal costs. The community health professionals consider the clinic a "thank you note" to a business that is vital to Louisiana and New Orleans, with its thriving traditions of jazz, rock, and other musical styles. Music sustains an estimated 50,000 jobs in Louisiana and pumps $2.2 billion a year into the economy.

Source: Sick musicians can get new gig: LSU medical clinic. (1998, May 2). The Clarion Ledger. Jackson, Mississippi, p. 5a.

covered that can be ironed out before the major investments of time, energy, and resources (Clark, 1996). Pilot studies often reveal that more training is needed, along with more or different types of resources and more time. Minor flaws can be corrected; feedback can be collected from the pilot participants with ideas about how the implementation might be changed or improved; and fine tuning can increase likelihood for success in the implementation (Schuster & Goeppinger, 1996). The following three boxes are all examples of community-focused interventions implemented through a **collaborative arrangement** between health professionals and community leaders.

Role of the Community Health Nurse

The roles of the community health nurse (CHN) and other professionals depend on the nature of the health problem, the community's ability to make decisions, and professional and personal

Gilpin County's Action Plan on Priority Health Problem: Substance Abuse.

ACTION PLAN
FOR
TASK FORCE ON GILPIN COUNTY'S
PRIORITY HEALTH PROBLEMS

Problem: Substance abuse, primarily alcohol abuse
Nature and extent:

The nature and extent of the substance abuse problem in Gilpin County may not be fully or accurately reflected in the data available because we have not yet found good measuring tools to use to get an accurate picture of the substance abuse problem in our community or any other.

BUT WE DO KNOW:

The community opinion survey revealed that substance abuse was the most common concern of the 98 people surveyed.

The key informant survey revealed that substance abuse was the most common concern of the 43 people interviewed.

The secondary data ranks Gilpin County 12th in the state for per capita sales in drinking places out of 64, 58th per capita retail sales in liquor stores, 19th for liquor licenses per 10,000 population, 2nd for DUI case filings per 1,000 and 7th for alcohol related fatal crashes per 10,000.

We had 1 drug abuse violation under the age of 18 in 1999.

We had 4 drug abuse violations over the age of 18 in 1999.

We had 2 accidental deaths for a rate of 105.2 compared to a state rate of 39.5–2 were motor vehicle deaths.

Alcohol related fatal crash rate for Gilpin County was .85 per 10,000.

Of the convicted DUI cases, approximately 80% are tourists, 20% locals.

We have lost two of our teenagers in the past 5 years to alcohol related fatal crashes.

The alcohol and drug counselor's caseload of 60 has two common denominators:

1.   All of the clients are from dysfunctional families
2.   All of the clients have underlying emotional problems which lead them to abuse alcohol/drugs.

Our community is a bedroom community which lacks a central focus, a common community meeting place, and community based, organized recreation opportunities. It is geographically isolated, has no public transportation and is a tourist attraction.

The local schools have some alcohol and drug education information in the curriculum, but Gilpin School does not have a K–12 health education curriculum.

According to Gilpin County Social Services, 7 Gilpin County youths were in alcohol and drug treatment inpatient programs from 1995 through 2000 at a cost of $53,040, 20% of which came from Gilpin County taxes and 80% from state taxes. This does not include school costs.

RESOURCES we have:

schools, clinics and alcohol and drug counselor, a mental health counselor, a library, private organizations like the Elks, the VFW, the American Legion, Lions, Masons, Alan Green Foundation, A.A., Alanon, natural outdoor; Al-ateen recreation activities and day care homes; We have some participation, S.A.D.D. chapters in both schools, scouts, PTO, Booster Club, churches, library, county nursing services, school nursing services E.N.T., Fire Department.

There are some things we could change:

1.   We could improve the organized recreation facilities.
2.   We could develop a community focus.
3.   We could secure public transportation.

Goals

1.   Improve the health status of the people of Gilpin County.
2.   Foster more community pride and concern for one another.
3.   Encourage healthy family functioning.
4.   Reduce the incidence of substance abuse among tourists and locals.
5.   Promote positive adult role modeling for our youth.

Process Objectives

1.   To annually offer a server intervention training course in Gilpin County.
2.   To encourage and support the development of a K–12 health education curriculum at the Gilpin school by September, 2000.
3.   To encourage the adoption of the policy at the school to make it a requirement for graduation to successfully complete a 1/2 credit course in health by September, 2000.
4.   To encourage and support the development of a "Natural Helpers" program at the school and to support the continuation of a peer counseling program in the local mental health department.

GILPIN COUNTY TASK FORCE ON PRIORITY HEALTH PROBLEMS

RANKED STRATEGIES

STRATEGIES

1. K-12 Health Education
2. Peer Counseling for Youth
3. Community Based Recreation Programs including equipment for the "WREC" Center
4. Drug Abuse Training for School Staff
5. Public Transportation
6. Buddy System for Safe Rides
6. Family Strengthening seminars
7. School based recreation events for the community
7. Public awareness campaign and neighborhood resource program using local newspaper and newsletter
8. Age-appropriate school and community library resources on health
9. Apprenticeship-mentorship program for youth
10. Resource list of People-Resources in Gilpin County
11. Collaborative program with local members of the community who will be trained in economic development skills

Source: Jeanne Nicholson, R.N., Colorado Department of Health and Environment, 1986.

5. To encourage curriculum development at both schools that promote enjoyment of outdoor activities natural to Gilpin County, i.e. fishing, cross country skiing, hiking, backpacking, etc. by September, 2000.

6. To encourage the availability of family strengthening seminars by October, 2000.

7. To encourage and support alternative drug free recreation activities by January, 2000.

8. To promote and support a public transportation system for Gilpin County residents by December, 2000.

9. To promote industrial growth in Gilpin County.

10. To continue to support human services in Gilpin County that provide mental health counseling for Gilpin residents.

Outcome Objectives

To reduce the incidence of alcohol related injuries and deaths by 10% by December of 2000.

To reduce the incidence of alcohol use among Gilpin youth by 10% by December of 2000.

FYI

Alaskans Race to Vaccinate: Children as a Population at Risk— A Community-Focused Intervention Implemented Through Collaboration between Health Professionals and Target Population

A population assessment revealed that only 52.7% of the young children in Alaska were fully immunized. Through collaboration with several groups, including the University of Alaska Anchorage School of Nursing, the Iditarod Trail Committee, and the Indian Health Service, the Alaska Nurses Association established the "I Did It By TWO Race to Vaccinate" as a health project analogous to the Iditarod Sled Dog Race. The original Iditarod, in 1925, was an appropriate focus because that relay, in which mushers and dogs carried antitoxin across 700 miles of Alaskan wilderness, halted a diphtheria epidemic. Alaska's "checkpoints" are two, four, and six months of age. The best possible "finishing time" is 12 to 15 months. Any child who reaches the long distance goal by age two wins an Iditarod certificate autographed by a musher. The Iditarod is the most famous sled dog race in the world, and the mushers who drive the sleds are influential spokespersons. The geographic outreach to connect with the target population was extensive, since the Iditarod Race runs from Anchorage to Nome, covering more than 1,049 miles. The immunization project has become the largest in the nation in conjunction with a sporting event. Outcome evaluation revealed first and second year immunization rates improved to more than 80% in targeted areas.

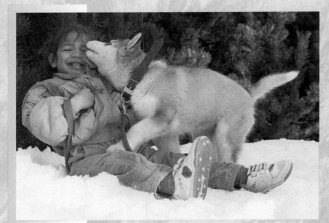

Alaskan child with husky puppy.

Carolyn Keil, PhD, RN
Associate Professor, University of Alaska Anchorage
Project Director, Race to Vaccinate, 1992–1996
Adapted from: Alaskans Race to Vaccinate. (1996). Reflections (4th Quarter).

FYI

Carter Center's Interfaith Health Program: Faith Population as Target Community, A Community-Focused Intervention Implemented Through a Collaborative Arrangement Between Health Professionals and Community Leaders

President Jimmy Carter and the Carter Center in Atlanta, Georgia, along with leaders from the Atlanta Interfaith Health Program, have developed a highly successful collaborative project to help faith communities nationwide to prevent disease and promote wellness in their congregations. Through this program, *Starting Point*, religious groups and health professionals work together to identify risk factors, such as economics or age, and link resources to the church congregations. Dr. Fran Wenger of the Emory School of Nursing in Atlanta is one of the original organizers of this program and is responsible for training lay church leaders in identification of risk and the development of interventions. Religious groups across the country are building an impressive network of leaders, scholars, and community activists who share a common goal: *to help people through their churches and religious groups lead more healthful lives.* This effort uses a step-by-step training program in which lay volunteers in the church are prepared to be "health promoters." These volunteers then help identify group needs and then work to find appropriate resources, such as the American Cancer Society or the local Red Cross, to meet them. Jimmy Carter sums up the program in this way: "The key to empowering any community, be it religious or otherwise, is team work and a strong spirit of collaboration."

Source: Starting Point: Empowering Communities to Improve Health. A Manual for Training Health Promoters in Congregational Coalitions. Interfaith Health Program. *(1997). Atlanta: The Carter Center.*

values and preferences. Also important is the history of the community's ability to solve its own problems. The nurse will play a different role in an established population where there is a history of successful health problem management, as opposed to one that is poorly organized and loosely connected to each other or that has vague community identity. In one case the nurse may serve only as advisor, whereas in another, the nurse must work with the community first to teach the community how to solve problems.

Social Change and Community Action

The age-old question of how to "teach an old dog new tricks" leads us inevitably to the process of change. There are two types of change: unplanned or spontaneous change and planned change. There is considerable debate about the ultimate benefits of unplanned change, but the CHN is most interested in planned and directed change. Such community changes imply that the activities of the CHN are directed toward some goal or goals set in the planning stage of the nursing process. Intervention activities based on the concepts of planned change center around conscious, deliberate, and intentional actions directed toward healthy change in the community (Chin & Benne, 1989). Several forces influence the process of creating meaningful change.

The CHN intervenes in changing attitudes, values, knowledge, and skills of the community or population. Kurt Lewin (1951), in his force field theory, postulated that there are always two types of forces that affect the likelihood of change in any situation: driving forces and restraining forces. These two types of forces work in opposition to each other, and Lewin theorized that it is the relative strength of each force that determines whether change will occur. Force field theory postulates that when driving forces are stronger than restraining forces, change occurs.

Driving forces are those influences that favor change. Restraining forces, by contrast, impede change. For example, a group of restless teens, frustrated with the lack of unorganized recreational settings, may be a driving force that motivates a community to establish safe socialization sites for teens to gather. However, the same teen population might feel threatened by adults making the decisions about how these safe socialization sites operate and would therefore serve as a restraining force operating against change.

The role of the CHN in promoting healthy change involves manipulating the driving and restraining forces in ways that increase the likelihood of positive changes in the population. This occurs by increasing the driving forces while minimizing the restraining forces. The nurse in the change agent role can promote these changes through an understanding of the process. An underlying assumption of this process is that the community or population must participate in the planning of change. Some resistance to change can be assumed in most situations. To counter this resistance, the nurse engages the population members in planning the change. Such participation can result in decreased resistance to that change (Lippitt, Langseth, & Mossop, 1985). You will learn more about change theory in chapter 18.

Lay Advisors

Community members who hold more status and prestige in the community and are looked to by community members as the "movers and shakers" are the lay advisors who can make or break community intervention. By promoting new ideas and representing positive change, lay advisors provide the connection to the community while often displaying natural leadership abilities that can be encouraged and reinforced by the community health nurse (McKinley, 1973).

Focus Groups

Small groups in the community are often the selected mechanism by which change is introduced and sustained. Existing community groups or new groups formed specifically around the community objectives are often successful in implementing healthy change. These groups link the individual to the community. Through formal groups such as church-related organizations or special interest groups, such as the Parent Teacher Organization, nurses can provide the leadership both in initiating healthy change and promoting the group's efforts toward autonomy and self-care.

Policy and Legislation

To effect change at the governmental level, collective needs must be translated into a grassroots power base of influence. Nurses are often unfamiliar with this level of intervention and often need to

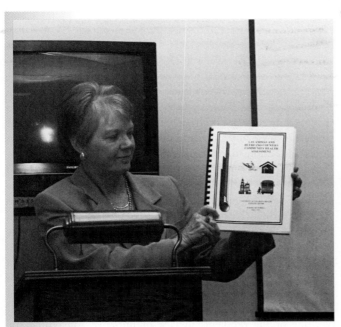

A community assessment report should be shared with target community. Dr. Judith Barton shares County Health Assessment with residents in rural Colorado.

seek coalition with other influential professional and organizational constituents to effect change. *Policy* refers to the principles and values that govern actions directed toward given ends; policy statements set forth a plan, direction, or goal for action. Because politics is always about scarce resources, the CHN involved in policy changes whether at the local, state, national, or global level effects healthy change in communities by influencing the distribution of resources, the amount of resources allocated, and the recipients of the allocated resources, that is, the target community (Chitty, 1997). Although different from politics, policy is shaped by politics (Mason, Talbott, & Leavitt, 1993).

Through the assessment process, the CHN identifies, along with the community or population, health needs or problems. Depending on the nature of the problem, the CHN can use his or her knowledge of the political process to influence the policy process, such as drafting legislation, providing formal testimony as an advocate for the community, and lobbying governmental officials to make certain that those health issues are a priority for action. All activities are done with the community, by serving as both advocate and educator for the population in efforts to meet those identified goals (Chitty, 1997).

Mass Media

The most common use of the mass media to promote healthy change in communities has been to communicate specific health information to larger audiences. Using a combination of media forms (television, radio, Internet, newspapers, newsletters, and magazines) provides a greater possibility for exposure and contact with the population. Some community members are more oral, whereas others read more, watch or view television, read newsletters, or notice posters in selected community sites. Some

population members might be more likely reached through the Internet. Web sites are the latest in media resources that can be successful communication tools for health issues.

Media coverage of health issues and events can be a successful strategy for informing and motivating large numbers of the population (Box 2-11). A well-constructed, focused media campaign can be an excellent means for disseminating and modifying values about health. Such activities can be as simple as a well-timed letter to the editor, which can provide an excellent forum for airing of health concerns and eliciting feedback from the community. Securing the local newspaper's editorial support can be a major factor in soliciting legislators' and other policy makers' attention, particularly with controversial community issues. Press releases should also be considered standard fare for most community projects that serve a targeted population (Box 2-12). In addition, feature writers for local and state newspapers are always looking for stories of interest. Novel approaches to community programs, even the community or population assessment itself, should be of interest to readers, particularly when the newspaper has a large readership. Other media tools include television talk programs, beginning with local television stations and expanding to the networks. The coverage of community health issues not only helps inform the population about health issues but also is an excellent way of promoting positive, accurate public images of nursing in a health promotion role. Publicizing these nursing roles, goals, concerns, and accomplishments in the policy arena will serve to increase the likelihood of public support of nurse-initiated policy recommendations (Hanley, 1984).

Media Advocacy

Media advocacy is the strategic use of the mass media to advance healthy public policy by applying pressure to legislators and other policy makers (Wallack, Dorfman, & Woodruff, 1997). By focusing the attention of those who have the power to change policy, the media become a powerful tool for drawing attention to the actions of a specific group (e.g., the town council, a governing body, or a planning commission). This can also occur when the news story alerts people in the target population to an issue or an action and mobilizes community and population support. The goal in media advocacy is to have the news story told from a public health perspective. This means emphasizing the public policy dimensions of prevention and shifting the focus away from the individual health behavior to the cultural, social, economic, and political context of health issues. When the health issue is visible to large numbers of people, the issue becomes part of the public agenda. Thus, once a health issue is on the public agenda, media advocacy helps advance the goals of community policy by directing public attention to the actions of those responsible for enacting or opposing the policy. For example, one of the problems in lack of initiative concerning the AIDS epidemic was the lack of media attention. The issue did not make it to the national policy agenda as a result of complicated influences, primarily because the population at perceived

---

BOX 2-11 STEPS IN USING THE MEDIA FOR A HEALTH POLICY INTERVENTION

1. Designate one member of the community team who has experience with media relations as spokesperson.
2. Identify health issues from goals that would be appropriately advanced in the media.
3. Work in conjunction with professional organizations and specialty groups to develop a media strategy.
4. Build coalitions with consumer groups and lay leaders in the community.
5. Go public through newspapers, television, radio spots, and Web sites.
6. Evaluate effectiveness through community response: letters to the editor, phone calls, chat groups on the Internet, and so on.

BOX 2-12 SAMPLE PRESS RELEASE

For immediate release. October is Breast Cancer Awareness month. The focus on breast cancer targets all age groups of women and their partners in an effort to educate the public about the importance of early detection and treatment of breast cancer. The American Cancer Society sponsors the national campaign, and local health organizations, schools of nursing, and voluntary health groups working with the American Cancer Society provide speakers, materials, promotional media messages, and community-focused events. The Breast Cancer Awareness Committee of the greater Hattiesburg, Mississippi, area is a group of representatives from health care agencies, voluntary agencies, schools of nursing, and health care consumers who develop various projects in the community to enhance the public's awareness about breast cancer survival in the Pine Belt. Students in the University of Southern Mississippi College of Nursing BSN and RN students are involved in this collaborative effort as part of their community health educational experiences in their senior course, community health nursing. They have developed activities and projects that raise awareness on the college campus about the importance of breast self-examination (BSE). The students learn about the use of the media in community health education. Activities include sorority and fraternity presentations, newspaper press releases, television interviews, a Web site devel-

opment focusing on men and breast cancer, and information booths at the student center and post office throughout the month of October.

Attachment: Fact Sheet
Contact Persons:
Breast Cancer Awareness Team, Chairperson, Karen Lundy, 601-266-4452
American Cancer Society Regional Director, Robert Nerraro, 601-254-6678

Fact Sheet for Press Release
Breast Cancer

In 1997, according to the National Breast Cancer Coalition, one in eight women living to age 85 will develop breast cancer. Statistics from 1997 show the following:

- A woman dies of breast cancer every 11 minutes.
- Approximately 43,9000 women and 400 men die from breast cancer.
- Breast cancer is the leading cause of death in women ages 15–34 and 35–54.
- Breast cancer is the second leading cause of death in women ages 55–74.
- If caught early, the disease can be treated effectively with surgery that preserves the breast.

According to the American Cancer Society, a 5-year survival rate after treatment for localized, early breast cancer is 93%.

---

risk was the male homosexual community, which had little success accessing the media. Without public attention on an issue or an event, the broader community remains in the dark, along with those who have the power to make the desired change (Wallack, Dorfman, & Woodruff, 1997). According to Daniel Schorr, National Public Radio commentator, "If you don't exist in the media, for all practical purposes, you don't exist" (Communications Consortium Media Center, 1991, p. 7). By using the media to promote healthy change, Flynn (1998) advocates that nurses continue to think "upstream" and focus on fairness and equity in targeting those populations at risk.

Education

Educational strategies are perhaps the most common strategies used by CHNs in promoting health and preventing illness in both individuals and communities. Educating the target popula-

tion about available knowledge and community resources is common. The purpose of educating the target population about health issues and possible solutions is ultimately to create greater self-sufficiency and a community that is better prepared to make appropriate health-related decisions in the future. These include decisions about personal health behaviors, decisions about the use of available health resources, and decisions about societal health issues (Clark, 1996). Education strategies take many forms, including formal presentations, printed materials, community billboards, media, and the Internet. When current information and research are provided about health issues, people can become more involved in their own self-care and make informed decisions regarding personal behaviors that promote health; for example, should ear protection be used by persons in a rifle club, or should teens be held to a higher standard regarding alcohol use and driving automobiles? Health education can be viewed as a means of freeing people in populations from influences that lead them to unhealthy behaviors. Education is much more than merely imparting knowledge and skills; it includes helping people change their attitudes to those more conducive to healthful behavior. People learning to use resources—learning not only what is available in the community but how to apply that knowledge in promoting healthy change—is an even more empowering strategy (Greenberg, 1989).

On a more global level, populations can be educated about decisions related to social health issues, such as AIDS or teen suicide risks. For example, educating the target population can assist people in determining whether they support legislation that requires motorcyclists to wear helmets or that bans smoking in senior centers. An informed population is better able to make decisions about major health issues that affect their lives (Clark, 1996).

Evaluation Phase

To evaluate the effectiveness of implementations, the nurse evaluates the responses of the community to the interventions, the progress that has been made in affecting outcome measures, such as statistical changes, and how well the efforts have fared in comparison to the goals and objectives. Evaluation data are collected in various formats and should come from diverse viewpoints, both from the target population and from the team members (Anderson & McFarlane, 1996). Because the nursing process is cyclical instead of linear, evaluation as the final step in the process ultimately affects the next assessment. In community health interventions, there rarely is a true end point, but rather there is a dynamic interplay of the steps in a process. The effectiveness of community nursing interventions depends on continuous reassessment of the community's health and on appropriate revisions in the planning interventions. Essentially, evaluation boils down to this: What has been the intervention's impact on the health of the target population or community? Because the community is so complex and so many variables affect the outcome of health measures, it is often difficult to measure all the variables, including the interventions, that shaped the

outcomes. The nurse must be cautious about attributing changes to the interventions, or denying influence because of lack of concrete evidence that changes occurred. Was it worth the time and effort and resources? What would or could be done differently in the future? Equally important, the community must have an opportunity to shape the evaluation conclusions. Before a final analysis and evaluation report is finished, the team should seek input from the community and population members. Does the community deem the process a success? After all, the perceived results are most important in the final analysis and should be reported in the formal conclusions.

The evaluation process entails both formative evaluation and summative evaluation. *Formative evaluation* measures focus on the process *during* the community interventions (Clark, 1996). For example, perhaps a strategy had been devised in which parents of young children would be offered a safety class on accident prevention at home. This class was initially offered on Saturday mornings. In the first two classes, only a few parents attended. It was discovered that Saturday mornings were often taken up with Little League sports and dancing lessons. The class was rescheduled for a weekday after work and attendance doubled within a week. In contrast, *summative evaluation* refers to the outcomes of the interventions, those measures that include end of intervention evaluations. Such measurements as satisfaction surveys, self-reports from parents of changes in their use of safety information in the home, or changes in the number of home accidents reported by the local hospital are all summative evaluation strategies (Benner & Meleis, 1978).

Putting the evaluation into lay terms in the final report to the community is expected of all community assessment team projects. The media (e.g., newsletters, local newspapers, and television stations) and churches are appropriate resources for distributing the final report to the community. Whatever the outcome, because of the community assessment process, both the team members and the target population are changed. Closure in the form of a final report can have a critical impact on the future of the population or community's response to health challenges and interventions.

CONCLUSION

Assessment of communities or populations will be a critical nursing skill in the rapidly evolving U.S. health care system. The need for nurses to be able to assess communities and populations as the focus of nursing care has always been an integral skill for public health nurses working in official public health agencies. With an increasing focus on keeping participants of health care plans healthy, an emphasis on health promotion and prevention will influence health plans (e.g., health maintenance organizations and preferred provider health plans) to place nurses in community- and population-focused care activities. In addition, health care agencies receiving federal funding to offset expenses incurred for treating the underinsured or noninsured are now required to assess the communities and populations they serve. In other words, there is a new emphasis on prevention rather than illness care pervading the U.S. health care system. Preparation in community/population assessment is a skill you will definitely want to master as you enter the professional practice of nursing.

CRITICAL THINKING ACTIVITIES

Population Assessment Guide For Community Health Nursing Students: An Introductory Field Experience for a Local Geopolitical Community

1. Before beginning your community assessment, identify the conceptual framework you would like to use in organizing your community assessment, for example, the GENESIS framework or the community-as-patient model. Remember, a conceptual framework for community assessment will help you in knowing what data to collect, how you should collect the data, and how to interpret the analysis of data for community planning.

2. Go to the local library and access census data for your community before going out to the community so that you have a feel for the social status of your community. Necessary demographic data to collect include the following:

   - Total population for catchment area
   - Racial composition (%) for catchment area
   - Ethnic composition (%) for catchment area
   - Age distribution (% by category) for catchment area
   - Educational attainment (% by category) in catchment area
   - % of all persons living below poverty level
   - % of children younger than age of 5 living below poverty level
   - % of persons 65 years and older living below poverty level
   - % of females 16 years and older who have children younger than 6 years of age and who work outside the home

   Use census data to compare to your catchment area.

3. Meet with a key informant at the designated time. Ask the key informant to tell you what he or she knows about the immediate community in which the health center is located. What kind of people live in the community? What are some of the health issues (views of health are broad, including economic, political, cultural, education issues)? What does the key informant see as a primary strength of the community?

Ask your key informant about specific gathering places within the community where you might talk to community members, such as fire stations, housing offices, recreation centers, and so on.

Ask your key informant if it would be okay if you talked to a few of the patients waiting in the clinic area. Explain that you will introduce yourself as a student nurse who is conducting a community health needs assessment and you will then ask the waiting patients to just describe what it is like to live in this community.

4. Spend a little time in the clinic setting meeting some of the patients in the waiting rooms. Many of the clerks working in these clinics live in the neighborhood, and they may also be willing to talk to you. Be brave! Find out all you can about what it is like to live in the community. What is a strength of the community? What is a need? How has the community changed across time (history)? What is currently happening in the community? These are general "round the world" questions that can open up a full discussion. Write down the questions mentioned in this guide on an index card. When in doubt as to what to say next, just ask the person to more fully describe what they are talking about. For example, if the person is talking about gang crimes in the neighborhood, you can ask, "Can you tell me some more about this problem with gangs?"

5. Gather outside the clinic and take a windshield survey of your community (census tract boundaries). Pay attention to environmental characteristics such as range of housing, industry, recreation facilities, and so on.

6. Spend some time talking to members of the community who are located outside the clinic area. For example, you may venture into the recreation center and talk to a few people. Venture into a day-care center and ask to talk to the workers, children, and parents. Ask again about what it is like to live in the neighborhood.

7. Review any secondary data (e.g., health status reports) you were able to obtain from your key informant or others in the community.

8. Meet for lunch or an afternoon snack to analyze the findings from the secondary and primary sources. As a group, brainstorm about strengths and needs of the community assembled from observations, interviews, census data, and any previous reports you have been able to obtain. Develop two to three community diagnoses. Decide on an outline for a written report on your community assessment, and write a report on your community assessment as a group or divide up the outline for section writing.

9. Do an oral presentation of your community assessment. Share your findings with the "target" community and with your classmates.

Source: Adapted from Barton, J. (1997). "Undergraduate Mini Community Health Assessment." University of Colorado School of Nursing Health Sciences Center.

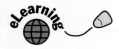

Explore Community Health Nursing on the web! To learn more about the topics in this chapter, use the passcode provided to access your exclusive web site: http://communitynursing.jbpub.com
If you do not have a passcode, you can obtain one at this site.

REFERENCES

Aiken, L. H. & Salmon M. E. (1994). Health care workforce priorities: what nursing should do now. *Inquiry, 31,* 318.

American Association of Colleges of Nursing (AACN). (1986). *Essentials of college and university education for professional nursing: Final report.* Washington, DC: Author.

American Nurses Association (ANA). (1986). *Standards of community health nursing practice.* Kansas City, MO: Author.

American Public Health Association (APHA), Public Health Nursing Section. (1981). *The definition and role of public health nursing in the delivery of health care. A position paper.* Washington, DC: Author.

Anderson, E. T., & McFarlane, J. (1996). *Community as partner: Theory and practice in nursing.* Philadelphia: Lippincott.

Association of Community Health Nursing Educators (ACHNE). (2000). *Essentials of baccalaureate nursing education for entry level practice in community health nursing.* Louisville, KY: Author.

Baldwin, J. H., Conger, C. O., Abegglen, J. C., & Hill, E. M. (1998). Population-focused and community-based nursing—moving toward clarification of concepts. *Public Health Nursing, 15*(1), 12–18.

Barton, J. A., Smith, M., Brown, N. J., & Supples, J. M. (1993). Methodological issues in a team approach to community health needs assessment. *Nursing Outlook, 41*(6), 252–261.

Basch, C. (1987). Focus group interview: an underutilized research technique for improving theory and practice in health education. *Health Education Quarterly, 14*(Winter), 411–448.

Benner, P., & Meleis, A. (1978). Process or product evaluation? *Nursing Outlook, 23,* 302–307.

Cassel, J. (1976). The contribution of the social environment to host resistance. *Am J Epidemiology, 104*(2), 107.

Chin, R., & Benne, K. D. (1989). General strategies for effecting changes in human systems. In W. L. French, C. H. Bell, & R. A. Zawacki (Eds.), *Organization development: Theory, practice and Research* (pp. 89–95). Homewood, IL: BPI Irwin.

Chitty, K. (1997). *Professional nursing: Concepts and challenges* (2nd ed.). Philadelphia: W. B. Saunders.

Clark, M. J. (1996). *Nursing in the community* (2nd ed.). Stanford, CT: Appleton and Lange.

Communication Consortium Media Center. (1991). *Strategic communication for non-profits: Strategic media—Designing a public interest campaign* (p. 7). Washington, DC: Benton Foundation and the Center for Strategic Communications.

Community Health Advisor Network. (1996). Hearts and hands for health. In *Community facilitator implementation manual.* Hattiesburg, MS: University of Southern Mississippi Center for Community Health.

Cottrell, L. S. (1976). The competent community. In B. H. Kaplan, R. N. Wilson, & A. H. Leighton (Eds.), *Further explorations in social psychology.* New York: Basic Books.

Eisen, A. (1994). Survey of neighborhood-based, comprehensive community empowerment initiatives. *Health Education Quarterly, 21*(2), 235–252.

Flynn, B. C. (1994). Partners for healthy cities. *Healthcare Forum Journal, 37*(3), 55–56.

Flynn, B. C. (1998). Communicating with the public: Community-based nursing research and practice. *Public Health Nursing, 15*(3), 165–170.

Flynn, B. C., & Dennis, L. I. (1996). Health promotion through healthy cities. In M. Stanhope, & J. Lancaster (Eds.), *Community health nursing: Promoting health of aggregates, families and individuals.* St. Louis: Mosby.

Flynn, B. C, Ray, D., & Rider, M. (1994). Empowering communities: Action research through healthy cities. *Health Education Quarterly, 21*(3), 395–405.

Gebbie, K. M. (1996, November 18). *Preparing currently employed public health nurses for changes in the health care system: Meeting report and suggested action steps.* New York: Columbia University School of Nursing Center for Health Policy and Health Sciences Research. (Report based on meeting in Atlanta, July 11, 1996.)

Glick, D. F., Hale, P. J., Kulbok, P. A., & Shettig, J. (1996). Community development theory: Planning a community nursing center. *Journal of Nursing Administration, 26*(7/8), 44–50.

Glittenberg, J. E. (1981). An ethnographic approach to the problem of health assessment and program planning: Project GENESIS. In P. Morley (Ed.), *Transcultural nursing: Developing, teaching, and practicing* (pp. 142–152). Salt Lake City: University of Utah Press.

Goeppinger, J. (1984). Primary health care: An answer to the dilemmas of community health nursing? *Public Health Nursing, 3,* 129–140.

Goeppinger, J., & Baglioni A. J. (1986). Community competence: a positive approach to needs assessment. *American Journal of Community Psychology 13,* 507.

Goeppinger, J., Lassiter, P. G., & Wilcox, B. (1982). Community health is community competence. *Nursing Outlook, 30*(8), 464.

Goeppinger, J., & Schuster, G. (1988). Community as client: Using the nursing process to promote health. In M. Stanhope, & J. Lancaster (Eds.), *Community health nursing: Process and practice for promoting health.* St. Louis: Mosby.

Gordon, L. J. (1990). Who will manage the environment? *American Journal of Public Health, 80,* 904–905.

Gordon, L. J. (1993). The future of environmental health and the need for public health leadership. *Journal of Environmental Health, 56*(5), 38–40.

Greenberg, J. S. (1989). *Health education: Learner-centered instructional strategies.* Dubuque, IA: W. C. Brown.

Hamilton, P. (1983). Community health diagnosis. *Advances in Nursing Science, 5*(3), 21–36.

World Health Organization. (1985). *Handbook of resolutions and decisions by the World Health Assembly and the Executive Board, 1972–1984* [Vol. 2(31), 42]. Geneva: World Health Assembly.

Hancock, T. (1993). The evolution, impact and significance of the Healthy Cities/Healthy Communities movement. *Journal of Public Health Policy, 14*(1), 5–18.

Hanley, B. (1984). Legislation and policy. In J. A. Sullivan, *Directions in community health nursing.* Boston: Blackwell.

Hegyvary, S. T. (1990). Education: Redefining community. *Journal of Professional Nursing, 6*(1).

Higgs, Z. R., & Gustafson, D. D. (1985). *Community as client: assessment and diagnosis.* Philadelphia: F. A. Davis.

Kauffman, K. S. (1994). The insider/outsider dilemma: Field experience of a white researcher "getting in" a poor black community. *Nursing Research, 43*(3), 179–183.

Keck, C. W. (1994). Community health: our common challenge. *Family and Community Health, 17*(2), 1–9.

Keller, L. O., Strohschein, S., Lia-Hoagberg, B., & Schaffer, M. (1998). Population-based public health nursing interventions: A model from practice. *Public Health Nursing, 15*(3), 207–215.

Kopf, E. W. (1986). Florence Nightingale as statistician. In B. W. Spradley (Ed.), *Readings in community health nursing.* Boston: Little, Brown.

Lalonde, M. (1974). *A new perspective on the health of Canadians—a working document.* Ottawa: Government of Canada.

Leininger, M. M. (1988). Leininger's theory of nursing: Cultural care diversity and universality. *Nursing Science Quarterly, 1*(4), 152–160.

Lewin, K. (1951). *Field theory in social science.* New York: Harper.

Lippitt, G. L., Langseth, P., & Mossop, J. (1985). *Implementing organizational change.* San Francisco: Jossey-Bass.

Lundy, K. S., & Barton, J. A. (1995). Assessment: Data collection of the community client. In P. J. Christiansen, & J. W. Kenney (Eds.), *Nursing process: Application of conceptual models* (4th ed.). St. Louis: Mosby.

Magilvy, J. K., McMahon, M., Bachman, M., & Evenson, C. (1992). The health of teenagers: A focused ethnographic study. *Public Health Nursing, 4*(1), 35–42.

Mason, D., Talbott, S., & Leavitt, J. (Eds.). (1993). *Policy and politics for nurses: Action and change in the workplace, government, organization and community* (2nd ed.). Philadelphia: W. B. Saunders.

McKinley, J. B. (1973). Social networks, lay consultation, and help-seeking behavior, *Social Forces, 53*(1), 275.

Mead, G. H. (1934). *Mind, self, and society.* Chicago: The University of Chicago Press.

Montero, L. A. (1985). Florence Nightingale on public health nursing. *American Journal of Public Health, 75*(2), 181.

Muecke, M. A. (1984). Community health diagnosis in nursing. *Public Health Nursing, 1*(1), 23–35.

Neuman, B. (1989). *The Neuman systems model: Application to nursing theory and practice.* Norwalk, CT: Appleton-Century-Crofts.

Reinhart, U. W. (1984). Rationing the health-care surplus: An American tragedy. *Nursing Economics, 1*(4), 210.

Rodgers, S. (1984). Community as client—a multivariate model for analysis of community and aggregate health risk. *Public Health Nursing, 1*(4), 210.

Ruth, J., Eliason K., & Schultz, P. R. (1992). Community assessment: A process of learning. *Journal of Nursing Education, 31*(4), 181.

Salmon, M. E. (1993). Public health nursing—the opportunity of a century. *American Journal of Public Health, 83,* 1674–1675.

Schultz, P. R., & Magilvy, J. K. (1988). Assessing community health needs of elderly populations: Comparison of three strategies. *Journal of Advanced Nursing, 13,* 192–202.

Schuster, G., & Goeppinger, J. (1996). Community as client: Using the nursing process to promote health. In M. Stanhope, & J. Lancaster, *Community Health Nursing: Promoting Health of Aggregates, Families and Communities* (pp. 289–314). St. Louis: Mosby.

Smith, M. C., & Barton, J. A. (1992). Technologic enrichment of a community needs assessment. *Nursing Outlook, 40*(1), 32–37.

Stoner, M. H., Magilvy, J. K., & Schultz, P. R. (1992). Community analysis in community health nursing practice: The GENESIS model. *Public Health Nursing, 9*(4), 222–227.

Sullivan, J. A. (1984). *Directions in community health nursing.* Boston: Blackwell.

Von Bertalanffy, L. (1968). *General systems theory.* New York: George Braziller.

Wallack, L., Dorfman, L., & Woodruff, K. (1997). Communications and public health. In Scutchfield, F. *ples of public health practice*. Albany, NY: Delmar.

Wallerstein, N., & Bernstein, E. (1994). Introduction to community empowerment, participatory education, *Quarterly, 21*(2), 141–148.

Watson, N. M. (1984). Community as client. In J. A. Sullivan (Ed.), *Directions in community health nursing*. B

Wax, R. H. (1986). Gender and age in fieldwork and field work education: "Not any good thing is done by one head, & M. E. Conaway (Eds.), *Self, sex and gender in cross-cultural fieldwork*. Urbana, IL: University of Illinois Pr

Williams, C. A., & Highriter, M. E. (1978). Community health nursing: population focus and evaluation. *Public I. (2–4)*, 197.

World Health Organization (WHO). (1976, October 11–15). Criteria to be considered in selecting a preventive health action. In *Report of the First Interdisciplinary Workshop on Psychosocial Factors and Health*. Stockholm: Author.

APPENDIX A

THE LUNDY-BARTON GENERAL SYSTEMS MODEL FOR COMMUNITY AND POPULATION ASSESSMENT AND INTERVENTION

The unique responsibility of community health nursing practice is defining problems and proposing solutions at the population level. The process of making this connection from the individual to the community has proven to be an especially difficult task for the nurse conducting a community or population assessment. The community health assessment process is based on the understanding of the community as client. Although nurses wouldn't consider the omission of individual client assessment and base intervention on intuition, this is almost precisely what happens when we fail to do a thorough assessment when planning and delivering health care services to community populations. For example, we would not ever consider just examining the arm of a patient and totally ignoring the rest of the body when we plan nursing interventions. And yet by looking at only one aspect of the community, such as the physical parameters, we are just examining the "arm" and ignoring the "body" of the community. One of the major difficulties in conducting a community assessment is that students and practicing nurses alike have often been limited to individualistic patient care. This focus on personal care sometimes presents difficulty in the transference of those skills to assessment and problem solving at the community level.

The Lundy-Barton Model uses familiar systems theory and the nursing process to guide the collection and interpretation of data, development of interests, and evaluation of nursing strategies to promote community health.

The Lundy-Barton Model includes a database, a needs list, assessment, and a plan to address each need with progress notes delineated for selected problems. Each of these components will be discussed in relation to community assessment with concurrent identification of the nursing process components.

DATABASE (ASSESSMENT PHASE: NURSING PROCESS)

The collection of data corresponds to the assessment phase of the nursing process. The collection of data has one primary goal—to learn about the client. The exploration of available data about the community can be general or quite specific, depending on the definition of the community or population as well as the purpose of the project. An example of how the definition of community can affect the assessment of a community can be illustrated by the distinction of munity as a *place* or *nonplace*. A *place* community, according to Anderson and Carter (1974), refers to a specific geographic locality, one that can be defined by physical boundaries. This definition is the one most often used in health planning projects for specific urban or rural locales. A *nonplace* community is defined as one based on cooperation and commitment by its members to common goals and ideologies. A nonplace community is in a sense a "mind" community, such as the academic community or the nursing community. The distinction can also be made on the degree of attachment to a specific locale and the scope of activities, interest, and needs. Place communities have the greatest attachment to a specific locality, whereas nonplace communities usually have limited geographic ties. Nonplace communities generally are narrow in their scope of activities, interests, or needs, whereas place communities have a wider scope of activities, interests, and needs. Defining the community as a place or nonplace will thus affect the direction and method of assessment (Anderson & Carter, 1974).

There are eight categories of data, which are presented in the following section and are considered necessary for the database of a community or population assessment.

COMMUNITY PROFILE

What makes the identified community different from any other community? The "community client" is somewhat harder to get to know than the individual client. Instead of using temperature, pulse, respiration, blood pressure, and so on, the indices of a community will take the form of *demographics* and *vital statistics*, such as morbidity/mortality rates, sex, age, ethnic and racial distributions, educational levels, occupation/employment patterns, and socioeconomic patterns. Mortality rates are important indices because they provide a picture of the health and living conditions of a community. The infant mortality rate is considered perhaps the most sensitive indicator of a community's health status. According to Taylor, "such indices require a basic readjustment in thinking. A woman is either pregnant or not pregnant; a community is about 3 per cent pregnant. A patient has or does not have heart disease; the community always has heart disease though the rate may go up or down" (Mattison, 1968).

Demographic data can be found in local and state health departments and on the Internet. United States census data are an excellent source for demographic data concerned with population density, population age distribution, occupational distribution, socioeconomic characteristics (income, education, employment), and marital status. Information concerning the kinds of family forms that are prevalent—young families with small children, percentage of women working, and so on—is also available through the U.S. Census and can provide useful information for the identification of family needs.

Information about how the population is distributed spatially is extremely important in considering the location, distribution, and delivery of health services. Whether a population is densely or sparsely populated has also been shown to affect other aspects of people's lives such as norms, values, and types of health problems. Population density can also affect behavior and the emotional health of residents.

Information about the percentage of persons in each age category contributes to the assessment of health needs. Many times, when the age distribution is examined in a historical context, it becomes evident that there has been a population shift over time.

Morbidity and mortality statistics can help provide a statistical picture of the community or population in terms of the incidence and prevalence of specific diseases and deaths within a community. These statistics can be obtained through local and state health departments and the CDC (for specific population groups such as teenagers) as well as from special interest groups, such as the American Cancer Society or the American Heart Association, or the various population interest groups such as women & HIV/AIDS. Most can be obtained from the Internet.

COMPARISON OF THE PROFILE

Demographics and other statistics *should be compared* with adjoining communities or similar populations, the state, and/or the nation to ascertain the relative significance of the statistics. Not only can these comparisons provide clues as to what kinds of health problems and needs exist in a particular community, but they can also provide an evaluation of the effectiveness of existing health services and programs.

Psychological Climate

Just as an evaluation of an individual client includes an examination of his or her psychological status, an assessment of the community is incomplete without evaluating the psychological aspects. There are three areas: (1) self-concept, (2) attitude toward health, and (3) history and changes over time. How the community views itself is usually based on history and traditions from the past. How does one find out what kind of *self-concept* the community or population has? Ask the members! Each community often thinks of itself in terms of descriptors such as, "we are a friendly-type place," or "we just leave each other well-enough alone," which can reflect whether the inhabitants see themselves as being connected to adjoining communities or separate from them. Listen to the people talking with each other—are the inhabitants proud of their community or are they somewhat distanced and seemingly apathetic? Does the population express powerlessness or worthlessness, such as women who have been abused by parents?

In addition to evaluating the community's self-image as an indicator of the psychological climate, it is useful to determine the *community's attitude toward health in general.* Is health care a priority in the community? Indicators such as safety and public service media messages (e.g., radio, television, billboards) are evidence of the degree of voluntary efforts for the development of health programs and should aid in the assessment of where health fits into the community priority structure. Populations have a wide variety of attitudes and values about health. Teens may have very little interest in health because of their developmental level of self-awareness.

A third area to assess in terms of the psychological database is information concerning the *historical changes that a community has experienced* and its response to those changes. Understanding the history of the community or population—how and when it came to be, how it has responded to

change (e.g., industrial growth, highway construction, rapid population growth or decline), and how it has dealt with health problems in the past—would all be helpful in planning realistically for health services. A community's experiences, its ability to mobilize resources, as well as dominant patterns of solutions to health problems all significantly affect how that community will respond to intervention. For example, the population of homosexual men has a long history of discrimination in the United States and may exhibit a distrust of the traditional health care system as a result. Knowledge about the community's past can give perspectives on the present and future.

Nutritional Evaluation

A history and evaluation of the community's nutritional status, as a part of the community assessment process, includes identification of sources of food (e.g., homegrown, imported into community, processed foods, fast foods), ethnic or regional food prevalence, and food preparation customs (e.g., vegetarian, seafood availability, red meat). Morbidity/mortality statistics related to nutritional status and resources (e.g., goiter, cardiac disease, cancer) are also vital information to include in the nutritional assessment. A population of truck drivers may have nutritional patterns of consumption related to their erratic pattern of eating on the run.

Physical Fitness

In examining the community's "fitness," the presence or absence of exercise/fitness facilities available and/or used by the public, such as jogging and bicycling trails, are most certainly a reflection of its inhabitants' interest in physical fitness. Although most communities do not fall into a clear-cut category of either sedentary or active, one pattern usually tends to dominate and can provide important health status information. As a population, elders tend to be more sedentary than their younger counterparts.

Physical Examination

A physical examination of the community client involves a hands-on type of approach. This obviously applies only to a geographic community. Shumway and Wisehart (1969) suggest using a walking tour to know a community at the resident level. They advise that getting "a feel for a community" involves a *systematic approach of observations* that can ultimately increase one's sensitivity to the surrounding ecological elements. If the community can be defined as a place community, the *geographic boundaries should be defined* and described as clearly as possible. Parameters can be defined in several ways: census tracts, natural boundaries (e.g., mountains, rivers), or roads and streets, specifically noting terrain, proximity to needed resources, and *isolation/proximity* to other communities. The *climate* has been demonstrated to have a significant effect on the health risks of a population. Whether the climate is desert or mountainous can affect the lives of the inhabitants in dramatic ways. Such factors as road conditions, animal vectors, housing conditions, and general appearances of the community should be noted in the physical assessment of the community.

REVIEW OF SYSTEMS

Once the "physical examination" has been done, it is important to conduct a review of systems within the community or population. This review should include an assessment of the services and facilities, human power, government (federal, state, county), and leadership (formal and informal) of both health and nonhealth systems that affect the population or community.

The *health system* should include all organizations and services that provide health care. The private health services and public health services should be examined not only for availability and quality, but also for the degree of coordination between the services. The availability of homes for the elderly, services for the disabled (including accommodation in the community, such as access ramps), and mental health services are examples of such services to be assessed. As community workers know all too well, it is often not a case of availability of needed services, but rather a lack of coordination within agencies, a lack of awareness of the services by the community members, an unwillingness by the members to use the facilities, or unacceptability of resources or services as a result of cultural differences. The source of health care is an-

other important aspect of this assessment of health care systems specific to the community. Particularly in rural communities, the local pharmacist may be the primary source for health information and should be included in the assessment. Most members of population seek health care and advisement on health issues from nonprofessionals daily. These sources should be identified in the assessment.

Nonhealth systems, such as the political system, the economic system, the educational system, and the religious system, should be assessed as critical influences on the health of a community. Health care does not exist in a vacuum apart from the other social structures within a community; it is influenced by and influences other systems within the community.

The *political system/atmosphere* of a community can be assessed through various sources: the local newspaper, community action groups, and/or previous history and political activities. The community should be assessed as liberal or conservative.

Klein (1965) identifies three important components of the political system that reflect interaction patterns of a community. This can also be applied to a population. *Authority* within a community can be often identified by the political leaders of a community—both elected, official leaders and nonofficial leaders (e.g., religious leaders). *Power* is often associated with authority but is not by any means limited to it. Power patterns in a community can often be identified by examining how formal decisions are made and who makes or vetoes them. *Prestige* is often based on social status, family class designation, and wealth. These three concepts, authority, power, and prestige, are closely linked.

The *social system* includes the prevalent norms and values as well as the dominant ethnic makeup of the community or population. Values influence norms and are often difficult to determine. Norms and values are intangible, so the community worker has to get a real feel for the group through direct involvement before they become apparent. Customs, specific town laws, and cultural patterns are reflective of that community's value system.

Communication patterns, both formal and informal, are an integral component of the social system.

Communication as a necessary process by which people exchange information and interact with each other is basic to community living. *Informal* communication tends to occur wherever people collect—post offices, local cafes, recreation centers, barbershops, and so on. How information is disseminated can be reflected in community bulletin boards, supermarket notice boards, and the like. Often, asking community residents where information is obtained will yield the most accurate information. The beauty shop or local bar might serve as the center for information dissemination. Without an understanding of who the key people and places are in terms of informal communication, meaningful, realistic programs can seldom be created.

Formal communication channels include all forms of media, including newspapers, television, radio, telephone, and postal systems. These channels of communication can be used very effectively in the dissemination of health information, as well as in the identification of community ideas, attitudes, and health knowledge.

Information about *educational systems* includes public and private educational facilities, libraries, special educational services (pregnant teens, handicapped, adult education), and available resources. The *economic system* includes major businesses and industries as well as the census information previously mentioned—median family income, unemployment rates, major occupations, and percentage of families living below the poverty level.

The *religious system* is an important part of the community and can have a major influence on the political ideology and social norms and values of a community. Major denominations should be identified along with the major religious leaders of a community. Services and community health programs sponsored by religious groups are an integral part of the community's health care delivery system.

PROBLEM LIST (NURSING DIAGNOSIS: NURSING PROCESS)

The problem list corresponds to the nursing diagnosis component of the nursing process. As with individual nursing diagnoses, community diagnoses should specifically indicate that (1) *no* problems exist that demand intervention by the nursing discipline or by any other members of the health team or (2) needs exist as stated in terms of community problems that have evolved when basic human needs are either not being met or are being met inadequately.

Nursing diagnoses on the community level (as with the individual) use a humanitarian approach when specifying basic human needs. Examples of nursing diagnoses at the community level are as follows:

- *Increased number of respiratory diseases related to air pollution*
- *Increased infant mortality rate related to increased teenage pregnancies*
- *Lack of neighborhood participation related to apathy*

PROBLEM ASSESSMENT AND PLAN FORMULATION (PLANNING: NURSING PROCESS)

The integration of the two problem-solving methods of Problem-Oriented Medical Recording (POMR) and the nursing process requires that the nurse reassess each community diagnosis using the SOAP format. During this phase, each problem is individually described and evaluated with an intervention plan formulated for each problem. The specific components of the SOAP format follow:

Subjective data: encompasses the community's point of view; how do persons in the community express the problem?

Objective data: a summarization of vital statistics, health statistics, review of systems, environmental realities, and so on related to identified problem

Assessment: includes an analysis of the identified needs or problem in terms of origination of the problem, overall impact, possible intervention points, and community parties that may have an interest in the problem and its solutions

Plan: further diagnostic plans or an initial intervention plan developed for the identified problem in terms of short- and long-term goals/objectives with specific actions to be taken in order to accomplish each objective; health team members, community members, or organizations are designated to carry out specific actions

After each problem has been reassessed using the SOAP format, the problems are then prioritized. A committee of community members, experts, and community leaders should be involved in problem prioritization.

PROGRESS NOTES (EVALUATION: NURSING DIAGNOSIS)

The evaluation of the community assessment process should be documented in the form of progress notes. Progress notes are simply an appraisal of the effects of some predetermined plan to accomplish some measurable objective. During this phase of the POMR, new objectives and plans for each problem may be determined.

REFERENCES

Anderson, R. E., & Carter, I. E. (1974). *Human behavior in the social environment: A social systems approach.* Chicago: Aldine.

Hunter, F. (1953). *Community power structures: A study of decision makers.* Chapel Hill, NC: University of North Carolina Press.

Klein, D. C. (1965). Community and mental health: an attempt at a conceptual framework. *Community Health Journal, 1,* 301–308.

Mattison, B. (1968, June). Community health planning and the health professions. *Journal of Public Health, 58,* 1015–1021.

Shumway, S. M., & Wisehart, D. (1969). How to know a community. *Nursing Outlook, 17,* 63–64.

LUNDY–BARTON GENERAL SYSTEMS MODEL FOR COMMUNITY AND POPULATION ASSESSMENT AND INTERVENTION

COMMUNITY/POPULATION

I. Database (Assessment Phase)
  A. Definition of community or population
  B. Profile
    1. Demographics (census data)
    2. Morbidity (illness patterns)
    3. Birth rate
    4. Death rates by age
    5. Mortality rate (death rate)
    6. Socioeconomic characteristics
      a. Occupation/employment patterns
      b. Median income
      c. Percent of families below poverty level income
  C. Psychological climate
    1. Self-concept
    2. Attitude toward health
    3. Historical changes of community over time
  D. Nutritional evaluations
    1. Sources of food
    2. Statistics related to nutritional status
  E. Physical fitness
    1. Facilities
    2. Attitudes of residents
  F. Physical examination (for geographic communities)
    1. Systematic observation of community
    2. Defined parameters/boundaries
    3. Climate
    4. Location, topography, rural/urban
    5. Area in miles
    6. Environmental conditions
      a. General description
      b. Housing, quality and condition
      c. Sanitation, water supply, sewage, and trash disposal
      d. Degree of pollution (air, water)
      e. Presence of vectors
      f. Safety/protection
        (1) Police
        (2) Fire
        (3) Other
      g. Transportation
  G. Review of systems
    1. Health system
      a. Private, public services
        (1) Hospitals
        (2) Long-term care
        (3) Ambulatory service
          (a) Primary care
          (b) Mental health/substance abuse
          (c) Home health
          (d) Public health
      b. Resources for specific health needs (e.g., elderly, teen parents)
      c. Human power—need versus availability, type (health workers)
      d. Other health care or related resources
        (1) Occupational health service
        (2) School health

(3) Voluntary agencies
(4) Welfare agencies
(5) Other
2. Nonhealth systems
  a. Political system/atmosphere
    (1) Dominant values
    (2) Authority formal, nonformal leadership
    (3) Current political issues in community
  b. Social system
    (1) Prevalent norms
    (2) Cultural patterns/variables
    (3) Dominate values
    (4) Customs
    (5) Recreational/social facilities/ activities
  c. Communication patterns
    (1) Informal and formal communication sources (e.g., newspapers, bulletin boards)
  d. Educational system
    (1) Public, private schools (number, type, student population, availability)
    (2) Values
    (3) Special educational services (e.g., pregnant teens, disabled, adult learners)

    (4) Libraries
  e. Economic system
    (1) Major businesses/industries
    (2) Marketing and shopping facilities
    (3) Leading occupations
    (4) Employment patterns
  f. Religious systems
    (1) Major denominations
    (2) Religious leadership
II. Problem List (Nursing Diagnosis)
  A. Identification of needs and assets from the assessment
III. Problem Assessment and Plan Formulation (Plan)
  A. Subjective data: community's point of view
  B. Objective data: nurse's point of view
  C. Assessment: interpretation of data
  D. Plan
    1. Short-term goals/objectives
    2. Long-term goals/objectives
    3. Specific actions for each objective/goal
  E. Prioritization of nursing diagnoses
IV. Progress Notes (Evaluation)
  A. Specification of any intervention implemented and evaluation of effectiveness
  B. Formulation of new objectives and plan

Chapter 3

History of Community Health and Public Health Nursing

Karen Saucier Lundy and Kaye W. Bender

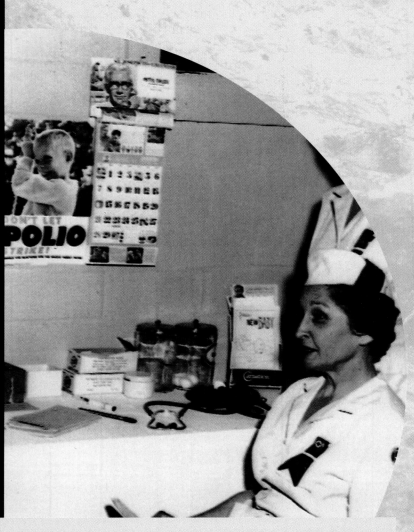

For as long as humanity has existed, so has the nursing of the sick. Health practices of early humans most likely evolved as a way for groups to survive. Many of these early causal links between humans and environment were attributed to superstition and religion. Early evidence from these primitive societies suggests that techniques such as mind-body connections (e.g., voodoo or spells), isolation or banishment from the group, and fumigation (e.g., smoke) were used to manage disease and protect the health of the community (Hanlon & Pickett, 1984).

CHAPTER FOCUS

QUESTIONS TO CONSIDER

After reading this chapter, answer the following questions:

1. When did humans first begin thinking about the causes of illness?
2. What were the contributions of the Greeks and Egyptians to our health practices today?
3. What are the origins of public health?
4. Who did the first home visits?
5. What were major health concerns of the Middle Ages?
6. What were Florence Nightingale's contributions to nursing as a profession?
7. What was the Chadwick Report and why is it significant to community health nursing?
8. What role did William Rathbone play in the evolution of community health nursing?
9. Who is Lillian Wald and why is she considered a prominent figure in the development of community health nursing in the United States?
10. What led to early standardization of public health nursing practice in the United States?
11. What are the major legislative events that occurred in the 1960s?

KEY TERMS

Air, Waters, and Places
Black Death
Case management
Chadwick Report
Deaconesses

District nursing
Florence Nightingale
Greek era
Health visiting
Industrial Revolution

John Snow
Lillian Wald
Nightingale School of
   Nursing
Plato

Roman era
Shattuck Report
St. Vincent de Paul
The Republic

Although a specialized nurse role per se had not been developed in early civilizations, human cultures recognized the need for nursing care. The truly sick person was weak and helpless and could not fulfill the duties that were normally expected of a member of the community. In such cases, someone had to watch over the client, nurse him or her, and provide care. In most societies, this nurse role was filled by a family member, usually female. As in most cultures, the childbearing woman had special needs that often resulted in a specialized role for the caregiver. Every society since the dawn of time seemed to have someone to nurse and take care of the mother and infant around the childbearing events. In whatever form the nurse took, the role was associated with compassion, health promotion, and kindness (Bulllough & Bullough, 1978).

Classical Era

More than 4,000 years ago, Egyptian physicians and nurses used an abundant pharmacological repertoire to cure the ill and injured. The Ebers Papyrus lists more than 700 remedies for ailments from snake bites to puerperal fever. The Kahun Papyrus (circa 1850 BC) identified suppositories (e.g., crocodile feces) that could be used for contraception (Kalisch & Kalisch, 1986). Healing appeared in the Egyptian culture as the successful result of a contest between invisible beings of good and evil (Shryock, 1959). The physician was not a shaman; instead there was specialization and separation of function, with physicians, priests, and sorcerers all practicing separately and independently. Some clients would consult the physician, some the shaman, and others sought healing from magical formulas. Many tried all three approaches. The Egyptians, quite notably, did not accept illness and death as inevitable but believed that life could be indefinitely prolonged. Because Egyptians blended medicine and magic, the concoctions believed to be the most effective were often bizarre and repulsive by today's standards. For example, lizard's blood, swine's ears and teeth, putrid meat and fat, tortoise brains, the milk of a lactating woman, the urine of a chaste woman, and excreta of donkeys and lions were frequently used ingredients. At least some explanation for these odd ingredients can be found in the following: "These pharmacological mixtures were intended to sicken and drive out the intruding demon which was thought to cause the disease. Drugs containing fecal matter were in fact used until the end of the eighteenth century in Europe as common practice" (Kalisch & Kalisch, 1986).

As early as 3000 to 1400 BC, the Minoans created ways to flush water and construct drainage systems. Circa 1000 BC, the Egyptians constructed elaborate drainage systems, developed pharmaceutical herbs and preparations, and embalmed the dead. The Hebrews formulated an elaborate hygiene code that dealt with laws governing both personal and community hygiene, such as contagion, disinfection, and sanitation through the preparation of food and water. Hebrews, although few in number, exercised great influence in the development of religious and health doctrine. According to Bullough and Bullough (1978), most of their genius was religious, giving birth to both Christianity and Islam. The Jewish contribution to public health is greater in sanitation than in their concept of disease. Garbage and excreta were disposed of outside the city or camp, infectious diseases were quarantined, spitting was outlawed as unhygienic, and bodily cleanliness became a prerequisite for moral purity. Although many of the Hebrew ideas about hygiene were Egyptian in origin, Moses and the Hebrews were the first to codify them and link them with spiritual godliness. Their notion of disease was rooted in the "disease as God's punishment for sin" idea.

The civilization that grew up between the Tigris and Euphrates Rivers is known geographically as Mesopotamia (modern Iraq) and includes the Sumarians. Disease and disability in the Mesopotamian area, at least in the earlier period, was considered a great curse, a divine punishment for grievous acts against the gods. Having such a curse of illness resulting from sin did not exactly put the sick person in a valued status in the society. Experiencing illness as punishment for a sin linked the sick person to anything even remotely deviant: Such things as murder, perjury, adultery, or drunkenness could be the identified sins. Not only was the person suffering from the illness, he or she was branded by all of society as having deserved it. The illness made the sin apparent to all; the sick person was isolated and disgraced. Those who obeyed God's law lived in health and happiness. Those who transgressed the law were punished, with illness and suffering thought to be consequences. The sick person then had to make atonement for the sins, enlist a priest or other spiritual healer to lift the spell or curse, or live with the illness to its ultimate outcome. In simple terms, the person had to get right with the gods or live with the consequences (Bullough & Bullough, 1978). Nursing care by a family member or relative would be needed in any case, regardless of the outcome of the sin/curse/disease–atonement/recovery or death cycle. This logic became the basis for explanation of why some people get sick and some don't for many centuries and still persists to some degree in most cultures today.

The Greeks and Health

In Greek mythology, the god of medicine, Asclepias, cured disease. One of his daughters, Hygeia, from whom we derive the word *hygiene,* was the goddess of preventive health and protected humans from disease. Panacea, Asclepias' other daughter, was known as the all-healing "universal remedy," and today is used to describe any ultimate "cure all" in medicine. She was known as the "light" of the day, and her name was invoked and shrines built to her during times of epidemics (Brooke, 1997).

During the **Greek era**, Hippocrates emphasized the rational treatment of sickness as a natural rather than god-inflicted phenomenon. Hippocrates of Cos (460–370 BC) is considered the father of medicine because of his arrangements of the oral and written remedies and diseases, which had long been secrets held by priests and religious healers, into a textbook of medicine that was used for centuries (Bullough & Bullough, 1978). Hippocrates' contribution to the science of public health was his recognition that making accurate observations of and drawing general conclusions from actual phenomena formed the basis of sound medical reasoning (Shryock, 1959).

In Greek society, health was considered to result from a balance between mind and body. A most important book, *Air, Waters and Places,* which detailed the relationship between humans and the environment, was written by Hippocrates. This is considered a milestone in the eventual development of the science of epidemiology as the first such treatise on the connectedness of the web of life. This topic of the relationship between humans and their environment did not reoccur until the development of bacteriology in the late 19th century (Rosen, 1958).

Perhaps the idea that most damaged the practice and scientific theory of medicine and health for centuries was the doctrine of the four humors, first spoken of by Empedocles of Acragas (493–433 BC). Empedocles was a philosopher and a physician, and as a result, he synthesized his cosmological ideas into his medical theory. He believed that the same four elements (or "roots of things") that made up the universe were found in humans and in all animate beings (Bullough & Bullough, 1978). Empedocles believed that man was a microcosm, a small world within the macrocosm, or external environment. The four humors of the body (blood, bile, phlegm, and black bile) corresponded to the four elements of the larger world (fire, air, water, and earth) (Kalisch & Kalisch, 1986). Depending on the prevailing humor, a person was either sanguine, choleric, phlegmatic, or melancholic. Because of this strongly held and persistent belief in the connection between the balance of the four humors and health status, treatment was aimed at restoring the appropriate balance of the four humors through the control of their corresponding elements. By manipulating the two sets of opposite qualities—hot and cold, wet and dry—balance was the goal of the intervention. Fire was hot and dry, air was hot and wet, water was cold and wet, and earth was cold and dry. For example, if a person had a fever, cold compresses would be prescribed for a chill and the person would be warmed. Such doctrine gave rise to faulty and ineffective treatment of disease that influenced medical education for many years (Taylor, 1922).

Plato, in *The Republic,* detailed the importance of recreation, a balanced mind and body, nutrition, and exercise. There was a distinction made among gender, class, and health as early as the Greek era; only males of the aristocracy could afford the luxury of maintaining a healthful lifestyle (Rosen, 1958).

In the *Iliad,* a poem about the attempts to capture Troy and rescue Helen from her lover Paris, 140 different wounds are described. The mortality rate averaged 77.6%, the highest as a result of sword and spear thrusts and the lowest from superficial arrow wounds. There was considerable need for nursing care, and Achilles, Patroclus, and other princes often acted as nurses to the injured. The early stages of Greek medicine reflected the influences of Egyptian, Babylonian, and Hebrew medicine. There-fore, good medical and nursing techniques were used to treat these war wounds: The arrow was drawn or cut out, the wound washed, soothing herbs applied, and the wound bandaged. However, in sickness in which no wound occurred, an evil spirit was considered the cause. For example, the cause of the plague was unknown, so the question became how and why affected soldiers had angered the gods. According to the *Iliad,* the true healer of the plague was the prophet who prayed for Apollo to stop shooting the "plague arrows." The Greeks applied rational causes and cures to external injuries, while internal ailments continued to be linked to spiritual maladies (Bullough & Bullough, 1978).

Roman Era

During the rise and the fall of the **Roman era** (31 BC–476 AD), Greek culture continued to be a strong influence. The Romans easily adopted Greek culture and expanded the Greeks' accomplishments, especially in the fields of engineering, law, and government. The development of policy, law, and protection of the public's health was an important precursor to our modern public health systems. For Romans, the government had an obligation to protect its citizens, not only from outside aggression such as warring neighbors, but from inside the civilization, in the form of health laws. According to Bullough and Bullough (1978, p. 20), Rome was essentially a "Greek cultural colony."

During the third century BC, Rome began to dominate the Mediterranean, Egypt, the Tigris-Euphrates Valley, the Hebrews, and the Greeks (Boorstin, 1985). Greek science and Roman engineering then spread throughout the ancient world, providing a synthesized Greco-Roman foundation for eventual public health policies (Bullough & Bullough, 1978).

Galen of Pergamum (129–199 AD), often known as the greatest Greek physician after Hippocrates, left for Rome after studying medicine in Greece and Egypt and gained great fame as a medical practitioner, lecturer, and experimenter. In his lifetime, medicine evolved into a science; he submitted traditional healing practices to experimentation and was possibly the greatest medical researcher before the 17th century (Bullough & Bullough, 1978). He was considered the last of the great physicians of antiquity (Kalisch & Kalisch, 1978).

The Greek physicians and healers certainly made the most contributions to medicine, but the Romans surpassed the Greeks

FYI

Did you know that engineers during the Roman era developed an aqueduct system capable of providing 40 gallons of water per person per day to its 1 million residents, comparable to our consumption rates today?

in promoting the evolution of nursing. Roman armies developed the notion of a mobile war nursing unit as their battles took them too far from home to be cared for by their wives and family. This portable hospital was a series of tents arranged in corridors; as battles wore on, these tents gave way to buildings that became permanent convalescent camps along the battle sites (Rosen, 1958). Many of these early military hospitals have been excavated by archaeologists along the banks of the Rhine and Danube Rivers. They had wards, recreation areas, baths, pharmacies, and even rooms for officers who needed a "rest cure" (Bullough & Bullough, 1978). Coexisting were the Greek dispensary forms of temples, or the *iatreia,* which started out as a type of physician waiting room. These eventually developed into a primitive type of hospital, places for surgical clients to stay until they could be taken home by their families. Although nurses during the Roman era were usually family members, servants, or slaves, nursing had strengthened its position in medical care and emerged during the Roman era as a separate and distinct specialty.

The Romans developed massive aqueducts, bath houses, and sewer systems during this era. At the height of the Roman Empire, Rome provided 40 gallons of water per person per day to its 1 million inhabitants, which is comparable to our rates of consumption today (Rosen, 1958). Even though these engineering feats were remarkable at the time, poorer and less fortunate residents often did not benefit from the same level of public health amenities, such as sewer systems and latrines (Bullough & Bullough, 1978). However, the Romans did provide many of their citizens with what we would consider public health services.

Middle Ages

Many of the advancements of the Greco-Roman era were reversed during the Middle Ages, after the decline of the Roman Empire (476–1453 AD). The Middle Ages, or the medieval era, served as a transition between ancient and modern civilizations. Once again, myth, magic, and religion were explanations and cures for illness and health problems. The medieval world was the result of fusion among three streams of thought, actions, and ways of life—Greco-Roman, Germanic, and Christian—into one (Donahue, 1985).

Nursing was most influenced by Christianity with the beginning of **deaconesses,** or female servants, doing the work of God by ministering to the needs of others. Deacons in the early Christian churches were apparently available only to care for men, while deaconesses cared for the needs of the women. This role of the deaconess in the church was considered a forward step in the development of nursing and in the 19th century would strongly influence the young Florence Nightingale. During this era, Roman military hospitals were replaced by civilian ones. In early Christianity, the *diakonia,* a kind of combination outpatient and welfare office, was managed by deacons and deaconesses and served as the equivalent of a hospital. Jesus served as the example of charity and compassion for the poor and marginal of society.

Communicable diseases were rampant during the Middle Ages, primarily because of the walled cities that emerged in response to the paranoia and isolation of the populations. Infection was next to impossible to control. Physicians had little to offer, deferring to the church for management of disease. Nursing roles were carried out primarily by religious orders. The oldest hospital (other than military hospitals in the Roman era) in Europe was most likely the Hotel Dieu in Lyons, France, founded about 542 by Childbert I, king of France. The Hotel Dieu in Paris was founded about 652 by St. Landry, bishop of Paris. During the Middle Ages, charitable institutions, hospitals, and medical schools increased in number, with the religious leaders as caregivers. The word *hospital,* which is derived from the Latin word *hospitalis,* meaning service of guests, was most likely more of a shelter for travelers and other pilgrims as well as the occasional person who needed extra care (Kalisch & Kalisch, 1986). Early European hospitals were more like hospices or homes for the aged, sick pilgrims, or orphans. Nurses in these early hospitals were religious deaconesses who chose to care for others in a life of servitude and spiritual sacrifice.

Black Death

During the Middle Ages, a series of horrible epidemics, including the **Black Death** or bubonic plague, ravaged the civilized world (Diamond, 1997). In the 14th century, Europe, Asia, and Africa saw nearly half their populations lost to the bubonic plague. According to Bullough and Bullough (1978), an interesting account of the arrival of the bubonic plague in 1347 claims that the disease had started in the Genoese colony of Kaffa in the Crimea. The story passed down through the ages was that the city was being besieged by a Mongol khan. When the disease broke out among the khan's men, he catapulted the bodies of its victims into Kaffa to infect and weaken his enemies. The soldiers and colonists of Kaffa carried the disease back to Genoa. Worldwide, more than 60 million deaths were eventually attributed to this horrible plague. In some parts of Europe, only one fourth of the population survived, with some places having too few people to bury the dead. Families abandoned sick children, and the sick were often left to die alone (Cartwright, 1972).

Nurses and physicians were powerless to avert the disease. Black spots and tumors on the skin appeared, and petechia and hemorrhages gave the skin a darkened appearance. There was also acute inflammation of the lungs, burning sensations, unquenchable thirst, and inflammation of the entire body. Hardly anyone afflicted survived the third day of the attack. So great was the fear of contagion that ships were set to sail with bodies of infected persons without a crew, drifting through the North, Black, and Mediterranean seas from port to port with their dead passengers (Cohen, 1989). Bubonic plague is caused by the bacillus *Pasteurella pestis,* which is usually transmitted by the bite of a flea carried by an animal vector, typically a rat. After the initial flea bite, the infection spreads through the lymph nodes, and the nodes swell to enormous size; the inflamed nodes are called *bu-*

bos, from which the bubonic plague derives its name. Medieval people knew that this disease was in some way communicable, but they were unsure of the mode of transmission (Diamond, 1997), hence the avoidance of victims and a reliance on isolation techniques. The practice of quarantine in city ports was developed as a preventive measure and is still used today (Bullough & Bullough, 1978; Kalisch & Kalisch, 1986).

The Renaissance

During the rebirth of Europe, great political, social, and economic advances occurred along with a tremendous revival of learning. Donahue (1985, p. 188) contends that the Renaissance has been "viewed as both a blessing and a curse." There was a renewed interest in the arts and sciences, which helped advance medical science (Boorstin, 1985; Bullough & Bullough, 1978). Columbus and other explorers discovered new worlds, and belief in an earth-centered rather than sun-centered universe was promoted by Copernicus (1473–1543); Sir Isaac Newton's (1642–1727) theory of gravity changed the world forever. Gunpowder was introduced, and social and religious upheavals resulted in the American and French revolutions at the end of the 18th century.

In the arts and sciences, Leonardo da Vinci, known as one of the greatest geniuses of all time, made a number of anatomical drawings based on dissection experiences. These drawings have become classics in the progression of knowledge about the human anatomy. Many artists of this time left an indelible mark and continue to exert influence today, including Michelangelo, Raphael, and Titian (Donahue, 1985).

The Advancement of Science and Public Health

It took the first 50 years of the 18th century for the new knowledge from the Enlightenment to be organized and digested, according to Donahue (1985). In Britain, Edward Jenner discovered an effective method of vaccination against the dreaded smallpox virus in 1798. Psychiatry developed as a separate branch of medicine, and instruments such as the pulse watch and the stethoscope were invented that measured and allowed for assessment of the body.

One of the greatest scientists of this period was Louis Pasteur (1822–1895). A French chemist, Pasteur first became interested in pathogenic organisms through his studies of the diseases of wine. His discovery that if wine was heated to a temperature of 55 to 60ºC, the process killed the microorganisms that spoiled wine, was critical to the wine industry's success in France. This process of pasteurization led Pasteur to investigate many fields and save many lives from contaminated milk and food.

Joseph Lister (1827–1912) was a physician who set out to decrease the mortality resulting from infection after surgery. He used Pasteur's research to eventually arrive at a chemical antiseptic solution of carbolic acid for use in surgery. Widely regarded as the father of modern surgery, he practiced his antiseptic surgery with great results, and the Listerian principles of asepsis changed the way physicians and nurses practice to this day (Dietz & Lehozky, 1963). Robert Koch (1843–1910), a physician known for his research in anthrax, is regarded as the father of microbiology. By identifying the organism that caused cholera, *Vibrio cholerae,* he also demonstrated its transmission by water, food, and clothing. Edwin Klebs (1834–1913) proved the germ theory, that is, that germs are the causes of infectious diseases. This discovery of the bacterial origin of diseases may be considered the greatest achievement of the 19th century. Although the microscope had been around for two centuries, it remained for Lister, Pasteur, and Koch—and ultimately Klebs—to provide the missing link (Dietz & Lehozky, 1963; Rosen, 1958).

The Emergence of Home Visiting

In 1633, **St. Vincent de Paul** founded the Sisters of Charity in France, an order of nuns who traveled from home to home visiting the sick. As the services of the sisters grew, St. Vincent appointed Mademoiselle Le Gras as supervisor of these visiting sisters. These nurses functioned as the first organized visiting nurse service, making home visits and caring for the sick in their homes. De Paul believed that for family members to go to the hospital was disruptive to family life and that taking nursing services to the home enabled health to be restored more effectively and more efficiently.

The Reformation

Religious changes during the renaissance were to influence nursing perhaps more than any other aspect of society. Particularly important was the rise of Protestantism as a result of the reform movements of Martin Luther (1483–1546) in Germany and John Calvin (1509–1564) in France and Geneva. Although the various sects were numerous in the Protestant movement, the agreement among the leaders was almost unanimous on the abolition of the monastic or cloistered career. The effects on nursing were drastic: monastic-affiliated institutions, including hospitals and schools, were closed, and orders of nuns, including nurses, were dissolved. Even in countries where Catholicism flourished, seizures of monasteries by royal leaders occurred frequently.

· ·

The reformation had a devastating effect upon nursing . . . imagine our situation in the United States if a decree went out that hospitals would be closed in two years. There would be no places available to care for the ill. Such were the conditions in England from 1538–1540 during the Reign of Henry VIII. No provision was made for the sick poor, there was no lay organization to replace those who had fled, and no one to develop or teach others to carry on.

Dietz & Lehozky, 1963

· ·

Religious leaders, such as Martin Luther in Germany, who led the Reformation in 1517, were well aware of the lack of adequate nursing care as a result of these sweeping changes. Luther advocated that each town establish something akin to a "community chest" to raise funds for hospitals and nurse visitors for the poor (Dietz & Lehozky, 1963). For example, in England, where there had been at least 450 charitable foundations before the Reformation, only a few survived the reign of Henry VIII, who closed most of the monastic hospitals (Donahue, 1985). Eventually, Henry VIII's son, Edward VI, who reigned from 1547 to 1553, was convinced and did endow some hospitals, namely St. Bartholomew's Hospital and St. Thomas' Hospital, which would eventually house the Nightingale School of Nursing later in the 19th century (Bullough & Bullough, 1978).

The Dark Period of Nursing

The latter half of the period between 1500 and 1860 is widely regarded as the "dark period of nursing" because nursing conditions were at their worst (Donahue, 1985). Education for girls, which had been provided by the nuns in religious schools, was lost. Because of the elimination of hospitals and schools, there was no one to pass on knowledge about caring for the sick. As a result, the hospitals were managed and staffed by municipal authorities; women entering nursing service often came from illiterate classes, and even then there were too few to serve (Dietz & Lehozky, 1963). The lay attendants who filled the nursing role were illiterate, rough, inconsiderate, and often immoral and alcoholic. Intelligent women and men could not be persuaded to accept such a degraded and low-status position in the offensive municipal hospitals of London. Nursing slipped back into a role of servitude as menial, low-status work. According to Donahue (1985), when a woman could no longer make it as a gambler, prostitute, or thief, she might become a nurse. Eventually, women serving jail sentences for crimes such as prostitution and stealing were ordered to care for the sick in the hospitals instead of serving their sentences in the city jail (Dietz & Lehozky, 1963). The nurses of this era took bribes from clients, became inappropriately involved with them, and survived the best way they could, often at the expense of their assigned clients.

Nursing had, during this era, virtually no social standing and no organization. Even Catholic sisters of the religious orders throughout Europe "came to a complete standstill" professionally because of the intolerance of society (Donahue, 1985, p. 231). Charles Dickens, in *Martin Chuzzlewit* (1910), created the immortal characters of Sairey Gamp and Betsy Prig. Sairey Gamp was a visiting nurse based on an actual hired attendant whom Dickens had met in a friend's home. Sairey Gamp was hired to care for sick family members but was instead cruel to her clients, stole from them, and ate their rations; she was an alcoholic and has been immortalized forever as a reminder of the world in which Florence Nightingale came of age (Donahue, 1985).

She was a fat old woman, this Mrs. Gamp, with a husky voice and a moist eye, which she had a remarkable power of turning up and showing the white of it. Having very little neck, it cost her some trouble to look over herself, if one may say so, to those to whom she talked. She wore a very rusty black gown, rather the worse for snuff, and a shawl and bonnet to correspond. . . . The face of Mrs. Gamp—the nose in particular—was somewhat red and swollen, and it was difficult to enjoy her society without becoming conscious of the smell of spirits. Like most persons who have attained to great eminence in their profession, she took to hers very kindly; insomuch, that setting aside her natural predilections as a woman, she went to a lying-in [birth] or a laying-out [death] with equal zest and relish.

Charles Dickens, 1910

Early Organized Health Care in the Americas: A Brave New World

In the New World, the first hospital in the Americas, *the Hospital de la Purisima Concepción,* was founded some time before 1524 by Hernando Cortes, the conqueror of Mexico. The first hospital in the continental United States was erected in Manhattan in 1658 for the care of sick soldiers and slaves. In 1717, a hospital for infectious diseases was built in Boston; the first hospital established by a private gift was the Charity Hospital in New Orleans. A sailor, Jean Louis, donated the endowment for the hospital's founding (Bullough & Bullough, 1978).

During the 17th and 18th centuries, colonial hospitals were often used to house the poor and downtrodden. Hospitals called *pesthouses* were created to care for clients with contagious diseases; their primary purpose was to protect the public at large, rather than to treat and care for the clients. Contagious diseases were rampant during the early years of the American colonies, often being spread by the large number of immigrants who brought these diseases with them on their long journeys to America. Medicine was not as developed as in Europe, and nursing remained in the hands of the uneducated. Average life expectancy at birth was only around 35 years by 1720. Plagues were a constant nightmare, with outbreaks of smallpox and yellow fever. In 1751, the first true hospital in the new colonies, Pennsylvania Hospital, was erected in Philadelphia on the recommendation of Benjamin Franklin (Kalisch & Kalisch, 1986).

By today's standards, hospitals in the 19th century were disgraceful, dirty, unventilated, and contaminated by infections; to be a client in a hospital actually increased one's risk of dying. As in England, nursing was considered an inferior occupation. After the sweeping changes as a result of the Reformation, educated religious health workers were replaced with lay people who were "down and outers," in prison, or had no option left but to work with the sick (Kalisch & Kalisch, 1986).

The Chadwick Report and the Shattuck Report

Edwin Chadwick became a major figure in the development of the field of public health in Great Britain by drawing attention to the cost of the unsanitary conditions that shortened the life span of the laboring class and the threats to the wealth of Britain. Although the first sanitation legislation, which established a National Vaccination Board, was passed in 1837, Chadwick found in his classic study, *Report on an Inquiry Into the Sanitary Conditions of the Laboring Population of Great Britain*, that death rates were high in large industrial cities such as Liverpool. A more startling finding, from what is often referred to simply as the **Chadwick Report**, was that more than half the children of labor-class workers died by age 5, indicating poor living conditions that affected the health of the most vulnerable. Laborers lived only half as long as the upper classes.

One consequence of the report was the establishment of the first board of health, the General Board of Health for England, in 1848 (Richardson, 1887). More legislation followed that initiated social reform in the areas of child welfare, elder care, the sick, the mentally ill, factory health, and education. Soon sewers and fire plugs, based on an available water supply, appeared as indicators that the public health linkages from the Chadwick Report had an impact.

In the United States during the 19th century, waves of epidemics of yellow fever, smallpox, cholera, typhoid fever, and typhus continued to plague the population as in England and the rest of the world. As cities continued to grow in the industrialized young nation, poor workers crowded into larger cites and suffered from illnesses caused by the unsanitary living conditions (Hanlon & Pickett, 1984). Similar to Chadwick's classic study in England, Lemuel Shattuck, a Boston bookseller and publisher who had an interest in public health, organized the American Statistical Society in 1839 and issued a census of Boston in 1845. Shattuck's census revealed high infant mortality rates and high overall population mortality rates. In his *Report of the Massachusetts Sanitary Commission* in 1850, Shattuck not only outlined his findings on the unsanitary conditions but made recommendations for public health reform that included bookkeeping of population statistics and development of a monitoring system that would provide information to the public about environmental, food, and drug safety and infectious disease control (Rosen, 1958). He also called for services for well child care, school-age children's health, immunizations, mental health, health education for all, and health planning. The **Shattuck Report** was revolutionary in its scope and vision for public health, but it was virtually ignored during Shattuck's lifetime. It was 19 years later, in 1869, that the first state board of health was formed (Kalisch & Kalisch, 1986).

The Industrial Revolution

During the mid-18th century in England, capitalism emerged as an economic system based on profit. This emerging system resulted in mass production, as contrasted with the previous system of individual workers and craftsmen. In the simplest terms, the **Industrial Revolution** was the application of machine power to processes formerly done by hand. Machinery was invented during this era and ultimately standardized quality; individual craftsmen were forced to give up their crafts and lands and become factory laborers for the capitalist owners. All types of industries were affected; this new-found efficiency produced profit for owners of the means of production. Because of this, the era of invention flourished, factories grew, and people moved in record numbers to the work in the cities. Urban areas grew, tenement housing projects emerged, and overcrowded cities became serious threats to well-being (Donahue, 1985).

Workers were forced to go to the machines, rather than the other way around. Such relocations meant giving up not only farming, but a way of life that had existed for centuries. The emphasis on profit over people led to child labor, frequent layoffs, and long work days filled with stressful, tedious, unfamiliar work. Labor unions did not exist, nor was there any legal protection against exploitation of workers, including children (Donahue, 1985). All these rapid changes and often threatening conditions created the world of Charles Dickens, where, as in *Oliver Twist*, children worked as adults without question.

According to Donahue (1985), urban life, trade, and industrialization contributed to these overwhelming health hazards, and the situation was confounded by the lack of an adequate means of social control. Reforms were desperately needed, and the social reform movement emerged in response to the unhealthy byproducts of the Industrial Revolution. It was in this world of the 19th century that reformers such as John Stuart Mill (1806–1873) emerged. Although the Industrial Revolution began in England, it quickly spread to the rest of Europe and to the United States (Bullough & Bullough, 1978). The reform movement is critical to understanding the emerging health concerns that were later addressed by Florence Nightingale. Mill championed popular education, the emancipation of women, trade unions, and religious toleration. Other reform issues of the era included the abolition of slavery and, most important for nursing, more humane care of the sick, the poor, and the wounded (Bullough & Bullough, 1978). There was a renewed energy in the religious community with the reemergence of new religious orders in the Catholic church that provided service to the sick and disenfranchised.

Epidemics had ravaged Europe for centuries, but they became even more serious with urbanization: Industrialization had brought people to cities, where they worked in close quarters (as compared with the isolation of the farm) and contributed to the social decay of the second half of the 19th century. Sanitation was poor or nonexistent, sewage disposal from the growing population was lacking, cites were filthy, public laws were weak or nonexistent, and congestion of the cities inevitably brought pests in the form of rats, lice, and bedbugs, which transmitted many pathogens. Communicable diseases continued to plague the population, especially those who lived in these unsanitary environments. For example, during the mid-18th century, typhus and typhoid fever claimed twice as many lives each year as did the Battle of Waterloo (Hanlon & Pickett, 1984). Through foreign trade and immigration, infectious diseases were spread to all of Europe and eventually to the growing United States.

John Snow and the Science of Epidemiology

John Snow, a prominent physician, is credited with being the first epidemiologist by demonstrating in 1854 that cholera rates were linked with water pump use in London (Cartwright, 1972). Snow investigated the area around Golden Square in London and arrived at the conclusion that cholera was not carried by bad air, nor necessarily by direct contact. He formed the opinion that diarrhea, unwashed hands, and shared food somehow played a large part in spreading the disease.

People around Golden Square in London were not supplied with water by pipes but drew their water from surface wells by means of hand-operated pumps. A severe outbreak of cholera occurred at the end of August 1853, resulting in at least 500 deaths in just 10 days in Golden Square. By using rates of cholera, Snow for the first time linked the sources of the drinking water at the Broad Street pump to the outbreaks of cholera. This proved that cholera was a waterborne disease. Dr. Snow's epidemiological investigation started a train of events that eventually would end the great epidemics of cholera, dysentery, and typhoid.

When Snow attended the now-famous community meeting of Golden Square and gave his evidence, government officials asked him what measures were necessary. His reply was, "Take the handle off the Broad Street pump." The handle was removed the next day, and no more cholera cases occurred (Snow, 1855). Although he did not discover the true cause of the cholera—the identification of the organism—he came very close to the truth (Rosen, 1958).

And Then There Was Nightingale . . .

Florence Nightingale was named one of the 100 most influential persons of the last millennium by *Life Magazine* (1997). She was one of only eight women identified. Of those eight women, such as Joan of Arc, Helen Keller, and Elizabeth I, Nightingale was identified as a true "angel of mercy," having reformed military health care in the Crimean War and having used her political savvy to forever change the way society views the health of the vulnerable, the poor, and the forgotten. She is probably one of the most written about women in history (Bullough & Bullough, 1978). Florence Nightingale has become synonymous with modern nursing.

Florence Nightingale was the second child born to the wealthy English family of William and Frances Nightingale on

FYI

Florence Nightingale never made a public appearance, never issued a public statement, and did not have the right to vote.

May 12, 1820, in her namesake city, Florence, Italy. As a young child, Florence displayed incredible curiosity and intellectual abilities not common to female children of the Victorian age. She mastered the fundamentals of Greek and Latin, and she studied history, art, mathematics, and philosophy. To her family's dismay, she believed that God had called her to be a nurse. Nightingale was keenly aware of the suffering that industrialization created; she became obsessed with the plight of the miserable and suffering. There existed conditions of general starvation that accompanied the Industrial Revolution, overflowing prisons and workhouses, and displaced persons in all sections of British life. She wrote in the spring of 1842, "My mind is absorbed with the sufferings of man, it besets me behind and before. . . . All that the poets sing of the glories of this world seem to me untrue. All the people that I see are eaten up with care or poverty or disease" (Woodham-Smith, 1951, p. 31).

For Nightingale, her entire life would be haunted by this conflict between the opulent life of gaiety that she enjoyed and the plight and misery of the world, which she was unable to alleviate. She was, in essence, an "alien spirit in the rich and aristocratic social sphere of Victorian England" (Palmer, 1977, p. 14). Nightingale remained unmarried, and at the age of 25, she expressed a desire to be trained as a nurse in an English hospital. Her parents emphatically denied her request, and for the next 7 years, she made repeated attempts to change their minds and allow her to enter nurse training. She wrote, "I crave for some regular occupation, for something worth doing instead of frittering my time away on useless trifles" (Woodham-Smith, 1951, p. 162). During this time, she continued her education through the study of math and science and spent 5 years collecting data about public health and hospitals (Dietz & Lehozky, 1963). During a tour of Egypt in 1849 with family and friends, Nightingale spent her 13th year in Alexandria with the Sisters of Charity of St. Vincent de Paul, where her conviction to study nursing was only reinforced. While in Egypt, Nightingale studied Egyptian, Platonic, and Hermetic philosophy; Christian scripture; and the works of poets, mystics, and missionaries in her efforts to understand the nature of God and her "calling" as it fit into the divine plan (Calabria, 1996).

The next spring, Nightingale traveled unaccompanied to the Kaiserwerth Institute in Germany and stayed there for 2 weeks, vowing to return to train as a nurse. In June 1851, Nightingale took her future into her own hands and announced to her family that she planned to return to Kaiserwerth and study nursing.

According to Dietz and Lehozky (1963, p. 42), her mother had "hysterics" and "scene followed scene." Her father "retreated into the shadows," and her sister, Parthe, expressed that the family name was forever disgraced (Cook, 1913).

In 1851, at the age of 31, Nightingale was finally permitted to go to Kaiserwerth and she studied there for 3 months with Pastor Fliedner. Her family insisted that she tell no one outside the family of her whereabouts, and her mother forbade her to write any letters from Kaiserwerth. While there, Nightingale learned about the care of the sick and the importance of discipline and commitment of oneself to God (Donahue, 1985). She returned to England and cared for her ailing father, from whom she finally gained some support for her intent to become a nurse.

In 1852, Nightingale wrote the essay "Cassandra," which stands today as a classic feminist treatise against the idleness of Victorian women. Through her voluminous journal writings, Nightingale reveals her inner struggle throughout her adulthood with what was expected of a woman and what she could accomplish with her life. The life expected of an aristocratic woman in her day was one she grew to loathe; throughout her writings, she poured out her detestation of the life an idle woman (Nightingale, 1979, p. 5). In "Cassandra," Nightingale put her thoughts to paper, and many scholars believe that her eventual intent was to extend the essay to a novel. She wrote in "Cassandra," "Why have women passion, intellect, moral activity—these three—in a place in society where no one of the three can be exercised?" (Nightingale, 1852, p. 37). Although uncertain about the meaning of the name "Cassandra," many scholars believe that it came from the Greek goddess Cassandra, who was cursed by Apollo and doomed to see and speak the truth but never to be believed. Nightingale saw the conventional life of women as a waste of time and abilities. After receiving a generous yearly endowment from her father, Nightingale moved to London and worked briefly as the superintendent of the Establishment for Gentlewomen During Illness, finally realizing her dream of working as a nurse (Cook, 1913).

The Crimean Experience: "I Can Stand Out the War with Any Man"

Nightingale's opportunity for greatness came when she was offered the position of female nursing establishment of the English General Hospitals in Turkey by the secretary of war, Sir Sidney Herbert. Soon after the outbreak of the Crimean War, stories of the inadequate care and lack of medical resources for the soldiers became widely known throughout England (Woodham-Smith, 1951). The country was appalled at the conditions so vividly portrayed in the *London Times*. Pressure increased on Sir Herbert to react. He knew of one woman who was capable of bringing order out of the chaos and wrote the following now-famous letter to Nightingale on October 15, 1854, as a plea for her service:

> There is but one person in England that I know of who would be capable of organising and superintending such a scheme. . . . The difficulty of finding women equal to a task

after all, full of horrors, and requiring besides knowledge and good will, great energy and great courage, will be great. Your own personal qualities, your knowledge and your power of administration and among greater things your rank and position in Society give you advantages in such a work which no other person possesses (Woodham-Smith, 1951, pp. 87–89).

Nightingale took the challenge from Sir Herbert and set sail with 38 self-proclaimed nurses with varied training and experiences, of whom 24 were Catholic and Anglican nuns. Their journey to the Crimea took a month, and on November 4, 1854, the brave nurses arrived at Istanbul and were taken to Scutari the same day. Faced with 3,000 to 4,000 wounded men in a hospital designed to accommodate 1,700, the nurses went to work (Kalisch & Kalisch, 1986). This is the scene that the nurses faced: There were 4 miles of beds 18 inches apart. Most soldiers were lying naked with no bed or blanket. There were no kitchen or laundry facilities. The little light present took the form of candles in beer bottles. The hospital was literally floating on an open sewage lagoon filled with rats and other vermin (Donahue, 1985).

The barrack "hospital" was more of a death trap than a place for healing before Nightingale's arrival. In a letter to Sir Herbert, Nightingale wrote with tongue in cheek, that "the vermin might, if they had but unity of purpose, carry off the four miles of beds on their backs and march them into the War Office" (Stanmore, 1906, pp. 393–394).

By taking the newly arrived medical equipment and setting up kitchens, laundries, recreation rooms, reading rooms, and a canteen, Nightingale and her team of nurses proceeded to clean the barracks of lice and filth. Nightingale was in her element— she set out not only to provide humane health care for the soldiers but to essentially overhaul the administrative structure of the military health services (Williams, 1961). Nightingale and her nurses were faced with overwhelming odds and deplorable conditions. No accommodations had been made for their quarters, so they ended up in one of the hospital towers, 39 women crowded into six small rooms. In addition to having no furniture, one of the rooms even had a long-neglected, forgotten corpse swarming with vermin! Ever the disciplinarian, Nightingale insisted on strict adherence to a standard nurse uniform: gray tweed dresses, gray worsted jackets, plain white caps, short woolen cloaks, and brown scarves embroidered in red with the words "Scutari Hospital" (Bullough & Bullough, 1978).

Florence Nightingale and Sanitation

Although Nightingale never accepted the germ theory, she demanded clean dressings; clean bedding; well-cooked, edible, and appealing food; proper sanitation; and fresh air. After the other nurses were asleep, Nightingale made her famous solitary rounds with a lamp or lantern to check on the soldiers. Nightingale had a lifelong pattern of sleeping few hours, spending many nights writing, developing elaborate plans, and evaluating implemented changes. She seldom believed in the "hopeless" soldier, only one that needed extra attention. Nightingale was convinced that most of the maladies that the soldiers suffered and died from were preventable (Williams, 1961).

Before Nightingale's arrival and her radical and well-documented interventions based on sound public health principles, the mortality rate from the Crimea War was estimated to be from 42% to 73%. Nightingale is credited with reducing that rate to 2% within 6 months of her arrival at Scutari. She did this through careful, scientific epidemiological research (Dietz & Lehozky, 1963).

According to Palmer (1982), Nightingale possessed the qualities of a good researcher: insatiable curiosity, command of her subject, familiarity with methods of inquiry, a good background of statistics, and the ability to discriminate and abstract. She used these skills to maintain detailed and copious notes and to codify observations. She relied on statistics and attention to detail to back up her conclusions about sanitation, management of care, and disease causation. Her now-famous "cox combs" are a hallmark of military health services management by which she diagrammed deaths in the Army from wounds and from other diseases and compared them with deaths that occurred in similar populations in England (Palmer, 1977).

Nightingale was first and foremost an administrator: She believed in a hierarchical administrative structure with ultimate control lodged in one person to whom all subordinates and offices reported. Within a matter of weeks of her arrival in the Crimea, Nightingale was the acknowledged administrator and organizer of a mammoth humanitarian effort. From her Crimean experience on, Nightingale involved herself primarily in organizational activities and health planning administration. It was through her success at Scutari that she began a long career of influence on the public's health through social activism and reform, health policy, and the reformation of career nursing. Palmer contends that Nightingale "perceived the Crimean venture, which was set up as an experiment, as a golden opportunity to demonstrate the efficacy of female nursing" (Palmer, 1982, p. 4).

• •

Many soldiers wrote about their experiences of the Angel of Mercy, Florence Nightingale. One soldier wrote perhaps one of the most revealing tributes to this "Lady with the Lamp":

What a comfort it was to see her pass even. She would speak to one and nod and smile to as many more, but she could not do it all, you know. We lay there by hundreds, but we could kiss her shadow as it fell, and lay our heads on the pillow again content.

Tyrell, 1856, p. 310

• •

An African nurse from Jamaica, Mary Grant Seacole, offered her services to Nightingale after hearing of the need in Scutari. Although Nightingale was unable to hire Seacole as a part of the nursing staff, Seacole volunteered her services without pay. Sea-

cole was so committed to providing care to the British military that she set up an inn that provided food and lodging near Scutari (Hine, 1989).

Scores have been written about this almost mythic figure in history; she truly was a beloved legend by the time she left the Crimea in July 1856, 4 months after the war. Longfellow immortalized this "Lady with the Lamp" in his poem of 1857, "Santa Filomena" (Longfellow, 1857).

• •

Miss Nightingale had stamped the profession of nurse with her own image . . . in the midst of the muddle and the filth, the agony and the defeats, she had brought about a revolution.

Woodham-Smith, 1951, p. 179

• •

Returning Home a Heroine: The Political Reformer

When Nightingale returned to London, she found that her efforts to provide comfort and health to the British soldier succeeded in making heroes of both Nightingale and the soldiers (Woodham-Smith, 1951). Both had suffered from negative stereotypes: The soldier was often portrayed as a drunken oaf with little ambition or honor, the nurse as a tipsy, self-serving, illiterate, promiscuous loser. After the Crimean War and the efforts of Nightingale and her nurses, both returned with honor and dignity, never more the downtrodden and disrespected.

After her return from the Crimea, Florence Nightingale never made a public appearance, never attended a public function, and never issued a public statement (Bullough & Bullough, 1978). She single-handedly raised nursing from, as she put it, "the sink it was" into a respected and noble profession (Palmer, 1977). As an avid scholar and student of the Greek writer Plato, Nightingale believed that she had a moral obligation to work primarily for the good of the community. Because she believed that education formed character, she insisted that nursing must go beyond care for the sick; the mission of the trained nurse must include social reform to promote the good. This dual mission of nursing—caregiver and political reformer—has shaped the profession as we know it today, especially in the field of community health nursing. LeVasseur (1998) contends that Nightingale's insistence on nursing's involvement of a larger political ideal in the historical foundation of the field distinguishes us from other scientific disciplines such as medicine.

How did Nightingale accomplish this? You will learn throughout this text how community health nurses effect change through others. Florence Nightingale is the standard by which we measure our effectiveness. She effected change through her wide command of acquaintances: Queen Victoria was a significant admirer of her intellect and ability to effect change, and she used her position as national heroine to get the attention of elected officials in Parliament. She was tireless and had an amazing capacity for work. She used people. Everyone who could be of service to her was enlisted in her goals. Her brother-in-law, Sidney Herbert, was a member of Parliament and often delivered her "messages" in the form of legislation. When she wanted the public incited, she turned to the press, writing letters to the *London Times* and having others of influence write articles. She was not above threats to "go public" by certain dates if an elected official refused to establish a commission or appoint a committee. And when those committees and commissions were formed, Nightingale was ready with her list of selected people for appointment (Palmer, 1982).

When Nightingale returned to London after the Crimean War, she remained haunted by her experiences related to the soldiers' dying of preventable diseases. She was troubled by nightmares and had difficulty sleeping in the years that followed. She wrote in her journal: "Oh my poor men; I am a bad mother to come home and leave you in your Crimean graves. . . . I can never forget. . . . I stand at the altar of the murdered men and while I live, I fight their cause" (Woodham-Smith, 1983, pp. 178, 193). Nightingale became a prolific writer and a staunch defender of the causes of the British soldier, sanitation in England and India, and trained nursing. She never gave up until she was in her 80s and unable to read or write.

As a woman, she was unable to hold an official government post, nor could she vote. Historians have had varied opinions about the exact nature of the disability that kept her homebound for the remainder of her life. Recent scholars have speculated that she experienced posttraumatic stress disorder from her experiences in the Crimea; there is also considerable evidence that she suffered from the painful disease brucellosis (Barker, 1989; Young, 1995). She exerted incredible influence through friends and acquaintances, directing from her sick room sanitation and poor law reform. Her mission to "cleanse" spread from the military to the British empire; her fight for improved sanitation both at home and in India consumed her energies for the remainder of her life (Vicinus & Nergaard, 1990).

The First School of Nursing: The Nightingale School

The British public honored Nightingale by endowing 50,000 pounds in her name upon her return to England from the Crimea. The money had been raised from the soldiers under her care and donations from the public. This Nightingale Fund eventually was used to create the **Nightingale School of Nursing,** which was to be the beginning of professional nursing (Donahue, 1985). Nightingale, at the age of 40, decided that St. Thomas' Hospital was the place for her training school for nurses. While the negotiations for the school went forward, she spent her time writing *Notes on Nursing: What It Is and What It Is Not,* published in 1859. The small book of 77 pages, written for the British mother, was an instant success. An expanded library edition was written for nurses and used as the textbook for the students at St. Thomas. The nursing students chosen for the new training school were handpicked; they had to be of good moral character, sober, and honest. Nightingale believed that the

strong emphasis on morals was critical to gaining respect for the new "Nightingale nurse," with no possible ties to the disgraceful association of past nurses. Nursing students were monitored throughout their 1-year program both on and off the hospital grounds; their activities were carefully watched for character weaknesses, and discipline was severe and swift for violators.

One of the most important features of the Nightingale School was its relative autonomy. Both the school and the hospital nursing service were organized under the head matron. This was especially significant because it meant that nursing service began independently of the medical staff in selecting, retaining, and disciplining students and nurses (Bullough & Bullough, 1978).

Nightingale and Military Reforms

The first real test of Nightingale's military reforms came in the United States during the war between the states. Nightingale was asked by the Union to advise on the organization of hospitals and care of the sick and wounded. She sent recommendations back to the United States based on her experiences and analysis in the Crimean, and her advisement and influence gained wide publicity. Following her recommendations, the Union set up a sanitary commission and provided for regular inspection of camps. She expressed a desire to help with the Confederate military also but unfortunately had no channel of communication with them (Bullough & Bullough, 1978).

· ·

Money would be better spent in maintaining health in infancy and childhood than in building hospitals to cure disease. (1894)

· ·

It is cheaper to promote health than to maintain people in sickness. (1894)

· ·

Preventable disease should be looked upon as a social crime. (1894)

· ·

I look to the day when there are no nurses to the sick but only nurses to the well. (1893)

Florence Nightingale
Seymer, 1954, pp. 312–318

· ·

William Rathbone and District Nursing

William Rathbone, a wealthy ship owner and philanthropist, is credited with the establishment of the first visiting nurse service, which eventually evolved into **district nursing.** He was so impressed with the private duty nursing care that his sick wife had received at home that he set out to develop a "district nursing service" in Liverpool, England. At his own expense, in 1859, he developed a corps of nurses trained to care for the sick poor in their homes (Bullough & Bullough, 1978). He divided the community into 16 districts; each was assigned a nurse and a social worker who provided nursing and health education. His experiment in district nursing was so successful that he was unable to find enough nurses to work in the districts. Rathbone contacted Nightingale for assistance. Her recommendation was to train more nurses, and she advised Rathbone to approach the Royal Liverpool Infirmary with a proposal for opening another training school for nurses (Rathbone, 1890). The infirmary agreed to Rathbone's proposal, and district nursing soon spread throughout England as successful "health nursing" in the community for the sick poor through voluntary agencies (Rosen, 1958). Ever the visionary, Nightingale contended that "Hospitals are but an intermediate stage of civilization. The ultimate aim is to nurse the sick poor in their own homes (1893)" (Attewell, 1996). She also wrote in regard to visiting families at home, "We must not talk *to* them or *at* them but *with* them (1894)" (Attewell, 1996). A similar service, **health visiting,** began in Manchester, England, in 1862 by the Manchester and Salford Sanitary Association. The purpose of placing "health visitors" in the home was to provide health information and instruction to families. Eventually, health visitors evolved to provide preventive health education and district nurses to care for the sick at home (Bullough & Bullough, 1978).

Florence Nightingale and Community Health Nursing

Although Nightingale is best known for her reform of hospitals and the military, she was a great believer in the future of health care, which she anticipated should be preventive in nature and would more than likely take place in the home and community. Her accomplishments in the field of "sanitary nursing" extended beyond the walls of the hospital to include workhouse reform and community sanitation reform. In 1864, Nightingale and Rathbone once again worked together to lead the reform of the Liverpool Workhouse Infirmary, where more than 1,200 sick paupers were crowded into unsanitary and unsafe conditions. Under the British Poor Laws, the most desperately poor of the large cities were gathered into large workhouses. When sick, they were sent to the workhouse infirmary. Trained nursing care was all but nonexistent. Through legislative pressure and a well-designed public campaign describing the horrors of the Workhouse Infirmary, reform of the workhouse system was accomplished by 1867. Although not as complete as Nightingale had wanted, nevertheless, nurses were in place and being paid a salary (Seymer, 1954).

Early efforts in community health nursing are evidence from Nightingale's views on "health nursing," which she distinguished from "sick nursing." She wrote two influential papers, one in 1893, "Sick-Nursing and Health Nursing" (Nightingale, 1893), which was read in the United States at the Chicago Exposition, and the second, "Health Teaching in Towns and Villages" in 1894 (Monteiro, 1985). Both papers praised the success of prevention-based nursing practice. Winslow (1946) acknowledged Nightingale's influence in the United States by being one of the first in the field of public health to recognize the importance of taking responsibility for one's health. She wrote in 1891 that "there are more people to pick us up than to help us stand on our own two feet" (Attewell, 1996). According to Palmer (1982), Nightingale was a leader in the high-level wellness movement long before the concept was identified. Nightingale saw the nurse as the key figure in establishing a healthy society. She saw a logical extension of nursing from acute hospital settings to the broadest sense of community that we use today. Clearly, through her *Notes on Nursing*, she visualized the nurse as "the nation's first bulwark in health maintenance, the promotion of wellness, and the prevention of disease" (Palmer, 1982, p. 6).

According to Monteiro (1985), two recurrent themes are found throughout Nightingale's writings about disease prevention and wellness outside the hospital. *The most persistent theme is that nurses must be trained differently and instructed specifically in district and instructive nursing.* She consistently wrote that the "health nurse" must be trained in the nature of poverty and its influence on health, something she referred to as the "pauperization" of the poor. She also believed that above all, health nurses must be good teachers about hygiene and helping families learn to better care for themselves (Nightingale, 1893). She insisted that untrained, "good intended women" could not substitute for nursing care in the home. Nightingale pushed for an extensive orientation and additional training, including prior hospital experience, before one was hired as a district nurse. She outlined the qualifications in her paper "On Trained Nursing for the Sick Poor," in which she called for a month's "trial" in district nursing, a year's training in hospital nursing, and 3 to 6 months training in district nursing (Monteiro, 1985). She said, "There is no such thing as amateur nursing."

The second theme that emerged from her writings was the focus on the role of the nurse. She clearly distinguished the role of the health nurse in promoting what we today call self-care. In the past, philanthropic visitors in the form of Christian charity would visit the homes of the poor and offer them relief (Monteiro, 1985). Nightingale believed that such activities did little to teach the poor to care for themselves and further "pauperized" them, keeping them unhealthy and prone to disease. The nurse then must help the families at home manage a healthy environment for themselves, and Nightingale saw a trained nurse as being the only person who could pull off such a feat. She stated, "Never think that you have done anything effectual in nursing in London, till you nurse, not only the sick poor in workhouses, but those at home."

· ·

There are five essential points in securing the health of houses:
   Pure air
   Pure water
   Efficient drainage
   Cleanliness
   Light

Florence Nightingale. (1860). *Notes on Nursing: What It Is and What It Is Not.* London: Harrison. Source: Cook, 1913, p. 133

· ·

To set poor people going again with a sound and clean house as well as a sound body and mind is about as great a benefit as can be given them—worth acres of relief. This is depauparizing them.

Rathbone, 1890, p. 84

My view you know is that the ultimate destination of all nursing is the nursing of the sick in their own homes. . . . I look to the abolition of all hospitals and workhouse infirmaries. But no use to talk about the year 2000.

Florence Nightingale, Letter to Henry Bonham Carter, 1867
Source: Woodham-Smith, 1950, p. 129

Nightingale died in her sleep on August 13, 1910, and was buried quietly and without pomp near the family's home at Embley, her coffin carried by six sergeants of the British Army. Only a small cross marks her grave: "FN. Born 1820. Died 1910." (Brown, 1988). The family refused burial at Westminster Abbey out of respect for Nightingale's wishes.

Community Health and Public Health Nursing in the United States

The pattern for health visiting and district nursing practice outside the hospital was similar in the United States to that in England (Roberts, 1954). American cities were besieged by overcrowding and epidemics after the Civil War. The need for trained nurses evolved as in England, and schools throughout the United States developed along the Nightingale model. Visiting nurses were first sent from philanthropic organizations in New York City (1877), Boston (1886), Buffalo (1885), and Philadelphia (1886) to care for the sick at home. By the end of the century, most large cities had some form of visiting nursing program and some headway was being made even in smaller towns (Heinrich, 1983).

Lillian Wald

Lillian Wald, a wealthy young woman with a great social conscience, graduated from the New York Hospital School of Nursing in 1891 and is credited with the title "public health nurse." After a year working in a mental institution, Wald entered medical school at Woman's Medical College in New York. While in medical school, she was asked to visit immigrant mothers on New York's Lower East Side and instruct them on health matters. Wald was appalled by the conditions there. During one now-famous home visit, a small child asked Wald to visit her sick mother. And the rest, as they say, is history. See Box 3-1.

What Wald found changed her life forever and secured a place for her in American nursing history. Wald said, "of all the maladjustments of our social and economic relations seemed epitomized in this brief journey" (1915, p. 6). Wald was profoundly affected by her observations; she and her colleague, Mary Brewster, quickly established the Henry Street Settlement in this same neighborhood in 1893. She quit medical school and devoted the remainder of her life to "visions of a better world" for the public's health.

The Henry Street Settlement was an independent nursing service where Wald lived and worked. This later became the Visiting Nurse Association of New York City, which laid the foundation for the establishment of public health nursing in the United States. At the Henry Street Settlement, nurses not only made family-oriented home visits, but the philosophy was truly one of holism as the basis for all care. The health needs of the population were met through addressing social, economic, and environmental determinants of health, in a pattern after Nightingale. The mission of Henry Street was to provide families with the education and tools to care for themselves. These nurses helped educate families about disease transmission and stressed the importance of good hygiene. They provided preventive, acute, and long-term care.

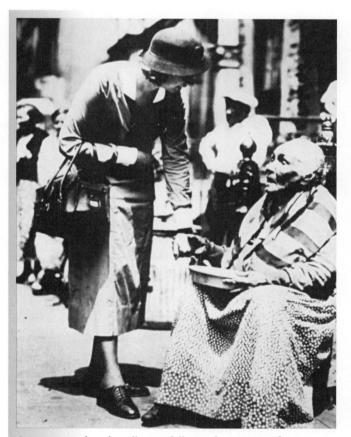

A nurse makes her "rounds" on the street of New York City for the Henry Street Visiting Nurse Services.

BOX 3-1 LILLIAN WALD TAKES A WALK

From the schoolroom where I had been giving a lesson in bed-making, a little girl led me one drizzling March morning. She had told me of her sick mother, and gathering from her incoherent account that a child had been born. I caught up the paraphernalia of the bed-making lesson and carried it with me.

The child led me over broken roadways . . . between tall, reeking houses whose laden fire-escapes, useless for their appointed purpose, bulged with household goods of every description. The rain added to the dismal appearance of the streets and to the discomfort of the crowds which thronged them, intensifying the odors which assailed me from every side. Through Hester and Division Streets we went to the end of Ludlow; past odorous fish-stands, for the streets were a market-place, unregulated, unsupervised, unclean; past evil-smelling, uncovered garbage cans . . .

All the maladjustments of our social and economic relations seemed epitomized in this brief journey and what was found at the end of it. The family to which the child led me was neither criminal nor vicious. Although the husband was a cripple, one of those who stand on street corners exhibiting deformities to enlist compassion, and masking the begging of alms by a pretense of selling; although the family of seven shared their two rooms with boarders—who were literally boarders, since a piece of timber was placed over the floor for them to sleep on—and although the sick woman lay on a wretched, unclean bed, soiled with a

hemorrhage two days old, they were not degraded human beings, judged by any measure of moral values.

In fact, it was very plain that they were sensitive to their condition, and when, at the end of my ministrations, they kissed my hands (those who have undergone similar experiences will, I am sure, understand), it would have been some solace if by any conviction of the moral unworthiness of the family I could have defended myself as a part of a society which permitted such conditions to exist. Indeed, my subsequent acquaintance with them revealed the fact that miserable as their state was, they were not without ideals for the family life, and for society, of which they were so unloved and unlovely a part.

That morning's experience was a baptism of fire. Deserted were the laboratory and the academic work of the college. I never returned to them. On my way from the sick-room to my comfortable student quarters my mind was intent on my own responsibility. To my inexperience it seemed certain that conditions such as these were allowed because people did not know, and for me there was a challenge to know and to tell. When early morning found me still awake, my naive conviction remained that, if people knew things—and "things" meant everything implied in the condition of this family—such horrors would cease to exist, and I rejoiced that I had a training in the care of the sick that in itself would give me an organic relationship to the neighborhood in which this awakening had come.

Source: The House on Henry Street. *(1915). New York: Henry Holt and Company.*

As such, Henry Street went far beyond the care of the sick and the prevention of illness: It aimed at rectifying those causes that led to the poverty and misery. Wald was a tireless social activist for legislative reforms that would provide a more just distribution for the marginal and disadvantaged in the United States (Donahue, 1985). Wald began with 10 nurses in 1893, which grew to 250 nurses serving 1,300 clients a day by 1916. During this same period, the budget grew from nothing to more than $600,000 a year, all from private donations.

Lillian Wald hired African American nurse Elizabeth Tyler in 1906 as evidence of her commitment to cultural diversity. Although unable to visit white clients, Tyler made her own way by "finding" African American families who needed her service. In 3 months, Tyler had so many African American families within her caseload that Wald hired a second African American nurse,

Edith Carter. Carter remained at Henry Street for 28 years until her retirement (Carnegie, 1991).

During her tenure at Henry Street, Wald demonstrated her commitment to racial and cultural diversity by employing 25 African American nurses over the years, and she paid them salaries equal to white nurses, and provided identical benefits and recognition to minority nurses (Carnegie, 1991). This was exceptional during the early part of the 20th century, a time when African American nurses were often denied admission to white schools of nursing and membership in professional organizations and were denied opportunities for employment in most settings. Because hospitals of this era often set quotas for African American clients, those nurses who managed to graduate from nursing schools found themselves with few clients who needed or could afford their services. African American nurses struggled for years

RESEARCH BRIEF

Mosley, M. O. (1996). Satisfied to carry the bag: Three black community health nurses' contributions to health care reform, 1900–1937. Nursing History Review, 4, 65–82.

Three exceptional African American nurses, Jessie Sleet, Elizabeth Tyler, and Edith Carter, are considered pioneers in community health nursing. This research article details how these three African American community health nurses made significant contributions to the development of New York City's community health nursing by providing much needed health care to unserved members of the African American community (1900–1937). They provided strong leadership in diverse roles, such as supervisors, administrators, and educators in clients' homes, babies' health stations, settlement houses, and clinics. Their work occurred during a period of rapid industrialization, immigration, and great population growth in the midst of teeming slums, disease, and death. In community health nursing history, it was a period of establishment, activism, expansion, and development. For these African American nurse pioneers, it was a time of significant challenges and growth. They faced educational, professional, and racial barriers and increased mortality among people of their own race. This research chronicles their brave and skilled efforts to transcend these barriers and improve the health of African American citizens during the early part of the 20th century.

for the right to take the registration examination available for white nurses.

Community organization became the means by which Wald and her nurses effected change in the social and political arenas. Community assessments were primary methods of data collection and provided Wald with the evidence that she needed when raising funds through private sources and convincing public officials of the efficacy of community nurses. As she said, "Nursing is love in action and there is no finer manifestation of it than the care of the poor and disabled in their own homes" (Wald, 1915, p. 14).

The Expansion of Community Health Nursing

Lillian Wald submitted a proposal to the city of New York after learning of a child's dismissal from a New York City school for a skin condition. Her proposal was for one of the Henry Street Settlement nurses to serve free for 1 month in a New York school. The results of her experiment were so convincing that salaries were approved for 12 school nurses. From this, school nursing

was born in the United States and became one of many community specialties credited to Wald (Dietz & Lehozky, 1963).

In 1909, Wald proposed a program to the Metropolitan Life Insurance Company to provide nursing visits to their industrial policyholders. Statistics kept by the company documented the lowered mortality rates of policyholders attributed to the nurses' public health practice and clinical expertise. The program demonstrated savings for the company and was so successful that it lasted until 1953 (Hamilton, 1988).

Industrial or occupational health nursing was first started in Vermont in 1895 by a marble company interested in the health and welfare of its workers and their families. Surveillance of communicable disease was a major role of early public health nurses. Tuberculosis (TB) was a leading cause of death in the 19th century, and once the tubercle bacillus was isolated in 1882 by Koch, prevention of transmission was a primary goal for the community health nurse. Nurses visited clients bedridden from TB and instructed persons in all settings about prevention of the disease (Abel, 1997).

Both voluntary visiting nurses and nurses eventually appointed by local and state agencies were employed as TB nurses (Wald, 1915). Wald also provided the impetus for the development of rural nursing in the United States through her work with the American Red Cross. The Town and Country Nursing Service, supported by voluntary and charitable organizations, supplied small towns and rural areas with trained public health nurses (Dock et al., 1922).

Wald's other significant accomplishments include the establishment of the Children's Bureau, set up in 1912 as part of the U.S. Department of Labor. She also was an enthusiastic supporter of and participant in women's suffrage, lobbied for inspections of the workplace, and supported her employee, Margaret Sanger, in her efforts to give women the right to birth control. She was active in the American and International Red Cross and helped form the Women's Trade Union League to protect women from sweatshop conditions.

Lillian Wald first coined the phrase "public health nursing" and transformed the field of community health nursing from the narrow role of home visiting to the population focus of today's community health nurse (Robinson, 1946). According to Dock and Stewart (1931), the title of public health nurse was purposeful: The role designation was designed to link the public's health to governmental responsibility, not private funding. Public health nursing, as has historically been the case, became so much in demand that a department of nursing and health was started at the Teachers College of Columbia University in New York in 1910. Students in this program did their clinicals in home visiting at the Henry Street Settlement. By 1912, the National Association of Public Health Nursing (NOPH) was formed, and Lillian Wald was elected the first president. A unique feature of this organization, as compared with other organizations for nurses, was that it was open to public health nurses and others in the community interested in promoting community health (Rosen, 1958).

As state departments of health and local governments began to employ more and more public health nurses, their role increasingly focused on prevention of illness in the entire community. A discrimination developed between the visiting nurse, who was employed by the voluntary agencies primarily to provide home care to the sick, and the public health nurse, who concentrated on preventive measures (Brainard, 1922).

Early public health nurses came closer than hospital-based nurses to the autonomy and professionalism that Nightingale advocated. Their work was conducted in the unconfined setting of the home and community, they were independent, and they enjoyed recognition as specialists in preventive health (Buhler-Wilkerson, 1983). Public health nurses from the beginning were much more holistic in their practice than their hospital counterparts. They were involved with the health of industrial workers, immigrants, and their families, and were concerned about exploitation of women and children. These nurses also played a part in prison reform and care of the mentally ill (Heinrich, 1983).

Considered the first African American public health nurse, Jessie Sleet Scales was hired in 1902 by the Charity Organization Society, a philanthropic organization, to visit African American families infected by TB. Scales provided district nursing care to New York City's African American families and is credited with paving the way for African American nurses in the practice of community health (Mosley, 1996).

Dorothea Linde Dix

Miss Dix, a Boston schoolteacher, became aware of the horrendous conditions in prisons and mental institutions when asked to do a Sunday school class in the House of Correction at Cambridge, Massachusetts. She was appalled at what she saw and went about studying if the conditions were isolated or widespread; she took 2 years off to visit every jail and almshouse from Cape Cod to Berkshire. With her statistics in hand and analysis completed she addressed the legislature of Massachusetts: "I proceed gentlemen, briefly, to call your attention to the *PRESENT STATE OF INSANE PERSONS CONFINED WITHIN THIS COMMONWEALTH, IN CAGES, CLOSETS, CELLARS, STALLS, PENS; CHAINED, BEATEN WITH RODS, AND LASHED INTO OBEDIENCE!*" (TIFFANY, 1890, P.76).

Her report was devastating. Boston was scandalized by the reality that the most progressive state in the Union was now associated with such appalling conditions. The shocked legislature voted to allocate funds to build hospitals. For the rest of her life, Dorothea Dix stood out as a tireless zealot for the humane treatment of the insane and imprisoned. She had exceptional savvy in dealing with legislators: She acquainted herself with the legislators and their records and displayed the "spirit of a crusader." For her contributions, she is one of the pioneers of the reform movement in the United States, and her efforts are felt worldwide to the present day (Dietz & Lehozky, 1963).

Dix was also known for her work in the Civil War, having been appointed superintendent of the female nurses of the Army by the secretary of war in 1861. Her tireless efforts led to the recruitment of more than 2,000 women to serve in the Union army during the Civil War. Officials had consulted with Nightingale concerning military hospitals and were determined not to make the same mistakes. Dix enjoyed far more sweeping powers than Nightingale in that she had the authority to organize hospitals, to appoint nurses, and to manage supplies for the wounded (Brockett & Vaughan, 1867). Among her most well-known nurses during the Civil War were the poet Walt Whitman and the author Louisa May Alcottt (Donahue, 1985).

Clara Barton

The idea for the International Red Cross was the brainchild of a Swiss banker, J. Henri Dunant, who proposed the formation of a neutral international relief society that could be activated in time of war. The International Red Cross was ratified by the Geneva Convention on August 22, 1864. Clara Barton, through her work in the Civil War, had come to believe that such an organization was desperately needed in the United States. However, it was not until 1882 that Barton was able to convince Congress to ratify the Treaty of Geneva, thus becoming the founder of the American Red Cross (Kalisch & Kalisch, 1986). Barton also played a leadership role in the Spanish-American War in Cuba, where she led a group of nurses to provide care for both U.S. and Cuban soldiers and Cuban civilians. At the age of 76, Barton went to President McKinley and offered the help of the Red Cross in Cuba. The President agreed to allow Barton to go with Red Cross nurses but only to care for the Cuban citizens. Once in Cuba, the U.S. military saw what Barton and her nurses were able to accomplish with the Cuban military, and American soldiers pressured military officials to allow Barton's help. Along with battling yellow fever, Barton was able to provide care to both Cuban and U.S. military personnel and eventually expanded that care to Cuban citizens in Santiago. One of Barton's most famous clients was young Colonel Teddy Roosevelt, led by his Rough Riders, who later became the President of the United States. Barton became an instant heroine both in Cuba and in the United States for her bravery, tenaciousness, and organized services for the military and civilians torn apart by war. On August 13, 1898, the Spanish-American War came to an end. The grateful people of Santiago, Cuba, built a statue to honor Clara Barton in the town square, where it stands to this day. The work of Barton and her Red Cross nurses spread through the newspapers of the United States and in the schools of nursing. A congressional committee investigating the work of Barton's Red Cross staff applauded the work of these nurses and recommended that the U.S. Medical Department create a permanent reserve corps of trained nurses. These reserve nurses became the Army Nurse Corps in 1901. Clara Barton will always be remembered both as the founder of the American Red Cross and

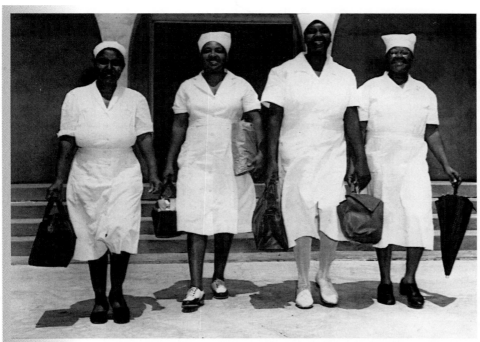

Nurse midwives in rural areas contributed to the decline in maternal and infant mortality during the 1950s.

the driving force behind the creation of the Army Nurse Corps (Frantz, 1998).

The Birth of the Midwife

Women have always assisted other women in the birth of babies. These "lay midwives" were considered by communities to possess special skills and somewhat of a "calling." With the advent of professional nursing in England, registered nurses became associated with safer and more predictable childbirth practices. In England and in other countries where Nightingale nursing schools were prevalent, most registered nurses were also trained as midwives with a 6-month specialized training period. In the United States, the training of registered nurses in the practice of midwifery was prevented primarily by physicians. U.S. physicians saw midwives as a threat and intrusion into medical practice. Such resistance indirectly led to the proliferation of "granny midwives" who were ignorant of modern practices, were untrained, and were associated with high maternal morbidity (Donahue, 1985).

The first organized midwifery service in the United States was the Frontier Nursing Service founded in 1925 by Mary Breckenridge. Breckenridge graduated from the St. Luke's Hospital Training School in New York in 1910 and received her midwifery certificate from the British Hospital for Mothers and Babies in London in 1925. She had extensive experience in the delivery of babies and midwifery systems in New Zealand and

Australia. In rural Appalachia, babies had been delivered for decades by granny midwives, who relied mainly on tradition, myths, and superstition as the bases of their practice. For example, they might use ashes for medication and place a sharp axe, blade up, under the bed of a laboring woman to "cut" the pain. The people of Appalachia were isolated because of the terrain of the hollows and mountains, and roads were limited to most families. They had one of the highest birth rates in the United States. Breckenridge believed that if a midwifery service could work under these conditions, it could work anywhere (Donahue, 1985).

Breckenridge had to use English midwives for many years and only began training her own midwives in 1939, when she started the Frontier Graduate School of Nurse Midwifery in Hyden, Kentucky, with the advent of World War II. The nurse midwives accessed many of their families on horseback. In 1935, a small 12-bed hospital was built at Hyden and provided delivery services. The nurse midwives under the direction of Breckenridge were successful in lowering the highest maternal mortality rate in the United States (in Leslie County, Kentucky) to substantially below the national average. These nurses, as at Henry Street Settlement, provided health care for everyone in the district for a small annual fee. A delivery had an additional small fee. Nurse midwives provided primary care, prenatal care, and postnatal care, with an emphasis on prevention (Wertz & Wertz, 1977).

Mary D. Osborne, who functioned as supervisor of public health nursing for the state of Mississippi from 1921 to 1946,

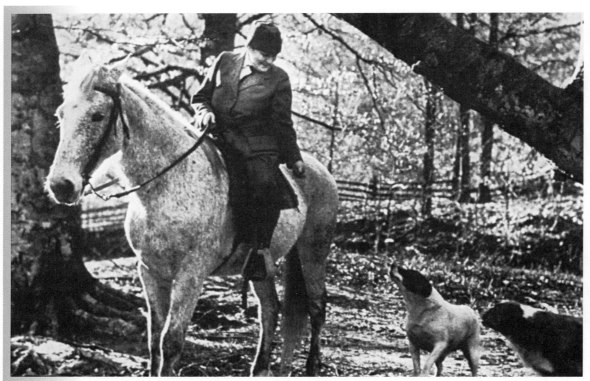

Mary Breckinridge, founder of the Frontier Nursing Service.

had a vision for a collaboration with community nurses and granny midwives, who delivered 80% of the African American babies in Mississippi. The infant and maternal mortality rates were both exceptionally high among African American families, and these granny midwives, who were also African American, were untrained and had little education.

Osborne took a creative approach to improving maternal and infant health among African American women. She developed a collaborative network of public health nurses and granny midwives in which the nurses implemented training programs for the midwives, and the midwives in turn assisted the nurses in providing a higher standard of safe maternal and infant health care. The public health nurses used Osborne's book, *Manual for Midwives,* which contained guidelines for care and was used in the state until the 1970s. They taught good hygiene, infection prevention, and compliance with state regulations. Osborne's innovative program is credited with reducing the maternal and infant mortality rates in Mississippi and in other states where her program structure was adopted (Sabin, 1998).

Early Education and Standardization of Practice of Public Health Nursing

After the turn of the century in the United States, infectious diseases such as smallpox, TB, malaria, cholera, and typhoid were

practice priorities for public health nurses. The public health nurse often initially detected an infectious disease, then referred those clients to physicians for treatment, provided follow-up care to clients when indicated, and tried through education and demonstrations to family and caregivers to prevent the spread of disease. Progress for early education efforts was largely gained through experience. A 3-month orientation and observation process was established in the early 1920s for nurses new to the concepts and policies of public health nursing. The philosophy was simple: Public health nursing was about prevention of disease, the promotion of health, care of the sick, and rehabilitation to productive life (Erickson, 1996).

By 1927, the Rockefeller Foundation provided private funding for a training station for health workers in conjunction with several local county health departments. Nurses, physicians, and sanitarians from many states and foreign countries received public health orientation and training through this initiative before it was discontinued in 1932. In 1929, The Rockefeller Foundation provided grants through the Rosenwald Fund designated for programs to improve the health and lower the death rates of the African American population in the South. These funds, used to establish permanent public health nursing positions for African American nurses, targeted children in areas where nursing and sanitation would make a profound impact on health and health practices (Forbes, 1946).

Challenges of the 1930s

In 1933, President Roosevelt initiated the New Deal to relieve the economic hardship of the country. The Social Security Act in 1935 (Public Law No. 99-271) provided funding to increase public health programs, particularly to extend services and improve health care for mothers and children in rural areas suffering from economic stress. State boards of health secured funds in 1934 through the Children's Bureau of the U.S. Department of Labor for state supervisory nurses, regional supervisory nurses, and local county nurses. The goal of this special project was to place at least one public health nurse in each county in every state. The efforts to reach this goal were remarkable, but qualified public health nurses continued to be few in number (ASTDN, 1993).

The United States Public Health Service, under the nursing consultation of Pearl McIver, provided leadership in the development of public health nursing services to the states. This effort was encouraged by the National Organization of Public Health Nursing and the Nursing Section of the American Public Health Association. Joint efforts between the federal public health nurses and those who were becoming organized in the states became the impetus for the growth of the specialty of public health nursing (ASTDN, 1993).

Another provision of the Social Security Act of 1935 was the establishment of Crippled Children's Services. Through this initiative, public health nurses were trained in rehabilitation nursing, primarily in orthopedics. These nurses visited crippled children in their homes, held conferences with parents, and assisted in the field clinics (Roberts, 1985a).

Syphilis had also been recognized as a major source of morbidity and mortality for many years. In 1938, the United States Public Health Service (USPHS) and state boards of health cooperated in a major project to attempt to conquer the disease through case finding, treatment, follow-up contact, and education. Public health nursing was in the vanguard of this effort. Educational conferences were planned so that all public health nurses would have an opportunity to attend. Prenatal screening of clients for syphilis was being introduced as a standard nursing intervention at this time. These efforts were particularly successful in the South (Erickson, 1940) (Box 3-2).

The country was gradually recovering from the Depression, and economic progress was accelerating. Farm production had broadened through diversification. New industries expanded the economy. The southern states, along with some of the eastern states, began to recognize the importance of nursing service in industrial hygiene programs. The United States Division of Industrial Hygiene asked for a public health nurse to visit plants and help institute nursing services. The prevention of disease, improvement of hazardous work conditions, promotion of health practices including nutrition, and first aid were the interventions to be provided through industrial nursing. As these nurses were employed, short-term educational and direct experience opportunities in areas with industrial nurses were planned so that the nurses could receive the best preparation possible for the role (Morton, Roberts, & Bender, 1993; Roberts, 1985a, 1985b; Smith, 1934).

Progressive Initiatives After the War Years

By 1942, state boards of health and education began to enter cooperative agreements to strengthen public health nursing services to the school-age population. The role of the public health nurse in the school was generalized, but much emphasis was placed on health promotion, immunizations, nutrition, and correction of physical defects. Landmark legislation was passed by the U.S. Congress in March 1943, establishing the Emergency Maternity and Infant Care (EMIC) program for the care of the dependents of enlisted men of the U.S. armed services. The program was designed to provide for maternity care and acute illness care of their infants and was administered through the United States Children's Bureau. In less than a month, the program was initiated in almost all states. Training for public health nurses was once again funded by the federal government, and the role of the public health nurse expanded to include mothers and babies in a more formal way (ASTDN, 1935–1993).

The USPHS Division of Public Health Nursing conducted research during the mid-1940s to study public health nursing. The most significant recommendations included the designation of public health nursing in states as a major division of nursing, the recognition of public health nursing as a service

---

BOX 3-2 PUBLIC HEALTH MILESTONES IN THE 1920S AND 1930S

1920s	Frost established epidemiology as science basic to community health
1920s	National Organization for Public Health Nursing formed
1920s	Public Health Nursing Section of American Public Health Association formed
1921	First federal monies allocated for health and social welfare
1923	Health Organization of League of Nations founded
1925	Frontier Nursing Service founded
1930s	Association of State and Territorial Directors of Nursing formed
1930	Crippled Children's Programs established
1930	National Institutes of Health established
1935	Social Security Act passed
1938	American Public Health Association set standards for school health

Source: APHA, 1997.

delivery system to all public health divisions and programs, and the importance of educational and practice issues related to professional nursing. The studies cited a low educational level for public health nurses and strongly recommended upgrading educational qualifications. The studies critiqued the established expenditure of nursing time and activities, determining that many duties carried out by public health nurses could be delegated to clerical staff and health aides. Health aides were introduced to the public health team with high school graduates employed to support public health nursing. These individuals quickly became a valuable resource and support to public health nursing, performing both clerical and clinical support activities (ASTDN, 1935–1993).

In December 1947, senior cadet nurses had a 6-month general training in public health and polio care through the training center of the state boards of health. The purpose of the Cadet Nurse Corp Program, funded through the USPHS, was to encourage young women to study nursing and to augment the supply of nurses in all health services.

Nurses were returning to work following the close of World War II, although the overall demand for nurses continued to exceed the supply. Newly constructed hospitals, industry, and public health agencies were all clamoring and vying for the short supply of nurses. While more active professional nurses and more students in schools existed by the early 1950s than at any previous time, the increase in numbers and caliber of nurses had not kept pace with the need for service (ASTDN, 1935–1993).

Throughout the 1950s, the nursing home industry began to emerge, with licensure requirements for standards of operation developed to ensure quality of services and care. Communities were accommodating an increase in the number of elderly persons living with chronic and degenerative diseases. Public health nurses provided training courses for nurses' aides employed in nursing homes. County public health nurses regularly visited the nursing homes within their communities, providing TB skin testing, administering flu vaccines, and providing technical assistance in nursing care. Nutritionists and physical therapists provided additional expertise to improve care processes and support public health nurses in the areas of rehabilitation and nutrition (Hanlon & Pickett, 1974; Morton, Roberts, & Bender, 1993).

A national trend began in the 1960s to release psychiatric clients from institutional care as improved psychotropic drugs and treatment modalities were available. Inadequate staffing at the state mental health institutions as a result of the nursing shortage was a complicating factor. The National Institute of Mental Health funded projects to study the impact that public health nurses might have on mental health care. A mental health nurse consultant was employed by many states to spearhead the research efforts of these projects. The project's public health nursing activity was defined as "aftercare" and was designed to determine the effectiveness of integrating follow-up services to mental health clients and their families into general public health nursing service. Public health nursing services included case finding and referral, hospital discharge planning, home and family assessments before and after discharge to the home, and medication monitoring (Amendt & White, 1965; Cottrell, 1948). Mental health services remained an integral part of public health service delivery throughout this decade, with new activities enhancing the community focus (Box 3-3).

Great emphasis was placed on child health, growth, and development in the early 1960s. Communicable disease, intestinal parasites, and physical defects that had been so prevalent in the school-age population were greatly diminished. Evaluations of this population found the new concerns to be dental and oral defects, vision and hearing defects, mental and emotional disturbances, accidents, and serious nutritional deficiencies. Continuing education was provided to enhance public health nurses' skills in observation, assessment, and nursing interventions in the care of children. Public health nurses began to be trained to assess developmental progress of children. Child health services provided by public health nurses included screening for physical defects, administration of immunizations, follow-up to correct physical defects, referral for mental health evaluations, consultation with teachers, and health promotion in nutrition, accident prevention, and mental health (Roberts, 1985).

An evaluation of the school health programs in the mid-1960s identified the need for additional nursing personnel to provide more direct preventive health services. Specialized federal funding through Title V grants was provided through the

---

BOX 3-3 PUBLIC HEALTH MILESTONES OF THE 1940S AND 1950S

1940s	Public health programs focused on health needs of the war period
1946	The Centers for Disease Control and Prevention established by Congress
1946	Mahoney introduced use of penicillin for treatment of syphilis
1948	National Heart, Lung, and Blood Institute established
1948	World Health Organization established
1950	Tuberculosis outpatient treatment becomes acceptable
1950	Introduction of the Salk vaccine
1950	White House Conference on Children and Youth
1950s	Policy emphases on health and federal funds for states, environmental health issues, housing, behavior, medical care, and children's health

Source: APHA, 1997.

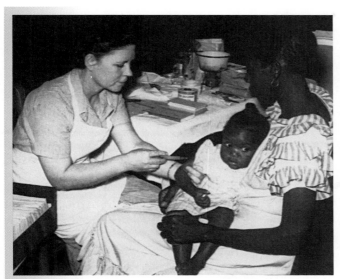

Public health nurses implemented the Salk vaccine beginning in 1955 in efforts to eradicate polio.

state departments of education to promote public health initiatives. Many schools recruited their nursing staff from the public health nursing workforce. Those public health nurses who went to schools took a broad view of child health and served as emissaries to school administrators and local boards' members. County public health nurses continued to serve as consultants to the schools in the areas of immunizations and communicable disease and as a referral source for Crippled Children's Services (Roberts, 1985).

Immunizations administered by public health nurses were proving effective, yet surveys showed that many preschool and school-age children were not completely immunized. Boards of health, continuing their vigilance regarding children's health status, received federal grants under the Vaccination Assistance Act. In 1965, public health nurses administered an increased number of immunizations. The oral polio vaccine, known as the Sabin vaccine, became available in a sugar cube administration form. A measles vaccine became available in 1966 and rubella in 1969. Following mass initial immunization campaigns for both measles and rubella, the new vaccines were incorporated into routine immunization schedules for children (ASTDN, 1935–1993).

By the mid-1960s, federal funding for maternal/child health services required the incorporation of contraceptive information and general reproductive health into public health services. The objective was to reduce maternal and infant mortality and to generally improve the health and well-being of mothers and children. Some states had already identified the health problems associated with multiple unplanned and unwanted pregnancies and had been early leaders in efforts to repeal federal and state laws restricting birth control services. By 1944, these efforts had resulted in integrated family planning counseling and issuing of select supplies with maternity and postpartum services into

many of the county health departments. Contraceptive supplies at that time included condoms and diaphragms. However, because of the wide divergence of public opinion, the development of the program was slow and unpublicized (ASTDN, 1935–1993; Morton, Roberts, & Bender, 1993).

Social and Political Influence of the 1960s and 1970s

By 1965, county health departments routinely provided contraceptive counseling and supplies. Oral contraceptives were also available by this time and gave women more convenient and accepted choices. Public health nurses promoted family planning and were key in identifying women at highest risk and need for such services. Family planning nursing visits increased across the country. Eventually, the federal government appropriated monies for additional education of public health nurses to function as family planning nurse practitioners.

Landmark legislation in 1965 amended the Social Security Act of 1935 by establishing Medicare, a health insurance plan for people 65 years of age and older and for those with long-term disabilities. The insurance plan included reimbursement for intermittent skilled nursing services provided to homebound persons. The purpose of home health services was twofold. Health care costs were beginning to skyrocket; home care would reduce costly hospitalization stays with the added benefit of clients' being in familiar home settings, enhancing quality of life. The goal of the program was to rehabilitate clients to their maximum potential and to teach families to care for the physical and emotional needs of clients.

Public health nurses had been providing home nursing services on a limited basis since the inception of public health nursing, but this would be the first reimbursement established for direct nursing services. In addition, the reimbursable home health nursing services to be provided would require public health nurses to learn new assessment and rehabilitative technical skills. Federal regulations established for certification were monumental, however. Continuing education for the nurses and nurses' aides who were directly providing care was just one of the regulations that in itself would be an immense task once service delivery was fully implemented (Buhler-Wilkerson, 1993; Erickson, 1993; IOM, 1988).

Federal grants through the USPHS were made available to support the implementation of home health. Nurse consultants, supervising nurses, and staff nurses attended university-supported educational offerings in rehabilitation care and techniques. Educational workshops were designed to upgrade nursing skills and techniques in rehabilitative care and on the conditions of participation for home health services. Additional workshop topics included documentation of skilled care and nursing care plans, medication administration and side effects, and the disease processes of many chronic health conditions.

After federal costs studies were implemented by the public health nurses in home health care, it was demonstrated that additional auxiliary staff, including health aides and clerks, would allow public health nurses more time for nursing activities. Action was taken to create additional clerical and aide positions to support the nursing staff.

More liberal social values emerged, and the 1960s became known for having spawned a sexual revolution. These effects were recognized by the early 1970s. Communities were faced with tremendous increases in sexually transmitted diseases and teen pregnancy rates. Social programs in response to these increases were initiated in the 1960s and were formalized in public and community health efforts in all states. The establishment of Medicaid through the amendment to the Social Security Act, Title XIX, enhanced the delivery of health care services to a wider range of recipients. The quantity and variance of activities in public health nursing continued to increase.

All the while, the traditional programs of health protection and disease control moved forward, many with an accelerated pace. Collaboration with other agencies, institutions, and groups continued at a high level in an effort to coordinate resources to achieve the best possible public health service delivery. Medicaid programs enhanced the expansion of Crippled Children's Services as a payment mechanism for many previously uncovered services. Additional screening and specialty treatment clinics for neurology, heart, and orthopedics were established throughout the United States. Other initiatives also centered around the delivery of child health services. Particularly in states with high infant mortality rates, state boards of health entered cooperative agreements in the 1970s to establish public health nursing positions in newborn intensive care units. The goal was to improve the communication, referral, and follow-up mechanisms for these high-risk infants after discharge from the hospital.

Title XIX of the Social Security Act (Medicaid) established Early Periodic Screening Diagnosis and Treatment (EPSDT) in 1969 to improve the access to preventive and primary health care for low-income children. State boards of health used this opportunity to strengthen the delivery of well child services. These physical screenings were made available primarily by public health nurses and were reimbursable nursing services, another recognition of the value of public health nursing service. The Denver Developmental Screening Test (DDST) was incorporated into the physical assessment, giving public health nurses a new tool to help find potential developmental delays and provide early intervention in the newborn to 6-year age groups. Workshops and in-services were conducted to teach the DDST standardized procedures.

Medical technology continued to advance rapidly, including advances in genetic diagnostics and treatment. Routine screening for sickle cell anemia was introduced and was integrated with EPSDT services. Other genetic technological advances determined that a contributing factor to the high incidence of mental retardation resulted from genetic disorders such as hypothyroidism and phenylketonuria. Medication and dietary treatments were developed for these genetic disorders that would im-

prove the quality of life and life expectancy. Nursing interventions included a home assessment, treatment modalities ordered by the attending physician, provision of dietary supplements, and teaching basic child health care and special health care based on the genetic diagnosis derived from the screening (ASTDN, 1935–1993; Hanlon & Pickett, 1974). Please refer to Box 3-4 for Milestones of the 1960s and 1970s.

A dramatic increase in home health nursing visits began at the close of the 1970s as a result of Medicare's implementation of diagnosis-related groups (DRGs), designed to lower costs through reduced institutionalization. Medicaid also reimbursed for home health services to eligible individuals not on Medicare and for some children with special health care needs. Private medical insurance plans and the Veteran's Administration were beginning to reimburse for home health services as well. Addi-

---

BOX 3-4 PUBLIC HEALTH MILESTONES OF THE 1960S AND 1970S

1960s	Public health policy issues focused on inequality, integration, poverty, "the pill," housing, environmental health, consumer protection, human rights, and peace
1960	Tuberculosis sanatoriums phased out and mainstream treatment begun
1961	First White House Conference on Aging
1961–1962	Sabin vaccine introduced
1962	National Institute of Child Health established
1964	Surgeon General's Report on Smoking and Health published
1965	Medicaid and Medicare programs enacted
1970s	Roe v. Wade
1970	Occupational Safety and Health Administration established
1973	HMO Act passed
1976	National immunization program for "swine flu"
1978	Association of Community Health Nursing Educators formed
1979	Last outbreak of poliomyelitis in the United States
1979	First Healthy People report

Source: APHA, 1997.

tional nursing positions were essential to meet the demand and to balance the quantity relationship with quality nursing care. As more acutely ill clients were cared for in the home and more advanced technological care was introduced into home health care, this specialty increased (ASTDN, 1935–1993).

Public Health Nursing Services in the 1980s and 1990s

As the 1980s began, the United States was experiencing an economic recession with skyrocketing interest rates and rising unemployment rates. National leadership was reducing funding for many of the social programs begun in the 1960s; the philosophy was that less governmental spending would enhance the national economy. The increased number of homeless persons became a national concern. Continuing concerns included illicit drug use, rising teen pregnancy rates, and alterations in family unit structures. Inadequate health care resources were also a continuing concern requiring cost containment, management of resources, and careful evaluation and incorporation of advancing technology. During this era, public health nursing services became varied throughout the country. In some states, basic services included both traditional preventive health services and family health services directed at high-risk mothers and babies and a reduction of unplanned pregnancies (ASTDN, 1935–1993).

Fortunately, public health nursing continued to grow and was a strong workforce in the country by the 1980s. Infant death rates declined significantly. Public health nurses participated in many research studies on public health problems such as congenital syphilis and TB preventive studies. Federal funding requirements changed from categorical grants to block grants. Categorical funding of the 1960s and 1970s had required that resources be restricted to the program that funded the resource; a nursing position funded by family planning, for example, was limited to family planning activities. Block funding allowed agencies more discretion on the use of these funds; therefore, services could be offered more efficiently to the public. Integrated public health nursing delivery systems were born. The integration of services allowed public health nurses to return to the more client-oriented or family-oriented care that had been the traditional philosophy of public health nursing (ASTDN, 1993; Buhler-Wilkerson, 1993).

Genetics screening programs expanded as a result of advanced technology in the early 1980s. The first initiative was newborn screening for sickle cell anemia. The goal was early detection of disease because early intervention could prevent common infections or premature deaths. State legislatures mandated hospitals to collect newborn screening specimens before infant discharge from the hospital. Screening included at least three genetic disorders: sickle cell anemia, phenylketonuria (PKU), and hypothyroidism. Public health nurses were given the responsibility for following up with the newborns with a questionable or positive screen. Questionable screens for PKU and hypothyroidism require prompt attention because early treatment with

diet and/or medication will prevent irreversible mental retardation and growth delay. The availability of public health nurses provided an effective means for timely follow-up of screenings and for the implementation of medical and nursing care plans when indicated (ASTDN, 1993).

A crucial indicator of any state's quality of life is infant mortality. Public health nursing became a viable resource during the 1980s for delivering services (either personal or preventive) aimed at reducing infant mortality. The major cause of infant mortality was prematurity. Contributing factors included poor nutrition, smoking, teen pregnancy, and inadequate prenatal care. Socioeconomic factors such as inadequate housing, drug abuse, and lack of education were also contributing factors. Maternal risk scoring and documentation to ensure referrals to appropriate levels of care were standards of care. Tracking systems were intensified to ensure adequate levels of care.

Family planning services during the 1980s were also identified as a priority to reduce infant mortality. Risk factors included age and/or inadequate income to purchase contraceptive supplies. Public health nurses continued to promote family planning services, provide health promotion and education in their communities, and intensify tracking systems of teens and others at risk. The Special Supplemental Food Program for Women, Infants, and Children (WIC) continued to address infant mortality. WIC certification and nutrition education were integrated into maternal and child health nursing services' standards of care.

Congressional authorization gave states the option to expand their Medicaid programs in 1987. The services' expansion included case management of high-risk mothers and infants to ensure comprehensive care as a reimbursable service. Nutritionists, social workers, and public health nurses formed teams to establish care plans and assume case manager roles based on the client's risk factors. Public health nursing activities included nursing assessments, home visits, health education, and communication with medical providers in an effort to improve the overall status of this high-risk population. Documentation of the care process was essential for continuity of care from the initial assessment and plan of care through implementation of services and ongoing evaluation.

Case management emerged during this decade as a new term, but the concept and the related activities of case management were the principles and foundations upon which public health nursing practice had been built. **Case management** is a program for intensive individual supervision, follow-up, and referrals to appropriate levels of care. Public health nurses had been providing a form of case management through the years to many clients, such as those receiving TB treatment, those receiving home health services, and children with special health care needs.

School health nurses also became stronger in this era. School nurses strengthened the educational process of students by assisting them in improving or adapting to their health status. School nurses were available during school hours to serve as counselors and to provide case finding and referral to physicians, health departments, and other agencies as appropriate to meet the needs of school-age children. Activities included general health screening and referral, hearing and vision screening, identification of suspected abuse and neglect, substance abuse counseling, and appropriate decision making and support. In addition, school nurses provided classroom presentations on health issues and provided emergency care for injuries and illnesses at school.

Communicable disease had renewed public health interest in the nation throughout the 1980s. Tuberculosis case rates were increasing. Measles cases were being reported among college-age students. New communicable disease concerns emerged in the 1980s, including increased incidence of hepatitis B, human immunodeficiency virus (HIV) infection, and acquired immunodeficiency syndrome (AIDS). Case conferences with private medical consultants were established on a district level for initiation and ongoing review of treatment plans carried out by public health nurses. Drug resistance and failure to take medication were identified as major hindrances to individual cure and subsequent eradication of TB. In 1986, public health nurses initiated directly observed therapy (DOT) for TB cases. Rather than self-administration, clients would present to the health department or the public health nurse would visit the home for administration of medications. Later in the decade, public health officials recognized that the increase in TB cases was, in part, associated with the emerging HIV and AIDS cases. HIV screening became a standard of nursing care for all active TB cases.

Many states took an early stance to address measles among the college-age population in the mid-1980s as a result of the increased incidence of disease reported throughout the nation. The college-age population was at greatest risk for disease because they had been immunized with less-than-effective immunizations in the late 1960s or had not received the immunization. Collaboration with state college boards resulted in requirement of measles and rubella immunity for college admission. Public health nurses reviewed immunization records, provided screening tests when indicated, and administered immunizations to assist in the control of measles.

The first cases of AIDS were diagnosed in the early 1980s. Research soon unraveled part of the mystery of the disease. Risk factors for transmission of disease were identified, and a screening test for HIV, the virus that leads to AIDS, was available. Screening provided a means to detect HIV infection earlier and to provide appropriate counseling and education to alter risk behaviors and reduce transmission. Education to the public and to high-risk individuals was the only effective weapon that public health had to address this disease. Public health nurses attended educational workshops to gain knowledge and skills for testing and counseling clients who requested testing. Health education materials were developed to support counseling and educational strategies. In addition, public health nurses implemented standards of care by integrating assessment of risk factors for clients receiving other public health services and by disseminating in-

formation through public presentations in schools and community organizations.

Progress continued for public health nurses during this era, yet dilemmas remain. A national nursing shortage was recognized, with all states feeling the effects. Public health felt the effects of the nursing shortage greatly with the vacancy rates reaching 20% at times. A commission on nursing was organized by the Secretary of the U.S. Department of Health and Human Services to examine and make recommendations regarding the nursing shortage. The commission's report, completed in 1989, cited the reality of the shortage and the impact on health care delivery. The shortage was determined to result from the increasing demand for nurses, and the report urged agencies to be attentive to using measures aimed at reducing the barriers to effective recruitment and retention (Department of Health and Human Services, 1988).

One of the commission's recommendations was that nursing should have greater representation in the policy and decision-making activities of health care institutions. Acting on this recommendation, both public health nurses and their administrations developed mechanisms whereby public health nurses moved into broader policy-making roles. At the close of the decade, public health nursing continued as a strong force in the delivery of health care in many states and in health promotion and disease prevention in others. Public health nurses were instrumental in establishing and integrating new initiatives in public health to combat old public health problems as well as to address new public health concerns. The value of public health nursing activities continued to be recognized as reimbursement for select activities and for nurse practitioner services were expanded.

The federal government's staggering budget deficits were the major national focus as the 1990s began. Health care costs were escalating, and governmental measures attempting to control increasing costs were not proving effective. The gloomy financial picture was exacerbated by Desert Storm, the U.S. military troops' assignment by President George Bush to protect Saudi Arabia and to retaliate for Iraq's invasion of Kuwait.

Current and emerging health care issues of the 1990s lay close to the heart of public health. The percentage of the population older than 65 continued to rise. Life expectancy in the United States had risen from 47 years in 1900 to 75 years in 1990. Infant mortality, although significantly declining through the years, required continued vigilance. The increased incidence of syphilis and other sexually transmitted diseases was of chief concern to public health. The number of persons infected with HIV and/or diagnosed with AIDS was increasing at alarming rates. Substance abuse continued to be a major problem, with studies reflecting it as a contributing factor in 50% of all traffic accidents, in the transmission of HIV infection, and in infant morbidity and mortality.

Yet federal funding reductions were inevitable for public health as a result of the sluggish national economy as the United

States entered the 1990s. Without significant infusions of money for additional staff, medications, vaccines, and health promotion/disease prevention activities, states faced increases in preventable diseases and deaths and a reversal of the recent favorable trends in lowering infant mortality and teen pregnancy. Difficult economic times resulted in the careful reviews of resources and the utilization of those resources. Focus was again directed toward enhancing nursing education and staff development, strengthening relationships with schools of nursing, and developing a quality assurance process for the integration of public health nursing services. Because of the large number of nurses employed, public health nurses were afforded greater access to approved continuing education opportunities specific to their area of practice. Select continuing education offerings, including TB updates, HIV testing and counseling courses, and community assessment, became required orientation for newly employed public health nurses (Gebbie, 1996).

The nation experienced a significant increase in the incidence of syphilis. Case rates were climbing and were higher than they had been since the late 1940s. Much of the increased incidence was associated with drug abuse—the exchange of sex for drugs. Congenital syphilis was again an issue of public health concern for infant morbidity and mortality. Public health nursing protocols included standards of care for infected maternity clients and follow-up for their newborn infants. Public health nurses increased their assessment for signs and symptoms of disease and for risk status of clients in their care, assisted disease intervention specialists with follow-up of clients with positive laboratory results, and assisted with accessing medical treatment.

The incidence of another communicable disease, hepatitis B, was also increasing. With the advent of hepatitis B vaccination, public health nurses implemented new protocols to screen maternity clients for hepatitis B and to provide follow-up and immunization administration to the infants of infected mothers. Standing orders were written to effectively carry out the immunization and follow-up of these infants. This was a major new public health initiative. See Box 3-5 for a summary of activities during the years.

Federal monies increased for public health to address preventive intervention strategies for persons infected with HIV during 1990s. States initiated programs to make select drugs available to clients. These programs required private physicians to submit medication orders for the client. Public health nurses assisted clients with completing application forms, consulting

---

BOX 3-5 PUBLIC HEALTH MILESTONES OF THE 1980S AND 1990S

1980s	Public policy centered around AIDS, Medicare, Medicaid, tobacco control, international health, minority health, national health care reform, and national health objectives
1982	Warning labels on aspirin for Reye's syndrome prevention
1986	First antitabacco initiative by public health community
1988	The Future of Public Health published by the Institute of Medicine
1989	Year 2000 Health Objectives published
1990	Healthy People 2000 Report published
1991	Healthy Communities 2000: Model Standards published
1993	AZT sanctioned as able to reduce perinatal HIV
1996	War and Public Health published
1997	Plans under way for modern microbiological/biomedical laboratory capabilities
2000	Healthy People 2010 published

Source: APHA, 2000.

---

private physicians regarding program guidelines, and administering medication.

Immunization administration had been a priority public health effort in for public health nurses since the early part of the century. A national emphasis reemerged in the early 1990s to meet a national objective to complete the immunization series of 90% of all children by 2 years of age. The Centers for Disease Control and Prevention (CDC) identified barriers to children receiving their basic immunization series. The national discussion provided public health nurses with current knowledge to guide their assessment of simultaneous administration of several vaccines when indicated and on contraindications for immunization administration (DHHS, 1992).

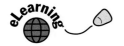

Explore Community Health Nursing on the web! To learn more about the topics in this chapter, use the passcode provided to access your exclusive web site: http://communitynursing.jbpub.com
If you do not have a passcode, you can obtain one at this site.

CONCLUSION

In 1993, public health nursing celebrated 100 years of phenomenal accomplishments in prevention of disease, promotion of health, rehabilitation, and care of disease and disability to individuals, families, groups, and communities since its organization in 1893. In celebrating these accomplishments, the nation's public health nurses were recognized for incorporating the tremendous scientific and technological discoveries and advances made in this century into their nursing practice. Public health nurses have remained alert to continued advances in technology and client care, as well as to other factors influencing the profession.

The history of public health and community health nursing informs the present by linking the social and political environment to the response of nursing in the community. Since the earliest accounts presented, health and health care have resulted from religious influences, available knowledge about disease causation, and the use of human expertise in managing health. By considering the historical context under which humans attempt to survive and stay healthy, community health nurses can more appropriately care for the present and future public health needs of the population.

CRITICAL THINKING ACTIVITIES

1. Take a walk through your neighborhood and college campus. Identify public health measures that exist that can be traced to the Greek and Roman eras.

2. How do you think Lillian Wald would react to present day public health departments?

3. How does the current interest in alternative and complimentary health care relate to the Greeks' ideas about health?

REFERENCES

Abel, E. K. (1997, November). Take the cure to the poor: Patients' responses to New York City's tuberculosis program, 1894–1918. *American Journal of Public Health, 87,* 11.

Amendt, J. A., & White, R. P. (July, 1965). Continued care services for mental patients. *Nursing Outlook,* pp. 57–60.

American Public Health Association (APHA). (1991). *Healthy Communities 2000: model standards* (3rd ed.). Washington, D.C.

American Public Health Association (APHA). (1997, November). *Public health milestones.* Washington, D.C. Unpublished paper.

Association of State and Territorial Directors of Nursing (ASTDN). (1993). *Historical summary of the Association of State and Territorial Directors of Nursing (1935–1993).* Unpublished manuscript.

Association of State and Territorial Directors of Nursing (ASTDN). *Selected reports from annual meeting and correspondence, 1935–1993.*

Attewell, A. (1996). Florence Nightingale's health-at-home visitors. *Health Visitor, 69*(10), 406.

Barker, E. R. (1989). Care givers as casualties. *Western Journal of Nursing Research, 11*(5), 628–631.

Boorstin, D. J. (1985). *The discoverers: A history of man's search to know his world and himself.* New York: Vintage.

Brainard, A. M. (1922). *The evolution of public health nursing.* Philadelphia: W. B. Saunders.

Brockett, L. P., & Vaughan, M. C. (1867). *Woman's work in the Civil War: A record of heroism, patriotism and patience.* Philadelphia: Seigler McCurdy.

Brooke, E. (1997). *Medicine women: A pictorial history of women healers.* Wheaton, IL: Quest Books.

Brown, P. (1988). *Florence Nightingale.* Herts, UK: Exley Publications.

Buhler-Wilkerson, K. (1985). Public health nursing: In sickness or in health? *American Journal of Public Health, 75,* 1155–1156.

Buhler-Wilkerson, K. (1993). Bringing care to the people: Lillian Wald's legacy of public health nursing. *American Journal of Public Health, 83*(12), 1778–1786.

Bullough, V. L., & Bullough, B. (1978). *The care of the sick: The emergence of modern nursing.* New York: Prodist.

Calabria, M. D. (1996). *Florence Nightingale in Egypt and Greece: Her diary and "visions."* Albany: State University of New York Press.

Carnegie, M. E. (1991). *The path we tread: Blacks in nursing 1854–1990* (2nd ed.) New York: National League for Nursing Press.

Cartwright, F. F. (1972). *Disease and history.* New York: Dorset Press.

Cohen, M. N. (1989). *Health and the rise of civilization.* New Haven, CT: Yale University Press.

Cook, E. (1913). *The life of Florence Nightingale* (Vols. 1 and 2). London: Macmillan.

Cottrell, H. (1948). *Mental health principles in the state and local health programs: A Commonwealth Fund demonstration* (Record Group 51, Vol. 36). Mississippi Department of Archives, Division of Public Health Nursing, Historical Files.

Department of Health and Human Services (DHHS). (December, 1988). *Final report of the Secretary's Commission on Nursing.* Washington, DC: DHHS.

Department of Health and Human Services, Public Health Services, Centers for Disease Control and Prevention. (May, 1992). *Standards for pediatric immunization practice.* Atlanta: Department of Health and Human Services, Public Health Services, Centers for Disease Control and Prevention.

Diamond, J. (1997). *Guns, germs, and steel: The fates of human societies.* New York: W. W. Norton.

Dietz, D. D. & Lehozky, A. R. (1963). *History and modern nursing.* Philadelphia: F. A. Davis.

Dickens. C. (1844). *Martin Chuzzlewit.* New York: Macmillan.

Dock, L. N., & Stewart, I. M. (1931). *A short history of nursing* (3rd ed.). New York: G. P. Putnam.

Dock, L., Pickett, S. E., Noyes, C. D., Clement, F., Fox, E., Van Meter, A. (1922). *History of American Red Cross nursing.* New York: Macmillan.

Donahue, M. P. (1985). *Nursing: The finest art.* St. Louis: Mosby.

Ercikson, G. P. (June, 1996). To pauperize or empower: Public health nursing at the turn of the 20th and 21st century. *Public Health Nursing, 13*(3), 163–169.

Erickson, P. (1940). *The role of the public health nurse in the syphilis research project in Washington County.* Presented at the 1940 annual meeting of the Mississippi Nurses Association, Jackson, MS.

Forbes, M. D. (1946). *Report of a review of public health nursing in the Mississippi Board of Health* (Record Group 51, Vol. 36). Mississippi Department of Archives, Division of Public Health Nursing, Historical Files.

Frantz, A. K. (1998). Nursing pride: Clara Barton in the Spanish-American War. *American Journal of Nursing, 98*(10), 39–41.

Gebbie, K. M. (1996, Nov. 18). *Preparing currently employed public health nurses for changes in the health care system: Meeting report and suggested action steps*. New York: Columbia University School of Nursing Center for Health Policy and Health Sciences Research. (Report based on meeting in Atlanta, GA, July 11, 1996).

Hamilton, D. (1988). Clinical excellence, but too high a cost: The Metropolitan Life Insurance Company Visiting Nurse Service (1909–1953). *Public Health Nursing, 5,* 235–240.

Hamilton-Gordon, S. (1906). *Sidney Herbert of Lea: A memoir* (Vol. 1). New York: E. P. Dutton.

Heinrich, J. (November/December, 1983). Historical perspectives on public health nursing. *Nursing Outlook, 32*(6), 317–320.

Hanlon, J. J., & Pickett, G. E. (1974a). Community nursing services. In *Public health administration and practice* (pp. 533–547). St. Louis: Mosby.

Hanlon, J. J., & Pickett, G. E. (1974b). Historical perspectives. In *Public health administration and practice* (pp. 22–44). St. Louis: Mosby.

Hanlon, J. J., & Pickett, G. E. (1984). *Public health administration and practice* (8th ed.). St. Louis: Mosby.

Health Resources and Services Administration, Division of Nursing (HRSA). (1993). *A century of caring: A celebration of public health nursing in the United States* (Pub. No.189301993). Rockville, MD: Author.

Heinrich, J. (1983). Historical perspectives on public health nursing. *Nursing Outlook, 32*(6), 317–320.

Hemphill, M. (1980). *Fevers, floods, and faith: A history of Sunflower County, Mississippi, 1844–1976* (pp. 598–631). Indianola, MS: Author.

Hine, D. C. (1989). *Black women in white: Racial conflict and cooperation in the nursing profession 1890–1950*. Bloomington, IN: Indiana University Press.

Institute of Medicine (IOM). (1988). *The future of public health*. Washington, D.C.: National Academy Press.

Kalisch, P. A., & Kalisch, B. J. (1986). *The advance of American nursing* (2nd ed.). Boston: Little, Brown.

LeVasseur, J. (1998). Plato, Nightingale, and contemporary nursing. *Image: Journal of Nursing Scholarship, 30*(3), 281–285.

Longfellow, H. W. (November, 1857) Santa Filomena, *Atlantic Monthly, 1,* 22–23.

The 100 People Who Made the Millennium. (1997). *Life Magazine, 20*(10a).

McNeill, W. H. (1976). *Plagues and peoples*. New York: Doubleday.

Monteiro, L. A. (1985). Florence Nightingale on public health nursing. *American Journal of Public Health, 75*(2), 181–185.

Morton, M., Roberts, E., & Bender, K. (1993). *Celebrating public health nursing: Caring for Mississippi's communities with courage and compassion. 1920–1993*. Jackson, MS: Mississippi State Department of Health.

Mosley, M. O. P. (1996). Satisfied to carry the bag: Three black community health nurses' contribution to health care reform, 1900–1937. *Nursing History Review, 4,* 65–82.

Nightingale, F. (1893). Sick-nursing and health-nursing. In *Women's mission* (pp. 184–205). Arranged and ed. by Baroness Burdett-Coutts. London: Sampson, Law, Marston and Co.

Nightingale, F. (1979). Cassandra. In M. Stark (Ed.), *Florence Nightingale's Cassandra*. Old Westbury, NY: Feminist Press.

Nutting, M. A., & Dock, L. L. (1937). *A history of nursing* (Vol. 1). New York: G. P. Putnam.

Palmer, I. S. (March/April, 1977). Florence Nightingale: Reformer, reactionary, researcher. *Nursing Research,* pp. 13–18.

Palmer, I. S. (1982). *Through a glass darkly: From Nightingale to now*. Washington, D.C.: American Association of College of Nursing.

Rathbone, W. (1890). *A history of nursing in the homes of the poor*. Introduction by Florence Nightingale. London: Macmillan.

Reverby, S. M. (1993). From Lillian Wald to Hilliary Rodham Clinton: What will happen to public health nursing? *American Journal of Public Health, 83*(12), 1662–1663.

Richardson, B. W. (1887). *The health of nations: A review of the works of Edwin Chadwick* (Vol. 2). London: Longmans, Green and Company.

Roberts, E. (1985a). *Highlights: Maternal and child health and crippled children's service, 1935–1985*. Jackson, MS: Mississippi Department of Health.

Roberts, E. (March, 1985b). *The role of the southern nurse in public health*. Symposium on Southern Science and Medicine at the Education and Research Center, Jackson, Mississippi. Education and Research Center.

Roberts, M. (1954). *American nursing: History and interpretation*. New York: Macmillan.

Robinson, V. (1946). *White caps: The story of nursing*. Philadelphia: J. B. Lippincott.

Rosen, G. (1958). *A history of public health*. New York: M.D. Publications.

Sabin, L. (1998). *Struggles and triumphs: The story of Mississippi nurses 1800–1950*. Jackson, MS: Mississippi Hospital Association Health, Research and Educational Foundation.

Seymer, L. (1954). *Selected Writings of Florence Nightingale*. New York: Macmillan.

Shryock, R. H. (1959). *The history of nursing: An interpretation of the social and medical factors involved.* Philadelphia: W. B. Saunders.

Smith, E. (1934). *Mississippi special public health nursing project made possible by federal funds.* Paper presented at the 1934 annual Mississippi Nurses Association meeting, Jackson, MS.

Snow, J. (1855). *On the mode of communication of cholera* (2nd ed.). London: Churchhill Publishers.

Stanmore, A. H. G. (1906). *Sidney Herbert of Lea: A memoir.* New York: E. P. Dutton.

Taylor, H. O. (1922). *Greek biology and medicine.* Boston: Marshall Jones.

Tiffany, F. (1890). *The life of Dorothea Linda Dix.* Boston: Houghton, Mifflin.

Thoms, A. B. (1929). *Pathfinders: A history of the progress of colored graduate nurses.* New York: Kay Print House.

Tyrell, H. (1856). *Pictorial history of the war with Russia 1854–1856.* London: W. and R. Chambers.

United States Public Health Service (USPHS). (July, 1979). *Healthy people: The Surgeon General's report on health promotion and disease prevention.* Washington, D.C.: Author

United States Public Health Service (USPHS). (September, 1990). *Healthy people 2000: National health promotion and disease prevention objectives.* Washington, D.C.: Author.

Van Doren, M. (1945). *Walt Whitman.* New York: Viking Press.

Vicinus, M., & Nergaard, B. (1990). *Ever yours, Florence Nightingale: Selected letters.* Boston: Harvard University Press.

Wald, L. D. (1915). *The house on Henry Street.* New York: Henry Holt.

Wertz, R. W., & Wertz, D. C. (1977). *Lying-In: A history of childbirth in America.* New Haven, CT: Yale University Press.

Williams, C. B. (1961, May). Stories from Scutari. *American Journal of Nursing, 61,* 88.

Winslow, C-E. A. (1946). Florence Nightingale and public health nursing. *Public Health Nursing, 38,* 330–332.

Woodham-Smith, C. (1951). *Florence Nightingale.* New York: McGraw-Hill.

Woodham-Smith, C. (1983). *Florence Nightingale.* New York: Atheneum.

Young, D. A. (1995). Florence Nightingale's fever. *British Medical Journal, 311,* 1697–1700.

Zerwekh, J. V. (1991). Tales from public health nursing: True detectives. *American Journal of Nursing, 91*(10), 30–26.

Zerwekh, J. V. (1993). Going to the people-public health nursing today and tomorrow. *American Journal of Public Health, 83*(12), 1676–1678.

Zerwekh, J, Primono, J., & Deal, L. (1992). *Opening doors: Stories of public health nurses.* Olympia, WA: Washington State Department of Health.

Chapter 4

Epidemiology of Health and Illness

Gail A. Harkness

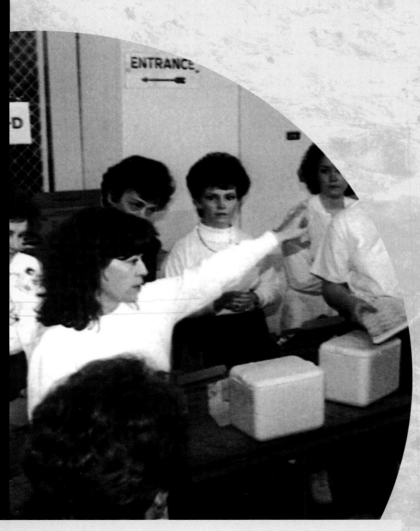

To understand the changes that can occur in the health of individuals or in various populations, it is necessary to identify the relationships between the biological and psychosocial phenomena that underlie health and illness. Epidemiology, the basic science of preventive medicine, has provided a process for understanding these relationships by studying different populations of people in various situations. Through study of health problems as they occur in groups or populations, many characteristics of specific illnesses or disabilities can be identified that may not be evident in the study of individuals alone.

Questions to Consider

After reading this chapter, answer the following questions:

1. What is the contribution of epidemiology to public health?
2. How do nurses use the principles of epidemiology?
3. How is the epidemiological process related to nursing and research?
4. What is the usefulness of rates in community health nursing?
5. What is the natural history of disease and levels of prevention?
6. What are *incidence* and *prevalence*?
7. What are the characteristics of a population by person, place, and time?
8. What are the characteristics of the four types of epidemiological research studies?
9. How can epidemiological research be used in community health nursing?

Key Terms

Adjusted rates	Epidemiological triad	Period prevalence	Retrospective
Case–control	Incidence	Point prevalence	Risk factors
Cross–sectional	Intervention	Primary prevention	Secondary prevention
Crude rates	Morbidity	Prospective	Specific rates
Epidemic	Mortality	Rate	Tertiary prevention
Epidemic curve			

INDIVIDUAL WITHIN THE FRAMEWORK OF LIFE.

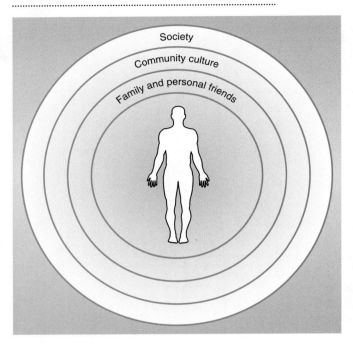

Health care for all individuals should be planned within the framework of family and personal friends, the immediate community culture where they live, and the larger world society. Any individual's health care needs cannot be completely or correctly defined unless these broader factors are analyzed and appropriately incorporated into a plan of care. Just as information must be collected about individuals in assessing health problems, data must be collected about groups, communities, and populations to assess the broader health needs of society.

For instance, the association between lung cancer and smoking might not have been ascertained by studying individual cases of lung cancer. Many smokers never develop lung cancer, and some nonsmokers do develop lung cancer. However, in 1950, Doll and Hill contrasted a group of lung cancer patients with a group of people who did not develop lung cancer. They clearly demonstrated that more people with lung cancer had smoked cigarettes than those people without the disease. This was substantiated by further research, and cigarette smoking is now considered a primary risk factor for lung cancer. This information has been the basis for national campaigns to decrease smoking among Americans. This example demonstrates the value of identifying certain characteristics or behaviors that increase risk of health problems even if the pathophysiology is not precisely known. Health care personnel can implement preventive health measures for both individuals and groups of people who are at high risk even if the causative factors are not known.

Epidemiology Defined

Epidemiology is the study of the distribution and the determinants of states of health and illness in human populations (Harkness, 1995). *Distribution* refers to the frequency of occurrence of states of health and illness; *determinants* refers to agents or factors that contribute to the cause of various states of health and illness. The word *epidemiology* is derived from the Greek word meaning **epidemic:** *epi*, upon; *demos*, people; and *logos*, treatise. The ultimate goal of epidemiology is to use the information obtained from the study of the distribution and determinants of states of health and illness to prevent or limit the consequences of illness and disability in humans and maximize their state of health. Although the influence of the environment on the occurrence of disease and the contagious nature of many diseases can be traced to Hippocrates, the techniques of modern epidemiological investigation were first developed in the mid-19th century.

William Farr, a physician from London, established the field of medical statistics. In 1839, he was appointed to the Office of the Registrar General for England and Wales. He set up a system for compilation of the numbers and causes of deaths and compared the deaths of workers in different occupations, the difference in mortality between men and women, and the effect of imprisonment on the frequency of death. He realized that studying the data from populations of people would provide much more information about human disease than studying individual cases (Humphreys, 1885).

During the mid-19th century, infectious diseases such as cholera and plague were still killing much of the population of Europe. The primary goal then was to limit the spread of these devastating diseases and prevent their recurrence. John Snow, another British physician, investigated the epidemic of cholera that took place from 1848 to 1854. His classic investigation of the outbreak clearly established the rate as a fundamental tool of epidemiology. Snow investigated cholera outbreaks associated with water supplied from two different water companies. He demonstrated statistically that cholera was associated with the water company that obtained their water from an area of the Thames River that was heavily polluted with sewage, and not with the company that obtained its water further upstream (Snow, 1855).

Florence Nightingale was a contemporary of Farr and Snow and was significantly influenced by their statistical methods. Nightingale is probably best known for her work at the British military hospital in Scutari. British and French troops had invaded the Crimea on the north coast of the Black Sea, supporting Turkey in its dispute with Russia. She and her 38 nurses found the conditions appalling. Buildings were infested with rats and fleas, streams of sewage flowed under the buildings, linens were filthy, and supplies were scarce. They initiated sanitary reforms, keeping records of illness and deaths. The following figure shows a polar-area diagram designed by Nightingale to dramatize the needless deaths that occurred during the war and the effect of her reforms (Aiken, 1988; Cohen, 1984).

As a result of these early investigations, epidemiology traditionally has been associated with infectious diseases, with a focus

NIGHTINGALE'S POLAR-AREA DIAGRAM.

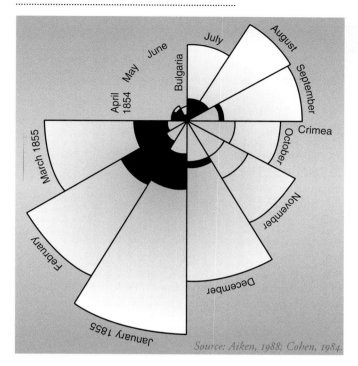

Source: Aiken, 1988; Cohen, 1984.

> ### FYI
>
> Florence Nightingale has been called one of the first epidemiologists as a result of her use of statistics to document health care needs.

on the **epidemiological triad**: agent, host, and environment. This model is based on the belief that health status is multifactorial, determined by the interaction of many agent, host, and environment characteristics, and not by any single factor. For example, factors influencing the development of a heart attack include heredity, high cholesterol levels, dietary excess, cigarette smoking, emotional stress, and many other factors. No one factor is considered a causative factor for the illness. Therefore, the epidemiological trial still remains a fundamental conceptual framework for the contemporary study of health problems.

Epidemiology can be considered both as a *methodology* used to study health-related conditions and as a *body of knowledge* that results from research into a specific health-related condition (Harkness, 1995). Using epidemiological research methodology to investigate health problems leads to the accumulation of a body of knowledge about that particular problem. (Epidemiological research methods are discussed later in the chapter.) Practitioners then can use this body of knowledge in their clinical decision mak-

THE EPIDEMIOLOGICAL TRIAD.

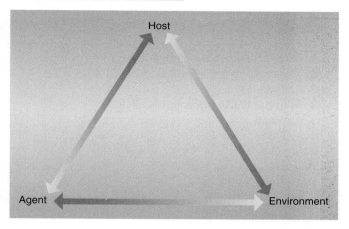

ing and in developing health services. For example, epidemiological research has associated hypertension, obesity, and smoking with increased incidence of heart disease. These are all potentially modifiable risk factors that often are associated with lifestyle and behavior choices. Nurses and other health professionals can use this information when assessing individual patients and helping them make choices about intervention techniques that may reduce their risk of heart disease. Also, community health nurses may initiate programs to identify hypertension at an early stage, to stop smoking, or to decrease weight in an attempt to decrease the risk of heart disease for the population as a whole.

Scope of Epidemiology

The scope of epidemiology has been expanded and therefore changed in recent years. Not only are the distribution and determinants of illness and disease investigated, but variables that contribute to the maintenance of health are also studied. The evolving changes in demographic characteristics, the patterns of disease, methods of control and prevention of health problems, and the need for maintaining wellness have contributed to this shift in the scope of epidemiology. *Healthy People 2010* uses determinants of health to derive the objectives for the nation. The depth of topics covered by the objectives reflect the diversity of critical influences that determine the health of persons who live in communities. Improved public health services, increased life expectancy, increased frequency of noninfectious disease and chronic degenerative conditions, and advances in technology are continually changing the health needs of society. (See Table 4-1 for a comparison of the leading causes of death in the United States over time.) Provision of present and future health care depends on (1) identifying health problems and needs, (2) collecting and analyzing data to identify factors that influence those health problems or needs, and (3) planning, implementing, and evaluating methods for prevention and control. These steps form the basis of the epidemiological process.

TABLE 4-1   COMPARISON OF THE LEADING CAUSES OF DEATH IN THE UNITED STATES BETWEEN 1900 AND 1996

1900	1996
1. Major cardiovascular-renal diseases	1. Diseases of the heart
2. Influenza and pneumonia	2. Malignant neoplasms
3. Tuberculosis	3. Cardiovascular accidents
4. Gastritis, duodenitis, enteritis, cholitis	4. Chronic obstructive pulmonary disease
5. Accidents	5. Accidents
6. Malignant neoplasms	6. Pneumonia and influenza
7. Diphtheria	7. Diabetes mellitus
8. Typhoid and paratyphoid fever	8. Other infections and parasitic diseases
9. Measles	9. Suicide
10. Cirrhosis of the liver	10. Chronic liver disease and cirrhosis

Bureau of the Census, 1998, p 100.

The Epidemiological, Research, and Nursing Processes

The epidemiological process, the research process, and the nursing process have all evolved from steps in the problem-solving process. All three processes have similar basic components: defining the problem, gathering data, analyzing the data, and evaluating the results. The research process focuses on obtaining new knowledge about a health condition. The epidemiological process and the nursing process are more focused on planning for control, for prevention, or for intervention activities that will help mediate a health condition (Table 4-2). The cyclical nature of the epidemiological process is illustrated in the following figure.

Natural History of Disease

In 1958, Leavell and Clark, two public health physicians, championed the cause of preventive medicine by emphasizing that prevention is required at every phase of the disease process. They called the course of any disease process as it develops in humans the "natural history of the disease" (see the figure

TABLE 4-2   SIMILARITIES BETWEEN THE EPIDEMIOLOGICAL PROCESS, THE RESEARCH PROCESS, AND THE NURSING PROCESS

EPIDEMIOLOGICAL PROCESS	RESEARCH PROCESS	NURSING PROCESS
Define problem	Define problem	**Assessment:**
Gather information from reliable sources	Review literature	Establish patient database
Describe problem by person, place, time	Conceptualize problem	
Formulate tentative hypothesis	Define variables	**Diagnosis:**
	Identify methodology	Interpret data
Analyze descriptive data to test hypothesis		Identify health care needs
		Select goals of care
Plan for control of the problem		**Planning:**
		Select process for achieving goals
Implement control plan	Collect data	**Implementation:**
		Initiate and complete actions to achieve goals
Evaluate control plan	Analyze data	**Evaluation:**
Prepare appropriate report	Publish report	Determine extent of goal achievement
Conduct further research	Conduct further research	

MODEL OF THE EPIDEMIOLOGICAL PROCESS.

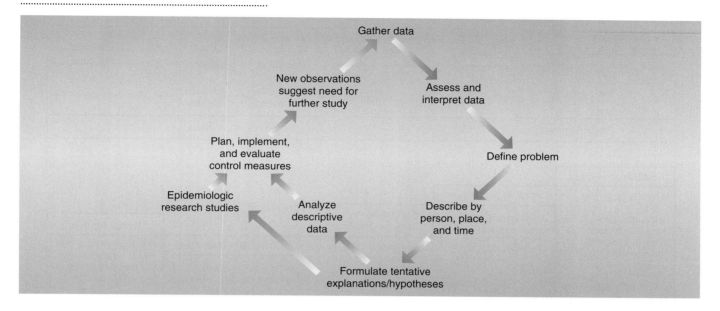

Gather data

Assess and interpret data

New observations suggest need for further study

Define problem

Plan, implement, and evaluate control measures

Epidemiologic research studies

Analyze descriptive data

Describe by person, place, and time

Formulate tentative explanations/hypotheses

on p. 106). During the prepathogenesis period, there are factors within individuals and their environments that may predispose or precipitate the disease. The initial interactions among agent, host, and environment occur during this period. For example, an individual may have an inherited predisposition to high cholesterol levels and may be obese, a smoker, and under excessive pressure at work in the prepathogenesis period. The period of pathogenesis begins when the host begins to respond with biological, psychological, or other changes. It is manifested by signs and symptoms that continue until the condition is resolved by recovery, disability, or death. If this individual is not able to modify the factors that predispose to disease, he or she is at high risk for a heart attack.

Leavell and Clark also identified levels of prevention for the prepathogenesis and pathogenesis periods: primary prevention, secondary prevention, and tertiary prevention.

Primary prevention includes activities that prevent a disease from becoming established and occurs during the prepathogenesis period. These activities include both health promotion activities and specific protection activities such as immunizations and protection from hazards and hygiene. Because no symptoms of illness exist, primary prevention programs are directed toward either the general healthy population or toward a group of healthy people who are known to be at high risk for a particular disease, illness, or injury. For example, public health organizations and voluntary agencies have emphasized the importance of regular exercise, a low-fat diet, and smoking cessation programs in an attempt to prevent coronary artery disease.

Secondary prevention includes activities designed to detect disease and provide early treatment. These activities involve early diagnosis, prompt treatment, and measures to limit disability. Screening programs for high cholesterol is an example of secondary prevention of coronary artery disease. If high levels are found, early treatment can be effective in lowering cholesterol levels.

Tertiary prevention includes the treatment, care, and rehabilitation of people with acute and chronic illness to achieve their maximum potential. If coronary artery disease is not prevented, a myocardial infarction may occur. A coronary artery bypass graft may be required, followed by a cardiac rehabilitation program.

Both secondary and tertiary prevention occur during the pathogenesis period. However, tertiary prevention is initiated after irreversible changes have resulted from the disease process. A detailed outline of the natural history can be created for any illness, and it becomes a helpful guideline for health professionals at all three levels of prevention.

Descriptive Epidemiology

Descriptive epidemiology focuses on the frequency and distribution of states of health within a population. By describing characteristics of groups of people who have or do not have certain illnesses, factors that are associated primarily with the people who have the illness can be identified. These are called **risk factors.** Generally, descriptive data can tell us what kind of people are at risk of developing certain health problems; what diseases, disabilities, or needs they have; how these problems are distributed in

LEVELS OF APPLICATION OF PREVENTIVE MEASURES IN THE NATURAL HISTORY OF DISEASE.

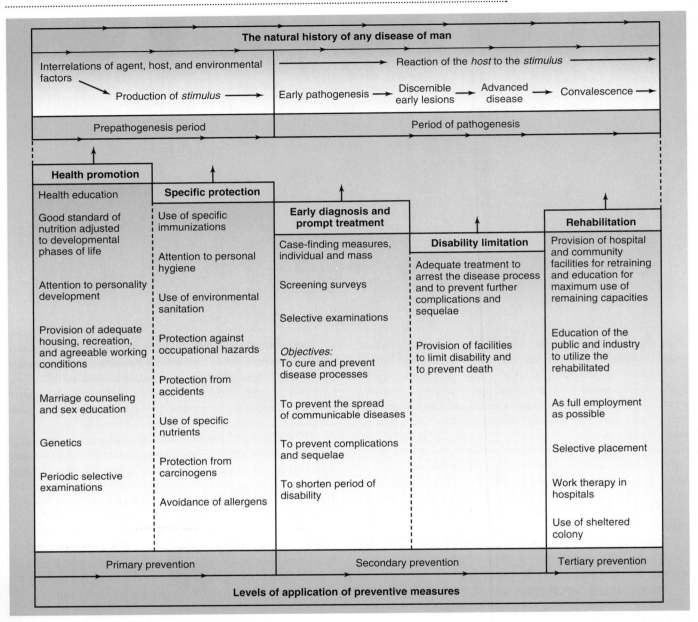

Source: Leavell & Clark, 1965.

the community; who goes where for different kinds of health service; and who provides the health services they need. Health professionals then use this information to set priorities for health programs, to find ways of using health resources more effectively, to plan strategies to meet emerging health care needs, and to evaluate the effectiveness of measures used to control or prevent specific disorders. However, it is important to emphasize here that descriptive epidemiology can be used to study states of wellness. For example, identifying factors such as diet and exercise that are

associated with healthy, community-dwelling elderly people older than 85 years of age can provide the information necessary to enhance wellness in other elderly populations.

Use of Rates

All epidemiological investigations depend on the ability to quantify the occurrence of a health problem. The most basic measure of frequency is to count the number of affected individuals. However, this may be misleading. The number of people in the population who could have been affected, but were not, should be taken into consideration. For example, five people in a community may have developed human immunodeficiency virus/ acquired immunodeficiency syndrome (HIV/AIDS). The implications of this event would be interpreted very differently if those people came from a community of 500 people versus a community of 100,000 people. Also, the time frame in which the problem has occurred is important. The use of ratios, proportions, and rates provide a more valid description of health problems.

A *ratio* is a fraction that obtained by dividing one quantity by another quantity; it represents the relationship between the two numbers. The numerator is not included in the denominator. For example, the number of boys on a pediatric unit could be contrasted with the number of girls on the same unit using a ratio: 10 boys and 5 girls would result in a 2:1 ratio of boys to girls. A *proportion* is a type of ratio that includes the quantity in the numerator as a part of the denominator. Therefore, it is the relationship of a part to the whole. Dividing the number of boys on the pediatric unit by the total number of boys and girls on the unit results in a proportion: 10 boys out of 15 boys and girls would result in a proportion of boys equal to 67%.

A **rate** is a proportion that includes the factor of time. It is a measure of the quantity of a health problem in a specific population within a given period. Rates are the best indicators of the probability that a disease, condition, or event will occur; therefore, rates are the primary measurements used to describe occurrence. By using rates, it is possible to compare events that happen at different times and places and with different people. For example, rates make it possible to compare the occurrence of HIV/AIDS in two or more locations.

A rate consists of two parts: a *numerator* and a *denominator*. The numerator is composed of the number of cases of the health problem being investigated within a given period. The denominator is the population at risk during the same period. If the period is long, the population at risk is often estimated at a midperiod, such as midyear. There are four basic principles that apply to the calculation of rates:

1. *The numerator should include all events being measured; therefore, adequate information must be available.*

2. *Everyone in the denominator must be at risk for the event in the numerator.*

3. *A specific period must be indicated during which observations are made.*

RESEARCH BRIEF

Cook, R. L., Royce, R. A., Thomas, J. C., & Hanusa, B. H. (1999). What's driving an epidemic? The spread of syphilis along an interstate highway in rural North Carolina. American Journal of Public Health, 89(3), 369–373.

The purpose of this research study was to determine whether county syphilis rates were increased along I-95 in North Carolina during a recent epidemic. Data on syphilis cases, demographics, drug activity, and highways were used to conduct a longitudinal study of North Carolina counties from 1985 to 1994. Crude and adjusted incidence rates were calculated and adjusted for sociodemographic factors and drug use. A cross-sectional design was used. Ten-year syphilis rates in the I-95 counties greatly exceeded rates in non–I-95 counties: 38 versus 16 cases per 100,000 persons) and remained high even after adjustment for race, age, sex, poverty, urban area designation, and drug activity. Syphilis rates were stable until 1989, but increased sharply in I-95 counties after 1989. Increased drug activity in I-95 counties preceded the rise in syphilis rates. The authors offer possible explanations for these results: spread of syphilis through contact between truck drivers and local sex workers at truck stops and rest stops; cocaine distribution; and the use of crack cocaine, which increases risky behaviors such as higher numbers of sexual partners and less frequent condom use, owing in part to the exchange of sex for drugs. Although the authors do not state specifically which factors were responsible for the increase in syphilis rates along I-95, cocaine distribution along the highway seems the most likely explanation. Further study is recommended to determine the specific associations along I-95. A better understanding of the cause of the association has public health implications where more resources and interventions can be focused.

FERTILITY RATE AND ABORTION RATIO AND RATE BY YEAR: UNITED STATES, 1972–1994.

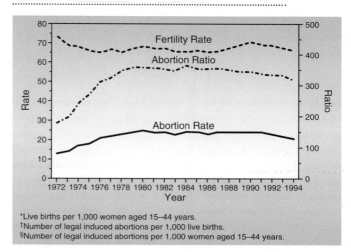

*Live births per 1,000 women aged 15–44 years.
†Number of legal induced abortions per 1,000 live births.
§Number of legal induced abortions per 1,000 women aged 15–44 years.

TABLE 4-3	HYPOTHETICAL EXAMPLE OF THE CALCULATION OF RATES THAT CAN BE COMPARED BETWEEN TWO CITIES

CITY A, 1998	CITY B, 1998
Number of hepatitis cases = 45	Number of hepatitis cases = 341
Population of City A = 153,000	Population of City B = 1,326,000
Hepatitis rate 45 × 100,000	Hepatitis rate 341 × 100,000
City A = 153,000	City B = 1,326,000
Hepatitis rate	Hepatitis rate
City A = 0.000294 × 100,000	City B = 0.00257 × 100,000
Hepatitis rate	Hepatitis rate
City A = 29.4 cases/100,000 people in 1998	City B = 25.7 cases/100,000 people in 1998

Counting only cases, City B has a higher frequency of hepatitis. However, when the population at risk is included in the rate calculation, City A has more cases per population than City B.

4. *To make the rate a reasonable size to interpret and remove decimal points, the rate is multiplied by a base, usually a multiple of 10. Any base multiple of 10 may be chosen that results in a rate above the value of 1.*

The formula for rate calculation follows. Table 4-3 illustrates the calculation of rates that can be compared between cities.

$$Rate = \frac{\text{Number of conditions or events occurring in a period of time}}{\text{Population at risk during the same period of time}} \times \text{Base multiple of 10}$$

An example of the difference between rates and ratios is shown in the figure on p. 107. Fertility rates are defined as live births per 1,000 women age 15 to 44 years. Women experiencing live births are in the numerator, and all women of childbearing age are in the denominator. The abortion ratio is the number of legal induced abortions per 1,000 live births. The numerator, the number of legal induced abortions, is not a part of the denominator, live births. Therefore, it is a ratio and not a rate. However, the number of legal induced abortions per 1,000 women of childbearing age is a rate, the abortion rate. The graph on p. 107 shows the changes in the rates and ratio over a 22-year period (CDC, 1997a).

Incidence Rates

Incidence or occurrence rates are a form of rate that measures the occurrence of new illnesses in a previously disease-free group of people within a specific time frame, often a year. Therefore, it is a measure of the probability that people without a certain condition will develop the condition over a period of time. The numerator of incidence rates include only the number of *new* conditions or events occurring within a period of time; therefore, the date of onset must be known. The general rules that apply to rates apply to incidence rates. Incidence rates and incidence ratios, especially **mortality** (death) rates, are often indices of the health of communities.

Incidence rates can be used to determine trends over time. For example, the following figure shows the rates of group B streptococcal (GBS) infection among infants in the United States (CDC, 1997c). This infection is the leading cause of bacterial disease and death among newborns in the United States and can cause illness and death in peripartum women and in adults with chronic medical conditions. Therefore, the incidence of this disease has been tracked in selected cities and their surrounding regions in different geographic locations. This incidence rate has

INCIDENCE RATE OF EARLY-ONSET GROUP B STREPTOCOCCAL (GBS) DISEASE BY YEAR AND SITE—SELECTED SITES, 1993–1995.

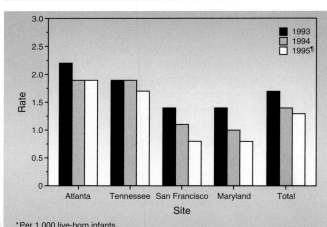

*Per 1,000 live-born infants.
†Defined as isolation of group B streptococci from a normally sterile site (e.g., blood or cerebrospinal fluid) from a resident of an area under surveillance. GBS cases were categorized as early-onset (illness onset at age <7 days) and late-onset (illness onset at age 7–90 days).
§The three-county San Francisco Bay area, California; four urban counties in Tennessee; the eight-county metropolitan area of Atlanta, Georgia; and the entire state of Maryland.
¶For San Francisco, Maryland, and total, p<0.01, chi-square for trend.

been calculated as the number of infants infected per 1,000 live births. The figure shows that there is a decreasing incidence of GBS, and it is believed to be the result of improved measures of surveillance and widely publicized state-sponsored prevention activities (CDC, 1997c).

FYI

The mortality rate of lung cancer has surpassed the mortality rate of breast cancer among women.

Prevalence Rates

Prevalence rates measure the number of people in a given population who have an existing health problem within a specified time frame. There are two types of prevalence rates. **Period prevalence** indicates the existence of a condition during an interval of time. **Point prevalence** refers to the existence of a condition at a specific point in time. Prevalence measures the amount of illness or **morbidity** that exists in a community as a result of the health problem under investigation. Many health care workers believe that prevalence rates are more important than incidence rates in determining the total burden of the illness on the community. Knowledge of the prevalence of a condition such as diabetes mellitus within a population can lead to the prioritizing of facilities, services, and manpower to meet the special needs of diabetics in the community.

Prevalence is influenced by two factors: the number of people who have developed the condition in the past and the duration of their illness. The longer the duration of a condition, the higher the prevalence rate in the community. This is best illustrated with

chronic diseases. For example, there are many more cases of diabetes in a community than would be indicated by calculation of the incidence rate, which reflects new cases only. Although the incidence rate for diabetes is low, people live for many years with the illness, and the duration is high. Therefore, in calculating prevalence rates, the numerator consists of the number of *existing* cases of the condition or event that occur within a specified period. For example, the existing cases of diabetes mellitus include new cases that were recently diagnosed plus those cases diagnosed in the past who are currently living with the illness.

Crude, Specific, and Adjusted Rates

Other common rates include crude, specific, and adjusted rates. **Crude rates** measure the experience of health problems in populations of designated geographic areas. These broad descriptive statistics may obscure significant differences in the risk of developing various conditions. Factors such as age, gender, ethnicity, and other demographic factors are not taken into consideration. Therefore, **specific rates** for subgroups of the population may be calculated. These more detailed rates are commonly calculated to describe the distribution of health problems by age, gender, ethnicity, and other demographic characteristics. **Adjusted rates** have been standardized, removing the differences in composition of populations, such as age. The following figure (part a) illustrates the prevalence of self-reported diabetes in three specific age groups. The rates are highest in those older than 65. Part b of the figure illustrates age-adjusted rates of self-reported diabetes by race (CDC, 1997f). In this example, age adjustment removes age as a factor in the calculation of the rates. Therefore, the differences shown reflect a rather dramatic increase in diabetes mellitus in African Americans. Knowledge of these factors can be helpful in assessing individual patients for their health care needs, as well as group needs for prevention and control programs.

AGE-ADJUSTED PREVALENCE OF SELF-REPORTED DIABETES BY RACE—UNITED STATES, 1980–1994.

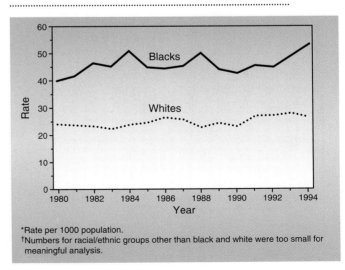

*Rate per 1000 population.
†Numbers for racial/ethnic groups other than black and white were too small for meaningful analysis.

PREVALENCE OF SELF-REPORTED DIABETES BY AGE GROUP—UNITED STATES, 1980–1994.

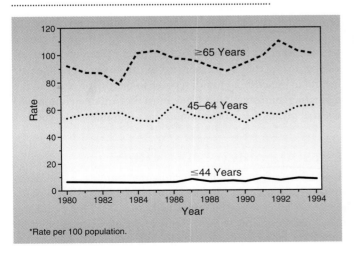

*Rate per 100 population.

Sources of Data

To describe a specific condition or event appropriately, it is necessary to collect data from reliable sources. Traditionally, epidemiologists have used the census of the population as a reliable source for the denominators in the calculation of rates. The census is required once every 10 years by the United States Constitution and is the basis for apportionment of seats in the House of Representatives. It has been performed every 10 years since 1790. The 21st census was completed in 1990. Through the years, the census has expanded, including characteristics of housing, nativity, migration, education, employment, income, and other information that is gathered from random samples of the population. Census information is analyzed and reported for the nation as a whole and in progressively small regions down to municipalities, census tracts, and blocks. Results are also reported in regions known as standard metropolitan statistical areas (SMSA). These regions are densely populated and are not necessarily bound by traditional state or county lines. The majority of the population of the United States lives within these areas.

BOX 4-1 COMMON REPORTABLE COMMUNICABLE DISEASES

AIDS	Malaria
Amebiasis	Measles
Anthrax	Meningitis
Botulism	Meningococcal
Brucellosis	infection
Campylobacteriosis	Mumps
Chancroid	Pertussis
Chickenpox–zoster	Plague
Chlamydia	Poliomyelitis
Cholera	Psittacosis
Diptheria	Rabies
Encephalitis	Reye's syndrome
Food-associated	Rocky Mountain
illnesses	spotted fever
Giardiasis	Rubella
Gonorrhea	Salmonellosis
Granuloma inguinale	Shigellosis
Hemophilus	Syphilis
influenzae	Tetanus
Hepatitis A, B, non-A,	Toxic shock syndrome
non-B, unspecified	Trichinosis
Legionellosis	Tuberculosis
Leprosy	Tularemia
Leptospirosis	Typhoid fever
Lyme disease	Typhus
Lymphogranuloma	Yellow fever
venereum	

Vital statistics are data collected from the continuous recording of events such as births, deaths, marriages, divorces, and adoptions, usually by state agencies. This information can be used to provide valid numerators and denominators for calculation of rates. The Centers for Disease Control and Prevention (CDC) in Atlanta collects all information regarding reportable diseases from state health departments. A sample of common reportable communicable diseases is found in Box 4-1. However, reportable diseases may vary somewhat from state to state. The CDC also collects information about other infectious and noninfectious health problems through a series of more than 100 national surveillance programs. The *Morbidity and Mortality Weekly Report (MMWR)* published by the CDC is the vehicle for distributing this information to health care professionals.

The National Health Survey, established in 1956, provides information about the health needs of the population of the United States. The National Center for Health Statistics is responsible for the ongoing surveys of households, physical examinations and laboratory reports, and health services providers. Most of this information is prevalence data and is the only nationwide source of data on chronic illness, minor conditions, and functional problems.

The Behavioral Risk Factor Surveillance System (BRFSS) was established in 1984 to collect, analyze, and interpret behavioral risk factor data from all states. Information is gathered about health behaviors such as obesity, lack of physical activity, smoking, safety belt use, and screening programs for breast cancer and elevated blood cholesterol. These BRFSS data were used in the formulation of both national and state objectives for the year 2000 and are being used for the development of 2010 objectives. Data are published regularly in the *MMWR*.

Any health-related information that has been collected about a group of people can be a source of data used to determine the distribution of states of health. Often, health-related information is found in databases from health care institutions, disease registries, insurance companies, industries, accident and police records, private doctors offices, local surveys, and any other place where information is gathered. Community health nurses are likely to use these data when planning programs for groups of people with specific health needs and information about the population is needed. These records reflect only those conditions or events that are characteristic of the people that sought the services of that agency or participated in the survey. These data are helpful in establishing health services to meet their needs and in evaluating outcomes, but data must be interpreted carefully when applying the information to the community as a whole.

Person, Place, and Time

One of the first steps in investigating the distribution and determinants of a health care problem is to describe the problem (*what occurs*) in terms of person, place, and time. Descriptive epidemiology deals primarily with the study of the distribution of health problems. However, research studies that attempt to identify the determinants of a problem (*why it occurs*) depend on the accurate collection of descriptive data. Examining the information about person, place, and time can help identify the characteristics of people who develop a disease or illness and those who do not.

Person

Describing the person characterizes *who* develops the health problem. There are many variations among people according to genetic factors, biological characteristics, behavioral choices, and socioeconomic conditions. Because so many variations exist, incidence and prevalence rates should be calculated according to these factors. This can be done by examining individual case data and examining specific and adjusted rates. Age is the most important characteristic affecting health status, followed by sex. Therefore, age-specific rates and sex-specific rates are usually calculated when describing a problem. Age-specific rates are calculated using the number of people in a given age group who have the problem being investigated in the numerator, and the population at risk in the given age group in the denominator.

An example of age-specific rates follows. The study was initiated following a 7-day period of intense environmental heat where maximum high daily temperatures in Dallas County, Texas, ranged from 101°F (38.3°C) to 106°F (41.1°C), and a series of deaths occurred. The figure above is a bar graph that demonstrates that the average rate of heat-related deaths each year is greatest in the newborn to 4, 75 to 84, and 85 age groups, as well as the very young and the elderly (CDC, 1997d).

Using this knowledge, community health nurses could initiate multiple actions, either for individuals in their care or for groups. When a heat wave is forecast, primary prevention messages about how to avoid heat-related illness should be disseminated to the public. The elderly should be encouraged to main-

AVERAGE ANNUAL RATE OF HEAT-RELATED DEATHS BY AGE GROUP—UNITED STATES, 1979–1994.

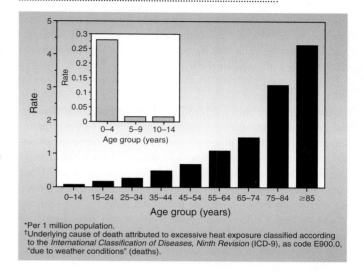

*Per 1 million population.
†Underlying cause of death attributed to excessive heat exposure classified according to the *International Classification of Diseases, Ninth Revision* (ICD-9), as code E900.0, "due to weather conditions" (deaths).

tain their fluid intake and assisted to increase their time in air-conditioned environments, making use of shopping malls and public libraries, even for part of the day. Alcohol consumption should be discouraged because it may cause dehydration and increase the risk for heat-related illnesses. Parents of young children should be educated about the increased heat sensitivity of young children and their need for adequate fluids. Day-care centers could be primary sites for dissemination of information.

Often, specific rates are presented in table form, combining characteristics of persons and changes over time. Table 4-4 indi-

---

TABLE 4-4   NUMBER OF REPORTED TUBERCULOSIS CASES, PERCENTAGE CHANGE IN NUMBER OF CASES, AND RATES*, BY SEX, AGE, AND YEAR—UNITED STATES, 1992 AND 1998

CHARACTERISTIC	NO. REPORTED CASES		% CHANGE FROM	RATE	
	1992	1998	1992 TO 1998	1992	1998
Sex†					
Male	17,433	11,413	−34.5%	14.0	8.6
Female	9,236	6,935	−24.9%	7.1	5.0
Age group (yr)†					
0–14	1,707	1,082	−36.6%	3.1	1.9
15–24	1,974	1,548	−21.6%	5.5	4.2
25–44	10,444	6,365	−39.1%	12.7	7.6
45–64	6,487	4,973	−23.3%	13.4	8.7
≥65	6,025	4,393	−27.1%	18.7	12.8
Total	26,673	18,361	−31.2%	10.5	6.8

*Per 100,000 population.
†Persons were excluded for whom sex (4 in 1992 and 13 in 1998) and age (36 in 1992) were not reported.

cates the number of reported tuberculosis cases, the age and sex characteristics of the cases, and the percentage change between 1992 and 1998 (CDC, 1999). This information shows that people older than 65 are the most vulnerable to tuberculosis. Nurses use this knowledge in establishing primary prevention programs and in assessing their elderly patients for signs and symptoms that may be indicative of the infection.

Place

Where the rates of the health problem are the highest or the lowest can be determined by examining the characteristics of place. Understanding where illness occurs is a primary factor to be considered in planning prevention and control measures and making decisions about distribution of health care resources. Place can be a neighborhood, a health care facility, a town, a region, a nation, or any other natural or political boundary. The identification of health differences between urban and rural sectors or between similar localities are often helpful in investigating specific health needs of a community.

Place often is illustrated through the use of maps. For example, in an attempt to monitor progress to reduce the risk of severe adverse effects in children of mothers who consume alcohol, the CDC published the prevalence by state of reported frequent alcohol consumption among women of childbearing age. The following figure illustrates the prevalence of this risk factor (CDC, 1997b). State health departments have used these data to determine priorities for their health objectives for 2010. For example, Michigan, Iowa, and Pennsylvania have the highest prevalence rates and should have targeted primary prevention programs toward this risk factor. Community health nurses would participate in the various efforts to reduce alcohol consumption in this age group.

Time

When health problems occur can be described by identifying short-term fluctuations measured in hours, days, weeks, or months; by periodic changes that are seasonal or cyclical; or by long-term changes over decades that reflect gradual changes. Describing the time of short-term outbreaks of infectious diseases is often performed by developing an **epidemic curve.** These graphs provide indications as to the mode of transmission and spread of the organism. The following figure is an example of an epidemic curve. It depicts an outbreak of viral gastroenteritis associated with eating oysters in Louisiana during December 1996 and January 1997 (CDC, 1997h). In this outbreak, 179 people became ill. The public health department was notified of the problem, contaminated oysters were identified, waterways closed, and the oysters recalled. The outbreak ended abruptly 2 days later. The only known source of the strain of gastrointestinal virus is feces from ill persons. Therefore, the probable source of the virus was oyster harvesters who admitted to routinely discharging sewage overboard. The oysters subsequently became contaminated with the virus and, after harvesting, were eaten by unsuspecting people in restaurants. Nurses working in public health agencies often are involved in identifying outbreaks such as this and may be involved in gathering and analyzing information and implementing control and preventive measures.

Periodic and *cyclical* changes also occur. For example, respiratory diseases are more common in the winter and spring (periodic), and hepatitis often increases in incidence every 7 to 9 years (cyclical). The figure on p. 113 (top, left) reflects both periodic and cyclical changes in pneumonia and influenza mortality (CDC, 1997g). A seasonal baseline is developed, and variations from this baseline determine whether an epidemic is occurring.

PREVALENCE OF REPORTED FREQUENT ALCOHOL CONSUMPTION AMONG CHILDBEARING-AGE WOMEN (18–44 YEARS)—UNITED STATES, BEHAVIORAL RISK FACTOR SURVEILLANCE SYSTEM, 1995.

Reported consumption level	Pregnant women					All women				
	1991 (n = 1,053)	(95% CI†)	1995 (n = 1,313)	(95% CI)	p value	1991 (n = 26,105)	(95% CI)	1995 (n = 30,415)	(95% CI)	p value
Any drinking§	12.4	(9.5–15.2)	16.3	(13.1–19.4)	0.07	49.4	(48.4–50.3)	50.6	(49.7–51.6)	0.02
<7 Drinks per week	12.2	(9.4–15.0)	14.6	(11.5–17.6)	0.27	43.9	(43.0–44.9)	45.7	(44.8–46.5)	0.01
7–14 Drinks per week	—¶		0.9	(0.0–1.8)	—	3.4	(3.1–3.8)	3.0	(2.6–3.3)	0.04
>14 Drinks per week	0.1	(0.0–0.3)	0.3	(0.0–0.7)	0.28	1.4	(1.2–1.6)	1.1	(0.9–1.3)	0.04
≥5 Drinks on occasion**	0.7	(0.2–1.2)	2.9	(1.5–4.3)	0.003	10.5	(10.0–11.1)	10.5	(9.9–11.1)	0.96
Frequent drinking††	0.8	(0.3–1.4)	3.5	(1.9–5.1)	0.002	12.4	(11.8–13.1)	12.6	(12.0–13.3)	0.67

*Because weighted data are used in this analysis, results for 1991 may be slightly different from those reported previously. For consistency, national analyses were restricted to the 47 states that participated in the BRFSS in both 1991 and 1995.
†Confidence interval.
§Levels of any drinking may not add to the total prevalence of any drinking because some women did not respond to questions about consumption frequency and amount. One additional state was eliminated from the breakdown of any drinking because questions regarding consumption frequency and amount were not asked in that state in 1995.
¶Too few observations to calculate a reliable estimate.
**Five or more drinks on at least one occasion during the preceding month.
††Consumption of an average of seven or more drinks per week or five or more drinks on at least one occasion during the preceding month.

NUMBER OF CASES OF GASTROENTERITIS ASSOCIATED
WITH EATING OYSTERS HARVESTED FROM LOUISIANA
WATERWAYS, DECEMBER 1996–JANUARY 1997.

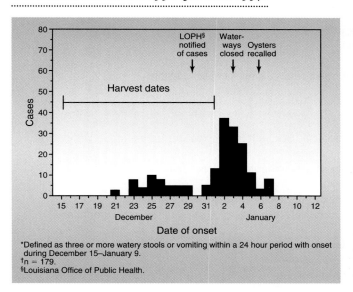

*Defined as three or more watery stools or vomiting within a 24 hour period with onset
  during December 15–January 9.
†n = 179.
§Louisiana Office of Public Health.

WEEKLY PNEUMONIA AND INFLUENZA (P&I) MORTALITY
AS A PERCENTAGE OF ALL DEATHS IN 122 CITIES—
UNITED STATES, JANUARY 1, 1993–FEBRUARY 15, 1997.

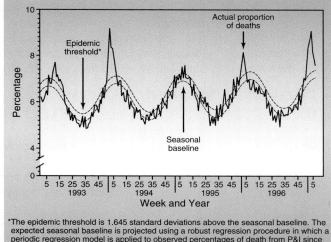

*The epidemic threshold is 1.645 standard deviations above the seasonal baseline. The
 expected seasonal baseline is projected using a robust regression procedure in which a
 periodic regression model is applied to observed percentages of death from P&I since
 1983.

These types of data are the evidence base for many of the control, prevention, and surveillance activities that are initiated by public health departments and community agencies initiated to keep the public healthy (see figure top, right).

Long-term changes or trends over time are shown in the following figure (CDC, 1997e). During the 20th century, significant changes in life expectancy at birth occurred. The figure includes gender, a characteristic of persons to make the graph more meaningful. In a similar manner, the changes in trends of the

mortality of various cancers can be seen when examined over decades (see figure below).

Analytic Epidemiology

Analytic epidemiology focuses on the determinants of health problems, or the *why*. When descriptive data are analyzed, the variations in person, place, and time often suggest tentative explanations or hypotheses. These hypotheses can then be tested through application of research methods in an attempt to find the reasons, or determinants, for these variations. This is a cyclical process because new knowledge may require further descriptive or analytic analysis. Four types of studies are used in epidemiological analytic investigations: **cross-sectional, retrospective, prospective,** and **intervention** (experimental) studies. The basic characteristics of these studies are outlined in Table 4-5.

LIFE EXPECTANCY AT BIRTH BY YEAR OF BIRTH AND SEX—
UNITED STATES, 1900–1996.

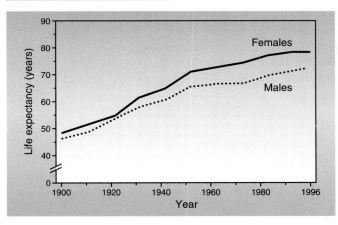

FYI

The Framingham Heart Study is a prospective study that has continued to follow the health characteristics of a community for more than 30 years. Much of the information about risk factors for coronary heart disease that underlies preventive programs was obtained from the results of this study.

TABLE 4-5   **CHARACTERISTICS OF EPIDEMIOLOGICAL ANALYTIC STUDIES**

CROSS-SECTIONAL SURVEYS

Purpose	Describe health states and look for tentative hypotheses
Design	All data is collected at the same time
Data collection	Interviews, observation, questionnaires
Advantages	Flexible, broad, economical, uncomplicated; rapid results, large samples possible
Disadvantages	Superficial, cannot infer cause and effect

CASE-CONTROL OR RETROSPECTIVE STUDIES

Purpose	Determine whether a group with a health problem (case) differs in exposure from a group without the problem (controls)
Design	Select case and control samples according to specific criteria. The dependent variable (case or not) has already occurred
Data collection	Trace past experience to determine relevant exposure factors (independent variables)
Advantages	First step in hypothesis testing, inexpensive, relatively small samples can be used, results obtained quickly
	Good design for studying rare or chronic conditions
Disadvantages	Information about past exposure may not be available
	Selection of appropriate control groups may be difficult
	Incidence can only be estimated
	Temporal association between exposure and outcome may be difficult to determine
	Potential selection, recall. and observation bias

PROSPECTIVE, COHORT, OR LONGITUDINAL STUDIES

Purpose	Determine whether the incidence of the health problem varies between the exposed and nonexposed
Design	Samples chosen and observed forward in time
Data collection	Information on outcome variables obtained at specific intervals
Advantages	Incidence rates can be calculated directly
	Time sequence easier to obtain
	Effects of rare exposure can be investigated
	Multiple outcomes may be studied
Disadvantages	May extend over a long period
	Expensive
	Cases lost to follow-up

THERAPEUTIC OR PREVENTIVE TRIALS, INTERVENTION STUDIES

Purpose	Determine whether a group with particular characteristics will benefit from interventions when compared with a group or groups who do not receive the intervention
Design	Randomly choose and assign groups to either a study group or comparison group
	Introduce an intervention (independent variable) to the study group
Data collection	Collect data prospectively on a number of dependent variables
Advantages	Cause and effect can be examined
Disadvantages	Control over confounding variables
	Can conduct with small groups
	Possible reactivity (Hawthorne effect)
	Possible noncompliance with study protocols
	Observation bias, placebo effect

Source: Modified from Harkness, 1995.

Ideally, the epidemiologist is seeking to establish a cause-and-effect relationship between the health problem or outcome that is being studied (dependent variable) and exposure factors (independent variables) that preceded it in time. Often, associations can be made between a condition and a specific factor, but a direct cause-and-effect relationship is weak or does not exist. More than one factor must be present for any illness to occur (multifactorial causation). Even in an infectious process, such as tuberculosis, presence of the organism alone is not sufficient to cause the disease. Characteristics of the agent, the host, and the environment all interact to determine the onset of the infection. The more factors that can be identified as contributors to a disease process, the weaker the cause-and-effect relationship will be.

RESEARCH BRIEF

Redelmeier, D. A., & Tibshirani, R. J. (1997). Association between cellular-telephone calls and motor vehicle collisions. The New England Journal of Medicine, 336(7), 453–458.

This epidemiological study of cellular phone use and motor vehicle collisions used a case-crossover design to study. The purpose of the research was to study whether using a cellular telephone while driving increases the risk of a motor vehicle collision. The sample included 669 drivers who had cellular phones and had been in accidents with significant property damage but no personal injury. Each person's cellular telephone calls on the day of the collision and during the previous week were analyzed using telephone bills.

A total of 26,798 cellular phone calls were made during the 14-month study period. The risk of a collision when using a cellular phone was four times higher than the risk when a cellular telephone was not being used. The relative risk was 4.3 (95% confidence level, 3.0 to 6.5). The relative risk was similar for drivers who differed in personal characteristics such as age and driving experience. Of note, cellular phone calls made close to the time of the collision were particularly hazardous (relative risk, 4.8 for calls placed within 5 minutes of the collision, as compared with 1.3 for calls placed more than 15 minutes before the collision). Hand-free units offered no protection over handheld units (3.9 relative risk). Of the drivers, 39% used the cellular phones to call for emergency services, providing some advantage after the accident. The use of cellular phones in motor vehicles is associated with a quadrupling of the risk of a collision during the brief period of a phone call. There are implications from this study for education about risk reduction and the use of this new technology.

CONCLUSION

Promoting and preserving the health of populations is a fundamental characteristic of community health nursing. Although nursing is a profession that focuses primarily on the individual, the person's health care needs cannot be completely or correctly defined unless family, personal friends, and the characteristics of the community and the society are considered. Epidemiology, the science of preventive medicine, provides a framework for studying and understanding these interactions. *Epidemiology* is the study of the distribution and the determinants of states of health and illness in human populations. The basic conceptual framework of epidemiology is the interaction among the agent, host, and environment—the epidemiological triad. Epidemiology is considered both as a methodology used to study health-related conditions and as an accumulated body of knowledge about a state of health. Nurses use the body of knowledge about a health problem in their clinical decision making and may become involved in epidemiological research methods to gather new health-related information.

Descriptive epidemiology examines the distribution of states of health in the population. The primary tool that is used in epidemiology is the rate, a proportion that includes the factor of time. Incidence rates measure the probability that people without a certain condition develop the condition during a specific time frame. The number of new conditions or events are measured. Prevalence rates measure the extent of an existing health problem within a specific period. These rates are often calculated according to characteristics of person (who), place (where), and time (when). Analytical epidemiology attempts to define the determinants of health problems (why) through rigorous research techniques. Types of analytical studies include cross-sectional, retrospective, prospective, and intervention studies.

CRITICAL THINKING ACTIVITIES

1. Using an example from your practice, identify two examples that illustrate how the epidemiological body of knowledge is used in clinical decision making.

2. Between January 1 and December 1, 1998, 25 new cases of tuberculosis were diagnosed in Boon Town, population 450,000. A prevalence survey taken the first week in January 1998 indicated that there were 250 cases on the list of active tuberculosis cases. There were 20 deaths due to tuberculosis recorded during this 1-year period. Using this information, calculate the following rates.

   - What was the incidence rate per 100,000 population for tuberculosis during 1998?

   - What was the prevalence rate per 100,000 population for tuberculosis during 1998?

   - What was the cause-specific death rate per 100,000 for tuberculosis in 1998?

3. Discuss how nurses could use the case-control research methodology to answer questions in their practice.

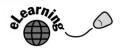 Explore Community Health Nursing on the web! To learn more about the topics in this chapter, use the passcode provided to access your exclusive web site: http://communitynursing.jbpub.com
If you do not have a passcode, you can obtain one at this site.

REFERENCES

Aiken, L. (1988). Assuring the delivery of quality patient care. State of the Science Invitational Conference: Nursing resources and the delivery of patient care (NIH Publication No. 89-3008, pp. 3–10). Washington, D.C.: U.S. Department of Health and Human Services, Public Health Service.

Bureau of the Census. (1998). Statistical abstracts of the United States, 1998, the national data book (118th ed., p 100). Washington, D.C.: U.S. Department of Commerce, Economics and Statistics Administration.

Centers for Disease Control and Prevention (CDC). (1997a). Abortion surveillance: Preliminary data—United States, 1994. *Morbidity and Mortality Weekly Report, 45*(51&52), 1123–1127.

Centers for Disease Control and Prevention (CDC). (1997b). Alcohol consumption among pregnant and childbearing-aged women—United States, 1991 and 1995. *Morbidity and Mortality Weekly Report, 46*(16), 346–350.

Centers for Disease Control and Prevention (CDC). (1997c). Decreasing incidence of perinatal group B streptococcal disease—United States, 1993–1995. *Morbidity and Mortality Weekly Report, 46*(21), 473–477.

Centers for Disease Control and Prevention (CDC). (1997d). Heat-related deaths—Dallas, Wichita, and Cooke Counties, Texas, and United States, 1996. *Morbidity and Mortality Weekly Report, 46*(23), 528–531.

Centers for Disease Control and Prevention (CDC). (1997e). Mortality patterns—preliminary data, United States, 1996. *Morbidity and Mortality Weekly Report, 46*(40), 941–944.

Centers for Disease Control and Prevention (CDC). (1997f). Trends in the prevalence and incidence of self-reported diabetes mellitus—United States, 1980–1994. *Morbidity and Mortality Weekly Report, 46*(43), 1014–1018.

Centers for Disease Control and Prevention (CDC). (1997g). Update: Influenza activity—United States, 1996. *Morbidity and Mortality Weekly Report, 46*(8), 173–176.

Centers for Disease Control and Prevention (CDC). (1997h). Viral gastroenteritis associated with eating oysters—Louisiana, December 1996–January 1997. *Morbidity and Mortality Weekly Report, 46*(47), 1109–1112.

Centers for Disease Control and Prevention (CDC). (1999). Progress toward the elimination of tuberculosis—United States, 1998. *Morbidity and Mortality Weekly Report, 48*(33), 732–736.

Cohen, B. (1984). Florence Nightingale. *Scientific American, 250*(3), 129.

Doll, R., & Hill, A. B. (1950). Smoking and carcinoma of the lung: preliminary report. *British Medical Journal, 2739.*

Harkness, G. A. (1995). *Epidemiology in nursing practice.* St. Louis, Mosby.

Humphreys, N. A. (1885). *Vital statistics: A memorial volume of selections from the reports and writings of William Farr, 1807–1183.* London: Sanitary Institute of Great Britain.

Leavell, H. F., & Clark, H. G. (1965). *Preventive medicine for the doctor in his community: an epidemiologic approach.* New York: McGraw-Hill.

Leavell, H. R., & Clark, H. G. (1958). *Preventive medicine for the doctor in his community,* 3rd ed. New York: McGraw-Hill.

Snow, J. (1855). *On the mode of communication of cholera.* London: Churchill. (Reproduced in *Snow on cholera.* [1965]. New York: Hafner.)

Chapter 5
Health Care Systems in Transition

Bonita R. Reinert

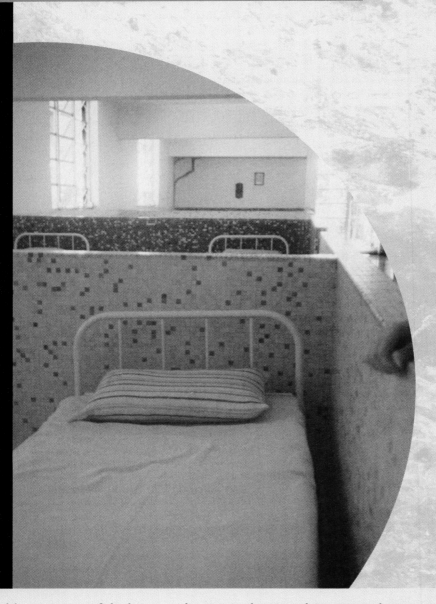

Health care is one of the largest industries in the United States, employing an esti-mated 10 million workers. The health care system in the United States includes the most technology-rich facilities and the most advanced practices in the world. The most well-educated physicians, nurses, and other health care workers use sophisticated treat-ments on a daily basis to prolong life and restore function.

CHAPTER FOCUS

Evolution of the U.S. Health Care Delivery System
- Private Health Care
- Public Health Care
- Military Health Care
- Health Care Reform

Current U.S. Health Care Delivery System
- Levels of Care
- Health Care Providers
- Health Care Settings
- Issues Affecting Delivery of Health Care Services

Managed Care
- Managed Care Delivery Systems
- Managed Care Organizations
- Patient Care Outcomes

Health Politics and Policy
- Government Policy
- Public Opinion and Special Interest Groups
- Nursing and Health Care Policy

New Nursing Opportunities
- Advanced Practice Nurses
- Entrepreneurs
- Data Management
- Research

QUESTIONS TO CONSIDER

After reading this chapter, answer the following questions:

1. How did the current U.S. health care system evolve to its present form?
2. What is the difference between private and public health care?
3. What are some of the current issues affecting health care delivery in the United States?
4. How do politics and policy influence the health care delivery system?
5. What are some of the current and evolving health care settings?
6. What impact is managed care having on health care delivery?
7. What are some potential roles for nurses within the changing health care system?

KEY TERMS

Capitation

Diagnosis-related groups (DRGs)

Fee-for-service

Health care delivery system

Health maintenance organizations (HMOs)

Integrated health care systems

Managed care

Managed competition

Point-of-service (POS) plans

Preferred provider organization (PPO)

Preventive care

Primary care

Prospective payment system (PPS)

Third-party payer

As a result of its cutting-edge nature, the U.S. health care system is the most costly, in terms of resources, in the world. Current patterns of health care delivery have resulted in an annual cost that exceeds $9.8 billion (HCFA, 1998), a figure that is significantly higher than that of any other industrialized nation. By the year 2008, it has been projected that health care costs in the United States could exceed $2.2 trillion, a figure that will represent more than 16.2% of the country's gross domestic product (HCFA, 1998).

Despite technological advances and high health care costs, clinical outcomes are not always significantly better in the United States when compared with other industrialized nations. For example, among the industrialized countries, the United States ranks 1st in health care technology but 17th in rates of low-birth-weight babies and 12th in life expectancy (Children's Defense Fund, 1998). Access to health care is believed to be one of the determinants of our less-than-auspicious health indicators.

A lack of access to quality health care services can take several forms. For example, needed services may simply not be available in an accessible location or during hours when individuals are able to use them. The health care site may not be organized in a user-friendly manner so that individuals can obtain timely and acceptable services. For example, providers may not be as culturally sensitive or as multilingual as is needed in certain locations of this country.

Routine health care may also not be accessible because of a lack of personal funds and/or insurance coverage. Medications and special treatments may be beyond the financial resources of the individual despite a provider's carefully developed plan of care. Finally, individuals may not have a regular provider and may have to receive care from a variety of providers in a number of unconnected facilities. Thus, care may not be comprehensive or timely.

Although leaders in government, health care, and consumer groups continue to express concern over access issues, inequities in the current system are readily apparent. By most accounts, more than 45 million (16%) Americans are uninsured. In addition, many more U.S. citizens are underinsured, and the figure is growing. Individuals working at part-time and minimum wage jobs make up a large part of the uninsured and underinsured in this country.

A lack of insurance often results in a lack of prevention services and early interventions. Lack of adequate prenatal care and infant immunizations, especially for the poor and minority populations, has led to illness, disability, and ultimately, increased financial demands on the public health care system. Statistically, African Americans fair worse in virtually every condition that affects health (U.S. National Center for Health Statistics, 1998). The rates of infectious disease such as tuberculosis, sexually transmitted diseases, and acquired immunodeficiency syndrome (AIDS) continue to rise, especially within at-risk populations. A lack of accessible community mental health services has resulted in a number of tragedies and untold stress for families.

Attempts to contain spiraling costs, deal with the dissatisfaction of consumers and providers, and address issues of uneven access and poor clinical outcomes have resulted in cost containment legislation, new configurations of providers, and new ways of providing care. Because nursing care holds the answer to many of the current dilemmas, the nursing profession appears to be poised at that edge of an exciting and challenging future.

Evolution of the U.S. Health Care Delivery System

The term **health care delivery system** refers to a multilevel industry that transforms various resources into essential services designed to meet the health care needs of a population. This transformation occurs through a complex set of interactions among consumers, providers, payers, employers, and the government. Resources include things such as physical structures, personnel, technology, supplies, and financing. The system is both guided and, in some instances, undermined by competition, demands for profit, technological innovation, standards, and government regulations.

Many critics suggest that the health care system in the United States is not actually a system at all because it is not a coordinated whole with interrelated parts. Instead, health care in this country often occurs as a series of fragmented episodes that may be isolated, unrelated, confusing, or even competing. Furthermore, in the United States, there is no single source of oversight, policies, or goals, nor is there a set of shared values and concerns among the various entities in the delivery system.

Services may be provided in traditional settings, such as hospitals or physicians' offices, and in less traditional settings, such as shelters, specially equipped vans, or shopping malls. Client care information may or may not be shared among the providers in the subsystems or even between providers at separate sites in a single subsystem. Furthermore, follow-up contact between providers and clients is rare.

Reimbursement may come from one or more of the following sources: private insurance companies, managed care organizations, government agencies, foundations, and the client. The client is often the one who has to decide who to bill, what to do when reimbursement is denied, or who to talk to when the bill is only partially reimbursed.

Finally, services may need to be accessed in private, public, and/or military health care systems. Each system has a unique set of rules and requirements. Coverage may be overlapping, costs of care are different, and reimbursement occurs in different ways.

Private Health Care

Our complicated private health care system has changed dramatically in the last 200 years. In the 19th century, family, servants, or close friends cared for clients in the home with physicians making visits as needed. Treatment involved medicinal herbs and comfort measures. Medical knowledge was limited, and most medical practitioners in the United States lacked a standardized education. Medical treatments were based on common sense, and physicians often lacked acceptance as professionals. Care was purchased out of private funds or provided on a charity basis. The few hospitals that existed basically served indigent clients, without family or support, who found themselves at death's door. Medical treatments performed in these early hospitals were often crude and seldom were very effective.

After the middle of the 19th century, large jumps in medical knowledge occurred that paved the way for significant gains in surgical interventions and the treatment of disease. The new, more sophisticated procedures required centralized facilities to house the new technology and train the personnel needed to provide client care. This resulted in an era of extensive hospital construction, the institutionalization of health care, and the establishment of the hospital as the center of health care delivery (see Box 5-1).

After World War I, the medical profession in this country grew in prestige and power. This transformation was based on trends such as the following: movement to cities away from family and friends, advances in medical science and technology, organization of medicine and adoption of state licensing requirements, establishment of worker's compensation and growth of health insurance, and educational requirements for providers (Shi & Singh, 1998).

To ensure that hospital bills would be paid, insurance companies such as Blue Cross were formed. With the establishment of broader health insurance coverage, providers were at less financial risk, and insurance policies provided for the reimbursement of increasing numbers of clients. Clients selected the provider. Providers simply decided on the appropriate course of care for the client, implemented that care, and then submitted

bills at the end of the illness episode. This form of payment was known as fee-for-service.

Fee-for-service is a form of retrospective payment for health care in which a facility or provider submits a bill for services rendered at the completion of the health care episode. An advantage of this type of billing is that care is reimbursed according to the acuity of the client based on the services required. However, some health care experts now believe that paying a fee for each service performed encourages unnecessary services and frequent return visits, which increases health care costs.

The Hill-Burton Act was passed in 1946 to help communities build hospitals. The National Institutes of Health became a major funding source for health care research in the 1950s. The Medicare Act was passed in 1965 to provide hospital insurance for the elderly. Each of these efforts increased the organizational strength of the health care system.

Two acts passed by Congress have significantly affected the methods by which hospitals are reimbursed for care. The Tax Equity and Fiscal Responsibility Act of 1982 (TEFRA) established a cost-per-case basis for Medicare-reimbursed inpatient services. The 1983 amendments to the Social Security Act established a prospective payment method of paying for inpatient services for Medicare clients based on a system of admitting diagnoses known as **diagnosis-related groups (DRGs)**.

Under the **prospective payment system (PPS)**, an annual fixed (prospective) rate was established for reimbursing providers for care based on 467 diagnoses or procedures. The prototype for the prospective payment system was developed at Yale University. Under the Yale program, reimbursement amounts bore "little or no relationship to length of stay, services rendered, or costs of care" (Williams & Torrens, 1999, p. 137). Rules stated that costs above the established amount for a given DRG would be absorbed by the hospital, but if the care was delivered for less than the established amount, the hospital could keep the difference and make a profit.

Third-party payers are agencies or organizations like insurance companies or health maintenance organizations that are responsible for all or part of an insured individual's health care costs. Third-party payers also adopted the DRG system as a part of their cost-saving measures. It has been suggested that prospective payment legislation introduced a new era of fiscal constraints, demands for accountability, and pressure to provide services in innovative ways. This new era involved the constant evaluation of practices, policies, and procedures to limit costs whenever possible and has resulted in concerns about access, equitable treatment decisions, and quality of care (Box 5-1).

As a result of the need to control costs, provide quality care, and meet the needs of increasing numbers of individuals, a variety of creative and innovative health care organizations have developed. Often called *alphabet health care,* acronyms such as HMOs (health management organizations), PPOs (preferred provider organizations), POS (point-of-service plans), and MCOs (managed care organizations) have become part of our

---

BOX 5-1 PHASES OF HEALTH CARE SYSTEM DEVELOPMENT

Development of the private health care delivery system occurred in four phases:

1. Prior to the 1850s: Illness and disability were handled at home. Few hospitals and clinics existed, and they provided mostly indigent care.

2. 1850–1930: Significant gains in medical knowledge occurred. Technological advances necessitated an increase in the number of hospitals and nurses.

3. 1930–1980: Health care became more organized. Insurance became available, so people were more likely to go to hospitals for care.

4. 1980 to present: Soaring costs resulted in reorganization, restructuring, reallocation of scarce resources, and difficult ethical decisions.

new health care vocabulary (Feldstein, 1999). With these new health care models have come some difficult ethical questions. Is health care a right? If a treatment or procedure is available and I want it, should my insurance pay for it? Who should decide on the appropriateness of medical treatment plans, the doctor or the insurance company? These questions are probably going to be with us for some time because there are no easy answers.

Public Health Care

"Public health can be defined as an effort organized by society to protect, promote, and restore people's health" (Fairbanks & Wiese, 1998). The U.S. public health system is an interwoven local, state, and national governmental agency designed to look at broad community-based health issues and protect the general public from the hazards that result from living in populated urban areas.

Massachusetts was the first state to establish a state department of health, modeled, in part, after the British General Board of Health. Lemuel Shattuck, from Massachusetts, produced a visionary report in 1850 titled *Report of the Sanitary Commission of Massachusetts*. In that report, he outlined the health needs of the state and offered recommendations related to the need for sanitary engineers, accurate vital statistics, inspectors, food and drug regulations, public health education, and routine preventive health care for all citizens. Despite its carefully written and documented recommendations, it was virtually ignored for almost 20 years.

In 1872, the Public Health Association was formed. Its membership focused on interdisciplinary efforts to improve health, and it developed a number of health promotion and illness prevention materials for the public. In the 1880s, based on work by Pasteur and Koch, public health moved from a narrow emphasis on environmental sanitation to a broader view that included bacteriology and immunology.

During the first decade of the 20th century, public health services began to expand. The Social Security Act of 1935 provided federal funding for support of local health departments and marked the first step toward the development of a nationwide network of public health agencies. Public health agencies were responsible for providing health care services to special populations such as urban poor, mothers, babies, Native Americans, and so on (Fairbanks & Wiese, 1998).

Today, public health agencies range in size and scope from local health departments to the Centers for Disease Control and Prevention (CDC) in Atlanta and focus on ensuring that the public health of the community is protected, promoted, and restored. To meet that goal, public health departments currently have a wide range of population-based goals (Box 5-2). To meet the goal of healthy communities, public health agencies have expanded their core functions to include community assessment, policy development, limited medical services (e.g., immunizations, well baby checkups, sexually transmitted disease treatment and surveillance), and program evaluation (Keck & Scutchfield, 1997).

BOX 5-2 PUBLIC HEALTH GOALS

The public health system is responsible for the following:

- Preventing epidemics and the spread of disease
- Reducing environmental hazards
- Preventing injuries
- Promoting healthy behaviors
- Providing disaster services
- Ensuring the quality and accessibility of health services

Source: Fairbanks & Wiese, 1998.

Military Health Care

One of the most important fringe benefits of military life is a system of well-organized, comprehensive health care services provided at little or no extra cost (Williams & Torrens, 1999). Military personnel are also covered for service-connected problems for life. Health care is always available when needed, although personnel may have little choice of provider. Finally, the military health care system emphasizes prevention in addition to illness care.

Ambulatory care is provided in base and regional clinics. Simple hospital services, including short-term stays, are available through base dispensaries or sick bays on-board ships. More advanced care is available in regional hospitals. Well-trained medics, nurses, and physicians, in facilities owned by the U.S. government, provide most of the care. The system of care is well organized, integrated, and sophisticated.

Dependents and families of active duty personnel are covered by an extensive health insurance plan known as the Civilian Health and Medical Program of the Uniformed Services (CHAMPUS). This program allows dependents and families to obtain health care from private clinics and practitioners, local hospitals, and HMOs when similar services are not available from a nearby military base.

A second program, the Veterans Administration (VA) health care system, is a hospital and long-term care system that exists to care for retired and disabled military personnel. A hospital clinic system is available for complicated ambulatory services, but most simple ambulatory services are obtained through other systems of care. The VA health care system is probably the largest long-term care provider in the United States and is funded through an annual appropriation from Congress.

Health Care Reform

The current health care delivery system is undergoing dramatic changes. Advances in research and technology have resulted in the most sophisticated care in the world, and the most costly. At the same time, millions of Americans have limited or no access to health care services. When the uninsured do receive care, it is often in costly emergency rooms and after the condition has become unnecessarily complex. Uncompensated care is on the rise, and many providers are limiting their numbers or refusing to care for uninsured or underinsured clients. Clients without a regular provider are often forced to seek care in emergency rooms, where care is often fragmented, after conditions have become serious. Consequently, it is not surprising that health care reform draws many supporters.

Health care reform is not a new issue. Major legislative initiatives directed at health care reform were proposed seven times during the 20th century. The administrations of Roosevelt, Truman, Kennedy, Nixon, Ford, Carter, and Clinton all attempted to design some type of health care reform. Only the Social Security Act, supported by President Kennedy before his death, passed successfully.

Each time, the need for health care reform was based on the need to control health care costs while providing access to quality health care services to increasing numbers of people. Before 1993, the prototypes for Clinton's health care reform bill had been debated through three elections and defeated by two legislatures because of concerns about increased costs and governmental control.

A massive reorganization attempt was started during the first year of President Clinton's administration under the direction of Hillary Clinton. The plan, based on the concept of **managed competition,** would have guaranteed all individuals access to a basic benefit package of selected primary and preventive services while ensuring cost containment and quality care. The benefits would have been financed by employers, individuals, or (in the case of unemployed, indigent individuals) the government.

The failure of the Clinton plan is generally attributed to a number of structural, strategic, and tactical mistakes (Shi & Singh, 1998). The opposition was well organized, the President had differences within his own party, the plan was too complex, the drafters of the plans were politically naive, and the President's political base of support was narrow. The arguments that were most often heard were that the plan was too expensive and too confusing and taxpayers did not want to pay for health care for poor people. The failure of the plan left the United States and South Africa as the only major industrialized nations in the world without some form of universal insurance coverage. Although the reform package was never passed, health care changes did occur.

Current U.S. Health Care Delivery System

In response to a need for change, a number of new and innovative organizations are emerging, and many traditional components of the system are in transition. A single hospital operating independently or a physician in an individual practice is becoming unusual. Hospitals, physicians, clinics, and other providers have been forced into a variety of interrelated systems. Growth and consolidation of smaller providers into larger organizations, horizontal and vertical integration of services within organizations, changes from government-owned facilities to private nonprofit and for-profit facilities, and diversification of traditional health care services are occurring at an amazing rate (Lee & Estes, 1997). Large purchasers of medical services are demanding wholesale prices for services and even dictating terms. Insurance coverage is constantly changing and client choices have been reduced.

Levels of Care

Our health care delivery system provides six basic levels of care: preventive, primary, secondary, tertiary, restorative, and continuing or long-term health care. Preventive care includes education and screening programs. Primary care includes services directed at reducing the potential for a disease through continuous, coordinated, and comprehensive care. **Preventive care** and **primary care** generally take place in the primary care provider's office. Secondary care is concerned with early detection and treatment of acute illness and injury to prevent disability and mortality. Secondary care usually occurs in the primary care provider's office or in a community hospital. Tertiary care is concerned with slowing the progression of established disease, preventing further disability, and improving the individual's degree of functioning. Tertiary care sometimes occurs in community hospitals and sometimes in large medical referral centers.

Restorative care includes hospice and chronic care and occurs in hospitals or special rehabilitation facilities. Long-term care occurs in long-term care facilities such as nursing homes and hospice facilities. Historically, this country has focused most of its resources on tertiary care provided in large medical care institutions.

Health Care Providers

Registered nurses and physicians are the two largest groups of health-care professionals, but as health care has become more complex, the number and variety of providers has increased proportionately. The American Medical Association identified 29 allied health training occupations accredited through the association's Committee on Allied Health Education and Accreditation, as described in the following sections.

Physicians

Physicians make up the second largest group of health care professionals. A total of 463,870 physicians are currently practicing in the United States (U.S. Department of Labor, 1998). They diagnose and treat clients in an attempt to cure or improve their clients' conditions. Physicians may be allopathic (MDs) or osteopathic (DOs). In the past, most physicians were in solo practice. Today, many physicians are joining group practices or contracting with health care corporations. By joining groups, physicians are able to spread their workload and their risks.

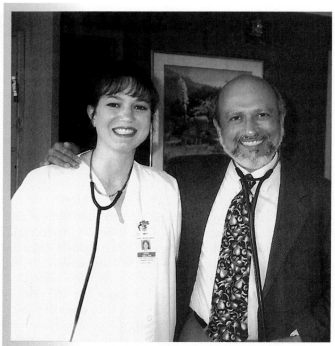

Physicians and nurses work in acute care settings in collaboration to improve health of clients.

Nurses

Nurses make up the largest group of health care providers. There are 2,007,030 nurses employed in the United States (U.S. Department of Labor, 1998). Approximately 66% of all nurses work in hospitals, 10% work in community/public health, 8% in ambulatory care, and 7% in nursing homes and extended care (ANA, 1998). Nurses both deliver and coordinate health care for clients within settings and across sites, collaborate with physicians, and carry out day-to-day treatments and care.

More than 140,000 registered nurses have the education and credentials to call themselves advanced practice nurses (ANA, 1998). The category "advanced practice nurse" contains several different specialty areas, including clinical nurse specialists, nurse practitioners, nurse midwives, and nurse anesthetists. These advanced roles have grown over the years, usually in response to a physician shortage or a physician maldistribution. Each role has its own certification, rules and regulations, and state recognition process. Nurses are at an important juncture in the development of the profession. They currently have the opportunity to show their value in providing quality care at a reasonable cost while obtaining positive client outcomes.

Physician Assistants

The physician assistant (PA) role is new to the health care delivery system. The first training program for PAs was started at Duke University in 1965. In 1995, there were 80 PA programs in the United States (Fowkes & Mentink, 1997). Approximately 35,898 PAs are currently practicing in the United States (AAPA, 1998). The PA training program is typically the last 2 years of an undergraduate degree program and focuses on medical science and clinical skills. PAs work directly under the supervision and license of physicians, who are responsible for their performance. PAs can provide various medical services, such as history taking and physical examinations, minor medical diagnosis and care, follow-up care for acute and chronically ill clients, hospital rounds, surgical assistance, and so on.

Specialized Care Providers

Within the health care delivery system, certain groups of professionals provide focused care services. Examples are clinical psychologists, dentists, podiatrists, and optometrists. These professionals are licensed, although standards vary from state to state. They are usually addressed as "doctor," and in some areas, they may have prescriptive authority and hospital privileges (i.e., they can admit and treat clients in a hospital setting). Their education is in depth in their specialty areas at a master's level or higher.

Technicians/Therapists

Many people who provide ancillary health care services are called *technicians* or *technologists;* examples include the medical laboratory technician or medical technologist, the medical record technician, the x-ray technician, and the dietary technician. Other ancillary health care professionals are called *therapists;* examples are respiratory, occupational, physical, mental health, and speech therapists. Each is educated and licensed to provide a specific service and are educated at a bachelor's level or higher.

Other Providers

Other providers include professionals such as pharmacists and social workers. Pharmacists are specialists in the science of drugs and can make recommendations about drug therapy. Most programs preparing pharmacists are 5 years long and include an internship. Pharmacists make up the third largest group of health care providers.

Social workers are assuming increasingly important roles in today's health care delivery system. These professionals counsel clients and families, often directing them to various health care resources, and may also be involved in discharge planning.

Chaplains address the spiritual and emotional needs of clients and families from a nondenominational perspective.

Health Care Settings

Services may be provided in traditional settings, such as hospitals, nursing homes, physicians' offices, ambulatory clinics, and homes. Today, services may also be provided in less traditional settings such as shelters, shopping malls, homeless shelters, pharmacies, schools, and job sites.

Acute Care Facilities

Hospitals, or acute care facilities, make up the largest component of the U.S. health care delivery system and account for 40% of the total personal health expenditures in 1991 (U.S. Department of Commerce, 1997). Hospitals include federal, state, and local government facilities and those owned by private organizations. Privately owned hospitals include voluntary (not for profit) or proprietary (for-profit) hospitals. Religious or charitable groups operate voluntary hospitals and may be independent or represent health maintenance organizations or cooperatives. Individuals, partnerships, or corporations own proprietary hospitals. The last decade has seen an increase in investor-owned hospital corporations; the stock of these large corporations is traded on the stock exchange.

In the current health care market, many hospitals have established home health agencies to help clients as they transition from the hospital to the home environment. Community health nurses can provide a critical link between hospital care and home care.

Short-Term Specialized Care Facilities

Some facilities, such as mental health centers, substance abuse facilities, and rehabilitation centers, offer very specialized services, and clients are admitted for a short-term stay to learn how to function with their disability(ies). Another example of a short-term facility is a respite care facility that provides temporary inpatient services for individuals who are usually cared for at home. The purpose of respite care is to offer relief to the informal caregiver, usually a family member.

Short-term facilities may be part of a network of coordinated services or a single independent entity. Centers may be staffed with a variety of health care providers, including physicians, nurses, and social workers.

Short-term specialized care facilities discharge clients into the community after short stays. Community health nurses could provide family and home assessments to determine the client's needs upon discharge and serve as a resource to clients once they are at home.

Long-Term Facilities

Long-term care may be defined as a wide range of social, personal, and health care services in addition to medical care. These services may include arranging social functions, exercise classes, and shopping trips to improve mental and physical function. The services might also include assistance with eating and bathing, arranging for therapy sessions, dental treatments, and visits by health care providers. These services may be needed by older individuals or individuals who have lost their ability to care for themselves through disease or injury. Long-term care focuses on maintaining as much function as possible and emphasizes activities of daily living (basic needs such as eating, dressing, bathing, and ambulating).

Most long-term care occurs in nursing homes but may also take place in a variety of other ways, such as assisted living facilities, hospice organizations, and home health care agencies. Community health nurses have excellent skills at assessing community resources and individualized client needs in each of these long-term care modalities.

Ambulatory Care Sites

Clients can receive care for conditions not requiring hospitalization at ambulatory care sites. Clinics and physicians' offices are the most common types of ambulatory sites, but this category would also include specially equipped trucks and buses that make scheduled stops in underserved areas. Many ambulatory care sites are affiliated with hospitals, but others operate independently. Traditional "walk-in" clinics have existed for many years and are often supported by government funding or charitable organizations. People often use the clinics in lieu of a personal physician. Centers may operate on an appointment or drop-in basis. Some clinics are specialized, such as family-planning clinics or those offering only women's health care services, and nurse practitioners or PAs often provide the care. Community health nurses can provide essential services in assisting clients while they try to meet their health care needs and stay at home.

Rural Health Centers

Rural health centers were developed as a result of federal funding and the need to provide care in rural, impoverished areas with few or no local physicians. Teams of residents and physicians from medical centers, along with nurse practitioners and PAs, often provide much of the care in rural health centers. These providers may cover several clinics on a rotating basis. Community health nurses play an important role in providing continuity in the care of clients who are often seen by many different providers.

Day-Care Centers

Day-care centers target specific client populations; for instance, many day-care centers serve elderly clients who cannot be left alone for long periods but who can carry out activities of daily living. Other day-care centers serve clients who are physically or mentally challenged, such as those with cerebral palsy or Down syndrome, or those who have chemical dependencies. These centers care for clients when family members are working and offer services such as meals, rehabilitation, and occupational therapy. Because the primary needs of these clients are in the area of personal care needs, nurses play an important role in these facilities.

Hospice

A hospice, run by public or private agencies, is designed to care for terminally ill clients and their families by providing noncuring, supportive, and palliative services. Many clients receiving these services have cancer, although conditions such as AIDS, multiple sclerosis, or end-stage renal disease may also require hospice care. Although nurses play the major role, a team approach, including physicians, therapists, volunteers, and clergy, is often used. Nursing activities focus on managing pain, treating symptoms, and preparing the client and family for death and bereavement.

Retirement Communities

In the last 20 years, the number of retirement communities in the United States has increased significantly. These communities take many forms, such as entire small towns, retirement subdivisions, apartments or condominiums, and continuing-care communities. Although the services vary, retirement communities usually provide a number of levels of care. In an arrangement known as assisted living, older people live independently but have care nearby if needed. A convalescent center may be associated with the facility, and services such as physical and occupational therapy may be provided. Other health care services such as dental care may also be available. Residents are guaranteed access to various health care services, and the financial responsibilities are spread over the entire community. Some of the fees, such as entry fees, must be prepaid and may be very expensive. Entry fees and monthly maintenance fees are often high, thus limiting access to some of these facilities to more affluent retirees.

Home Health Care

As prospective payment has forced clients to be discharged from hospitals earlier, home health care has become an essential part of the health care delivery system. Care is provided by registered nurses skilled in assessment and practical nurses and aides trained to provide safe client care. Agencies receiving Medicare reimbursement must be certified and must meet certain conditions and federal standards.

Technology, previously found only in hospitals, is now provided by home care agencies. Treatments may include such things as intravenous feedings and medications, ventilators, portable dialysis machines, and cardiac monitoring. Although home health care has changed dramatically, it is still the traditional practice area for community health nurses. In addition to skilled nursing care, home health care may include services such as physical, occupational, or speech therapy, homemaker services, and home-delivered meals.

Alternative Health Care

Alternative health care involves nontraditional treatments such as acupressure, acupuncture, therapeutic touch, herbal treatments, hypnosis and imagery, and homeopathy. Alternative health care treatments are now being studied to see how they can be used to support more traditional medical plans of care. Congress established the Office of Alternative Medicine in 1992 to sponsor research in this field to attempt to determine the value of nontraditional treatments on client outcomes. Nurses have often been supportive of and practiced alternative health care. Current research has recently focused more attention on some of these modalities and made them more acceptable in mainstream health care.

Issues Affecting Delivery of Health Care Services

Many issues have contributed to the growth, complexity, and expense of our health care delivery system such as deregulation, consumerism, technology, the graying of America, and our litigious society. Local, state, and federal governments have attempted to address these issues at one time or another. However, short-term fixes for any one factor have had little impact on the overall problem.

Deregulation

In the last few years, the United States has experienced deregulation of health care. The result has been a proliferation of facilities and technology (e.g., computed tomography [CT] scans and magnetic resonance imaging [MRI]) in some urban areas, which has resulted in excess capacity and, in turn, increased expensive competition. This expense is passed along to the clients, and maldistribution of essential services is seen in underserved areas. Competition as a price control strategy has not helped control health care costs. Americans still want the specialist, the newest technology, the cutting edge treatment, and the hospital that looks like a four-star hotel. They simply hope their insurance will pay for it.

Focus on Secondary and Tertiary Health Care Services

Historically, we have allocated the majority of our resources to the care that occurs after the client has become critically ill. Vast amounts of money are spent on critical care units, technical procedures, and sophisticated surgical techniques, but little money has been spent preventing the illness in the first place. Education and screening services are often not reimbursed by third-party payers and are undervalued by busy providers. Although MCOs often say they value what these preventive services can accomplish, the cost is often more than they wish to pay. As a result, managed care often makes decisions about which preventive services are the most valuable and ignore the rest.

Increasing Consumerism

Health care consumerism is the public's involvement in determining the type, quality, and cost of their health care. Today, consumers are reading, looking up information, subscribing to newsletters specializing in their health care problem, and attending support groups. They are better informed and are asserting their right to have an active part in decisions related to their care.

In the past, the poor often either went without health care or had to be satisfied with a lesser quality of care. However, values are changing, and equal access to health care is now viewed by many as a right.

Technological Advances

Advances made in technology have drastically changed health care and altered how physicians treat hospitalized clients. For example, the life expectancy of a client with diabetes has increased considerably. New chemotherapy treatments have extended cancer clients' lives and, in some cases, greatly increased the quality of their lives. Heart, lung, and liver transplants, unheard of three decades ago, have become commonplace. The latest antibiotic therapies ward off deadly diseases. All these advances have reduced hospital stays and allowed people to live longer.

The new technology is expensive, and some advances have raised formidable ethical questions. If you can extend the life of an 80-year-old man for a short time by putting him on a ventilator, should you do it? If you can keep a premature baby alive on life support but you know that the child has multiple irreparable problems that will result in incredible future costs, should you do it? For the cost of the care of one elderly man on a ventilator for several weeks, you could provide prenatal care to a large group of pregnant women.

Increasing Longevity of Americans

Americans born in 1995 can expect to live an average of 76 years (men 73, women 80), compared with 47.3 years for those born in 1900 (U.S. Department of Commerce, 1997). The fastest-growing age group is people 85 and older. Because the heaviest users of health services are the elderly, more emphasis is being placed on their needs, the need for services has increased, and gerontology has become a significant branch of medicine and nursing. Topics such as living wills and powers of attorney are becoming more widely discussed as people become concerned about their ability to maintain life, as well as the quality of that life.

Defensive Medicine and Government Regulation

The cost of defensive medicine and government regulations has been a major factor affecting the delivery of health care in this country. Physicians are often forced to pay extremely high costs for malpractice insurance and attorney fees when they are sued. As a result, some physicians have simply stopped offering high-risk services such as obstetrics or they have stopped providing care to indigent clients as a way to increase their profits.

Physicians also tend to practice defensive medicine by ordering more tests or more expensive treatments. In addition, increased government regulation has caused many physicians to increase their office staff, reduce their client load, or join health care systems where billing services are provided. The results of the increased costs are that the physician must become much more cost conscious and health care has become a business rather than a service.

> **BOX 5-3 FACTORS AFFECTING HEALTH CARE DELIVERY**
>
> - Failure of competition as a strategy following deregulation of health care
> - Emphasis on secondary and tertiary health care instead of prevention
> - Increasing consumerism
> - Escalating cost of technology
> - Aging of the population
> - Cost of defensive medicine
> - Government regulation and administrative costs

Managed Care

Total integration of services is expected to be the future economic structure of the health care delivery system. Networks are expected to compete for clients by becoming more efficient, charging lower prices, offering a wider range of services, and ensuring quality care for a fixed cost for the individual. They will maintain a central database to ensure comprehensive care as the client moves from provider to provider within the system. These networks are called managed care.

Managed Care Delivery Systems

The concept of **managed care** encompasses a wide variety of organizational structures and is quickly becoming the dominant management strategy of our health care delivery system. By definition, *managed care* refers to a system that, for a set fee, assumes responsibility and accountability for the health of a population through the use of effective, responsible, and cost-efficient care.

> Managed care integrates the financing and delivery of health care services to covered individuals, most often by arrangements with providers. These systems offer packages of health care benefits, explicit standards for the selection of health care providers, formal programs for ongoing quality assurance and utilization review, significant financial incentives for its members to use providers, and procedures associated with the plan (ANA, 1998).

MCOs made their appearance in the 1970s and 1980s as the insurance industry was faced with employers starting to self-insure and health care costs that were soaring. The huge reserves of money that insurance companies had previously invested were being depleted. Strategically thinking insurance companies redefined their market and began developing managed care organizations. Today, managed care involves some 70 million Americans (Herzlinger, 1997).

The goals of managed care are achieved by keeping clients healthy and treating them in the lowest-cost setting using providers that have also agreed to provide services at a reduced rate. Under this system, primary care replaces the hospital as the center of care. The goal is to keep people out of the hospital, not to keep the hospital beds full. More treatments and care are provided in clinics and physicians' offices. Ambulatory clients go home to recover from surgery rather than upstairs for a leisurely recovery in a private room.

Managed care has transformed health care from a service industry into a competitive, market-driven business. The question now is whether health care decisions are made based on the client's needs or the need to show a profit for the organization and its stakeholders. Who is making the decisions about treatment options, and who is caring for the client with complex, multisystem problems? Is the cheapest treatment the best treatment? All of these questions are currently without answers.

If managed care looks at the long-term answer to client care questions, the answer lies in the premise that a healthy client is cheaper to care for that an unhealthy one. Therefore, preventive care is the only answer. If managed care looks at the short-term answer, then cheaper is better.

Managed Care Organizations

The majority of MCOs can be categorized into three basic types: HMOs, PPOs, and PSOs. **Capitation** refers to the amount of money that is paid to an HMO to cover the cost of health care for a group of clients. An agency or organization representing a group of individuals seeking health care contracts with a group of providers and pays a predetermined fee periodically, usually quarterly.

Health Maintenance Organizations

Federally recognized **health maintenance organizations (HMOs)** are prepaid health management plans that offer an organized system for providing a predetermined set of health care services in a geographic area to a voluntarily enrolled group of people for an established fee. This system combines traditional insurance and health care delivery in one organization and provides a wide range of services, including inpatient and outpatient hospital care, infertility and mental health services, therapeutic x-ray treatments, alcohol and drug addiction treatment, and physical therapy.

HMOs were first established in 1973 under a federal program. The number of HMOs in existence grew from 175 in 1976 to 556 in 1992 (U.S. Department of Commerce, 1997). Enrollment is voluntary; members have the option to select another plan. Because the fee paid by members is fixed annually, the organization tries to minimize costs. To do this, HMOs must place greater emphasis on health promotion and disease prevention. Some HMOs hire providers as employees and some contract with providers for services.

Preferred Provider Organizations

A **preferred provider organization (PPO)** is a type of managed care plan composed of a group of physicians, and possibly one or more hospitals, that get together and offer a prepaid health care plan to employers. In preferred provider arrangements, clients select their health care providers from the list of preferred providers and receive services at a discounted cost. If a consumer chooses to seek services from a provider who has not contracted with the plan, a substantial deductible fee is assessed or the service is not covered. In the future, PPOs are likely to grow larger with a wider range of providers.

Point-of-Service Plans

Point-of-service (POS) plans are also known as open-ended HMOs. POS plans provide a set of services that are covered under the established fee, but members are also given the choice of going out of the network for services. Members share in costs with the HMO if they decide to go out of the network for care.

Multilevel Integrated Systems

Integrated health care systems consist of a mix of many types of health care facilities and providers connected through different types of contractual arrangements. These complex systems will be able to supply a broad range of services, from in-house care to outpatient and from traditional to nontraditional care, within their own system (vertically integrated) or will arrange for the services to be provided by other systems (horizontally integrated). Primary care providers, hospitals, retirement communities, wellness centers, pharmacies, health food outlets, rehabilitation centers, counseling centers, and many other types of providers from a large geographical area will be connected and accessible to members.

The process of changing traditional systems into new, multilevel integrated systems is often complicated and emotionally difficult. The literature is full of words designed to make the transformation process sound less cold and calculating. The first term to appear was *downsizing,* which immediately was changed to *rightsizing.* This term simply refers to cutting the number of funded positions to decrease costs. *Redesigning* was the next term to make an appearance. Redesigning referred to the process of examining all job descriptions for equitable distribution of activities, role overlap, excess specialization, and waste. The next term to appear was *restructuring.* Restructuring refers to an assessment of the overall organizational structure in an attempt to improve productivity. Finally, *reengineering* refers to a comprehensive and often radical process to look at jobs and organizational structure as a way to form new relationships, new visions, and improved functioning and productivity. Future integrated health care systems will be larger and more comprehensive

Patient Care Outcomes

The term *patient care outcomes* refers to the consequences of care that the client receives or does not receive. Outcome studies are becoming very popular in MCOs as a way to predict and provide effective client care. Outcome studies look for trends over time in client status and adverse events. Adverse patient care outcomes are occurrences that are not expected as a result of the client's disease process or treatment. Data obtained from client care studies are used as a basis for decisions, the development of policies and procedures, and changes in health care practice.

Improved patient care outcomes involve assessing individual clients' care and recovery as well as large data sets from across the country and world. Large national databases will be used in the future to provide predictive information on which to base treatments, types of care, lengths of care, and level of provider needed to achieve positive outcomes.

Health Politics and Policy

How did our health care delivery system become so expensive? Who should pay for the ever-increasing costs of health care and hospitalization? These questions have become the basis for untold numbers of legislative reports, articles, studies, and documentaries. The astronomical cost of some forms of treatment has made it impossible for the average client to pay personally for needed medical, surgical, and nursing services. Single illness episode bills well above $10,000 are no longer the exception.

Many people rely on government interventions to help with soaring costs and inaccessible services.

Government Policy

Health insurance provides protection against the high cost of medical care and hospitalization arising from illness or injury. Most Americans look to their jobs for health insurance, but increasingly, insurance benefits are not available at work sites. The number of Americans who are uninsured or underinsured is increasing at an alarming rate. Americans have appealed to their legislators for help.

Government policy focuses on health care on several levels. Legislation establishes boards to govern the practice of health care professionals and health care agencies, establishes commissions to examine health care delivery and make recommendations, and sets guidelines for the payment of Medicare benefits. Medicare guidelines affect the entire health care industry because the government is the third-party payer for more than 40% of all expenditures in health care (U.S. Bureau of the Census, 1995).

The publication of *Healthy People 2010,* based on the progress made under *Healthy People 2000* goals, again moved forward the agenda of disease prevention and health promotion for all citizens (APHA, 1998). The majority of the goals for the year 2010 still fall into three categories: increasing the healthy life span, reducing health disparities, and increasing access to services. Before the publication of *Healthy People 2000,* these goals were not central in health legislation. However, in a time of increasing fiscal austerity, these goals make increasing sense. Keeping people well is much less costly then trying to cure or rehabilitate them.

Finally, there have been many debates about whether the United States should adopt a national health insurance plan or support market competition. Under a national plan, taxpayers would pay the government for the coverage, much as insurance companies currently collect funds from subscribers, and everyone would be covered at a predetermined basic level of services. The disadvantage is that government plans rarely operate very efficiently, and many people believe that it is inappropriate for government to meddle in individuals' health care decisions.

Market competition has been promoted as another way to keep health care costs at a reasonable level while ensuring quality care. Under this system, the government would allow a rivalry between health care providers for the purpose of attracting clients. However, an unequal distribution of the most ill clients might keep corporations from wanting to insure the very clients who need care the most.

Public Opinion and Special Interest Groups

Public opinion expressed through special interest groups is very influential in the development of public policy. Many special interest groups, such as the American Hospital Association, the American Medical Association, and the American Insurance Association, spend huge amounts of time and money providing legislators with information on which to base health care decisions. Many legislators lack an in-depth understanding of health care issues. As a result, information provided by special interest groups often serves as a basis for health care decisions. When that happens, decisions may fail to reflect the best interests of the majority.

Nursing and Health Care Policy

As the largest health care provider group, it is important for nurses to be both a visible and vocal advocate for quality health care. To meet that important goal, the American Nurses Association (ANA) has worked tirelessly over the years to develop an effective special interest group infrastructure. In response to the health care reform issue, the ANA formulated a position paper

RESEARCH BRIEF

Blegen, M., Goode, C., & Reed. L. (1998). Nurse staffing and patient outcomes. Nursing Research, 47(1), 43–50.

Hospitals today are faced with critical staff mix decisions. However, few studies have examined the effects of decreased numbers of staff registered nurses (RNs) on patient care outcomes. The purpose of this study was to examine the relationships among total hours of nursing care, registered nurse skill mix, and adverse patient care outcomes. Adverse outcomes were defined as unit rates of medication errors, client falls, skin breakdown, client and family complaints, infections, and deaths. Study sites included 42 inpatient units. The correlation among the variables were determined after controlling for client acuity.

Units with higher average client acuity had lower rates of medication errors and client falls but higher rates of the other adverse outcomes. With average client acuity on the unit controlled, the proportion of hours of care delivered by RNs was inversely related to the unit rates of medication errors, decubiti, and client complaints. Total hours of care by other nursing personnel were directly related to increased rates of decubiti, complaints, and mortality. An unexpected finding was that the relationship between the RN proportion of care was curvilinear; as the RN proportion increased, rates of adverse outcomes decreased up to 87.5%. Above that level, as RN proportion of care increased, the adverse outcome rates also increased. This finding was likely related to client acuity. The conclusion of the study was that the higher the RN skill mix, the lower the incidence of adverse occurrences on the client care unit.

that states that the U.S. health care system needs restructuring, wellness promotion must become our emphasis, and universal access to health care services must be developed.

The ANA has been politically active in several other areas, including health care rationing. With limited resources, the question of health care rationing must be addressed. Those with adequate insurance worry about restrictions, and the uninsured or underinsured worry that they will be excluded. Rationing can mean limiting access to care or limiting contact to the more expensive providers.

Through the years, the ANA and state organizations have continued to support legislation that ensures basic health care services for everyone. To influence policy, nurses need to vote and be politically active in their states and know what bills are being considered. To be politically active, you can work on someone's campaign, run for political office, support candidates financially, or simply stay in contact with elected state and federal officials and provide them with information when needed.

New Nursing Opportunities

As health care changes, the practice of nursing must also change. Nurses must stay knowledgeable about health care trends to make decisions about future careers. Those trends include growth in the health care workforce, economics as a driving force, changing demographics of the United States, transformation of individual providers into multilevel corporations with physicians becoming employees, the philosophical move from "everything for a few" to "an adequate amount for many," and the increased importance of ambulatory care and home health care (Huston & Fox, 1998). Some of the nursing roles related to these trends are discussed next. However, many future roles are yet to be created.

Advanced Practice Nurses

Advanced practice nursing is not a new category of nurses, but many of the traditional roles are changing. Nurse practitioners are moving into specialized areas such as geriatrics, acute care, and correction facilities health care. Clinical nurse specialists are becoming experts in case management, genetics, and comprehensive cancer care. Nurse anesthetists and nurse midwives are managing clients with specialized needs. Advanced practice nurses are prepared to work *with* physicians, not *for* them. As specialties develop, nurses are finding ways to become experts in those areas, and as more emphasis is placed on controlling health care costs, more providers will look to advanced practice nurses as providers of effective, quality, lower-cost care.

Entrepreneurs

In the future, more nurses than ever before will own nursing businesses. In areas like home health, health care management, insurance evaluation, nursing clinics, environmental evaluation, workplace health care, caregiver support, program evaluation, and respite care, the opportunities are endless. Nurses will be in a position to contract with larger systems for consulting services and the application of specialized knowledge and skills.

Data Management

Public and private agencies are looking for nurses who are skilled at creating and managing large databases containing client information. This field is known as *informatics*. Every health care organization is struggling with the need to maintain information in a safe but easily accessed manner. Data must be available for evaluation and decision making. Nurses with an understanding of client care data coupled with a working knowledge of computers, the workings of databases, and the use of evaluative statistics will be in the perfect position to fill these critical slots.

Research

We can no longer make decisions on the basis of what we have done before or what we think will work. Decisions must be based on data that can be seen, measured, and reproduced as needed integrated with sound clinical practice experience. We are moving into an age of evidence-based client care. Consequently, client care research is more important today than at any time in the past. Nurse researchers try to develop an understanding of essential client care issues on which to base practice. They may be employees of an organization or working on research project funded by the government or other organizations. Their work provides the structure for future practice that will "identify and apply the most efficacious interventions to maximize the quality and quantity of life for individual clients" (Sackett et al., 1997).

....

Our ancestors tithed in the hope of life after death; we hope for more and better life before death.

Robert G. Evans

....

....

I don't know the key to success, but the key to failure is trying to please everybody.

Bill Cosby

....

CONCLUSION

Some critics suggest that our health care system, which is supposed to guarantee access, innovation, and quality care, has instead become a system in crisis. A crisis exists in several areas: cost, availability, equity, efficiency, and responsiveness to public needs. This chapter contains a discussion of the history of our health care delivery system and descriptions of the changing components of that system. New roles for nursing are emerging as our health care system moves from one that was measured by the cost of its components to a system measured by the effectiveness of the care provided by its components.

CASE STUDY

A pregnant woman with severe epilepsy has presented to the health department from a local obstetrical practice. She had been working part-time at a local grocer until her seizures became unmanageable, and she is no longer employed. The client has been referred to the health department so that she can qualify for state funds for high-risk maternity care. The client's husband works for a local manufacturing company and has HMO coverage for both himself and his wife through a company-sponsored managed care plan. The deductible and co-payment are more than the couple can afford to pay, and they would like to find other resources to pay for the additional services needed to manage the epilepsy. The public health nurse checks with the state high-risk maternity care program and finds that the couple exceeds the income criteria and most likely will not qualify.

1. What are possible health and economic consequences if the client's health is not managed appropriately during pregnancy?

2. What system problems can you identify from the situation that result in ethical issues of treatment and care?

3. Who is responsible for seeing that this client receives appropriate care at an affordable cost?

CRITICAL THINKING ACTIVITIES

1. You are a 28-year-old single mother with three children. You are having pain in your stomach and trouble sleeping. You have no money and no insurance. How will you get someone to help you? What will you do if you need medication?

2. You are a 22-year-old single parent with two children ages 1 and 3. Your mother is unemployed and watches the children while you work. Your job does not provide you with insurance. Your pay is too high to allow you to be eligible for Medicaid and too low to allow you to afford insurance. What types of services do you need from the Health Department?

3. In a world of limited resources, developing equitable health policies involves many difficult decisions. How would you answer the following questions?

   - Should an 85-year-old man with debilitating emphysema be placed on a respirator?

   - Should a 78-year-old woman with breast cancer be put on chemotherapy?

   - Should major health insurance plans reimburse for experimental treatments?

   - Should an insurance plan be required to pay for a liver transplant for an alcoholic?

   - Should a baby with multiple incurable birth defects be placed in a neonatal intensive care unit?

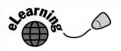

Explore Community Health Nursing on the web! To learn more about the topics in this chapter, use the passcode provided to access your exclusive web site: http://communitynursing.jbpub.com
If you do not have a passcode, you can obtain one at this site.

REFERENCES

American Academy of Physician Assistants. (1998). *Physician assistants—statistics.* www.aapa.org

American Nurses Association (ANA). (1998). Managed care: challenges and opportunities for nursing. *Nursing facts.* www.nursingworld.org/readroom/fsmgdcar.htm

Children's Defense Fund (1998). *Children's Defense Fund: Healthy start FAQs.* www.childrensdefense.org/facts_america98.html

American Public Health Association (APHA). (1998). *Healthy people 2010 objectives.* Washington, DC: Author.

Fairbanks, J., & Wiese, W. H. (1998). *The public health primer.* Thousand Oaks, CA: Sage Publications.

Feldstein, P. (1999). *Health care economics.* Albany, NY: Delmar Publishing.

Fowkes, V. K., & Mentink, J. (1997). Nurses and physician assistants: issues and challenges. In J. C. McCloskey & H. K. Grace (Eds.), *Current issues in nursing.* St. Louis: Mosby.

Herzlinger, R. (1997). *Market driven health care: who wins, who loses in the transformation of America's largest service industry.* Redwood City, CA: Addison-Wesley.

Health Care Financing Agency (HCFA). (1998). *National health expenditures projections: 1998–2008.* www.hcfa.gov/stats/nhe%2Dproj/proj1998/hilites.htm

Huston, C., & Fox, S. (1998). The changing health care market: Implications for nursing education in the coming decade. *Nursing Outlook, 46,* 109–114.

Johnson, C., & Broder, D. (1996). *The system: The American way of politics at the breaking point.* Boston: Little, Brown.

Keck, C. W., & Scutchfield, F. D. (1997). *Principles of public health practice.* Albany, NY: Delmar Publishers.

Lee, P. R., & Estes, C. L. (1997). *The nation's health* (5th ed.). Sudbury, MA: Jones and Bartlett.

Sackett, D. L., Rosenbergm W. C., Grant, J. A., Haynes, R. B., & Richardson, W. S. (1997). In P. R. Lee & C. L. Estes (Eds.), *The nation's health* (5th ed.). Sudbury, MA: Jones and Bartlett.

Salmon, M. (1997). Nursing practice in a political era. In J. C. McCloskey & H. K. Grace (Eds.), *Current issues in nursing.* St. Louis: Mosby.

Shi, L., & Singh, D. (1998). *Delivering health care in America: a systems approach.* Gaithersburg, MD: Aspen Publishers.

U.S. Bureau of the Census. (1995). Health insurance coverage by selected characteristics. *Annual demographic survey.* http://ferret.bls.census.gov/macro/031996/health/2_000.htm

U.S. Department of Commerce. (1997). *National health expenditures.* www.hcfa.gov/stats.nhe%2Doact/nhe.htm

U.S. Department of Labor. (1998). *1997 National employment and wage estimates.* http://stats.bls.gov/oes/national/oes_prof.htm

U.S. Health and Human Services. (1999). *National health expenditures projections: 1998–2008.* www.hcfa.gov/stats/nhe%2Doact/nhe.htm

U.S. National Center for Health Statistics. (1997). *National health statistics.* www.cdc.gov/nchswww/default.htm

U.S. National Center for Health Statistics. (1998). *National health statistics.* www.cdc.gov/nchswww/default.htm

Williams, S., & Torrens, P. (1999). *Introduction to health services.* Albany, NY: Delmar Publishers.

Chapter 6
Managed Care
Ann H. Cary

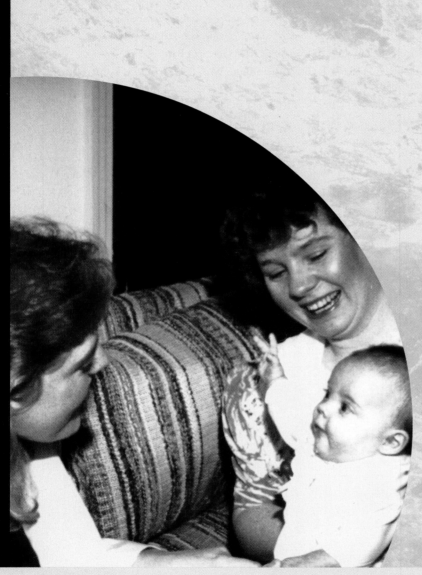

Nursing is managed care . . . Since the beginning of the century, expert nurses have been shepherding the care of acute and chronic patients in homes, clinics, and hospitals. Much has changed since those early days, but much has stayed the same. It's our job as nurses to develop a strong enough understanding of the needs of the system, of our own skills and strengths and those of our communities, that we can— collectively and individually—actively help craft the emerging system.

B. B Gray in Turner, 1999a, p. xii

QUESTIONS TO CONSIDER

After reading this chapter, answer the following questions:

1. What are the forces driving the development of managed care delivery systems?
2. What are the key principles of managed care?
3. What are the differences among managed care delivery models?
4. What are the requirements for credentialing for delivery systems?
5. What are the roles/skills of nurses working in managed care?
6. How can information about managed care be accessed via web sites?

KEY TERMS

Benefits interpreter
Capitated payment
Case or care manager
Community nursing
organizations (CNOs)
Co-payments
Deductibles
Fee-for-service plans
Gatekeeper

Health maintenance
organization (HMO)
Health plan employer
data and information
set (HEDIS)
Indemnity plans
Managed care
National Committee on
Quality Assurance (NCQA)

Pathfinder
Patient advocate
Physician hospital
organization (PHO)
Point-of-service plan
Preferred provider
organization (PPO)
Primary care provider

Provider liaison
Quality Compass
Risk manager
Safety net system
Self-insured plans
Triage nurse
Utilization and resource
reviewer

What Is Managed Care?

Managed care is a health care system that incorporates both financing and delivery of services. Typically, individuals join, enroll, or subscribe to a managed care plan. These individuals are known as the *covered lives* or *population* of the managed care organization (MCO). Subscribers or enrollees have health services provided by the organization in accordance with the coverage (services) identified in their contracts.

Financing and payment for managed care is typically prepaid so that a specific dollar amount is established to cover the projected costs of all health care for the enrollee. Payment to the plan/provider may be on a monthly or annual basis. In return for the **capitated payment** (per person payment fee) arranged between the plan/provider and the payer (employer, government funder, and/or self-payer) enrollees receive a package of health care benefits, standardized selection processes for their providers, quality and utilization management reviews of their care, and financial incentives for using the plan procedures (ANA, 1995; May, Schraeder, & Britt, 1996).

Managed care systems are clothed in many different costumes and called by a variety of names. As a consumer of health services at the turn of the century, you have likely used managed care services in at least one of its many forms. Likewise, as a health professional employed in delivery systems, you will need to know the expectations for your practice. Managed care clearly targets a population of patients who are enrolled in or subscribed to a particular system and values population-based outcomes by providers. Examples of this view of population-practice as a defining characteristic of managed care employers may include immunization and mammogram rates, access to primary care practitioners, and arrangements with public health, educational, and social service organizations (HEDIS, 1999).

Health care delivery continues to respond to market demands and state and federal policies. It is likely that health care systems in your community may look different from systems in other states or communities. Managed care systems have not appeared overnight and have been shaped by many architects. These systems are responding to employer demand to reduce the costs of the health care benefit for employees. Federal and state funding of Medicare and Medicaid services have followed the lead of non-government employers to demand cost effective and quality access to appropriate health services. Consumers in communities without managed care systems have seen out-of-pocket expenses for their own care needs rise. Health care system boards and corporate stockholders have argued for the financial health of the corporation as well as corporate investment in the community.

The values of these stakeholders have encouraged the presence of managed care in communities; however, the degree of penetration or market presence of managed care is dissimilar, especially relative to the Medicaid population. While costs of health services are the initial drivers of managed care systems, only those that provide cost-effective, quality plans will remain viable to the community. Clearly, nurses play a role in designing, implementing, and evaluating health care services for managed care populations

In contrast, the prevailing system prior to managed care is known as the *fee-for-service system*. In **fee-for-service plans,** providers deliver a service, set a fee for the service, and receive reimbursement from a payer (health insurance company, individual, or government) for the fee charged or allowed. These health insurance plans are traditionally called **indemnity plans.** The incentive to fee-for-service providers is to increase revenues by charging higher fees and generating more services. For example, the more a patient visits a physician, the more money that physician makes. Fee-for-service provider reimbursement has encouraged more billable services than may have been appropriate and increased the administrative cost of health care as a result of billing, review, and payment activities to each provider, for each patient served, for each visit.

The fee-for-service system, dominant in the 20th century, has been viewed as a major force in escalating costs and strained employer, government, and individual budgets. Managed care, initiated in the 1920s, has moved from a gradual to a frantic pace in U.S. health care in the 1990s and is now a corrective force for reestablishing a balance in cost, quality, and access to services for patients, payers, and providers. For example, in 1997 more than 75% of employees received care from managed care plans. Additionally, legislation has been passed to provide incentives for Medicare and Medicaid enrollees to access managed care systems (Rapaport, 1997).

Principles of Managed Care

The following are the fundamentals of managed care systems:

1. *All health care choices have a price, and choices for service are made by providers, clients/consumers, and administrators of health plans. All parties who choose are held accountable for the financial burden of the resources chosen. The more one party exercises the freedom of choice in health-related services (or selects services outside those services covered by an insurance plan), the greater the cost to that party (Packard, 1997; Spitzer-Lehmann, 1996).*

2. *Care is population based. The health status and actuarial data of enrolled and targeted populations support the structure and process of health care delivery. For example, the construction of health care teams and use of disease management protocols will be influenced by the number of diabetics or asthmatics represented in the health plan. Population-based outcomes such as* **health plan employer data and information set (HEDIS)** *measures are inherent values of mature managed care providers and credentialing bodies (Spitzer-Lehmann, 1996).*

3. *An MCO uses financial, clinical, community, policy, personal, and administrative information as the basis for en-*

suring quality and value (Spitzer-Lehmann, 1996). Obtaining and managing information is critical.

4. *Primary care is central. Clients must seek referrals from a primary care provider who is responsible for coordinating care before receiving services of a medical specialist (Spitzer-Lehmann, 1996).*

5. *Integration and interdependence from a systems perspective is critical (e.g., provider mix, seamless information flow, coordination). Continuity and integration of clinical and financial services is important to strong managed care.*

6. *Financing and delivery are linked in managed care systems (Spitzer-Lehmann, 1996).*

7. *Consumers have rights in managed care systems. In December 1997, President Clinton's Advisory Commission on Consumer Protection and Quality in the Health Care Industry issued its* Principles and Consumer Bill of Rights, *which are now incorporated in all federally supported health care activities. Four principles guiding the* Consumer Bill of Rights and Responsibilities *in accessing and receiving health care include the following:*

   • *All health care consumers are created equal.*

   • *Quality comes first in health care.*

   • *The parts of the health care system that work are preserved.*

   • *Costs matter and must be identified and related to outcomes of health care.*

Box 6-1 lists the eight rights and responsibilities of consumer health care services that support the principles of managed care noted by Spitzer-Lehman (1996).

Beck and Demsey (1996) reveal that successful managed care models are noted for pricing practices, defined provider networks, risk-sharing of costs, and care management techniques. For instance, when an MCO sets prices, it may use mathematical models to predict what costs will be influenced by the cost of living data for the region, will use and encounter patterns of enrollees, will determine age and sex of enrollees, and will examine the nature of health care management in the system. Discounts are typically applied to providers in the system because this is a method to increase volume or reduce the chance of losing volume of payment. Managed care models use capitation pricing to pay providers a fixed amount per member per month to provide all defined services. Providers may be protected from situations where premiums do not cover costs, such as in catastrophic cases (e.g., patients with human immunodeficiency virus [HIV], transplants, multisystem failure), with the MCO agreeing to pay the provider by a fee-for-service method above a certain amount (e.g., $15,000). Conversely, providers (physicians and nurse practitioners) share in the risks of using more resources than forecasted or budgeted by having payments withheld from them; however, when the MCO has a financial surplus, providers may share in the distribution of bonuses or stock. For the MCO to provide for all needed services, it contracts with myriad providers

---

BOX 6-1 CONSUMER BILL OF RIGHTS AND RESPONSIBILITIES, 1997

Consumers rights in health care include the following:

• Accurate, literacy-appropriate information

• Choice of provider sufficient to ensure quality care

• Access to appropriate (a prudent layperson's definition of) emergency care

• Participative decision making relative to health care options

• Respectful and nondiscriminatory care

• Confidentiality and access to own health information

• Fair and efficient process for complaints/appeals

• Assumption of responsibility for health, decision making, and treatment plans

Source: Advisory Commission on Consumer Protection and Quality in the Health Care Industry. (1997). Consumer bill of rights and responsibilities: Report to the President of the United States. *Washington, D.C.: U.S. Government Printing Office.*

(psychiatrists, home health agencies, pharmacies, durable medical equipment suppliers) to guarantee coverage for benefits.

Care management techniques examine the use of services, costs, and performance measures of providers. Some of these measures include controls on referrals, preauthorization for services (e.g., for diagnostics and emergency care), number and costs of prescriptions written, and frequency of office visits. As is apparent, each of these activities require capabilities in database information development and management to provide answers to the following questions: What do we provide; to whom; what are the outcomes; how do we compare; what do patients think of services; how can we perform consistent with our targets; and what are our trends?

Managed Care Models
Health Maintenance Organizations

The **health maintenance organization (HMO)** is a type of managed care system that provides or arranges designated services requested by members for a fixed (capitated/prepaid) premium. In accordance with the Health Maintenance Organization Act, an HMO has three required characteristics:

1. *An organized system for providing or ensuring health care in a geographic area*

2. A set of basic and supplemental health maintenance and treatment services

3. Voluntarily enrolled populations (May, Schraeder, & Britt, 1996)

Even within this description of the HMO, there are at least four types of HMO models (ANA, 1995):

1. Staff model, in which providers are salaried employees of the organization.

2. Independent practice associations (IPA), which are separate legal entities that contract with an HMO for fees but continue to provide care in the individual or group practice to non-HMO enrollees. HMO enrollees must select only among IPA providers.

3. Group models, which negotiate with a multispecialty group of providers to deliver care to HMO members. These non-HMO-employee providers receive fees at a negotiated rate.

4. Network models, which contract with two or more independent group practices to provide care at a capitated rate.

Preferred Providers Organizations

A second model of managed care is the **preferred provider organization (PPO),** which contracts with independent providers for a negotiated, discounted fee-for-service to its members. The providers under contract are called *preferred providers.* Should the member use the PPO provider, the out-of-pocket expenses are much lower than when using a nonparticipating provider. Physician and advanced practice registered nurse (APRN) providers in these systems practice solo or in group settings. The quality of practice is monitored, and cost and patient satisfaction data to support "best practices" are collected (May, Schraeder, & Britt, 1996).

Physician Hospital Organizations

The third model is the **physician hospital organization (PHO),** which is a legal entity owned by one or more hospitals and physicians responsible for negotiating with third parties for contracts

RESEARCH BRIEF

Cheney, K. (July, 1997). How to be a managed care winner. Money, pp. 122–131.

Cheney advises consumers to sharpen their product-savvy analysis when shopping for a managed care plan. The article describes plans in clear terms, identifies expected costs of the typical MCO plan type, and provides advice on selecting a plan: "You should join if . . ." Also included is a sample appeal letter for those experiencing care/treatment denials, and a problem-action format illustrating common problems experienced by consumers, as well as describing possible solutions.

and serving as a marketing unit. The PHO as a single entity agrees to provide services to subscribers. Physicians typically maintain ownership of their practices in this model (Huntington, 1997; Managed Care Resources, 1997; May, Schraeder, & Britt, 1996).

Point-of-Service Plans

The fourth model is the **point-of-service (POS) plan,** also known as the open-ended HMO. Each time a member/enrollee seeks care, options are given to use the managed care program or the out-of-plan program, for which substantially higher costs are incurred by the enrollee in the form of premiums, **co-payments,** and **deductibles.** This allows enrollees to opt out of the managed choice plan—a choice that incurs greater financial risk for the enrollee. POS has been used by HMOs to ease the transition to strict managed care plans (ANA, 1995; May, Schraeder, & Britt, 1996).

Community Nursing Organizations

Although not widely identified in health systems and health services literature, **community nursing organizations (CNOs)** constitute a new experimental type of managed care. In 1987, Congress authorized through budget act legislation (the Omnibus Reconciliation Act [OBRA]) the funding of a CNO demonstration project composed of four national sites, which remain in existence today: Carle Clinic, Carondolet Health Services, Visiting Nurse Service of New York, and Living at Home/Block Nurse Program. This project examines the role of nursing in providing high-quality care with capitated payments for Medicare beneficiaries through a nurse-centered managed care model of financing and delivery at each site. The goals of these CNOs are to prevent unnecessary institutionalization, provide preventive and health promotion services, coordinate care to promote continuity, and demonstrate effective use of prospective (prepaid) and capitation payment methods. Medicare recipients must agree to obtain all nonemergency services through the CNO, which may include home health services (nursing, therapies, aides, supplies, dressings); prosthetics and durable medical equipment; ambulance service; outpatient visits to physical therapists, clinical psychologists, or social workers; primary nursing services (in-person consultations, care plan development, coordination of services, care monitoring); consultations with family and physicians; and homemaker/personal care (May, Schraeder, & Britt, 1996).

In these CNOs, the nurse partner and nurse case manager are key. Nurse partner caseloads are linked with primary care physicians to optimize collaboration on enrollees' health care plans. This collaboration attempts to achieve efficiency and effectiveness of service type, level, intensity, and frequency. The nurse case manager authorizes any CNO service for the patient. Because community-based services are important to reduce inappropriate institutionalization, the CNO nurse partner manages transitional services among sites and supports member access to little-known community resources. Nurse partners strongly emphasize health promotion activities for improved lifestyles and recommend prevention activities. In a research study by O'Grady (1999), the nursing interventions provided with the greatest frequency to CNO, community-based patients included those of teaching and empowerment. In this capitated funding method, both clinical and financial responsibility remain with the nurse to provide cost-effective, appropriately planned, well-executed services to the well population (Lamb & Zazworsky, 1997; May, Schraeder, & Britt, 1996).

Examples of nursing actions in the CNO environment include assessment of health status and authorization for service; phone calls to monitor care; education by telephone, face to face, and mail; use of advocacy skills to initiate and monitor referrals with patients; and evaluations of caseloads and individuals based on service authorization and use to establish improved practice patterns. Many of these functions are considered case management activities.

Management Mechanisms

Managed care models embrace a large variation in organizational structure, consumer choices, financial risks, consumer rights,

RESEARCH BRIEF

Weinrick, R. M., Zuvekas, S. H., & Drilea S. K. (1997). Access to health care—sources and barriers: 1996. MEPS Research Findings No 3 (AHCPR Pub No. 98-0001). Rockville, MD: Agency for Health Care Policy & Research.

Access to Health Care: Service and Barriers

According to the 1996 Medical Expenditure Panel Survey the picture of access to health care in the United States looked like this:

* *Approximately 12% of American families experienced barriers to receiving needed health care because of inability to afford medical care and insurance-related problems.*

* *Almost 18% of Americans reported no usual source of care, which represents 46 million of the U.S. population.*

* *Groups at risk for experiencing no usual source of care included Hispanic Americans (30%), uninsured, younger than 65 (38%), and young adults ages 18–24 (34%).*

* *Families in which all members were insured were two to three times more likely to receive needed health care than families in which one or more members lacked health insurance.*

Regardless of the expansion of managed care in Medicaid, Medicare, and employee populations, access to health care and the need for safety net providers and systems remains an important issue for U.S. citizens.

and grievance procedures. However, all use one or more management mechanisms to regulate incentives and behavior:

* *Contracts between insurers and providers to ensure comprehensive services but only necessary treatments*
* *Utilization and quality control activities*
* *Explicit provider selection standards and financial incentives for consumers to use designated providers*
* *Direct contracting with cost-effective providers*
* *Discounted provider reimbursement*
* *Cost-sharing by enrollees for more expensive services*

Nurses employed in these systems must be able to assess the effectiveness and efficiency of these services and be advocates for the benefit of all populations under the nurse's care (Packard, 1997). As consumers and employees are provided regular options to change enrollment among the managed care plans, they are increasingly challenged to compare benefit and liability implications as well as judgments of quality performance among providers.

Credentialing: Regulation and Accreditation

Organizations and systems delivering health care services are subject to oversight activities by external bodies. Typical regulatory oversight includes licensure by the state, certification by a government agency, and/or accreditation by a voluntary accrediting organization. Each oversight mechanism requires that certain conditions must be met. The aim of the regulatory mechanism is to ensure integrity of the organization and activities as well as the safety of the publics' health.

Organizational credentialing is required in addition to the credentialing of an individual provider required by the practice discipline. Credentialing of providers is an important legal obligation of the MCO. Credentialing can include verification of provider's license, certification, malpractice coverage, charting procedures, and admitting privileges, to name a few. As you may recall, nurses are licensed by the state and may be certified in an area of specialty practice by voluntary professional organizations. To meet regulatory standards, organizations typically require that health professional employees (e.g., nurses) hold current licensure and certification credentials to practice in that system.

Several voluntary organizations offer accreditation processes (organizational credentialing) and designations to managed care plans and networks:

The **National Committee on Quality Assurance (NCQA)** is a nonprofit organization created to improve patient care quality and health plan performance in conjunction with managed care plans, purchasers, consumers, and the public. In some states, NCQA accreditation of managed care plans is mandated. Although its standards do not yet focus on nurse-specific outcome measures for patients, the process targets quality improvement, credentialing, members' rights and responsibilities, utilization management, preventive services, and medical records. NCQA has constructed a national database of information on the quality of managed care plans so that performance and accreditation information for each plan can be compared by the public. Managed care plans submit data congruent with the NCQA-sponsored **HEDIS**, which contains at least 50 measures (HEDIS, 1999). As an example, eight clinical HEDIS measures that reflect important performance contributions to the health status of U.S. consumers include (1) advising smokers to quit, (2) initiating beta-blocker treatments, (3) screening for breast cancer, (4) screening for cervical cancer, (5) monitoring cesarean section rates, (6) performing childhood immunization, (7) performing diabetic eye examinations, and (8) delivering first trimester prenatal care.

Data on HEDIS measures provide a global performance picture for clinical quality in general and for specific plans for which the public may query. The *Healthy People 2000* and *2010* objectives can serve as a national gold standard against which clinical HEDIS measures are designed, monitored, and evaluated (e.g., immunization rates). The NCQA **Quality Compass** is the name of the database that contains accreditation and HEDIS information from more than 300 health plans. Updated CD-ROMs for Quality Compass are available periodically to provide current

information from existing and new participants. These statistics are important to employers and consumers in choosing among managed care plans. The data also assist managed care plans to set performance goals and monitor improvement and accountability (ANA, 1995; NCQA, 1997). To date, the ANA Nursing Report Card indicators are not used in the managed care industry.

Other accreditation bodies offering credentialing to various types of managed care plans include the Utilization Review Accreditation Commission (URAC) and the Joint Commission on Accreditation of Health Care Organizations (JCAHO) for integrated delivery networks and health plans (JCAHO, 1998; May, Schraeder, & Britt, 1996). (See Box 6-2 for a comprehensive list.)

It is interesting to note that as managed care penetration has increased nationally, consumer advocates, the media, and lawmakers have voiced issues of clinical integrity, access, and satisfactory performance within the mantra of public safety. Although HMOs are heavily regulated by state and federal legislation, PPOs and others are less stringently regulated or largely unregulated to date. The debate concerning whether voluntary accreditation mechanisms are sufficient to ensure the health of the "enrolled" public has generated a demand for legislative regulation of the managed care industry. In 1996 and

---

BOX 6-2 PUBLIC/PRIVATE CREDENTIALING OF MANAGED CARE

AAAHC: *American Association for Ambulatory Health Care is a private organization that conducts voluntary quality reviews of ambulatory health centers including HMOs.*

CHAP: *Community Health Accreditation Program is a private voluntary accreditation program for home care agencies and community nursing organizations.*

HCFA: *Health Care Financing Administration is a government agency that reviews federally qualified HMOs under the Federal HMO Act.*

JCAHO: *Joint Commission on Accreditation of Healthcare Organizations conducts a voluntary, private accreditation for health care networks.*

MQC: *Medical Quality Commission is funded by major HMOs and corporations to promote quality research in health care and establish accreditation for prepaid medical group practices and IPAs that provide services to members of HMOs.*

NAIC: *National Association of Insurance Commissioners is a private organization that publishes a model act to help state legislatures adapt licensure laws for HMOs.*

NCQA: *National Committee for Quality Assurance (see text).*

OPM: *Office of Personnel Management audits HMOs and health plans under Federal Employees Health Benefits Programs.*

PROs: *Peer review organizations provide mandatory quality reviews of inpatient and outpatient care for Medicare beneficiaries enrolled in Medicare risk contracting HMOs.*

State licensure of PPOs: *Many states require the PPO and PPO-like plans to go through a licensure process.*

URAC: *Utilization Review Accreditation Commission is a private organization made up of health care associations and labor groups whose goal is to improve the quality and efficiency of interactions among the utilization review industry, providers, payers, and purchasers of health care. Primarily it provides accreditation of PPO and POS networks (Rapaport, 1997).*

Source: ANA, 1996.

1997, more than 2,200 managed care bills to regulate health care delivery were introduced in the states (Gaffney, 1997). A Presidential Advisory Commission on Consumer Protection and Quality in the Health Care Industry issued the *Patient's Bill of Rights* in 1997, and federal legislative efforts addressed issues of preexisting conditions, transportable health insurance coverage for uninsured children ($24 billion), and changes in Medicare to encourage more elderly patients to seek managed care. Internally, health industry leaders are attempting to ensure voluntary compliance with quality standards as an alternative to additional government regulations for the industry. Clearly, there is not consensus that voluntary standards are sufficient in the absence of a regulatory framework. Such a framework in the future may include government oversight and/or quasi-governmental bodies as regulatory structures (Kertesz, 1997).

Ethical Issues

Four major stakeholders are typically impacted by managed care systems. Situations abound in which the goals among stakeholders conflict, resulting in ethical issues and dilemmas not easily resolved to the satisfaction of all parties. Stakeholders include patients, providers, investors/stockholders, and

RESEARCH BRIEF

Silva, M. C. (1998). Ethics and managed care: A select annotated bibliography. Ethics Forum, 8(2), 1–4.

The author presents a collection of article annotations published since 1995 concerning ethical issues in managed care. These articles focus on consumer rights, access to care, the moral imperative of rehabilitation institutions, quality and ethics concept integration, and a principles, values, and ethics approach to managed care nursing.

the community. Silva (1998) identifies six problem areas related to MCOs:

1. *Limited numbers of within-system providers*
2. *Financial penalties for out-of-network provider use*
3. *Imposition of gag rules to limit information on choice of treatments*
4. *Restrictive formularies for drugs*

CASE STUDY

Maintaining Sean's Functional Status: Managed Costs, Managed Care, or Both?

Sean is a disabled skier living in Vermont and working at Maple, Inc. His employer provides two options for health plans, MAC-MCO and SHMO-MCO, both managed care entities. Sean has worn a high leg prosthesis since adolescence, when he lost his left leg in an auto accident. Lately Sean has sensed that the bearings on his prosthesis are disintegrating, causing difficulty in functioning. He contacts his primary care provider at MAC-MCO Systems and both agree to an evaluation for replacement. Sean asks the managed care plan to cover the services of Eli Prostotic, of Prostotic, Inc., because Eli crafted and fit his original and subsequent prostheses and accomplished a perfect fit each time.

1. Initially MAC-MCO denied the referral to Prostotics because it was an out-of-network provider. Sean wrote a letter of appeal. You

are the nurse in charge of the appeals section at MAC-MCO.

- What type of evidence would you require in the appeal letter to justify coverage of Sean's out-of-network referral?

2. Based on the estimate $32,950 submitted by Prostotic, Inc., for the prosthetic device and services, you recognize this is 20% higher than your network provider. You authorize half the payment by MAC-MO and half paid by Sean. Sean appeals this decision.

- What type of evidence would you require in the second appeal letter to justify MAC-MCO expending $32,950 on this prosthesis?
- What other negotiations would you orchestrate to meet the financial guidelines of Sean's benefit under the MAC-MCO contract?
- Who are the parties who will be financially impacted by these negotiations for a new prosthesis?
- Which aspects of patient advocacy conflict with your role as systems allocator?

Source: Adapted from Cheney, 1997.

5. *Lack of accountability of MCO to external assurance organizations or regulators*

6. *Inadequate appeals procedures for complainants*

In addition, MCO saturation in a market may rob the community of resources to deliver uncompensated care. For example, physicians in a community may not be able to provide as much uncompensated care because of the decline of their own incomes when they become employers in managed care systems. The **safety net system** of providers in voluntary and public health systems are then stressed to provide additional services. Another concern is price competition, which requires sacrificing quality to meet price requirements that cannot be met except through denial of appropriate care. Finally, MCOs may engage in deceptive advertising and enrollment strategies, selecting and aggressively enrolling only healthy participants. These examples illustrate the ethical dilemmas for communi-

ties when cost and market share are the overriding values in market competition.

Within MCOs, nurses simultaneously fulfill the role of **patient advocate** as well as system/services allocator. As a nurse fulfilling these dual roles, you may confront dilemmas in practice when you implement or witness the activities within the MCO system. Cary (1998) notes the conundrums apparent when the allocator and advocate roles work discordantly with client care and systems resources. Box 6-3 highlights the barriers to access for enrollees based on systems resource constraints.

Nurses' Roles in Managed Care

When you explore the systems of managed care as your potential employer, the roles of the managed care nurse will have likenesses and dissimilarities to nurses seeking employment in acute care,

---

BOX 6-3 BARRIERS TO ACCESS/UTILIZATION IN MANAGED CARE: ADVOCACY AND ALLOCATION DILEMMAS

- Few choices of plans and no point-of-service options in a benefit package
- Absence of services in a plan
- Employees limited to choice of providers selected by the insurer
- Providers excluded or rotated from panels for reasons unrelated to quality performance/efficiency measures
- Provider behaviors predicated on economic incentives and threats
- "Gag" rules for providers (withholding information)
- Administrative rules that limit visit times, services, and referrals
- Administrative controls on providers to reduce utilization
- Waste in administrative activities and duplication in clinical processes
- Culturally insensitive providers of care
- Inadequate staffing
- Less-than-competent provider substitution
- Lack of communication between and within information systems
- Providers who fail to assert the ethical guidelines and codes of the profession

Source: Adapted from Cary, 1998.

RESEARCH BRIEF

Buerhaus, P. I. & Staiger, D. O. (1997). Future of the nurse labor market according to health executives in high managed-care areas of the United States. Image, 29(4), 313–318.

Future of the Nurse Labor Market According to Health Executives in High Managed Care Areas of the United States

In survey research of 62 health executives in 11 states with major managed care enrollments in HMOs, researchers asked about changes in nurse employment, earnings, collective bargaining, benefits, nurse's roles, provider substitutions for registered nurses (RNs), patient severity, quality of patient care, and expectations for nurse employment during the remainder of the decade.

Executives reported that the nurse labor market would be positive and fast changing. Concerns were expressed about the aging RN workforce, possible developments of an RN shortage, and the linking of quality patient care to provision of nursing services. In addition, executives challenged nurse educators to adapt quickly to the changing employer needs for nurses prepared to meet the new systems' demands. Finally, expectations for the workforce include new jobs in home care; RN delegation of activities to lesser trained personnel; greater responsibilities in care management and technology; health care emphasis in wellness; and prevention, case-finding, and triage. All settings will use continuing education and retraining to upskill to employment needs.

long-term care, and other health care settings. However, the use of a systematic process of care management based on the context of biopsychosocial, environmental, informatics, and organizational theories as applied through the nursing process reflect the strength of nursing to ensure managed care successes. Opportunities and specific skills for nurses working with managed care systems are listed in Box 6-4.

As an additional resource, the ANA describes eight roles and subsequent functions of nurses in managed care as explicated below (ANA, 1995):

1. *Benefits interpreter:* This role is key to the education of members in managed care organizations so that they clearly understand the benefits available to them. Likewise, the nurse explains the grievance procedures available to clarify or dispute in-

---

BOX 6-4 NEW OPPORTUNITIES AND THE ACCOMPANYING SKILLS

Nurses can position themselves to accept the emerging roles in managed care systems. To assist in this process, the following seven areas of opportunity for nurses in a managed care environment and the skills needed to take on these new roles have been identified.

CONSUMER ADVOCACY

- Use of decision trees/tools
- Projection of statistical probabilities
- Negotiation skills
- Group interaction and facilitation
- Patient teaching using new media
- Understanding of principles of ethics

CHANGE AGENT

- Understand chaos theory/change theory
- Leadership skills vs. management skills
- Self-managed team abilities
- Grasp of organizational behavior and development theory

INDIVIDUAL GROWTH

- Self-empowerment
- Professional image
- New self-accountability for life-long learning and relevancy in a changing environment
- Computer literacy
- Networking ability
- Business-related skills: verbal and written presentation skills, communication technology familiarity, publication/media production, economics/finance forecasting skills
- Sensitivity to cost and quality, total quality management process, benchmarking, utilization management cost analysis, data integrity, tracking and manipulation, "best practices"

COMMUNITY-BASED CARE

- Cultural competence
- Assessment
- Population-focused care
- Innovative approaches to enhancing health of a community
- Epidemiology and environmental health
- Understanding concepts of risk

INFORMATION SYSTEMS

- Computer-related skills
- Informatics
- Decision support systems
- Ability to access and process data

ENTREPRENEURS/INTRAPRENEURS

- Understanding of contracts
- Abilities in innovative program development
- Marketing/selling
- Program budgeting
- Business plan development
- Problem identification and costing of solutions

PUBLIC HEALTH POLICY AND REGULATORY BODIES

- Legislative skills
- Knowledge of civics
- Understanding of administrative, legislative, and judicial roles of government
- Knowledge of key regulatory bodies related to nursing and health care
- Basic skill in legal interpretation and drafting

Source: ANA, 1996, p. 19.

terpretations. Because member satisfaction is a critical component of stable enrollment, the effectiveness of the nurse as a benefits interpreter is essential to the organization.

2. *Client advocate and educator:* Of all disciplines employed in managed care, nurses with their educational background in clinical and behavioral science can ensure a variety of skillful educational and empowerment strategies in working with clientele. Advocacy helps identify needed care and education, including prevention of diseases, promotion of health, and the protection of groups of people from environmental risks. Advocacy activities may entail educating clientele on the existence and use of covered services, educating management on the collective and exceptional needs of enrollees, and educating payers and communities about the emerging gaps in essential and supportive services that can undermine a population's health status.

3. *Triage nurse:* Triaging is an activity that directs access to services so that they are efficiently and effectively used. Nurses may use telecommunications to process inquiries as well as on-site visits for complex, sudden, or acute events. Anchored in a firm knowledge base of clinical health and disease states and established best practice guidelines, the triage nurse assists the patient to identify problems and symptoms, reviews the medical record, provides clinical decisions on appropriate options, advises clients, and secures appropriate services. In many cases, the triage nurse is the first point of contact for entry to a service of the health plan.

4. *Utilization and resource reviewer:* Utilization managers help control health care costs by assessing the appropriateness of care and ensuring use of the least costly treatments known to be effective. Utilization review includes a number of data-gathering activities that measure the appropriateness, necessity, and quality of care. Mechanisms of review may include preadmission certification, concurrent review with discharge planning, retrospective review of care, length of stay, site of care, and treatment appropriateness. Nurses have been historically employed in this role for insurance companies.

5. *Risk manager:* The risk manager's goal is to decrease the occurrence of unintended adverse events and outcomes for clients and the organization. In achieving risk management outcomes, the nurse identifies potential risk factors and situations detrimental to clients' health; analyzes patterns and frequencies of events to detect system, structure, and process deficits; evaluates alternative approaches to reducing risks; and implements corrective action. Monitoring sentinel events/patterns are essential to this role of detecting emergent disease patterns or risks to quality in the system.

6. *Provider liaison:* The administrative, clinical, and financial structures and processes in a managed care organization require collaboration, teaming, cooperation, and coordination among providers to achieve clear intended outcomes. The role of provider liaison requires the nurse to provide information and to interact with a variety of health professionals. This ensures that clients understand the functions and responsibilities of each

team member as they receive coordinated care from interdisciplinary providers at different sites of care.

7. *Primary care provider:* In this role, the nurse is the first point of contact and identifies further steps to manage a client's presentation of complaints and history as well as initiates referrals to other providers or specialists. Terms that are used for this role are **gatekeeper, pathfinder,** or provider of first contact. Because of the advanced clinical skills required in this role, MCOs may employ advanced practice registered nurses to fill these roles and positions.

8. *Case or care manager:* "If you have seen a case manager you have seen one case manager." The roles of case managers vary considerably among different systems. Some case managers monitor the long-term needs of enrollees while others manage the current episode of care. Case managers use critical pathways, care maps, and disease management protocols to identify key events that must occur to achieve outcomes. This ensures that the patient progresses through the restoration/maintenance goals appropriately or adjustments in the plan are made.

In community-based case management, the role of case manager requires a comprehensive knowledge of complementary community resources, eligibility requirements, and expected outcomes. For catastrophic illnesses, closely managed care provides patients with appropriate monitoring, the matching of resources to the stage of illness, monitoring of financial impact, and utilization of the right service at the right time for the desired outcome. Highly developed communication skills, multimethod assessment and monitoring tools to gauge need and progress, negotiation and advocacy strategies, information management, and financial forecasting are essential. The ultimate risks to be avoided by case managers include fragmentation or

RESEARCH BRIEF

Wrinn, M. M. (1998). Stepping up to the plate in 1998: Case management faces opportunities and challenges. Continuing Care, 17(1), 16–21.

The role of case manager in managed care organizations is central to successful financial and clinical outcomes. Case management is a nucleus of the continuum of care with case managers as orchestrators of services in precise and synchronous fashion. The author reminds the reader that the primary objective of the case manager in these systems is to be an advocate for the patient. Learning needs for case managers in the 21st century include knowledge of regulatory issues for all venues of care; disease management; guidelines and standards; technology; performance outcomes; and data identification, retrieval, analysis, and dissemination.

duplication of service, inappropriate utilization of providers and intensity of service, and denial of appropriate care (Cary, 1996, 1998; Steinhauser, 1999).

Managed Care and Healthy Communities: Nursing's Approach

In the absence of a policy of universal access to health care in the United States and the emergence of market-based health care, certain populations continue to need public support to obtain necessary health and social services. The term *health care safety net* includes the institutions, programs, and professionals who harness resources to serve the uninsured or the socially disadvantaged. Typical providers include urban public hospitals, community health centers, inner-city teaching hospitals, and local health departments. Populations in our communities using the safety-net systems include the uninsured, Medicaid, persons with acquired immunodeficiency syndrome (AIDS), substance abusers, frail elderly, children from low-income families, low-income pregnant women, the homeless, and the mentally ill (Baxter & Mechanic, 1997).

RESEARCH BRIEF

Gordon, S. (1997). Managed care or damaged care: The challenge for nursing. Clinical Excellence for Nurse Practitioners, 1(5), 333–336.

The major tenets of the corporatization of health care, as played out by the introduction of managed care systems, are discussed by the author. Concerns are raised about the intense structure of competitive systems that pit providers against one another to provide services to a predictable population as well as ensure provider income. On one level, the market competition positions clinician economic self-interest against patient well-being. On another level, competition raises the incentives to provide highly regarded quality care and ensure intended clinical outcomes. Nurses are challenged to help consumers understand the significance of the new market implications through their intrinsic roles as educators, leaders, and advocates on behalf of costs, quality, and access to care.

RESEARCH BRIEF

Agency for Health Care Policy and Research (AHCPR). (January, 1998). Research Activities, 212, 1–32.

This monthly publication is a digest of research findings typically produced with financial support from AHCPR. The particular issue is a collection of research findings based on studies predominately inclusive of managed care. Studies include access, primary care in managed care, costs of home care, methodology comparisons, referral patterns, special service and treatment utilization, efficacy, and general announcements.

There are major concerns in communities where managed care reduces the revenue streams for safety-net systems and providers. These cross-subsidies that have supported the safety-net services are in danger of disappearing. This means that fewer of the most vulnerable, who are in most need of services, will be able to obtain care from a shrinking safety net of community services and providers. The impact of market-driven managed care on the safety-net options for health and social services in a community must be monitored by community health nurses, who often serve on the front line of providing care to marginalized populations.

In 1998, the ANA issued a guide for nurses endorsing principles of managed care on which policies and social action could be interpreted. Within the emerging systems of managed care in our communities and with large numbers of both acute and community-based nurses encountering the challenges of delivering appropriate health care, these principles offer an emphasis for patient advocacy and consumer protection, enhanced quality of care accountability, and increased access to an appropriate array of services (ANA, 1998).

Market-driven managed care will ultimately survive only if consumers and providers work to achieve quality outcomes substantiated by evidenced-based practices with populations. Nurses working in MCOs and with patients covered by MCO and/or safety-net providers must maintain the broad view of health to include environments for education, behavior, income, housing, sanitation, and social services. Nurses must remain responsive to community needs and faithful to the application of principles that support health care access, quality, and cost efficiencies in an effort to achieve healthy communities.

CONCLUSION

Managed care delivery systems have swept across the United States; there is even evidence in Europe, the Middle East, and Malaysia to suggest that managed care is being implemented alongside existing delivery systems. Clients enrolled in managed care systems are likely to experience fewer medical procedures, greater standardization of care, less opportunity to select a provider of choice without personal financial risks, shorter hospital stays, and greater numbers of outpatient and ambulatory care procedures. Nurses employed in these systems are offered greater staff development and continuing education opportunities as organizations attempt to "right-skill" their employees. New skills in technology, information systems, case management, delegation of patient care activities, performance assessment and improvement activities, advocacy, and allocation functions will be required of nurses employed by these systems.

There are many structures and types of managed care organizations operating in communities. Nurses must understand the structure, processes, goals, and outcomes expected by the MCO seeking to employ a nurse. Additional skill development may enhance a nurse's competitive chance for employment positions in these systems. Opportunities to apply clinical and program development skills in wellness and prevention are expected to rise in MCOs. However, nurses must be alert to ethical dilemmas that occur when access to care is prescribed by organizational financial goals in contrast to a patient's need for appropriate services. Nurses will hold roles as both patient advocate and service allocator in these new systems of care to communities.

CRITICAL THINKING ACTIVITIES

1. You are a nurse employed by Start-Up managed care attempting to sell the Start-Up managed care plan to the local cabinet production company (CPC) in your community. This employer will have 35,000 potential covered lives if you are successful in securing a contract.

   - Explain the Wellness Program and Services (WPS) feature of your benefit plan. What types of services are offered? Why would CPC be interested in the WPS feature of your plan? What data could you provide to convince the CPC health benefits administrator of the value of WPS for the company, for employees, for the community?

   - Discuss four "rights" that clients of managed care organizations can expect to receive.

   - Discuss two "rights" that stockholders and/or investors in managed care organizations can expect to be honored by MCO corporations.

   - Discuss three "rights" that providers in managed care organizations can expect to be honored by MCO corporations.

   - Name three potential conflicts in "rights" among the clients, stockholders, and providers in managed care organizations.

   - Explore one of the web sites listed in the text's web site or the web site of a managed care company serving your community. Make a presentation to your classmates of the scope of information in the web site that would be useful to clients, providers, employers, and potential consumers. What additional information should be added to make the web site more informative?

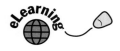

Explore Community Health Nursing on the web! To learn more about the topics in this chapter, use the passcode provided to access your exclusive web site: http://communitynursing.jbpub.com
If you do not have a passcode, you can obtain one at this site.

REFERENCES

Agency for Health Care Policy & Research. (January, 1998). *Research Activities, 212,* 1–32.

American Nurses Association (ANA). (1995). *Nursing facts.* Washington, D.C.: Author.

American Nurses Association (ANA). (May/June, 1996). *Task force on standards and regulation of managed care report* (pp. 11–13, 82, 86). Washington, D.C.: Author.

American Nurses Association (ANA). (1998*). Managed care: Nursing's blueprint for actionæ principles.* Washington, D.C.: Author.

Baldwin, F. D. (May/June, 1997). Helping yourself: Where to find good information. *Consumer Digest,* pp. 82, 86.

Baxter, R. J., & Mechanic, R. E. (1997). The status of local health care safety nets. *Health Affairs, 16*(4), 7–23.

Beck, D. F., & Dempsey, J. (1996). The managed care time clock: What's making it tick? *Health Care Supervisor, 14*(3), 1–12.

Buerhaus, P. I., & Staiger, D. O. (1997). Future of the nurse labor market according to health care executives in high managed-care areas of the United States. *Image, 29*(4), 313–318.

Cary, A. H. (1996). Case management. In Stanhope, M., & Lancaster, J. (Eds.), *Community health nursing* (4th ed., pp. 357–374). St. Louis: Mosby.

Cary, A. H. (1998). Advocacy or Allocation? *Nursing Connections, 11*(1), 1–4.

Cheney, K. (1997, July). How to be a managed care winner. *Money,* pp. 122–131.

Gaffney, T. (1997). *Managed care trends in the states.* Unpublished paper delivered at managed care workgroup meeting. Washington, D.C.: American Nurses Association.

Gordon, S. (1997). Managed care or damaged care: The challenge for nursing. *Clinical Excellence for Nurse Practitioners, 1*(5), 333–336.

Health Plan Employment Data and Information Set (HEDIS). (1999). *Reporting set measures by domain.* www.ncqa.org/news/h99meas.htm

Hager, M. (May/June, 1997). Inside "managed" care. *Consumers Digest,* pp. 37–40.

Huntington, J. A. (1997). Glossary for managed care. *On-line Journal of Issues in Nursing.* www.nursingworld/ojin/tpc2_gls.htm

Joint Commission on Accreditation of Health Care Organizations (JCAHO). (1998). Accreditation manual for health care networks (AMHCN). Chicago: Author.

Kertesz, L. (May, 1997). HMO makeover: Are managed care's efforts to overhaul its image too little, too late? *Modern Healthcare,* pp. 36–38, 42–46.

Lamb, G. S., & Zazworsky, D. (1997). The Carondelet model. *Nursing Management, 28*(3), 27–28.

Managed Care Resources, Inc. (1997). *Managed care terms and definitions.* www.mcres.com

May, C. A., Schraeder, C., & Britt, T. (1996). *Managed care and case management: Roles for professional nursing.* Washington, D.C.: American Nurses Publishing.

Mechanic, D. (1998). Topics for our times: Managed care and public health opportunities. *American Journal of Public Health, 88*(6), 874–875.

Miller, R. H., & Luft, H. S. (1997). Does managed care lead to better or worse quality of care? *Health Affairs, 16*(5), 7–25.

National Committee on Quality Assurance (NCQA). (February, 1997). *NCQA releases Quality Compass update.* www.NCQA.org/news/qcrel3.htm

O'Grady, E. T. (1999). *The community organization demonstration: An analysis of interventions.* Unpublished doctoral dissertation. George Mason University, Fairfax, VA.

Packard, N. J. (1997). The price of choice: Managed care in America. *Nursing Administration Quarterly, 17*(3), 8–15.

Rapaport, M. G. (May/June, 1997). Choosing a health plan. *Consumers Digest,* pp. 42–44.

Remler, D. K., Donelan, K., Blendon, R. J., Lundberg, G. D., Leape, L. L., Calkins, D. R., Binns, K., & Newhouse, J. P. (1997). What do managed care plans do to affect care? Results from a survey of physicians. *Inquiry, 34,* 196–204.

Rosenthal, A. (May/June, 1997). How to save on health insurance. *Consumers Digest,* pp. 44–46.

Silva, M. C. (1998). Ethics and managed care: A select annotated bibliography. *Ethics Forum, 8*(2), 1–4.

Spitzer-Lehmann, R. (September, 1996). A new framework for managed care: Marrying finance and service delivery. Paper presented at the pre-conference meeting of the Nursing Management Congress, Chicago.

Steinhauser, E. K. (1999). Developing a strategy to win with a difficult load. *Continuing care, 18*(5), 20–25, 32.

Turner, S. O. (1999a). *The nurse's guide to managed care.* Gaithersburg, MD: Aspen.

Turner, S. O. (1999b). *Essential readings in nursing managed care.* Gaithersburg, MD: Aspen.

Weinick, R. M, Zuvekas, S. H., & Drilea, S. K. (1997). *Access to health care-sources and barriers: 1996* (MEPS Research Findings No. 3). Rockville, MD: AHCPR.

Wrinn, M. M. (1998). Stepping up to the plate in 1998: Case management faces opportunities & challenges. *Continuing Care, 17*(1), 16–21.

Unit II
Influences on a Community's Health

Chapter 7

Economics of Health Care

Sherry Hartman

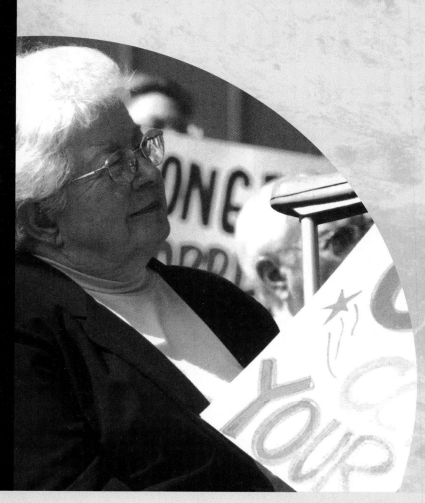

Not very long ago, economic concerns were not considered an appropriate topic for basic nursing education or perhaps even for advanced nursing. In-depth knowledge was essential only for nurse administrators who needed to deal with budgets and financial resources. In today's health care environment, however, nurses need to understand health care problems from many approaches and viewpoints. The science of economics is one of those approaches that has become increasingly important. Even though "money concerns" have traditionally been resisted by practitioners whose focus has been on meeting client needs, most now acknowledge the impact of economics on health care problems and solutions. All care providers need at least a rudimentary understanding of the economic workings of the system in which they practice at the institutional, national, and sometimes even global levels. Controlling costs while maintaining quality and access has become the major challenge of the new century. To do this, an understanding of economic descriptions and explanations of the health care market are necessary.

CHAPTER FOCUS

An Economic Approach to Health Care
    Competition in the Market
    Competition versus Regulation
    Market Failure in Health Care

Rising Costs and Today's Health Care System
    From Private Pay to Government Involvement
    Increased Costs: The Economic Indicators
    Decreased Access: The Economic Barriers
    Influences on Costs and Access

Paying for Health Care
    Direct Payments by Consumers and Charity
    Health Insurance
    Publicly Funded Insurance and Direct Care Programs

Cost Containment, Cost Analysis, and Quality

Public Health, Managed Care, and the Economics of Prevention
    Opportunities for Collaboration
    Counterforces to Collaboration
    Prevention and Alternative Therapies

Significance of Economics for Community Health Nursing Practice

Healthy People 2010: Objectives Related to Access

QUESTIONS TO CONSIDER

After reading this chapter, answer the following questions:

1. Why is the U.S. health care market referred to as an *imperfect market*?
2. What are the major roles of government and private enterprise in the U.S. health care market?
3. What factors are contributing to high and rising health care costs?
4. What are the strategies used for cost containment of national health expenditures?
5. What are the financing, eligibility, and covered benefits of Medicare and Medicaid?
6. What other health care financing is covered by the government?
7. Why is it that despite public and private health insurance programs, some U.S. citizens are without any coverage?
8. How and why might public health and managed care organizations collaborate?
9. How are community health nurses affected by the economic environment of their practice?

KEY TERMS

Benefit period	Demand	Inflation	Regulation
Categorical programs	Entitlement	Market	Relative value scale
Categorically needy	Experience ratings	Market failure	Self-insurance
Community ratings	Free market competition	Market justice	Social justice
Cost-benefit analysis	Gross domestic product	Medically needy	Supplier-influenced
Cost containment	(GDP)	Medigap insurance	demand
Cost-effectiveness	Health care market	Resource utilization	Supply
analysis	Health insurance	groups, version 3	Technology assessment
Cost of illness studies	purchasing cooperatives	(RUG-III)	Welfare
Cost sharing	(HIPCs)		

Nurses usually don't think in market (and particularly for-profit market) terms; rather we think in terms of profit or benefit for people.

Carole A. Anderson, Editor, *Nursing Outlook*, 1997

Several chapters in this text, describing the context of and influences on health care practice, also highlight aspects of health problems from an economic point of view rather than strictly a biological or psychosocial perspective. Health care system analysts are concerned with the best structures for delivering the various needed health care services; health policy makers are concerned with deciding the best actions to take from among possible alternatives; health economists are concerned with the distribution of scarce resources among a defined population. These areas are interrelated: Economic analysis influences policy decisions, which often drive the health care delivery structures. In turn, the resultant structures are analyzed in terms of how efficiently they distribute resources.

This chapter provides a basic understanding of the economic approach to health problems. After an explanation of economic theory and principles applied to health care, the current state of financing of health care in the United States is considered along with some of the history that has brought us to today's increased consideration of market economics in health care. The many sources of funding for health care are explained. Approaches to cost containment and methods of economic analyses are described, followed by a look at the opportunities for collaboration between managed care and public health. Finally, some of the implications of economics for community health nursing are summarized.

An Economic Approach to Health Care

Competition in the Market

Like most sciences, economics is complex and broad in its scope. It looks at how finite goods and services are distributed to those who want or need them. A major way of conceptualizing this process is to see it as a **market.** In a marketplace, those who have something to sell and those who have needs or wants come together to make exchanges. There are various markets depending on the commodity being exchanged: for example, the automobile market, the entertainment market, housing market, and the **health care market.** In health care the market includes all health care–related services that need to be distributed among the total U.S. population. Within that overall market are specific markets: the health care labor market, home health care market, hospital care market, pharmaceuticals market, personal health insurance market, employer-paid health insurance market, and so on. A single hospital can also focus on its market: those potential users

of its service and competing sellers in its service area. A market could also be defined geographically, such as the home health care market within a certain region. Whatever organization a nurse works in, and particularly in a for-profit system, firms are concerned with their position and success in the market, and nurses play a key role in their quality and financial outcomes. At the broadest levels, market mechanisms are important to understanding the total health care picture of a single state and of the whole nation.

The essence of any market is buyers and sellers. There is a particular amount of a product or service such as health care that buyers are willing and able to purchase and consume, which is referred to as the **demand** for the product. There is a certain amount that sellers or providers are willing to make available, which is referred to as the **supply** of the product. In both cases the amount demanded or supplied is related to the price (or cost) of the health product. Competition is the key to understanding why some policy makers and health care leaders desire more free market mechanisms in health care. Competition in the market is the mechanism for setting price and quality. Suppliers compete for buyers of their products. Those that operate most efficiently (by satisfying buyers with the quality they want at the lowest possible cost) flourish, and those who do not have satisfied consumers close down. Price is most commonly the basis for competition, but it can also be based on technical quality, amenities, access, or other factors if prices become stabilized.

Competition Versus Regulation

Market mechanisms are not the only way for goods to become distributed. Centralized decision making may determine the distribution of goods and services, as a central authority determines how sellers and buyers make their exchanges. The central authority may be the only producer/seller and therefore may control all exchanges. This was the means of allocation in the Soviet Union and Eastern European nations until just over 10 years ago. Since the collapse of the communist block, capitalist, free market economics as practiced in the West now dominate in most developed countries.

The strong values of **free market competition** have influenced U.S. methods of distribution of health services. In contrast to many other developed nations, the United States has never adopted a national health care system with a global budget or centralized decision making. The United States mainly has a private system of financing as well as delivering health services. Private sources provide payment for 53% of health care products and services, and 47% comes from government sources; most hospitals, physicians, and other health care providers are private businesses. However, even though the origins and values lie with the free market, the 20th century was marked by increasing government involvement in health care. From the earliest origins in a free market of direct exchange between individuals and their private physicians, the U.S. system of health care moved slowly to more centralized decisions through government **regulation.**

For example, federal and state governments determine public sector expenditures and reimbursement rates for Medicare and Medicaid services. They regulate by setting standards of participation for certification to provide services for Medicaid and Medicare clients. Such government regulations become the minimum standards of quality in other, private sectors of the health services market (Shi & Singh, 1998).

During the Reagan presidency of the 1980s there was growing interest in more market-oriented approaches in many sectors of the economy. The free market is thought to be efficient for all goods and services in dispersing scarce resources. Following this thought, many economic theorists claim to show the superiority of free market competition over government regulation for allocating scarce health care resources (Rice, 1998). Responding to escalating health care costs, in 1981, among many changes in the health care industry, came the announcement from the Reagan administration that competition in the market, not governmental regulation, would be allowed to shape health care delivery (McKenzie, 1997).

Other countries with more centralized health care systems have since looked to the United States's changes and introduced more market mechanisms as well (Chen & Mastilica, 1998; Jerome-Forget, White, & Wiener, 1995; Le Grand, 1999). Issues of costs, cost cutting, and sources of funds to cover costs became and remain the dominant subjects of policy decisions in health care (Pulcini & Mahoney, 1998). More private and public money being spent on health care means less money available to spend on other wants or needs. In the public sector, spending more on health care leaves less to spend on education, the military, the environment, and other needed public goods. Increasing taxes to cover costs is not a popular option. Policy-making tensions for **cost containment** are between regulation by the government—for example, the failed Clinton plan for universal health coverage—and reliance on market competition to distribute health care services, such as competitive bidding for Medicare managed care contracts. Government regulation continues to play a large role at the same time that there is increasing reliance on the private sector and a competitive, cost-driven market. Between these two forces, some predict that market forces in the health care delivery industry will continue to have more rapid, extensive, and influential effects than any initiatives from state or federal sources of regulation (Sultz & Young, 1997). The appropriateness of these forces in the health care setting is considered in the next section.

Market Failure in Health Care

Those who believe in the superiority of competitive marketplaces base their preference on what would happen in an ideal, pure market. In an ideal market the following occurs: On the demand side, consumers have a variety of choices in goods and services to purchase. For individual consumers these include choices among doctors, hospitals, home health agencies, pharmacies, medical equipment suppliers, and so on. Consumers maximize their sat-

isfaction through self-motivated behavior and pick the quality they want for the price they are willing to pay. Income, tastes, preferences, and information about the product influence their choice. Consumers' choices tell suppliers whether their products are priced right and have the right quality. Suppliers then adjust price and quality to satisfy consumers. For suppliers in a competitive industry, there are strong incentives to minimize the costs of making their products and service. They can then be priced competitively to sell in the marketplace. Suppliers must be innovative and respond to customers' perceptions of quality. These two behaviors—benefit-maximizing behaviors of consumers and profit-maximizing behaviors of suppliers—through the mechanism of the market, produce the best patterns of production and consumption.

For the market to operate ideally as just described, certain conditions must exist. These are underlying assumptions and must hold true for the market to work as described in theory. Economists recognize that the realities of the market often violate the basic assumptions and create what is referred to as **market failure**. In a failed market the necessary competition does not occur as it should. It fails to produce the best outcomes for achieving the best use of resources. Fair allocation, quality and cost control, and setting of social priorities that enhance social welfare, all of which are the supposed gains of an effective market, are not realized. Box 7-1 lists some of the key conditions necessary for a classic, ideal free market to exist. Each of these is discussed in the following paragraphs, with examples to indicate how the U.S. health care market fails to operate under the forces of ideal free market factors.

In a free market, *consumers have full information about the nature of the services they require, the results of their decisions, and the benefits they can obtain.* The complexity of medical care itself and of the health care system makes informed choices difficult for

---

BOX 7-1 FACTORS NECESSARY FOR A FREE MARKET IN HEALTH CARE WITH OPTIMAL OUTCOMES

- Consumers have full information about the nature of the services they require, the results of their decisions, and the benefits they can obtain.
- Consumers and buyers act independently.
- Consumers bear the financial impact of their decisions and are aware of price differences.
- There is unrestrained competition regarding price and quality among providers.
- No single provider has monopoly power.
- Providers of services seek to operate efficiently to maximize profits.

clients. Consumers cannot know if a prescription or surgery is the better buy for their illness. There are so many choices of treatment—perhaps an acupuncturist would be a better buy. Treatment is sometimes urgently needed. Clients often do not have the time, skills, or resources to find needed information, and such information can be costly. In choice of health plan coverage, consumers do not know the differences between plan characteristics that indicate quality, convenience, flexibility, and extent of coverage. Even after a choice is made, consumers often cannot know if they made the right decision or what would have happened under other circumstances. Did the care cause the improvement or would it have happened anyway? What would have happened if another provider or treatment had been chosen?

In a free market, consumers and providers must act independently. Because of the "asymmetries of information" (Blumenthal, 1994, p. 252) in our health care market, health care consumers must depend on and accept the word of providers. Indeed, the words and advice of providers are as much the product being purchased as the examination or treatment. In a truly free market, the power lies with the consumer. However, physicians (suppliers) often are viewed as agents acting on behalf of clients. Thus, consumer demand is subject to artificial demand, which is commonly called **supplier-influenced demand** (Shi & Singh, 1998). In some cases, physicians own laboratories and invest in health care organizations, which may affect their ability to be impartial in recommending the use of these resources. On the other hand, some managed care firms limit the choices physicians can offer clients, which puts limits on demand.

In a free market, consumers bear the financial consequences of their purchase decisions and are aware of price differences among products. Most Americans rely on reimbursement by third parties, who bear the financial impact of decisions to receive care. This can cause them to not be sensitive, to act as if care is free, to believe that they should get their money's worth for premiums paid, and to have no incentive to "shop around" for better prices. In general, most health consumers are not aware of prices for services, variations in prices between suppliers, and the relationship between price and quality. Even if consumers do want to compare prices for products, it is often difficult because of item-based pricing. Surgery, for example, includes charges for a surgeon, supplies, use of facilities, and services of an anesthesiologist and possibly a pathologist. Exact use of each of these items sometimes cannot be anticipated, making it difficult to determine a price before receiving the service and compare it with a competitor's price. Even though health plans now negotiate fees for "packages" of services or benefits in order to overcome the pricing problems, these are not standardized and thus are still difficult to compare.

In a free market, there is unrestrained competition among providers. Unrestricted access to the market is blocked in several ways for some health care providers. An example is the case of advanced practice nurses, who have not been free to set up primary care practices as they wish. Many states require medical oversight of nursing practice, such as permission for prescription privileges of nurse practitioners. Most third-party payment has not provided direct payment for nursing care. Payment for most nursing care is included in hospital or clinic charges. If consumers must directly bear the cost for any nursing services they might receive, then services that could be offered by nurses will have a limited demand in the market. Limits on entering the market for nurses as well as for some complementary or alternative health practitioners is the same as giving physicians control over competitors. The results are lack of competition based on lower prices or on quality (Rambur & Mooney, 1998).

No single provider in a free market has monopoly power. In response to pressures for cost reduction from health plans, providers are forming alliances and integrated delivery systems. Consolidation among health care networks of hospitals and multispecialty group practices give very large market shares to these groups. In certain geographic areas of the United States, a single large medical system has taken over as the sole provider of major health service, restricting competition (Rice, 1998; Shi & Singh, 1998). The mergers create massive local market leverage that gives them absolute control over local services pricing. In some markets, newly formed local provider monopolies have created price increases of 20% to 50%. For example, after consolidation of most of the oncology groups in one local market into a single group, the cost of 1-hour chemotherapy rose 51%, from $95.76 to $145 (Halvorson, 1999).

Providers of services in the free market seek to operate efficiently to maximize profits. Many of the providers in health care operate as nonprofit organizations. Their only constraint is to make their budgets balance such that expenditures equal revenues. Some may have goals beyond maximizing services, such as extending high salaries and benefits to administration or improving organizational status with expensive equipment regardless of the majority of clients' needs for such technology. Workers in organizations may have adverse incentives from a firm's goal of profit. In the case of physicians, such conflicting goals can be seen when they seek to exhaust every possibility in client diagnosis and order many costly tests. This has been a motivation for instituting capitated payment systems of managed care, which can encourage less spending on care to realize higher retained profit. This can inhibit quality.

As the preceding examples show, the current delivery and consumption of health care in the United States occur in what has been called a *quasi-market* or an *imperfect market* (Shi & Singh, 1998). Much of the controversy over introducing more market mechanisms into health care delivery is related to how poorly the U.S. health care system measures up to the assumptions for an efficient free market. Chapter 6 discusses and lists access and utilization barriers to managed care. Compare those with the problems with the free market in health care. Many problems of access to managed care are economic problems in that they limit access to the free market and thus its efficient functioning. Although we may have success applying free market principles to the place (market) where automobiles, condos, and refrigerators are exchanged for cash, they seem less appropriate for health care. The place where relief of pain, care of infections, and comfort of the spirit are exchanged for cash is thought to be very different (Rambur & Mooney, 1998). For this reason, we have both competition and intricate governmental and social structures to regulate our market systems.

Rising Costs and Today's Health Care System

From Private Pay to Government Involvement

In the past the client or family was expected to pay for their own health care. In 1940, 81.3% of health care was paid by the individual or the family, and 18.7% was financed by some intermediary third party. Of that 18.7%, 2.6% was from private insurance and 16.1% from public funding (Gibson & Waldo, 1982). The value system of the United States has long resisted strong government intervention in health care. Values of individualism, freedom, and protection of privacy underlie this resistance. Even though the idea of a national system of health services has long been present and has been implemented in much of the rest of the world, such is not the case in the United States. Instead, health care originated in the private sector, and only in times of exceptional need has the government intervened with social programs. Chapter 9's appendix lists major legislative actions related to health that have been taken by the federal government. The legislation marks the evolution of the government from a minimal provider of services and protector of public health to that of a major financier for a public enterprise whose controls have

grown over the autonomy of providers and the choices of providers of care (Litman & Robins, 1991).

The Social Security Act of 1935 established Social Security but failed to include health care. The existence of the first indemnity insurance plans, Blue Cross for hospital care and Blue Shield for physician care, diffused political moves for compulsory health insurance (Pulcini & Mahoney, 1998). In 1959, with the Federal Employees Health Benefit Act, Blue Cross negotiated to provide health insurance coverage for federal employees and set the stage for later involvement in Medicare and Medicaid. In the 1960s, during a period of relative prosperity and a growing concern for poor and elderly populations, Medicaid (Title XIX) and Medicare (Title XVIII) programs were passed as amendments to the Social Security Act. At the same time, the federal government became more involved in health care, with legislation establishing regional medical programs, comprehensive health planning, and extensive educational aid to medical and related health professions. In 1997, payment sources were completely the reverse of 1940: Individuals paid directly for 17.2% of their care, and 82.8% was paid by a third party (36.5% by private insurance sources and 46.4% from public funds). The figure below (left) displays these changes.

It was soon evident that the costs of health care were escalating. When the government paid for more health care expenses, the effect was as though individuals had more money to pay for care. As economic theory predicts, increased sources of funds led to increased demand and the revenues of the industry increased as well. Government intervention had contributed to rising costs

SOURCES OF PAYMENT FOR HEALTH CARE, 1940 AND 1997.

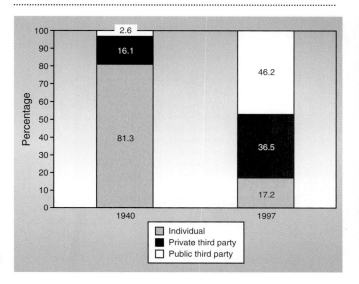

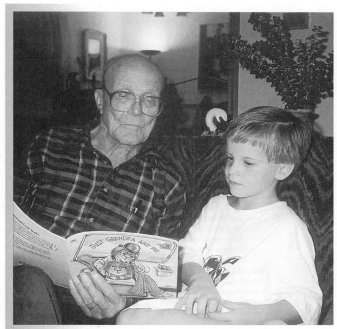

Children and elders often compete for resources in the U.S. health care system.

(Finkler & Kovner, 1993, p. 80). The inability of society or government to limit the rising costs is one of the roots of our present fiscal difficulties in health care.

Increased Costs: The Economic Indicators

One indicator of the United States' high spending is its spending in comparison to other industrialized nations. The United States spends close to a third more on health care than the next highest ranked country (see the figure below).

A more commonly cited indicator is related to the U.S. gross domestic product. **Gross domestic product (GDP)** is the monetary total of all finished goods and services (public and private) produced within a nation in 1 year. Health care expenditures (which means all funds private and public spent on health care) as a percentage of the GDP is a standard measure for comparing and tracking changes in expenditures (Jacobs, 1996).

In the United States, health care has had a long history of escalating costs and an increasing share of the GDP. The figure on the right (top) indicates the rising amounts in all areas with a continuing greater share being paid by private sources but a narrowing of the gap between government and private funding. Private funding paid for 53.6% of health care ($585.3 billion), down from 59.5% in 1990. Currently, most people are still covered by employer-based health insurance. Health care expenditures as a percentage of the GDP grew at an alarming rate for more than 30 years. In the early 1990s, policy makers predicted that, unchecked, health care spending would reach 19% of GDP by 2000 (White House Domestic Policy Council, 1993). The second figure shown on the right shows this trend through the early 1990s, when at last there was a sustained level of low growth for nearly 5 years.

Health care spending grew faster than the GDP for the past three decades as well. The figure on p. 157 (top) depicts the leveling off that led to the situation in 1996 in which the growth

NATIONAL HEALTH EXPENDITURE BY SOURCE OF FUNDS 1960 TO 1997.

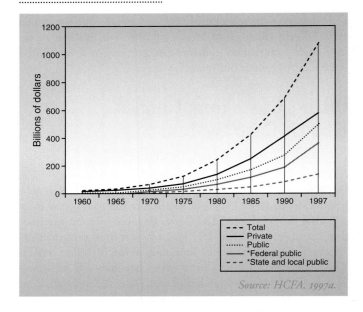

Source: HCFA, 1997a.

rate of the overall economy exceeded the growth rate of health care expenditures. The second figure on p. 157 also shows this mid-1990s trend toward slowed growth as the amount of change in per capita health care expenditures fell.

In 1997, health care expenditures represented 13.5% of the GDP and totaled $1092.4 billion, health care's smallest claim on the nation's resources in 5 years (HCFA, 1998a). U.S. health care spending was predicted to top $1 trillion by 1995 (Standard and

U.S. SPENDING ON HEALTH CARE IN 1995: COMPARISON OF THE UNITED STATES WITH OTHER DEVELOPED COUNTRIES.

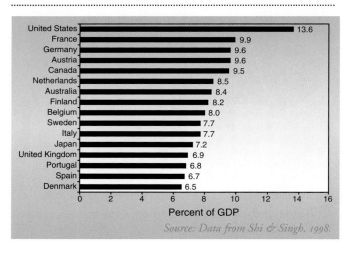

Source: Data from Shi & Singh, 1998.

ACTUAL AND PREDICTED NATIONAL EXPENDITURES AS A PERCENTAGE OF THE GDP 1960 TO 2007.

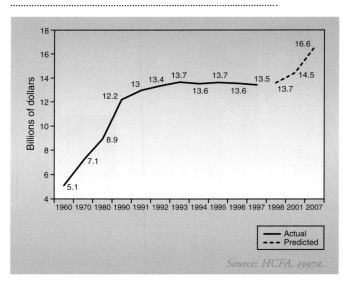

Source: HCFA, 1997a.

ANNUAL CHANGE IN NATIONAL HEALTH EXPENDITURES AND THE GDP 1961 TO 1997.

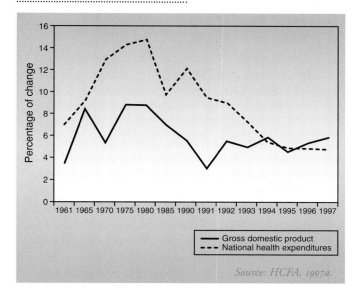

Source: HCFA, 1997a.

Poor's Corporation, 1992), but with the slower rate of growth, it was 1996 before the trillion dollar mark was passed. The more recent progress in reducing the rate of spending growth has been unexpected. Analysts disagree over the reasons for the slowed rate, but many believe the efficiencies introduced by increased market competition and managed care are responsible. However, economic analysts are reluctant to view these lowered rates as a permanent trend. The limits of realizing improved efficiency without harming quality may have been reached as many factors

ANNUAL CHANGE IN THE PER CAPITA HEALTH CARE EXPENDITURES 1990 TO 1997.

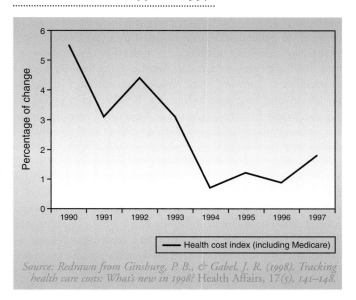

Source: Redrawn from Ginsburg, P. B., & Gabel, J. R. (1998). Tracking health care costs: What's new in 1998? Health Affairs, 17(5), 141–148.

continue to affect costs. For example, Halvorson notes that surgery fees "have been negotiated down 30-40% in many markets during the past four years. For these rock bottom fees, there is no where to go but up" (1999, p. 28). Projections continue to show future rates of growth in the 8% to 10% annual range (Bishop, 1998; Halvorson, 1999). Looking back to the figure on p. 156 (bottom right) shows that predictions in the late 1990s were that the rate of growth would again begin to climb in the early 2000s (Smith, Freland, Heffler, McKisick, & the Health Expenditures Projection Team, 1998).

Decreased Access: The Economic Barriers

Services offered by the U.S. health care system are undoubtedly the best anywhere in the world. Yet the United States is often below other developed countries in health status indicators. One author has described it thus: "It is a healthcare system focused on providing excellent care for the individuals within it, while virtually ignoring the more basic health service needs of the larger populations outside of it" (Sultz & Young, 1997, p. 46). Even though superior services are present, the dark side of the situation is that they are not accessible to all. Access to care means that people can get health care when they need it. Inadequate access for millions of Americans is a core problem and has led to the concern about health care in the United States.

The concept of access to health care has long been recognized as an issue and a responsibility for nurses (Stevens, 1992). Gulzar (1999) examined the concept of access to health care from a nursing perspective and delineated its many dimensions. She defined access to health care as "the fit among personal, sociocultural, economic, and system-related factors that enable individuals, families and communities to have timely, needed, necessary, continuous, and satisfactory health services" (p. 17). These include, for example, age, gender, ethnicity, and culture appropriateness, understandable language, health care providers and facilities near where people live, available transportation, timeliness, and affordability.

Economically, the major barrier to health care access, which is closely associated with the concern of rising costs, is the inability to pay (Bodenheimer & Grumbach, 1995). Very few people can afford to pay out of pocket for the tremendous costs of an illness episode or for the ongoing expenses of a chronic illness, and long-term institutional care is far beyond most individuals' ability to pay. In 1996, 41.7 million Americans (15.6% of the population) were without health insurance, an 14.8% increase over 7 years (from 1989) (Carrasquillo, Himmelstein, Woolhandler, & Bor, 1999). Without coverage, people either do not seek needed care or do not pay for the care they do receive. The poor and working poor without adequate access do not lack emergency or urgent care because no one needing such care is turned away if they go to a hospital. It is primary care such as checkups, screenings, chronic illness follow-ups, and prenatal care that they lack, leaving many of them eventually needing more costly and less timely treatment.

NUMBER OF UNINSURED PERSONS IN THE UNITED STATES 1984 TO 1996.

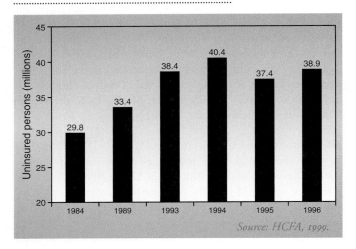

Source: HCFA, 1999.

A CONVERSATION WITH...

HEALTH POLICY AND ETHICS ANALYST EMILY FRIEDMAN

There is a new and growing class of uninsured people. Women aged 50 to 64 are disproportionally likely to be uninsured, often because they are not covered through spousal benefits that have ended because of loss of a job.... Older women ... have been thrown into the individual health insurance market and can't afford coverage. I know a little about this first-hand. I am self-employed and buy my own health insurance. When I turned 50, my insurance sent me a birthday present of a 22% rate increase. That was followed this year with a 9% increase. There's a 14% rate increase on the way. When I am 55, I will be paying twice what I am paying now. I have a $500 deductible and have never filed a claim. I can afford it. But many cannot. I have friends who are working, yet who have sold belongings to pay for health care. The situation is very serious and it is happening to middle class people.

—Emily Friedman,
Health Policy and Ethics Analyst
Source: Brown, 1999.

From the 1930s to mid-1970s, the numbers of insured grew as a result of growth in private insurance and passage of Medicare and Medicaid, but since 1976, the numbers of *uninsured* have been growing (see the figure above).

Although the numbers of people covered by Medicare and Medicaid have grown, there has been a drop in the number covered by private health insurance. Today approximately 41.7 million Americans lack insurance at any given time (Sultz & Young, 1997) and as many as 50 to 60 million are without it at some time during the year (Rowland, Lyons, Salganicoff, & Long, 1994). Lack of insurance is not just a problem of the poor; the numbers are growing among the middle class. Many are especially concerned about children's access to care. Recent reports show that more than 10 million children in the United States (14.2% of those younger than 15 years of age) are without insurance and another 5 million are underinsured (Alpert, 1998). The proportion covered by private employment-based insurance has declined. Almost 25% of children in families where a parent is working full-time are without employment-based insurance, and 12% had no insurance (Havens & Hannon, 1997). Most of the uninsured do not qualify for Medicaid. Because states set their own standards for eligibility, there are wide differences in poor people (those with incomes below the federal poverty level) who are covered by Medicaid. These range from a high in Washington, D.C., of 60% of poor people covered by Medicaid to a low of 29% of the poor covered in Nevada. Many of the newly uninsured are employed or are dependents of those who are employed.

Recent research has shown that even though more employers are offering insurance, fewer employees are purchasing it (Cooper & Schone, 1997; Ginsberg, Gabel, & Hunt, 1998). One factor explaining this is the rise in the proportion of premiums that the employee must pay. Another is the long-term trend of premiums increasing more rapidly than earnings, especially for low-income employees (Ginsberg, 1998). Higher premiums are also harder for employers to pay, especially in smaller firms. Furthermore, there has been a shift in workers to the service industry, with low-wage, part-time, nonunion jobs that are less likely to offer them coverage (Levit, Olin, & Letsch, 1992).

Having private insurance does not guarantee financial access to care. Research has shown that one in six people have insurance policies that do not protect them from difficulties in getting needed care (Himmelstein & Woolhandler, 1995). Based on surveys of those who were asked if they had needed but did not receive any of seven preventive services during a year, an estimated 6.3 million people reported that they did not get needed care.

The uninsured were twice as likely not to receive care, but three fourths of those who went without were insured, and 46% had private insurance. Those who had Medicaid were as likely to go without care as the uninsured. Many physicians do not accept the coverage offered by Medicaid. Both the insured and the uninsured cited cost as the major barrier to care (Himmelstein & Woolhandler, 1995). Other studies have cited cost and lack of employer-provided coverage as reasons for having no coverage (Donelan, Blendon, Hill, Hoffman, Rowland, Frankel, & Altman, 1997).

Public programs are generally considered inadequate for prenatal care (Hughes & Runyan, 1997) and mental health pro-

grams (Mechanic & Rochefort, 1997), and contractual arrangements for home health care can restrict needed visits in home health care services (Shaughnessy, Schlenker, & Hittle, 1995). Private coverage restricts access because of high out-of-pocket expenditures of co-payments and deductibles, fixed indemnity (maximum payment allowed), and exclusions, such as for preexisting conditions. Such an exclusion may be for a set time after enrollment or may be permanent. Changing jobs can trigger this restriction. Most Americans are underinsured for preventive services, catastrophic illness, and long-term care (Harrington & Estes, 1997, p. 2). *Healthy People 2010* objectives that address access issues are listed below.

HEALTHY PEOPLE 2010

OBJECTIVES RELATED TO ACCESS

Access to Quality Health Services

Clinical Preventive Care

1.1   Increase the proportion of persons with health insurance.

1.2   Increase the proportion of insured persons with coverage for clinical preventive services.

Primary Care

1.3   Increase the proportion of persons who have a specific source of ongoing care.

1.4   Increase the proportion of persons with a usual primary care provider.

1.5   Reduce the proportion of families that experience difficulties or delays in obtaining health care or do not receive needed care for one or more family members.

Educational and Community–Based Programs

7.9   Increase the proportion of hospitals and managed care organizations that provide community disease prevention and health-promotion activities that address the priority health needs identified by their community.

Family Planning

9.13   Increase the proportion of health insurance policies that cover contraceptive supplies and services.

Oral Health

21.12   Increase the proportion of children and adults under age 19 years at or below 200% of the federal poverty level who received any preventive dental service during the past year.

Public Health Infrastructure

23.16   Increase the proportion of federal, tribal, state, and local public health agencies that gather accurate data on public health expenditures, categorized by essential public health service.

Source: DHHS, 2000.

Numerous negative outcomes for those who are uninsured or underinsured and thus lack access have been documented. These negative outcomes include increased economic burdens and worsened health and mortality (Donelan et al., 1997). Chapter 25 discusses in more depth the vulnerability of the medically indigent.

Influences on Costs and Access

No single factor explains why health spending has grown at the rate it has, but several influences collectively contribute to the situation. As discussed earlier, there was an economic effect of increased demand as a result of greater sources of funds from government. In addition, as listed in Box 7-2, increases over the last few years have resulted from several sources.

Inflation, which is indicated by the rising consumer price index, has continued for all goods and services in the United States, but prices have increased at an even greater rate for health care services. The figure to the right shows the relative shares of some health care expenditures in 1997.

Physicians and hospitals account for the greatest proportion by far. Expenditures for public health services, as shown in the figure on the right, account for only a little more than 3% of overall spending. Drug costs increased 15% to 20% in the late 1990s and are expected to continue to rise. Halvorson (1999) gives two reasons for the increases. Drug companies market new, very expensive drugs directly to consumers, who then request them from their physicians. In addition, companies raise the prices on older drugs that research shows to be most effective.

Most advanced technology is expensive. New and costly methods of care push prices up. One of the major contributors to health care services inflation is increased technology, which introduces newer and costlier treatments and methods of care. An excellent example is the availability of new treatment for infertility. Infertility treatments can cost up to $20,000, and $500,000 to $1 million can be spent on premature (or multiple) infants (Halvorson, 1999). As newer technologies are introduced, doctors and nurses become dependent on their use. Increased technology requires more highly trained personnel to run it, and its complexity contributes to specialization among health care

BOX 7-2 INFLUENCES ON RISING HEALTH CARE COSTS

- Increased government funding
- Inflation
- Rising drug costs
- Increased use of expensive technology
- Increased wages of health care personnel
- Population changes
- Administrative and medical excess

THE NATION'S HEALTH DOLLAR: 1997. WHERE IT WENT. (Other includes dentists, other professional care, durable medical products, research, and construction.)

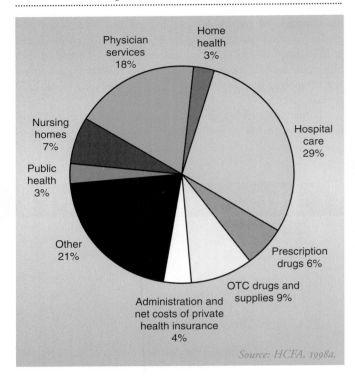

Source: HCFA, 1998a.

providers. This contributes to higher personnel wages and benefit costs. Consumers are also used to increasing technology and want the very latest in methods and equipment.

Another obvious factor in rising costs is the change in population demographics. The overall population is growing, partly as a result of immigration. Immigrants who enter the United States are often poor and have many health problems. Giving access to these groups increases costs. Large population numbers alone can mean greater costs, but costs per capita (per person) in the United States have grown as well. In 1960, the health care costs per capita were $143, and today they are close to $4,000. Costs per person can be partially explained by the changing demographics of an aging population. High-tech medicine and other factors have prolonged life. In the year 2000, it is estimated that 13% of the population is older than 65 years of age. New terms, such as the *old old* and the *young old*, have come into use as the population lives longer and *old* has new meanings. The over-85 group is growing at a rapid rate. Older persons require more health resources as a result of normal processes associated with aging as well as longstanding chronic illness. The need for more long-term care resources and personal health services are increasing proportionately with the aging population.

Even though some in the United States are deprived of needed health care, there is also the factor of excess in the system. Excess comes in a variety of forms. High-tech equipment is expensive, as is the investment in spaces to house it. It often becomes used more often than necessary to justify its high cost. In a society where providers fear litigation, even when less expensive options may be equally effective, high-tech procedures may be overused, resulting in medical excess that is referred to as *defensive medicine*. Many argue that excessive and unwanted measures are used to prolong life past the ability to have quality of life for both the terminally ill and the elderly.

Administrative excess contributing to increased costs includes both inefficiencies in systems of care and high administrative costs. Inefficient systems of care can be inferred from the patterns of differentiation in treatment and costs across geographic service areas, for example. These differences, unexplained by other factors, are attributed to disagreement on "best practices" among direct care providers. Some practices are more expensive. For instance, the benefits of coronary artery bypass surgery over more conservative and less costly treatment are questioned. Greater numbers of hysterectomies and cesarean sections for women in some areas are explained by practice patterns that may not be cost-effective. Even with similar population attributes and illnesses, more days are spent in the hospital in some areas than others. All this points to the need to look for more cost-effective clinical practices. Administrative costs, while accounting for a small proportion of the health care dollar, still come under criticism. The U.S. General Accounting Office estimated that in 1991, $67 billion of administrative spending was unnecessary (Bodenheimer & Grumbach, 1995).

Closely associated with clinical practice patterns has been the emphasis on cure over prevention of illness. Practice is often guided by reimbursement patterns, and payment from most sources in the recent past has been made only when illness is present. Many economic analyses indicate that preventing illness is more cost-effective than waiting for costly illness to be diagnosed, treated, and monitored. Managed care systems that focus on cost-effectiveness have begun to emphasize preventive care. The relationship of managed care and public health concerns for health promotion and disease prevention is addressed in detail later in this chapter.

Paying for Health Care

Access to health care is determined by financing. Thus, demand in the marketplace is directly related to the amount of financing. Services and treatments that are covered by a source of payment have greater demand than if those services were not covered. Financing of health care in the United States is complex. There are multiple sources of funds for health care. These funds, both public and private, are dispersed in a variety of programs and health plans through which resources are used to purchase services. The figure above indicates the major sources of funds spent on personal health care in 1997. Private sources accounted for 54.7% while public funding paid for 46.3%.

THE NATION'S HEALTH CARE DOLLAR: 1997. WHERE IT CAME FROM.

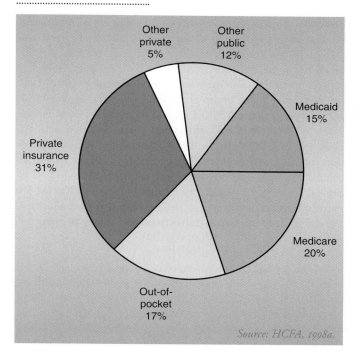

Source: HCFA, 1998a.

Direct Payments by Consumers and Charity

Funds that are paid directly by individuals are sometimes called *out-of-pocket payments*. Some individuals or families assume all their own costs for health care services. This is possible when costs are low. A common example is the purchase of over-the-counter drugs. However, this is the least common method of paying for services. With most individuals covered by either private or public insurance, the more common out-of-pocket expenses are in the form of **cost sharing**. These expenses include insurance premiums, insurance deductibles, co-payment of a percentage of medical costs, costs above fixed payments, and noncovered services. Because so many consumers are unable to meet the costs of services they need and because providing health care to the suffering is seen by some as a moral imperative in modern societies, charity, insurance, and government sources provide funds in varying degrees (Wesson, 1999). Those who cannot afford to pay for needed care often turn to care financed by charity. Charity care has been seen as a religious duty or vocation, and various religious as well as secular organizations have offered care to the needy for little or no charge. Many physicians and other providers have also cared for the needy, either for free or based on a sliding scale. Philanthropic organizations financed by donors have established institutions to offer charitable care and special services. Another form of nongovernmental funds for health care is expenditures covering health care services provided for employees in industrial settings.

Health Insurance

Risk is a notion central to the concept of insurance. Risk is the possibility of a substantial financial loss from costs of a health event that has a small probability of occurring. Health insurance is a contractual agreement for payment of such health care costs and protection from the risk. For a prepaid premium, specific benefits or protections are covered. When the insurance company collects premiums from many subscribers, the risk is shifted from the individual to the group by pooling resources. Health insurance is highly regulated by federal and state governments. For example, significant federal reform was passed in 1996 with the Health Insurance Portability and Accountability Act. Key provisions of the act were portability of health insurance (if certain conditions of prior coverage are met), mental health parity as regards lifetime limits, mandatory minimum length of stay for obstetric clients, the creation of tests of new funding methods (medical savings accounts), and further fraud and abuse sanctions.

Private

Individual private health insurance is purchased by many Americans. Those who work in businesses that do not offer health insurance, the self-employed (including farmers), new college graduates, and early retirees are examples of those younger than 65 who purchase their own private insurance. These types of policies do not spread risk as in group insurance, but rather base premiums on each individual's health risk.

Employment Based

The most common kind of insurance is employer-provided insurance. The employer pays all or most of the insurance premium as an employment benefit. In 1994, the average of premiums paid by employers was 72%; the remaining 28% was paid by employees. Health insurance as a fringe benefit became popular during World War II, when wages were frozen but benefits could be given. It still is favored by tax policy, which does not apply income or social security tax to benefits. Premiums paid through employment are determined by group risks. **Experience ratings** are based on a group's own health insurance claims experience. One group may be at greater risk as a result of occupational hazards or susceptibilities. Their premiums will be higher because they can be expected to use health care services more often. In contrast, **community ratings** base premiums on the utilization experience of a whole community, so rates are the same for everyone regardless of indicators of risk such as age or occupation.

As health care costs have risen, employers' insurance costs have risen also. After salaries and raw materials, health care is the third largest cost category for U.S. corporations (Loubeau & Maher, 1996). Employers who compete in the global market are especially concerned because competitors in other countries with government-funded health care do not have the same costs and thus can set lower prices. Employers have initiated more and more cost containment strategies. Generic-only prescriptions, second opinions, preadmission testing, and more outpatient surgery are some of the employer strategies. For some employers (as well as individuals) **health insurance purchasing cooperatives (HIPCs)**, organizations that represent a number of employers, help lower costs. By consolidating purchasing power and realizing efficiencies in enrollment and premium collection, they can help small employers get lower rates than they could alone (Chollet, 1996). However, a main strategy has been to offer managed care plans as an exclusive or alternative health plan. Managed care plans cover nearly 75% of employees with health insurance in small as well as large firms (Shi & Singh, 1998).

Some employers with large workforces have begun to rely on **self-insurance.** Instead of paying premiums to an insurance plan, they assume health care cost risks by budgeting for medical claims from their employees. Government policy stimulated this option when it passed the Employee Retirement Income Security Act of 1974, which allowed self-funded, nonprofit health plans by corporations. Such plans were exempted from taxes and certain mandatory benefits required of regular plans (Health Insurance Association of America, 1991). For large employers, self-insurance was a better economic alternative. For employees, coverage can be less certain and they may have less recourse for appealing claims that are not covered.

Some of the political debate over health care funding has centered around whether health insurance coverage should be mandated for all firms with workers. The proponents believe it is sound business and will attract a stable workforce. Those opposed, mostly small business leaders, believe that the expense would cause small businesses to fail and jobs would be lost.

Publicly Funded Insurance and Direct Care Programs

Public financing supports **categorical programs** that are developed to benefit a certain category of people. The largest of these are Medicare for the elderly and Medicaid for the indigent. The

FEDERAL ENTITLEMENT AND WELFARE PROGRAM EXPENDITURES, 1998.

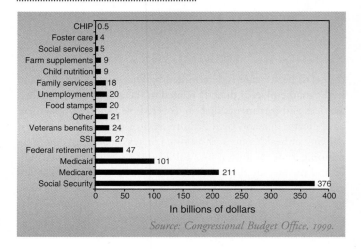

Program	In billions of dollars
CHIP	0.5
Foster care	4
Social services	5
Farm supplements	9
Child nutrition	9
Family services	18
Unemployment	20
Food stamps	20
Other	21
Veterans benefits	24
SSI	27
Federal retirement	47
Medicaid	101
Medicare	211
Social Security	376

Source: Congressional Budget Office, 1999.

balance of government support goes to U.S. public health service hospitals, services of the Veterans Affairs hospitals and health services, the Department of Defense for military personnel and dependents, the Indian Health Service, state and local support for inpatient psychiatric and other long-term care facilities, workers' compensation, public health activities, and other grants and initiatives. In most cases the government provides the financing but obtains insurance and health care services through the private sector. Payments are disbursed in programs of reimbursements, direct payment, grants, matching funds, and subsidies. Some programs combine federal and state funds. The figure on p. 162 shows the amounts of federal money spent on U.S. entitlement and welfare programs.

The large impact of Medicaid, Medicare, and Social Security compared with other programs can be seen.

Medicare

Title XVIII of the Social Security Act, titled "Health Insurance for the Aged and Disabled," is commonly know as Medicare. Its beginning in 1966 was a historical benchmark. By giving health insurance to everybody older than 65 years of age who are covered by Social Security, it signaled a giant step for government entry into personal health care financing. In 1973, other groups became eligible for benefits: persons entitled to Social Security or Railroad Retirement disability benefits for at least 24 months, persons with end-stage renal disease (ESRD) requiring continuing dialysis or kidney transplant, and certain otherwise noncovered persons who elect to buy into Medicare. The Health Care Financing Administration (HCFA) is responsible for overseeing the total program. Medicare covers approximately 50% of the medical expenses of the elderly (Bodenheimer & Grumbach, 1995).

Medicare consists of two parts, which differ in sources of funding and benefits. These are hospital insurance (HI), known as *Part A,* and supplementary medical insurance (SMI), known as *Part B.* A third part of Medicare, established by the Balanced Budget Act of 1997, is the Medicare+Choice program, known as *Part C,* which began to provide services on January 1, 1998. In 1998, almost 39 million persons were enrolled in one or both of Parts A and B. Some HI and/or SMI service was used by about 87% of all Medicare enrollees in 1997.

Hospital insurance, Part A of Medicare, is mandatory. It provides benefits for care provided in the hospital, outpatient diagnostic services, extended care facilities, and short-term care at home required by an illness for which the client was hospitalized. HI is financed primarily by payroll taxes collected for Social Security from employees and self-employed workers. The tax is 1.45% of earnings paid by both employers and employees, as well as 2.9% for the self-employed. Before 1994, there was a ceiling on income taxed for Medicare, but in 1993, the Omnibus Budget Reconciliation Act of 1993 (OBRA-93) made all earnings subject to Medicare tax. Part A hospital insurance has limits on care and requires deductibles and co-payments based on the duration of services.

The following is an overview of the health benefits covered by Medicare's hospital insurance:

- Inpatient hospital care *covers a semiprivate room, meals, regular nursing services, operating and recovery rooms, intensive care, inpatient prescription drugs, laboratory tests, x-ray examinations, psychiatric hospital stays, inpatient rehabilitation, and long-term care hospitalization when medically necessary, as well as services and supplies used in the hospital. A maximum of 90 days is allowed per benefit period. Past 90 days, there is a lifetime reserve of 60 inpatient days. A **benefit period** is an episode of illness starting with hospitalization and ending when the beneficiary has not been a patient in a hospital or skilled nursing facility for 60 consecutive days. There is no limit on the number of benefit periods.*

- Skilled nursing facility (SNF) care *is covered only if it follows within 30 days of a hospitalization of 3 days or more, not including the day of discharge. Up to 100 days of care can be covered. Nursing facility care is not covered unless the required care is for skilled nursing or rehabilitation care.*

- Home health agency (HHA) care, *including care by a home health aid, can be provided intermittently in the residence of a home-bound beneficiary. Again, skilled care must be necessary. Some supplies and equipment may be provided. There are no time or visit limits. Full-time nursing, food, drugs, and blood are not covered as HHA services.*

- Hospice services *for terminally ill clients are covered for Medicare-certified hospices. The client must have a life expectancy of less than 6 months and forgo benefits for traditional medical treatment for the terminal illness. Covered care includes pain relief, supportive medical and social services, physical therapy, nursing services, and symptom management.*

Supplemental medical insurance, Part B, is available to almost all residents and certain immigrants age 65 and older, even if they are not entitled to HI services, and disabled persons who are eligible for HI. Coverage is voluntary and is financed by general tax revenues as well as a required monthly premium. Premiums are currently set at a level ($48.80/month) that covers 25% of the national expenditures for the aged beneficiaries. Although the majority of coverage goes to physician fees, SMI also covers many nonphysician services. To be covered, all services must either be medically necessary or be one of the prescribed preventive benefits (e.g., flu vaccinations). Special payment rules, including deductibles, maximum amounts payable, or higher cost sharing, apply to certain services and care. A yearly deductible ($100 in 1998) and a co-insurance of 20% of allowed charges is paid by the beneficiaries.

Medicare+Choice was created through the Balanced Budget Act of 1997. This option increases the managed care plans available to Medicare beneficiaries. Beneficiaries are given the option of a variety of risk-based plans, including coordinated care plans such as health maintenance organizations (HMOs), provider-sponsored organizations (PSOs), and preferred provider organizations (PPOs), as well as other approved alternatives to traditional Medicare. From the beginning of Medicare, alternative payment methodologies have existed for HMO-type providers. However, in 1995, less than 8% of the total Medicare population was enrolled in such plans. The goal has been to expand the number of managed care options and increase the number of contractors (Vladeck & King, 1997). The Medicare+Choice program offers beneficiaries a broad range of health plan options similar to those available in the private sector.

Market principles are evident in Medicare's performance as both a purchaser as well as regulator of managed care. Beneficiaries are given information to allow them to compare their choices and make a selection based on individual preferences and market conditions. The Medicare Compare Database Web site, provided by HCFA, encourages Medicare consumers to "comparison shop" and gives detailed information on Medicare's health plan options for costs and benefits effective January 1, 2000.

Electing to participate in managed care plans may serve as an alternative to purchasing **Medigap insurance,** which is desired if the beneficiary has traditional fee-for-service coverage. Medicare can leave beneficiaries with substantial out-of-pocket-costs. Because Part B excludes coverage for prescription drugs, glasses, dentures, hearing aids, yearly physical examinations, routine foot care, and dental care, many individuals supplement their Medicare benefits. Only 12% qualify for Medicaid to pick up these extra expenses, and some retirees have employer plans that cover extra expenses. The term *Medigap* is used to mean private health insurance that pays most of the health care service charges not covered by Parts A and B of Medicare. Such policies, offered by Blue Cross and Blue Shield and commercial health insurance companies, must meet federal standards.

Methods of payment to providers of services for Medicare beneficiaries continue to change as cost-containment incentives are encouraged. Currently, hospitals are paid on a prospective payment system of fixed price per case for clients in 468 diagnosis-related groups (DRGs). Just as DRGs were implemented to contain hospital costs, **resource utilization groups, version 3** (RUG-III) were launched in July 1998 to contain costs in SNFs. They are designed to differentiate clients by their levels of resource use. Payment is made on a per diem rate that varies according to client RUG-III category. The goal is to relate pay to client care requirements and to pay SNFs with different client caseloads equitably. The new payment system is to be phased in over 3 years and is expected to have a profound effect on SNFs (Shi & Singh, 1998). Likewise, HCFA has developed ambulatory patient groups (APGs) based on the same goals, which are to be used in clinic settings. These have not been used in Medicare reimbursement yet, but some states have adopted the classification system for Medicaid programs (Shi & Singh, 1998).

Reimbursement for physicians before 1992 was for a "reasonable charge," which was the lowest of actual charge, customary charge, or prevailing charge in the area. This has changed to payments based on lowest of submitted charges or a fee schedule based on a **relative value scale.** The relative values are based on the time, skill, and intensity it takes to perform a service. The scale places more value on care received through primary care physicians and emphasizes prevention and health promotion. Less value is placed on surgeries and use of high technology. Fees for nurse practitioners and clinical nurse specialists are set at 85% of what a physician would be paid under the Medicare fee schedule. Outpatient and home health services are currently reimbursed on a reasonable cost basis, but the 1997 Balanced Budget Act provided for implementing a prospective payment system for these services in the future. Claims for both HI and SMI are processed by nongovernmental organizations that contract to serve as the fiscal agent between the federal government and providers. They function locally to apply coverage rules and are known as *intermediaries* and *carriers*.

Medicaid

Because people have contributed to Medicare through taxes, it is considered an **entitlement** program due to them regardless of their wealth. Medicaid, however is a **welfare** program representing funds transferred from more economically affluent individuals to those in need. Title XIX of the Social Security Act is a federal-state matching funds program with the intent to provide basic health care services to the economically indigent. The federal government provides matching funds based on the per capita income of each state. By law, it cannot be more than 83% or less than 50% matching funds. There is no set limit on total federal outlays. Within broad national guidelines, which the federal government provides, each state (1) establishes its own eligibility standards; (2) determines the type, amount, duration, and scope of services; (3) sets the rate of payment for services; and (4) administers its own program. Policies vary greatly from state to state; therefore, a person who is eligible for Medicaid in one state may not be eligible in another state. In addition, eligibility and services in a state can change during a year. The broad federal guidelines include certain mandated coverage. These include inpatient and outpatient hospital services, skilled nursing care, physician services, home health care, family planning services, and early and periodic screening, diagnosis, and treatment services for eligible individuals younger than 21 years of age.

Recipients must establish their eligibility for Medicaid based on income and assets. In 1996, more than 36 million individuals were provided health care assistance at a cost of $160 billion ($91 billion in federal and $69 billion in state funds) (Waid, 1998). Individuals younger than 21 made up 46% of that number. The Medicaid program provides services to two broad groups of persons: the categorically needy and the medically needy. For the **categorically needy,** federal funds are matched for mandatory eligibility groups, which include people receiving Supplemental Security Income (SSI) in some states; those who meet the requirements for Aid to Families with Dependent Children (AFDC) that were in effect in their state prior to July 16,

1996; children younger than 6 and pregnant women whose family income is below 133% of the federal poverty level (FPL); and all children born after September 30, 1983, who are younger than 19 and living in families whose income is at or below the FPL. For children, this means that by 2002, all poor children younger than 19 will be eligible. In 1999, the poverty level for the 48 contiguous states for a family of four was $16,700; for Hawaii it was $19,210, and for Alaska it was $20,880 (Department of Health and Human Services, 1999). States also have the option of providing coverage to specified other categorically related groups, for example, the **medically needy** (those persons who incur medical expenses beyond the scope of their income). These groups may then receive matching federal funds.

In 1996, the Personal Responsibility and Work Opportunity Act made sweeping welfare reforms that have had consequences for the Medicaid program. Changes in eligibility for SSI had an impact. For immigrants who lost SSI, Medicaid can continue only if they qualify under some other eligibility status. The new legislation ended the original foundation of the welfare system, AFDC, and replaced it with Temporary Assistance for Needy Families (TANF). TANF is a block-grant program that limits lifetime cash welfare benefits to 5 years (or less at a state's option). Welfare funds are no longer unconditionally guaranteed to eligible poor families, but states are allowed to impose a wide range of other restrictions as well. For example, if recipients are not involved in work-related activities by the end of their second year on welfare, they forfeit future benefits. Single mothers have an automatic 25% reduction in benefits if they refuse to help establish the paternity of their children. Of significance for Medicaid was the delinkage of its benefits from welfare cash assistance. The law does not require persons covered by TANF to receive Medicaid. However, under the reform, those eligible for Medicaid under AFDC requirements in effect on July 16, 1996, are generally still eligible.

Because Medicaid eligibility is no longer linked to welfare, it is necessary to reach needy families and children who are outside of as well as in the welfare system to ensure that as many children and families as possible obtain health insurance coverage. Following the initiation of TANF, some states saw a drastic reduction in children enrolled in Medicaid. Many believed that families were losing Medicaid as they transitioned off welfare (Mississippi Health Advocacy Program, 1998). Guidelines for protecting and expanding health coverage in the post-welfare reform world have been developed by the HCFA (HCFA, 1999a).

Other developments in Medicaid services are related to long-term nursing home care. Increasing numbers of elderly citizens, added to the excessively high expense of long-term institutions and home-based care, have created an increasing number of new eligible recipients for Medicaid coverage. Many with modest resources rapidly use them up in paying for nursing homes or home care. Nursing home expenses normally reach $30,000 to $40,000 per year. Middle-class individuals paying these costs quickly become medically needy and meet state guidelines for Medicaid. With Medicare coverage limited to only 3 months and little private in-surance coverage for nursing home care, Medicaid currently funds almost half of annual nursing home care expenditures. Out-of-pocket payments make up the next largest percentage of funds. A very small amount of both institutional and home-bound long-term care services are paid by private insurance. Insurance for long-term care has been difficult to market. Younger, healthier groups whose enrollment would spread the risk and costs generally do not enroll. Therefore, long-term care insurance rates stay high and policies cover only a portion of expenses. Long-term care is expected to be an increasingly utilized provision of Medicaid, with efforts focused on more community-based long-term care alternatives (Shi & Singh, 1998; Sultz & Young, 1997; Waid, 1998).

Reimbursement under Medicaid is made directly to providers. Rate-setting formulas, procedures, and policies vary widely among states. Fee-for-service systems of payment have dominated. However, federal waivers allow states to develop innovative delivery or reimbursement systems. The last few years have seen a growth in enrollment of Medicaid beneficiaries in managed care from 9.5% of beneficiaries in 1991 to 53.6% in 1998. As with Medicare, public policy makers have been eager to realize the cost savings reported by private buyers of managed health care services. Competitive bidding strategies allow bids to be made by provider plans. Several states have converted their entire Medicaid programs to managed care.

Children's Health Insurance Program

The Children's Health Insurance Program (CHIP) is a new program that was initiated by the Balanced Budget Act of 1997. CHIP provides federal funds of approximately $24 billion over 5 years for states to expand Medicaid eligibility to include more uninsured children. These are mostly low-income children who would not qualify for Medicaid based on the plan in effect on April 15, 1997, but whose families cannot afford private insurance. In 1999, it was estimated that 3.1 million uninsured children would be eligible for CHIP. In addition, 8.8 million children with private insurance would qualify based on family income alone (Seldon, Banthin, & Cohen, 1999). Coverage can be provided by states through Medicaid expansion, separate CHIP program, or a combination. Under a separate CHIP program, states can establish more flexible eligibility requirements. In some cases, states can implement coverage for low-income families, not just children, under CHIP. Also, eligibility for coverage can be expanded to up to 200% of the poverty level. By September 1999, 56 state and territory plans had been submitted for implementing CHIP expansion. For these plans, an estimated 2.7 million enrollments were expected by September 2000 (HCFA, 1999c). As with Medicare and Medicaid, managed care options were being offered.

CHAMPUS and Direct Care Programs

Another category of persons who have publicly funded health care insurance is military personnel and dependents. The Military Health Services System, funded under the Department of

Defense, operates to provide medical services to active and retired members of the armed forces and their dependents. Care is provided through military facilities, including hospitals and clinics, and is supplemented by services purchased from civilian systems and paid for by the Civilian Health and Medical Program of the Uniformed Services (CHAMPUS). Services are free at military facilities, but when care is received from civilian providers who are paid through CHAMPUS, there is cost sharing (deductibles and co-insurance) by the families. CHAMPUS does not cover active duty service members (who receive all their care from the military facilities), only retirees and dependents.

Linked to the military health care system is the Veterans Administration (VA) health care system. Through this system, the federal government acts as a direct supplier of services to veterans for both war-related injuries and disabilities. For poor servicemen, care is also given for illnesses not related to military service. The system is composed of more than 173 hospitals, 401 clinics, and 133 nursing homes (Inglehart, 1996). The cost of this system in 1995 was $16.1 billion (National Center for Health Statistics, 1997).

The federal government is also involved in direct care to Native Americans living on reservations. The Indian Health Service (IHS) provides both inpatient and ambulatory clinic services in 50 hospitals, 158 health clinics, and several ambulatory clinic facilities. These facilities operate at the local level to serve 1.1 million American Indians with expenditures of $1.4 billion.

In 1976, tribal governments were granted authority to operate IHS facilities, which are often in remote areas and have low volume. The recent trend has been to refer to and contract with private providers for specialty care and diagnostic services.

Other Public Sources of Health Care Funding

The government funds numerous health programs for specific populations and specific health problems. Many of these have come about through amendments to the Public Health Service Act of 1994. The programs in place at most local health departments come from this funding and assist vulnerable at-risk groups (Gerber & McGuire, 1995). These programs cover immunizations, tuberculosis, venereal diseases, and family planning, along with other services. Rural health clinics, migrant health clinics, and community health centers also are publicly funded. Community health centers (685 in 1996) operate with 28% of their funds authorized from the Public Health Services Act. These clinics, which pioneered the employment of nurse practitioners, serve as the primary safety net for the poor and underserved in both rural and inner-city settings (Shi & Singh, 1998).

Cost Containment, Cost Analysis, and Quality

Costs must be contained for the public to get maximum returns on prepaid private insurance, employer-sponsored insurance, and taxes paid toward health care programs. The maze of interconnecting factors related to the causes of high and rising health care costs, of course, guide the mechanisms chosen for controlling them. Mechanisms for cost containment include policy decisions at federal, state, local, and organizational levels. The forces influencing how these decisions are made are complex, as described in chapter 9. Reform proposals described by Reinert in chapter 5 show the policy makers' quandary in trying to rectify the cost and quality problems of our system. Proposals are for either total or incremental system changes or for changes in the financing of health care. As has been pointed out, economic trends related to costs in the last few years have so far shown results that encourage the strategy of market competition (although predictions of ability to sustain the trends vary). To quote a health services researcher, "The effects of what is now referred to as 'market driven' reform being played out through the proliferation and increasing gains by managed care in controlling costs are pervasively evident throughout virtually every component of the delivery system" (Sultz & Young, 1997, p. 196). The managed care solution is covered in detail in chapter 6, and its relation to prevention and cost control is discussed later in this chapter.

Both regulatory and competitive strategies to control costs have been mentioned throughout the previous discussion in this chapter. Box 7-3 summarizes some of the methods of these two strategies. One economic strategy that has become increasingly important for nurses and other providers is economic evaluation, which contributes to finding the most cost-effective ways of delivering care and treatments. At the level of both practice guidelines and social policy, economic evaluation is essential. Economic evaluation can be used to help in resource allocation in delivery of nursing care and to improve the overall quality of clinical care (Stone, 1998).

Where once the focus of health decision making was only on the effectiveness of treatments and interventions, under competition providers are now competing for contracts with consumers. Consumers look around and make choices based on information about price, quality indicators, and levels of users' satisfaction. Insurers want to know what services to cover and how much to cover. Those who pay often make the treatment decisions. Policy makers want to know how to control public expenditures. Cost evaluation assessments can be expensive, but for stakeholders, competition provides the incentive to invest in the needed cost-effectiveness and quality outcomes data they provide. The data are used for internal decisions and now, more and more often, for letting potential buyers know about the "product" they are buying for "marketing" purposes.

A number of analytic techniques can be used to focus on quality and include cost in the analysis. These techniques include cost of illness studies, cost-benefit analysis, and cost-effectiveness analysis. **Cost of illness studies** estimate the total monetary effects of a specific disease or condition. They consider all the resources used by physicians to diagnose and treat the condition, as well as resources used to help clients and their families cope with the illness (Max, 1997). In California, for example, the cost per case of cerebral palsy in the state was estimated

BOX 7-3 COST-CONTAINMENT STRATEGIES

Controlling quantity of supply:

- Incentives to decrease numbers of specialist physicians
- Certificate of need to limit technology duplication

Controlling price:

- Reimbursement for lower-cost providers such as nurse practitioners
- Reimbursement caps; for example:
  - DRGs—diagnosis-related groups
  - RBRVU—resource-based relative value units
  - APGs—ambulatory patient groups
  - RUGs—resource utilization groups

Controlling quantity of demand:

- Patient cost sharing; for example:
  - Increased proportion of premiums
  - Co-payments
  - Deductibles
- Managed care to provide only necessary and appropriate services

Competition:

- Insurers to shop for best benefit plans
- Managed care plans to shop for best provider contracts

Prioritizing through cost analysis:

- Focus on prevention
- Reduced inefficiency of interventions

RESEARCH BRIEF

Windsor, R.A., Lowe, J. B., Pekins, L. L., Smith-Yoder, D., Artz, M., Crawford, M., Amburgy, K., & Boyd, N. R. (1993). Health education methods for pregnant smokers: Behavioral impact and cost benefit. American Journal of Public Health, 83, 201–206.

This study was conducted from 1986 to 1991 at the four highest census maternity clinics, representing 85% of the cohort, of a county health department in Birmingham, Alabama. The sample consisted of 814 pregnant smokers, 400 in the experimental group and 414 in the control group. All the clients received standard information from the nurse on the risks and importance of quitting smoking during a 30-minute group prenatal education class. The intervention group also received a three-component intervention: (1) a 15-minute risk counseling session teaching a 7-day cessation program with a written guide, (2) a letter sent to the client in 7 days, and (3) social support in form of a buddy letter, contract, and tip sheet, as well as newsletters with testimonials on successful quitting. Total intervention cost, including salary and materials, was computed at $6 per client. Behavioral change was computed as quit rates. Benefit was defined as the estimated number of low-birth-weight (LBW) infants preventable by cessation of smoking by the mother. It was computed as the incremental costs of an LBW birth and was based on a statewide dissemination of the intervention.

The study confirmed an additional 6% to 12% quit rate was achievable in public health clinics with the intervention. The cost-benefit ratio if disseminated statewide was $1:$17.90 in favor of the intervention.

---

at $445,000 (Waitzman, Romano, & Scheffler, 1994). **Cost-benefit analysis** (CBA) uses such measures to compare benefits, in terms of disease prevention, with the costs of a program. In this technique, benefits are measured in monetary terms. CBA is the principal method used to evaluate decisions involving public expenditures. Decisions are based on alternatives providing the greatest net benefit, the greatest level of economic efficiency (Moore, Laufer, & Conroy, 1998). The research brief above is an example of a cost-benefit study. The drawback of this method in health care is the difficulty of placing a dollar value on outcomes like pain or grief or premature loss of life. The methods for determining such costs are developed in economics but are controversial (Thompson, 1999).

Cost-effectiveness analysis (CEA), sometimes considered a more acceptable health care alternative, calculates a ratio in which health outcome is measured in health units, such as cases avoided or years of life saved. Cost of treatment or intervention

is measured in dollars. Thus, results are presented in terms of cost per case prevented or cost per life saved. The purpose of CEA is to compare the relative value of different interventions in creating better health and/or longer life. Costs of alternative programs are compared based on a single nonmonetary outcome. CEA furnishes information that is useful in a variety of settings. In a managed care setting, an organization may wish to know the cost savings per low-birth-weight birth avoided as a consequence of a prenatal care outreach program. In addition, the organization could ask the cost of the program per year of life saved for its enrolled population. Analysis for a state health department might look at different strategies to control tuberculosis in the population. It could compare the cost-effectiveness of screening all community members versus screening only those at high risk based on history and exposure. In a larger context, the department might evaluate the costs of an educational program aimed at housing repair to reduce dust and peeling paint per case of high blood lead level avoided.

One other area in which cost-benefit and cost-effectiveness are used is in the broader field of technology assessment. **Technology assessment**, a form of policy research, helps decision makers deal with developing and using expensive health care practices and technologies. It is assessment that includes CBA and CEA. In addition, it also analyzes safety and the social impact of technologies (Thompson, 1999).

CEA assists in setting priorities for the use of scarce resources. For instance, research was done on the use of cholesterol-modifying agents to compare cost-effectiveness of primary prevention with secondary prevention of heart disease. Primary prevention was administration of the drug to those who had never had heart disease, and secondary prevention was administration of the drug to those who had a history of angina or myocardial infarction. In primary prevention the cost per year of life saved was more than $50,000, whereas in secondary prevention there was actually a cost savings for some groups. Recommendations were to give priority to secondary intervention when resources are scarce (Buerhaus, 1998). Even though the influence of CEA on policy is not well documented, it is believed to have played a key role in some major decisions. Medicare's first preventive service, coverage of the pneumococcal vaccine, was based on a CEA done by the Office of Technology Assessment. Cancer screening recommendations of the American Cancer Society are based on CEA studies (Buerhaus, 1998; Gold, Siegel, Russell, & Weinstein, 1996).

Public Health, Managed Care, and the Economics of Prevention

The current economic environment has had consequences for the public health sector, which focuses on health and well-being for the entire nation, vulnerable populations, prevention, non-biological determinants of health, and safety-net primary care. Along with market forces playing a greater role in the total health care system, there has been a redefinition of the government role. Even though government is a key instrument in community action, taxpayers appear unwilling to pay more money for publicly funded health programs (Lasker & Committee on Medicine and Public Health, 1997). With costs rising, a tightening of public funds is the result. Support is threatened for the health system's public goods: research, education of health professionals, population-based programs, and safety-net care for the uninsured and underinsured. Five mechanisms for federal cost cutting have been moving authority and monetary responsibility for programs to states and local governments, downsizing, reorganizing, privatizing, and linking funds to documented results. Personnel, program budgets, and whole programs have been cut (Lasker & Committee, 1997).

Opportunities for Collaboration

Despite the concerns about the effects of cost cutting on public health program delivery and the threats of an imperfect market of privatized managed care, there are reasons for community health nurses to be encouraged by the rapid growth of managed care. One of the commonalties among all the payers of health care services has been cost-containment efforts through increased enrollment of their beneficiaries in managed care plans. In Medicaid the federal government has signed waivers to allow states to move people into managed care, and in Medicare there has been an acceleration of people into managed care as a matter of policy (Shalala & Reinhardt, 1999). Enrollment is encouraged and steadily increasing for employee-sponsored insurance as well. The positive element is the population orientation of managed care and the potential it provides to strengthen public health efforts.

Managed care links both the insurance and the delivery of services by paying care providers a set amount for all the services of their insured population. Thus, the care providers share the financial risk of the enrolled population's health status. The incentive is to keep the population healthy.

Managed care organizations providing health care become linked in two ways to public health efforts. First, they share the interest in using population-based methods of epidemiology to study, track, and understand their enrolled populations and to keep those populations healthy. Second, to keep their enrolled populations healthy, they are aware of the benefits of collaboration in the wider public health efforts that focus on preventing illness for the total population. Their enrolled populations are a part of the total population. The total population achieves better outcomes with environmental protections, greater health awareness, early detection of disease, and improved health behavior. If the total population remains or becomes healthier, their enrolled populations do the same and the managed care organizations realize the benefits of decreased use of expensive services for preventable illnesses. Plans that can improve population health will control their costs and thus have a major advantage in a competitive market.

Before managed care, the influence and prestige of health care professionals outside public health disciplines did not guide public opinion or government action toward prevention and health. The emphasis on cure of diseases over which there was more biological control left the social and behavioral issues of health, such as drugs, alcohol, cigarettes, acquired immunodeficiency syndrome (AIDS), violence, and so on, with less attention and less funding. As noted earlier, a very small percentage of our national health care expenditures goes to public health activity (slightly more than 3%). The cost-effective methods of prevention and public health have not been recognized or valued by most individuals, groups, and governments in the United States.

The more cost-effective prevention strategies are less dramatic, and as Sultz and Young observe, "Unlike the recipients of heart transplants, . . . the media cannot show pictures of the hundreds of thousands of children who have *not* been crippled and

FYI

Insurance and Prevention

Contraceptives are cost effective: for every $1 public health funds invested in family planning, $4 to $14 of public funds is saved in pregnancy and health-care related costs.

The vast majority of private insurers cover prescription drugs, but may exclude coverage for prescription contraceptives. Similarly most policies cover outpatient medical services but often exclude outpatient contraceptive services for coverage.

Health insurance companies are more likely to cover sterilization or abortion services than contraceptives. This indicates the insurance community's tendency to pay for surgical services and not preventive care.

The Institute of Medicine Committee on Unintended Pregnancy recently recommended that "financial barriers to contraception be reduced by increasing the proportion of all health insurance policies that offer contraceptive services and supplies."

Source: APHA, 1998.

have *not* died due to poliomyelitis since the successful programs have been initiated" (1998, p. 267). Many believe that the new market incentives that led to managed care as a means of cost control will provide powerful economic incentives for a stronger alliance between managed care organizations and public health initiatives at all levels—federal, state, and local (Mechanic, 1998; Robbins & Freeman, 1999).

The shift in incentive from acute services as profitable to disease prevention as profitable is changing both who provides care as well as how care is provided (Shi & Singh, 1998). In contrast to most indemnity plans of insurance, managed care plans and providers are increasing preventive services such as screening, immunizations, and counseling for high-risk conditions. They encourage preventive services by increasing access to primary care providers. By making the providers accountable to the populations they care for and linking reimbursement for prevention to attaining certain goals, managed care methods could enhance the delivery of preventive services. If organized managed care plans, especially those enrolling public beneficiaries such as Medicaid, assume the services that have been offered by state and local health departments and publicly financed community health centers, these public services are affected. By losing Medicaid

and other primary care clients to managed care plans, they must deal with shrinking budgets. Community health centers have reacted to competition by forming health plans of their own (Shi & Singh, 1998). Public health agencies are regrouping and devoting their resources to the core public health functions. If they are no longer competing for clinical patients and payments, they can focus on surveillance, communitywide interventions, and ensuring and enhancing access (Robbins & Freeman, 1999).

Some see these changes as encouraging and an imperative for collaboration and cooperation through partnerships between managed care organizations and public health agencies. The Centers for Disease Control and Prevention (CDC) has brought together members of the public health and managed care sectors at national conferences that focus on prevention (CDC, 1995). In addition, the CDC has formed partnerships with the American Association of Health Plans and The HMO Group, which have encouraged the managed care community's concern with public health and preventive measures (Schauffler & Scutchfield, 1998).

The Committee on Medicine and Public Health reported on its mission and initiatives to join medical care and public health care (Lasker & Committee, 1997). Through their work, funded by both private and public funds, the committee found and examined 414 examples of collaborative efforts. They described the projects and how the collaborative work was done. Benefits accrued to both health sectors as public health agencies gain from the prevention efforts of managed care organizations and the organizations benefit from the expertise of public health practitioners. Managed care organizations are learning to conduct health assessments of the communities they serve and to identify areas where they can have a large influence on improving the communities' health (Shi & Singh, 1998). The collection and analysis of population-based data are the skills of public health, which makes collaboration welcome. Robbins and Freeman (1999) report the initiation of a New England joint venture between the not-for-profit managed care organizations of six states and those states' public health services. The goals they believe will be achieved are improved health and efficiency to reduce health care costs, and thus an increase in the political resolve to provide coverage for everyone.

Counterforces to Collaboration

The opportunities are not without problems, however, and the interface of public health with the new organized systems for delivering clinical care is evolving. One pressing issue is who will care for the individuals who remain uninsured? Even with policy efforts to increase coverage for all and especially for children, there still is not access for all. If health departments are expected to be the safety net, then they must be funded to do so. With Medicaid clients moving to managed care plans, they can no longer cross-subsidize uninsured primary and preventive care with Medicaid funds. Another issue for health departments is the "dumping" of services covered by private managed care plans.

Plans may cover immunizations in their capitated fee, yet still send their enrollees to a health department for immunizations without reimbursing the department. Coordination of state reporting for notifiable diseases, directly observed therapy, and sexually transmitted disease (STD) contact tracing may be problematic, with managed care organizations seeing clients formerly seen by the departments. Health departments must be able to obtain such client enrollment and encounter information for surveillance and epidemiological studies. Clarification of these and other roles and responsibilities must be addressed in the midst of the new forces at work in the total system (Rosenbaum & Richards, 1996; Schauffler & Scutchfield, 1998).

Another barrier to collaboration is the nature of for-profit firms. Not-for-profit providers are converting to for-profit at an increasing rate. With accountability to their stockholders as their priority, their motivation is to seek short-term advantages that reflect a positive bottom line. An advantage could be realized in the short term from cutting preventive measures and increasing profits. Many know that their enrollees may change plans often and will not remain their financial responsibility if illness occurs in the future (Mechanic, 1998). Profit maximization can be socially undesirable when there are product quality effects. Clearly, withholding preventive services has an effect on individuals as well as the larger public. With the public criticizing these and other business practices, they want for-profit plans in health care to be accountable for social responsiveness and social trust that any course in business ethics would encourage (Arrow, 1997).

Prevention and Alternative Therapies

Among the many changes driven by economics that are of import for community health nursing has been the increased acceptance of alternative therapies. Insurance plans and managed care organizations driven by consumer demand and the search for less costly services for their populations have discovered alternative care methods. The economic impact of alternative care was realized with the publication of the landmark study by Eisenberg. Although the study included only 1,539 individuals, extrapolation of the results to the larger population indicated that more visits were made to alternative providers than to conventional primary care providers; $13.7 billion was spent, mostly out of pocket; and dollars spent exceeded out-of-pocket costs for hospitalization (Weeks, 1997). These numbers indicated a potential market for insurers and managed care.

Driven by the realization of economic benefit, health plans have begun to include alternative therapy providers and treatment modalities in their plans (Box 7-4). Alternative therapies most often are focused on holistic, wellness approaches that realize the benefits of prevention. Surveys of clients of alternative providers show that there are effects on use of conventional pharmaceuticals, necessity of conventional surgeries, development of self-care abilities, and reduced visits to conventional physicians after self-care education (Weeks, 1997).

Providing a popular source of care in their plans may be a multiple strategy to (1) increase market share by meeting a con-

sumer demand, (2) realize the cost savings of lower technology treatments for illnesses, and (3) use fewer services because of increased wellness. Including alternative approaches to health in a particular program, there are possibilities for linkages and collaboration with public health. In Washington state, an integrated natural medicine/conventional medicine clinic is offered as a part of county services. There are indications that it may be expanded, and other states are interested in setting up such clinics

CASE STUDY

One of your clients at the clinic where you work comes in for a routine visit regarding her hypertension. In the midst of her visit she tells you, "I am so confused. I have to make a decision about what Medicare plan to choose. I've only been on Medicare for two years and I've just begun to understand how it works and what they will really pay. There are gaps, but it is pretty good for me. Now they tell me I have a choice of changing plans. But I don't know what to do. How can I decide which is best for me? Surely you know more about these things than I do. What should I do?"

1. What is your role in such a situation? How would you respond?

2. What might you consider in educating this client about care plans?

3. Are there resources you could refer her to?

(Weeks, 1997). Washington was also the first state to mandate health plan coverage of the full range of state-licensed providers such as naturopaths, acupuncturists, and chiropractors (Hamilton, 1996).

Plans that are beginning to create benefit packages for people interested in alternative care cover such alternatives as chiropractors, naturopathy, reflexology, rolfing, herbs, acupuncture, clinical nutritionists, massage, yoga, biofeedback, and chelation (Hamilton, 1996; Weeks, 1997). For managed care organizations there are issues with safety and efficacy documentation, which is not available in most cases.

Significance of Economics for Community Health Nursing Practice

This chapter has examined the implications of economics for individuals, families, and communities for whom nurses care. It is easy to become immersed in the immediacy of individual nursing roles and remain unaware of the outside forces affecting practice. Today, economics more than social and political demands drives our practice and the results for our clients. Who gets seen? What treatment can they get? Who will treat them? What will the setting be? Who will you work with? Who will pay you? The answers to all these questions are influenced by economic considerations of financing of health and welfare services, reimbursement rates, insurance mechanisms, and means of delivery. In many ways today's environment has become favorable for community nurses as care moves into the community, population-focused skills are needed, and prevention is valued. Following are just some of the other implications for current practice in a rapidly changing environment.

Perhaps one of the most valuable interactions with clients addresses their needs as consumers. As stated earlier, informed consumers are vital in a market situation. They need education, advocacy, and assistance. Beyond educating clients about their health or illness needs, nurses need to educate them to make informed choices about their care. Even though Medicare covers screening mammograms, most beneficiaries do not get them (Vladeck & King, 1997). Clients need assistance to increase their self-care knowledge, reinforce effective self-care, and partner with health care providers. Nurses can also reinforce the trend for consumers to be active and more informed about their health care options, including alternative therapies. The Internet is playing a large role for seniors, who have said that the primary reason they access the Internet is to get health information (Licht, 1999).

Nurses can help consumers understand price and quality issues in services. Educating and informing clients about complicated health plans, payment systems, restrictions, and options will benefit them in the market. In addition to educating them to meet their own needs, consumers need referrals, advocacy in appeals processes, and good documentation to ensure reimbursement. When considering consumers in the marketplace, there are also opportunities as a nurse provider to inform health plan purchasers about the needs of their populations and how best to meet them. Currently, most employer health plans look only at cost and do not consider quality in making plan decisions (Dentzer, 1998). Nurses have this knowledge and can purposefully encourage quality choices.

Dynamic changes are occurring in the nursing labor market. Reimbursement patterns and cost control are moving jobs into the community, seeking to replace or substitute nurses with cheaper labor sources, and creating new roles. Demand management, through telephone triage positions staffed by nurses, is eliminating unnecessary visits to clinics and emergency rooms (Larson-Dahn, 1998). In market settings, positions of case management, risk management, provider liaison, benefits coordinator, utilization review, quality assurance, and positions using population assessment skills are needed. There are new opportunities in prevention counseling services, and adding alternative therapies to practice options is encouraged with new reimbursement trends.

Perhaps one of the most important labor market changes for nurses is gaining third-party reimbursement for advanced practice nurses (ANA, 1997a). There had been reimbursement in specific rural areas, but the Balanced Budget Act of 1997 gave Medicare coverage to nurse practitioners and clinical nurse specialists for any service that would be covered under Medicare Part B when provided by a physician, regardless of geographic area. Nurses' reimbursement is at 80% of the physician rate. Direct reimbursement removes some of the barriers to entering the market, and the lower price for services makes nurses more competitive.

Community health nurses can optimize client care by using economic information in building coalitions, performing research, lobbying, negotiating with insurers, and influencing policy on health care allocation. In speaking the language of the marketplace, nurses can be more persuasive by having a broadly accepted reference point. In policy issues, nurses need to continually evaluate new or needed legislation that will affect client care as well as themselves as consumers. A current example is the rapid conversion of nonprofit hospital systems and health plans to private for-profit entities. The American Nurses Association issued a position statement recognizing the impact of these conversions and the need for regulation and oversight of the conversions (ANA, 1997b). Continued access for the affected communities and safeguards for the rights and benefits of employees need to be protected. Nurses can participation in collecting, analyzing, and interpreting data for policy decisions. Understanding economic evaluation methods such as cost-effectiveness analysis adds to nurses' ability to explain the value-adding contribution of nursing services. CEA techniques have the potential to refine practice and lead to nursing interventions that get the best return in terms of health. Measures of effectiveness alone will not be as relevant for management and policy decisions (Siegel, 1998).

CONCLUSION

Even with the opportunities outlined previously, much in the current nursing literature reflects the uneasiness that nurses have with a health care system in which some are provided care and others, for lack of resources, go without. Historically, as well as during the recent failed Clinton health reform, nurses have been advocates for access to quality, cost-effective health care services for all. The gaps in access in our current system are evident. Nurses have also expressed misgivings about referring to those they care for as *customers, buyers,* or *consumers.* For some, the philosophy of health care as a business threatens the human interactions of nursing and creates an environment that restricts understanding of nursing's value and purpose (David, 1999).

Nurses worry about the safety of vulnerable clients caught in cost-cutting efforts. Nurses also question a system in which savings from cost cutting go into the pockets of high-salaried executives and stockholders (Gordon, 1997). Is managed care an ethically supportable response to rising costs and giving of quality care? For community health nurses, the system can seem at odds with the nation's public health goal of attaining the highest levels of health and welfare for its citizens. Nurses appear to be struggling, as do other citizens, with the contrasting basic principles of justice underlying the production and distribution of health care resources. In broad contrast, these are market justice and social justice.

Approaching distribution by relying on capitalism and private for-profit enterprise is the **market justice** approach. Favoring the market is at the heart of the American traditions of individualism and limited government. The market solution is based on people's willingness and ability to pay. Those who cannot pay have individual accountability and do not receive services. People have the right to purchase the health goods they value. They purchase these goods with resources earned from their own efforts. The ideal result is economic efficiency. Market justice emphasizes individual rather than collective responsibility for health.

In contrast, a **social justice** approach holds health care to be a social good that should be collectively financed and available to all citizens regardless of ability to pay. Social justice favors societal responsibility for health care, to be achieved through government initiative. Elements of both market justice and social justice are present in our system, but market justice dominates

(Shi & Singh, 1998). If the United States has embraced the market system in health care, does this mean that collectively we believe only those who can pay should receive care or that people can only get the amount of care they can afford? As the only developed country in the world without some measure of universal health care coverage, it would seem so. Why we have adopted such a national stance has been the subject of debate for decades. Our policies may be accurately reflecting the ethic of the U.S. citizenry (Rice, 1998). One survey reported that only 23% of Americans agreed with the statement, "It is the responsibility of the government to take care of the very poor people who cannot take care of themselves." The U.S. response was considerably lower than that of the citizens of other countries (Blendon, Benson, Donelan, Leitman, Taylor, Koeck, & Gitterman, 1995). This ethic would explain the present inability of our policy makers to decide who, if anyone, is to provide health care to those who do not have economic access.

Although the two differing ethics reflect our values and beliefs about what is good or best, both beliefs seem to have flaws. Dowd (1999) suggests that the question we really are facing is one of whether our problems are best solved by "imperfect government or imperfect markets" (p. 269). The United States is not alone in the struggle to deal with the economic challenges of health care. What is emerging internationally is discussion about a fundamentally different "third way" in health care—a middle road between a centrally planned system and one based on market principles (Center for Economic and Social Justice, 1998; Le Grand, 1999).

Nurses can better contribute to the ongoing dialog if they understand both the opportunities and the downfalls of the two economic approaches as they operate in our present system. Nurses can look back as far as Florence Nightingale and find the origins of our public involvement in what is good for society. LeVasseur (1998) describes the Nightingale legacy as a "guardian-like stamp on nursing" (p. 281). She says, "Nightingale showed a strong sense of responsibility to her society and a passion for reform. . . . It was not enough for Nightingale to have knowledge of the good, but it was important to put that knowledge into action as a guardian of the people" (p. 281). Nurses today need not and should not be passive participants in the broad marketplace of ideas about what our society values in health care.

CRITICAL THINKING ACTIVITIES

1. Explain how under imperfect market conditions, both prices and quantities of health care are higher than they would be in a highly competitive market.

2. Two emergency room nurses are debating the issue of access to health care. One is concerned about the stigma of those who are uninsured and claims that people without health insurance receive less health care and have poorer health than those with insurance. The other disagrees, claiming that hospitals, doctors, and public health clinics deliver large amounts of charity care, which allows uninsured people to have the services they need. Who has the stronger case? What does research tell us?

3. The following is a dialog with Health and Human Services Secretary Donna Shalala and Princeton Economist Uwe Reinhardt:

   Shalala: In fact, Medicare is the best payer in the system: It pays more quickly and better than most private systems do.

   Reinhardt: And it operates more cheaply. Medicare passes through much more money, about 97 cents of every premium dollar, because its administrative costs are so low. No private insurer can match that record. Most providers don't know this.

   Shalala: People just can't get the stereotype of big bureaucracy out of their heads. And the idea that Medicare's administrative expenses are 3 or 4 percent while the private sector spends 12 percent just doesn't register with many people, particularly those who see health care as a business.

   (Shalala & Reinhardt, 1999)

   Why might the difference exist between government and private spending? How might someone in a for-profit organization respond to this conversation?

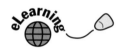

Explore Community Health Nursing on the web! To learn more about the topics in this chapter, use the passcode provided to access your exclusive web site: http://communitynursing.jbpub.com
If you do not have a passcode, you can obtain one at this site.

REFERENCES

Alpert, J. J. (1998). Editorial: Serving the medically underserved. *American Journal of Public Health, 88,* 347–348.

American Nurses Association (ANA). (1997a). *Medicare reimbursement for NPs and CNSs:* www.nursingworld.org/gova/federal/agencies/hcfa/medreimb.htm.

American Nurses Association (ANA). (1997b). *Position statement on privatization and for-profit conversion:* www.nursingworld.org/readroom/position/practice/prprivat.htm.

American Public Health Association (APHA). (1998). *Fact sheet: Prescription contraceptive equity:* www.apha.org/legislative/factsheets/fs2.htm.

Anderson, C. A. (1997). The economics of health promotion. *Nursing Outlook, 45,* 105–106.

Arrow, K. J. (1997). Social responsibility and economic efficiency. In T. Donaldson & T. W. Dunfee (Eds.), *Ethics in business and economics.* Brookfield, VT: Ashgate.

Bishop, C. E. (1998). Health cost containment: What will it mean for workers and local economies? *Public Health Reports, 113*(3), 204–213.

Blendon, R. J., Benson, J., Donelan, K., Leitman, R., Taylor, H., Koeck, C., & Gitterman, D. (1995). Who has the best health care system? A second look. *Health Affairs, 14*(4), 220–230.

Blumenthal, D. (1994). The vital role of professionalism in health care reform. *Health Affairs, 13*(1), 252–256.

Bodenheimer, T. S., & Grumbach, K. (1995). *Understanding health policy: A clinical approach.* Stamford, CT: Appleton and Lange.

Brown, C. (1999). Ethics, policy, and practice: Interview with Emily Friedman. *Image: The Journal of Nursing Scholarship, 31,* 259–262.

Buerhaus, P. I. (1992). Nursing competition and quality. In M. Johnson & J. McClosky (Eds.), *The delivery of quality health care.* St. Louis: Mosby.

Buerhaus, P. I. (1994). Managed competition and critical issues facing nurses. *Nursing and Health Care, 15*(1), 22–26.

Buerhaus, P. I. (1998). Milton Weinstein's insights on the development, use and methodological problems in cost-effectiveness analysis. *Image: The Journal of Nursing Scholarship, 30*(3), 223–227.

Carrasquillo, O., Himmelstein, D., Woolhandler, S., & Bor, D. (1999). Going bare: Trends in health insurance coverage, 1989 through 1996. *American Journal of Public Health, 89*(1), 36–41.

Centers for Disease Control and Prevention (CDC). (1995). Prevention and managed care: Opportunities for managed care, purchasers of health care, and public health agencies. *Morbidity and Mortality Weekly Report, 44,* 1–12.

Center for Economic and Social Justice. (1998). *The third way: Is it for real?:* www.cesj.org/thirdway/press_club.htm.

Chen, M., & Mastilica, M. (1998). Health care reform for Croatia: For better or for worse? *American Journal of Public Health, 88*(8), 1156–1160.

Chollet, D. J. (1996). Redefining private insurance in a changing market structure. In S. H. Altman & U. E. Reinhardt (Eds.), *Strategic choices for a changing health care system.* Chicago: Health Administration Press.

Congressional Budget Office. (1999). Homepage. www.cbo.gov/index.html.

Cooper, P. F., & Schone, B. S. (1997). More offers, fewer takers for employment-based health insurance:1987–1996, *Health Affairs, 16*(6), 142–149.

Cowley, G., King, P., Hager, M., & Rosenberg, D. (1995, June 26). Going mainstream. *Newsweek,* pp. 56–57.

David, B. A. (1999). Nursing's conflicting values in competitively managed health care. *Image: The Journal of Nursing Scholarship, 31*(2), 188.

Dentzer, S. (1998, January–February). A guide to managed care, part 2. *Modern Maturity,* pp. 35–41, 43.

Department of Health and Human Services (DHHS). (1999). *Annual update of the HHS poverty guidelines:* http://aspe.os.dhhs.gov/poverty/poverty.htm.

Donelan, K., Blendon, R., Hill, C., Hoffman, C., Rowland, D., Frankel, M., & Altman, D. (1997). Whatever happened to the health insurance crisis in the United States? Voices from a national survey. In P. Lee & C. Estes. (Eds.), *The nation's health.* Sudbury, MA: Jones and Bartlett.

Dowd, B. (1999). An unusual view of health economics. [Review of The economics of health reconsidered]. *Health Affairs, 18*(1), 266–269.

Finkler, S. A., & Kovner, C. T. (1993). *Financial management for nurse managers and executives.* Philadelphia: W. B. Saunders.

Gerber, D. E., & McGuire, S. L. (1995). Understanding contemporary health and welfare services: The Social Security Act of 1935 and the Public Health Service Act of 1944. *Nursing Outlook, 43*(6), 266–272.

Gibson, R. M., & Waldo, D. R. (1982). National health expenditures, 1981. *Health Care Financing Review, 4*(1), 1–35.

Ginsberg, P. B. (1998). Health system change in 1997. *Health Affairs, 17*(4), 165–169.

Ginsberg, P. B., Gabel, J. R., & Hunt, K. A. (1998). Tracking small firm coverage: 1989–1996. *Health Affairs, 17*(1), 167–171.

Gold, M. R., Siegel, J. E., Russell, L. B., & Weinstein, M. C. (1996). *Cost-effectiveness in health and medicine.* New York: Oxford University Press.

Gordon, S. (1997). Advocating for nursing. In C. Harrington & C. L. Estes (Eds.), *Health policy and nursing. Crisis and reform in the U.S. health care delivery system.* Sudbury, MA: Jones and Bartlett.

Gulzar, L. (1999). Access to health care. *Image: The Journal of Nursing Scholarship, 31*(1), 13–19.

Halvorson, G. C. (1999). Health plans' strategic responses to a changing market place. *Health Affairs, 18*(2), 28–29.

Hamilton, J. (1996, May). Insurance for alternative treatments. *American Health,* p. 44.

Harrington, C., & Estes, C. L. (1997). *Health policy and nursing.* Sudbury, MA: Jones & Bartlett.

Havens, D. M., & Hannon, C. (1997). Children first: Expanding health insurance coverage for children. *Journal of Pediatric Nursing, 11,* 85–88.

Health Care Financing Administration (HCFA). (1998a). *National health expenditures tables:* www.hcfa.gov/stats/nhe-oact/tables/tablist.htm.

Health Care Financing Administration (HCFA). (1998b). Highlights, national expenditures, 1997. www.hcfa.gov/stats/nhe%2Doact/hilites.htm.

Health Care Financing Administration (HCFA). (1999a). *Supporting families in transition. A guide to expanding health coverage in the post-welfare reform world:* www.hcfa.gov/medicaid/wrdl3229.htm.

Health Care Financing Administration (HCFA). (1999b). *Medicaid managed care enrollment report:* www.hcfa.gov/medicaid/omchmpg.htm.

Health Care Financing Administration (HCFA). (1999c). *Children's Health Insurance Program status report as of September 7, 1999:* www.hcfa.gov/init/chstatus.htm.

Health Insurance Association of America. (1991). *Source book of insurance data.* Washington, DC: Author.

Himmelstein, D., & Woolhandler, S. (1995). Care denied: U.S. residents who are unable to obtain needed medical services. *American Journal of Public Health, 85*(3), 341–344.

Hughes, D., & Runyan, S. (1997). Prenatal care and public policy: Lessons for promoting women's health. In C. Harrington & C. L. Estes (Eds.), *Health policy and nursing: Crisis and reform in the U.S. health care delivery system* (2nd ed.). Sudbury, MA: Jones and Bartlett.

Inglehart, J. K. (1996). Reform of the Veterans Affairs health care system. *New England Journal of Medicine, 335,* 1407–1411.

Jacobs, P. (1996). *The economics of health and medical care* (4th ed.). Gaithersburg, MD: Aspen.

Jerome-Forget, M., White, J., & Wiener, J. (Eds.). (1995). *Health care reform through internal markets.* Washington, DC: The Brookings Institution.

Larson-Dahn, M. (1998). An innovative approach to appropriate resource utilization. *Nursing Economics, 16*(6), 317–319.

Lasker, R. D., & the Committee on Medicine and Public Health. (1997). *Medical and public health: The power of collaboration.* New York: The New York Academy of Medicine.

Loubeau, P. R., & Maher, V. F. (1996). Any-willing provider laws: Point and counterpoint. *Medicine and Law, 15*(2), 219–226.

Le Grand, J. (1999). Competition, cooperation, or control? Tales from the British National Health Service. *Health Affairs, 18*(1), 27–39.

LeVasseur, J. (1998). Plato, Nightingale, and contemporary nursing. *Image: The Journal of Nursing Scholarship, 30*(3), 281–285.

Levit, K., Olin, G. O., & Letsch, S. W. (1992). American's health insurance coverage 1980–1991. *Health Care Financing Review, 14,* 31–57.

Licht, J. (1999, August). Seniors eager to log on. *Washington Post:* www.washingtonpost.com/wp-srv/health/daily/aug99/webseniors0831.htm.

Litman, T. J., & Robins, L. S. (Eds.). (1991). *Health politics and policy* (2nd ed.). Albany, NY: Delmar Publishers.

Max, W. (1997). Economic analysis in health care. In C. Harrington & C. L. Estes (Eds.), *Health policy and nursing. Crisis and reform in the U.S. health care delivery system* (2nd ed.). Sudbury, MA: Jones and Bartlett.

McKenzie, J. F. (1997). *An introduction to community health.* Sudbury, MA: Jones and Bartlett.

Mechanic, D. (1998). Topics for our times: Managed care and public health opportunities. *American Journal of Public Health, 88,* 874–875.

Mechanic, D., & Rochefort, D. (1997). A policy of inclusion for the mentally ill. In C. Harrington & C. L. Estes (Eds.), *Health policy and nursing: Crisis and reform in the U.S. health care delivery system* (2nd ed.). Sudbury, MA: Jones and Bartlett.

Mississippi Health Advocacy Program. (1998). *What welfare advocates need to know about low income families' eligibility for and entitlement to Medicaid—Action alert:* www.mhap.org.

Moore, S., Laufer, F. L., & Conroy, M. B. (1998). The economics of health care. In D. J. Mason & J. K. Leavitt (Eds.), *Policy and politics in nursing and health care* (3rd ed.). Philadelphia: W. B. Saunders.

National Center for Health Statistics. (1997). *Health: United States, 1996–1997.* Hyattsville, MD: Public Health Service.

Pulcini, J., & Mahoney, D. (1998). Health care financing. In D. J. Mason & J. K. Leavitt (Eds.), *Policy and politics in nursing and health care* (3rd ed.). Philadelphia: W. B. Saunders.

Rambur, B., & Mooney, M. M. (1998). A point of view: Why point-of-care places are not free marketplaces. *Nursing Economics, 16*(3), 122–124, 146.

Rice, T. (1998). *The economics of health reconsidered.* Chicago: Health Administration Press.

Robbins, A., & Freeman, P. (1999). How organized medical care can advance public health. *Public Health Reports, 114,* 120–125.

Rosenbaum, S., & Richards, T. B. (1996). Medicaid managed care and public health policy. *Journal of Public Health Management Practice, 2*(3), 76–82.

Rowland, D., Lyons, B., Salganicoff, A., & Long, P. (1994) Profile of the uninsured of America. *Health Affairs, 13*(2), 283–287.

Schauffler, H. H., & Scutchfield, F. D. (1998). Managed care and public health. *American Journal of Preventive Medicine, 14*(3), 240–241.

Seldon, T. M., Banthin, J. S., & Cohen, J. W. (1999). Waiting in the wings: Eligibility and enrollment in the state children's health insurance program. *Health Affairs, 18*(2), 126–133.

Shalala, D. E., & Reinhardt, U. E. (1999). Viewing the U.S. health care system from within: Candid talk from HHS. *Health Affairs, 18*(3), 47–55.

Shaughnessy, P. W., Schenkler, R. E., & Hittle, D. F. (1995). Case mix of home health patients under capitated and fee-for-service payments. *Health Services Research, 30*(1), 1–8.

Shi, L., & Singh, D. A. (1998). *Delivering health care in America: A systems approach.* Gaithersburg, MD: Aspen.

Siegel, J. E. (1998). Cost-effectiveness analysis and nursing research—is there a fit? *Image: The Journal of Nursing Scholarship, 30*(3), 221–222.

Smith, S., Freland, M., Heffler, S. McKisick, & The Health Expenditures Projection Team (1998). The next ten years of health spending: What does the future hold? *Health Affairs, 17*(5), 128–140.

Standard and Poor's Corporation. (1992). U.S. grapples with health care crisis. *Health Care Industry Surveys,* H15–H17.

Stevens, P. E. (1992). Who gets care? Access to health care as an arena for nursing. *Scholarly Inquiry for Nursing Practice, 6*(3), 185–200.

Stone, P. W. (1998). Methods for conducting and reporting coat-effectiveness analysis in nursing. *Image: The Journal of Nursing Scholarship, 30*(3), 229–234.

Sultz, H. A., & Young, K. M. (1997). *Health care USA: Understanding its organization and delivery.* Gaithersburg, MD: Aspen.

Thompson, K. M. (1999). Economic issues in health care. In L. Y. Kelly & L. A. Joel (Eds.), *Dimensions of professional nursing* (pp. 220–241). New York: McGraw-Hill.

Vladeck, B. C., & King, K. (1997). Medicare at 30: Preparing for the future. In C. Harrington & C. Estes (Eds.), *Health policy and nursing: Crisis and reform in the U.S. health care delivery system.* Sudbury, MA: Jones and Bartlett.

Waid, M. O. (1998). *Brief summaries of Medicare and Medicaid. Title XVII and Title XIX of the Social Security Act. Report prepared for Health Care Financing Administration, DHHS:* www.hcfa.gov/medicare/ormedmed.htm.

Waitzman, N. J., Romano, P. S., & Scheffler, R. M. (1994). Estimates of the economic costs of birth defects. *Inquiry, 31,* 188–205.

Weeks, J. (1997). The emerging role of alternative medicine in managed care. *Drug Benefit Trends, 9*(4), 14–16, 25–28.

Wesson, A. F. (1999). The comparative study of health reform. In F. D. Powell & A. F. Wesson (Eds.), *Health care systems in transition* (pp. 3–24). Thousand Oaks, CA: Sage Publications.

White House Domestic Policy Council. (1993). *Health security: The President's report to the American people.* Washington, DC: U.S. Government Printing Office.

Windsor, R. A., Lowe, J. B., Pekins, L. L., Smith-Yoder, D., Artz, M., Crawford, M., Amburgy, K., & Boyd, N. R. (1993). Health education methods for pregnant smokers: Behavioral impact and cost benefit. *American Journal of Public Health, 83*(2), 201–206.

Chapter 8
Politics and the Law

Sharyn Janes, Karen Saucier Lundy,
and Heather Rakauskas Sherry

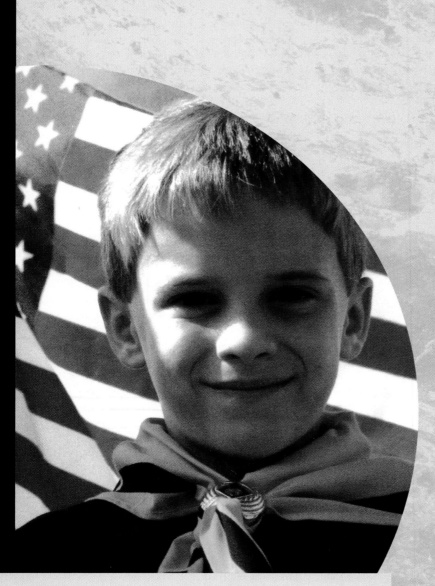

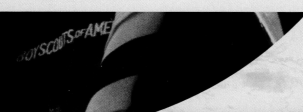

*Never doubt that a small group of thoughtful, committed citizens
can change the world; indeed, it's the only thing that ever does.*
Margaret Mead

CHAPTER FOCUS

Government Authority
  Protection of the Public's Health
  Power, Authority, and the Health of the Public
  Evolution of the Government's Role in Health Care

Government
  Federal Government
  State Government
  Local Government
  Different Types of Law
  How an Idea Becomes a Law

Regulation and Licensing of Nursing Practice
  The Regulatory Process
  Licensure

Nursing Practice and the Law
  Nursing Practice in Correctional Settings
  Forensic Nursing: An Emerging Nursing Role

Healthy People 2010: Objectives Related to Law

QUESTIONS TO CONSIDER

After reading this chapter, answer the following questions:

1. What is the role of the government in the health of its citizens?
2. How do the concepts of power and authority relate to public health regulation?
3. What is the history of governmental roles in health care?
4. What are the three branches of the federal government? What does each do in relation to health?
5. How is state government organized? How does it relate to health care?
6. What are the different kinds of laws?
7. What are the steps in the development of laws?
8. How can nurses be involved in the development of law and policy?
9. What are the primary issues related to regulation and licensure of nursing practice?
10. What settings are more likely to be influenced by legal issues in the practice of community health nursing and why?
11. What is the role of the nurse in correctional settings and in forensics?

KEY TERMS

Bill of Rights
Coercive power
Connection power
Constitutional law
Correctional nursing
Democracy
Equality
Executive branch
Expert power
Federal Register

Forensic nursing
Freedom
Information power
Judicial branch
Judicial or common law
Legislative branch
Legitimate power
Licensure
Lobbying

Malpractice
Negligence
Nurse Multistate
  Licensure Mutual
  Recognition Model
Nurse practice act
Police power
Political action
  committees (PACs)

Political power
Power
Preamble of the U.S.
  Constitution
Referent power
Regulatory process
Reward power
Statutory law
U.S. Constitution

While the political efforts of movers and shakers like Florence Nightingale, Lillian Wald, and Margaret Sanger are well documented, politics and policy have been historically seen as "outside" the scope of nursing. For most nurses, "political activism" meant voting in national and state elections. By the closing years of the 20th century, however, nurses began to realize that they could influence public policy by using nursing knowledge and skills. In 1992, acknowledging that decisions affecting nurses and their clients were being made in the national political arena, the American Nurses Association (ANA) moved its national headquarters to Washington, D.C. (Milstead, 1999).

Government Authority

Protection of the Public's Health

The early American colonists viewed health as controlled by divine intervention. They believed it was a result of self-care, and minimal governmental intervention was expected. Because health care was not a power granted to the federal government (such as defense or printing money), it developed into a power of the states or was left to the people themselves. Governmental health care and policies to provide funding and resources for health care were, for all practical purposes, nonexistent in the early days of the United States (Turnock, 1997).

As each new American colony was founded, the way in which it would be governed was a primary consideration. The specific problems and situations that each new colony faced varied so widely that each developed its own procedures and laws based on its own needs. From this evolved the idea of states' rights, which continues to play a critical role in the governance of health care policies, such as seat belt laws and immunization laws. Any attempts to limit the power of the states, either by the federal government or other states, is usually strongly opposed. Most states, for instance, will have similar laws about school attendance, drinking age, and immunizations, but the regulations themselves will vary considerably.

Federal law is based on the **U.S. Constitution,** which was ratified in 1789. The creators of the Constitution were careful to limit the federal government's involvement in the daily lives of citizens. The word *health* was never mentioned in the U.S. Constitution, making health care legislation problematic, because the Constitution therefore grants limited power in the creation of health laws. The Constitution has been amended 26 times. The first 10 amendments, known as the **Bill of Rights,** were adopted within 3 years of the Constitution's ratification. The Bill of Rights focuses on the protection of our most basic value: freedom. Freedom of speech, freedom of the press, and due process are all included. In recent years, the constitutional amendments have had relevance to health care issues. For example, the Fourteenth Amendment provides protection of personal liberty, such as a woman's right to choose to have an abortion. It is important to note, however, that neither the U.S. Constitution nor state constitutions guarantee access to health care. States retain whatever power the U.S. Constitution does not specifically define in federal law. State power concerning health care is termed **police power.** The state can use its power to protect the health, welfare, and safety of its citizens by establishing boards of nursing and medicine and passing immunization laws (Kelly & Joel, 1996).

Power, Authority, and the Health of the Public

Politics is always about **power**—who gets it, how it is obtained, how it is applied, and to what purposes it is used (Bacharach & Lawler, 1980). The German sociologist Max Weber defined power as the ability to control the behaviors of others, even in the absence of their consent (Weber, 1947). Power then is the capacity to participate effectively in a decision-making process. If citizens cannot or do not affect the process, they are powerless (Lenski, 1984).

Power can be classified as either legitimate or illegitimate. Power is considered legitimate if people recognize that those who apply it have the right to do so. This includes elected government officials, aristocracy, and those believed to be inspired by God. Weber referred to legitimate power as authority (Bacharach & Lawler, 1980). A simple illustration of this authority is that if the police stop you for speeding and levy a fine against you, you will recognize the law and the person carrying out the law as legitimate and you will probably obey. A political system can exist only if the people see the authority as legitimate. Most persons must see it as desirable, workable, and better than alternatives. We may complain about our legal system and its excesses or our Congress members and their self-serving interests, but most of us believe that the system works to our benefit most of the time. Once the bulk of citizens in any society no longer consider the political system legitimate, it is doomed, for its power can then rest only on coercion, which will eventually fail. Most revolutions, such as the French Revolution, the Iranian Revolution, and the American Revolution, were preceded by an erosion of the legitimacy of the existing political system (Robertson, 1981).

....

Among the Indians there have been no written laws. Customs handed down from generation to generation have been the only laws to guide them. Every one might act different from what was considered right if he choose to do so, but such acts would bring upon him the censure of the Nation. . . . This fear of the Nation's censure acted as a mighty band, binding all in one social, honorable compact.

George Copway (Kah-ge-ga-bowh), Ojibwa Chief, 1818–1863

....

Concepts of Power

Political power is defined by Hewison (1994) as the "ability to influence or persuade an individual holding a governmental office to exert the power of that office to [effect] a desired change" (p. 1171). What allows some people to have more influence than others? Where does such power come from? Nurses can benefit from understanding these sources of power. French and Raven (1959) identify five power bases:

1. **Coercive power,** *which is the use of force to gain compliance, often born out of real or perceived fear or threat to self. Police often use coercive power.*

2. **Reward power,** *which involves giving something of value for compliance. Compliance then results from the perceived potential for reward or favor of someone in power. A politician may help constituents obtain money for a new hospital in exchange for their political support.*

3. **Expert power,** *which results from expert knowledge or skills. Bill Gates has considerable expert power because of his expertise in computers and systems.*

4. **Legitimate power,** *which results from a title or position, such as an elected judge or the surgeon general.*

5. **Referent power,** *which results from being closely associated with someone who is powerful; for example, the aide or spouse of a senator. This can also be referred to as* reflected power.

Hersey, Blanchard, and Natemeyer (1979) added two additional sources of power:

6. **Information power,** *which results from the desire for information held by one person from one who does not have access to the information. This is commonly seen in the diplomatic corps of the United States.*

7. **Connection power,** *which results from the belief that a certain person has a special connection to a person or organization believed to be powerful. Lobbyists often use this kind of power when working with legislators' staff assistants (Helvie, 1998).*

One primary way of gaining power as a nurse is through knowledge. Nurses can use their knowledge of politics, power, and the change process to introduce change favoring health in the legislative process. Nurses have historically had very little interest in achieving power. Others have too long been the "voice" of nursing, and nurses and their clients have suffered through lack of appropriate nurse advocacy (Huston, 1995).

Another way that nurses can achieve power is through affiliating with others who have similar interests in health. Through networking and using the power of numbers, nurses can effect change through those in power positions. Coalitions of people and organizations are most effective in bringing about change (Helvie, 1998).

. . . .

When nurses fully understand the impact of policy in the health care arena, when nurses fully understand the importance of tying outcomes research to public policy and when nurses fully understand the politics of health care, and mobilize their numbers and influence behind the political process, only then will the health system thrive and with nurses as key players.
Betty Dickson, Mississippi Nurses Association
Executive Director and Lobbyist

. . . .

The idea of a nation-state is relatively new. The concept emerged in Europe only a few centuries ago, then spread to the Americas, and spread to most parts of Africa and Asia only during the 20th century. In the founding of the United States, a representative democracy was a new idea. **Democracy** comes from a Greek word meaning "rule of the people," and this is no doubt what Abraham Lincoln had in mind when he defined democracy as "government of the people, by the people, and for the people." Democracy in the United States requires that we recognize the powers of the government as being derived from the consent of the governed. We elect representatives who are responsible for making political decisions. According to Robertson (1981), "Representative democracy is historically recent, rare and fragile" (p. 488).

There are five basic conditions that must exist for a democracy to thrive:

1. Advanced economic development: *This almost always involves an urbanized, literate, and sophisticated population that expects and demands participation in the political process.*

2. Restraints on government power: *This involves institutional checks on the power of the state (Robertson, 1981).*

3. *Consensus on basic values and a widely held commitment to existing political institutions.*

4. *Tolerance of dissent.*

5. Access to information: *A democracy depends on its citizens to make informed choices. There must be a free press.*

. . . .

Give me liberty or give me death!

Patrick Henry, 1775

. . . .

Freedom versus Equality

Freedom is defined in the United States as freedom "of"—freedom of speech, freedom of the press, and so on. In more socialist societies, freedom is defined as freedom "from"—freedom from hunger, freedom from unemployment, freedom from exploitation by people who want to make a fortune. In the United States, we equate freedom with "liberty." Socialist societies equate freedom with **"equality."** In general, the more liberty that exists in a society, the less equality. Your liberty to be richer than anyone else violates other people's right to be your equal; other people's right to be your equal violates your liberty to make a fortune. In the United States, we have chosen to emphasize liberty, which evolves from our value system. This emphasis can lead only to social inequality. Socialist societies emphasize equality, thus limiting personal liberty (Robertson, 1981).

In health care we often fail to understand why laws cannot be easily passed to impose penalties on persons who engage in risky behavior, such as requiring helmets for motorcyclists or tubal ligations for women who have injured their children through neglect or abuse. The answer lies in our emphasis on freedom in the United States and the limited power of the state. Recognizing and understanding these basic concepts about our government can help us use our skills and resources in the political process much more efficiently.

. . . .

Eternal vigilance is the price of liberty.

Wendell Phillips, 1852

. . . .

Evolution of the Government's Role in Health Care

The **Preamble of the U.S. Constitution** states that one of the purposes of the federal government is to "promote the general welfare" of the people. This can be found in Article 1, Section 8. The federal government derives its power to become involved in health care activities from this simple declaration. Because of this very general statement, the degree of health care services provided by the federal government is often a source of conflict among the various constituents and political parties. As a capitalistic society, and lacking clear direction from the U.S. Constitution, the provision of health services for the general population has historically been the concern of private enterprise. Private physicians delivered services to clients, and clients in turn paid a fee for that service. This concept has been the foundation of medical care provision in the United States since the beginning (Miller, 1992).

The first involvement of the federal government in health care was highly specialized for government employees. As early as 1796, the Marine Hospital Service was established to provide care for sick and disabled seamen. In 1852, St. Elizabeth Hospital in Washington, D.C., was established to provide health care for federal employees. A landmark study, the Shattuck Report, written in 1850, recommended measures such as the creation of local and state boards of health; collection of vital statistics; and supervision of housing, factories, sanitation, and communicable disease control. Soon health departments in major cities became common. The Shattuck Report is considered the basis for the development of local and state health departments (see chapter 3). Military personnel were soon cared for through the federal government, which eventually led to the Veterans Administration (VA). The VA is currently the largest health care system in the United States.

It was not until after World War II that the federal government ventured into health care and community health programs for the general population. In 1946, the Hill-Burton Act provided funds for building hospital facilities in many communities. Government funding for specific treatments for disease did not happen until the 1960s. Before the 1960s, the federal government primarily provided programs for the economically disadvantaged populations. The social welfare programs of the 1960s brought about the most dramatic changes in federal involvement in health care. The establishment of Medicare in 1965 was sig-

---

BOX 8-1 1965: WHAT A YEAR FOR HEALTH LAW IN THE UNITED STATES!

- Drug Abuse Control Amendments of 1965 (Public Law No. 89-74)
- Federal Cigarette Labeling and Advertising Act (Public Law No. 89-92)
- Construction Act Amendments of 1965 (Public Law No. 89-105)
- Community Health Services Extension Amendments of 1965 (Public Law No. 89-109)
- Health Research Facilities Amendments of 1965 (Public Law No. 89-115)
- Water Quality Act of 1965 (Public Law No. 89-234)
- Heart Disease, Cancer, and Stroke Amendments of 1965 (Public Law No. 89-239)
- The Clean Air Act Amendments and Solid Waste Disposal Act of 1965 (Public Law No. 89-272)
- Health Professions Educational Assistance Amendments of 1965 (Public Law No. 89-290)
- Medical Library Assistance Act (Public Law No. 89-291)
- Appalachian Regional Development Act of 1965 (Public Law No. 89-4)
- Older Americans Act (Public Law No. 89-73)
- Social Security Amendments of 1965 (Public Law No. 89-97)
- Vocational Rehabilitation Act Amendments of 1965 (Public Law No. 89-333)
- Housing and Urban Development Act of 1965 (Public Law No. 89-117)

Source: Forgotson, 1967.

---

nificant in that it became the first program to provide health services to citizens other than federal employees. The basic purpose of Medicare was to provide health care for the elderly. The Medicaid program was developed in 1965 and provided health care for low-income individuals. See Box 8-1 for a list of the most significant health legislation acts passed during the "turning point decade" of the 1960s.

The Civil Rights Act of 1964, although not directly related to health, provided fair access to health facilities for all races and genders. The Environmental Protection Agency (EPA) was created through the National Environmental Policy Act and is historically one of the most significant pieces of U.S. environmental health policy. In recent years, significant legislation has been passed, including the Americans with Disabilities Act in 1990. This act increased the opportunities for Americans with disabilities to be integrated into mainstream society by removing physical barriers and improving public accommodation and services.

Government

Federal Government

The federal government consists of three separate branches—Executive (Office of the President), Legislative (Congress), and Judicial (federal court system). All three branches have a powerful impact on the health care delivery system and nursing practice. Nurses should be aware of how the different branches of the government affect health care policy and the ways that nurses can have a voice.

Executive Branch

The **Executive branch** consists of the president, the vice president, the Office of Management and Budget, and the cabinet departments, whose leadership is appointed by the president and approved by Congress. The cabinet departments that have the greatest effect on health care policy and nursing education, research, and practice are the Department of Health and Human

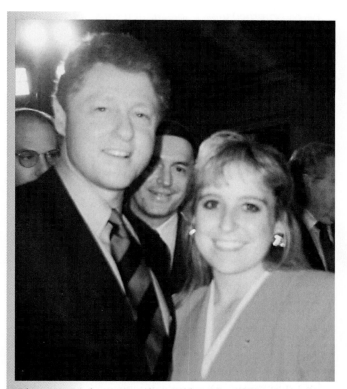

Chapter author, Heather Rakauskas Sherry, and President Bill Clinton.

Services, the Department of Education, and the Department of Labor.

The Department of Health and Human Services

The Department of Health and Human Services (DHHS) is the federal agency most concerned with protecting the health of all Americans and providing essential human services, especially for those who are least able to help themselves. There are more than 300 programs under DHHS supervision, with a wide spectrum of activities and services. Some of these services include the following (DHHS, 1999):

- *Medical and social science research*
- *Communicable disease prevention, including immunization services*
- *Financial assistance for low-income families*
- *Child abuse and domestic violence prevention*
- *Medicare and Medicaid*
- *Child support enforcement*
- *Food and drug safety*
- *Maternal and infant health improvement*
- *Services for older Americans*
- *Substance abuse treatment and prevention*

Box 8-2 lists a few of the health offices and services under the umbrella of DHHS.

U.S. Public Health Service.

The U.S. Public Health Service (PHS) is responsible for the administration of many of the most familiar federal health care agencies and services. The PHS is headed by the surgeon general of the United States, who is appointed by the president. The 200th anniversary of the PHS was celebrated in 1998. In 200 years, the PHS has grown from a handful of contract physicians to eight operating divisions within the DHHS, with more than 50,000 health care professionals and

---

BOX 8-2 U.S. DEPARTMENT OF HEALTH SERVICES

Office of the Secretary of Health and Human
 Services
Office of the Assistant Secretary/Surgeon General
 Administration on Aging
 Administration for Children and Families
 Health Care Financing Administration
 Social Security Administration
 Public Health Service

Agency for Health Care Policy and Research

Food and Drug Administration

Agency for Toxic Substances and Disease Registry

Health Resources and Services Administration

Substance Abuse and Mental Health Services Administration

National Institutes of Health

Centers for Disease Control and Prevention

Indian Health Service

a 6,000-member, all-officer Commissioned Corp (Satcher, 1998). The operating divisions of the PHS are outlined in Box 8-3 and described below. Many nurses are employed by all divisions of the PHS, including a chief nurse, who holds the rank of rear admiral.

The mission of the Agency for Health Care Policy and Research (AHCPR) is to generate and distribute information that improves health care delivery. AHCPR funds cross-cutting research on health care systems, health care quality and cost issues, and effectiveness of medical treatments (DHHS, 1999). Along with the American Academy of Nursing, the AHCPR sponsors a nursing scholar in the agency to study the integration of clinical nursing care with issues of cost and access to health care (Bednash, Heylin, & Rhome, 1998).

The Agency for Toxic Substances and Disease Registry (ATSDR) monitors and funds research programs and interventions aimed at preventing health-related problems associated with exposure to toxic substances. Working with states and other federal agencies, the ATSDR conducts public health assessments, health studies, surveillance activities, and health education programs in communities near waste sites on the EPA's National Priorities List. Toxicological profiles have been developed for hazardous chemicals found at these sites (DHHS, 1999).

Services to prevent and treat mental health problems and substance abuse are provided through the Substance Abuse and Mental Health Services Administration (SAMHSA). Funding is provided through block grants to the states for substance abuse and mental health services, including treatment for more than 340,000 Americans with severe substance abuse problems (DHHS, 1999). Funding for education and research is disbursed through SAMHSA's Center for Mental Health Services, Center for Substance Abuse Treatment, and Center for Substance Abuse Prevention (Bednash, Heylin, & Rhome, 1998).

The Centers for Disease Control and Prevention's (CDC) mission is to promote health and quality of life by preventing and controlling disease, injury, and disability. The CDC employs more than 7,000 people in 192 different occupations (CDC, 1998). The focus of the CDC is on the community as the client, allowing nurses to make significant contributions in a variety of areas. Nurses are involved in the establishment of infection control guidelines and the prevention of substance abuse, human immunodeficiency virus (HIV), and other sexually transmitted diseases, as well as in the areas of violence, adolescent and school health, women's health, infants' and children's health, and immunization (Bednash, Heylin, & Rhome, 1998). The CDC also guards against international disease transmission with CDC personnel stationed in more than 25 foreign countries (USDHHS, 1999).

The mission of the U.S. Food and Drug Administration (FDA) is to ensure safe food and cosmetics, safe and effective medicines and medical treatments, and safe products such as microwave ovens (Bednash, Heylin, & Rhome, 1998). FDA approval is needed before any experimental drugs can be tested or sold in the United States.

The Health Resources and Services Administration (HRSA) helps provide health resources for medically underserved populations. HRSA consists of the Office of Rural Health, the Bureau

A CONVERSATION WITH . . .

At no other time in our nation's history has our country so needed the expertise of nurses in the development of health policy. As our nation struggles to reverse the tide of rising numbers of uninsured children and adults, to increase consumer involvement in health choices, and to care for our expanding aging population, we must turn to the expertise of our nation's nurses.

I have spent many years with nurses. In Congress, I worked closely with the American Nurses Association on issues of pay equity and equal rights. In 1984, ANA was the first group to endorse my candidacy for Vice President. In my 1992 race for the U.S. Senate, I reached out to a nurse, Judy Leavitt, to work on health policy and be a leader in my campaign. And again, in 1998, I turned to the nurses for their expertise in my U.S. Senate campaign.

—Geraldine Ferraro,
former member of the U.S. House of Representatives (D-New York) and 1984 U.S. Vice Presidential Candidate

Source: Mason, D. J., & Leavitt, J. K. (Eds.). (1998). Policy and politics in nursing and health care. Philadelphia: W. B. Saunders.

of Primary Care, the Bureau of Maternal and Child Health, the Office of Minority Health, and the Bureau of Health Professions. The Bureau of Health Professions contains the Division of Nursing, which oversees funding for undergraduate and graduate nursing education programs (Bednash, Heylin, & Rhome, 1998). A nationwide network of HRSA community and migrant health centers, as well as primary care programs for the homeless and residents of public housing, serve more than 8 million Americans each year. HRSA provides services to persons with HIV or acquired immunodeficiency syndrome (AIDS) through the Ryan White CARE Act programs, oversees the organ transplant system, and works to decrease infant mortality and improve child health (DHHS, 1999).

The Indian Health Service (IHS) provides comprehensive health services to Native Americans and Alaska Natives primarily living on reservations. In 1999, the IHS had 37 hospitals, 60 health centers, 3 school health centers, and 46 health stations. In addition, the IHS provided assistance to 34 urban Indian health centers. Services are provided to nearly 1.5 million Native Americans and Alaska Natives of 557 federally recognized tribes (DHHS, 1999).

The National Institutes of Health (NIH) funds and conducts health research through 19 different institutes and centers, including the National Institute of Nursing Research (NINR). The National Institute of Nursing Research began as an NIH center in 1986 and was elevated to institute status in 1993. The research funded through NINR focuses on health promotion and disease prevention, acute and chronic illness, and nursing systems (Bednash, Heylin, & Rhome, 1998).

Department of Education

The U.S. Department of Education provides billions of dollars each year for postsecondary education, including nursing education. Federal Family Education Loans (Stafford Loans), Pell Grants, Perkins Loans, and Federal Work Study programs are just a few of the sources of funding provided (Bednash, Heylin, & Rhome, 1998).

Department of Labor

The U.S. Department of Labor is responsible for enforcing the Fair Labor Standards Act (minimum wage and overtime), the Employee Retirement Income Security Act (employee benefit and retirement plans), and the Occupational Safety and Health Act (OSHA) (job safety and health). All these are important to nursing practice. The ANA has worked closely with the Department of Labor for nearly 20 years to ensure adequate funding for the health and safety of nurses in the workplace through enforcement of OSHA standards (Bednash, Heylin, & Rhome, 1998).

Legislative Branch

The U.S. Congress is the **legislative branch** of the federal government. Congress has two houses with equal power: the Senate

---

BOX 8-4 RESPONSIBILITIES OF THE U.S. CONGRESS

- Conduct hearings on issues that may generate federal legislation.
- Draft legislation.
- Estimate cost of proposed legislation.
- Enact legislation to create programs.
- Review legislated program operations.
- Determine the federal budget.
- Appropriate funds for federal operations.
- Decide entitlement policy (e.g., Medicare, Medicaid, Social Security).
- Confirms or rejects presidential nominations for high-level federal positions (e.g., cabinet members, federal judges).

Source: Bednash, Heylin, & Rhome, 1998.

---

and the House of Representatives. The Senate has 100 members, two from each state. The House of Representatives membership varies according to the population. A representative is elected to represent a specific number of constituents, so states with larger populations have more representatives. The number of representatives a state has increases or decreases with corresponding changes in the state's population. The House of Representatives currently has more than 400 members. The sole legislative power of the federal government lies with the two houses of Congress. A partial list of the responsibilities of the U.S. Congress is outlined in Box 8-4.

Judicial Branch

The **judicial branch** of the federal government, known as the U.S. court system, consists of 94 federal district courts, 13 circuit courts of appeals, the U.S. Supreme Court, and several specialized courts to address customs, patents, military issues, and so on. A Supreme Court justice generally keeps his or her appointment until retirement or death. At that time, a replacement is appointed to the position by the president and approved by Congress.

Although the judicial branch of the government is not involved in making policy, the way in which the courts interpret the law may have a profound effect on health care, including nursing practice. Nurses can affect the outcome of court cases by serving as expert witnesses or legal consultants (Bednash, Heylin, & Rhome, 1998).

State Government

Although the role of the federal government is in the forefront of American politics, the truth is that most of the policies and laws

In 1991 I received a telephone call from Geraldine Ferraro asking me to come to New York City to be interviewed for a leadership position on her campaign for a United States Senate seat representing the state of New York. How did Gerry find me and why did she want a nurse to work on a major national campaign?

My connection to Gerry followed one of the most important principles of political involvement and influence—"use your connections." I had spent a sabbatical year at the ANA working in the governmental affairs department. While there, I collaborated with one of the women who had been involved in Gerry's nomination for vice president of the United States in 1984. She knew Gerry was considering a run for the U.S. Senate, so she called her to recommend my political skills to her. Gerry indicated a strong interest in working with me because of my involvement with ANA, the first group to endorse her candidacy for vice president. Gerry called me and hired me a week later.

For a year and half I worked as the upstate campaign coordinator. I was responsible for 54 of the 62 counties in the state, an area that covers over 40,000 square miles. I started with nothing except a great candidate. I had to organize an office, create a database of contacts, organize a grassroots network, raise thousands of dollars, and create fundraising and media events. Although I had been an active volunteer in numerous congressional and state legislative campaigns, I had never been a paid staff member. I did not have an appointed position in the political party, so I had to use all my communication skills, organizational skills, and nursing intuition to create a campaign presence in every one of the 54 counties under my leadership.

It helped to have a candidate with name recognition. When I called major democratic leaders and potential supporters I didn't have to introduce my candidate. I used my connections and those of Gerry to build a grassroots structure. I focused on women's organizations, women leaders, nurses and their organizations, other health professionals, and any other men and women throughout the state who wanted to volunteer for Gerry. Gerry's candidacy energized and excited the electorate, as it had when she ran for vice president. It wasn't hard getting volunteers; it was only

difficult organizing them to contribute in meaningful ways. Whether it was organizing events for fundraising, working with the media, conducting voter registration drives, or soliciting political endorsements, it took incredible planning and organizational skill and thousands of volunteer hours. I planned it all—over 200 events—supported by a grassroots structure of over 5000 volunteers from every profession, occupation, and interest group who held campaign events, gave money, and worked for Gerry in their home communities.

The nurses came out in droves. Nurses who had never been involved politically suddenly wanted to help Gerry and listen to her message. Because I had been active in both the ANA-PAC and New York State political activities, I was able to help Gerry receive an early endorsement by the ANA-PAC and encourage New York State Nurses Association to mobilize their members.

What was it like to work so closely for such a national and international "celebrity"? It was fun, grueling, exciting, challenging, and a once in a lifetime experience. What made it easy was Gerry. She was personable, caring, and in many ways very much like her constituents. She had experienced poverty as well as success; she was a

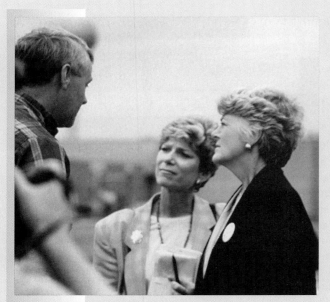

Judy Leavitt and 1984 vice presidential candidate, Geraldine Ferraro.

teacher and a lawyer; she was a mother, grandmother, and wife—so she knew about the issues and could relate to people throughout the country. She used me to draft her health platform and respected my expertise in teaching her about the issues. In addition, Gerry was able to bring the best political and media consultants to work with me and the campaign staff. Traveling with Gerry was the most fun of the entire year and a half. We would often spend two or three days alone traveling throughout the upstate counties, affording us an opportunity to become good friends. I was the oldest staff person, much closer in age to Gerry. That created a special bond that enabled me to have access to her and engendered mutual respect. At each event, I would sometimes look around as she was speaking and think how lucky I was to be able to have the opportunity to help elect someone whom I admired and believed could have been a fine senator. Unfortunately that never happened. Gerry lost in the primary election by less than 10,000 votes out of 4 million cast. The country lost the chance to have a great senator. I gained a friend and stories for a lifetime.

—Judy Leavitt,
MEd, RN, Campaign Manager for Geraldine Ferraro,
Candidate for U.S. Senate in 1992

related to nursing practice are created at the state level. The creation and enforcement of nurse practice acts and the regulation of nursing practice through licensing occurs at the state level. In 1996, more than 100,000 bills were introduced in state legislatures across the country, with about 25% of them affecting nurses and nursing practice (Gaffney, 1998). State governments consist of the same three branches as the federal government: executive, legislative, and judicial.

Executive Branch

The executive branch of state government consists of the governor, the lieutenant governor, and the attorney general. Most governors are elected to 4-year terms and are eligible for reelection. The governor is responsible for presenting the state budget to the legislature and overseeing state spending. The governor's policy initiatives are often presented as part of the state budget proposal and may contain health-related programs. The lieutenant governor presides over state affairs in the absence of the governor and can influence health and social policies within the state. The attorney general represents the public's interests in legal cases coming before the court, not including the state supreme court. The attorney general's office is often called on to interpret the nurse practice act to clarify the intent of legislation or regulations (Gaffney, 1998).

State Agencies

State agencies may be divided into five different categories:

1. *Agencies led by elected officers such as secretaries of state, treasurers, and attorney generals*

2. *Agencies led by officers appointed by the governor or independent boards, such as secretaries of human services and commissioners of health*

3. *Professional licensing and regulatory boards, such as boards of nursing*

4. *Public authorities and corporations, such as higher education assistance authorities*

5. *Independent boards and commissions, such as councils of higher education and public utilities commissions*

The Department of Health is a state organization whose primary purpose is to oversee and maintain the health of the community. The director of the state department of public health is appointed by the governor. There are many different divisions within the department of public health, which may include data collection and surveillance, administration of Medicaid and other federally funded programs, public health programs, and hospital regulation (Gaffney, 1998).

Legislative Branch

State legislatures are the oldest part of the American government, existing long before the drafting of the U.S. Constitution. In fact, the Declaration of Independence was signed by representatives of the legislatures of the 13 colonies that became the original 13 states. State legislatures levy taxes, appropriate funding, and create and monitor agencies to carry out state business (Gaffney, 1998). Patterned after the federal legislature, all state legislatures (excluding Nebraska) are comprised of two houses: a Senate and a House of Representatives. In each state, the House of Representatives is larger than the Senate because senators represent larger districts within the state than members of the House. Therefore, each senator has a greater number of constituents.

Judicial Branch

State judicial systems are similar to that of the federal system. The state supreme courts serve to interpret the language of their state constitutions and apply it in the courtroom. In recent years, there has been an upheaval in state law related to health care.

Many more malpractice suits are being brought against physicians, nurses, and hospitals by people who believe that they have been injured as a result of negligence or inappropriate action (Gaffney, 1998).

Local Government

Local governments are the link between citizens and the state and federal governments. Local governments distribute billions of federal and state dollars to local community agencies to provide services. The quality of life in a community is determined by how local government officials make decisions about the delivery of services. Some of the services provided and monitored by local governments are public health, public education, drinking water, sewage disposal, police protection, and solid waste management (Majewski & O'Brien, 1998).

The number, size, and type of local government varies throughout the country depending on state and regional culture, economics, and geography. The U.S. Census Bureau has divided local governments into four categories: counties, municipalities, towns and townships, and special districts (Majewski & O'Brien, 1998). Local governments are divided into the same branches of government (with variations) as the federal and state governments.

Different Types of Law

According to Webster's New World College Dictionary (Neufeldt, 1996), a law is a rule of conduct established and enforced by the authority, legislation, or custom of a given community, state, or other group. There are three types of laws in the United States: constitutional law, legislation and regulation, and judicial or common law.

Constitutional law is derived from federal and state constitutions and is the supreme law of the land. The U.S. Constitution is the highest legal authority that exists, and no other law, state or federal, may overrule it. A state constitution is the highest state law authority, but any provisions that conflict with the federal constitution will be invalidated by the courts. It is not considered a conflict, however, if state constitutions provide more expansive individual rights than those guaranteed by the federal constitution (Kaplan, 1985).

Legislation and regulation, known as **statutory law,** is established through formal legislative processes. Each time the U.S. Congress or state legislatures pass legislation, the body of statutory law grows (Betts & Waddle, 1993). Statutes are enacted by both federal and state governments. Local statutes, called *ordinances,* are enacted by local governing bodies, such as city and county councils (Kaplan, 1985).

Judicial or common law, known as case law, is derived from decisions made in the courtroom. Common law is based on the principles of justice, reason, and common sense rather than rules and regulations (Guido, 2001). Each time a judge or a jury makes a decision, the body of common law grows (Betts & Waddle, 1993). Decisions are made based on decisions from previous similar cases. Judges are bound by previous decisions (i.e., prece-

dents) unless it can be shown that the previous rulings are no longer valid. Therefore, a decision made in a case with no predecessors is critical because it becomes a precedent-setting case.

Common law can be categorized as either civil or criminal. Civil law protects individuals and involves the enforcement of rights, duties, and other legal relations between private citizens (Betts & Waddle, 1993). For example, an individual can sue another individual or a company for not fulfilling the terms of a legal contract. Criminal law is a crime against the state and involves public concerns against unlawful behavior that threatens society (Betts & Waddle, 1993). Murder is an example of criminal law. Although the crime was committed against an individual, it threatens the security of society as a whole.

How an Idea Becomes a Law

In today's climate of health care reform, nurses must understand the legislative process to be able to influence the development of sound health care policy for their clients and for the profession of nursing (Abood & Mittelstadt, 1998). Because the legislative process is similar at both the state and federal levels, it is described at the state level in this chapter. Although the legislative pathway may differ slightly from state to state, the basic process is the same (Abood & Mittelstadt, 1998). The state of Florida is used as the example.

A bill can be introduced only by a member of the legislature. Legislators introduce bills for many reasons, which may include pleasing a constituent or a special interest group, declaring a position on an issue, getting publicity, or simply avoiding a political attack (Abood & Mittelstadt, 1998). Companion bills (or twin bills) are sometimes introduced by legislators in the Senate and House of Representatives to increase the likelihood that the bill will pass and become law.

During a legislative session, the House and Senate meet separately and attempt to pass legislation that has previously been considered by a number of legislative committees. Committees are often referred to as the "heart of the legislative process" because they allow legislators to break down into smaller groups to discuss pertinent issues (Florida Legislature, 1994a). This enables members to have more in-depth discussions than would be possible if all issues were discussed by the entire legislature. Committees are established by authority of rules, which are adopted separately by the House and the Senate. The Speaker of the House and the President of the Senate, both of whom are elected by each body and represent the majority party, designate a chair and a vice-chair for each committee and appoint legislators to serve as committee members. Legislators usually serve on more than one committee.

There are three basic kinds of committees: standing, select, and conference committees. Standing committees are established by both the Senate and the House of Representatives to manage their business. They can be distinguished from each other by the kind of issues that they consider. For example, the Florida House of Representatives has a standing committee on health care licensing and regulation, which is responsible for considering bills relating to that particular area. The staff of this committee is responsible for doing the fact-finding groundwork for legislation that is referred to the committee for consideration. For example, if the committee were considering a bill proposing a change in the requirements for registered nurse (RN) licensure, it would study the current licensure requirements, find out why the sponsor of the bill (one or more of the representatives) believes the change is necessary, examine what the effects of the proposed change might be, and hear testimony from nurses, as well as the broader health care community, to gain insight about how they feel about the proposed change. Once all these things are considered, the committee passes judgment on the proposed legislation.

If the bill passes the committee, it travels either to the next committee of reference (if there is more than one) or to the floor of the House or Senate to be voted on by the respective body as a whole. If the committee does not pass the proposed legislation (reports unfavorably on the bill), the legislation will die unless two thirds of the members vote to reconsider it. This is a very high percentage, and further consideration is unlikely to occur in this situation.

Committees wield significant power in the legislative process. The chair of each committee has a great deal of influence over legislation because he or she decides which bills will be heard by the committee. If a bill is not heard, it cannot be voted on and therefore cannot be passed. Committees also have the authority to amend proposed legislation, so the original bill may look very different by the time it reaches the floor of the House or Senate.

A second type of committee is the select committee. These types of committees are appointed to perform certain tasks and may last anywhere from a few minutes to several years. For example, on the opening day of each legislative session, the Senate president will appoint a select committee to inform the House of Representatives that they are ready to begin conducting business. The Speaker of the House will appoint a similar committee that completes the ritual. These select committees complete their ceremonial function in a few minutes. On the other hand, when an issue arises that merits special consideration, a select committee may be established to consider that particular issue in depth. For example, the 1999 Florida Legislature had to consider a comprehensive legislative package introduced by Governor Jeb Bush regarding education. Rather than refer the large number of bills to different standing committees, the Speaker of the House of Representatives appointed a Select Committee on Transforming Florida's Schools to consider the bills as a complete educational package. This committee consisted of members of the House of Representatives (from both political parties) and was chaired by the member who sponsored the legislation. It met for 2 weeks immediately before the legislative session, heard testimony from supporters and opponents, and was responsible for amending and voting on the bills in the package.

The third type of committee is a conference committee. Before the functions of this kind of committee can be described, it is necessary to further explain the process of how a bill becomes a law. For a bill to be signed into law and become an act that is sent to the governor for consideration, it must pass both houses of the legislature in identical form. This is often more difficult than it sounds. First, the bill must have a sponsor in both the House and the Senate. These "companion" bills may be identical, similar, or very dissimilar. When a bill makes it through the committee process and is considered on the floor of the House or Senate, it goes through an amendatory process. Once amended, the bill requires a majority vote to pass.

Let's use RN licensure requirements as a hypothetical example. The House bill, after completing the committee process, increases both the level of education needed to obtain an RN license and the competencies required to pass the licensure exam. On the floor, House members amend the bill to add two more competencies. The bill, as amended, passes with a majority vote and is sent to the Senate for consideration. The Senate takes up the House bill and agrees with the increased educational requirements but decides to amend the bill because it does not agree with the competencies that the House has chosen. In the amendatory process, the Senate removes three of the competencies required in the House bill and adds two new competencies from the original Senate bill. The House bill, as amended by the Senate, then passes the Senate with a majority vote and is sent back to the House. If the House does not agree with the changes made by the Senate, they may reach an impasse. This often results in the bill's demise. However, if the proposed legislation is important to the leadership in each house, the presiding officers may appoint a conference committee in an attempt to reach a compromise agreement.

If differences cannot be reconciled through the conference committee, the proposed legislation will fail. If the conference committee can reach an agreement, the House and Senate must vote on the compromise "as is," and no amendments can be offered. Usually, conference reports are submitted during the waning hours of a session, when time is short and legislators are unlikely to reject conference committee recommendations because it will most likely result in the failure of the bill (Florida Legislature, 1994a).

It is important to realize that many bills make it through the committee process but never get heard on the floor of the House or Senate. The presiding officers of each house, through the

FYI

A conference committee is appointed every legislative session to consider the budget. This committee is always important because the budget is the only bill that the legislature is *required* to pass.

standing committees on rules and calendar, have control over which bills will be considered by the full House or Senate. Just as in committee, if a bill is not heard on the floor, it cannot be voted on and therefore cannot pass.

If a bill makes it through the committee process and passes both houses in identical form, it is called an *act*. Each act is sent to the governor for consideration, and he or she may either sign it into law, allow it to become law without his or her signature, or veto it. If an act is vetoed, the legislature may override it with a two-thirds vote in both houses. However, because the governor does not consider the acts until after the legislative session has adjourned, the legislature would be forced to either call a special session or wait until the next session to take action.

How Nurses Can Get Involved

Nurses can become involved in the political process at various levels. The first and most important thing is to be an informed voter. Nurses should watch the news, read the newspaper, surf the Internet, and be aware of what the candidates stand for on the national, state, and local levels. Nurses should also find out where candidates stand on the issues that are important to them as nurses. This can be accomplished with just a minimal amount of investigation. Nurses can contact the professional organizations to which they belong to find out which candidates they support. If a candidate is an incumbent, his or her voting record on issues of importance should be checked. Nurses must make phone calls, write letters, and ask questions!

Once legislators are in office, nurses should get to know them and make themselves and their views known to them. Box 8-5 contains some tips for effectively communicating ideas to legislators.

To have one of your ideas introduced as a bill, you must first find a sponsor in both the House and the Senate. The best scenario would be to approach a potential sponsor who is influential among legislators and who has a record of sponsoring successful legislation in your area of interest. This person will be likely to have more success in building coalitions among members than a less experienced legislator. It is also helpful if the legislator feels strongly about the issue because he or she will be more likely to fight for the proposed legislation.

Some legislative bodies place limits on the number of bills that can be filed by a particular member. It is necessary to investigate whether limitations exist and, if so, approach potential sponsors early. Timing can be crucial, especially if the issue of concern is a highly publicized one. Be aware of media coverage and strategically plan your moves.

Lobbying

The 1999 Florida Guide to Legislative Lobbyist Registration defines **lobbying** as "influencing or attempting to influence legislative action or non-action through oral or written communication or attempting to obtain the goodwill of a member or employee of the Legislature" (p. 2). A lobbyist is a person who is employed and receives payment for the primary purpose of lob-

---

BOX 8-5 TIPS FOR EFFECTIVE COMMUNICATIONS WITH LEGISLATORS

- Know who your legislators are and know how to contact them.
- Have a clear understanding of the legislative process.
- Contact your legislator about an issue that concerns you before the legislature takes action on it. (Although the legislative session may not begin until March, the committee process begins during the fall months. It is important to remember that all bills must first go through the committee process.)
- Use a variety of communication methods to contact your legislator, including telephone calls, letters, e-mail, fax, office visits, and so on. Be extremely careful to use correct spelling and grammar so that you do not lose your audience.
- Be polite, even if you disagree with the legislator's viewpoint on the issue. Your ability to effectively communicate your concerns diminishes if you go on the attack.
- Be prepared! Share with your legislator facts and figures that demonstrate the effect that a particular bill might have on your profession. Your opinions must be backed up with facts to be given any credence. You are the expert. Show it.
- Be concise and specific. It is important to remember that legislators must consider a large range of issues. Their time and attention are limited.
- Suggest a course of action and offer assistance. It is always beneficial to leave a one-page summary of your ideas with your legislator so that he or she may refer back to it or pass it on to legislative staff or other members.
- Establish a rapport with legislative aides and committee staff. These are the people who have direct and frequent contact with legislators and are responsible for providing them with a great deal of information.

Source: Florida Legislature, 1994b.

---

bying on behalf of another person, group, or governmental entity. Most states, if not all, require lobbyists to be registered as such. This registration allows citizens to be informed about activities that are aimed at influencing government decision making. For example, when major legislation relating to health care is being considered, it may be beneficial to know which groups

CASE STUDY

Two Mississippi Nurses Lead the Way

Deborah Konkle-Parker, MSN, FNP

As a nurse practitioner working in an outpatient HIV clinic in Jackson, Mississippi, Debbie Konkle-Parker and other providers depended on the federal Ryan White AIDS Drug Assistance Program (ADAP), administered by the Mississippi Department of Health (MSDH), to help many of their clients get medicines. ADAP was used primarily to help clients who had no health insurance or whose medications exceeded the Mississippi Medicaid limit of five prescriptions per month.

In early April 1997, after several years of uneventful program usage, word was received from the health department that the Ryan White program was not accepting any more referrals for ADAP assistance. The recent addition of expensive protease inhibitors to the treatment regimen for HIV had depleted the entire year of federal ADAP funding by mid-March. This news came suddenly, without warning, and with no back-up plan for those with no other resources.

This sudden news sent providers and clients reeling, with no way to deal with this shortfall in services. A week later, there was a meeting of health care providers at the Mississippi Department of Health. At this meeting, the health care providers were informed that those individuals who were already receiving a protease inhibitor from ADAP would continue to receive medications, but all others would be cut off from the program. No more referrals were being accepted. This could literally mean the difference between life and death for many clients.

To deal with the problem, Debbie Konkle-Parker organized a problem-solving session to determine a way to cope with this change. She sent letters to concerned individuals, requesting their presence at a networking meeting. The meeting was attended by health care providers representing all disciplines, representatives from MSDH, representatives from the pharmaceutical industry, and persons with HIV/AIDS. The discussion at the meeting revealed that although most states provided funding from their state budgets to augment the federal ADAP dollars, Mississippi did not. It was decided that to change this policy, it was im-

portant to become an organized body to influence the legislators. The Mississippi HIV/AIDS Assembly was formed, with Debbie Konkle-Parker as its chair. The Mississippi HIV/AIDS Assembly consisted of two committees: (1) the AIDS Aware committee for mobilizing grassroots lobbying efforts around the state and (2) the Health Provider Network of interdisciplinary health care providers who could mobilize organizational lobbying efforts. Shortly after this meeting, the Mississippi State Department of Health found a way to temporarily redirect some of the money from other parts of the Ryan White program to re-enroll some clients who had been dropped from the program. But that effort was only putting a "Band-Aid" on the problem until further funding could be obtained.

The Health Provider Network set about the task of determining the direction of the work of the assembly, and the AIDS Aware committee gathered grassroots support for their efforts. The highest priority goal was supporting the Health Department's request of $500,000 from the state budget for ADAP. Although this amount was much less than what was actually needed, it was determined that politically this was an amount that reasonably could be requested by the Health Department. The Mississippi AIDS Assembly requested $2 million from the legislature, which was the estimate of how much money was actually needed to meet the extent of the problem in Mississippi.

Through these two committees, several different actions were taken, including providing speakers to bring attention to the issue for the public; maintaining a "silent" presence, including media coverage at a key budget hearing meeting; attending a meeting of the legislature's public health committee where bills were decided on before being brought to the floor; and applying consistent pressure on legislators to consider this issue. Multiple mailings went out to individuals throughout the state, encouraging personal communication with their legislators and a "spreading of the word."

The result of this year-long work was the first-ever state dedication of $750,000 to the Mississippi Ryan White AIDS Drug Assistance Program, with more to follow each year. This funding allowed a return of new referrals to the program and an immediate lessening of the waiting list of individuals needing medications.

Continued

CASE STUDY—cont'd

Connie Thompson, BSN, RN

As the infection control coordinator of a medical center in Jackson, Mississippi, Connie Thompson played a big role in the efforts of the Mississippi HIV/AIDS Assembly and eagerly joined in the excitement surrounding its legislative victory. But after the excitement faded away, Thompson realized that this was only the beginning. More funding and services were needed, not only for persons living with HIV/AIDS, but for persons living with any chronic disabling disease.

In August 1998, under the leadership of Thompson, a variety of Mississippi organizations and agencies joined forces in an effort to influence legislative health care issues for disabled persons. Eventually this group formed a coalition of more than 50 organizations and agencies known as the Coalition for Uninsured Mississippians, representing thousands of Mississippians with disabilities or chronic illnesses who are denied access to health insurance each year. These individuals—persons with cancer, heart disease, HIV,

diabetes, asthma, lupus, arthritis, and other diseases—earn a little more money, either from disability payments or job income, than the maximum allowed to qualify for Medicaid. However, they don't make enough money to be able to afford expensive private health insurance.

As a result, these men, women, and children are forced to make frequent visits to hospital emergency rooms for basic health care. Or worse, they do not seek care at all until a crisis occurs that requires inpatient hospitalization. Proper disease management with regular clinic visits for appropriate follow-up and networking for client care and services would maintain optimal health standards for these individuals. Quality of life for these persons would greatly improve and health care would be more cost-effective if they had access to health insurance.

The timing for the work of the coalition was a critical factor. The Federal Balanced Budget Act of 1997 offered states the option of allowing citizens with disabilities to purchase Medicaid on a sliding fee scale according to their income. In August 1998, the U.S. Department of Health and Human Services urged state governors, state legislators, and Medicaid directors to take advantage of this important new option. The Coalition for Uninsured Mississippians sought support from Mississippi's citizens for a legislative bill that would allow disabled persons with incomes below 250% of the federal poverty level to buy in to Medicaid coverage. The purchase of this coverage would

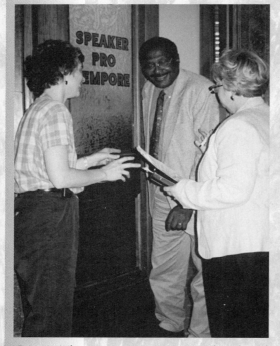

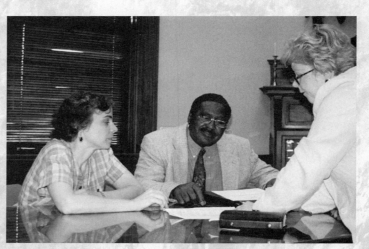

Connie Thompson, BSN, RN, and Deborah Konkle-Parker, MSN, RN, FNP, work with Robert G. Clark, Mississippi State Representative.

be based on a sliding scale fee. Both the Balanced Budget Act of 1997 and the encouragement from the U.S. Department of Health and Human Services were used to support the coalition's action.

Within 2 months of the coalition's initial meeting a petition supported by thousands of Mississippians had been sent to the co-chairs of the joint subcommittees of health and welfare of the state legislature. A statewide Forum for Effective Advocacy of Chronic Illnesses and Disabilities was held to discuss the issues, and a task force was formed to meet with the director of the division of Medicaid to look for solutions. Connie Thompson, as the facilitator of the Coalition for Uninsured Mississippians, was invited to serve on the attorney general's Partners for a Healthy Mississippi task force.

As a result of the coalition's efforts, a bill to expand Medicaid coverage by authorizing a buy-in opportunity to workers who are disabled and earning less than 250% of the federal poverty was drafted and signed into law by the Mississippi legislature and the governor during the 1999 legislative session.

In both of the above scenarios, nurse-led public policy strategies, starting with simple problem-solving meetings, have achieved the goal of improving health care for some of Mississippi's poor and vulnerable citizens.

have hired lobbyists to promote their interests and monitor their activities and expenditures.

For example, home health agencies may hire lobbyists whose principal responsibilities are to represent the organization's interests to the legislature and other government agencies. Nurses employed by a home health agency would not be considered lobbyists unless their most significant work responsibility dealt with governmental affairs. However, this does not mean that the nurses cannot contact their legislators and actively support or oppose legislation that affects their home health agencies. It simply means that the nurses are not be required to register because they do not receive payment for the purposes of lobbying.

Lobbyists must adhere to many rules and regulations, which may vary widely from state to state. Therefore, it is important that nurses be aware of the rules, if any, that apply in their states. Regulations may also change from year to year, which makes it necessary to keep current. For example, in Florida, rules and regulations regarding the receipt of gifts from lobbyists are established in statute (Section 112.3148, Florida Statutes). Other states may not be so proscriptive and may outline rules only in policy manuals or employee handbooks. Some states may not even have rules for lobbyists, but most have some kind of regulation.

Best practices for lobbying as well as for concerned constituents include being aware of all applicable rules and restrictions, establishing a good rapport with legislators and legislative staff, and always backing up your position with hard data. If nurses adhere to these principles, their likelihood of successfully communicating their ideas will greatly increase.

Political Action Committees

Through the years, the ANA and various other specialty health organizations have taken leadership roles in mobilizing nurses in grassroots lobbying. This has required a significant effort to educate nurses about the political process and how to remain cognizant of the political issues that affect nursing and health. Because federal law requires that campaign contributions be kept as a separate fund and that no organizational membership be used for this purpose, many groups have created separate organizations for political activities. These organizations are referred to as **political action committees (PACs).** Their work is completely separate from the rest of the organization's work. The primary

RESEARCH BRIEF

Monardi, F., & Glantz, S. A. (1998). Are tobacco industry campaign contributions influencing state legislative behavior? American Journal of Public Health, 88(6), 918–923.

This study examined the influence of tobacco industry campaign contributions on state legislators' tobacco voting records in six states. Data on campaign contributions to state legislators and legislators' tobacco control policy scores were analyzed using multivariate simultaneous equations regression models. The data analysis revealed that as tobacco industry contributions increase, the calculated policy scores tended to decrease (i.e., state legislators become more supportive of the tobacco industry's political agenda). These results were significant even after controlling for partisanship, majority party status, and leadership effects. The conclusion of the study was that tobacco industry campaign contributions significantly influence state legislators in terms of tobacco control policy making.

purpose of a PAC is to endorse and support candidates for public office who support the legislative agenda of the organization or group making the endorsement (Curtis & Lumpkin, 1998). Nursing PACs exist at the federal and state level, most often through the ANA (ANA-PAC) and state nurses associations. ANA-PAC is the 30th largest federal PAC and in 1995 was identified as the second fastest growing federal health care PAC in the nation (Kelly & Joel, 1996).

Regulation and Licensing of Nursing Practice

The Regulatory Process

Although it is important for nurses to be involved in the legislative process, it is equally important for nurses to understand the **regulatory process**. According to Webster's New World College Dictionary (Neufeldt, 1996), *regulation* is "the act of controlling, directing, or governing according to a rule, principle, or system" (p. 1131). Once bills are passed into law by the legislative branch of government, they must be implemented by the administrative agencies of the executive branch (Abood & Mittelstadt, 1998; Loquist, 1999). Legislation is purposely expressed in broad terms to provide flexibility and adaptability of laws over time. Regulation is expressed in very specific terms describing how the administrative agency with jurisdictional authority will implement the law (Loquist, 1999). The legislative process is used to create policy and laws to address a particular issue when none exist. Regulation is used to clarify and interpret existing policy and laws and decide what methods will be used to enforce them (Loquist, 1999).

Regulations frame the way health policy is transposed into services and programs. Although regulations are a direct result of passed legislation, they are shaped into their final forms by the ongoing involvement of health care professionals and their professional organizations, third-party payers, consumers, and other special interest groups. Before a federal agency can implement a law, it must publish the proposed regulation or set of regulations in the *Federal Register*. The publication of the proposed regulations affords anyone with any interest in the regulations the abil-

HEALTHY PEOPLE 2010

OBJECTIVES RELATED TO LAW

3.14   Increase the number of states that have a statewide population-based cancer registry that captures case information on at least 95% of the expected number of reportable cancers.

6.13   Increase the number of tribes, states, and the District of Columbia that have public health surveillance and health-promotion programs for people with disabilities and caregivers.

13.9   Increase the number of state prison systems that provide comprehensive HIV/AIDS, sexually transmitted diseases, and tuberculosis (TB) education.

13.10   Increase the proportion of inmates in state prison systems who receive voluntary HIV counseling and testing during incarceration.

15.24   Increase the number of states and the District of Columbia with laws requiring bicycle helmets for bicycle riders.

18.11   Increase the proportion of local governments with community-based jail diversion programs for adults with serious mental illnesses.

23.15   Increase the proportion of federal, tribal, state, and local jurisdictions that review and evaluate the extent to which their statutes, ordinances, and bylaws assure the delivery of essential public health services.

27.14   Reduce the illegal buy rate among minors through enforcement of laws prohibiting the sale of tobacco products to minors.

Source: DHHS, 2000.

ity to react to them before they become finalized. Commenting on proposed regulations before they are finalized is one of the most important, but often neglected, parts of the legislative process (Abood & Mittelstadt, 1998).

The U.S. Constitution dictates that the government has a duty to protect its citizens. The Tenth Amendment to the U.S. Constitution provides the states with all the powers not specifically reserved for the federal government. Regulation of health care professions is one way that each state exercises its responsibility to protect the health, safety, and welfare of its residents.

Nursing practice in each state is governed by a **nurse practice act,** which includes the laws and regulations that control the requirements for entry into practice, the standards for acceptable practice, the standards for continuing competence, and the disciplinary actions taken for misconduct (Loquist, 1999). The state nurse practice act is the most important piece of legislature for nurses because it governs every facet of nursing practice (Guido, 2001).

Each state legislature designates a board of nursing to administer the nurse practice act. There are 61 boards of nursing in the United States and its territories. The most critical role of the board of nursing is to ensure the safety of the public by monitoring the competency of practicing nurses through licensure (Loquist, 1999).

Licensure

A license is "a formal permission authorized by law to do something" (Neufeldt, 1996, p. 779). Nurses must be licensed in a state in order to work as an RN, licensed practical nurse (LPN), or vocational nurse (LVN). **Licensure** provides the public with the greatest level of protection because it protects the title of RN or LPN and delineates the scope of nursing practice (Loquist, 1999). Requirements for licensure include proof of graduation from an approved academic program, a passing score on the licensing examination, and personal qualifications such as citizenship or visa permits, good physical and mental health, and good moral character (Barnum, 1997; Guido, 2001; Loquist, 1999).

All states administer licensing examinations using a standardized national test developed and administered by the National Council of State Boards of Nursing (NCSBN). Licensing examinations are called the National Council Licensing Examination for Registered Nurses (NCLEX-RN) and the National Council Licensing Examination for Practical Nurses (NCLEX-PN). Traditionally, nurses have been required to be licensed in the state in which they practice. If a nurse moves to a different state, he or she must obtain a license from the new state. A national examination makes seeking reciprocity (recognition of licensure from one state to another) an easy process if the nurse has a valid license in one state (Betts & Waddle, 1993; Guido, 2001).

In recent years, the use of telecommunication technology has transformed the health care delivery system and challenged the individual state licensing system. Mergers of health care systems have produced giant corporations that operate across state lines. Nurses serve as case managers for clients living in many different states and staff regional or national telephone advice and consultation hot lines (Hutcherson & Williamson, 1999; Loquist, 1999; Wakefield, 1999). As nurses began practicing in several states at the same time, separate licenses had to be obtained from each state. This policy is impractical and expensive.

In response to the licensing dilemma, the NCSBN adopted a new model for nursing regulation called the **Nurse Multistate Licensure Mutual Recognition Model.** According to the ANA, multistate licensure allows a nurse to practice in several states while holding a license in only one state. States enter into interstate compact agreements to coordinate activities associated with licensure. This mutual recognition model allows nurses to practice in states that have adopted an interstate compact with each other. The nurses are held accountable for compliance with the laws and regulations of each state's nurse practice act (ANA, 1998). In March 1998, Utah became the first state to pass legislation to adopt the Mutual Recognition Model (ANA, 1998). Other states are following, but not without controversy. Many nursing organizations, concerned with client safety and nursing standards, are questioning the appropriateness of the model (King, 1999).

State boards of nursing are responsible not only for ensuring the competency of nurses entering into practice, but also for monitoring the competence of those nurses already in practice. Most nurse practice acts have provisions that require employers to report any violations. Procedures for reporting misconduct, conducting investigations, and issuing sanctions are outlined in the regulations of each state's or territory's nurse practice act. Licensed nurses are responsible for knowing the laws and regulations that govern nursing practice in their states (Loquist, 1999).

Nursing Practice and the Law

The most common lawsuits filed against health care professionals involve the principles of **negligence** and **malpractice,** which fall under the classification of tort law. Torts are legal wrongs committed against another person or against the property of another person. The wrongdoing may be intentional or unintentional and must result in physical, emotional, or economic harm (Betts & Waddle, 1993; Guido, 2001).

Although the terms *negligence* and *malpractice* are often used interchangeably, there is a fine distinction between them. *Negligence* is a general term that describes the failure to act as any prudent or reasonable person would act in a specific circumstance. *Malpractice* is a more specific term that considers a professional standard of care as well as the professional status of the health care provider. To be liable for malpractice, the person committing the misconduct must be a professional acting in a professional role. Professional misconduct includes either doing something that should not be done (commission) or not doing something that should be done (omission) (Betts & Waddle, 1993; Guido, 2001).

For a nurse to be found guilty of malpractice in a court of law, the following must have existed:

- *A duty was owed to the client.*
- *There was a breach of the duty owed to the client.*
- *Harm was caused to the client.*
- *The harm was foreseeable.*
- *The action or inaction of the nurse caused the harm (Guido, 2001).*

Nursing Practice in Correctional Settings

The role of the community health nurse in correctional settings is relatively new. Health care for this population has unique challenges for the nurse in this specialized legal setting (Box 8-6). The basis of correctional health care is providing primary care for inmates from the time of entry into the system, through transfers to other facilities, and to final release from custody back to the community (Earley, 1999). Nurses in correctional facilities provide health care to populations incarcerated in jails, prisons, juvenile detention facilities, and similar settings. Ages range from youths to aged adults. Women, although representing a small minority of the incarcerated population, make up a growing number of persons in correctional facilities (ANA, 1995).

Although often not fully realized by the general population, the existence of health care in correctional facilities is based on the Eighth Amendment of the U.S. Constitution, which prohibits "cruel and unusual punishment" of those convicted of crimes. Furthermore, as a public health concern, correctional institutions are reservoirs of physical and mental illness, which constantly spill back into the community. Appropriate treatment must be provided, with a focus on prevention of transmission of communicable disease. The health of the general community is affected as the inmate population continues to increase.

The consequences of untreated illness in the system are not just for the inmate or even just to the correctional system. These are public health problems that require effective management and close collaboration between correctional health and the public health system (Conklin, Lincoln, & Flanigan, 1998).

Incarcerated populations have greater health risks than the general population for communicable disease, especially HIV and tuberculosis, violence-associated risks, decreased educational levels, substance abuse, and poverty. Not only do inmates have higher risks for many of these health problems upon admission, but environmental conditions within the correctional facility and behaviors associated with incarceration lend themselves to the spread of communicable disease. The nurse in the correctional setting can provide interventions aimed at interrupting the chain of contagion and can educate the inmates about self-care and protection from these risks. Inmate education is an essential function of **correctional nursing.** The goals are for inmates to remain healthy while incarcerated and to return to the community properly educated about remaining free of communicable disease, as well as to prevent others from becoming infected. Peer education groups have been an effective strategy in the correctional system (Conklin, Lincoln, & Flanigan, 1998).

The first standards for nursing practice in correctional settings, the *ANA Scope and Standards of Nursing Practice in Correctional Facilities*, were developed and approved by the ANA in 1985 and revised in 1995. These standards address the scope of nursing practice in correctional settings as well as standards of care and standards of professional performance (ANA, 1995).

. . . .

Prisons do not exist in a vacuum: they are part of a political, social, economic, and moral order.

James B. Jacobs, 1977

. . . .

Forensic Nursing: An Emerging Nursing Role[1]

Forensic nursing, although relatively new in the United States, has been a recognized subspecialty of nursing in other parts of the world for several years. Forensic nursing derives its role and

[1]This section on forensic nursing was authored by Margaret M. Aiken, PhD, RN, Sexual Assault Nurse Examiner (SANE), Memphis Sexual Assault Resource Center, Memphis, Tennessee.

BOX 8-6 LEVELS OF PREVENTION ACTIVITIES IN CORRECTIONAL FACILITIES		
PRIMARY PREVENTION	**SECONDARY PREVENTION**	**TERTIARY PREVENTION**
Stress reduction education	Treatment of infections	Injury rehabilitation
Prenatal care	Trauma care for injuries	Diabetes foot care
Immunizations	Screening for suicide risk	Stroke rehabilitation
Violence prevention	Disaster and emergency care	

functions from the gap that exists between criminal justice/law enforcement and health care for victims of crime.

In 1992, a group of nurses, most of whom were sexual assault nurse examiners (SANEs), met in Minneapolis, Minnesota. As a result of this meeting, it was decided that nurses involved in an array of roles that interacted with the criminal justice system would operate under the "umbrella" of forensic nursing. Another result of the Minneapolis meeting was the formation of the International Association of Forensic Nursing.

In 1996, the ANA recognized forensic nursing as a subspecialty in nursing practice. This was significant because it enabled and allowed the practitioners to define the scope of practice and determine standards of practice and care. The *ANA Scope and Standards of Forensic Nursing Practice* were approved and published in 1997. A major function of forensic nursing, especially in cases of interpersonal violence (i.e., rape assault), is the assessment and documentation of injury and the appropriate collection, packaging, and storage of physical and biological evidence. Forensic nurses can be found functioning in rape crisis centers, emergency departments, and nursing homes. In some regions of the United States, forensic nurses are coroners and death investigators assisting the police with homicide cases and cases of unexplained death.

The Memphis Sexual Assault Resource Center came in to existence in the mid-1970s. It was one of the first programs of its type in the United States. In those early years the client population consisted mainly of adult women. Later, changes in child abuse law precipitated an exponential increase in the number of children evaluated. In the late 1990s, services were expanded to the collection of biological evidence from those suspected of crimes (sexual offenses, homicide, and driving under the influence [DUI]).

CONCLUSION

Nurses in the community must remain current and informed about politics and law as related to public health nursing practice. The political system is ultimately about the distribution of power through formalized and complex systems of law, policy, and regulatory control mechanisms. Settings within the community have legal implications for the nurse, and there are emerging opportunities for nurses within the political/legal community, such as correctional and forensic nursing. Furthermore, for nurses to maintain control of professional nursing practice, understanding and applying political knowledge helps secure our future in the health care delivery system.

CRITICAL THINKING ACTIVITIES

1. Do all three types of law apply to professional nursing practice? In what ways?
2. In what ways can nurses influence legislation that affects nursing practice?
3. What types of nursing situations may lend themselves to malpractice suits?
4. What steps can you take to avoid a lawsuit?
5. Is there a particular "type" of client that will sue? What makes you think so?

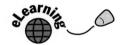

Explore Community Health Nursing on the web! To learn more about the topics in this chapter, use the passcode provided to access your exclusive web site:
http://communitynursing.jbpub.com
If you do not have a passcode, you can obtain one at this site.

REFERENCES

Abood, S., & Mittelstadt, P. (1998). Legislative and regulatory processes. In D. J. Mason & J. K. Leavitt (Eds.), *Policy and politics in nursing and health care* (3rd ed., pp. 384–396). Philadelphia: W. B. Saunders.

American Nurses Association (ANA). (1995). *Scope and standards of nursing practice in correctional facilities.* Washington, DC: Author.

American Nurses Association (ANA). (1998). *Multistate regulation of nurses:* www.nursingworld.org/gova/multibg.htm.

Bacharach, S. B., & Lawler, E. J. (1980). *Power and politics in organizations.* San Francisco: Jossey-Bass.

Barnum, B. S. (1997, August 13). Licensure, certification, and accreditation. *Online Journal of Issues in Nursing:* www.nursingworld.org/ojin/tpc4/tpc4_2.htm.

Bednash, G. P., Heylin, G. B., & Rhome, A. M. (1998). Federal government. In D. J. Mason & J. K. Leavitt (Eds.), *Policy and politics in nursing and health care* (3rd ed., pp. 436–457). Philadelphia: W. B. Saunders.

Betts, V. T., & Waddle, F. I. (1993). Legal aspects of nursing. In K. K. Chitty (Ed.), *Professional nursing. Concepts and challenges.* Philadelphia: W. B. Saunders.

Centers for Disease Control and Prevention (CDC). (1998). *Fact book FY 1998* (DHHS Publication No. 1998-638-018). Washington, DC: U.S. Government Printing Office.

Conklin, T., Lincoln, T., & Flanigan, T. (1998). A public health model to connect correction health care with communities. *American Journal of Public Health, 88*(8), 1249–1251.

Curtis, B. T., & Lumpkin, B. (1998). Political action committees. In D. J. Mason & J. K. Leavitt (Eds.), *Policy and politics in nursing and health care* (3rd ed., pp. 546–554). Philadelphia: W. B. Saunders.

Department of Health and Human Services (DHHS). (1999). *Greetings from the Secretary. Donna Shalala:* www.hhs.gov/about/greeting.html.

Earley, J. (1999, Spring/Summer). Nursing behind bars. *Minority Nurse,* pp. 22–25.

Florida Legislature, Office of the Clerk. (1994a). *Citizen's guide to the legislature. How the committee process works:* www.leg.state.fl.us/citizen/documents/howcomm.html. Accessed May 1999.

Florida Legislature, Office of the Clerk. (1994b). *Citizen's guide to the legislature. Getting your voice heard: Tips for effectively communicating your ideas:* www.leg.state.fl.us/citizen/documents/howwrite.html. Accessed May 1999.

Florida Legislature, Office of the Clerk. (1994c). *Citizen's guide to the legislature. How an idea becomes a law:* www.leg.state.fl.us/citizen/documents. Accessed May 1999.

Forgotson, E. H. (1967). 1965: The turning point in health law—1966 reflections. *American Journal of Public Health, 57*(6), 934–935.

French, J. R., & Raven, B. (1959). The basis for social power. In D. Cartwright (Ed.), *Studies in social power.* Ann Arbor: University of Michigan Press.

Gaffney, T. (1998). State government. In D. J. Mason & J. K. Leavitt (Eds.), *Policy and politics in nursing and health care* (3rd ed., pp. 417–427). Philadelphia: W. B. Saunders.

Guide to Legislative Lobbyist Registration. (1999). Tallahassee, FL: Lobbyist Registration Office.

Guido, G. W. (2001). *Legal issues in nursing* (3rd ed.). Upper Saddle River, NJ: Prentice Hall.

Helvie, C. O. (1998). *Advanced practice nursing in the community.* Thousand Oaks, CA: Sage.

Hersey, P., Blanchard, K., & Natemeyer, W. (1979). Situational leadership: Perception and impact of power. *Group Organizational Studies, 4,* 418–428.

Hewison, A. (1994). The politics of nursing: A framework for analysis. *Journal of Advanced Nursing, 20,* 1170–1175.

Hutcherson, C., & Williamson, S. H. (1999, May 31). Nursing regulation for the new millennium: The mutual recognition model. *Online Journal of Issues in Nursing:* http://nursingworld.org/ojin/topic9/topic9_2.htm.

Huston, C. J. (1995, Fall). Nursing and political action in the twentieth century: From separation to fusion. *Revolution: The Journal of Nurse Empowerment,* 50–53.

Kaplan, W. A. (1985). *The law of higher education* (2nd ed.). San Francisco: Jossey-Bass.

Kelly, L. Y., & Joel, L. A. (1996). *The nursing experience* (3rd ed.). New York: McGraw-Hill.

King, S. E. (1999, May 31). Multistate licensure: Premature policy. *Online Journal of Issues in Nursing:* www.nursingworld.org/ojin/topic9/topic9_3.htm.

Lenski, G. E. (1984). *Power and privilege.* Chapel Hill, NC: University of North Carolina Press.

Lobbyist Registration Office. (1999). *Guide to legislative lobbyist registration 1999.* Tallahassee, FL: Florida Legislature.

Loquist, R. S. (1999). Regulation: Parallel and powerful. In J. A. Milstead (Ed.), *Health policy and politics. A nurse's guide* (pp. 105–146). Gaithersburg, MD: Aspen.

Majewski, J. V., & O'Brien, M. C. (1998). Local government. In D. J. Mason & J. K. Leavitt (Eds.), *Policy and politics in nursing and health care* (3rd ed., pp. 405–416). Philadelphia: W. B. Saunders.

Miller, D. F. (1992). *Dimensions of community health.* Dubuque, IA: Wm. C. Brown.

Milstead, J. A. (1999). Advanced practice nurses and public policy, naturally. In J. A. Milstead (Ed.), *Health policy and politics. A nurse's guide* (pp. 1–41). Gaithersburg, MD: Aspen.

Neufeldt, V. (Ed.). (1996). *Webster's new world college dictionary* (3rd ed.). New York: Macmillan.

Robertson, I. (1981). *Sociology* (2nd ed.). New York: Worth.

Satcher, D. (1998, May/June). Public Health Service: On the job for 200 years. *Public Health reports, 113,* 201–203.

Turnock, B. J. (1997). *Public health: What it is and how it works.* Gaithersburg, MD: Aspen.

Wakefield, M. K. (1999). Have license, will travel. *Nursing Economics, 17*(2), 114–116.

Weber, M. (1947). *The theory of social and economic organization* (ed. and trans. A. M. Henderson & T. Parsons). New York: Oxford University Press.

Chapter 9
Health Policy
Nancy Milio

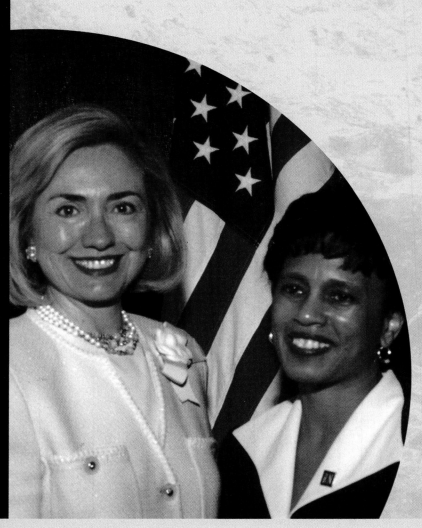

To meet the social responsibility of the health professions to promote and maintain health in all segments of the population, our knowledge and skill must go beyond the biomedical and psychosocial aspects of health and illness. Today, nurses' competence requires understanding health policy—what it is and how it is made. This chapter provides an overview of health policy and its relationship to the public's health. It outlines policy-making activities and the governmental and other "players" (or stakeholders) that influence those processes. It is important for nursing as a profession and for those in practice to understand policy development in local, state, and national contexts to recognize when community health might be affected and to find ways to influence policies to promote and protect health. This awareness can guide nursing's contribution to policy action on behalf of people's health.

QUESTIONS TO CONSIDER

After reading this chapter, answer the following questions:

1. What is health policy and how is it related to the health care system?
2. What are the purposes of health policy?
3. How have health policies been developed from a historical perspective in the United States?
4. Why is health policy needed in the United States?
5. What is the policy-making process?
6. How can the tobacco control health issue be used to illustrate successful public health policy making?
7. How are policies developed and by whom?
8. How are policies evaluated in the United States?
9. Who are stakeholders and how do they influence policy development?
10. What is the role of community health nurses in the health policy-making process?

KEY TERMS

Appropriations	Fiscal policy	Outputs	Public policy
Authorization	Health policy	Policy environment	Rule making
Bargaining	Impacts	Policy instruments	Stakeholders
Collaboration	Organization policy	Public health prevention	Strategic information
Cooperation	Outcomes	policies	

Policy is like a play in many acts, which unfolds inevitably once the curtain is raised. To declare then that the performance will not take place is an absurdity. The play will go on, either by means of the actors or by means of the spectators who mount the stage.

Klemens von Metternich, 1880

Health Policy and Public Policy

Health policy is public (governmental) policy that affects health and health care in national, state, and local arenas. It covers a broad range, including economic, housing, environmental, budgetary, and health services policy. Typically, the public, politicians, press, and professionals see health policy to include mainly those that finance and organize the delivery of personal health services; more than 90% of total U.S. national health expenditures—about $1 trillion a year—is devoted to supporting such services. However, much more than health services policy affects people's health (Lasker, 1997; Vincenzino, 1997).

Manner of living, wages, the condition of industry and commerce, public administration, years of abundance and those of famine—everything that contributes to affluence and civilization—produce great variations in death rate. Affluence and wealth . . . is in truth the most important of all hygienic factors, namely that which best assures the very preservation of life.

Rene Villerme, mid-19th century

Like all **public policy,** health policy is a guide to government action to alter what would otherwise occur, seeking more desirable or acceptable prospects. It points the way and enables effective action to coherent activity by public and private institutional systems. It is a decision about amounts and allocations (or distribution) of resources in organizations and governments.

The overall amount (i.e., the budget of governments or institutions) is a statement of commitment to a certain area of social or community or organizational relevance or concern, like health services or education. The distribution of that amount within the budget is a statement of the true priorities of the decision makers regardless of their statements about goals or mission. Together, the total amount and its allocation are called **fiscal policy.**

Goals and Policies

Goals, by themselves, are not policies. Although policies have goals, they are much more than that. For example, the goals of *Healthy People 2000* were not a policy because they had no instruments or resources specifically allocated to carry them out, other than having national health agencies monitor national progress toward the goals. The document did not carry the force

of law, which derives from one of the three constitutional sources of policy: Congress (legislation), the Executive branch (the president's executive orders, which remain in force throughout his or her term of office and apply only to the Executive branch), or independent regulatory agencies, created by Congress, having a specific jurisdiction, such as the U.S. Food and Drug Administration and the Environmental Protection Agency. None of these institutions is absolute; all are subject to constitutional checks and balances. The job of the courts is to interpret, not create, policy; however, in doing so, they inevitably influence policy, as do myriad organizations and groups in and outside government.

None of these three types of policy bodies at the national level, nor their counterparts in states and localities, is required to follow statements about national goals. Goals are useful as a framework and a source for policy ideas but are not in themselves sufficient for effective policy. They must first be fully formulated and adopted in legislation, executive order, or regulation, which are accompanied by the broad methods (or legal instruments discussed in the following) and authorized funds to carry them out. Otherwise, they remain at a voluntary level of action, dependent on the willingness of relevant groups to invest their own resources to follow them.

For example, by the late 1990s, states had adopted only some of the *Healthy People* goals and were either unwilling or unable to track more than 40% of them, quite apart from authorizing funds to achieve them. In some states this monitoring capacity actually declined as a result of funding cutbacks. In addition, monies allocated to use the data often did not have high priority: Just 6 in 10 states included some environmental health objectives in their public health planning and fewer than 10 states provided air-quality data, taking more than 2 years to distribute it; fewer than half the states provided childhood poverty data and took more than 4 years to give it to local health departments; and fewer than 25 states collected data on injuries (Krieger, Chen, & Ebel, 1997; NACCHO, 1998; Public Health Foundation, 1998).

The clearest and most accurate sign or indicator to determine whether actual policy change has occurred in any governmental body or other organization—health center, school, home care agency—is a change in the size and/or allocation of its resources: money, the authority and responsibilities vested in certain positions (e.g., staff nurses), and other resources. When organizations, as a result of policy changes, conduct their services differently, as staff do things differently, consumers can also behave differently: Patterns change. **Organization policy** is that of a single organization or a type of organization (e.g., public schools), either public (e.g., health department) or private (e.g., churches or child care centers or corporations), and it is closely tied to governmental policy changes.

Purpose of Public Policy

So the purpose of policy making is to shape the direction and pace of change in a preferred direction by modifying current patterns of action. It is not to change the behavior of every individual, each of whom is free to follow a policy or not, perhaps with possible personal consequences, such as refusing a vaccine or driving faster than the speed limit at the risk of injury or fine.

Rather, the aim of policy making is to change the decisions of organizations about their use of resources. This, in turn, changes the activities of managers and staff, clients, and customers from former patterns toward new patterns in governmental agencies, nonprofit organizations, and commercial organizations, whether construction firms, restaurants, regulatory agencies, schools, or clinics. A school board policy requiring the availability of healthy foods in cafeterias will change the types of foods that schools buy, the menus and methods of preparation by kitchen staff, and the pattern of foods that students and teachers will eat, thereby promoting health.

Choosing Policies

To address any health problem, there are always several choices (including doing nothing). We know, for example, that about 900,000 mostly low-income children in the United States have health-damaging blood levels of lead, mainly from exposure to lead-based paint in old houses and environmental contamination. The problem is five times worse in African American children, even when they are not living in old housing and are not in the lowest income bracket, indicating discrimination in the choice of neighborhoods available to some African American

families (GAO, 1998; Krieger et al., 1997). Here are the policy choices:

- *Health care systems can conduct outreach, screening, and treatment.*
- *Community coalitions can form to conduct outreach, screening, and treatment.*
- *State Medicaid agencies can require Medicaid contractors to provide and report on these services for their enrollees.*

These policy changes—with their goals, means, and accompanying shift in budget and program resources—would result in secondary prevention, that is, finding and treating the health problem after it exists, whether or not overt symptoms are evident. This is basically an individual and clinical perspective.

To adopt a public health, population-oriented, primary preventive policy approach—to prevent the problem before it begins—additional choices are possible:

- *Require lead paint removal and environmental code enforcement after providing information to landlords, polluting organizations, tenants, and homeowners.*
- *Develop safe, affordable housing.*
- *Provide for safe and effective schools and schooling, including job training and jobs development.*
- *Work for procommunity/antidiscrimination changes.*

STRATEGIES FOR PREVENTION AND HEALTH PROMOTION BASICALLY AIM AT EITHER (1) CHANGING INDIVIDUALS' BEHAVIOR OR PHYSICAL CONDITION THROUGH INFORMATION/EDUCATION OR CLINICAL MEANS (OR CHANGING INDIVIDUAL PRACTITIONERS) OR (2) CHANGING THE DECISIONS OF ORGANIZATIONS ABOUT THEIR USE OF RESOURCES THROUGH POLICY EFFORTS. THIS, IN TURN, CHANGES THE ACTIVITIES OF MANAGERS AND STAFF, CLIENTS AND CUSTOMERS IN POLICY AND SERVICE ORGANIZATIONS IN THE PUBLIC AND PRIVATE SECTORS.

Intervention Strategy	Focus
Individual-directed, information-mediated change	• Homes and communities (e.g., computers, TV campaigns, health fairs) • Organization settings (e.g., counseling; computers; small-group training of patients, clients, customers, health care practitioners, librarians, teachers, clergy)
Organization-directed	• Policy bodies: – Congress, legislatures – Independent regulatory agencies – Government Administration (e.g., executive orders, rule making) • Specific organizations: – Government organizations (e.g., health departments, housing, schools) – Nongovernment organizations (e.g., managed care organizations, community health centers, companies, retailers)

We all declare for liberty; but in using the same word, we do not all mean the same thing. With some the word liberty may mean for each man to do as he pleases with himself, and the product of his labor; while with others the same may mean for some men to do as they please with other men, and the product of other men's labor. Here are two, not only different, but incompatible things, called by the same name—liberty.

Abraham Lincoln

All this effort would require entry by health proponents into the complex and long-term processes that result in organizational and public policy change. Policy does not just happen. It is determined by organized groups in and outside government and therefore can be observed, analyzed, and understood well enough to promote health-supporting development. Policy-making processes shape policy content as groups that are affected by them (stakeholders) attempt to influence policy development to favor their own needs and priorities.

The results often have indirect or direct impact on population health. Indirect effects include access to the conditions for healthful living, such as housing, jobs, information and education, health care, protective environments, tax equity, and civil rights (Milio, 1997). The coalition of environmental health organizations, for example, worked to influence the Congress in the 1970s to pass historic laws protecting air, water, and habitats. The laws have been effective in directly improving the health of millions of Americans and indirectly affecting health by preserving the viability of agricultural land needed for sustaining food and nutrition for future generations.

There is nothing more difficult to plan, more doubtful to success, nor more dangerous to manage than the creation of a new system.

Machiavelli, *The Prince*, 1512

History of Health Policy in the United States

Historically, the United States has enacted broader health policies than those in recent years. During much of the 1990s, health policy had been viewed narrowly, focusing on health services delivery and the economics of it, while weakening environmental health, healthful living conditions, and primary public health prevention legislation (Center for the Future of Children, 1997; DHHS, 1995).

Some of the major steps in health policy since the start of the nation include the first national health service and national health insurance program set up before the end of the 18th century. This was, and in modified form continues to be, a system of government health care paid by private employer insurance for

the U.S. Merchant Marine. A larger and fully tax-supported national health service is the one provided to Congress and the president, the only fully socialized medical system in the United States today. These are national governmental health care systems that are available to everyone in special groups. Most advanced countries have national systems available to their entire population, including immigrants.

The master of every ship of the United States arriving from a foreign port . . . shall pay . . . twenty cents per month for every seaman employed . . . to provide for . . . the sick or disabled seamen in [government] hospitals . . . now established in the several ports.

The U.S. Fifth Congress, July 16, 1798

Constitutional provisions in our national and state governments to protect the health, safety, and welfare of people authorize, but do not require, governments to use legal tools to realize these purposes. For example, if health were part the Bill of Rights, governments would be legally required, would be liable, to protect health.

Other national health policies include the Pure Food and Drug Act (1906); Social Security Act and its income support for the poor, blind, disabled, and elders and health services for mothers and children (1935); and the first environmental law, the Water Pollution Control Act of 1948. The Economic Opportunity Act was to develop poor communities and end poverty (1964); the National School Lunch and Child Nutrition Amendments included the Women, Infants, and Children's Supplemental Food Program (WIC) (1972) (Weissert & Weissert, 1996). Also see Box 9-1 for a list of federal health legislation that has been passed.

RESEARCH BRIEF

Louis, B., & Lewis, M. (1997). Increasing car seat use for toddlers from inner-city families. American Journal of Public Health 87(6):1044–1045.

Effective and simple public health policies can prevent injury. Illustrating the effectiveness of relatively low-cost incentives, health departments that gave low-income urban families toddler car seats to randomly selected groups of parents (one group with and one without additional education by a safety expert), there was a dramatic increase in the use of the equipment, which continued a year later, regardless of the education component.

BOX 9-1 SELECTED MILESTONES IN FEDERAL HEALTH LEGISLATION

Pure Food and Drug Act, 1906

Maternity and Infancy Act, 1921

Social Security Act, 1935

Nurse Training Act, 1941

Public Health Services Act, 1944

Hospital Survey and Construction Act (Hill-Burton), 1946

Water Pollution Control Act, 1948

National Health Survey Act, 1956

Grants-in-Aid to Schools of Public Health Act, 1958

Federal Employee Health Benefits Act, 1959

Health Service for Agricultural Migratory Workers Act, 1962

Mental Retardation Facilities and Community Mental Health Centers Construction Act, 1963

Health Professions Educational Assistance Act, 1963

Economic Opportunity Act, 1964

Appalachian Redevelopment Act, 1965

Older Americans Act, 1965

Federal Cigarette Labeling and Advertising Act, 1965

Economic Opportunity Act Amendments (neighborhood health centers), 1966

Highway Safety Act, 1966

Child Nutrition Act, 1966

Comprehensive Health Planning Act, 1966

Federal Coal Mine Health and Safety Act, 1969

National Environmental Policy Act, 1969

Comprehensive Drug Abuse Prevention and Control Act, 1970

Occupation Health and Safety Act, 1970

National School Lunch and Child Nutrition Amendments (WIC), 1972

Consumer Product Safety Act, 1972

Health Maintenance Organization Act, 1973

Toxic Substances Control Act, 1976

Rural Health Clinics Act, 1977

Omnibus Health Act (Medicaid expansions), 1986

Americans with Disabilities Act, 1990

Year 2000 Health Objectives Planning Act, 1990

Preventive Health Amendments Act, 1992

RESEARCH BRIEF

General Accounting Office. (1992). Early interventions: federal investments like WIC can produce savings. *Washington, DC: U.S. Congress.*

Prevention of prenatal and newborn health problems was successful through the Women, Infants and Children Supplemental Food Program (WIC) for at-risk and low-income women. The $3 to $4 saved in health care costs were invested in the program for each public dollar. A related voucher program increased fresh fruit and vegetable intake for the vast majority of participants.

Present Need for Public Health Policy

Although overall U.S. death rates are declining, continuing gaps in health between disadvantaged and other populations are increasing in many respects. In addition, disability from chronic illness is widespread (Cutler & Sheiner, 1999). Health inequalities in morbidity, mortality, and disability are strongly related to poverty and income inequality. Gaps in health between low- and high-income groups can be expected to increase further as wealth inequalities continue to grow; this asset gap is now largest since the 1920s (Kaplan, 1996; Montgomery, Kiely, & Pappas, 1996; Wolff, 1996).

Widening health gaps are not accounted for by biomedical and behavioral risk factors alone. Rather, they are affected by a complex web of linked living standards as experienced in jobs and workplaces, homes, and communities. In turn, these are related to how supportive public policies are in these sectors (Link & Phelan, 1995). Virtually all measures of health and illness are worse among poor people compared with their better-off counterparts, regardless of ethnicity, gender, or age. Because of the breadth of the determinants of health, much has been written about the need for broad social and economic policies to promote health (Krieger, 1994).

Evidence shows that public health–oriented public policies make a difference. For example, Social Security retirement income has been the single most important policy to reduce poverty in the United States, especially among elders, thereby contributing to healthful living standards for millions of people. In recent years, a special tax credit for full-time working parents who earn poverty level wages has been the most important policy to prevent several million children from living in poverty (National Center for Children in Poverty, 1998).

Despite this, the tax credit was not enough to prevent an overall increase in child poverty since the 1980s because of low-wage jobs and national and state policies that cut back resources available to poor families. Economic penalties are placed on poor mothers under welfare reform laws; for example, if they are unable or unwilling to adhere to rules that are not required of other mothers, they are penalized. Requirements for mothers receiving welfare include the following:

- *Getting children's immunizations—in 17 states*
- *Making other pediatric visits—in 7 states*
- *Obtaining family planning information and/or services—in 5 states*
- *Having no more children—in 23 states*
- *Naming the child's father—in 21 states*
- *Stopping child school absenteeism—in 17 states*

Gotta feed the kids,
never see the kids
Gotta feed the kids,
never see the kids

(Graffitti rap, Chapel Hill, NC, 1998)

Public Health and Public Policy

Public health is a governmental (public) responsibility embodied in federal and state agencies, including the national Centers for Disease Control and Prevention, the Environmental Protection Agency, and state and local health departments. They are, in principal, accountable for the health of all the people, extending beyond the health of particular individuals, as is done in personal health services.

Public health policy involves promoting and protecting health, preventing disease, and preserving life through policies that ensure the determinants of health for all segments of the population (Rose, 1985, 1990). When it is effective, it makes healthy choices equitably available to all groups—about where to live, work, learn, obtain needed services and information, and participate in public life in safe, supportive, and sustainable environments.

In the words of the Institute of Medicine (1998):

[The mission of public health is] . . . fulfilling society's interest in assuring conditions in which people can be healthy . . . to generate organized community efforts to address the public interest in health by applying scientific and technical knowledge to prevent disease and promote health. . . . [It] is addressed by private organizations, but the governmental public health agency has a unique function: to see to it that vital elements are in place and that the mission is adequately addressed.

This echoes the historic understanding of the public health mission:

Public health is the science and art of preventing disease, prolonging life and promoting health . . . through organizing community efforts for sanitation of the environment, the control of communicable infections, the education of the individual in personal hygiene, the organization of medical and nursing services for the early diagnosis and preventive treatment of disease, and the development of the social machinery to ensure everyone a standard of living adequate for the maintenance of health, so organizing these benefits as to enable every citizen to realize his [*sic*] birthright of health and longevity (Winslow, 1920).

This public health enterprise, undertaken by government agencies and other allied groups, ranging from local health centers to national voluntary organizations like the American Health Association and public interest groups such as Handgun Control, Inc., requires organizational and organized action directed toward all types of entities, including policy bodies and the public. This historic approach of public health during most of its first century resulted in major successes, such as regulating sewage, water supplies, and housing conditions, decades before vaccines were discovered (Institute of Medicine, 1988).

As illustrated earlier, policies change organizations (and their resource allocations and programs) so that populations can have more healthful choices about where and how to live. Examples of **public health prevention policies** include tobacco control, for example, higher cigarette taxes of 50 cents in Oregon reduced smoking by 18% in youth; communicable disease prevention, as when public and private provider subsidies produced large increases in immunization rates, especially among poor and minority children; abortion funding for poor women, which resulted in an increase in early prenatal care, fewer teen births, and lower rates of low-birth-weight babies and infant death; and containment of alcohol liberalization, handgun controls, and motorcycle safety measures, all of which achieved widespread long-term health benefits (Center for Health Economics Research, 1993; Kraus, Peek, & Williams, 1995; National Cancer Institute, 1991; Office of Disease Prevention, 1993; Pentz, Brannon, Charlin, Barrett, MacKinnon, & Flay, 1989; Teh-Wei, Hai-Yen, & Keeler, 1995).

Policy Development

What follows is first an overview of the policy-making process and then an illustration of each step in policy development.

Policy Environment

Policy development does not occur on a clean slate. It always has precursors in earlier eras, deriving from experience with similar issues and societal assumptions about the role of government (Laumann & Knoke, 1987). Most importantly, it is formed in a context of near-term limiting and enabling circumstances. These are important to be aware of to plan effective strategies to influence policy making.

The following figure depicts the connections between policy making and health (Milio, 1976, 1986, 2000). It shows how policy works through organizational action, which shapes community environments, living patterns, and ultimately population health. This occurs in a **policy environment** or context that encompasses circumstances affecting whether and how policy making proceeds regardless of the type of policy in question. Important factors include the demographic and epidemiological nature of the population (e.g., an aging population, high rates of smok-

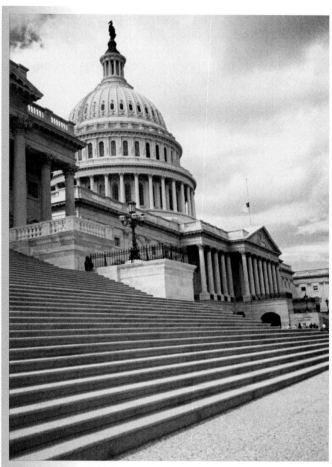

U.S. Senate Building.

ing), the economy and technology (e.g., inflation, unemployment, extent of information technology), the socioeconomic and ethnic makeup of communities (e.g., poverty and discrimination), the distribution of resources (e.g., homelessness and extremes in wealth), political party agendas, organizational hierarchies (e.g., dominant interest groups), and even sudden disasters—national emergencies from weather or war, for example, can stop all policy development as policy makers attend to (costly) emergency measures. All these things must be considered to some extent by policy participants. All this information is available and needed for effective policy work by interested nurses and is best done on an organized and thought-out basis.

Yet, however rapidly changing and uncertain the environment is, the policy making time clock is ticking, and the electoral calendar moves on. To be effective, policy action and influence must be exerted in time and be timely, in tune with the environment.

The media are in a unique position among organizations; they are not only channels for information. They also create and shape issues (Minkler, 1997), such as portraying teen violence as a parental problem rather than a public health problem that can be effectively addressed by, among other things, elimination of handguns. For example, Japan, where handguns are banned, had two handgun killings in 1997, whereas the United States had 9,400 and Canada had 100. Media portrayals set up ideas and expectations about the kinds of solutions needed to address problems (Dorfman, Woodruff, Chavez, & Wallack, 1997; Frost, Frank, & Maibach, 1997).

DEPICTION OF THE CONNECTIONS BETWEEN POLICY MAKING AND HEALTH. IT SHOWS HOW POLICY WORKS THROUGH ORGANIZATIONAL ACTION, WHICH SHAPES COMMUNITY ENVIRONMENTS, AFFECTING LIVING PATTERNS AND ULTIMATELY POPULATION HEALTH. THE CHANGES THAT RESULT IN ALL THESE AREAS THEN FEED BACK *(DOTTED LINES)* AND ARE TAKEN INTO ACCOUNT IN ONGOING EFFORTS TO FIND ACCEPTABLE AND EFFECTIVE WAYS TO DEAL WITH PUBLIC HEALTH PROBLEMS.

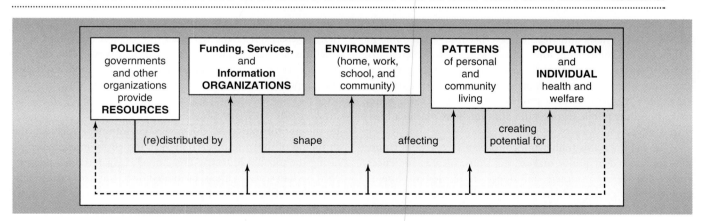

THE MEDIA ARE NOT ONLY CHANNELS FOR INFORMATION; THEY ALSO CREATE AND SHAPE ISSUES. MEDIA PORTRAYALS SET UP IDEAS AND EXPECTATIONS ABOUT THE KINDS OF SOLUTIONS NEEDED TO ADDRESS PROBLEMS. OTHER PLAYERS IN THE POLICY ARENA ACTIVELY ATTEMPT TO USE THE MEDIA FOR STRATEGIC PURPOSES. ORGANIZED INTEREST GROUPS IN AND OUTSIDE GOVERNMENT CAN INDIRECTLY REACH POLICY MAKERS AND THE PUBLIC THROUGH THE MASS MEDIA. THE "PUBLIC" IS ACTUALLY SEVERAL POPULATIONS THAT ARE AFFECTED BY POLICY MAKERS' DECISIONS, E.G., AUDIENCES, VOTERS, TAXPAYERS, CONSUMERS, AND DONORS TO PARTIES AND INTEREST GROUPS.

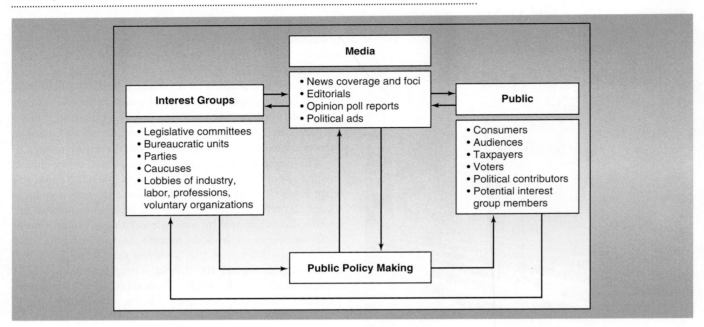

Will Gresham's law operate in the broadcasting and political worlds, wherein the bad inevitably drives out the good? Will the politician's desire for reelection—and the broadcaster's desire for ratings—cause both to flatter every public whim and prejudice—to seek the lowest common denominator of appeal—to put public opinion at all times ahead of the public interest?

John F. Kennedy, 1960

As global, profit-making corporations, the media seek to attract audiences and advertisers and often shape programming with this aim—news and weather have become "infotainment" rather than accurate and sometimes unpleasant depictions of complex realities (Cappela & Jamieson, 1996). Other players in the policy arena actively attempt to use the media for strategic purposes. Organized interest groups can indirectly reach policy makers and the public through the mass media (Columbia Institute, 1995).

The public in this framework consists of several populations that are affected by policy makers' decisions, such as audiences, voters, taxpayers, consumers, and donors to parties and interest groups. Policy choices set the parameters for health in the form of access to services, products, processes, prices, taxes, and information. Most of the public are not active members of interest

groups. Through these complex processes, then, ongoing outcomes of policy making create the conditions for the health of populations, especially of disadvantaged subgroups.

Public Health Advocacy and Action
The Case of Tobacco Control: A Success Story

Antismoking policy development in the United States in the 1980s and 1990s offers many lessons in public health policy making. (Heiser & Begay, 1997; Jacobson, Wasserman, & Raube, 1993) Some states passed strong laws (e.g., widespread bans on smoking in public places and private work sites and large penalties), whereas others enacted weaker legislation (e.g., narrow restrictions, smokers' rights clauses, minor penalties). More effective policy making involved legislative leadership, strong coalitions, and support by top public health and government officials.

Environmental Context

In the antitobacco case, the policy environment includes the shrinking of the U.S. tobacco market and costly legal challenges facing the tobacco industry. This impelled cigarette manufacturers to seek overseas markets, facilitated by liberal world trade policies. This offshore shift of production and marketing is weakening the once-firm alliance between cigarette manufacturers and tobacco farmers. The number of growers is shrinking, resulting in a less influential political constituency. These and other aspects of the environment make the industry increasingly vulnerable and present an opening for action by health advocates.

Successful policy-making activity must propose policies that fit the circumstances of the day. Thus, health proponents must be aware of current and changing circumstances (Rochefort & Cobb, 1993).

Policy Shape and Setting

Health-supporting policy action also depends on how the policy issue is framed. For example, the tobacco-control issue could be framed by public health advocates in the health field and allied groups as an environmental and child health issue, or by proto-bacco groups as one of smokers' right to take personal risks in using a legal product. The policy outcome could be very different depending on who defines the problem.

The policy arena, that is, where the action takes place—in local, state, or national jurisdictions, is another consideration. Successful tobacco control advocates used the open arenas of legislatures or the public referendum process and sought news media coverage to amplify their position in contrast to the highly paid, behind-the-scenes activities and television advertising of the industry.

For example, for some antitobacco campaigns, local ordinances rather than state law may be more readily enacted, despite the narrower public health impact at local levels. Sufficient community-level action can be a learning laboratory and can create political conditions for stronger statewide policies. Nurses, as members of health or other groups, can be part of any or all such efforts and may be able to get their own agency to publicly support tobacco control legislation.

Policy Goals, Tools, and Resources

The design of an effective policy includes goals and the means to reach the goals. The goals should eventually be specified as measurable objectives to help focus activity and to track progress. The strength (or absence) of means are important for the forward movement and implementation of a policy. Without measurable objectives, progress toward health goals becomes contentious; without sound means and resources, little program action is likely to occur.

Policy effectiveness depends on adequate financing and the choice of legislative tools used. The means to achieve policy goals involve a limited list of **policy instruments** (legal tools) that are used by most governments. These tools include economic incentives (e.g., tax breaks, subsidies) to businesses, governments, and taxpayers; mandates and regulation; and the development and provision of information, education, training, and services. Others are modeling, that is, becoming exemplars (e.g., not allowing smoking in government facilities) and market power or market management (Kessler, Witt, Barnett, Zeller, Natanblut, Wilkenfield, Lorraine, Thompson, & Schultz, 1996).

Tools, such as market management or market power, are used when, for example, governments buy public employee health insurance plans that cover only smoking cessation programs and collaborate with public health organizations in passing clean indoor air laws (Sofaer et al., 1997) When governments buy only recycled paper or healthy foods, the market price is often lowered for everyone.

Some of these tools are clearly more powerful than others in their potential effectiveness; for example, economic and regulatory instruments are more effective than information and education to ensure healthful changes in organizations and individuals: Smoking rates drop faster with a high tobacco tax and no-public-smoking rules than by information on health effects alone, especially among teens. However, the more effective means are the most difficult to get adopted because they have a higher political cost—that is, it is riskier to offend commercial groups by using economic instruments such as a tobacco tax increase than to simply inform the public of health risks through warning labels on cigarettes. This was clear in tobacco-control cases.

The Players as Stakeholders

Policies develop through the actions of the players and their relationships as they try to shape decisions about who pays and who gets what of the determinants of health. The players are the organized groups—**stakeholders**—whose interests are affected by current and prospective policies. They include political parties, the media, bureaucracies, voluntary and commercial organizations, public interest groups, and professional associations.

A policy issue draws the attention of public and private stakeholders who view a policy change as important to their interests. These stakeholders perceive themselves to be importantly affected by a change in policy. Their interests are the things they need to survive, including finances—from grants, contracts, dues, or sales—facilities, staff, authority, control, status, legitimacy, and image. In turn, these resources affect a group's bargaining power. Stakeholders include elected or other officials, legislative committees, parties, and bureaus; commercial, scientific, and medical groups; and voluntary nonprofit organizations, including public interest groups (DiMaggio & Anheier, 1990; Feldstein, 1996; Jasanoff, 1993; Warner, 1991).

The underlying interest of political and other governmental leaders is to retain power and authority. For businesses, increased profits and market share are important. Professionals want to acquire grants, higher career status, and control over their practice. Voluntary organizations must please their boards and donors; advocacy groups must satisfy their supporters (e.g., governing board, funders, membership), both existing and potential. Each group attempts to engage in political activity in ways that will shape any particular policy to favor its own interests (Benjamin, Perfetto, & Greene, 1995).

In the case of tobacco policy, the involvement of major health-related organizations illustrates these self-regarding calculations and accounts for their sometimes sideline roles in the policy-making process. Neither state health departments, public health associations, medical societies, nor large voluntary organizations did more than lend their names to the antitobacco coalitions that were fighting for strong tobacco-control legislation. Each of these mainline organizations had competing priorities, such as fears of budget cuts from opposition lawmakers, lack of staff, or legal restrictions in some local health departments. The medical societies chose to use their political capital to seek better clinical payment rates, and the large nonprofit groups feared a backlash from some donors. These organizational decisions about public health advocacy were strategic choices made by each organization that took into account the tradeoffs in resources for the group and its purposes. In one state, "risk protection" was required before a state chapter of the American Cancer Society publicly agreed to lead a tobacco taxation campaign (Heiser & Begay, 1997).

••••••••••••••••••••••••••••••

Each of us must choose whether to live our lives narrowly, selfishly and complacently or to act with courage and faith. We are not governed by fate or mysterious forces of history. It is the sum of our choices that will determine the kind of America and the kind of world in which we live.
    Madeleine Albright, U.S. Secretary of State
George Washington University Commencement, May 21, 2000

••••••••••••••••••••••••••••••

Player Connections

Alliances are more reliable and long-lasting when they are based on written agreements, agreed rules, or intense resource exchange. **Collaboration** differs from **cooperation** by the exchange of tangible assets (e.g., part-time staff or use of printing equipment in the former, as contrasted with the verbal support and good will in cooperative ties). For example, the California Nurses Association gained much more public support than it could have otherwise in a recent referendum on state health care reform by allying with labor unions and others and sharing staff.

To influence decision makers in the face of competition by well-financed, large-scale commercial interests, as in tobacco control, requires strategic planning, continuous management, and joint efforts, despite the difficulties of coalition formation (Heiser & Begay, 1997; Kegler, 1995).

••••••••••••••••••••••••••••••

The most impressive aspect of the law of the jungle is not ruthless competition and destruction, but rather interdependence and coexistence.
    Rene Dubos, *Man, Medicine, and Environment,* 1968

••••••••••••••••••••••••••••••

Information for Action

Information is basic to policy making. It is used to monitor, analyze, evaluate, report, and critique an issue. It becomes action-oriented when used for informing, educating, persuading, mediating, activating, or mobilizing others to act (Lindblom & Cohen, 1979).

The strategic problem for proponents of health-supporting policy is to use selected types of information to convince target groups that their policy position is economically feasible (to its supporters and users), politically acceptable (to the more powerful groups affected by it), socially approved within the milieu in which it is to operate, and administratively and technologically possible (Milio, 2000). To do this, a wide range of **strategic information** is needed—about the policy environment and the problem, as well as the purposes, interests, and tactics of the players, and the degree of support among constituencies, as gauged by polls and endorsements. This must be sought and developed by policy proponents, thus the need for an organized and sustained effort.

Studies can stimulate new ways to conceive policy problems and solutions and occasionally are directly incorporated into policy development, such as the knowledge that high tobacco taxes are the most effective way of reducing smoking in young people (Beyer & Trice, 1982; Brewer & De Leon, 1983; Brint, 1990; Webber, 1987). But science information is useful mainly when it is part of strategic information (Brown, 1997).

This wide array of information goes far beyond typical health status data and includes a variety of material available from all the social-political-economic disciplines and policy think tanks (institutes and centers). This information is often available on the Internet. The task then is to effectively use that information to influence policy making in language, formats, and amounts that are suited to each target group, including the press and the public.

••••••••••••••••••••••••••••••

Scientists are in general remarkably objective in reporting what they observe and measure; but the selection of their objects of study is profoundly influenced by the social environment in which they work and by the spirit of the age.
    Rene Dubos, *Man, Medicine, and Environment,* 1968

••••••••••••••••••••••••••••••

Policy Development Strategies

The most effective policy-making activities, demanding the most resources, include lobbying legislative or bureaucratic policy makers directly or through their constituents; ensuring the election or appointment of supportive political leaders; and engaging in litigation. Less effective means, often used by small groups, involve developing publicity through the media and organizing demonstrations, conferences, and public education programs (Walker, 1991). All such activities have long been on the agendas of national, state, and to some extent, local nursing organizations. Their voice is always stronger when allied with other groups, as occurred in the national health care reform effort of 1993–1994.

Bargaining

The central strategic activity to influence policies and move them through the phases of policy making is negotiation. This always involves compromise. Effective **bargaining** requires taking account of the interests of governments and other target groups and being willing to trade away some less valued interests to gain

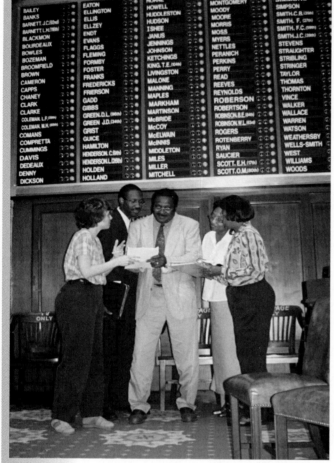

Nurses and other lobbying groups work to influence health policy through legislation.

others in the foreseeable future, such as agreeing to a 50-cent tobacco tax instead of a dollar so that political support for adoption is easier to gain.

Public distortion of facts by opponents requires prompt public rebuttal by health proponents, as when tobacco proponents maintained that there is no scientific proof of the health effects of smoking (Heiser, 1997). By contrast, to obtain political and organizational endorsement, proponents must demonstrate the political support needed by elected and bureaucratic officials, for example, by providing credible evidence of support from opinion polls and sponsorship by local groups and agencies. This involves developing information on group support for proponents' policy preferences or offering a promise by coalition members of future support for the policy maker's agenda.

Information Through the Mass Media

People's information is obtained directly from experience or through various interpersonal and technological channels. All such conduits select and shape the information they pass on according to their own priorities (Minkler, 1997). The new media mix includes TV networks, cable, satellite, VCRs, videos, CD-ROMs, as well as the print press, all merging on the Internet. This rapidly sprouting web has implications for both policy development activities and health information/education. The interplay between information and media in policy-making arenas is another important facet that can be used to promote public policy for health.

Mass media affect policy making in many ways. They convey information and messages that influence perspectives and actions, depending on when, how, and in what social and information contexts they are received. These messages flow not only through news channels, but also through programming, videos, talk shows, and advertising, by both expression and exclusion (Cappella & Jamieson, 1996).

The media set the agenda, telling people what issues are important to think and talk about. They also frame or focus certain aspects of issues, helping shape how people and policy makers understand them. This is especially true for the formation of short-term public opinion about public health issues, such as environmental pollution and poverty. When media attention wanes, public opinion drops (McCombs & Shaw, 1993).

As commercial organizations, the media depend on advertisers. They select content and target audiences to attract viewers for their sponsors. Larger audiences mean higher prices for advertising and higher revenues. Prime time news media focus on mainstream issues, as when they took 4 years before covering HIV/AIDS, believing that it was a minor problem of interest only to homosexuals and intravenous drug users but not to a large general audience (Edgar, Fitzpatrick, & Freimuth, 1992).

The media in this way reinforce mainstream views and set expectations about reality, including racial and gender stereotypes. For example, heavy viewers—those who watch more television (or videos) daily than others (more than 4 hours)—are more likely to overestimate the prevalence of divorce, illegitimacy, abortions, STD, and crime (Edgar, 1992). This perception clearly has implications for the kinds of demands the public makes (or indicates in polls) for public policy action.

• •

Where is the wisdom we have lost in knowledge?
Where is the knowledge we have lost in information?

T.S. Eliot, *The Rock*

• •

Health Information

Education and information are part of the package of useful policy tools and are longer lasting when accompanied by other stronger tools. Public health media campaigns are usually limited to attempts to influence *individual* behavior rather than to mold public opinion about policy issues. As costly as they are, however, these health education campaigns by themselves mainly affect knowledge or awareness, and only occasionally do they influence short-term behavior (Office of Technology Assessment, 1991; Rice & Atkin, 1994).

Several conditions must be in place to translate awareness of a health problem into changes in personal behavior, especially for the long term. The message must have the following characteristics:

- *Targeted and attractive for specific groups*
- *Conveyed over multiple channels long enough for "saturation" of the target groups*
- *Integrated with local interpersonal communication*
- *Supported by environmental, organizational, and policy changes to ensure long-term behavior change, such as increases in tobacco tax and laws against smoking in public places*

Mass Media and the Case of Health Care Reform: A Cautionary Tale

Policy issues raised in the mass media can have adverse public health policy effects. Issues are often defined too simply, solutions too superficially, and legitimacy conferred on only selected groups because of what "sells" to audiences and advertisers. This in itself suggests the need for greater attention to the electronic world by the public health community as the experience of health care reform portrays.

A series of studies covering the introduction and failure of the Clinton health care plan from September 1993 to July 1994 demonstrate how mass media are woven into policy-making processes and show how important it is to take the media into account in health policy development (Braun, 1995; Cappella & Jamieson, 1994, 1996; Columbia Institute, 1995). Findings show the following:

- *Although the media devoted much time and space to health care reform, two thirds of all coverage was on political strategy, not content, the pros and cons of each major proposal, or areas of agreement.*
- *Coverage was not balanced, giving more attention to the president's plan while others, like the single payer bill, had no real public airing. Without public knowledge about options, there was little likelihood of support for a compromise bill.*
- *The tone of the stories was that politicians act out of self-interest rather than commitment to the public good. Randomized viewer studies showed that strategy-based (versus issue-centered) stories created perceptions of policy makers to be posturing, deceptive, self-interested, and unconcerned with the welfare of citizens. Groups viewing only issue-centered stories were less cynical.*
- *News coverage of political advertising, by emphasizing the attack and controversial nature of the ads, dramatically enlarged the ads' audiences and collectively aired an additional 15 minutes of free nationwide television exposure. The ads' sponsors then had incentive to prepare ever more extreme ads, costing more than $50 million. These ads suc-*

ceeded in reaching legislators on key committees and their media market viewers.

- *The public was found to be generally poorly informed (e.g., 75% did not know the administration was the main proponent of an employer mandate requiring them to offer insurance to workers [favored by a majority of people]); fewer than half had heard of the single payer bill; and they wanted much more information and blamed the media for not providing it.*
- *Reporting of opinion polls was uncritical; it magnified the impact of uninformed opinion, creating "news" out of uninformed opinion (failing to qualify the results according to people's depth of knowledge) and influencing the actions of leading congresspersons and perhaps also of undecided viewers.*
- *The advertising, polls, and media coverage of them ultimately had an impact on Congress' rejection of major reform. Leaders said that public opinion was as influential in the debate as the administration itself, that interest group advertising (mainly by health insurance and business interests) was persuasive, that the public was not well informed on the issues, and that the media had done a poor job of helping people understand the issues. Despite this, leading members and staff of the House and Senate said their main sources of information about public opinion were the polls (mainly reported in the media), the trade group lobbies, and the media (Columbia Institute, 1996).*

Implementation

Congressional adoption of policies, known as **authorization**, only begins the next major phase of policy making: making a policy effective in the real world. Policies require **appropriations**, approved amounts of funds to be available over 1 year or more, to put the policy into effect. To complete the task, the monies must be allocated (i.e., distributed by an authorized agency, usually a government bureau, in the form of grants, contracts, or other payments).

Prior to this dispersal of funds, the policy must be interpreted in specific terms, known as **rule making**; opened to public comment for 30 to 60 days (always published in the weekly *Federal Register*); finalized; and then publicized to eligible recipient organizations, such as state agencies and community groups, including health centers and home health agencies. These potential users must apply for the funds by proposing what programs they will conduct with the monies. The awardees then implement programs, such as community or employee tobacco education, smoking cessation programs, or payment for the costs of setting up smoke-free workplaces.

Finally, the authorized agencies must monitor and enforce the rules that guide application of the policy and eventually feed this information back into the final phase of policy making: evaluation. At any point in implementation, groups may contest the

RESEARCH BRIEF

Goggin, M. (1987). Policy design and the politics of implementation. Knoxville, TN: University of Tennessee Press.

A successful policy requires effective policy execution. A detailed study of the implementation of the Medicaid program in California showed that certain features of the law, and possibly of any social welfare policy, promote successful implementation:

- The absence of a welfare stigma
- Consistency with existing beliefs and practices
- The absence of a threat to existing power arrangements
- A law that is clear
- Benefits that are perceived as health rather than welfare
- A law with inclusive eligibility requirements
- A single source of funds
- A law that includes provision for providers' rewards and/or penalties

The two indicators basic of success or failure for such programs are (1) the percentage of those eligible for services who actually receive them during a given period and (2) in the particular case of child health programs, the referral rate and the resultant changes in health status among members of the screened population.

process in court if they think it is proceeding too slowly or too quickly, fairly or unfairly.

* * *

In this and like communities, public sentiment is everything. With public sentiment, nothing can fail; without it, nothing can succeed.

Abraham Lincoln, 1858

* * *

The complexity of policy implementation processes, as federal and state funds are dispersed into programs across communities, means that there are infinite ways for opponents to change the pace and direction of a policy. For example, in both Massachusetts and California, where tobacco-control coalitions succeeded in passing tobacco tax referenda against strong industry lobbying, the actual use of the millions of new dollars became another source of contention. Rather than the intended use of the funds for antitobacco programs, policy makers attempted to use the monies for other, sometimes political, purposes such as financing hospital care in response to the hospital lobby (Begay & Glantz, 1997).

In one state, the antitobacco coalition sued the state in court and won, requiring authorization and allocation of the funds for the stated smoking prevention and control purposes. In the other

state, the coalition negotiated a compromise on the use of the funds, but this resulted in a decline in appropriations for tobacco control over the next several years. Analysis of such experiences can help inform future public health policy efforts.

* * *

Where there is no vision, the people perish.

Proverbs, *The Bible*

* * *

Evaluation

Research findings (i.e., science-based information)—in contrast to opinions and impressions—are often not available or are not used much by policy makers. Studies must be translated first into the organizational or political priorities of decision makers. The timing of findings makes a difference too in whether they are used, for instance, before interest groups have developed around a policy issue, or much later, when social acceptance improves (Brint, 1990).

Most evaluation consists of the impressions of user groups and program reports on **outputs,** such as numbers of people served, numbers reached by public education campaigns, new smoke-free workplaces, the decline of cigarette sales, and financial reports. Policy **impacts** include the indirect effects of a policy, sometimes unintended or unwanted. For example, when strict local no smoking laws were passed in California, bars and restaurants did not lose business as the tobacco industry had warned (Biener & Siegel, 1997). Or, when the WIC program was implemented, it created new local food retail jobs and improved local economies (National Farmers Association, 1996).

Outcomes, that is, changes in people's health, are more rare, sometimes because they can be seen only after a longer period of time than policy makers are willing to wait (such as a decline in lung cancer); sometimes because health indicators often require additional spending for evaluation research, monies that are often not available. Evaluation is thus both a political and scientific process, and its results determine whether a policy will be revised, cut back, or repealed (Zervigon-Hakes, 1995).

* * *

People don't eat in the long run—they eat everyday.

Harry L. Hopkins, 1933

* * *

The lesson is clear: Policy making for health continues long after adoption and requires that proponents continue to monitor the processes and to take action to preserve the health effectiveness of any specific policy. This kind of "watchdog" activity is often done by public interest groups, such as the Coalition on Smoking and Health; Handgun Control, Inc.; and the Center for Public Environmental Oversight in Washington, D.C. Governments also have monitoring agencies, including the General Accounting Office of the Congress to oversee legislative results, and the Office of Management and Budget, which oversees the effectiveness of most Executive branch agencies for the White House.

Nurses in Communities, Public Health Policy, and Primary Prevention

The tobacco coalitions all succeeded to some degree in obtaining public resources to prevent the biggest single cause of death in populations. Yet the largest risk factor threatening health and life, one not often discussed or addressed by the health sector, is the gross and growing disparity in social and economic determinants of health between the nation's disadvantaged communities and others (Krieger, 1994; Link & Phelan, 1995). It is possible for the public health community to initiate and work with coalitions in local, state, and national strategies to improve the conditions in which people live. This includes nurses, who see the effects of poverty and discrimination based on ethnicity, age, and other factors. They have been and, to fulfill their professional duty, should continue to be involved at every level, either through their practice settings, nurse groups, or by joining allied groups. To promote primary prevention policies, it is necessary to involve a wide range of organizations that affect living conditions and to focus on priority public, institutional, or corporate policies.

Among the many community conditions needed to support population health are housing, child welfare, and access to comprehensive primary care (Federman, Garner, Short, Cutter, Kiely, Levine, McGough, & McMillen, 1996; Montgomery, Kiely, & Pappas, 1996). With the kind of policy groundwork outlined previously, these issues can become priorities for health departments and other parts of the health community. Policy proposals can then be developed to ensure more healthful living conditions. A few examples follow.

Neighborhoods with high rates of unemployment, poverty, high rent, and crowded housing are associated with a high incidence of low-birth-weight babies. Adverse living situations predispose people to toxicities, infections, contagions, accidents, strains on eyesight, unhealthy food storage and use, and mental health stresses from lack of privacy, the ability to work at home, and recreation opportunities (Martin, 1977; Roberts, 1997).

The availability and adequacy of housing significantly affect health through the following strategies:

- *The siting of housing—whether near polluting industries or near transportation routes to access job opportunities, education and health services, and stores*
- *Local environmental controls and maintenance, such as water supply and waste management*
- *Housing structure involving overcrowding, ventilation, lighting, and temperature control*

Thus, legitimate public health activities include improved zoning, environmental regulations, and building codes; the development of adequate low-rent housing and transportation systems; support for tenant organizations and citizen grievance processes; and open hearings on housing issues. Although not under the direct control of health departments, community health organizations and agencies can form coalitions and raise these issues by defining the type and scope of health issues and the policy changes needed to support health, as well as through work with local and state organizations in housing, economic development, land use, and the environment to advise on and advocate changes (Hardy & Satterthwaite, 1987; Slater & Carlton, 1985).

On a smaller scale, taking account of commercial establishments' interest in safe and expanding markets, local governments and community organizations, led by health departments or other health advocacy groups can use their market power to influence the proportion of healthy foods of the local food supply as well as limit access to tobacco (CDC, 1999). For instance, they could require that cafeterias in their facilities contain low-fat, high-fiber food choices. This would encourage food suppliers to change their supplier contracts to retain their own contracts, with ripple effects on food processing corporations. The new options in these facilities would result in changes in eating habits for clients and employees while at the same time suggesting an exemplary "healthful practices" model for the public and the media. Nurses, for example, could propose healthy food options in their work site cafeterias in state and local health agencies, schools, hospitals, health maintenance organizations, prisons, military installations, vending machines, and so on.

With rising child impoverishment and lack of health care, child health and welfare are at risk. Specific, focused policies proposed by nurses allied with child welfare proponents (Deal & Shiono, 1998) that are worthy of advocacy efforts include the following:

- *An increase in cigarette excise taxes*
- *Strong indoor and outdoor air quality control and enforcement*
- *An above-poverty-level minimum wage*
- *Antihandgun measures*
- *Repair of the welfare and prevention safety net*
- *Comprehensive maternal-child care and child day care*

Advocacy Tools of the Future

Electronic networks are a potential new set of tools to extend the sources of support and strengthen the advocacy efforts for the public's health. Community-based groups, allied with the public health community, can raise and amplify issues, propose solutions, establish their legitimacy, and join larger coalitions. These advocacy networks, linked to national and local watchdog groups, can supply timely and accurate information not only about problems, but also about program and policy solutions and sources of technical assistance. Perhaps most importantly, these electronic links can coordinate joint advocacy efforts and alert local groups to timely actions in local, state, and national policy arenas, including coordination of e-mail, fax, phone, or letter-writing campaigns to pass, for example, a tobacco tax or ban handguns.

•••••••••••••••••••••••••••••

The new technologies hold promise for a greatly enhanced system that can meet the changing needs of an information-based society. At the same time, these technologies will generate a number of significant social problems. How these technologies evolve, as well as who will be affected positively or negatively, will depend on decisions now being made in both the public and private sectors . . . making choices about universal service is essentially making choices about equality of opportunity. Defining universal service is, in effect, making choices about the nature of society itself.

Office of Technology Assessment, U.S. Congress,
Critical Connections, 1990

•••••••••••••••••••••••••••••

The case has been made in public health forums and studies for electronic networks to link public health and other community organizations to improve community health, especially in poor areas. This collaboration could support core public health functions through strengthening services delivery, education, environmental health, community mobilization, and policy advocacy (Lasker, Humphreys, & Braithwaite, 1995; Milio, 1995, 1996). Nurses are in a position to point out the importance of electronic linkages with community organizations to develop and reinforce health and community partnerships.

RESEARCH BRIEF

Birckmayer, J., & Hemenway, D. (1999). Minimum-age drinking laws and youth suicide, 1970-1990. American Journal of Public Health, 89*(4), 1365–1368.*

The reported study examined the association between the minimum legal drinking age (MLDA) and suicide rates among young persons 18 to 20 years old. There is a well-documented relationship between suicide and alcohol consumption, with between one third and two thirds of all adolescent suicide victims having a measurable blood alcohol content. A cross-sectional design was used drawing data from the 48 contiguous states. Between 1970 and 1990, the suicide rate of 18 to 20 year olds living in states with an MLDA of 18 years was 8% higher than the suicide rate among 18- to 20-year-old youths in states with a higher MLDA of 21 years. The authors conclude that lowering the drinking age from 21 to 18 years in all states would lead to an annual increase of approximately 125 suicides among this age group. Lower legal drinking ages also correlate with increased motor-vehicle fatalities (of which some may indeed be suicidal in nature), which may further support maintaining the higher MLDA as public health policy.

CONCLUSION

An understanding of health policy making and the mission of public health is not merely an academic exercise. It is essential to the health professions and their institutions because practitioners in nursing and other health fields are in applied, not academic, disciplines. Our privileges are derived from our social responsibility to ensure the health of all populations. An awareness of the health effects of a wide range of public and corporate policies, the public reporting of these effects, and efforts to promote health-supporting policies fall within the scope of the health community and in our activities with other groups. Participation in any aspect of these complex and ongoing policy processes can engage us as individuals. But more often, policy work requires action through organizations to sustain the necessary long-term effort to ensure effective health-supporting policies.

The leaders in nursing of the past 150 years were great women with broad vision and understanding of the issues of their day. They engaged political, social, and health care groups in improving both the health care system and the health of all the people, especially the rural and urban poor, immigrants, and other vulnerable groups. The new century is at least as challenging and requires comparable vision, commitment, and energy.

FYI

The word *health* does not appear anywhere in the U.S. Constitution or Bill of Rights.

CRITICAL THINKING ACTIVITIES

1. Select a community health problem, such as teen suicide or school violence. Chapter author, Dr. Milio, contends that "Media are not only channels (p. 205) for information . . . they also create and shape issues." Think of several examples from the media in which your selected health issue is presented as a problem or a solution. Who is blamed for the problem? Are there solutions identified? Who are the stakeholders in any policy making related to your identified problem?

2. If you could design a Web site that influences health policy for children with learning disabilities, what components would you include? How would you include the public in its development and implementation? Who would you include as experts on your Web site? Decide how you could link your Web site to other advocacy groups. Design an evaluation of this project as related to effectiveness in policy making.

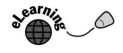

Explore Community Health Nursing on the web! To learn more about the topics in this chapter, use the passcode provided to access your exclusive web site: http://communitynursing.jbpub.com
If you do not have a passcode, you can obtain one at this site.

REFERENCES

Begay, M., & Glantz, S. (1997). Question 1 tobacco education expenditures in Massachusetts, USA. *Tobacco Control, 6,* 213–218.

Benjamin, K., Perfetto, E., & Greene, R. (1995). Public policy and the application of outcomes assessments: Paradigms vs politics. *Medical Care, 33*(4), AS299–AS306, supple.

Beyer, J., & Trice, H. (1982). The utilization process: A conceptual framework and synthesis of empirical findings. *Administrative Science Quarterly, 24*(4), 591–622.

Biener, L., & Siegel, M. (1997). Behavior intentions of the public after bans on smoking in restaurants and bars. *American Journal of Public Health, 87*(12), 2042–2044.

Braun, S. (1995, March/April). Media coverage of health care reform. A content analysis. *Columbia Journalism Review,* Supplement, 1–8.

Brewer, G., & De Leon, P. (1983). *Foundations of policy analysis.* Homewood, IL: Dorsey.

Brint, S. (1990). Rethinking the policy influence of experts: From general characterizations to analysis of variation. *Sociological Forum, 5*(3), 361–385.

Brown, L. (1997). Knowledge and power: Health services research as a political resource. In Ginzburg, E. (Ed.), *Health services research: Key to health policy* (pp. 20–45). Cambridge, MA: Harvard University Press.

Cappela, F., & Jamieson, K. (1996). *Media in the middle: Coverage of the health care reform debate of 1994.* Research report. Philadelphia: Annenberg School of Mass Communications.

Cappella, J., & Jamieson, K. (1994). *Public cynicism and news coverage in campaigns and policy debates: 3 field experiments.* Research report. Philadelphia: Annenberg School for Communication.

Center for Health Economics Research. (1993). *Access to health care: Indicators for policy.* Princeton, NJ: Robert Wood Johnson Foundation.

Center for the Future of Children. (1997, Spring). Welfare to work. *The Future of Children, 7,* 1.

Centers for Disease Control and Prevention (CDC). (1999). *Physical activity and good nutrition.* Atlanta: Author.

Columbia Institute. (1995, May). *What shapes lawmakers' views? A survey of members of Congress and key staff on health care reform.* Washington, DC: Author.

Cutler, D., & Sheiner, L. (1999). *Demographics and medical care spending: standard and non-standard effects.* Unpublished paper. Harvard School of Public Health.

Deal, L., & Shiono, P. (1998). Medicaid managed care and children: An overview. *The Future of Children, 8*(2), 93–104.

Department of Health and Human Services (DHHS). (1995, April). *Personal Responsibility Act of 1995. Preliminary impacts.* Washington, DC: Author.

DiMaggio, P., & Anheier, H. (1990). The sociology of non-profit organizations and sectors. *Annual Review of Sociology, 16,* 137–159.

Dorfman, L., Woodruff, K., Chavez, V., & Wallack, L. (1997). Youth and violence on local TV news in California. *American Journal of Public Health, 87*(8), 1311–1316.

Edgar, T., Fitzpatrick, M. A., & Freimuth, V. S. (1992). *AIDS: A Communication Perspective.* Hillsdale, NJ: Lawrence Erlbaum.

Federman, M., Garner, T. I., Short, K., Cutter, W. N. IV, Kiely, J., Levine, D., McGough, D., & McMillen, M. (1996, May). What does it mean to be poor in America? *Monthly Labor Review, 119*(5), 3–17.

Feldstein, P. J. (1996). *The politics of health legislation. An economic perspective.* Chico, CA: Health Administration Press.

Frost, K., Frank, E., & Maibach, E. (1997). Relative risk in the news media: a quantification of misrepresentation. *American Journal of Public Health, 87*(5), 842–845.

General Accounting Office (GAO). (1998). *Blood lead levels in children.* Washington, DC: U.S. Congress.

Hardy, J., & Satterthwaite, D. (1987). Housing and health. *Cities, 4,* 221–235.

Heiser, P., & Begay, M. (1997).Campaign to raise the tobacco tax in Massachusetts. *American Journal of Public Health, 87,* 968–973.

Institute of Medicine. (1988). *The future of public health.* Washington, DC: National Academy Press.

Jacobson, P., Wasserman, J., & Raube, K. (1993). Politics of antismoking legislation. *Journal of Health Policy, Policy & Law, 18,* 787–818.

Jasanoff, S. (1993). *The fifth branch: Science advisors as policymakers.* Cambridge, MA: Harvard University Press.

Kaplan, H. (1996). Inequality in income and mortality in the US: analysis of mortality and potential pathways. *British Medical Journal, 312,* 999–1003.

Kegler, M. (1995). *Community coalitions for tobacco control: Factors influencing implementation.* Chapel Hill: The University of North Carolina School of Public Health. PhD dissertation.

Kessler, D. A., Witt, A. M., Barnett, P. S., Zeller, M. R., Natanblut, S. L., Wilkenfield, J. P., Lorraine, C. C., Thompson, L. J., & Schultz, N. B. (1996). The Food and Drug Administration's regulation of tobacco products. *New England Journal of Medicine, 335*(13), 988–994.

Kraus, J., Peek, A., & Williams, S. (1995). Compliance with the 1992 California motorcycle helmet use law. *American Journal of Public Health, 85*(3), 96–99.

Krieger, N. (1993). Racism, sexism, and social class: implications for studies of health, disease, and well-being. *American Journal of Preventive Medicine, 9*(S2), 82–122.

Krieger, N. (1994). Epidemiology and the web of causation. *Social Science & Medicine, 39,* 887–903.

Krieger, N., Chen, J. T., & Ebel, G. (1997). Can we monitor socioeconomic inequalities in health? A survey of US health departments' data collection and reporting practices. *Public Health Report, 112*(6), 481–491.

Lasker, R. (1997). *Medicine and public health.* New York: New York Academy of Medicine.

Lasker, R., Humphreys, B., & Braithwaite, W. (1995, July). *Making a powerful connection: The health of the public and the national information infrastructure. Report of the Public Health Data Policy Coordinating Committee, U. S. Public Health Service.* Washington, DC: U.S. Government Printing Office.

Laumann, E., & Knoke, D. (1987). *The organizational state.* Madison, WI: University of Wisconsin Press.

Lindblom, C., & Cohen, D. (1979). *Useable knowledge.* New Haven, CT: Yale University Press.

Link, B., & Phelan, J. (1995). Social conditions as fundamental causes of disease. *Journal of Health & Social Behavior, 2*(Special Issue), 80–94.

Martin, A. (1977). *Health aspects of human settlements: A review.* Geneva: World Health Organization.

McCombs, M., & Shaw, D. (1993). The evolution of agenda-setting research. *Journal of Communication, 43*(2), 58–67.

Milio, N. (1976, March). A framework for prevention: Changing health damaging to health generating life patterns. *American Journal of Public Health, 66,* 35–38.

Milio, N. (1986). *Promoting health through public policy.* Ottawa: Canadian Public Health Association.

Milio, N. (1995). Beyond informatics: Community electronic networks and public health. *Journal of Public Health Management & Practice, 2*(3), 6–11.

Milio, N. (1996). *Engines of Empowerment: Using information technology to create healthy communities and challenge public policy.* Chico, CA: Health Administration Press.

Milio, N. (1997). Case studies in nutrition policymaking: How process shapes product. In Garza, B. (Ed.), *Beyond nutrition information.* Ithaca, NY: Cornell University Press.

Milio, N. (2000). Evaluating health promotion policies: tracking a moving target. In Rootman, I., Goodstadt, M., Potvin, L., & Springett, J. (Eds.), *Evaluation of health promotion: Principles and perspectives.* Copenhagen: World Health Organization.

Minkler, M. (Ed.). (1997). *Community organizing and community building for health.* New Brunswick, NJ: Rutgers University Press.

Montgomery, L., Kiely, J., & Pappas, G. (1996). Effects of poverty, race, and family structure of us children's health: Data from the National Health Interview Survey, 1978 through 1980 and 1989 through 1991. *American Journal of Public Health, 86*(10), 1401–1405.

National Association of City and Council Health Officials (NACCHO). (1998). *NACCHO study of electronic communication capacity of local health departments.* Washington, DC: NACCHO.

National Cancer Institute. (1991). *Strategies to control tobacco use in the United States: A blueprint for public health action in the 1990s.* Smoking and Tobacco Control Monographs 1. Bethesda, MD: Author.

National Center for Children in Poverty. (1998). *Young children in poverty.* New York: Columbia University School of Public Health.

National Farmers Association Market Nutrition Programs. (1996). *Program impact report.* Washington, DC: Author.

Office of Disease Prevention & Health Promotion. (1993). *For a healthy nation: Returns on investment in public health.* Washington, DC: U.S. Public Health Service.

Office of Technology Assessment. (1991). *Adolescent Health* (vol. 1). Washington, DC: U.S. Congress.

Pentz, M., Brannon, B. R., Charlin, V. R., Barrett, E. J., MacKinnon, D. P., & Flay, B. P. (1989). The power of policy: The relationship of smoking policy to adolescent smoking. *American Journal of Public Health, 79*(7), 857–862.

Public Health Foundation. (1998). *Measuring health objectives and indicators: 1997 state and local capacity survey.* Washington, DC: Author.

Rice, R., & Atkin, C. (1994). Principles of successful public communication campaigns. In J. Bryant & D. Zillman (Eds.), *Media effects: Advances in theory and research* (pp. 365–387). Hillsdale, NJ: Lawrence Erlbaum.

Roberts, E. (1997). Neighborhood social environments and the distribution of low birth weights in Chicago. *American Journal of Public Health, 87,* 597–603.

Rochefort, D., & Cobb, R. (1993). Problem definition, agenda access, and policy choice. *Policy Studies Journal, 21*(1), 56–71.

Rose, G. (1985). Sick individual and sick populations. *International Journal of Epidemiology, 14,* 32–38.

Rose, G. (1990). Future of disease prevention: British perspectives on the US Preventive Services Task For Guidelines. *Journal of General Internal Medicine, 5,* S128–S132.

Slater, C., & Carlton, B. (1985). Behavior, lifestyle, and socioeconomic variables as determinants of health status: Implications for health policy development. *American Journal of Preventive Medicine, 1,* 25–33.

Sofaer, S., et al. (1997). *Models for assessing the impact of changes in health care delivery and financing on community tuberculosis prevention and control programs.* Research report. Washington, DC: George Washington University Center for Health Outcomes Improvement Research.

Teh-Wei, H., Hai-Yen, S., & Keeler, T. (1995). Reducing cigarette consumption in California: Tobacco taxes vs an anti-smoking media campaign. *American Journal of Public Health, 85,* 1218–1222.

Vincenzino, J. (1997, July–September). Trends in medical care costs. *Statistical Bulletin,* 1–7.

Walker, J. (1991). *Mobilizing interest groups in America: Patrons, professions, and social movements.* Ann Arbor: University of Michigan Press.

Warner, K. (1991). Tobacco industry scientific advisors: Serving society or selling cigarettes? *American Journal of Public Health, 81*(7), 839–842.

Webber, D. J. (1987). Factors influencing legislators' use of policy information and implications for promoting greater use. *Policy Studies Review, 6*(4), 64–80.

Weissert, C., & Weissert, W. (1996). *Governing health. The politics of health policy.* Baltimore: Johns Hopkins University Press.

Winslow, C. E. A. (1920, March). The untilled field of public health. *Modern Medicine,* 183.

Wolff, E. (1995). *Top heavy: A study of the increasing inequality of wealth in America.* New York: Twentieth Century Fund.

Zervigon-Hakes, A. (1995). Translating research into public programs and policies. *The Future of Children, 5*(3), 175–191.

Chapter 10

Transcultural Nursing Care in the Community

Madeleine Leininger

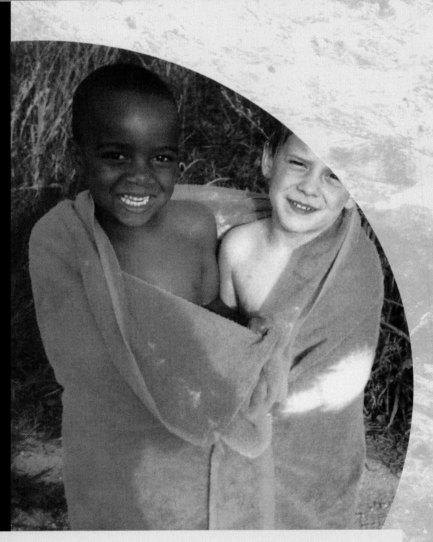

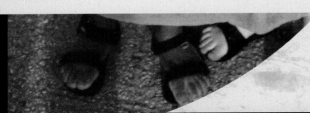

Establishing new knowledge and practice pathways is always a major challenge, for new pathways may create fears and uncertainty; yet these pathways are essential to meet community, societal, and global human needs.

CHAPTER FOCUS

Community-Based Transcultural Nursing

Scope of Transcultural Nursing

Transcultural Nursing Principles

Transcultural Concepts

Leininger's Theory of Cultural Care Diversity and Universality
- Development of the Theory
- Goal of the Theory
- Assumptions and Premises
- The Sunrise Model: A Visual Guide for the Theory
- Application of the Theory and Model

Healthy People 2010: Objectives Related to Cultural Diversity and Care

QUESTIONS TO CONSIDER

After reading this chapter, answer the following questions:

1. What is community-based transcultural nursing?
2. What are the principles of transcultural nursing?
3. What is culturally competent nursing care?
4. What is the theory of culture care diversity and universality?
5. How did the theory of culture care diversity and universality develop?
6. How is the sunrise model used as a guide for the Theory?
7. How are the theory of culture care diversity and university and the sunrise model used to provide culturally competent nursing care?

KEY TERMS

Caring	Cultural ignorance	Cultural variation	Etic view
Cultural backlash	Cultural imposition	Culturally competent care	Generic care
Cultural barriers	Cultural lifeways	Culture	Immigrants
Cultural bias	Cultural pain	Culture bound	Professional care nursing
Cultural blindness	Cultural shock	Emic view	Refugees
Cultural clashes	Cultural values	Ethnocentrism	Stereotyping

> **BOX 10-1 DEFINITIONS**
>
> **Culture:** *The learned, shared, and transmitted values, beliefs, norms, and lifeways of a particular group that guide their thinking, decisions, and actions in patterned ways.*
>
> **Cultural values:** *The powerful directive forces that give order and meaning to people's thinking, decisions, and actions.*
>
> **Cultural variations:** *The subtle or obvious variables among and between cultures that make them unique with respect to traditional or nontraditional ways of living.*
>
> **Cultural lifeways:** *The patterned ways of living of a particular individual or group.*
>
> **Cultural imposition:** *The tendency to impose one's beliefs, values, and lifeways on another individual or culture, due largely to ignorance about a culture.*
>
> **Ethnocentrism:** *The belief that one's own ways of living or doing are the best, most preferred, or superior to others.*
>
> **Stereotyping:** *The undesirable tendency to prejudge and fix cultures into rigid and biased ways, due largely to ethnocentrism and racism.*
>
> **Cultural blindness:** *The inability to recognize one's own values and lifeways or those of another culture, making culture invisible.*
>
> **Cultural clashes:** *Major conflicts in valuing and understanding differences between cultures and variability among or within cultures.*
>
> **Caring:** *Actions and activities directed toward assisting, supporting, or enabling another individual or group with evident or anticipated needs to improve a human condition or lifeway, or to face death.*
>
> **Nursing:** *A learned humanistic and scientific profession and discipline focused on human caring.*
>
> **Emic view:** *The insider's or local perspective about cultures, families, lifeways, and health care.*
>
> **Etic view:** *The outsider's or external perspective about cultures, families, lifeways, and health care.*
>
> **Culturally competent care:** *The deliberate and creative use of transcultural nursing knowledge and skills to assist or facilitate individuals or groups to maintain their well-being, recover from illness, or face a disability or death.*

Nursing is entering a new century and a new millennium with many new challenges, pathways, and opportunities. In the 21st century, nurses are and will continue to be involved with many immigrants, refugees, travelers, and strangers coming from many different places. Many nurses will live in a variety of different geographic locations and practice nursing in largely unfamiliar cultural and physical environments.

Today's nurses are learning to use transcultural nursing concepts, principles, and practices to help them function in different community and cultural contexts. Transcultural nursing has become one of the most essential and relevant pathways to meet the holistic and special needs of people from diverse and similar cultures. As nurses learn about the essential and desired care expectations of different cultures, they become aware of different ways to provide culturally competent and sensitive care. Transcultural nursing focuses on holistic and comprehensive ways to know and serve people of diverse cultures throughout the life cycle. The primary goals of *transcultural community-based nursing* are to help people of different and similar cultures maintain their health, prevent illnesses or disabilities, and die in culturally congruent and meaningful ways. Nurses in the 21st century are challenged to adopt this perspective to become better professional nurses.

Transcultural community-based nursing is essential for the future of the profession. Along with transcultural definitions, concepts, principles, and practices, a brief history of transcultural nursing is provided in this chapter to describe the growth of the field over the past five decades. The theory of culture care diversity and universality is presented in the final section of this chapter as an important perspective from which transcultural nursing can be studied and assessed. The theory can be used to assist nurses in providing culturally safe, effective, and congruent nursing care. Throughout this chapter, some reflective questions and examples are posed to help nurses reflect on the cultural beliefs, values, and lifeways that exist in different cultures. Because transcultural community-based nursing is the goal for the 21st century, some definitions of common terms related to the field of transcultural nursing are outlined in Box 10-1 (Leininger, 1995).

Community–Based Transcultural Nursing

Community-based transcultural nursing refers to the creative use of transcultural nursing concepts, principles, research, knowledge, and practices that focus on large overall designated communities or geographic contexts in order to provide culturally competent nursing care. Most communities have many diverse cultural groups with some similar, and some sharply diverse cultural lifeways.

The following fundamentals describe the nature, characteristics, and power of cultures, the concept of care, and transcultural nursing:

OBJECTIVES RELATED TO CULTURAL DIVERSITY AND CARE

Access to Quality Health Services

1.8 In the health professions, allied and associated health professions, and the nursing field, increase the proportion of all degrees awarded to members of underrepresented racial and ethnic groups.

Educational and Community-Based Programs

7.11 Increase the proportion of local health departments that have established culturally appropriate and linguistically competent community health-promotion and disease-prevention programs for racial and ethnic minority populations.

Mental Health and Mental Disorders

18.13 Increase the number of states, territories, and the District of Columbia with an operational mental health plan that addresses cultural competence.

Source: DHHS, 2000.

- *Cultures tend to be stable, yet they may change over time in beliefs, values, and cultural lifeways.*

- *Cultural patterns, norms (rules), and practices are powerful influences on human care and transcultural community practices.*

- *Cultural values and beliefs vary between and within cultures and must be understood to develop culturally congruent care practices.*

- *Cultural rituals, symbols, taboos, and practices are important to identify and understand for transcultural nursing.*

- *Transcultural nursing necessitates studying the total lifeways of people, including influences on care related to religion or spirituality, politics, economics, technologies, kinship ties, environment, and specific values and practices.*

- *Different modes of communication; use of space, land, and property; and use of home remedies are all part of discovering the transcultural nursing care needs of people.*

- *Different cultures in a community have different lifeways that must be considered by nurses.*

- *Different cultures have different caregivers to heal, cure, or assist their people.*

- *Cultural gatekeepers are found in communities that protect, defend, and uphold cultural values, beliefs, and desired lifeways.*

- *Transcultural care needs and expectations vary among communities and cannot be assumed to be alike.*

- *In every community there will be subcultures that are slightly different from the dominant culture and that require attention from the transcultural nurse. These subcultures include the* homeless, homosexuals, gangs, drug users, individuals from poor and affluent social classes, and others.

Although nurses have traditionally worked with people in communities, providing care in homes, schools, industrial plants, clinics, and other settings, the major missing dimension has been knowledge of the cultural background of the people and how to care for them in that context. Cultural factors have been taken for granted and often viewed as less important or not even recognized. With the advent of transcultural nursing came a new and heightened awareness of the importance of culturally based knowledge. It was soon discovered that nurses prepared in transcultural community-based nursing were able to demonstrate the use of their knowledge with specific cultures in beneficial ways. Nurses working in community or public health settings found that transcultural nursing concepts were important in providing effective care. In fact, nurses who were skilled and prepared to work with different cultures realized the unique care needs of clients and became confident with individuals, groups, families, and communities (Leininger, 1981, 1988, 1995).

Beginning in the mid-1970s, community health nurses encountered many new cultural strangers, such as immigrants, refugees, migrant workers, and others, and felt helpless in knowing how to understand and help them. That is when many community nurses began to enroll in transcultural nursing courses. The need for transcultural community-based care was clearly evident as they told their stories about trying to help cultural strangers who seemed to suddenly come into their nursing world. Some nurses did not understand why some

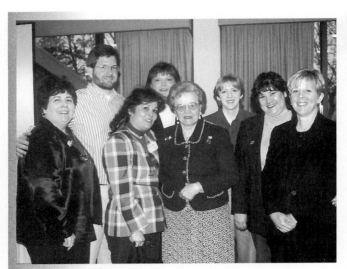

Dr. Madeleine Leininger (center), founder of Transcultural Nursing, with members of the Mississippi Chapter of the Transcultural Nursing Society.

Jemmott, L. S., Maula, E. C., & Bush, E. (1999). Hearing our voices: Assessing HIV prevention among Asian and Pacific islander women. Journal of Transcultural Nursing, 10(2), 102–111.

RESEARCH BRIEF

This study was conducted to (1) assess the impact of human immunodeficiency virus/acquired immunodeficiency syndrome (HIV/AIDS) on the Asian/Pacific Islander community and to determine whether there were any changes in behavior as a result of HIV; and (2) identify their perception of risk, HIV risk behaviors, factors contributing to risk behaviors, barriers to HIV prevention, and kinds of prevention programs that would benefit their communities. The study also described culturally competent considerations when designing HIV prevention strategies for Asian/Pacific Islander women. The participants consisted of 22 low-income women, ages 18 to 44, living in a large metropolitan area. They were divided into two different groups and interviewed using focus interviewing techniques guided by the health belief model. The women had numerous concerns about their risk for HIV related to their cultural taboo about discussing sexual issues and condom use. Both groups stated that HIV prevention efforts must be tailored to the cultural needs of Asian/Pacific Islander women if they were to be successful.

clients wanted their children to be cared for before any adults. Other nurses were baffled by strange terms such as *susto, evil eye,* and *sacred objects to heal* because they were terms specific to cultures and to cultural health care practices. Without understanding these terms and many others, nurses were disadvantaged. Many nurses said they had to almost completely relearn nursing from a different perspective, because many of their previous nursing ideas did not fit with specific cultures. Indeed, some nursing knowledge learned earlier was counter to what some cultures needed (Leininger, 1988, 1995). Some nurses became excited and developed creative ways to use transcultural nursing knowledge and skills in community contexts. They became firm advocates of transcultural nursing and encouraged other nurses to learn how to care for diverse cultures in their community experiences.

What are some of the major reasons why transcultural nursing is important today? What transcultural nursing concepts, principles, and research findings can help community nurses? First, any human community has people who are born, live, become ill or maintain health, and die within a community perspective (Leininger, 1981, 1988, 1995). Humans are culturally rooted, acting and making decisions daily that are based on largely unspoken values, beliefs, and cultural community lifeways (Leininger, 1970, 1978). Moreover, most cultures have beliefs about the way they prefer caregivers to care for them. They have ideas that certain decisions and actions can lead to their health and well-being or help them face ill-

nesses, disabilities, and death. Such community beliefs and expectations are extremely important to families and individuals. Although individuals or families may not always be willing to talk openly or directly with the nurses, their expectations still exist.

As a nurse enters the home of an individual or a family, the people remain alert to see whether he or she will be responsive to their cultural beliefs, values, mannerisms, dress, language, and symbols. For example, a community nurse who was knowledgeable about Vietnamese culture allowed a young Vietnamese mother to demonstrate how she cared for her infant's upper respiratory infection. The nurse was readily accepted by the mother, the family, and the community because she understood and respected traditional Vietnamese infant care.

People do not always consciously make known their cultural values, beliefs, and lifeways to others in daily conversations. However, if important cultural practices are violated or neglected, they will often speak out. They often go back to their cultural history to support their actions and beliefs and may say thing like "Well, it has always been this way" or "This is how we have always believed and lived and my grandparents have lived that way too." Sometimes, a nurse may not like to be told how to do things by nonprofessionals and may view the family as uncooperative, resistant, or difficult to work with when they fail to respond to the nurse's expectations. When resistance is met, the nurse should stop, listen, and learn from the people who understand cultural care decisions and actions. There are many examples of why families of specific cultural backgrounds are not willing to yield to an outsider's views. Transcultural nursing gives active and serious attention to the people's views, while the professional's views are secondary.

· ·

It is utterly exhausting being Black in America—physically, mentally, and emotionally. While many minority groups and women feel similar stress, there is no respite or escape from your badge of color.

Marian Wright Edelman
Source: Edelman, M. W. (1992). *The measure of our success. A letter to my children and yours.* Boston: Beacon Press.

· ·

Integrating transcultural knowledge and skills into community nursing is related to the principle that cultures have a right to have their cultural values known, respected, and appropriately used in nursing and related health care services (Leininger, 1970, 1988, 1995). Humans have a right to physical and psychological health care, and their cultural care needs should be treated with equal importance because cultural factors greatly influence how people act, feel, and perceive their environment.

However, the physical and mental needs of clients are generally emphasized more in nursing education and practice than the cultural needs. A person's culture often receives limited attention or is avoided by nurses because they do not understand it. Community nurses who have been oriented to transcultural nursing are alert to cultural care factors and use specific strategies and principles to help those of different cultural backgrounds living in a community. Cultural care needs are emphasized, and physical and emotional needs are met within a cultural perspective (Leininger, 1978, 1996).

Culturally congruent care provides culture-specific care decisions and actions for therapeutic benefits that fit with the cultural needs and expectations of clients. Transcultural nursing knowledge can assist nurses in providing culturally congruent care for individuals and families in different communities. Nurses must remain cognizant of culture-specific care that is compatible with the values and beliefs of individual cultures. This can be accomplished by being attentive to subtle differences and similarities among cultures and recognizing care differences and similarities among clients in various living or working contexts. Maintaining a comparative perspective and not assuming all cultures are alike is important. There often is a tendency to label and lump all members of a particular culture together when considering health care needs. However, there is great variability between and within cultures and among individuals and families, and these differences must be considered when providing culture-specific and culturally congruent care. To assume that all people in a particular culture are the same is stereotyping and leads to negative outcomes. For example, to avoid stereotyping, one should not assume that all Chinese men are stoic and fit clearly into one

CASE STUDY

As a community health nurse you are making home visits twice a week to Mrs. Mendoza, who lives in a rural community. Mrs. Mendoza is an 82-year-old Mexican American woman with a below-the-knee amputation of her left leg related to her diabetes mellitus. She lives with her 50-year-old son and two teenage grandsons. It is difficult to communicate with Mrs. Mendoza or to do any diabetic teaching because you do not speak Spanish and no one in the Mendoza household speaks English. During your first five visits, the neighbor who lives down the road was willing to come to Mrs. Mendoza's house during your visits to serve as your interpreter. However, on your sixth visit, you discover that the neighbor is not at home. *Because you are unable to communicate with Mrs. Mendoza you go to each of her neighbors' houses looking for someone who can speak English but find none of them at home. Frustrated and behind schedule, you return to Mrs. Mendoza's house to learn that her son, who has been at home during all of your visits, is able to speak English fluently.*

1. How do you feel when you learn that Mrs. Mendoza's son can speak English?

2. Why do you think he did not tell you he could speak English earlier?

3. What could you have done to make the situation different?

particular behavior style. Instead, it is recommended that one observe the actual behaviors and subtle impressions that do not place the Chinese man in a rigid position at all times.

Providing culturally based community caring is directly related to the nurse's intent or desire to heal clients, prevent unnecessary illnesses, and support people in achieving their daily living goals and needs. It is impossible to achieve such important goals unless the nurse knows and practices holistic culturally based care. Holistic culturally based care includes assessing the influences of religion, politics, technology, education, kinship (family), and specific cultural values and beliefs within the client's own environment. All these factors can and do influence the client's way of living and responding to nursing care. The theory of culture care diversity and universality provides this holistic, yet specific, care perspective to heal and help people in congruent or meaningful ways. Clients have a right to have these diverse factors influencing their well-being understood and respected by health care providers. For example, if a nurse fails to explore the social and religious concerns of a Mexican American client's family, the client might report that he or she received no nursing care at all.

Health care in the future will become more community focused and will emphasize maintaining health and preventing as well as treating illnesses. As the largest group of health care providers, nurses will be extremely important in providing care to various cultural groups. The ways in which different cultures prevent illnesses and maintain health will be a major focus of community health nursing in the 21st century and beyond. The community will be recognized as the natural and familiar context for all human caring and health services, becoming the dominant mode over hospital care by the year 2010 (Leininger, 1995, 1997b). Hospital services will decrease and will largely focus on treating special diseases, chronic illnesses, and acute emergencies with costly high-tech equipment. Clients from various cultural groups will have more power in regulating health care as they gain cultural strength and visibility.

Providing transcultural community-based and community-focused care helps professional nurses gain satisfaction and rewards from their important nursing contributions to society. As community nurses incorporate transcultural nursing into their work roles, the public will more easily recognize their significant and unique contributions. Traditional community and public health principles blended with transcultural nursing principles will take on new meaning and relevance in growing multicultural communities (DeSantis, 1997; Horn, 1979; Leininger, 1988; Luna, 1998).

Culturally competent care is both a message and a frame for patient care delivery. It is a concept which respects and engages people within the context of individual lifestyles, cultural heritages, and ethnic pride.
Deborah Washington, MSN, RN, Director of Diversity, Patient Care Services, Massachusetts General Hospital, Boston. Source: MGH Patient Care Services. (1997). *Caring Headlines, 3*(21), 4.

SCOPE OF TRANSCULTURAL NURSING CULTURES.

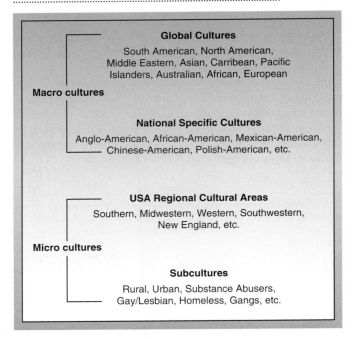

Scope of Transcultural Nursing

There are various types and sizes of community cultures. Some communities are very large (macroculture) and others are considerably smaller (microculture) (see the figure above). Nurses should make an effort to grasp the nature and scope of the communities in which they are working and be aware of the different microculture and macrocultures that exist within a particular environment.

Transcultural Nursing Principles

One of the most important goals of transcultural nursing is to enter the client's world and assist in therapeutic and beneficial ways. Providing culturally congruent care to people in a community first necessitates a careful assessment of the cultural needs of the people. After analyzing the cultural assessment data, the nurse should use transcultural principles, concepts, and research to develop and implement a culturally congruent plan of care. Working with different cultures requires that the nurse have "holding" (prelearned) knowledge about specific cultures. It is important that the nurse be able to carefully blend his or her *etic* (or professional knowledge) with the client's *emic* (or traditional and folk knowledge). These two categories of knowledge sometimes come together, but great discrepancies can exist and need to be resolved for the safety and health of the client. Rather than focus on medical treatments that may not fit the cultural needs of clients and may be useless or even detrimental, transcultural nursing focuses more on the information, beliefs, and practices of those being treated. Clients expect that their traditional beliefs and practices will be respected and that

BOX 10-2 TRANSCULTURAL NURSING PRINCIPLES

1. All human cultures have diverse living, caring, and healing modes that nurses need to study and understand to work effectively with people of different cultures.

2. Care is a basic human need, and it is the essence and dominant focus of the nursing profession.

3. Understanding one's own culture is the first essential expectation to understand other cultures or subcultures.

4. People have the right to have their cultural values known, respected, understood, and used appropriately in nursing and health care services.

5. Transcultural nursing is concerned with the comparative values, beliefs, and practices of specific cultures in order to provide meaningful, safe, and specific health care practices.

6. Nurses use humanistic and scientific cultural care knowledge as they provide care to different cultures. Humanistic care aspects make people remain human, and scientific research findings about cultures and care guide nurses' decisions and actions.

7. Understanding culture care differences and similarities enables the nurse to respect clients and assist them to grow, function, maintain their well-being or health, and prevent illnesses and premature death.

8. Willingness to enter the client's world and become an active and interested participant is essential in maintaining effective nurse-client or nurse-family relationships.

9. Listening, respecting, and being attentive to what clients of different cultures say or do are essential to understanding them and providing meaningful and beneficial nursing services.

10. A nurse's ability to speak the client's cultural language opens the door to understanding what the client is seeking or experiencing.

11. If the client's cultural lifeways, values, and caring expressions do not immediately "make sense," the nurse must continue to make an effort to understand them.

12. In every culture, care, healing, and health practices are greatly influenced by clients' worldviews, environmental context, and social structure features (including the religious or spiritual beliefs, kinship ties, political-legal views, economic aspects, technologies, and specific cultural historical values).

13. Every culture usually has two major types of health care systems: generic (indigenous, traditional, folk) and professional (learned in schools). Nurses need to understand these to provide culturally congruent care.

14. Cultures have their own culturally defined ways to promote and maintain health, face death, and deal with unfavorable sociocultural conditions and crises.

15. Health care practices in Western and non-Western cultures have major differences that need to be understood when planning and providing care to clients.

Source: Leininger, 1995.

appropriate rituals will be used to assist them in recovery or death within their cultural environment. Therefore, when possible, culturally appropriate interventions should be the preferred treatment, which may create a challenge for health care professionals. Understanding general transcultural nursing principles can help nurses bridge the gap between emic and etic points of view (Box 10-2).

Transcultural Concepts

To understand transcultural nursing as used within community nursing contexts, knowledge of several major concepts is essential. Some of these concepts come from anthropology, but others have been developed as basic transcultural nursing concepts. Although a few basic definitions were presented at the beginning of this chapter, there are some that merit further clarification with clinical examples to illustrate them.

Because an important goal of transcultural nursing is to provide culturally competent care, it needs to be considered at the outset. **Culturally competent care** refers to the use of culturally based knowledge in creative, congruent, and meaningful ways to provide beneficial and satisfying health care to diverse cultures. As nurses work with other cultures, they combine their clients' traditional knowledge with their own professional nursing knowledge to provide meaningful, safe, and responsible care. The nursing interventions must fit, or be reasonably tailored to incorporate, cultural values, beliefs, and practices to be effective and acceptable to the people. Nurses should encourage all members of the health care team to consider the cultural values of their clients when making decisions related to their health care.

The concept of cultural values is critical in health care because all cultures want their values and beliefs respected and upheld. **Cultural values** are the powerful directive forces that give order and meaning to why people think, act, and make decisions. For example, the extended family of an African American pregnant woman living in the rural South told the visiting nurse about their culture and what they valued. Several of the women said, "We value our greens, soul food, peas, pork, and special pregnancy foods." These mothers made clear the cultural values that needed to be considered by the nurse for the family's general nutrition and for the mother during pregnancy. The foods were viewed as essential for their health care, so the nurse included as many of these foods as possible in the nutritional plan for the pregnant mother, making modifications only where necessary.

Two concepts that are extremely helpful to nurses are emic and etic views. **Emic view** refers to what the local people or the "insiders" hold as important to know and believe. For example, a Philippine elderly mother and family believe that when the grandmother gets old, she should not live in a nursing home. Instead, they hold the emic view that the sons, daughters, and grandchildren should care for their elders. This emic or local Philippine view is different from Anglo-American families, who often believe that their elders will probably go to a nursing home for care and protection.

Etic view refers to an external or outsider's view of a culture. For example, many Anglo-American nurses believe that when Philippine elders reach about 80 years old, they should consider being placed in a nursing home so that they will not be a burden to other family members. This etic or outsider's view is very different from what the Philippine families value, wanting their elders to be cared for by family members in their homes and not in institutions such as nursing homes. The Philippine emic view and the Anglo-American nurses' etic views are very different and can often be a source of cultural conflicts and stresses.

Generic and professional care are related to emic and etic views. **Generic care** is the folk, naturalistic, or traditional health practices that cultures have known and used over time. In contrast, **professional care** is what is learned from nursing, medicine, and other health care education programs. Generic and professional care practices often have many differences that must be recognized and addressed. For example, several Mexican American families visited by a community health nurse wanted the nurse to know and integrate their generic (folk or naturalistic) care with the professional nursing care. They also wanted the community nurse to acknowledge that Mexican fathers are the ones responsible for major family decisions, such as signing treatment consents for family members. Respecting these important generic or folk family considerations was essential for the nurse to provide culturally congruent care.

Another set of closely related concepts is ethnocentrism and cultural imposition. **Ethnocentrism** refers to the belief that one's own ways are the best, most superior, or preferred ways of acting, believing, or valuing something. An example of this concept is Anglo-American nurses who contend that managed care is the best way to provide health services. Nursing students may also be ethnocentric, believing that faculty lectures are the best way to help students learn about nursing and therefore rejecting other methods of teaching. Ethnocentrism takes a strong position that there is only one "right" way to do things.

Cultural imposition refers to one group of people forcing their cultural beliefs, values, and patterns of behavior on others as a result of ethnocentrism, cultural biases, ignorance, or various other reasons. An example is an Anglo-American nurse who imposes her beliefs that women should be equal partners with their husbands in making health care decisions for the family on a Mexican American mother. This can create conflict within the family, causing difficulty for the woman and possibly leading to the family's total rejection of the nurse's care. Cultural imposition practices are one of the most common nursing care problems encountered with clients from different cultures.

Cultural ignorance refers to insufficient knowledge about a specific culture to provide safe and meaningful care. This chapter includes many examples of cultural ignorance as a major problem in nursing practices. Lack of knowledge often leads to destructive care practices and nontherapeutic outcomes for clients.

Cultural bias refers to a strong position that all decisions must be based on one's own values and beliefs. For example, nurses who firmly value nursing homes at the end of life, with no other alternative plan, can be considered culturally biased. It is a largely one-sided, rigid, and persistent stance. If nurses are not able to recognize and understand their cultural biases, these biases can greatly interfere with clients' choices, interests, and even therapeutic care practices. Both nurses and clients may have biases that should be recognized and discussed so that acceptable compromises can be reached.

Cultural shock refers to a state of being disoriented or unable to respond appropriately to a situation or person because of complete strangeness or unfamiliarity with what was seen or experienced. This concept is often seen between nurses and clients from different cultures. For example, a community nurse entered the home of a very poor Native American family and found there were six children (ages 3 to 10 years) sleeping on the floor with dirty blankets. The nurse also discovered that the children ate only bread and beans each day and that the house was very dirty. The nurse was shocked by the conditions and did not know what to say or do, so she left the home. She reported that she found an "unbelievable home situation" and became helpless and confused. Because of her cultural shock, she was not able to assess the overall health of the children or work with the family to meet their health care needs.

Cultural pain refers to the considerable discomfort, suffering, or unfavorable response experienced by an individual or group belonging to a particular culture when insulting and offensive comments are made by an outsider. Cultural pain is more common than realized among health personnel (Leininger, 1997a). For example, an African American family experienced cultural pain when an Asian American community health nurse showed facial disgust when she saw the family eating "chitlins" (choice intestinal animal products). The nurse emphatically said, "That food is not good for you and you should not be eating such food." She also referred to the family as a "Negro" family, which was most offensive to them. As a consequence, the African American family experienced cultural pain from the nurse's gestures and comments.

Cultural variation refers to the slight or marked variability among or between cultures that makes them unique or different. This variability is often due to differences between traditional and nontraditional lifeways over time. For example, Mexicans, Puerto Ricans, and Cubans show slight or major cultural variability in beliefs and lifeways because of different historical and cultural backgrounds, yet some similarities in language, values, and beliefs have been identified that results in them being known collectively as Hispanics or Latinos. Likewise, many Native Americans show cultural variability among the nearly 540 Native American nations in the United States. Nurses need to learn about variations between and among cultures and if there are changes in these cultures over time.

Cultural barriers refer to obstacles that interfere with cultures accessing or achieving their desired goals or opportunities. This concept was evident when an Anglo-American community nurse always made an appointment to care for an Arab-Muslim family at noon, which was their prayer time. The nurse insisted that the family members see her at noon, when it was convenient for her to give a special medication and check the father's blood pressure. Coming at noon was a culture barrier to the Arab-Muslim family because it is their prayer time, so they refused the community nurse's services.

Stereotyping refers to putting a label on members of a culture or subculture that reflects fixed characteristics perceived as belonging to that particular group without considering individual or group differences or cultural variability. For example, a nurse may stereotype Native Americans as "lazy and unreliable alcoholics" or label Vietnamese as "passive, unwilling to learn English, and too difficult to understand and help." Anglo-American clients may be labeled as "pushy, selfish, and materialistic." Such rigid stereotyping statements are imprecise and crude labels that cause cultural pain and inaccurate assessments. Stereotypes are usually negative, but positive generalizations may also be harmful. For example, some nurses may assume that all Asian Americans are high achievers or that all Jewish people are wealthy. All professional nurses should be keenly aware of stereotyping to avoid its potentially negative consequences.

Culture bound refers to specific care, health, and illness conditions that are unique or particular to a culture and often exist within a specific geographic area. For example, Kuru is a condition observed in the Eastern Highlands of New Guinea. It is culture bound and unique to the geographic area and female gender (Leininger, 1995). Some New Guinea women who are pregnant become weak and anorexic and die within 9 to 10 months. Other examples of cultural-bound conditions, such as

Arctic hysteria, running amok, *susto,* and mushroom madness, are found with specific cultures in certain geographic areas. Often, there may be no medical cure, but nursing care is essential.

Cultural backlash is a phenomenon that occurs when a culture has been "bought" or encouraged to use another culture's values, material goods, beliefs, and lifeways. This often proves to be unsuitable and leads to serious unfavorable outcomes. Taking on another culture's values or material goods leads to anger and disappointment because the other ideas or things do not fit the culture. For example, using self-care theory and practices in a non-Western culture may contradict cultural beliefs and lifeways. Western nursing faculty or practitioners may impose their practices on a non-Western culture, but the ideas and practices are not congruent with the cultural lifeways. As a consequence, non-Western nurses or clients may turn against the Western nurses as a cultural backlash for imposing their ideas or values on them. Cultural ignorance, cultural imposition, and culturally imperialistic behavior are often the factors contributing to cultural backlash. This is a serious and growing problem in cultural education as well as in nursing practice and exchange.

Immigrants and **refugees** are two different groups of people who are often confused with each other. An immigrant is a person who voluntarily chooses to come to another country for various reasons, which may include seeking new opportunities for employment. For example, Europeans immigrated to America in the early colonial days and started life anew. Today thousands of immigrants continue to come to the United States each year. In contrast, refugees are people who have been suddenly forced to leave their homeland and come to another country for survival because of political oppression, social injustices, destructive war conditions, or other threatening circumstances. For example, in the 1970s and 1980s, many Vietnamese, Cambodians, and Philippines left their homeland to escape oppressive war forces and/or because they were suddenly driven out of their country (Leininger, 1995). Nurses need to understand the historical shifts of different immigrants and refugees because their care and health needs are different. The community nurse is expected to understand and care for these strangers almost overnight as newcomers to the community.

Basic transcultural nursing ideas should be used to guide community nurses in their assessment and understanding of families and individuals from diverse cultures. All nurses should understand these fundamental concepts before beginning to

FYI

In Japan a bow is part of a typical greeting. The depth of the bow is determined by how much respect the person bowing wishes to convey.

work in the community so that they can avoid cultural clashes, cultural imposition, and other potentially negative outcomes with clients. It is a nurse's ethical and moral responsibility to study transcultural nursing principles before working with clients of diverse cultures and not to assume one can "luck it out" (Leininger, 1990). Self-awareness, along with the use of transcultural knowledge, can lead to successful and effective culturally congruent nursing care.

Leininger's Theory of Culture Care Diversity and Universality

Development of the Theory

The development of the theory of culture care diversity and universality began in the mid-1950s in the search for a body of transcultural nursing knowledge to guide nursing decisions and actions in the care of the culturally different (Leininger, 1991, 1995). As in any discipline or profession, theories are used to discover, explain, predict, and generate new knowledge or reaffirm existing knowledge. Without theories, nursing would have no scientific way to explain or interpret what happens and why. Nursing theories and clinical practices are interdependent because clinical practices need theories, and theories use clinical data to examine outcomes. These ideas led to the development of the theory of culture care diversity and universality as the scientific base for the substantive body of knowledge known as transcultural nursing (Leininger, 1970, 1991, 1995).

Interestingly, in the 1950s, there were virtually no nursing theories, and none that were focused on culture and caring phenomena. In that era nurses were preoccupied in meeting the post–World War II medical disease symptoms and treatment regimes prescribed by physicians. Very few nurses were interested in developing nursing theories to advance nursing knowledge. There were nurses interested in research, borrowing research methods from other disciplines, but few were thinking about nursing theories and nursing research methods that would focus on specific culture care phenomena. There was a need to focus on care as the essence of nursing with a transcultural nursing perspective and to develop a theory that (1) focused on culture and caring, (2) was a holistic theory that would include the total human being in a cultural context, (3) would generate practical knowledge to guide nursing care decisions and practices related to specific cultures, and (4) would provide a new kind of comparative nursing care that would be meaningful to different cultures and have healing or beneficial outcomes (Leininger, 1991, 1995).

The theory of culture care diversity and universality was the first nursing theory to focus on culture and care in different cultures with multiple holistic factors influencing care (Leininger, 1991). The theory helps nurses discover and use culture care findings in community-based practices in primary, secondary, or tertiary care settings. It is useful in community

nursing because it is practical and comprehensive regarding culture and care aspects. It is a theory that can be used with individual cultures or with several cultures, depending on the nurse's practice or research interests. In using the theory, nurses search for care meanings that can be used to provide culturally congruent care.

In developing the theory, it was assumed that there were cultural differences (diversities) as well as some universals (commonalities) that could be found in different cultures in which nurses were expected to provide care. It was further assumed that factors such as worldview and social structure features (e.g., religion and spirituality, kinship, philosophy of life, economics, politics, education, technology, and specific cultural values, beliefs, and lifeways) would significantly influence culture and care in different environmental contexts. In addition, transcultural nursing care would be influenced by both generic (folk or local) and professional care practices. Finally, there would be three major modes to guide cultural care decisions and actions, which would include (1) culture care preservation or maintenance, (2) culture care accommodation or negotiation, and (3) culture care structuring or repatterning (Leininger, 1991).

Goal of the Theory

The goal of the theory is to discover ways to provide culturally congruent and responsible transcultural nursing care (Leininger, 1991, 1995). The purpose of the theory is to discover, document, explain, and interpret culturally congruent care with individuals or groups under study (Leininger, 1991). The theory provides research findings that are tailored to meet the clients' holistic cultural needs and expectations. As a new theory, it brought together synthesized research knowledge of culture care that had not been previously discovered and had been neglected in nursing practice. Many cultures are pleased to learn that their cultural values and beliefs are used in transcultural nursing.

. . . .

In a real sense all life is interrelated. All men are caught in an inescapable network of mutuality, tied in a single garment of destiny.

Rev. Martin Luther King, Jr.

. . . .

Assumptions and Premises

To fully understand the theory and its relationship to transcultural community-based nursing, the following assumptions and premises that guide nurses in the use of the theory must be examined. They are specifically focused on community-based transcultural nursing care to help community nurses use the assumptions in meaningful ways (Leininger, 1991).

- *Community culture care is the essence and central focus of nursing actions and decisions for the healing and well-being of individuals and groups of diverse cultures.*

- *Transcultural community-based nursing care is essential for health, growth, and survival, as well as to help clients face death and disabilities.*

- *Culturally based community care is the broadest and most comprehensive means to discover, explain, and guide nursing care decisions.*

- *Transcultural community-based nursing combines generic (folk, local, and naturalistic) care with professional nursing care.*

- *Culture care values, beliefs, and practices are influenced by factors such as the client's worldview, language, philosophy, religion (spirituality), kinship (social ties), politics views, education, and ethnohistory within different environmental contexts.*

- *Culturally congruent nursing care can only occur when the client's cultural care values, patterns, and practices are known and appropriately used in culturally specific ways.*

- *Cultural conflicts, imposition practices, cultural stresses, and cultural pain can be anticipated when care fails to fit the client's lifeways, values, and beliefs.*

- *Cultural care differences and similarities in any community-based context are identifiable and can be used to develop culturally congruent, safe, responsible, and specific care.*

The Sunrise Model: A Visual Guide for the Theory

The sunrise model was developed to visualize the different dimensions of the theory as nurses study different cultures (see the figure on p. 230) (Leininger, 1991 1995). Nurses can use this conceptual model to see the different areas that need to be examined in assessing and planning care for clients of different cultures. Although the model is *not* the theory, it is a valuable guide to grasp the holistic aspects of humans living in a particular culture. This model can be used by community nurses to assess the cultural care factors of clients (individuals and groups, especially families) to get a holistic or complete picture of the client's cultural world. By using this model, nurses avoid partial or incomplete assessments that fail to know the clients and their total reality in a cultural context. Clients who have had nurses who used this model often say, "At last, nurses are looking at my total life and not just my body, diseases, emotional symptoms, or other pieces of me." Clients want nurses to know what guides their daily living along with their cultural values, beliefs, and practices.

By using the sunrise model, nurses remain focused on the theory to identify differences and similarities of care dimensions as expressed and practiced in the culture. Whether working with individuals, families, or groups, nurses should be aware that the traditional physical, psychological, and social components of care are not specifically identified in the sunrise model because these factors are embedded within the social structure and worldview and are included in both the generic and professional aspects of care. Moreover, gender, class, sexual orientation, and other factors are likewise an integral part of the areas identified in the model, but they are not specifically labeled. The environmental, historical, and language contextual aspects are given attention in the model as they provide holistic ideas relative to community-based transcultural nursing and health practices.

Community nurses generally use this model to assess clients' needs. Nurses can start anywhere in the model with what clients want to talk about. It is the clients or families who take the lead to tell their health or illness story. The nurse is expected to follow their lead. In so doing, the nurse gets access to emic client information and does not push for etic data or professional information alone. As the nurse assesses the client, the goal is to enter the world of the client rather than the world of the nurse. This allows the client to tell his or her story and explain how health, illness, and care are known to him or her. This ethnonursing, people-centered approach has been developed to characterize transcultural nursing as an approach truly interested in discovering the person's worldview and other aspects influencing one's well-being (Leininger, 1985, 1991, 1995). It allows the nurse to discover the meaning and experiences of care and health and identify what factors are cultural facilitators or barriers to good health.

The ethno (people) nursing approach to health assessment requires that the nurse understand his or her own culture before trying to discover another culture. If the nurse is not first aware of his or her own culture, cultural clashes, cultural imposition, and other problems may occur. With this people (ethno) approach, the nurse strives to get the emic or the client's worldview. The nurse is an active observer of the clients or families in their homes or local environments. This natural context provides rich and accurate data that are usually different from data obtained in an unnatural or unfamiliar environment such as a hospital or clinic. As the nurse actively listens to the client, he or she becomes attuned to the client's ways of thinking and knowing. For example, if the client wants to talk about family and health care, the nurse should pursue this focus because it is of interest to the client. Gradually, with several visits, the nurse addresses the different dimensions in the sunrise model. If the client did not address some areas, the nurse carefully asks the client to "tell me about" these aspects. Initially, clients like to talk about what interests them most or what they are most comfortable talking about. Once a trusting relationship develops, clients will become more comfortable talking about topics that are more sensitive.

Nurses should try to obtain in-depth, rather than superficial, knowledge about clients and work to identify what care factors seem to have the most influence on their health and illness status. This process is done in a co-participant (nurse with client) way to arrive at accurate assessments or research findings. By constantly reflecting on what is being stated and clarifying the clients' views and experiences using the different dimensions of the sunrise model, nurses usually discover some entirely new or

LEININGER'S SUNRISE MODEL.

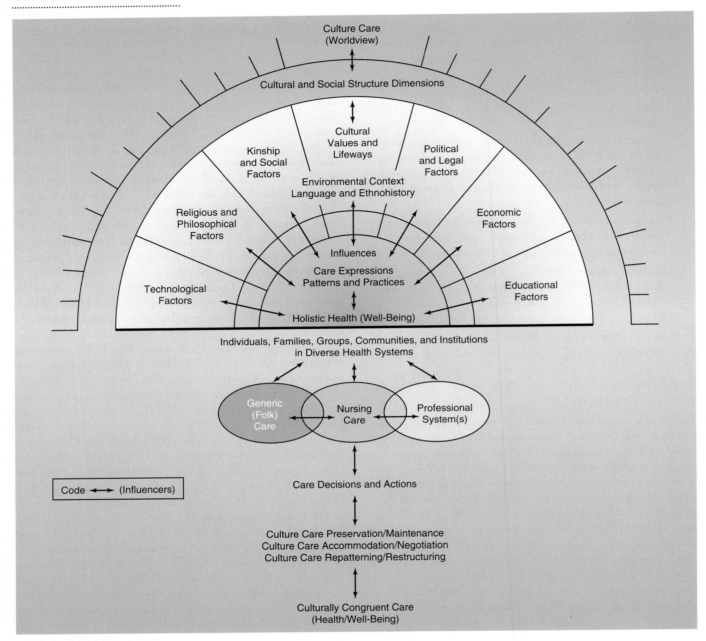

Culture Care
(Worldview)

Cultural and Social Structure Dimensions

Kinship
and Social
Factors

Cultural
Values and
Lifeways

Political
and Legal
Factors

Environmental Context
Language and Ethnohistory

Religious and
Philosophical
Factors

Economic
Factors

Influences

Care Expressions
Patterns and Practices

Technological
Factors

Educational
Factors

Holistic Health (Well-Being)

Individuals, Families, Groups, Communities, and Institutions
in Diverse Health Systems

Generic
(Folk)
Care

Nursing
Care

Professional
System(s)

Code ◄────► (Influencers)

Care Decisions and Actions

Culture Care Preservation/Maintenance
Culture Care Accommodation/Negotiation
Culture Care Repatterning/Restructuring

Culturally Congruent Care
(Health/Well-Being)

different knowledge that has not been taught or addressed in nursing textbooks.

Application of the Theory and Model
Greek American Families

A Greek American family was very pleased when visited by a nurse in their home because they could share many ideas about their generic herbs (folk practices) and how herbs were used to treat "little or big illnesses." They showed the nurse where the herbs grew in their home environment (backyard) and how and why they used herbs to "keep well." The Greek American family members talked about caring practices at home (emic) and how different they were from hospital (etic) care. The family said, "We do not like to go to the hospital unless desperately ill because the hospital is a sick place and they use medicines and foods that are not good for us. They do not understand what Greek people need to keep them well." In their kitchen, they showed the nurse what foods they thought were good to eat and shared folk practices that they use when they become ill. They explained to the nurse how they would like to be cared for as Greek clients in the hospital and stated that they believed that nurses could provide quality care for them if they understood Greek culture (Leninger, 1991, 1995, 1996).

As other transcultural nurses studied Greek American families, data were obtained from several Greek families who had lived in the United States and Canada for 20 years but had never shared their culture and health care practices with health professionals because "no one seemed interested in Greek beliefs, values, and caring" modalities (Leininger, 1991). Rosenbaum's (1990) transcultural nursing research has provided in-depth data about Greek Canadian widows and care. From several studies, the following culture care values were identified that are used today as a guide for nurses in the care of Greek American families: (1) Prevent illnesses with proper Greek foods and exercise and avoid hospitals, (2) keep active with family and religious services, (3) assist other Greek families with herbal remedies to prevent illnesses, and (4) show hospitality to strangers as a caring action. In all these Greek studies, the dominant factors that influenced the Greek families in the United States were their worldview, religion, kinship, specific cultural family values, generic care practices, and ethnohistory.

Phillipine American Families

To get a comparative cultural view, an example of Philippine Americans can be offered. Both Greek and Philippine cultures in the United States are good examples to teach nurses that cultural values and lifeways do not change readily. Nurse researchers studied several Philippine families in an urban context over a 2-year period and discovered culture care meanings and desired actions that should be considered by nurses and other health professionals. The Philippine families had lived in Midwestern, urban America for approximately 20 years, but their traditional cultural values, beliefs, and lifeways were still more apparent than Anglo-American values and lifeways. It was determined that the provision of culturally congruent care for Philippine families should include (1) maintaining smooth relationships with the family *(Pakikisama),* (2) remaining alert to "saving face" by avoiding shame and being demeaning in public talk, (3) showing respect for and deference to authority (especially elders), (4) showing mutual reciprocity by sharing between people *(Utang Na Loob),* (5) knowing how to provide holistic caring practices, (6) demonstrating gentle and tender ways of caring, and (7) remaining pleasant when caring for others, especially family members (Leininger, 1991).

These care meanings fit well with the dominant Philippine cultural values of (1) family unity and closeness, (2) respect for authority and elders, (3) leaving oneself to God *(Behala Na),*

(4) use of hot/cold theory in care and health practices, (5) folk foods and care practices, (6) the importance of religion in caring practices (the majority are Roman Catholics), and (7) nurses showing an obligation to family members when caring for them.

Using the sunrise model as a guide, kinship (family and social) ties, religion, cultural values, environment, generic herbs and treatment, and historical factors all need to be considered to get a holistic care perspective. Although the research with the Greek American and Philippine American families identified distinct differences between the two cultures, there were many commonalities, such as an emphasis on religion, family ties, historical factors, generic care, and use of their home environment resources. In working with these two cultures, professional nursing and medical practices were not relied on entirely, but rather the inclusion of generic family care with folk care practices was important to maintain and preserve the families' well-being.

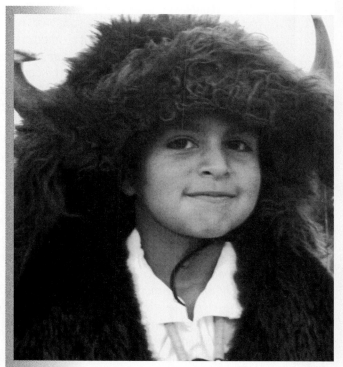

It is important for children to learn the ceremonies and rituals of their culture to develop a healthy sense of "self."

CONCLUSION

As we enter the 21st century, the theory of culture care diversity and universality has become a major theory to guide nurses in arriving at community-based transcultural nursing. It is the only theory that has an explicit nursing research method designed to tease out relevant and appropriate culture care data. All too often, borrowed theories and methods from other disciplines fail to tap nursing care phenomena, and the methods often prove to miss the cultural, environmental, and historical factors that hold special meaning and are stated in the people's language modes (Leininger, 1985, 1991, 1995). Moreover, in the past four decades, transcultural nursing researchers have found that qualitative research methods, such as ethnonursing, provide a wealth of rich culture and care data that are meaningful, specific, and appropriate in providing transcultural nursing care. It should be noted that research studies done in hospitals and clinics tend to reveal less opportunity for cultural informants to be heard or to get care that is culture specific and culturally congruent, unless the nurse is prepared in transcultural nursing and is a strong leader to support clients.

" A CONVERSATION WITH... "

Nursing students and others frequently ask me: How did transcultural nursing get started? In the 1950s I envisioned the field of transcultural nursing as an important and neglected area of study and practice. I was working as a child psychiatric clinical nurse specialist in a child guidance agency and discovered that children and families who came from different cultures could not be cared for or treated in the same way. I observed that children of African, Appalachian, German, Jewish, and other cultures clearly revealed differences in their eating, sleeping, playing, interaction, and sociocultural patterns. Because nurses were the major direct and continuous health care providers, they needed to understand these differences. I realized that my basic nursing program failed to prepare me to effectively deal with different cultures and types of care. I was culturally ignorant of the values, beliefs, and lifestyle practices of people. I had no idea how cultures could exert such a powerful force on people's health and well-being. I soon realized that nursing and other health care providers tended to treat all people alike, treating people as if they were mainly biophysical and psychological beings who were devoid of culture. Health care providers acted with limited knowledge and cultural influences on healing and well-being.

These realities led me to pursue graduate study in anthropology so that I could learn from scholars who had been studying cultures around the world for over 100 years. After learning from the experts in anthropology, I faced the challenge of how to develop the new field of transcultural nursing. One of the first tasks was to establish courses and programs in transcultural nursing, which entailed preparing faculty and practitioners to become transcultural nurse generalists and

specialists in a field unknown to nurses. It also involved stimulating nursing leaders and organizations, as well as nursing students, to become interested in transcultural nursing knowledge and practices.

Almost five decades later, transcultural nursing knowledge is recognized as essential for teaching, research, practice, and consultation worldwide. Nursing students have been the strongest and most persistent promoters of transcultural nursing, along with patients who recognize that they have a right to have their cultures respected and given attention in health services. Schools of nursing, as well as many hospitals, clinics, and community agencies, are giving attention to diverse cultures in education and clinical services. This attention is necessary to meet accreditation requirements. Community health nurses continue to see the urgent need for transcultural nursing as they care for many families of different cultures. Since patients are increasingly dismissed from hospitals early, it is the role of community health nurses to maintain care services and relationships with cultural groups, including many new immigrants, refugees, and other newcomers to their communities.

In the early years there were nurses who were resistant to transcultural nursing. They were afraid to deal with cultural factors and wanted to protect themselves by not getting involved in areas they did not understand. Transcultural nursing education has helped many nurses face their fears and move forward to become more competent practitioners.

Transcultural nursing concepts, principles, theories, and research findings are guiding nurses to provide transcultural nursing services in the community, hospitals, clinics, hospices, and many other settings where nurses work. The Journal of Transcultural Nursing was established in 1988 and provides a rich source of transcultural nursing research findings and other information. In addition, many books, articles, and other publications focus on transcultural nursing to guide nurses in their practices.

The Transcultural Nursing Society, established in 1974, offers regional, national, and global conferences where nurses can meet with other transcultural nurses to share ideas and experiences and expand their world-view. In 1988 the Transcultural Nursing Society began to certify nurses to ensure that they could provide safe, competent, and effective care to people of diverse cultures. Today there are over 100 certified transcultural nurses (CTN), but many more are preparing themselves to meet the certification requirements. The Transcultural Nursing Society became the first organization to provide certification of nurses worldwide, which is a hallmark for future nursing directions.

—Madeleine Leininger

CRITICAL THINKING ACTIVITIES

1. How many different cultural groups are there in your community? Who are they?
2. What are some of their traditions and values?
3. How are they different from you?
4. How are they like you?

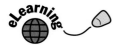

Explore Community Health Nursing on the web! To learn more about the topics in this chapter, use the passcode provided to access your exclusive web site:
http://communitynursing.jbpub.com
If you do not have a passcode, you can obtain one at this site.

REFERENCES

DeSantis, L. (1997). Building healthy communities with immigrants and refugees. *Journal of Transcultural Nursing, 9*(1), 20–31.

Horn, B. M. (1979). Transcultural nursing and child-rearing of the Muckleshoot people. In M. M. Leininger (Ed.), *Transcultural nursing: Proceedings from four transcultural nursing conferences* (pp. 57–69). New York: Masson.

Jemmott, L. S., Maula, E. C., & Bush, E. (1999). Hearing our voices: Assessing HIV prevention needs among Asian and pacific Islander women. *Journal of Transcultural Nursing, 10*(2), 102–111.

Leininger, M. (1970). *Nursing and anthropology: Two worlds to blend.* New York: John Wiley & Sons. (Reprinted in 1994 by Greyden Press, Columbus, OH).

Leininger, M. (1978). *Transcultural nursing.* (Reprinted in 1994 by Greyden Press, Columbus, OH).

Leininger, M. (1981). *Care: An essential human need.* Thorofare, NJ: Charles B. Slack.

Leininger, M. (1985). *Qualitative research methods in nursing.* New York: Grune & Stratton.

Leininger, M. (1988). *Care: Discovery and uses in clinical and community nursing.* Detroit: Wayne State University Press.

Leininger, M. (1990). *Ethical and moral dimensions of care.* Detroit: Wayne State Press.

Leininger, M. (1991). *Cultural care diversity and universality: A theory of nursing.* New York: National League for Nursing Press.

Leininger, M. (1995). *Transcultural nursing: Concepts, theories, research, and practice.* Columbus, OH: McGraw-Hill.

Leininger, M. (1996). Quality of life from a transcultural nursing perspective. *Nursing Science Quarterly, 9*(2), 71–78.

Leininger, M. (1997a). Cultural pain. *Images of Nursing.* (Summer Edition), 19–20.

Leininger, M. (1997b). Future directions in transcultural nursing in the 21st century. *International Nursing Review, 44*(1), 19–23.

Luna, L. (1998). Culturally competent health care: A challenge for nurses in Saudi Arabia. *Journal of Transcultural Nursing, 9*(2), 8–15.

Rosenbaum, J. (1990). Culture care of older Greek-Canadian widows within Leininger's theory of culture care. *Journal of Transcultural Nursing, 2*(1), 3–9.

Washington, D. (1997). Enriching our clinical practice through culturally competent care. *MGH Patient Care Services. Caring Headlines, 3*(21), 4.

Chapter 11
Ethics and Health
Pat Kurtz and Ronald L. Burr

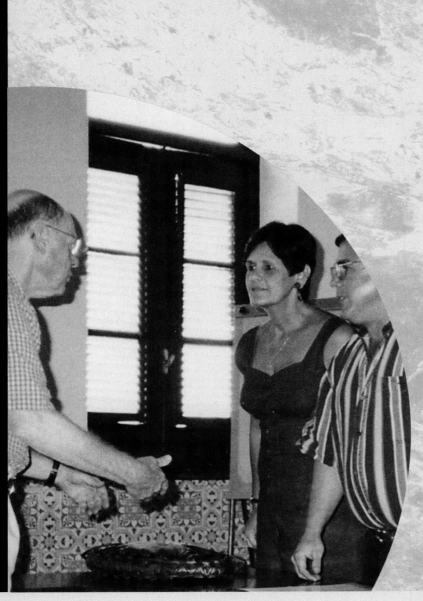

A state legislature allotted its state health department $750,000 to match Ryan White federal funding for medication sufficient to treat 20 clients with acquired immunodeficiency syndrome (AIDS). However, there were 100 clients who needed the help. How should the money (medications) be distributed? How, if at all, should community health nurses be involved in making such a decision? A terminally ill cancer client who is in great pain begs the nurse for more medication than the physician has ordered. What should the nurse do?

QUESTIONS TO CONSIDER

After reading this chapter, answer the following questions:
1. What is bioethics, and why is it important to the community health nurse?
2. What are virtue ethics according to Aristotle's philosophy?
3. What are the virtues that are considered primary to the ethics of health care professionals?
4. What is principle-based ethics? What are the differences in the two major principle-based approaches?
5. What is deontological theory, and how does it apply to community health nursing?
6. What are the duties and obligations for ethical nursing practice?
7. Why was modern bioethics developed, and what were the major changes?
8. What are the principles of nonmaleficence and beneficence?
9. When is it ethical not to treat? Why?
10. How are scarce resources of health care distributed justly, and what is the role of the community health nurse?
11. What is the theory behind the ethics of care, and how does it apply to the community health nurse?
12. What are the common steps in the process of ethical decision making?
13. What is service learning, and how does it apply to community health nursing?

KEY TERMS

Autonomy	Deontology	Ethics	Service learning
Beneficence	Discernment	Informed consent	Trustworthiness
Bioethics	Ethic of caring	Integrity	Utilitarianism
Categorical imperative	Ethical decision making	Justice	Values
Compassion	Ethical dilemma	Nonmaleficence	Virtues
Consequentialism			

One of the dilemmas of today's health care debate is that medical ethics, as currently structured and interpreted, is bad public policy and actually counterproductive to the total well-being of society.
Richard Lamm, Executive Director, Center for Public Policy and Contemporary Issues, and former governor of Colorado

Although very different situations, both examples in the introductory paragraph represent ethical dilemmas for the people who must make those decisions. We can assume that the decision makers in both situations want to do the "right" thing, but how can they know what that right thing is?

The situations we encounter as health care professionals are complex and puzzling and deal with serious issues of life and death. Our early experiences are usually of little help in guiding our actions in such complex situations. The philosophical discipline of **ethics** is the study of how we should behave, or how to determine the correct thing to do. **Bioethics** is one name for the study of ethics as it relates to health and the ethical problems that arise as a result of advances in health technologies and our increasing ability to do more to treat illness and prolong life. The theories resulting from ethical study provide a guide to examine ethical situations and to articulate preferred ways of living and behaving as health care practitioners. We must, however, remain aware that differences of opinion exist among those well versed in bioethics regarding which theories best fit which cases, as well as the role that character development plays in preparation for acting ethically as a health care professional.

As our understanding of the universe, the nature of human behavior, and societal relationships has increased or changed, theories about ethical behavior have been modified and new theories developed. One essential difference in the various approaches to ethical decision making has to do with the target of the action. For whom or what are we interested in doing the right thing—ourselves, a co-worker, an individual client, a family, an organization, a community, or a nation? Unfortunately, what may seem to be the right thing to do for one person or group may not be right for another. Being faced with a situation in which there are conflicting rights or obligations is known as an **ethical dilemma**.

Because of the variety of settings in which nurses practice and the philosophical assumption of the nursing community that nurses care for the whole person, nurses are often involved in all aspects of the client's life as it relates to health. Bishop and Scudder (1990) point out that a major characteristic of nursing is that nurses practice "in-between." By this they mean that in addition to the direct care nurses give the client, they must also manage and coordinate other aspects of the client's care. This management includes advocating for the client with the physician and other health care providers, interpreting the client's needs to the agency, and interpreting agency policy and other constraints to clients and families. For a community health nurse, it may also mean advocating for agencies and policies in the political arena.

For the nurse practicing in the community, there is the addition of the community itself as an interested party in the client's health care. Fry (1996) points out that in addition to the moral accountability of nurses for individual clients, community health nurses have a moral accountability for "how they provide health services to maximize total net health in population groups" (p. 108).

Everywhere, it appears, health care workers consider that the "best" health care is one where everything known to medicine is applied to every individual by the highest trained medical scientist in the most specialized institutions.
M. Charlesworth, past director of the World Health Organization, 1993

A different way of thinking about right and wrong actions may be needed in working with aggregate populations. The situation becomes complex when we attempt to weigh individual rights and privileges against assessments of what is best for a larger group. Horn (1999) suggests some considerations that compete in our conscientious ethical leanings and our ethical decision procedures: justice in distribution, client's comfort level or happiness, client's wishes, expense of services, client's responsibility in acquiring a condition, social role of client, and others.

In the situation about funding for AIDS medication, spreading the medications equitably among all clients would mean that no one gets a full, effective regimen. To give it only to people younger than 25 years of age, for example, may not be fair to others who may have productive years left before death and may exclude them from taking advantage of new procedures or medications as they arise. To give them only to people who are newly diagnosed to support a longer quality of life will mean abandoning clients with an earlier diagnosis who have been receiving medication.

This position that Bishop and Scudder (1990) describe of being "in-between" the client or at-risk populations and the multiple individual people and agencies involved in the client's care or at-risk populations' welfare exposes nurses to countless situations with ethical implications. You might wonder how to begin improving your abilities to act honorably and ethically in such situations. One place to begin is with the familiar. Nurses need to be aware of and clarify their own values as a first step in making ethical decisions for themselves and to understand the ethical positions of others in the health care arena.

Steele and Harmon (1983) and Uustal (1991) have developed strategies to aid in values clarification. The steps in the clarification process help people discover which values they hold and how strongly they hold them in relation to others. **Values** form the basis of ethical theories. Values often are the result of years of weighing the importance of one point of view against another, such as a mother's rights to control of her own body against the rights of an unborn fetus. Awareness of your own value system and understanding ethical theories will help you to recognize and deal with ethical situations.

This chapter presents basic principles of classical ethical theories (virtue or character ethics, deontology or formalism, and utilitarianism or consequentialism), as well as more recent formulations of biomedical ethics and the ethics of care. Examples show how these approaches may be used to view ethical dilemmas and provide direction for action.

Virtue or Character Ethics

One of the earliest philosophical approaches to correct behavior was that of virtue ethics. In this approach, it is thought that if a person has a "good" character, that person will behave ethically. Virtue ethics is based on the philosophy of Aristotle (384–332 BCE) and others. Aristotle believed that there was general agreement among people that everyone has a "life goal" and that the ultimate life goal could only be "happiness." Although each person has a different definition of happiness, Aristotle believed that happiness is achieved by "excellence in performing rational activities" (thinking), which includes "excellence in choosing."

Behavioral choices lie on a continuum between ultimate extremes. Gluttony and self-denial might be the two extreme ends of a continuum representing eating or any other behavior relating to meeting physiological or psychological needs. Foolhardiness and cowardice, for example, might represent the extremes of a continuum of risk-taking. Aristotle argued that the best choices lie between the two extremes, preferably in the middle, known as the *golden mean.* The person who selects and acts on these middle-ground choices is virtuous. A person who does so with a pattern of consistency born of practice is thought to have good character. The public records we have of admirable people, along with their exemplary patterns of decisions and behavior that lie between extremes, Aristotle termed **virtues.**

Burkhardt and Nathaniel (1998) point out that Aristotle believed becoming a virtuous person was a matter of habit and could be learned over time. The more one acts virtuously, the stronger the character trait becomes. For Aristotle, having good character would be superior to thinking that a single decision-making method would both work in every case and be remembered in, for example, the heat of crisis. In this view, the student would best begin practicing a life of moderate choices along the lines of the choices they believe an ethically ideal role model would make. Continuing to practice in this vein is believed to foster good habits that have the best likelihood of leading to right actions. That is, the virtuous nurse would simply be disposed to do the ethically right thing, rather than having to reason to an ethical solution by some procedure. The word *ethics* actually stems from a Greek word, *ethos,* which indicates well-developed habits.

Like many other experiences in life, a given behavior may or may not be considered virtuous, depending on the culture of the individual. Honesty is often considered a virtue. However, if you belong to a criminal community or to a poverty-stricken family or community, honesty may not be valued in the same way it is in a community of middle-class property owners. Likewise, not all virtues are ethical in nature. Cheerfulness may be considered a virtuous social trait, but it is ethical only when displayed within an ethical situation. Even a right action is not ethical by itself, according to Aristotle, unless the action comes from ethical motivation. In other words, to be considered virtuous, not only must the behavior be the right action, purposefully done, but it must also come from an ethically appropriate inner urge to do the right thing (Beauchamp & Walters, 1999). Box 11-1 lists the virtue ethics according to Aristotle.

Characteristic of certain roles, occupations, and professions are expectations that its practitioners will have character and virtues beyond those required of other people. In the case of nursing, there is an expectation by both society and the nursing profession that nurses will be (possess the virtue of) caring and will express that caring in all aspects of client-nurse interaction. As a virtue, caring may be considered a mean between extremes on a continuum of attention to and feeling for others' well-being. Too little attention and feeling for others would be callous, whereas an inappropriately great amount would be overly indulgent. From a client's point of view, appropriate caring includes or implies other virtues. For example, if nurses are caring, they are also trustworthy and can be depended on to give fitting priority to the client's welfare.

The Florence Nightingale Pledge identifies some virtues that were expected of nurses in the past. These virtues include purity, obedience, loyalty, and willingness to assume the handmaiden role to the physician (Davis & Aroskar, 1991). Changes in societal expectations of the role of women in general and expectations from within nursing have devalued some of those historical virtues and

---

BOX 11-1 VIRTUE ETHICS: ARISTOTLE

1. The ultimate goal of life is to achieve happiness, which comes from excellence of thinking.

2. An important aspect of excellence of thinking is excellence in choosing virtuous action—the golden mean.

3. A virtuous action is moral only when it is done from a motivation to do the right thing.

4. Virtue, for those of good character, is learned over time by the practice of acting in virtuous ways.

5. Virtues are partly discerned from instances of sustained exemplary behavior by role models.

replaced them with virtues of assertiveness, loyalty to and advocacy for the client, and willingness to take appropriate risks.

It is not uncommon for nurse educators and other nurses to question the virtuousness of today's nursing students and novice nurses. They complain that some nurses today are joining the profession for high salaries and job security and do not show the ethical character traits of caring and the strict honesty that they believe are required of nurses. Faculty members wonder how they can verify or promote the appropriate ethical virtues in students.

Beauchamp and Childress (1994) have identified four virtues that they consider primary to the ethics of health professionals. These virtues are compassion, discernment, trustworthiness, and integrity. **Compassion,** a notion related to caring, includes a concern for others and awareness of their pain or suffering. The compassionate person is disposed to respond with appropriate feelings of sympathy and mercy, as well as a desire to help decrease pain and other suffering. Ethically, being so disposed to show these compassionate feelings also may be a critical factor in a client's perception of being cared for.

Although compassion has a strong emotional component, **discernment** is an intellectual trait. The discerning person is able to take decisive action based on insight resulting from a history of clear judgment and understanding. The person is able to make ethical judgments without being unduly influenced by other personal or political factors. The person sees to the heart of the matter without the bias of personal involvement or personal feelings, without the common ethical flaw known as *conflict of interest.* The discerning individual is able to see what needs to be done when and in what way in situations involving ethical considerations.

Trustworthiness is a character trait that gives other people the confidence that the individual will consistently do the right thing for the right (ethical) reasons. Beauchamp and Childress (1994) believe that a lack of trustworthiness may be the most influential factor in whether a relationship continues between a client and a caregiver. Horn (1999) reinforces the strong obligation of providers to meet reasonable trust expectations in professional-client relationships. Peplau (1952), in her nursing theory of interpersonal relationships, identified trust as the basis for establishing therapeutic relationships with clients. Establishing this relationship may be complex, given the different ways in which humans learn to trust.

For example, the predominant male pattern of developing trust assumes that the trust is between equals. This pattern, prevalent for both men and women in traditionally male-oriented, free market and political organizations, may not be appropriate to understanding how an individual identified as a client may develop trust. Hartman and Burr (1997) propose that females have traditionally understood trust as developing among unequals in relation to their abilities to do good or harm to another, such as a child to a mother or traditional wife to traditional husband. Some balanced sense of these predominantly male or female ways of trusting may be needed to understand a client's relationship of unequal power to caregivers, although the balance

may shift in the relationship of community health nurses to groups they seek to influence. For example, in a more political arena, the male mode of relying on one's integrity or making good agreements with equals and keeping agreements may rise in importance.

Integrity exists when an individual habitually behaves in a way that is consistent with that individual's core values and beliefs. Persons of integrity, so to speak, "walk their virtuous talk." Integrity may be disturbed when the individual must compromise some beliefs and values. People are said to have integrity when they are known not to compromise their ethical principles. As equals, we are more likely to trust someone we believe has integrity.

As mentioned earlier, a community health nurse's ethics may be conflicted in complex situations involving individuals and aggregates. Such conflicts occur both for character or virtue ethics as well as for principle-based ethical decision-making procedures. A person of high character or virtue may have divergent, conscientious, ethical urges about how to treat an individual client and how to promote the health of a greater number. For example, in the case of the need to restrict the freedom of a person with an infectious disease, a compassionate nurse may have difficulty choosing between expressing compassion for the individual client (who may be personally known) and the less personally known aggregate.

Principle-Based Ethics— Developing Moral Rules

In principle-based ethics, the right or ethical action is determined not by the virtues (or habits) of individuals but by the support of a set of beliefs developed by careful reasoning. Such beliefs include, for example, ideas about who has what kinds of rights and which rights or obligations have priority over other rights and obligations. For example, who has the right to make a decision about a client's health care and in what way are health care providers obligated to support a decision they disagree with? The two major principle-based approaches are utilitarianism and deontology.

Utilitarian Theories—Doing the Most Good for the Most People

The primary belief of people who have adopted the utilitarian position is that the most ethical action is that which results in the greatest good (happiness) for the greatest number. A corollary to this would be that the best action causes the least harm to the fewest people. The philosophers who are most often cited as proponents of **utilitarianism** are John Stuart Mill (1806–1873) and Jeremy Bentham (1748–1832).

To a utilitarian, the important thing is not so much your good will toward others, but rather what consequences result from your action. Utilitarianism is known also as **consequen-**

tialism. Determining which action to take requires that all possible actions in the situation and the potential outcomes of each be examined for every person or group who may be involved. After the different outcomes are weighed and balanced, the action that leads to the best outcome for the most people is selected (Davis & Aroskar, 1991).

Some states, such as Oregon, have developed detailed considerations about how to use health care resources when those resources cannot meet every individual demand. Such considerations include providing preventive care (immunizations, perinatal care) rather than care designed to prolong life for the terminally ill. Such utilitarian considerations can and have seemed reasonable and even compassionate. This public policy approach to health care may generate ethical conflict for the nurse who, for example, values the elderly and seeks to support them and at the same time values prevention services.

. . . .

It has become appallingly obvious that our technology has exceeded our humanity.

Albert Einstein

. . . .

There are obvious limitations to the utilitarian approach. The first that may come to mind is the problem of how we can know what the outcomes will be for all the persons involved, because many factors beyond our control, or even beyond our knowledge, influence outcomes. Beauchamp and Childress (1994) suggested that three additional problems exist. One is that the preferred behavior and outcome may themselves be unethical. An example would be falsifying records in a home health agency so that the insurers will continue to pay for visits to otherwise ineligible clients. If the purpose of the falsification was to continue needed services to clients who would otherwise not receive them, the consequence is positive; however, the means are still unethical (as well as illegal).

The common expression for this criticism of the utilitarian approach is "the ends justify the means." To avoid this problem of justifying unethical or illegal means to achieve a good outcome, there must be general agreement about the ethical appropriateness of the action and outcomes.

A second problem is that a true utilitarian approach may not be practical for the average person. The principle of maximizing benefit or minimizing harm for the greatest number may place the individuals making the decision in a position of always having to sacrifice their own preferences for the greater good. This self-sacrifice may be too difficult for the average person and raises questions about the limits of our obligation to maximize benefits. Can someone truly make ethical decisions about a situation in which they may be harmed or benefited? For example, suppose that you are asked to support legislation that would provide increased health benefits for you and your family. After examining the proposed legislation, you realize that it will exclude many

needy people who are benefiting from current legislation. In this instance, opposition to the proposed legislation would benefit more people at your expense.

The third issue is the implication that maximizing good for the largest number gives undue advantage to the majority population. For example, legislation that mandates increased health benefits (e.g., mammography) for participants in a health maintenance organization (HMO), Medicaid recipients, or those who have other private insurance will benefit a large number of people. However, it excludes those without insurance who may have more need for the services and decreased ability to lobby for them. The criterion of justice (discussed later), so important in other approaches, is missing from the utilitarian approach. Box 11-2 lists the criteria of utilitarianism/consequentialism.

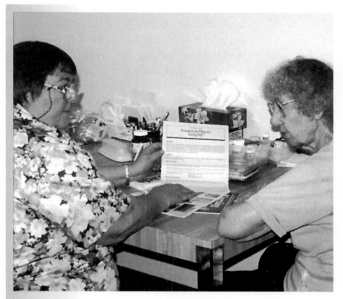

Dr. Pat Kurtz, chapter author, counseling elder client about Living Will.

Stason, W. B., & Weinstein, M. C. (1977). Public-health rounds at the Harvard School of Public Health. Allocation of resources to manage hypertension. New England Journal of Medicine, 296(13), 732–739.

RESEARCH BRIEF

Stason and Weinstein (1977) studied the cost-effectiveness of screening and treating hypertension using data from the Framingham longitudinal study and results of other hypertension studies. They projected various models of cost from initial screening to long-term treatment, considering such factors as dropout; nonadherence to medication; side effects; probability of more expensive events, such as stroke and myocardial infarction; and age. Based on their findings, they recommended that if funds are limited, it is more cost-effective to fund programs to increase adherence to the treatment regimen for those already in treatment than to institute extensive screening to identify new cases. They also found that it is more cost-effective if hypertensive men start treatment when they are young, but women when they are older. The implication is that if screening is instituted, the focus should be on these two groups, young men and older women.

What are the disadvantages to this utilitarian approach? Do you agree or disagree with this approach? Why?

BOX 11-3 DEONTOLOGICAL ETHICS: KANT

- Individuals establish their own moral rules based on the criterion that the generalized intention of their action could apply to everyone—could become a "law."
- The rules apply to every similar situation.
- People must be treated as ends and not means (given respect as autonomous persons).

A major area in which utilitarianism aids decision making is in public policy development, wherein it is alternatively referred to as *cost-benefit analysis*. It is the presumed goal of policy makers that whatever money is appropriated or whatever regulations are adopted is for the general good of society. Developing public policy requires the careful examination of possible options and the probable consequences of each. It is not uncommon that legislation is passed with good intentions, only to find later that a group of people has been left out, that the new legislation conflicts with other important practices, or that poor or fraudulent practices are encouraged. It is important that nurses be at the decision-making table to provide data about these options and consequences from their perspectives as caregivers and advocates. Further information about how to be effective in public policy and legislation is found in chapter 8.

Deontological Theories—Balancing Rights and Obligations

Ethical theories categorized as deontological uphold the position that whether an action is ethical depends on the action itself, principally the motivational basis for the action. The word *deontological* was originally meant to differentiate an ethic of duty from the more utilitarian ethic of consequences. Today any mixture of considerations that places emphasis somewhere other than simply on outcomes will be deemed deontological. In these theories, the results of the action are not a direct consideration. Immanuel Kant (1724–1804) is the philosopher who is credited with the major formulations of deontological theory.

Deontology proposes that ethical behavior is based on one or more rational rules that become what Kant referred to as a **categorical imperative**, an unconditional ethical "law." *Law* here means the generalized reason for an action, which would hold universally and which everyone must follow. If a rule meets that criterion, it will always be true for every similar instance, and the individual is therefore obligated to follow the rule in every instance.

For example, you might want to determine whether it is ethical to lie to a client about a diagnosis or prognosis. Based on Kant's imperative, you would first determine whether lying could be universally acceptable ethical behavior. Rationally, you would have to conclude that it could not; otherwise, no relationships that required trust could be developed. Therefore, lying is not ethical and is not acceptable in any situation. However, it could be argued that health care clients are a special case and that it is more important to prevent harm to them than to tell the truth. In that instance, it would be thought more ethical to lie than to tell clients facts about their illnesses that might demoralize, depress, or create anxiety.

Beauchamp and Walters (1999) point out that Kant added a second formulation of his imperative—that everyone should be treated as ends and not as means. Modern versions of deontological theory all include this second imperative in rules related to respect for individuals (the principle of **autonomy**). Box 11-3 lists the deontological ethics according to Kant.

We have many examples of other approaches to this rule-based deontological ethics. Western civilization has had the Judeo-Christian ethic, which includes the Ten Commandments, universal rules proposed for all humankind. Other religions have similar rules for behavior. Codes of ethics for professional groups are also examples of this approach.

Nursing's Code of Ethics

The current *Code for Nurses with Interpretive Statements* (1985), developed by the American Nurses Association (ANA), was the last of several suggested and adopted nursing codes over the years, beginning with the Nightingale Pledge in 1893. Each of these codes has reflected the developmental level of the profession and the social influences of the time. Interpretive statements elaborate the meanings and circumstances of the application of the code. The code itself is a set of 11 statements of duties and obligations related to ethical nursing practice. Box 11-4 lists the duties and obligations for ethical nursing practice.

Fowler (1999) has suggested that the code needs updating to reflect the changes in nursing, medicine, and society over the last 15 years. She believes that the code needs to reflect recent concerns for feminist ethics and global responsibilities. She asserts that the focus on ethical principles needs to include virtue and communitarian approaches (consensus-building approaches acceptable to all parties). The effects of the business world on the nursing workplace and more attention to the social conditions related to health and health care are also in need of examination. As in the past, changes will be made around the core values that have served nursing so well.

Modern Bioethics

Modern bioethics is a form of the deontological approach to ethics. Two events have influenced the development of modern

bioethical theory: the medical experiments of German physicians during World War II (Davis & Aroskar, 1991) and the increasing development and use of technology in medicine (Beauchamp & Childress, 1994). In the first instance, interest in gaining new knowledge that would be helpful in the Nazi war effort, together with a disrespect for certain groups of people (Jews, gypsies, mentally handicapped), motivated the Nazi doctors to perform experiments that were excruciatingly painful, degrading, and murderous. Revelation of these experiments at the Nuremberg trials following the war shocked the world community and increased awareness of humankind's capacity for inflicting harm. Further awareness and shock came with the revelation of inhumane research being conducted in the United States. Some, like the Tuskegee syphilis study being conducted on southern, African American men, was supported by the U.S. Public Health Service. The results of these and other revelations were a series of national and international codes of ethics for the conduct of research.

Increasingly more sophisticated technology over the last 30 years has enabled health care providers to perform complicated surgical procedures, such as heart bypass and organ transplants; to keep premature infants alive; to identify genetic abnormalities in a fetus; and to maintain nutrition, hydration, and respiration in clients in irreversible comas. In the struggle to find the right actions in these and other situations, solutions for many ethical dilemmas were eventually sought from the courts.

Situations that were once ethical problems have become case law. One well-known case is that of Karen Ann Quinlan, a young woman in an irreversible coma who was maintained on artificial feedings and a ventilator. When the parents were convinced that there was no hope of recovery, they requested that the ventilator be discontinued because they believed it to be hurtful. When the physicians refused to remove the ventilator, the parents sued. The issues in this case related primarily to the issue of autonomy. Without evidence that the client would have wanted lifesaving measures discontinued, it was assumed that she would have and that the parents were not necessarily adequate surrogates for her wishes. Eventually, the court ruled that there was enough evidence that Karen would not have wanted to prolong her life in this situation, and the ventilator was removed. Karen lived another 10 years. The courts have ruled on diverse situations, such as the autonomy of individuals in coma, obligations to continue treatment, restriction of freedom, and consent for treatment.

Beauchamp and Childress (1994) have identified four principles they consider essential to a theory of modern bioethics: respect for autonomy, nonmaleficence, beneficence, and justice (Box 11-5). Other principles, such as sanctity of life, truthfulness, confidentiality, and gratitude, are sometimes added to this list (Burkhardt & Nathaniel, 1998; Uustal, 1993). Some ethicists prioritize these principles, saying, for example, that when there is a conflict between principles, the principle of autonomy will take precedence over the others. Others believe that none of the obligations that arise in the course of relationships are primary. Each may be overridden in a situation of conflict with another ethical obligation. Beauchamp and Walters (1999) have stated that specifying those principles used to resolve such conflicts of obligations may be more important to bioethics than anything else.

Respect for the Autonomy of the Individual

Beauchamp and Childress (1994, p. 121) define personal autonomy as "personal rule of the self that is free from both controlling interferences by others and from personal limitations that prevent meaningful choice, such as inadequate understanding." Having respect for an individual's autonomy means understanding and acting on the belief that people have the right to make decisions and take actions based on their own beliefs and value systems.

The concept of autonomy is further elaborated by arguing that respect for autonomy is not just the negative action of not interfering, but also includes the obligation to take positive actions to promote the individual's capacity to be autonomous. An example of a positive action might be to provide care that will restore the individual's capacity to think clearly after a period of confusion. Working with family members to limit their pressure on the client for a particular decision or providing information an individual needs to make a good decision about treatment are other examples. From a community health perspective, it might include those policy decisions, taken at the community (perhaps state or national) level, that render individuals economically capable enough to have full political standing or autonomy.

Discussions in the literature about autonomy include issues related to privacy and confidentiality, the criteria for informed consent for treatment or research participation, and whether a person is mentally competent to make decisions. Autonomous decisions require that people be mentally competent to understand the information and to reason about the information in relation to their beliefs and the intended outcome. In addition, they must be able to communicate their beliefs and decisions to the caregiver or researcher. For individuals who are deemed incompetent or who are vulnerable to coercion (e.g., children and persons who are developmentally handicapped, mentally ill, demented, or imprisoned), ethics (and law) require special protections.

Principles of privacy and confidentiality both are derived from respect for autonomy. The belief that people should be allowed to control their own lives implies that others should not interfere and should not make information about them public. Confidentiality is particularly problematic for health care providers who learn many things about clients that the clients would not want others to know. The need to communicate with other health care providers opens many opportunities for loss of confidentiality. A recent case in point is knowledge that an individual has human immunodeficiency virus (HIV). Such considerations require a community health professional to think in increasingly complex ways in order to fulfill their duty to their clients' autonomy as persons.

Informed consent refers to the agreement of a client or research subject to undergo a medical or nursing treatment or to participate in a research study. There are guidelines to determine whether the consent given is actually "informed" consent (Box 11-6).

There are still many unanswered questions relating to informed consent. How much information should be given and in what detail? Can an ordinary person without a medical background really understand the potential consequences of a proposed treatment? To what extent do stress and anxiety about the diagnosis and prognosis interfere with rational thinking and understanding of the information?

Nonmaleficence

"First, do no harm" has been part of the Hippocratic Oath taken by physicians for centuries and has been a cornerstone of ethical practice in medicine and nursing. For some (Frankena, 1973), the principles of **nonmaleficence** and **beneficence** are the ends of a continuum relating to harm and obligations to help. In this context, the principle with the highest priority of obligation is that of inflicting no harm. The second priority of obligation is that a person should prevent harm. The third priority is that of removing harm, and fourth, that you should do or promote good. Practically speaking, it may be difficult to separate the ideas of prevention and removal of harm from that of doing no harm—a point of view of some relevance in community health functions relating to prevention.

Beauchamp and Childress (1994) cite Davis (1980) in a listing of rules that might emerge from the principle of nonmaleficence. These rules include not killing, not causing pain or suffering, not incapacitating others, not offending others, and not depriving others of "the goods of life." Major ethical issues related to nonmaleficence deal with prolonging the life of individuals and include the following:

- *Use of appropriate standards of care, such as not taking undue risks or performing procedures for which the person is not qualified*

- *Ethical differences between withholding treatment and terminating treatment once it has begun*

- *Whether a treatment is "normal" or extraordinary in relation to the medical condition; ordinary in this case has been considered those "treatments" that are obtained and used without undue pain, expense, and so on; extraordinary "treatments" are contrary and do not offer a reasonable hope of benefit*

- *The level of persons' "quality of life"*

- *The act of keeping someone alive by food and water treatment versus technology and other treatments*

- *Physician- and nurse-assisted suicide*

The focus of discussion and debate in all of these issues has to do with defining what constitutes "harm," defining treatment, and determining the conditions under which there is an obligation to provide treatment measures. Court decisions and ethical analyses have identified several instances in which it is legally and morally acceptable for providers not to institute treatment (see Box 20-12) (Cassel & Neugarten, 1991). However, we should remain aware that there are arguments against these instances and that not all ethicists agree. Box 11-7 lists these instances.

One of the more difficult problems in interpreting these instances is that of identifying levels of quality of life. The individuals making treatment decisions based on quality of life must be careful to look at the issue from the client's perspective, no one else's. One way to look at quality of life as a measure of whether to treat is to weigh the burdens of the treatment (excessive pain, diminished mental alertness) against the projected quality of life (ability to enjoy, relate to family, be aware of surroundings, be continent).

BOX 11-7 INSTANCES WHEN IT IS ETHICALLY RIGHT NOT TO TREAT

1. When treatment is futile or pointless—no benefit to the client

2. When the burdens of the treatment outweigh the benefits

3. When the quality of life is very low or nonexistent

RESEARCH BRIEF

Tsevat, J., Dawson, N. V., Wu, A. W., Lynn, J., Soukup, J. R., Cook, E. F., Vidaillet, H., & Phillips, R. S. (1998). Health values of hospitalized patients 80 years or older. HELP investigators. Hospitalized Elderly Longitudinal Project. Journal of the American Medical Association, 279(5), 371–375.

To assess the health values of older, hospitalized persons and compare their values with their surrogate decision makers, Tsevat et al. studied 414 clients, age 80 years and older. The clients provided self-ratings of their current quality of life and willingness to give up living time in exchange for excellent health. The surrogates were asked to rate how they thought the clients would reply. They found the following:

- *Current quality of life was rated as excellent or good by 31%.*

- *Sixty-nine percent were willing to give up only 1 month of every 12 to have excellent health the other 11 months.*

- *Twenty-five percent were willing to live only 2 weeks or less in excellent health rather than a year in their current state of health.*

- *Surrogates overestimated their client's trade-off time by 25%, believing they would trade 3 months rather than the 1 month most actually chose.*

- *Those who wanted longer life, regardless of the level of health, also wanted more life-extending procedures such as resuscitation.*

Contrary to some general beliefs, quality of life may not be the important issue in decisions about treating or not treating. Recent research has indicated that most elderly individuals, if given a choice, would prefer to live longer with ill health than to give up years of life and be healthy (Tsevat, Dawson, Wu, Lynn, Soukup, Cook, Vidaillet, & Phillips, 1998). Another study (Carmel, 1998) found that medical students underestimated the will of elderly clients to live and to receive life-sustaining treatments. These findings caution us about projecting our own ideas about the importance of quality of life onto others when making ethical decisions about treatment.

Beneficence

The principle of beneficence has to do with obligations to act in ways that would benefit or provide some good to others. Beauchamp and Childress (1994) focus on two aspects of beneficence: positive beneficence and utility. Positive beneficence provides rationale for a number of specific moral rules generally accepted by our society (Box 11-8).

BOX 11-8 RULES OF POSITIVE BENEFICENCE

- Protect and defend the rights of others.
- Prevent harm from occurring to others.
- Help persons with disabilities.
- Rescue persons in danger.

Beauchamp & Childress, 1994, p. 262.

Theoretical arguments about beneficence have to do with specific versus general beneficence and the extent to which we are obligated to people who are not in a special relationship with us, as are children, parents, and friends. In other words, are we obligated only to special people or to everyone? Formalized relationships between health care providers and clients is an example of a special relationship that obligates the provider.

A recurring dilemma among health care providers is what they believe to be the obligation of respecting the autonomy of individuals, including the right to know and make decisions about their health choices, and the obligation to prevent harm. Health care providers often believe that knowing a diagnosis and/or prognosis will cause psychological harm to clients and that "for their own good" clients should be denied that knowledge. This act of paternalism has been strongly objected to by nurses who believe that an individual's autonomy has too often been subordinated for the sake of someone else's concept of beneficence (Burkhardt & Nathaniel, 1998).

The utility aspect of beneficence rests on balancing the benefits against the risk of probable harms for the individual. Utility beneficence of an event or procedure is often determined by formulas that describe cost-effectiveness, cost-benefit, and risk assessment. This approach to ethics, which was discussed earlier in the utilitarianism section, is often thought to be at odds with a caring approach to ethics. However, we see that such an approach often presents itself, especially for a community practitioner.

In the research on costs of hypertension screening and treatment described in the Research Brief on p. 240, the authors identified very few benefits from large-scale screening. They predicted that there would be only a small number of individuals who would be found to be hypertensive on initial screening, who would undergo a second screening for verification, and who would then adhere to the treatment regimen. Because younger men would benefit more than younger women, screening might be more cost-effective for that subpopulation. The potential harm in a decision to focus on increasing adherence among people already diagnosed with hypertension is that those few people who ultimately would have benefited from the screening might suffer cardiovascular events and premature deaths. Community

health nurses are involved in decisions about screening programs and use research findings to support decisions about where to focus resources.

We should be wary, however, about relying only on the results of quantitative measures. These quantitative measures overlook other considerations, such as quality of life and the importance we place on the rescue of individuals from danger and threats to life. Some people would argue that however few individuals benefit from the screening, to extend the quality of life, and life itself, for those individuals, is worth the cost. From a practical point of view, it might be said, "Because everyone is going to die someday, we should spend our limited funds where they will be of the most use."

Justice

Justice may be defined generally as "fair, equitable, and appropriate treatment in light of what is due or owed to persons" (Burkhardt & Nathaniel, 1998, p. 57). The major focus of ethical theories of justice in relation to health care is the concept of "right to health care," meaning the right to government-subsidized health care for everyone. The arguments for or against the existence of such a right is consistent with various philosophical and political belief systems regarding the role of government in the lives of individuals.

One approach, the egalitarian view, is supported by Rawls (1971), who takes the position that not everyone has the same advantages in life—there is an "unequal playing field." Individual characteristics are a result of chance, and no one person is more deserving than another because both advantages and disadvantages are equally undeserved. Advantages and disadvantages include such things as ethnicity, gender, social status, place of birth, genetic inheritance, prenatal environment, and family structure.

Rawls advocates deliberate, unequal distribution of funds and services to compensate for the barriers resulting from the disadvantages. For example, Rawls would support providing more health care and other facilities for persons with disabilities to remove the initial disadvantages and to move toward achieving a satisfying life.

Scarcity of goods, in this case health care and/or the money to finance health care, requires hard decisions, both to stay within reasonable limits and to apply what is available with justice. It is easy to dismiss these issues of health care financing and justice in the delivery of health care as political in nature and unrelated to the everyday ethics of community health nursing. On the contrary, Aroskar (1998) has stated that all nurses, but particularly community health nurses, have an ethical responsibility to be actively involved in promoting legislation, planning for the community, and electing officials for the best possible use of public funds. Allocation of resources influences nurses' relationships with clients, thereby altering the ethical issues involved in treatment.

Ethics of Care

The theories of utilitarianism and deontology have in common the use of moral principles to guide behavior. These theories are concerned with the rights of individuals within a society and the obligations of individuals to others and to society. A more recently developed theory, known as the **ethic of caring**, takes a different position. More important than rights and obligations or outcomes are relationships and responsibilities. In this approach, the primary focus is on the well-being of the whole person. This means that the nurse is concerned with all aspects of the client's well-being, not merely the disease process. Care is designed for needs in all realms—physical, psychological, social, and spiritual—with an understanding that each affects the other and the totality of health. The broader social environment that affects the client is also of concern, such as the family. Nursing actions are deemed ethical when they take into consideration this whole person labeled *patient* or *client*. They are unethical when they focus on the disease process or anomaly.

There is also a component of compassion, which is a precursor to caring. The nurse who practices from this care approach will be concerned with developing personal characteristics and taking actions that will best show caring. This ethical approach is still developing to a large extent within nursing, where care has always been central. There are many barriers in the present health care system that interfere with care for the whole person, such as technology, managed care, and specialization (Purtilo, 1999).

The ethic of care rings true for many nurses who believe that it describes the context of and their feelings about their work. It is the connectedness and responsibility for having met the needs of individuals under their local or extended community care that give satisfaction. Benner (1984) provides many examples from her interviews that support this view. Bishop and Scudder (1996), in their discussion of nursing ethics, characterize the practice of nursing itself as a moral endeavor. "When nurses are attentive, efficient, and effective in their practice, they are being morally good persons, because they are fulfilling the moral sense of nursing by fostering the well-being of patients" (p. 112).

The person living a caring ethic bases actions on the needs of those for whom the individual cares, either naturally or in a formal caring relationship. For the community health nurse, the focus changes from the individual to the aggregate, but responding to needs at all levels remains the same (Box 11-9).

Ethical Issues for Community–Based Nursing

Community health nurses face many of the same ethical issues as acute care nurses. Respecting the client's wishes about the treatment/care process is sometimes in conflict with the nurse's concern for the client's welfare when the client is unable to make competent decisions, for example, when the client is taking several potent medicines and has some memory loss. Again, some clients are not physically able to adequately care for themselves and therefore are at risk for infection, falls, and exacerbation of their illnesses.

Although no serious harm may come to a client because of inadequate funding of health care services, the nurse whose ethical perspective includes strong obligations to do good or who practices an ethic of care will experience barriers that prevent carrying out those urges.

An additional problem may exist for community nurses. Aroskar (1995) pointed out the need for community nurses to shift from a focus on treatment of the individual to that of the implementation of public health goals, early screening, and prevention. Adopting the perspective that individual needs and rights are secondary to those of the aggregate may be uncomfortable. Other common problems that nurses face in the community include the limited reimbursement; disagreements with clients, family, and/or the physician about treatment decisions; and abuse or misuse of medication (Aroskar, 1995).

Ethical Decision Making

There are dozens of institutes and centers for the study of bioethics, most of these associated with universities. Some universities offer degree programs in ethics and clinical ethics. More and more often, health care agencies are using qualified ethicists on their ethics committees as consultants to help them with ethical problems. In larger agencies, nurses are able to consult ethicists to help them with **ethical decision making.**

However, nurses themselves often must reason through their ethical problems. Several authors have presented decision-making models (Aroskar, 1995; Burkhardt & Nathaniel, 1998; Fry & Spradley, 1990; Uustal, 1993). The common steps in the process include the following:

1. First, assess the situation. The nurse should identify the health problems and determine how those problems affect the autonomy and quality of life of the individual. For example, is the person mentally competent? Is the health problem life-threatening? Is the individual able to communicate and relate to others? To what extent can the person care for himself or herself? Is the problem likely to get

---

BOX 11-9 THE ETHIC OF CARE

- The focus is on the whole individual.
- The caregiver has a responsibility to meet the needs of those for whom the individual cares.
- There is an affective element of compassion in the relationship.

worse? What kinds of treatments are available, proposed, usual? Are the treatments likely to have a positive outcome? How painful or intrusive are they? What information does the person have about the problem?

2. *Second, identify the ethical issues separately from those of a strictly medical nature and determine which individuals and groups will be affected by the decision. For example, what is important for the client? What principles are involved: respecting the person, preventing harm, doing good, providing justice, maximizing outcomes for the greater number? Who are the "stakeholders" in this situation? Family, hospital or agency administration, physicians, nurses, the community?*

3. *Third, identify and understand the values of those who will be affected, including the values of the nurse. What do the individuals involved think about relevant issues, such as quality of life, prolonging life at all costs, autonomy in the face of increased risks, suffering, and the responsibilities of caring?*

4. *Fourth, develop alternative options and weigh them in the light of the rights and obligations of all concerned. What harms and benefits accrue to each of the stakeholders in relation to each option? If a client refuses chemotherapy, for example, does this decision conflict with the physician's belief that it will be beneficial? Will a family member feel guilty because "everything possible" wasn't done? Is there financial savings for third party payers?*

5. *Finally, decide on a course of action and later evaluate the outcome.*

Part of the decision-making process includes determining who should make the decision. It could be one of a variety of people, such as the client, a relative, the physician, or the ethics committee. In taking this approach, we should remain sensitive both to those who think that ethics is a decision-making process and those who believe that developing character is the salient feature of ethics.

Service Learning: Discovering the Self and Developing Community Values[1]

One skill needed for developing ethical responses is what is called a *moral imagination.* In Kohlberg's terms, the imagination develops with moral growth. This imagination gives one the ability to see the moral dimensions of more situations and to empathize with more issues, sides, and sentiments. Such an active imagination is developed with experience and contact with events, situ-

ations, and other's ideas. What are your beliefs about the importance and impact of your own personal decisions and actions in the world of nursing and society? How might you find out? What are your values, positions, and beliefs about those people beyond your familiar community? How have you learned those values? Might they change? Do you really know your community? Whom do you want to include or exclude from your personal community and why? What are the experiences of those different from you? The more these questions are asked and reflected on, the greater the moral imagination.

Even though learning by experience has always been a part of nursing through clinicals, practicuums, and laboratory assignments, a new interest has grown in a different form of experiential learning called **service learning.** Service learning is different because it emphasizes needs and benefits to an actual group of persons or a community versus focusing only on student academic and career learning. It is also distinguished by having an overt goal of developing a social consciousness, values, and skills regarding civic responsibility. In addition, to truly be service learning, there must be included a strong emphasis on personal insight, with planned methods and scheduled time for self-reflection and self-discovery. The focus is on the lessons learned and insights gained from performing service work, not just a clinical or professional intervention. The learner in performing a service is a "servant" to others. Many in nursing believe that service learning can help nursing students develop and strengthen the legacy of values believed to underlie both nursing and public health. Service learning lets students face situations in which they foster intangible qualities and values such as empathy, self-awareness, self-confidence, a caring activism to advocate for health, a sense of democratic civic responsibility, a global ecological awareness, cultural competence, and social justice. These are learned in such a way as to become a part of the student's life experience. These are the experiences that develop the moral imagination.

Even if your university does not have a service learning program, you can apply some of the methods yourself. When working in community settings such as day-care centers, Meals on Wheels, senior centers, youth services, soup kitchens, drug education programs, and so on, think beyond immediate health concerns. Think also about what it feels like to see yourself as "serving" them. Is "serving" a positive image for nurses? How can a group or community best be "served?" What is their best interest? What gets in the way of meeting their needs? How can they be empowered to help themselves? What organizational policies, local policies, state, or federal policies need to be changed to assist them? How do you feel about the needy? What did you or anybody else do to contribute to their situations? What are your beliefs about them and their situations? Are justice and care present in their lives? How much are you influenced by the beliefs of your friends, family, church, and the dominant society? Do you have any obligations to them beyond their physical health concerns? Would your personal beliefs and values ever make a difference?

[1]This section was authored by Dr. Sherry Hartman, Associate Professor, University of Southern Mississippi College of Nursing.

CASE STUDY

The Need for Home Care

Lila S., age 68, was referred to a home health agency after discharge from an acute care agency, where she had been hospitalized for pneumonia and stabilization of her diabetes with insulin regulation. She lived with her 6-year-old granddaughter in a small, grimy, cluttered trailer. The whereabouts of the girl's father were unknown, and her mother was in and out of drug treatment units. Lila's poor eyesight from cataracts made it difficult to test her blood glucose or measure her insulin. Painful leg ulcers and arthritis made it difficult to walk. Medicaid allowed four home visits by the nurse. This nurse had made home visits to Lila in the past and saw that her ability to care for herself had decreased and that she would need more help in the future. Lila S. has always been quite independent and does not agree that she is not taking care of herself well. She believes it is important that she maintain a home for her granddaughter.

Medical Issues

- It is important that Lila S.'s glucose be monitored and that her insulin dosage be adjusted accordingly. Her diabetes is fairly stable but needs careful monitoring because of the severe episode of hyperglycemia that accompanied the pneumonia.

- Lila S.'s poor eyesight increases the probability that she will make errors in her diabetes regimen.

- Leg ulcers require care and should be monitored by a knowledgeable person.

- Diminished mobility decreases her ability to go to sources of help.

Based on her assessment, the nurse decides that Lila S. needs a nurse to visit several times a week to monitor the glucose readings and help her adjust dosage and inject her insulin. Ideally, these visits should be done every day. An appeal made to the Medicaid reviewer for additional visits was denied, and the home health agency closed the case.

Ethical Issues

The nurse understood that the agency must have reimbursement for the services it provides; however, she believed that she and the agency had an obligation to continue care that they had begun for this client who was obviously in need and whose lack of care might be life-threatening. Legally, there is no obligation. Various possibilities were discussed with the client, including trying to find someone she could live with or who could live with her, or going to a nursing home. The client was insistent that she remain at home and care for her granddaughter. The ethical issues involved in this situation are as follows:

- The right of the client to decide how she wants to live (autonomy)

- The responsibility of the nurse to do no harm or to prevent harm by not abandoning the client (maleficence) or causing harm to the granddaughter

- The responsibility of the nurse to provide competent care, directly or indirectly, to the client (beneficence)

- The justice of a health care system that will not pay for needed health care that would be less expensive and likely prevent the otherwise high probability that the client will need more expensive care later

Utilitarian Approach

Utilitarians would start with the question, "Who would be affected by decisions in this instance?" The person most affected is the client herself and next most affected is the granddaughter. The nurse and the home health agency have some stake, and finally, society in general may be affected. In determining what would accomplish the most good for the most people, the effect of the decision on society would have the highest priority. Continuing home care to this client might be expensive at the time, but the long-range projection is that without the immediate care, the client will probably need much more expensive treatment and additional hospitalizations later. Based on concrete information about costs, the utilitarians would most likely decide in favor of continuing visits. They may also attempt to change the laws or regulations that tend to prohibit the more cost-effective solution.

Deontological Approach

The deontology, rule-based approach would examine the rights and obligations of the participants and determine which had priority. The foremost right is the right of the client to make her own decisions based on her own values. The providers are obligated to determine whether the client is competent to make rational decisions.

Continued

CASE STUDY—CONT'D

There is no reason to believe that Lila is incompetent, except for her unawareness that she is less able to care for herself. She values her independence and should be allowed to remain in her home. The providers are then obligated to allow and, preferably, support that choice by providing services to help her remain at home.

Another right of the individual is that of not being harmed by others. The health care providers must examine the medical and social information to determine whether the actions they take will be harmful in any way. Given the current situation, two alternatives present themselves. First, Lila remains in her home. It is probable that her diabetes will again go out of control. She will need hospitalization and may possibly need amputations. In this instance, she remains autonomous but incurs harm in the progression of her health problems. A second alternative is that she is persuaded to enter a nursing home where she can get daily help with her medical and physical needs. The harm in this scenario is that her sense of self as an independent person may be damaged, and she may feel guilty for not taking care of her granddaughter. Whether the deontologist values autonomy or nonmaleficence most, the preferred solution for Lila would be continuing the home visits.

Additional harm may be incurred by separating the granddaughter from her grandmother, who has provided a stable home and, presumably, love. If the granddaughter were older, she might be enlisted to help with the insulin injections, and perhaps the grandmother will not suffer any serious problems until the granddaughter is of an age to help.

The justice consideration is evident in this case in that what would seem to be a decent minimum of care cannot be provided because the woman is poor. It is not clear that Lila was born disadvantaged, except that diabetes has a large genetic component. Being poor does mean you may not get the early health care you need and may suffer more negative consequences than others.

Caring Approach

The major focus of the caring approach to this ethics problem will be the responsibilities of the nurse to the client with whom she has a formal caring relationship. The legal contract for the relationship stipulates a certain number of visits, but the emotional contract has a broader scope. The client will expect that the nurse will do everything possible to help her achieve her health goals. These expectations may include not abandoning her while she still needs help.

The nurse will respond to these expectations and try various avenues to enlist the help Lila needs to remain at home. If all else fails and the agency cannot continue visits, the Medicaid administration will not change the ruling, and no relatives, friends, or neighbors can be found to help, there is one last solution. The nurse may decide to utilize personal time, such as lunch hours, to provide the needed nursing care. This kind of devotion is above and beyond what is expected legally or ethically, but the feelings of responsibility for some client may generate this kind of behavior.

In all of the approaches described for this case, the issue of financial support is important. If finances were not a barrier, Lila would get all the help she needed to maintain herself and her granddaughter at home and satisfactorily manage her health needs. It is impossible to consider health care for individuals or groups without considering the benefits and cost to society. Even though a person may take a deontological or a caring approach to ethical decision making, most of the time the ultimate financial outcome must be considered.

CONCLUSION

Because of the special relationship nurses have as care providers to their clients, they are frequent participants in ethical decision making relating to clients, families, and the community. Expectations of the community and of the profession require that nurses possess certain virtues that will promote trust in all their professional relationships. Ethical decision making is based on the particular values individuals have acquired as children and as thinking adults.

Most decisions are based on three major ethical approaches: utilitarian, deontological, and caring. Some ethicists believe that developing virtuous habits, that is, having a character of moderation, minimizes or eliminates the need for decision theories. The utilitarian approach seeks to do the most good for the greatest number of people. The deontological approach attempts to balance competing rights of individuals with corresponding obligations. The caring approach utilizes a perspective of responsibility and caring on both a personal and professional level. Nurses may use any or all of these approaches depending on the situation. Their own character or integrity may be their guide.

In addition to the usual ethical situations that confront all nurses, community health nurses must also consider ethics from a larger, community perspective in the care of aggregate populations. Issues of distributive justice and ultimate outcomes balanced against available resources requires that nurses become involved in the arenas where policy is determined and funds allocated.

CRITICAL THINKING ACTIVITIES

1. It is commonly known that some nursing students cheat on some examinations. Should instructors assume that these individuals do not possess the character trait of honesty and that if they will cheat on examinations, they cannot be trusted to be honest about what they do or do not do for clients? That they will lie to protect themselves about a medication error or record that a treatment has been done when it was not? If students are dishonest, should they be dismissed from nursing school and refused admission to the profession? If nursing students cheat on examinations, what, if any, is the ethical responsibility of other students who know about it—considering that the health, even lives, of future clients may depend on their action?

2. What virtues are likely to contribute to ethical actions? To what extent is it reasonable to expect that ordinary nurses will possess these virtues? To what extent do you believe you possess these virtues?

3. How have your virtuous character traits determined your actions in ethically demanding situations?

4. In an effort to reduce costs and maintain the solvency of a health care agency, the administrator has, over the objections of the nurse administrator, reduced the number of professional nurses assigned to a community health field staff of which you are a part. In your opinion, the quality of care has decreased to the point that you believe it is unsafe. What personal and professional virtues do you believe are involved in responding to this situation?

5. A 14-year-old student sought an appointment with the school nurse and revealed that she was sexually active and wanted a mechanism for contraception. She had seen many of her contemporaries become pregnant and stated she was not ready for that, but planned to continue her sexual activity. The nurse was aware of the high pregnancy rates (and sexually transmitted disease rates) at the school, but she was ethically opposed to contraception and did what she could to convince the student to discontinue the sexual activity, refusing any contraceptive counseling or other aids. Is the student competent to make decisions that would lead to

CRITICAL THINKING ACTIVITIES—CONT'D

pregnancy and possible health problems? Is the nurse endangering the student in any way? Does the *Code for Nurses* provide any guidance for what the nurse should do in this instance?

6. A 40-year-old woman with adult-onset asthma presented to the emergency room with severe respiratory distress and panic level anxiety. Her physician met her there, as he had several times recently, to treat her. After providing emergency treatment, he offered her the opportunity to participate in a drug study, saying, "This new drug shows a great deal of promise in relieving and preventing asthma symptoms." The woman responded, "Anything to get some relief," and signed consent forms. Does this situation meet the criteria for informed consent? Does it make any difference that the client was a nurse? What barriers may have limited her autonomy?

7. Use the following case scenario to apply the steps in ethical decision making:

   John J., age 32, is known to the public health clinic staff from his visits for intramuscular Haldol injections. He spent some time in the state hospital 2 years ago and was diagnosed as having paranoid schizophrenia. He was stabilized on medication and discharged to live with his sister, who is married and has four children. He stayed with her only 2 weeks. He now lives under a bridge. He eats irregularly and has poor hygiene. The original plan was for him to be seen regularly at the mental health clinic, but he refuses to go there. Most of the time his sister is able to persuade him to get his medication at the public health clinic. Recently, his sister reported that he is thin and appears ill. He refuses to return to her home and when pressed becomes angry and shouts that he wants to be left alone. The sister has appealed to the clinic staff to do something.

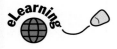

Explore Community Health Nursing on the web! To learn more about the topics in this chapter, use the passcode provided to access your exclusive web site:
http://communitynursing.jbpub.com
If you do not have a passcode, you can obtain one at this site.

REFERENCES

American Nurses Association (ANA). (1985). *Code for nurses with interpretative statements.* Kansas City, MO: Author.

Aroskar, M. (1995). Exploring ethical terrain in public health. *Public Health Management Practice, 1*(3), 16–22.

Aroskar, M. (1998). Ethical issues: Politics, power, and policy. In D. Mason & J. Leavitt (Eds.), *Policy and politics in nursing and health care* (pp. 241–248). Philadelphia: W.B. Saunders.

Beauchamp, T., & Childress, J. (1994). *Principles of biomedical ethics* (4th ed.). New York: Oxford University Press.

Beauchamp, T., & Walters, L. (Eds.). (1999). *Contemporary issues in bioethics* (5th ed.). Belmont, CA: Wadsworth, pp. 89–98.

Benner, P. (1984). *From novice to expert: Excellence and power in clinical nursing practice.* Menlo Park, CA: Addison-Wesley.

Bishop, A. H., & Scudder, J. (1990). *The practical, moral, and personal sense of nursing: A phenomenological philosophy of practice.* Albany: NY: State University of New York Press.

Bishop, A. H., & Scudder, J. (1996). *Nursing ethics. Therapeutic caring presence.* Sudbury, MA: Jones & Bartlett.

Burkhardt, M., & Nathaniel, A. (1998). *Ethics & issues in contemporary nursing.* Albany, NY: Delmar.

Carmel, S. (1998). Medical students' attitudes regarding the use of life-sustaining treatments for themselves and for elderly persons. *Social Science Medicine, 46*(4–5), 467–474.

Cassel, C., & Neugarten, B. (1991). The goals of medicine in an aging society. In *Too old for health care? Conservatism, medicine, law, economics and ethics.* Baltimore, MD: Johns Hopkins University Press.

Charlesworth, M. (1993). *Bioethics in a liberal society.* New York: Cambridge University Press.

Davis, A., & Aroskar, M. (1991). *Ethical dilemmas and nursing practice.* Norwalk, CT: Appleton & Lange.

Frankena, W. (1973). *Ethics* (2nd ed.) Englewood Cliffs, NJ: Prentice Hall.

Fry, S. (1996). Ethics in community health nursing practice. In M. Stanhope & J. Lancaster (Eds.), *Community health nursing practice. Health of aggregates, families, and individuals* (4th ed., pp. 93–116). St. Louis: Mosby.

Fry, S., & Spradley, B. (1990). Values and ethical decision making in community health. In B. Spradley (Ed.), *Community health nursing: Concept and practice* (4th ed., pp. 163–187). Glen View, IL: Scott, Foresman/Little, Brown.

Fowler, M. (1999). Ethics. Relic or resource? The code for nurses. *American Journal of Nursing, 99*(3), 56–58.

Hartman, S., & Burr, R. (1997). Trust in organizations: A cross gender approach to the ethics of developing a culture of trust in relationships. In *Ethics and relationships: Community, character, and career. Book of Proceedings. 8th Annual National Conference on Applied Ethics.* California State University, Long Beach, pp. 237-243.

Horn, P. (1999). *Clinical ethics casebook.* Belmont, CA: Wadsworth.

National Commission for the Protection of Human Subjects. (1978). *The Belmont report* (DHEW Publication No. 78-0012).Washington, DC: U.S. Government Printing Office.

Peplau, H. (1950). *Interpersonal relations in nursing.* New York: G. P. Putnam.

Purtilo, R. (1999). *Ethical dimensions in the health professions* (3rd ed.). Philadelphia: W. B. Saunders.

Rawls, J. (1971). *A theory of justice.* Cambridge, MA: Harvard University Press.

Steele, S., & Harmon, V. (1983). *Values clarification in nursing* (2nd ed.). Norwalk, CT: Appleton-Century-Crofts.

Tsevat, J., Dawson, N. V., Wu, A. W., Lynn, J., Soukup, J. R., Cook, E. F., Vidaillet, H., & Phillips, R. S. (1998). Health values of hospitalized patients 80 years or older. HELP investigators. Hospitalized Elderly Longitudinal Project. *Journal of the American Medical Association, 279*(5), 371–375.

Uustal, D. (1991). *Values and ethics in nursing: From theory to practice* (4th ed.). East Greenwich, RI: Educational Resources in Nursing and Wholistic Health.

Uustal, D. (1993). *Clinical and ethical values: Issues and insights.* East Greenwich, RI: Educational Resources in Health Care.

Chapter 12

Environmental Health

Carol J. Nyman, Patricia Butterfield,
and Jean Shreffler

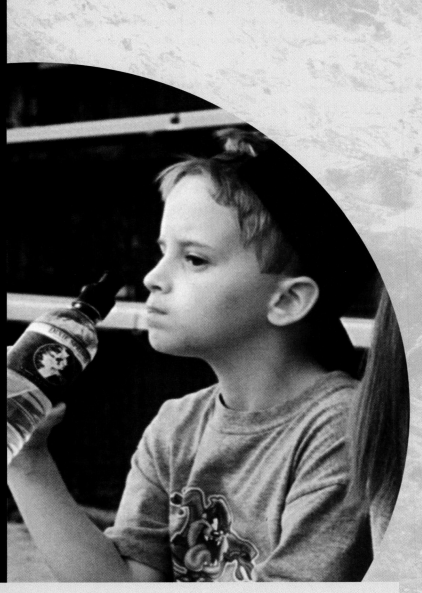

Only after the last tree has been cut down,
Only after the last river has been poisoned,
Only after the last fish has been caught,
Only then will you find that money cannot be eaten.

Cree Indian Philosophy

QUESTIONS TO CONSIDER

After reading this chapter, answer the following questions:

1. What specific global environmental threats impact public health?
2. What are current trends in disease and exposure in the environment?
3. What is the history of environmental health in the United States?
4. What is environmental health policy?
5. How does environmental health policy evolve?
6. What is the government's role in environmental health policy?
7. What are the specific roles of the community health nurse in promoting a healthy environment?
8. What is an exposure assessment, and how is it conducted?
9. What is the role of effective communication in the education of community residents?
10. What is upstream thinking, and how is it related to environmental health?
11. What are the key ethical principles related to the environment?
12. How does a community health nurse develop a clinical practice in environmental health?

KEY TERMS

Environmental health	Risk assessment	Social justice	Toxicology
Environmental justice	Risk management	Thinking upstream	Toxins

The impact of environmental agents on human health becomes fairly obvious when exposure levels are high and their effect on health is immediate. Nurses are most likely to observe such situations in emergency rooms and poison control centers. A frantic parent might call to report that their 3-year-old daughter was found playing with a bag of fertilizer in the garage. A young father, stripping woodwork in a spare basement room, is brought into the emergency room by his wife after being overcome by fumes from paint stripper. An elderly woman is found unconscious in her home after using her gas stove burners to heat her small apartment. In each situation, nurses and other health professionals organize a collective response to an immediate health crisis precipitated by an environmental agent. Detoxification procedures are initiated, and clinical efforts are focused on projecting target organ systems and maintaining system integrity.

In the previous scenarios, the link between environment and human health is readily apparent. It is easy to see that unfavorable consequences can result from a single exposure to a toxic agent. However, acute exposures comprise only the tip of the iceberg in the domain of environmental health. In most situations, associations between disease occurrence and exposure to one or more environmental factors are not easily traced; years or decades may have elapsed between exposure to the agent of concern and subsequent health effects. In addition, exposures may have occurred in small doses over time or may involve contact with a variety of compounds that interact with each other to cause incremental changes that ultimately culminate in disease. An additional complicating factor is that, for many environmental factors, incomplete and inconclusive science characterizes associations between exposure and the development of disease. Because of these and other considerations, environmental health is one of the most challenging and rapidly developing areas of community health nursing. Fortunately, for many nurses, it is also one of the most rewarding areas of practice.

Trends in Exposure and Disease

Health professionals and members of the general public are generally aware of the delicate balance that exists between the environment and global health. A goal of policy makers, both in the United States and elsewhere, has been to increase technology and encourage creative potential without compromising public health and safety. Unfortunately, despite our knowledge of the association between environmental contaminants and adverse health effects, our society continues to manufacture, use, and dispose of many potentially hazardous chemicals. In 1991, the U.S. industry reported the release of 3.39 billion pounds of potentially toxic chemicals into the air, water, and soil (EPA, 1993). The widespread use of chemicals with toxic effects highlights the importance of educating nurses who can formulate prevention programs to reduce opportunities of exposure in homes, workplaces, and public areas. Many cases of environmentally induced illness can be prevented, but this requires actions that have not traditionally been recognized as within the scope of nursing (Kleffel, 1991, 1996).

••••••••••••••••••••••••••••••

I have therefore come to believe that the world's ecological balance depends on more than just our ability to restore a balance between civilization's ravenous appetite for resources and the fragile equilibrium of the earth's environment; it depends on more, even, than our ability to restore a balance between ourselves as individuals and the civilization we aspire to create and sustain. In the end, we must restore a balance within ourselves between who we are and what we are doing. Each of us must take a greater personal responsibility for this deteriorating global environment; each of us must take a hard look at the habits of mind and action that reflect—and have led to—this grave crisis.

Al Gore, *Earth in the Balance: Ecology and the Human Spirit*, 1992

••••••••••••••••••••••••••••••

The recently documented increases in the prevalence of asthma, in both children and adults, have been attributed to increasing air pollution in many urban areas. Approximately 50% of waterborne disease cases have been found to be due to chemical contamination (DHHS, 1991). New cases of renal and liver disease are diagnosed annually in this country with no known cause; organic solvents and heavy metals are both known to cause damage to these organs. These same agents have been implicated as neurotoxins causing central nervous system damage and have been hypothesized to contribute to the occurrence of several types of neurodegenerative and neurobehavioral disorders. About 200,000 infants are born annually with some form of birth defect; the cause of many of these defects is unknown. Although it is inappropriate and alarmist to suggest that environmental agents are the cause of increased disease throughout the world, it is equally inappropriate to fail to consider the single and multiple effects of environmental agents as potential agents in changing global disease patterns. Part of the role of professional nursing is to participate in research that helps further the scientific community's understanding of the cause and pathogenesis of cancer, neurological conditions, autoimmune disorders, and other diseases.

A World View

Citizens' concerns addressing environmental health issues have been voiced at a global level over the past decade. Depletion of the ozone layer, the greenhouse effect, acid rain, deforestation, and weather changes are now understood as problems for the world that no single nation can hope to address alone (Last, 1993). The relationships of industrialization and deforestation to the emergence of new diseases, and the reemergence of diseases previously thought to be under control (e.g., tuberculosis), is of special concern.

Emerging health concerns have been hypothesized to result from the consequences of natural environmental changes (e.g., warming Pacific coastal waters secondary to El Niño weather changes), intentional environmental manipulation (e.g., deforestation, amateur irrigation projects), and the introduction of new species to a geographic area (e.g., livestock into rainforest areas). Recent ecological changes associated with human health problems include the following:

- *Population movements and the intrusion of humans into new habitats, particularly tropical forests*
- *Deforestation, with new forest-farmland margins that expose farmers to new vectors of disease*
- *Irrigation, especially primitive systems that serve as breeding areas for arthropods*
- *Rapidly expanding urbanization, with vector populations finding urban breeding grounds in standing water and sewage*
- *Changes in technology and industrial practices, such as the overuse of antibiotics in modern medicine or the use of antimicrobial-supplemented animal feeds and their contribution to the development of drug-resistant microbes*

It is apparent that these problems will require a perspective that transcends country or provincial boundaries and mobilizes global concern and cooperation. Import policies in developed nations need to address the transfer of natural resources from developing countries, such as mineral wealth, oil, and exotic lumber. Environmentally sound practices in the mining, agriculture, and forestry industries need to be enhanced through cooperative efforts between industry and citizen groups. Several disease surveillance organizations have requested additional funding for the development of a system that coordinates global reporting of disease surveillance and control efforts. Better diagnostic techniques, prevention strategies, and risk factor analysis must be taught to health care professionals worldwide. More funding for basic and applied research related to the environment and infectious diseases can yield significant improvements in public health. Education for a global perspective is needed to address the issue of infectious disease within the context of shared environmental responsibility. As our planet moves from a national to an international perspective on health problems, it is easier to see that environmentally destructive practices in one country can eventually culminate in health problems in many other countries throughout the world.

A summary of an outbreak of Hantavirus, an emerging viral condition, is presented in Box 12-1. This outbreak has been partially attributed to the unseasonably wet spring that occurred in the western United States during 1993. In New Mexico and several other states, rainfall patterns lead to a significant increase in the deer mice population, which leads to an increased risk of exposure to Hantavirus for persons residing in rural areas. Some scientists have hypothesized that global changes in weather patterns will lead to critical changes in disease occurrence over the next few decades.

The Environment and Health

Although many definitions of environment are used in the scientific literature, in this chapter the term *environment* refers to all external conditions or influences affecting living things (Valanis, 1996). Within this context, *environment* refers to more than biological and chemical hazards, including also dimensions of the social and cultural milieu. **Environmental health** refers to freedom from illness or injury related to toxic agents and other environmental conditions that are potentially detrimental to human health (Pope, Snyder, & Mood, 1995). Health care providers' roles in environmental health are expanding to include diagnosing and caring for people with exposures to chemical and physical hazards in their homes, workplaces, and communities through contaminated air, water, and soil.

Because environment is such a broad and pervasive concept, it can be difficult to define the boundaries of environmental health. The application of environmental health in clinical practice ranges from descriptions of hospital rooms to international and global perspectives on the health of the planet. Although a hospital room differs from a global ecology perspective in complexity as well as other dimensions, both views can provide insights into opportunities for health at the individual and collective level. Just as the scope of clinical practice varies from individual emergencies to situations in which a health care provider is charged with the health assessment of populations, so too must the scope of environmental health assessment vary across situations.

Environmental Health Policy: Historical Perspectives

Consumer activism has resulted in the passage of laws and the establishment of regulatory agencies to safeguard public health. In the United States, examples of such agencies include the federal Committee on Consumer Interests, the Consumer Advisory Committee, and legislation addressing child safety and hazardous household products (Fine, 1988). Consumer advocate groups also initiated the formation of coalitions to inform and mobilize

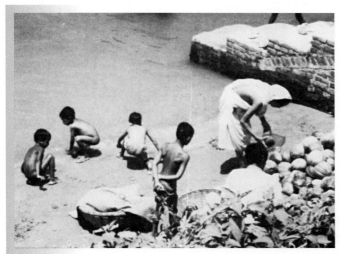

Children play in contaminated water of the Ganges in India.

BOX 12-1 AN OUTBREAK OF HANTAVIRUS

In May 1993, a healthy, athletic 21-year-old Navajo woman living on the reservation in New Mexico died from a respiratory ailment of acute onset. Five days later, on the way to her funeral, her 19-year-old fiancé, who had been feeling ill for several days, went into respiratory failure and could not be resuscitated. In late May, the woman's brother, who lived in a trailer near one the couple had shared, died of acute onset of a similar illness, as did his wife 5 days later. By early June, 24 cases with similar symptoms, including 12 deaths, had been reported in the area. Alert Indian Health Service personnel and Department of Health officials took immediate action, requesting assistance from the Centers for Disease Control and Prevention (CDC). Thanks in part to proactive epidemiology efforts and advances in molecular biology, within 4 weeks the CDC was able to identify the cause of death as pulmonary Hantavirus. This condition had not previously been seen in North America. The overall case fatality rate was 76%, with deaths in 13 of the first 17 confirmed cases (Duchin et al., 1994).

One of the strongest explanations for the appearance of this new and severe disease is environ-mental. The El Niño weather pattern had brought unusually wet weather to the area in the early 1990s. For 5 years, there had been a severe drought in the area, but in the winter of 1992-1993, there had been record snowfall followed by a rainy spring. The piñon nut harvest was unusually large, as was the mouse population. The University of New Mexico had done an ecological survey of the area that spring and was impressed to note a sudden population explosion among the deer mice—a tenfold increase since the previous year. The CDC discovered that deer mice were carriers of the Hantavirus, passing it in their urine and feces. With their numbers greatly increased, the deer mice were making more contact with humans by invading their homes, establishing a lethal connection with a new disease. The epidemiologist who did a survey of the initial victims' home after their deaths reported the presence of numerous mouse droppings (Garrett, 1994). Hantavirus may have been present in North America before 1993, but notable environmental and weather changes that occurred that year created a situation that brought humans, mice, and virus together in a profound way, allowing for the disease's presentation in humans.

citizens around environmental health issues. Significant legislation and the establishment of federal and state agencies with the goals of protecting and improving the health of the environment also resulted from this movement. Examples of legislation passed during the 1960s and 1970s include clean air and water acts, occupational health and safety acts, toxic substances control acts, and the Poison Prevention Packaging Act. During these two decades, the Environmental Protection Agency (EPA), Occupational Health and Safety Administration, and Nuclear Regulation Commission were also established (Stevens & Hall, 1997).

Public and governmental actions addressing environmental health continue to this day, although some observers believe that responses have not been sufficient to reduce the health risks in the environment. Community right-to-know federal legislation, enacted in 1987, authorizes citizens' access to information addressing the presence, management, and release of hazardous chemicals in their community. Information addressing the storage and use of more than 300 chemicals was collected by the EPA, assembled into databases titled the Toxic Release Inventory, and made available to the public. The Pollution Prevention Act of 1990 authorized data collection activities addressing toxic chemicals that leave a community facility. These recent govern-mental efforts have greatly enhanced the ability of citizens to gain access to environmental data in their region. Such data can empower citizens to be vigilant on behalf of their community and respond quickly and effectively in the event of a hazardous materials incident or spill.

· ·

They paved paradise and put up a parking lot.
Joni Mitchell, 1970

· ·

However, despite recent advances in environmental information access, some environmental advocates point out that although some environmental risks have been minimized or eliminated, new risks have been identified but not sufficiently addressed. Citizen's advocacy groups have observed that regulatory and safety measures taken in the past have not been uniformly implemented or enforced; loopholes exist in others. In addition, some policy makers and legislators believe that environmental initiatives and laws are not in the best interests of the economy; thus, laws, standards, or initiatives have been cancelled, weakened, or not provided the support required to be effective.

Recent Environmental Health Issues

In the second half of the 20th century, awareness of the damage to the environment and its return impact on health grew dramatically. Population growth (see the following figures), urban spread, advanced technology, industrialization, and modern agricultural methods were the source of great progress but led to the creation of environmental hazards that may not have been observed previously. Each year, the EPA receives approximately 1,500 notices of intent to manufacture new substances. These new products are added to the EPA's inventory of toxic chemicals, which currently includes more than 65,000 chemicals (U.S. Congress, Office of Technology Assessment, 1990).

Although the health effects of many chemicals have been documented, many others have not been thoroughly studied. Of additional concern is the cumulative effect of multiple chemicals on the human body over a lifetime. Studies of environmental carcinogenesis have primarily been conducted using animal bioassays to determine the incidence of cancer associated with exposure to a single agent (Garte, 1992). Although such tests have provided the bulk of scientific understanding of the dangers of selected agents, such as benzene, nitrosamines, and vinyl chloride, broader concerns exist about combinations of agents in the environment and possible synergism among health effects from multiple agents (Steingraber, 1997).

However, probably because of the rapid increase in chemical production and use since World War II, synthetically derived chemicals are often subject to irrational thinking about their dangers. Each environmental agent must be studied and understood; it is a profound mistake to conclude that all synthetic products are dangerous and those that are natural are safe. Some of the biggest threats to human health throughout the world originate from substances that predate the Industrial Revolution, including lead, mercury, and arsenic. Furthermore, chemical agents are often considered the sole source of environmental health threats; however, the scientific community has determined that physical agents (e.g., noise, vibration, ionizing radiation) and biological agents (e.g., bacterial contamination, fungal spores, viruses) also play significant roles in health problems of environmental etiology.

Historical Perspective on Environment and Health

The science of epidemiology has been closely linked to environmental health since the original work of John Snow in 1854. The same deductive processes in inquiry that Snow used to link cholera deaths to ingestion of contaminated Thames River water have since been duplicated countless times over the past century to link environmental agents with disease occurrence. Because the basic tenets of descriptive epidemiology (i.e., time, person, and place) have been so powerful a tool in establishing links between environmental agents and disease, this approach to scientific inquiry has stood the test of time for investigations of environmentally induced diseases at both local and global levels.

Some argue that epidemiological methods have been more effective in addressing infectious and acute diseases than chronic conditions. There may be some validity to this position, because links between exposure and disease are most easily made when

ESTIMATES OF WORLD POPULATION.

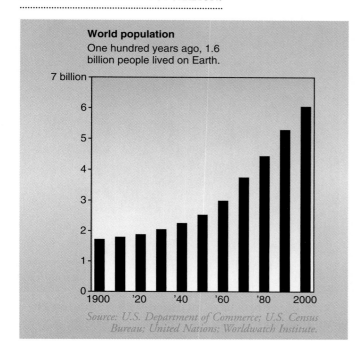

Source: U.S. Department of Commerce; U.S. Census Bureau; United Nations; Worldwatch Institute.

YEARS TAKEN TO REACH BILLION MARKERS.

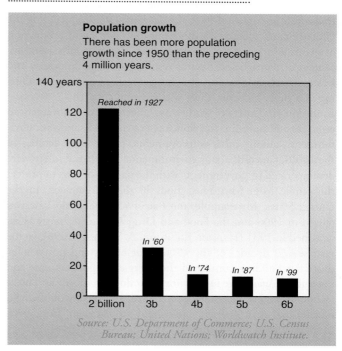

Source: U.S. Department of Commerce; U.S. Census Bureau; United Nations; Worldwatch Institute.

the induction period is relatively brief. However, in recent years, chronic disease epidemiology has played an important role in furthering an understanding of relationships between environmental exposures and several types of cancer, neurological impairment, and autoimmune conditions. Examples in this area include associations between the following:

- *Asbestos and mesothelioma*
- *Prenatal exposure to diethylstilbestrol (DES, a form of estrogen given to pregnant women in the 1950s and 1960s to prevent miscarriage) and a rare form of cervical cancer*
- *Occupational exposure to vinyl chloride (used in the manufacture of polyvinyl chloride plastic pipe) and the development of liver cancer*

One of the biggest challenges in the area of chronic disease epidemiology is to establish evidence of exposure and exposure dosage for agents without biomarkers (i.e., a physiological fingerprint of exposure such as an elevated serum lead level indicating recent lead exposure). In these cases, exposure is most often estimated by using a questionnaire or interview guide. This method of ascertaining exposure can be problematic for exposures that may (or may not) have happened years or decades ago. Despite this and other challenges, epidemiological approaches to inquiry have been effectively used to explore associations between exposure and disease for many environmentally induced conditions both acute and chronic in nature.

Origins of Environmental Health Policy

Although concerns for environmental risks to health and safety have existed to some extent for centuries, the current widespread awareness and concern about these risks among public and private sectors is a relatively recent phenomenon. With the industrial revolution in the 1800s, the developed world, including the United States, focused on modernization and rapid production of goods and services. Concerns about depletion of natural resources or damage and hazards resulting from the products and wastes of industrialization were not yet realized or acted on. During this time, however, there was growing concern for working conditions and safety of workers, as reflected in the movement to organize and unionize the workforce to demand safe work environments, among other improvements. In the early decades of the 1900s, concerns about environmental health and safety were demonstrated by governments with the passage of laws to protect the public from hazardous goods in the marketplace. In the United States, for example, the Pure Food and Drug Law was passed in 1906 and the Food and Drug Administration was established in 1931 (Henson, Robinson, & Schmele, 1996). In the next several decades of the 1900s, war efforts and postwar industrial rebuilding consumed the energies of governments and the public. Again, the international production of war and postwar goods and services took precedence, and the lay public held a belief that their governments would protect them from environmental risks and hazards.

The birth of the consumer-driven environmental movement that continues today can be traced to the 1960s and 1970s. Multiple trends and events served to raise international consciousness that some aspects of the environment had become a growing risk to public health and safety. Disenchantment with postwar living conditions and the realization of the environmental effects of nuclear proliferation and war occurred after World War II. Public cynicism toward the government and other institutions occurred in this country during and after the Vietnam War era. Several widely read exposes of environmental hazards also were published during this time. One influential publication, *Silent Spring* (Carson, 1962), predicted the poisoning and destruction of the natural environment in the name of progress with the use of pesticides. Rachel Carson's book was history making in its effect on thought and policy making following its publication. Consumerism gained momentum during this time as a result of the efforts of national leaders and consumer advocate groups. All of these trends and events resulted in public concern and activism followed by governmental responses to citizens' growing environmental awareness.

Environmental Policy: Governmental and Public Roles

One of the primary purposes of government in a democratic society is to protect and safeguard the governed or the public. To fulfill this purpose, the government passes laws and enacts rules and regulations to prevent and reduce risks to the public. Government agencies and offices have been created to identify and monitor risks and hazards, monitor compliance with rules, and gather data to inform policy makers. Government initiatives

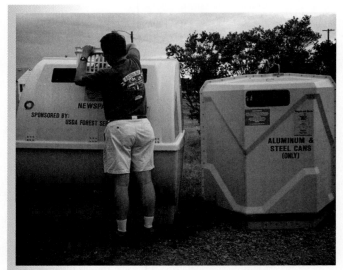

Recycling efforts have increased with significant environmental benefits.

have been implemented because of priorities of elected or appointed officials as well as in response to pressures from an environmentally conscious public.

Despite all of this governmental activity, our environment still poses hazards to the safety and health of the public, and in many cases, the dangers are more complicated now than ever before. Reasons for that increased risk include the following:

- *Environmental health has been addressed in a piecemeal fashion instead of in a potentially more effective comprehensive plan.*

- *Proposed policies and laws that improve the health of the environment are often perceived to be in conflict with what is in the best interests of business and the economy.*

- *Laws and policies cannot solve all environmental problems and risks without voluntary actions by individuals, groups, and organizations.*

- *Science has not been able to keep pace with potential environmental hazards and pollutants.*

- *In a world of finite resources, the costs of cleaning and protecting the environment are in competition with the costs of other desired and needed social programs.*

A discussion of nurses' actions to change local health policy on behalf of a disenfranchised group is summarized in the Case Study below.

At both the local and national levels, policy makers set national and state priorities among competing social programs, establish

CASE STUDY

Health Policy Actions Result from Community Involvement

Pam and Steven are registered nurses practicing at a mobile clinic that provides health care for migrant farm workers and their families in a midwestern state. They discuss the numerous children with skin and respiratory complaints that they have recently seen at the clinic. A review of clinic records reveals that more than twice the expected number of children had been seen in the clinic presenting with skin irritations, headaches, or abdominal cramping. The nurses begin to gather more detailed interview data from mothers who bring their children to the clinic with these symptoms. They learn that mothers are bringing their infants to the fields because there is no affordable day care available in this area. Older children work with their parents picking vegetables. They discuss their observations with the clinic's medical director and a toxicology consultant from the Migrant Council. They learn that the symptoms they have observed are common in pesticide exposure or poisoning.

A team from the clinic and Migrant Council visit the local vegetable fields and find multiple exposure risks for children. Some mothers carry infants into the fields in cloth carriers as they pick crops. Other infants are left at the edges of the crop rows in child carriers and strollers. Children as young as 4 years old pick vegetables next to their parents. Rubber gloves *and other protective coverings are not available in sizes small enough for child workers. Some children are observed picking pesticide-dusted vegetables and eating them unwashed for lunch. On review of applicable federal and state laws, they find that while regulations protecting children from pesticides in foods are strict and clear, they are much less clear regarding protection of adults or children who harvest that food. Laws regulating or providing for safety for agricultural child workers are also not clear.*

The team meets to examine the data collected and formulate an approach. They decide that an immediate priority is to reduce the potential pesticide exposures in this local area. They plan to work with farm owners to provide low-cost or no-cost day care and child-sized protective equipment. They also plan educational programs for migrant parents, offered after hours in their housing areas, focused on reducing exposures. Because migrant workers travel after harvest to other agricultural areas, reducing the problem in this area alone will not protect the children as they move to other areas. The team identifies informal leaders in the group of migrant workers and provides them with training in community development so that they will be better able to advocate for safe working conditions on behalf of their group wherever they work. The team also contacts legislators and policy makers to advocate for improved regulations to protect migrant workers and their families from pesticide exposures.

Source: Adapted from Crenson, 1997.

standards for environmental hazards and risks, take action against those who violate standards, and allocate billions of federal and state funds according to these established priorities. A broad set of population health goals to be achieved by the year 2000 was established by the U.S. Public Health Service (USPHS) 20 years ago and was reaffirmed with the publication of *Healthy People 2000* (DHHS, 1991) and *Healthy People 2010* (DHHS, 2000). The *Healthy People 2010* objectives, which include environmental health as one of 28 priority areas, is the basis for federal and state policy formulation and action; selected objectives related to the environment are listed in the *Healthy People 2010* box below.

The public plays an important role in setting the stage for policy decisions by expressing its values and in the actions it takes as an electorate. Policy makers are also influenced by organized interest groups and elected and appointed officials who represent these interests. In the environmental health arena, these groups have traditionally been organized into two factions:

(1) businesses and industries that depend on the environment for raw materials and/or disposal of waste and (2) citizen groups and voluntary organizations that have an interest in preventing or limiting the extraction of raw materials or disposal of waste. Nurses can work to foster health communication between groups and direct the dialog to areas of common ground. In addition to participation of citizens, nurses can enlarge their role in environmental health policy making by increasing their political expertise and activity as professionals.

In the United States, policy makers and the public alike trust the nursing profession to be advocates for clients and to speak and act on behalf of the health of the population. Nurses are reliable and trustworthy sources of information about threats to health and also represent the largest group of health care professionals among the voting age population. By staying informed of current and accurate information on environmental risks, organizing and becoming actively involved with

HEALTHY PEOPLE 2010

Objectives Related to Environmental Health

Outdoor Air Quality

8.1   Reduce the proportion of persons exposed to air that does not meet the U.S. Environmental Protection Agency's (EPA's) health-based standards for harmful air pollutants.

8.4   Reduce air toxic emissions to decrease the risk of adverse health effects caused by airborne toxics.

Water Quality

8.5   Increase the proportion of persons served by community water systems who receive a supply of drinking water that meets the regulations of the Safe Drinking Water Act.

8.8   Increase the proportion of assessed rivers, lakes, and estuaries that are safe for fishing and recreational purposes.

Toxics and Waste

8.11   Eliminate elevated blood lead levels in children.

8.12   Minimize the risks to human health and the environment posed by hazardous sites.

Healthy Homes and Healthy Communities

8.16   Reduce indoor allergen levels.

8.20   Increase the proportion of the nation's primary and secondary schools that have official school policies ensuring the safety of students and staff from environmental hazards, such as chemicals in special classrooms, poor indoor air quality, asbestos, and exposure to pesticides.

Infrastructure and Surveillance

8.27   Increase or maintain the number of territories, tribes, and states, and the District of Columbia that monitor diseases or conditions that can be caused by exposure to environmental hazards.

Global Environmental Health

8.29   Reduce the global burden of disease due to poor water quality, sanitation, and personal and domestic hygiene.

Source: DHHS, 2000.

groups of nurses and others around environmental issues, and actively communicating with and lobbying policy makers as well as organized interest groups, nurses can effectively influence public policy. In the practice arena, nurses can also inform and mobilize citizen groups and other professionals to become actively involved in communicating and lobbying policy makers about environmental issues of concern to themselves and their communities.

Nursing and the Environment

Nursing's efforts to promote health by influencing environmental conditions predate the modern environmental movement by more than a century. Florence Nightingale, the founder of modern nursing, developed her theory of nursing with a strong emphasis on the individual's environment. Although the term *environment* did not appear in her published works, she addressed health using five environmental dimensions: (1) pure, fresh air; (2) pure water; (3) efficient drainage; (4) cleanliness; and (5) light, that is, direct sunlight (Nightingale, 1969/1860). To Nightingale, the environment was the surrounding context in which the individual lived; a person's health or illness was a direct result of environmental influences. Deficiencies in any of the five factors produced a health deficit. Nightingale also stressed the importance of a comfortably warm, noise-free environment and a good diet. Although originally written for a hospital environment, her concepts were broad enough to serve as a basis for public health nursing also and remain integral parts of nursing and health care.

. . . .

Within the last few years, a large part of London was in the daily habit of using water polluted by the drainage of its sewers and water closets. This has happily been remedied. But, in many parts of the country, well water of a very impure kind is used for domestic purposes. And when epidemic disease shows itself, persons using such water are almost sure to suffer.

Florence Nightingale, 1860

. . . .

Nursing has long noted the influence of the environment on health and has assumed the role of managing the interaction between clients and their environments. Often, nursing's approach has been to assist the client to adapt to the environment; thus, the focus for intervention was changing the individual or community client to facilitate a better match with the environment. An emerging role for nursing today is to intervene directly in environmental factors in an attempt to change unhealthy conditions and mobilize individuals or communities to do the same. Nurse scientists are conducting studies on environmental factors directly, such as water and air quality, policies, laws that influence health of the population, and conditions in workers' environments to improve understanding of healthful/unhealthful environmental conditions and the interventions that can improve them.

Just as it is a challenge to draw a circle around the concept of environmental health, so too is it difficult to delineate the unique role of nursing in addressing environmental health issues. Many professional disciplines, from wildlife biologists to microbiologists to engineers, consider environmental health problems within their domain of expertise. Environmental health is an area in which many different professionals are needed to prevent, minimize, and improve environmental problems. Both basic and applied research efforts are required to understand all of the implications of environmental health problems. Professional nurses are well suited to participate in collaborative efforts because they have historically functioned at the center of the health care team. However, nursing efforts are focused exclusively on human health, in contrast to some professions, whose efforts are directed toward other species such as fish, large mammals, and plant life. Nursing interventions are directed toward preventing and minimizing the effects of environmental health problems on persons of all ages. That does not mean, however, that concerns about animal and plant life are dismissed or that health connections between species are not recognized.

Community health and occupational health are the nursing practice specialties often associated with health hazards in the physical environment. In view of the universal presence of environmental hazards, it is critical that nurses in all practice specialties have an understanding of environmental health (Pope, Snyder, & Mood, 1995). As client advocates, all nurses need to be concerned about the health of the environment because it is a major determinant of their clients' health.

It is important to consider the depth of inquiry when addressing the role of nursing in environmental health. What areas of inquiry contain the dimensions of environment that fall within the scope of nursing? Surely, given enough time and paper, one could generate a seemingly endless list of questions that relate human health to the environment. The challenge then lies in the ability to focus nursing assessment activities into areas that are most obvious to the clinical or research area of interest. One would expect to see overlapping areas of focus between environmental health, as it relates to professional nursing, and other professions such as **toxicology**, pharmacology, and the behavioral sciences. The goal then is not to stake out a new specialty area for nursing practice, but rather to integrate knowledge from nursing and other disciplines and apply this knowledge to the clients' needs for health promotion or restoration. A research study directed by nursing scientists is discussed in the Research Brief on p. 262.

Looking at the environment from a broad view, environmental factors are involved in almost all disease risks and include areas such as housing, nutrition, socioeconomic status, and lifestyle. Even the health of persons with genetic disorders can often be enhanced through nursing actions addressing personal and societal aspects of the environment. For community health nursing, environmental health goes beyond assessing the individual and a household and includes the need to assess the larger community, even the global community, to ensure the well-being of all. Environmental health includes a concern for not only the physical environment, but also the interrelated social,

RESEARCH BRIEF

Amaya, M. A., Ackall, G., Pingitore, N., Quiroga, M., & Terrazas-Ponce, B. (1997). Childhood lead poisoning on the US-Mexico border: A case study in environmental health nursing lead poisoning. Public Health Nursing, 14, 353-360.

Amaya and colleagues have documented high rates of exposure to lead, trace elements, and pesticides in Hispanic persons residing in United States–Mexico border communities. As one part of a larger study examining the serum lead levels in pregnant Hispanic women, a case investigation of a family with two children with elevated lead levels was conducted. Dust samples were collected both inside and outside the residence; additional samples were taken from water, paint, and cookware in the home. The evidence supported a hypothesis that primary exposure occurred from battery recycling and burning of electrical wire conducted on the premises by the father and grandfather of the children. Steps to ameliorate exposure pathways were undertaken by community health nurses working with the family. Monthly lead levels taken on both children declined over the next 4 months. Unfortunately, the family moved away without notice and was lost to follow-up 9 months after the initial event.

Such investigations capitalize on the risk communication skills of nurses working in border communities. Nurses' abilities to locate and intervene effectively with disenfranchised families are unsurpassed among health professions. Case-series and case-control studies by nurse scientists can yield important findings at the local and national levels, while furthering the role of nursing in the environmental health sciences. Elevated blood lead levels have been reported in approximately 8% of low-income children in El Paso County, Texas. Nursing research addressing the areas of risk communication, health care access, and intervention strategies with families at risk for lead exposure can lead to a significant reduction of persons affected by this serious health problem.

economic, psychological, and political environments. Such conditions as poverty, powerlessness, social injustice, and racism that arise from diverse environmental factors can reduce opportunities for health and contribute to illness just as certainly as do chemical or physical agents. A central goal of this chapter is to provide information that allows for a richer understanding of the connectedness among many features of the environment. Although information addressing physical agents predominates in this chapter, it is important to understand that aspects of the social and economic environment are also centrally linked to opportunities for health in civilizations throughout the world.

Roles of the Community Health Nurse

Nursing has a long history of identifying health risks and intervening directly on behalf of client health. The role of the nurse in providing pure water, a restful setting, and a hygienic hospital environment were among the early environmental concerns of the nursing profession. By the late 1800s and early 1900s, nursing became concerned with identifying and resolving communicable disease outbreaks, improper food handling, inadequate disposal of wastes, and unsafe water supplies (Tiedje & Wood, 1995). During the growing environmental awareness of the 1960s and 1970s, nursing expanded its environmental concerns to include identification and interventions related to exposures to **toxins** and chemicals from the home and community environments. More recently, nursing has acknowledged that the environment relevant to our clients' health is larger and more multifaceted than appreciated before. Accordingly, nursing's concerns have expanded to regional, national, and global physical environmental hazards as well as influences arising from the social, economic, psychological, and political environments.

Identification of Risks

Community health nurses often emphasize primary prevention activities that address environmental health because many environmentally induced illnesses are preventable through risk management activities. In concert with other professionals, community health nurses often conduct a systematic review of risks known as a quantitative **risk assessment.** Risk is the probability of injury, disease, or death for individuals or populations exposed to hazardous substances. It may be expressed numerically (e.g., "one in 1 million"), but this is often impossible and therefore risk may be expressed using terms such as *high, medium,* or *low.* The steps involved in a risk assessment are outlined in Box 12-2. **Risk management** involves developing and evaluating possible regulatory actions guided by the risk assessment plus other ethical, political, social, economic, and technological factors (U.S. Congress, Office of Technology Assessment, 1990).

BOX 12-2 STEPS IN AN ENVIRONMENTAL RISK ASSESSMENT

1. Hazard identification: Does the agent cause the adverse effect?
2. Exposure assessment: What exposures are currently experienced or anticipated?
3. Dose-response assessment: What is the relationship between the dose and incidence?
4. Risk characterization: What is the estimated incidence of the adverse effect in a given population?

Comprehensive Exposure Assessment

Community health nurses often participate in exposure assessments following the development of a case or suspected cluster of disease. Because of their methodical skills in home assessment, nurses are often called on to conduct comprehensive exposure assessments in homes or occupational settings. Strong interview, observation, and family assessment skills are needed by nurses to collect these data in a clear and systematic manner. Clues to potential solutions to environmental risks may occur during the course of community or home assessments, although the resolution of some risks may require the expertise of non-nursing professionals. Home visits often require follow-up conversations with toxicologists, industrial hygienists, or other scientists who have expertise with the exposures of interest.

Exposure assessments are much simpler when clients present with an acute illness, such as acute pesticide poisoning or inhalation fever. Assessments become much more complex when the specific types of agents have not been considered a priori or when the induction period between exposure and disease occurrence is unknown. The greatest challenges occur in persons with chronic disease or disease of unknown cause or when exposure to small doses of multiple agents has occurred over years or decades. In these types of clinical situations, it is very unusual to make a link between disease and a specific type of exposure with a high degree of confidence. Unusual conditions and rarer forms of cancer, such as the association between asbestos and development of mesothelioma, are the exception and can often be narrowed down to a specific place and time in a one's life. Box 12-3 includes basic

---

BOX 12-3 CONDUCTING A HOME ASSESSMENT AND ENVIRONMENTAL EXPOSURE HISTORY

AREAS OF VISUAL INSPECTION

Examine areas in the immediate vicinity of the home for the presence of the following:

- Water hazards
- Automobile, farm, or other large equipment
- Garbage/waste storage containers
- Garages, sheds, or other outbuildings for safety hazards
- Chemical storage areas
- Pets or livestock
- Areas where rats or mice could live around home or outbuildings
- General age and condition of home (e.g., presence of peeling paint, metal edges from siding)

Consider whether any of the aforementioned items constitute a health threat to any family members or to the community in general.

QUESTIONS TO CONSIDER IN ASSESSING ENVIRONMENTAL AGENTS IN THE HOME

Ask family members about the following areas:

- Hobbies or crafts involving potential for lead exposure (e.g., stained glass, ceramic glazing)
- Potential for significant exposure to gasoline or diesel exhaust from car repair activities or from nearby traffic

- Safe storage of food (stored where vermin cannot contaminate food) and proper cooking and refrigeration facilities
- Storage and use of insecticides, lawn care products, fertilizers
- Home heating—type of furnace, use of wood stoves
- Use of cleaning products that are strong irritants
- Fumigants or other products used for tick or flea control in the home
- Storage of food in copper or brass containers (can contaminate food with lead or copper)
- Exposure to wood preservatives (e.g., pentachlorophenol) in log homes
- Potential for lead exposure through lead-based plumbing
- Source of water (municipal or private well)
- Any seasonal changes in water sources during the year (e.g., private well during the winter and water delivered to a cistern during the summer months)
- Recent home renovation activities such as sanding or stripping of old paint that could result in lead exposure to family members

QUESTIONS ADDRESSING SYMPTOMS RELATED TO ENVIRONMENTAL AGENTS IN THE HOME

Does any member of the family have symptoms that they attribute to an environmental exposure? If so, elicit

Continued

BOX 12-3 CONDUCTING A HOME ASSESSMENT AND ENVIRONMENTAL EXPOSURE HISTORY—CONT'D

the nature of symptoms, duration, fluctuations in symptoms over the day and from week to week, seasonal changes, related symptoms in other family members or others who spend extended time in the home.

ASCERTAINING AGENT-SPECIFIC DATA FROM INDIVIDUALS

Exposures

- Concurrent and past exposures to metals, dust, fibers, fumes, chemicals, biological hazards, radiation, noise, vibration
- Typical work day (job tasks, location, materials, agents used)
- Changes in routines or processes
- Other employees or household members similarly affected

Health and safety practices at work site

- Ventilation
- Medical and industrial hygiene surveillance
- Employment examinations
- Personal protective equipment (e.g., respirators, gloves, coveralls)
- Lockout devices, alarms, training, drills
- Personal habits (smoking, eating in the work area, handwashing with solvents)

Work history

- Description of all prior jobs, including short-term, seasonal, or part-time employment and military service
- Description of present job(s)

Environmental history

- Present and prior home locations
- Jobs of household members
- Home insulating, heating and cooling system
- Home cleaning agents
- Pesticide exposure (e.g., pet flea treatments, roach and ant sprays)
- Water supply
- Recent renovation/remodeling
- Air pollution, indoor and outdoor
- Hobbies: painting, sculpting, welding, woodworking, piloting, autos, firearms, stained glass, ceramics, gardening
- Hazardous wastes/spills exposure

Medical history

- Past and present medical problems
- Medications

Source: Adapted from Agency for Toxic Substance and Disease Registry, 1992.

---

information addressing the components of a home assessment and environmental exposure history. As one would expect, data collection is customized to address the unique aspects of the exposures, setting, and persons involved in the situation.

Communicating Risk

Often, the most successful strategies for responding to environmental risks affecting a community involve empowering citizens to address the problem. If successful, these strategies result not only in the resolution of the immediate problem but also in the creation of a group able to address future threats. Nurses should be encouraged to become familiar with the principles of environmental risk communication. An increased availability of information to the public increases the possibility that the community health nurse will be sought for advice and further information. Nurses are trusted in a community, and the public values their

opinions. It is professionally responsible to share science-based information with persons most affected. Nurses should understand the influence of the environment and environmental agents on human health based on knowledge of relevant epidemiological, toxicological, and exposure factors. Basic principles of risk communication can be used in many environmental health situations, ranging from a toxic spill incident to a neighborhood meeting to discuss groundwater contamination. Overall, risk communication focuses on telling citizens what is known about a risk situation in a clear and forthright manner. In addition, it is important to directly explain what information is not currently known and the process by which additional information will be communicated to all parties. Basic guidelines addressing the principles of risk communication are listed in Box 12-4.

Infants and children have a unique vulnerability to being exposed to chemical agents. Communicating a balanced view of

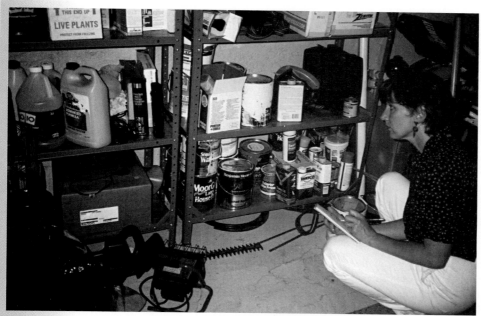

Chapter author, Dr. Patricia Butterfield, conducting a home environment exposure assessment.

BOX 12-4 BASIC GUIDELINES FOR RISK COMMUNICATION

Don't confuse people's understanding a risk with their acceptance of it—anger and resentment are often expressed when people are unwittingly exposed to an environmental hazard and feel that they have no control over the situation.

Avoid trivializing the risk or minimizing people's concerns. Frustration needs to be heard and acknowledged, not suppressed. It is important to listen attentively and respectfully to all concerns and respond in a clear manner with whatever information is currently available. Say what is known; also say what is not known. Gaining trust from the audience in a public meeting will not usually occur if people perceive that they are being patronized or placated. It is best to say what is currently known about the situation of concern and what is not known.

Often, health providers do not have all the information at hand or are waiting for additional information to come in (e.g., laboratory values or diagnostic tests from exposed persons). State clearly what information is not currently available and when that information will be available.

Respond to the different needs of different audiences. In an incident that involves a pesticide spill at a local school, the parents of schoolchildren will probably have different concerns than the janitor and physical facilities staff at the school. Think about your audience in advance—try to anticipate what questions you would have if you were in the audience and direct the discussion from that perspective.

Recognize that input from the public can help your agency make better decisions. Holding private meetings or trying to avoid public input is likely to fuel distrust in community members. By building in opportunities for affected persons to help remedy an environmental hazard situation, those persons gain a sense of control over the situation and feel like they are helping themselves and others. Think broadly about how to use citizens' help to get mailings out, set up phone trees, and form advocacy groups. If you do not allow citizens to work with you and your agency, they may begin to work against you.

Source: New Jersey Department of Environmental Protection, 1990.

these risks to parents is a challenge for nurses in the community. An example of this challenge involves the practice of breast-feeding. For many years, nurses have played a significant role in policies and clinical actions that support breast-feeding practices in new mothers. This advocacy role has been based on scientific findings that breast milk is the ideal infant food because of the easy digestibility of milk proteins, the presence of maternal antibodies, and safety from contamination through the use of improperly sanitized bottles. However, over the past two decades, scientists have become increasingly aware that human breast milk also carries a host of potentially serious risks to infant health. The greatest area of concern has been physiological evidence that many chemicals to which the mother has been exposed are transferred into breast milk. Of special interest are the findings from studies that examine the metabolism and fate of chemicals that have extremely long half-lives (i.e., years and decades) within human populations. Such agents include polychlorinated organic pollutants, including organochlorine pesticides, polychlorinated biphenyls (PCBs), and polychlorinated dibenzodioxins and dibenzofurans (PCDDs/PCDFs), as well as some forms of metals such as methylmercury. In most cases, persons ingest these agents in their diets, usually from contaminated fish and animal products such as meats, fats, cheese, and eggs. In large doses, many pesticide products and mercury compounds have affected neurobehavioral, neuromotor, and speech development (Kimbrough, 1995). Unfortunately, much less is known about the long-term effects of low-dose exposure in breast milk. For a variety of feasibility and methodological reasons, scientific studies of low-dose and early life exposures are extremely difficult to conduct. Such studies often help in the incremental advancement of scientific understanding but are not able to yield clear-cut answers to clinical questions (Gladen, Monaghan, Lukyanova, Hulchiy, Shkyryak-Nyzhnyk, Sericano, & Little, 1999; Hooper, 1999).

Infants and children are particularly susceptible to the toxic effects of chemical exposure for a number of reasons. Pound for pound of body weight, a child eats much more food than an adult. Youngsters between the ages of 1 and 5 years eat and drink three to four times more food and water than adults. In addition to increased food intake, there is evidence that compared with adult bodies, the metabolic pathways of children have a diminished ability to metabolize or detoxify chemical agents effectively. There is increasing evidence that children's daily activity patterns, such as playing on the ground and hand-to-mouth behavior, can also increase their exposure to environmental toxicants. Because of incomplete scientific evidence about the long-term consequences of exposure to chemical agents, primary prevention activities that reduce the opportunity of exposure provide the first and most important line of defense on behalf of children's health (Schmidt, 1999).

Assessment and Referral

A critical piece of comprehensive nursing practice is the identification of high-risk clients so that they can be referred for further evaluation and follow-up. To provide such care for these clients, nurses must have a good understanding of environmental health resources located within their geographic area. In many communities, professionals with environmental health expertise, such as industrial hygienists, physicians, and toxicologists, are located in the state health department. Other experts may be located in occupational health clinics in both hospital and community settings. For nurses working in agricultural communities, expertise in environmental health may often be found through contacts with county extension agents, pest management specialists, migrant and seasonal farm worker clinics, or agricultural medicine programs (Shreffler, 1996). It is essential that clients be referred to resources that are culturally and socioeconomically appropriate (Pope & Rall, 1995).

There is some evidence from applied research studies that both pediatric and adult clients are falling through the cracks of the health system when they are in need of specialized environmental health services. In a review of children residing in New York City, Markowitz, Rosen, and Clemente (1999) estimated that only 60% of high-risk children were being screened for lead poisoning; of those children who were found to have elevated lead levels, nearly 60% were not receiving timely follow-up by health care providers. In another recent study addressing the health consequences of lead exposure, elevated values were associated with an increased risk for hypertension later in life (Korrick, Hunter, Rotnitzky, Hu, & Speizer, 1999). A third environmental health study focused on persons at increased risk of developing lung cancer caused by both household radon exposure and cigarette smoking. Researchers developed statistical models of risk and determined that the most effective strategy to reduce the risk of radon-related cancer was smoking cessation. Stopping smoking was more effective in reducing cancer risk than directly reducing the levels of radon in the home (Mendez, Warner, & Courant, 1998). Although it is always optimal to reduce disease risk through all possible means (e.g., smoking cessation as well as radon reduction interventions), this study demonstrates the importance of addressing both environmental and behavioral means to minimize disease risk in exposed persons. Community health nurses are the health providers most familiar with their clients' home setting, lifestyle, work habits, and environmental exposures. Because of their unique presence in a variety of client settings, nurses may become aware of clients' environmental health risks and work toward directing them to an appropriate source of evaluation and treatment. A Case Study reflecting the need for ongoing assessment and education for families with asthma is presented in the box on p. 267.

Upstream Thinking: Making Connections Between Environmental and Human Health

One of the most challenging areas in environmental health is linking a past exposure from 10 to 20 years ago with the development of a health problem. Even though we are intellectually

CASE STUDY

Asthma Management in a Young Girl

A public health nurse working in an urban area has been coordinating services with the school nurse practitioner at Northside Elementary, a primary school located in a low-income neighborhood. The nurse practitioner calls to request a home assessment for 7-year-old Lateesha. Lateesha is in the second grade, and the teacher notes that she has performed poorly in the classroom compared with her skill level during the previous year. In a phone interview, the mother states that she thinks the child's inattentiveness in the classroom results primarily from several recent colds that required Lateesha to miss school. The mother notes that Lateesha has missed 8 days of school so far this year and has had some difficulty with the make-up work following these absences.

When the nurse visits the home, she notes that Lateesha's mother, brother, sister, and grandmother live in a three-bedroom apartment near the school. When entering the home, the nurse notes that the room is very warm and sees an older model space heater in the kitchen area. The mother explains she wants to keep it warm for Lateesha's little sister, a 4-year-old who has complained that the apartment is too cool during winter. The nurse also notes several ashtrays in the living room and the presence of Tigger, the family cat. The mother informs the nurse that Lateesha has had four severe colds since October and that the last physician they saw at the clinic suggested that Lateesha has asthma. The mother received two types of inhalers for Lateesha following this clinic visit but notes that no one explained whether Lateesha is to use the inhalers every day or only after she develops a cold or breathing difficulties.

1. What should be the focus of the interventions of the community health nurse with this family?

FYI

National Perspectives on Asthma Incidence in Urban Areas

A remarkable decrease in the incidence of many childhood communicable diseases has occurred during this century in U.S. populations; these conditions include diphtheria, pertussis, and polio. Unfortunately, this progress against many communicable diseases has been offset by an equally remarkable increase in asthma occurrence in both pediatric and adult populations in industrialized nations throughout the world. Overall asthma prevalence has increased by 58% since 1980; the mortality rate has increased by 78%. Children from urban areas and racial/ethnic communities have experienced the greatest increases in both prevalence and mortality. Hospitalization and morbidity rates for nonwhite children are almost twice those for white children. Asthma symptoms are caused by hyperresponsiveness of the airway to a number of common environmental allergens, including dust mites, animal dander, cockroaches, fungal spores, and pollens. Exacerbation of asthma has also been associated with air quality problems such as increased levels of sulfur dioxide, nitrogen dioxide, and ozone. Cigarette smoking as well as exposure to secondhand smoke also contribute to exacerbation of several childhood conditions such as otitis media, pneumonia, bronchitis, and asthma. Currently, approximately 30% of American preschoolers are exposed to residential tobacco smoke. Just as the precipitating factors for asthma are multiple, so too must be prevention efforts by nurses and other health providers. These efforts need to address household and community-based patterns of exposure as well as continuity of care and ongoing management for affected persons.

Source: Eggleston, Buckley, Breysse, Wills-Karp, Kleeberger, & Jaakkola 1999; Clark, Brosn, Parker, Robins, Remick, Philbert, Keeler, & Israel 1999.

aware that some agents have health consequences that may not be seen for years or decades, it can be difficult to take such a distant and uncertain threat seriously. One conceptual approach that has been used in interdisciplinary public health efforts, referred to as *upstream thinking,* uses the analogy of a river to demonstrate connections between preceding exposures and later health consequences. This approach is based on an article by

McKinlay (1979), who tells the story of a physician friend and his struggle to keep from feeling overwhelmed by the enormity of health problems that he encounters in clinical practice. The friend notes that he feels as if he is so caught up in rescuing individuals from the river that he has no time to look upstream to see who is pushing them in. In this analogy, the river represents illness and health providers' efforts to rescue people from illness.

However, in this portrayal no one receives care until they are downstream in the river of illness, which precludes efforts to intervene before illness develops. McKinlay challenges providers to look upstream, where the real problems lie. The river analogy includes many concepts in community health nursing, including the natural history of disease and levels of prevention. The power of the upstream conceptualization of health lies in its simplicity and the ease with which one can connect the causes of disease with their consequences.

Upstream thinking lends itself well to health problems of environmental origin and can be helpful in guiding practice decisions that have long- and short-term consequences for our clients. Examples of environmental upstream nursing actions include the following:

- *Instructing a client to wear a respirator when stripping paint from an old home*
- *Encouraging farmers who work with pesticides to refrain from wearing their work boots into the house*
- *Developing a school policy to establish waiting periods for children to be off the playground following applications of fertilizers and herbicides*

In each situation, the nurse is acting from a primary prevention viewpoint to prevent or minimize the occurrence of an exposure. It is not even necessary to know the toxicology of all of the agents involved. Nurses can initiate an action and then seek guidance from experts in toxicology or other disciplines. The goal is to minimize the opportunity for harm by linking an understanding of nursing actions today with the prevention of harmful health effects in the future (Butterfield, 1990).

Ethical Principles Addressing Environmental Health Nursing

Nurses have a duty to safeguard clients from environmental hazards and risks regardless of clients' income, insurance status, or lack of access to care. The nurses' code of ethics addresses responsibilities to collaborate with other health professionals and citizens in promoting community and national efforts to meet the health needs of the public (ANA, 1985).

Justice is a highly valued ethical principle in most societies today and is one of the beliefs that guide the practice of nursing. The concept of fairness of opportunity is a value in the United States that is supported in laws that forbid discriminatory treatment that limits one's opportunities on the basis of unchangeable characteristics such as gender, race, or socioeconomic status. **Social justice** means fairness or equality in the distribution of the benefits and burdens of society. According to the principles of social justice, no one person or group should have a disproportionate share of the benefits available to a society nor of the burdens that are present.

When applied to environmental health, principles of social justice suggest that the ability to live in a healthy environment as part of the process for attaining or maintaining health should be available to all. Because health is of fundamental importance to having opportunities for life, liberty, and the pursuit of happiness, environmental risks that take place or are allowed to persist differentially that are based on gender, race, or socioeconomic status would not be consistent with justice or fairness of opportunity (Daniels, 1985). Justice is not served when some persons or groups have disproportionate shares of the benefits of healthy

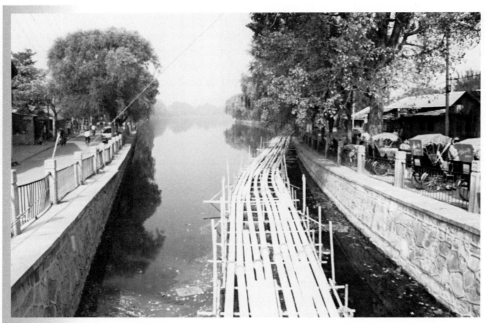

River in Hutong neighborhood in Beijing, China, demonstrating global clean-up efforts.

environments and others have disproportionate shares of the burdens of contaminated ones.

Most environmental hazards do not pose uniform or equal risks to the health of an entire population. Some widespread hazards, such as global warming, acid rain, and air or water pollution, involve an entire region or country, but most environmental health concerns involve different exposures within the same population. Some exposures occur because of behaviors or practices that could be considered changeable as a result of choices the individual makes. The decision to not wear protective gear when applying pesticides is an example of a choice that could easily be changed from health damaging to health protecting. Some exposures occur, however, because of unchangeable characteristics or circumstances of some individuals in the population, such as socioeconomic status, race, powerlessness, age, or gender. Lead exposure, for example, is most common in children who live in low-income housing. The disposal of toxic waste into sites located near low-income neighborhoods whose residents lack the financial resources and power to prevent it is another example of disproportionate exposure to environmental hazards (Bullard, 1990, 1993).

The distinction between changeable and unchangeable courses of action may not always be clear-cut. For example, the training one receives about pesticide safety and the availability of safety equipment may affect the use of safety measures more than personal choice. Many environmental risks occur from exposures to toxic substances on the job. Some individuals may have the ability to change occupations to reduce risks, but many others cannot reasonably entertain such an option. It also may be possible to alter some risks such as living in low-income housing with lead-based paint. In this example, although residents' incomes and ability to relocate may be unchangeable, they can work to improve the safety in their current housing and influence landlords to correct or reduce environmental hazards such as removal of lead-based paint.

FYI

In a nationwide survey more than 86,000 school children were asked what they worry about the most. Their answer? The environment!

Source: Environmental and Occupational Sciences Institute, Public Health and Risk Communication Division

Nurses play a role in promoting **environmental justice** in several ways. Educating individuals on ways to reduce exposure to toxic substances is important. Giving information about contacts in health departments or work safety committees is helpful to individuals and groups. Helping groups organize and present a united voice to industries and politicians is important to people who may otherwise have been powerless to protest. Community health nurses know the strengths of their communities and are able to identify the people who could provide leadership to the group. Community health nurses are also already sensitive to their community's cultural or ethnic attributes, which may affect the process of seeking environmental justice. Activists concerned about environmental hazards and social justice have also begun to work with and for disadvantaged groups to increase their awareness of unequal environmental risks and possible strategies to improve them. Disadvantaged at-risk groups in a particular area may not be organized into a functioning community or have community or neighborhood organizations that can be readily mobilized for action. In this case, activists work with whatever organizations exist or form an informal group of concerned residents who may get others involved over time. An environmental hazard close to where people live is an issue that can be effective in organizing and mobilizing citizens to work together as a group.

CONCLUSION

The role of community health nurses in environmental health is evolving in several ways:

- *From illness treatment to illness recognition and prevention*
- *Toward a multidisciplinary foundation of basic and applied science*
- *Toward an emphasis on activities in which nursing excels, such as risk communication, community-based investigations, and client advocacy strategies*
- *Toward an integration of environmental health principles into all domains of nursing practice and research*

Knowledge of pollutants, whether physical, chemical, or biological, is characterized by incomplete science. The field is constantly changing, with the discovery of new hazards, but also innovative ways of minimizing hazard use and exposure.

Nurses can participate in advancing environmental health science by participating in applied research activities on behalf of vulnerable groups or those disproportionately exposed to agents of concern.

Nurses have functioned at the fringe of power and politics, which has often been detrimental to the nursing profession, perhaps even to health care. In the field of environmental health, nurses are capable of making great contributions to the social, political, and economic forces that presently guide environmental health care policy. By broadening nurses' understanding of environment, new horizons in environmental health can be developed and expanded on behalf of the health of our clients, our nation, and our planet. The Case Study below uses a **thinking upstream** approach to explore nursing actions addressing social, economic, and political factors that culminate in the development of lead intoxication in children.

CASE STUDY

Broadening Nurses' Expertise in Environmental Health Clinical Practice—Thinking Upstream

Over the course of several years, a public health nurse was asked about water quality issues by clients attending the well-child clinic. These questions most commonly addressed parents' concerns about potable water contamination, and the nurse believed she was unqualified to answer these types of questions. After spending a few hours at home reviewing water quality information on the EPA's Internet home page, the nurse decided to seek some advice from the health department director about her lack of preparation to respond to clients' questions regarding environmental health. The director suggested that the nurse spend some time with a water quality specialist, who was located within another department, and authorized time for the nurse to work 1 week in that department. During her week with environmental health personnel, the nurse worked in the field when the environmental engineer inspected the installation of a private well west of town. She made a special ef-

fort to talk with all of the people in the environmental health department so that she had a better understanding of the full range of expertise within the department. After working in the field, she visited the laboratory to observe testing procedures for water quality and to learn about the different water tests available to the public.

When she returned to the well-child clinic the following week, the nurse decided to allocate at least half an hour per day to developing a resource library on water quality issues in the clinic. She obtained educational brochures from the environmental health department; in addition, she established a system where nurses could give interested clients a plastic bottle for water sampling and have them send it directly to the laboratory for analysis. The nurse also asked the environmental engineer to make his phone number available to respond to any questions from clients about their water and septic systems.

Over the next year, the nurse provided continuing education for the nursing staff until they became more comfortable providing clients with specific information about water quality and differentiating between questions they could answer and those that were best re-

CASE STUDY—CONT'D

ferred to the engineers and scientists in the other department. Nurses came to understand that the prevention of problems held the key to long-term sustainability of water quality in their community and ecosystem. Many of the same principles of prevention that were so familiar to them in public health nursing could be applied equally well to actions to reduce opportunities for water pollution.

During the next few months, the nursing staff reached beyond its original contacts with the environmental health department and extended further into partnerships with other environmental information and advocacy groups in the area. They worked with the local university's pollution preven-

tion program to display and educate clients about the safe disposal of household products and solvents, to reduce solid waste, and to increase participation in recycling of paint and motor oil. Nurses found that they could often incorporate several minutes of "pollution prevention" instruction into many well-child visits and that parents were often appreciative of this information. The nurses worked to make other health departments aware of their efforts and presented a summary of their program at their annual public health association conference. As a culmination of their work, the nurses developed an Internet site to educate professional colleagues throughout the nation on their growing expertise in water quality and pollution prevention.

BOX 12-5 RESOURCES FOR ENVIRONMENTAL HEALTH INFORMATION

Agency for Toxic Substances and Disease Registry (ATSDR): Part of the U.S. Public Health Service. It conducts public health assessments, health consultations and investigations, health education, applied research, and emergency response. It maintains an exposure registry and toxicological profiles.

ATSDR
1600 Clifton Rd. NE (E-60)
Atlanta, GA 30333
(404) 639-0500
(404) 639-6204 (Division of Health Education)

Association of Occupational and Environmental Clinics: Conducts information sharing, education, and research through a network of clinics. It provides professional training, community education, exposure and risk assessment, clinical evaluations, and consultation services.

AOEC
1010 Vermont Ave NW
Suite #513
Washington, D.C. 20005
(202) 347-4976

Fax: (202) 347-4950
E-mail: aoec@dgs.dgsys.com
http://occ-env.med.mc.duke.edu/oem/aoec.htm

Nurses Environmental Healthwatch: Involved in educating nurses about environmental concerns and nursing's role in bringing about a safe, healthy environment.

Nurses Environmental Healthwatch
181 Marshall Street
Duxbury, MA 02332

Centers for Disease Control and Prevention (CDC): Protects the public health of the nation by providing leadership and direction in the prevention and control of diseases and other preventable conditions. It also responds to public health emergencies.

CDC
1600 Clifton Road, NE
Atlanta, GA 30333
(404) 639-3286

Consumer Product Safety Commission: Provides information on health and safety effects related to consumer products. This agency has direct

Continued

BOX 12-5 RESOURCES FOR ENVIRONMENTAL HEALTH INFORMATION—CONT'D

jurisdiction over chronic and chemical hazards in consumer products.

Consumer Product Safety Commission
East West Towers
4340 East West Highway
Bethesda, MD 20814
(301) 504-0580
(800) 638-2772

Environmental Protection Agency (EPA): Responsible for coordinated and effective governmental action on behalf of the environment.

EPA
401 M Street SW
Washington, D.C. 20460
(202) 260-2090

National Center for Environmental Health (NCEH): Preventing or controlling disease or injury related to the interactions between people and the environment outside the workplace.

NCEH
Mailstop F29
4770 Buford Highway NE
Atlanta, GA 30341-3724
(404) 488-7003

National Institute of Environmental Health Sciences (NIEHS): Principal federal agency for biomedical research on the effects of chemical, physical, and biological environmental agents on human health and well-being.

NEIHS
P.O. Box 12233
Research Triangle Park, NC 27709
(919) 541-7825

Pesticide Education Center: Seeks to educate the public about the hazards and health effects of pesticides. Works with the individuals or groups, conducts workshops.

PEC
P.O. Box 420870
San Francisco, CA 94142-0870
(415) 391-8511

Society for Occupational and Environmental Health (SOEH): Includes scientists, academicians, and industry and labor leaders seeking to improve the quality of working and living places.

SOEH
6728 Old McLean Village Drive
McLean, VA 22101
(703) 556-9222

CRITICAL THINKING ACTIVITIES

1. Take a walk or a drive around your own neighborhood and identify any potential environmental health risks. What kind of prevention interventions can be done to minimize exposure to these hazards? As a nursing student, what role can you play?

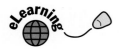

Explore Community Health Nursing on the web! To learn more about the topics in this chapter, use the passcode provided to access your exclusive web site:
http://communitynursing.jbpub.com
If you do not have a passcode, you can obtain one at this site.

REFERENCES

Agency for Toxic Substances and Disease Registry. (1992). *Case studies in environmental medicine (No. 26)—Taking an exposure history.* Atlanta: Author.

Amaya, M. A., Ackall, G., Pingitore, N., Quiroga, M., & Terrazas-Ponce, B. (1997). Childhood lead poisoning on the US-Mexico border: A case study in environmental health nursing lead poisoning. *Public Health Nursing, 14,* 353–360.

American Nurses Association (ANA). (1985). *Code for nurses with interpretive statements.* Kansas City, MO: Author.

Bullard, R. D. (1990). *Dumping in Dixie: Race, class, and environmental quality.* Boulder, CO: Westview Press.

Bullard, R. D. (1993). *Confronting environmental racism: Voices from the grassroots.* Boston: South End Press.

Butterfield, P. G. (1990). Thinking upstream: Nurturing a conceptual understanding of the societal context of health behavior. *Advanced Nursing Science, 12*(2), 1–8.

Carson R. (1962). *Silent spring.* Boston: Houghton Mifflin.

Clark N. M., Brosn, R. W., Parker, E., Robins, T. G., Remick, D. R. Jr., Philbert, M. A., Keeler, G. J., Israel, B. A. (1999). Childhood asthma. *Environmental Health Perspectives, 107*(Suppl. 3), 421–429.

Crenson, M. (1997, December 28). Kids at work in fields of unseen danger. *Missoulian,* p. A4.

Daniels, N. (1985). *Just health care.* Cambridge, MA: University Press.

Department of Health and Human Services, Public Health Service (DHHS). (1991). *Healthy people 2000* (Publication No. PHS-91-50212). Washington, DC: U.S. Government Printing Office.

Department of Health and Human Services, Public Health Service (DHHS). (2000). *Healthy People 2010. Conference edition.* Washington, DC: U.S. Government Printing Office.

Duchin, J. S, F. T. Koster, C. J. Peters, G. L. Simpson, B. Tempest, S. R. Zaki, T. G. Ksiazel, P. E. Rollin, S. Nichol, E. T. Umland, et al. (1994). Hantavirus pulmonary syndrome: A clinical description of 17 patients with a newly recognized disease. *New England Journal of Medicine, 330*(14), 949–955.

Eggleston, P. A., Buckley, T. J., Breysse, P. N., Wills-Karp, M, Kleeberger, S. R., Jaakkola, J. J. (1999). The environment and asthma in U.S. inner cities. *Environmental Health Perspectives, 107*(Suppl. 3), 439–450.

Environmental Protection Agency (EPA). (1993). *1991 toxics release inventory: Public data release* (EPA Pub. No. 745-R-93-003). Washington, DC: Office of Pollution Prevention and Toxics, EPA.

Fine, R. B. (1988). Consumerism and information: Power and confusion. *Nursing Administration Quarterly, 12*(3), 66–73.

Garrett, L. (1994). *The coming plague: Newly emerging diseases in a world out of balance.* New York: Penguin Books

Garte, S. J. (1992). Environmental carcinogenesis. In Rom, W. N. (Ed.), *Environmental and occupational medicine* (2nd ed., pp. 105–123). Boston: Little, Brown.

Gladen, B. C., Monaghan, S. C, Lukyanova, E. M., Hulchiy, O. P., Shkyryak-Nyzhnyk, Z. A., Sericano, J. L., & Little, R. E. (1999). Organocholines in breast milk from two cities in Ukraine. *Environmental Health Perspectives, 107*(6), 459–462.

Gore, A. (1992). *Earth in the balance: Ecology in the human spirit.* Boston: Houghton Mifflin Co.

Henson, R. H., Robinson, W. L., & Schmele, J. A. (1996). Consumerism and quality management. In Schmele J. A. (Ed.), *Quality management in nursing and healthcare.* Albany, NY: Delmar.

Hooper, K. (1999). Breast milk monitoring programs (BMMPs): World-wide early warning systems for polyhalogenated POPs and for targeting studies in children's environmental health. *Environmental Health Perspectives, 107*(6), 429–430.

Kimbrough, R. D. (1995). Polychlorinated biphenyls (PCBs) and human health: An update. *Critical Review Toxicology, 25,* 133–163.

Kleffel, D. (1991). Rethinking the environment as a domain of nursing knowledge. *Advanced Nursing Science, 14*(1), 40–51.

Kleffel, D. (1996). Environmental paradigms: Moving toward an eccentric perspective. *Advanced Nursing Science, 18*(4), 1–10.

Korrick, S. A., Hunter, D. J., Rotnitzky, A., Hu, H., & Speizer, F. E. (1999). Lead and hypertension in a sample of middle-aged women. *American Journal of Public Health, 89*(3), 330–335.

Last, J. M. (1993). Global change: Ozone depletion, greenhouse warming, and public health. *Annual Review of Public Health, 14,* 115–136.

Markowitz, M., Rosen, J. F., & Clemente, I. (1999). Clinician follow-up of children screened for lead poisoning. *American Journal of Public Health, 89*(7), 1088–1089.

McKinlay, J. B. (1979). A case for refocusing upstream: The political economy of illness. In Jaco E. G. (Ed.), *Patients, physicians, and illness* (3rd ed., pp. 9–25). New York: The Free Press.

Mendez, D., Warner, K. E., & Courant, P. N. (1998). Effects of radon mitigation vs. smoking cessation in reducing radon-related risk of lung cancer. *American Journal of Public Health, 88*(5), 811–812.

New Jersey Department of Environmental Protection. (1990). *Improving dialogue with communities: A risk communication manual for government*. New Brunswick, NJ: Author.

Nightingale, F. (1969). *Notes on nursing*. New York: Dover. (Originally published by D. Appleton and Company, 1860).

Pope, A. M., & Rall, D. P. (Eds.). (1995). *Environmental medicine: Integrating a missing element into medical education*. Washington, DC: National Academy Press.

Pope, A. M., Snyder, M. A., & Mood, L. H. (Eds.) (1995). *Nursing, health and the environment: Strengthening the relationship to improve the public's health*. Washington, DC: National Academy Press.

Schmidt, C. W. (1999). Poisoning young minds. *Environmental Health Perspectives, 107*(6), A307–307.

Shreffler, M. J. (1996). An ecological view of the rural environment: Levels of influence on access to health care. *Advanced Nursing Science, 18*(4), 48–59.

Steingraber, S. (1997). *Living downstream: An ecologist looks at cancer and the environment*. Reading, MA: Addison Wesley.

Stevens, P. E., & Hall, J. M.(1997). Environmental Health. In J. M Swanson & M. A. Nies (Eds.), *Community health nursing: Protecting the health of aggregates* (2nd ed., pp. 736–765). Philadelphia: W. B. Saunders.

Tiedje, L. B., & Wood, J. (1995). Sensitizing nurses for a changing environmental health role. *Public Health Nursing, 12*(6), 356–365.

U.S. Congress, Office of Technology Assessment. (1990, April). *Neurotoxicity: Identifying and controlling poisons of the nervous system* (Publication No. OTA-BA-436). Washington, DC: U.S. Government Printing Office.

Valanis, B. (1996). *Epidemiology in nursing and health care* (3rd ed.). Norwalk, CT: Appleton & Lange.

APPENDIX

ENVIRONMENTAL AGENTS AND THEIR ADVERSE HEALTH EFFECTS

Note: This table is not meant to be comprehensive, but to provide examples of several types of agents.

AGENT	EXPOSURE	ROUTE OF ENTRY	SYSTEM(S) AFFECTED	PRIMARY MANIFESTATIONS	AIDS IN DIAGNOSIS	REMARKS
METALS AND METALLIC COMPOUNDS						
ARSENIC	Alloyed with lead and copper for hardness; manufacturing of pigments, glass, pharmaceuticals; byproduct in copper smelting; insecticides; fungicides; rodenticides, tanning	Inhalation and ingestion of dust and fumes	Neuromuscular Gastrointestinal Skin Pulmonary	Peripheral neuropathy, sensory-motor Nausea and vomiting, diarrhea, constipation Dermatitis, finger and toenail striations, skin cancer, nasal septum perforation Lung cancer	Arsenic in urine	
ARSINE	Accidental byproduct of reaction of arsenic with acid; used in semi-conductor industry	Inhalation of gas	Hematopoietic	Intravascular hemolysis; hemoglobinuria, jaundice, oliguria or anuria	Arsenic in urine	
BERYLLIUM	Hardening agent in metal alloys; special use in nuclear energy production; metal refining or recovery	Inhalation of fumes or dust	Pulmonary (and other systems)	Granulomatosis and fibrosis	Beryllium in urine (acute); Beryllium in tissue (chronic); chest x-ray; immunological tests (such as lymphocyte transformation) may also be useful	Pulmonary changes virtually indistinguishable from sarcoid on chest x-ray
CADMIUM	Electroplating; solder for aluminum; metal alloys, process engraving; nickel-cadmium batteries	Inhalation or ingestion of fumes or dust	Pulmonary Renal	Pulmonary edema (acute); Emphysema (chronic) Nephrosis	 Urinary protein	Also a respiratory tract carcinogen
CHROMIUM	In stainless and heat-resistant steel and alloy steel; metal plating; chemical and pigment manufacturing; photography	Percutaneous absorption, inhalation, ingestion	Pulmonary Skin	Lung cancer Dermatitis, skin ulcers, nasal septum perforation	Urinary chromate (questionable value)	
LEAD	Storage batteries; manufacturing of paint, enamel, ink, glass, rubber, ceramics, chemical industry	Ingestion of dust, inhalation of dust or fumes	Hematological Renal Gastrointestinal Neuromuscular	Anemia Nephrotoxicity Abdominal pain ("colic") Palsy ("wrist drop") Encephalopathy, behavioral abnormalities	Blood lead Urinary ALA Zinc proto porphyrin; free erythrocyte protophyrin	Lead toxicity, unlike that of mercury, is believed to be reversible, with the exception of late renal and

Source: Tarcher, A. B. (Ed.). (1992). Principles and practice of environmental medicine. *New York: Plenum Press.*

Continued

AGENT	EXPOSURE	ROUTE OF ENTRY	SYSTEM(S) AFFECTED	PRIMARY MANIFESTATIONS	AIDS IN DIAGNOSIS	REMARKS
METALS AND METALLIC COMPOUNDS—cont'd						
LEAD cont'd			Central nervous system (CNS) Reproductive	Spontaneous abortion (?)		some CNS effects
MERCURY Elemental	Electronic equipment; paint; metal and textile production; catalyst in chemical manufacturing; pharmaceutical production	Inhalation of vapor; slight percutaneous absorption	Pulmonary CNS	Acute pneumonitis Neuropsychiatric changes (erethism); tremor	Urinary mercury	Mercury illustrates several principles. The chemical form has a profound effect on its toxicology, as is the case for many metals. Effects of mercury are highly variable. Though inorganic mercury poisoning is primarily renal, elemental and organic poisoning are primarily neurological.
MERCURY Inorganic	Agricultural and industrial poisons	Some inhalation and gastrointestinal (GI) and percutaneous absorption	Pulmonary Renal CNS	Acute pneumonitis Proteinuria Variable	Urinary mercury	The responses are difficult to quantify, so dose-response data are generally unavailable.
Organic		Efficient GI absorption, percutaneous absorption, and inhalation	Skin CNS	Dermatitis Sensorimotor changes, visual field constriction, tremor	Blood and urine mercury (?sensitivity)	Classic tetrad of gingivitis, sialorrhea, irritability, and tremor is associated with both elemental and inorganic mercury poisoning; the four signs are not generally seen together. Many effects of mercury toxicity, especially those in CNS, are irreversible.
Nickel	Corrosion-resistant alloys; electroplating; catalyst production; nickel-cadmium batteries	Inhalation of dust or fumes	Skin Pulmonary	Sensitization dermatitis ("nickel itch") Lung and paranasal sinus cancer		
ZINC OXIDE	Welding byproduct; rubber manufacturing	Inhalation of dust or fumes that are freshly generated		"Metal fume fever" (fever, chills, and other symptoms)	Urinary zinc (useful as an indicator of exposure, not for acute diagnosis)	A self-limiting syndrome of 24-48 hours with apparently no sequelae

Agent	Exposure	Route of Entry	System(s) Affected	Primary Manifestations	Aids in Diagnosis	Remarks
HYDROCARBONS						
BENZENE	Manufacturing of organic chemicals, detergents, pesticides, solvents, paint removers; used as a solvent	Inhalation of vapor; slight percutaneous absorption	CNS Hematopoietic Skin	Acute CNS depression Leukemia, aplastic anemia Dermatitis	Urinary phenol	Note that benzene, as with toluene and other solvents, can be monitored via its principal metabolite
TOLUENE	Organic chemical manufacturing; solvent; fuel component	Inhalation of vapor, percutaneous absorption of liquid	CNS Skin	Acute CNS depression Chronic CNS problems such as memory loss Irritation dermatitis	Urinary hippuric acid	
XYLENE	A wide variety of uses as a solvent; an ingredient of paints, lacquers, varnishes, inks, dyes, adhesives, cements; an intermediate in chemical manufacturing	Inhalation of vapor; slight percutaneous absorption of liquid	Pulmonary Eye, nose, throat CNS	Irritation, pneumonitis, acute pulmonary edema (at high doses) Irritation Acute CNS depression	Methylhippuric acid in urine, Xylene in expired air, xylene in blood	
KETONES Acetone(Methyl ethyl Ketone-MEK, Methyl n-proply Ketone-MPK, Methyl n-butyl Ketone-MBK, Methyl iso-butyl Ketone-MIBK	A wide variety of uses as solvents and intermediates in chemical manufacturing	Inhalation of vapor, percutaneous absorption of liquid	CNS Peripheral nervous system (PNS) Skin	Acute CNS depression MBK has been linked with peripheral neuropathy Dermatitis	Acetone in blood, urine, expired air (used as an index for exposure, not for diagnosis)	The ketone family demonstrates how a pattern of toxic responses (i.e., CNS narcosis) may feature exceptions (i.e., MBK peripheral neuropathy)
FORMALDEHYDE	Widely used as a germicide and a disinfectant in embalming and histopathology, for example, and in the manufacture of textiles, resins, and other products	Inhalation	Skin Eye Pulmonary	Irritant and contact dermatitis Eye irritant Respiratory tract irritation, asthma	Patch testing may be useful for dermatitis	Recent animal tests have shown it to be a respiratory carcinogen. Confirmatory epidemiological studies are in progress
TRICHLORO-ETHYLENE (TCE)	Solvent in metal degreasing, dry cleaning, food extraction; ingredient of paints, adhesives, varnishes, inks	Inhalation, percutaneous absorption	Nervous Skin Cardiovascular	Acute CNS depression Peripheral and cranial neuropathy Irritation, dermatitis Dysrhythmias	Breath analysis for TCE	TCE is involved in an important pharmacological interaction. Within hours of ingesting alcoholic beverages, TCE workers experience flushing of the face, neck, shoulders, and *Continued*

Agent	Exposure	Route of Entry	System(s) Affected	Primary Manifestations	Aids in Diagnosis	Remarks
HYDROCARBONS—cont'd						
TRICHLORO-ETHYLENE (TCE) cont'd						back. Alcohol may also potentiate the CNS effects of TCE. The probable mechanism is competition for metabolic enzymes
CARBON TETRACHLORIDE	Solvent for oils, fats, lacquers, resins, varnishes, other materials; used as a degreasing and cleaning agent	Inhalation of vapor	Hepatic Renal CNS Skin	Toxic hepatitis Oliguria or anuria Acute CNS depression Dermatitis	Expired air and blood levels	Carbon tetrachloride is the prototype for a wide variety of solvents that cause hepatic and renal damage. This solvent, like trichloroethylene, acts synergistically with ethanol
CARBON DISULFIDE	Solvent for lipids, sulfur, halogens, rubber, phosphorus, oils, waxes, and resins; manufacturing of organic chemicals, paints, fuels, explosives, viscose rayon	Inhalation of vapor, percutaneous absorption of liquid or vapor	Nervous Renal Cardiovascular Skin Reproductive	Parkinsonism, psychosis, suicide Peripheral neuropathies Chronic nephritic and nephrotic syndromes Acceleration or worsening of atherosclerosis; hypertension Irritation; dermatitis Menorrhagia and metrorrhagia	Iodine-azide reaction with urine (nonspecific since other bivalent sulfur compounds give a positive test); CS_2 in expired air, blood, and urine	A solvent with unusual multi-system effects, especially noted for its cardiovascular, renal, and nervous system actions
STODDARD SOLVENT	Degreasing, paint thinning	Inhalation of vapor, percutaneous absorption of liquid	Skin CNS	Dryness and scaling from defatting; dermatitis Dizziness, coma, collapse (at high levels)		A mixture of primarily alpha-tic hydrocarbons, with some benzene derivatives and naphthalenes
ETHYLENE GLYCOL ETHERS (Ethylene glycol monoethyl ether-Cellosolve, Ethylene glycol monoethyl acetate-Cellosolve acetate, Methyl- and butyl-substituted compounds such as ethylene glycol mono-methyl ether-methyl Cellosolve	The ethers are used as solvents for resins, paints, lacquers, varnishes, gum, perfume, dyes, and inks; the acetate derivatives are widely used as solvents and ingredients of lacquers, enamels, and adhesives. Exposure occurs in dry cleaning, plastic, ink, and lacquer manufacturing, and textile dying, among other processes.	Inhalation of vapor, percutaneous absorption of liquid	Reproductive CNS Renal Liver			Ethylene glycol ethers, as a class of chemicals, have been shown in animals to have adverse effects including reduced sperm count and spontaneous abortion, as well as CNS, renal, and liver effects

Agent	Exposure	Route of Entry	System(s) Affected	Primary Manifestations	Aids in Diagnosis	Remarks
HYDROCARBONS—cont'd						
ETHYLENE OXIDE	Used in the sterilization of medical equipment, in the fumigation of spices and other foodstuffs, as a chemical intermediate	Inhalation	Skin	Dermatitis and frostbite		Recent animal tests have shown it to be carcinogenic and to cause reproductive abnormalities. Epidemiologic studies indicate that it may cause leukemia in exposed workers
			Eye	Severe irritation; possibly cataracts with prolonged exposure		
			Respiratory tract	Irritation		
			Nervous system	Peripheral neuropathy		
DIOXANE	Used as a solvent for a variety of materials, including cellulose acetate, dyes, fats, greases, resins, polyvinyl polymers, varnishes, and waxes	Inhalation of vapor, percutaneous absorption of liquid	CNS	Drowsiness, dizziness, anorexia, headaches, nausea, vomiting, coma		Dioxane has caused a variety of neoplasms in animals
			Renal	Nephritis		
			Liver	Chemical hepatitis		
POLY-CHLORINATED BIPHENYLS (PCBS)	Formerly used as dielectric fluid in electrical equipment and as a fire retardant coating on tiles and other products. New uses were banned in 1976, but much of the electrical equipment currently used still contains PCBs	Inhalation, ingestion, skin absorption	Skin	Chloracne	Serum PCB level for chronic exposure	Animal studies have demonstrated that PCBs are carcinogenic. Epidemiological studies of exposed workers are inconclusive
			Eye	Irritation		
			Liver	Toxic hepatitis		
IRRITANT GASES						
AMMONIA	Refrigeration; petroleum refining; manufacturing of nitrogen-containing chemicals, synthetic fibers, dyes, and optics	Inhalation of gas	Upper respiratory tract	Upper respiratory irritation		
			Eye	Irritation		
			Moist skin	Irritation		
HYDROCHLORIC ACID	Chemical manufacturing; electroplating; tanning; metal pickling; petroleum extraction; rubber, photographic, and textile industries	Inhalation of gas or mist	Upper respiratory tract	Upper respiratory irritation		
			Eye	Strong irritant		
			Mucous membranes, skin	Strong irritant		

Continued

AGENT	EXPOSURE	ROUTE OF ENTRY	SYSTEM(S) AFFECTED	PRIMARY MANIFESTATIONS	AIDS IN DIAGNOSIS	REMARKS
IRRITANT GASES—cont'd						
HYDROFLUORIC ACID	Chemical and plastic manufacturing; catalyst in petroleum refining; aqueous solution for frosting, etching, and polishing glass	Inhalation of gas or mist	Upper respiratory tract	Upper respiratory irritation		In solution, causes severe and painful burns of skin and can be fatal
SULFUR DIOXIDE	Manufacturing of sulfur-containing chemicals; food and textile bleach; tanning; metal casting	Inhalation of gas, direct contact of gas or liquid phase on skin or mucosa	Middle respiratory tract	Bronchospasm (pulmonary edema or chemical pneumonitis in high dose)	Chest x-ray, pulmonary function tests	Strong irritant of eyes, mucous membranes, and skin
CHLORINE	Paper and textile bleaching; water disinfection; chemical manufacturing, metal fluxing; detinning and dezincing iron	Inhalation of gas	Middle respiratory tract	Tracheobronchitis, pulmonary edema, pneumonitis	Chest x-ray, pulmonary function tests	
OZONE Chlorine combines with body moisture to form acids, which irritate tissues from nose to alveoli.	Inert gas-shielded arc welding; food, water, and air purification; food and textile bleaching; emitted around high-voltage electrical equipment	Inhalation of gas	Lower respiratory tract	Delayed pulmonary edema (generally 6-8 hours following exposure)	Chest x-ray, pulmonary function tests	Ozone has a free radical structure and can produce experimental chromosome aberrations; it may thus have carcinogenic potential.

Agent	Exposure	Route of Entry	System(s) Affected	Primary Manifestations	Aids in Diagnosis	Remarks
IRRITANT GASES—cont'd						
NITROGEN OXIDES	Manufacturing of acids, nitrogen containing chemicals, explosives, and more; byproduct of many industrial processes	Inhalation of gas	Lower respiratory tract	Pulmonary irritation, bronchiolitis fibrosa obliterations ("silo filler's disease"), mixed obstructive-restrictive changes	Chest x-ray, pulmonary function tests	
PHOSGENE	Manufacturing and burning of isocyanates, and manufacturing of dyes and other organic chemicals; in metallurgy for one separation; burning or heat source near trichloroethylene	Inhalation of gas	Lower respiratory tract	Delayed pulmonary edema (delay seldom longer than 12 hours)	Chest x-ray, pulmonary function tests	
Isocyanates TDI (toluene diisocyanate) MDI (methylene diphenyldiisocyanate) Hexamethylene diisocyanate and others	Polyurethane manufacture; resin-binding systems in foundries; coating materials for wires; used in certain types of paint	Inhalation of vapor	Predominantly lower respiratory tract	Asthmatic reaction and accelerated loss of pulmonary function	Chest x-ray, pulmonary function tests	Isocyanates are both respiratory tract "sensitizers" and irritants in the conventional sense.
ASPHYXIANT GASES (simple asphyxiants: nitrogen, hydrogen, methane, and others)	Enclosed spaces in a variety of industrial settings	Inhalation of gas	CNS	Anoxia	O_2 in environment	No specific toxic effect; act by displacing O_2

Continued

Agent	Exposure	Route of Entry	System(s) Affected	Primary Manifestations	Aids in Diagnosis	Remarks
CHEMICAL ASPHYXIANTS						
CARBON MONOXIDE	Incomplete combustion in foundries, coke ovens, refineries, furnaces, and more	Inhalation of gas	Blood (hemoglobin)	Headache, dizziness, double vision	Carboxy-hemoglobin	
HYDROGEN SULFIDE	Used in manufacturing of sulfur-containing chemicals; produced in petroleum product use; decay of organic matter	Inhalation of gas	CNS Pulmonary	Respiratory center paralysis, hypoventilation Respiratory tract irritation	PaO$_2$	
CYANIDE	Metallurgy, electroplating	Inhalation of vapor, percutaneous absorption, ingestion	Cellular metabolic enzymes (especially cytochrome oxidase)	Enzyme inhibition with metabolic asphyxia and death	SCN in urine	
PESTICIDES						
ORGANOPHOS-PHATES (malathion, parathion, and others)		Inhalation, ingestion, percutaneous absorption	Neuromuscular	Cholinesterase inhibition, cholinergic symptoms: nausea and vomiting, salivation, diarrhea, headache, sweating, meiosis, muscle fasciculations, seizures, unconsciousness, death	Refractoriness to atropine; plasma or red cell cholinesterase	As with many acute toxins, rapid treatment of organophosphate toxicity is imperative. Thus diagnosis is often based on history and a high index of suspicion rather than biochemical tests. Treatment is atropine to block cholinergic effects and 2-pyradine-alsoxine methiodide (2-PAM) to reactivate cholinesterase

Agent	Exposure	Route of Entry	System(s) Affected	Primary Manifestations	Aids in Diagnosis	Remarks
PESTICIDES—cont'd						
CARBAMATES: (carbaryl [Sevin] and others)		Inhalation, ingestion, percutaneous absorption	Neuromuscular	Cholinesterase inhibition, cholinergic symptoms: nausea and vomiting, salivation, diarrhea, headache, sweating, meiosis, muscle fasciculations, seizures, unconsciousness, death	Plasma cholinesterase; urinary 1-naphthol (index of exposure)	Treatment of carbamate poisoning is the same as that of organophosphate poisoning except that 2-PAM is contra-indicated
CHLORINATED HYDRO-CARBONS chlordane DDT heptachlor chlordecone (Kepone) aldrin dieldrin uridine		Inhalation, ingestion, percutaneous absorption	CNS	Stimulation or depression	Urinary organic chlorine, or p-chlorophenol acetic acid	The chlorinated hydrocarbons may accumulate in body lipid stores in large amounts.
BIPYRIDYLS paraquat diquat		Inhalation, ingestion, percutaneous absorption	Pulmonary	Rapid massive fibrosis, only following paraquat ingestion		An interesting toxin in that the major toxicity, pulmonary fibrosis, apparently occurs only after ingestion.

Unit III
Care of Communities and Populations

Chapter 13

Health Promotion and Wellness

Joan H. Baldwin and Cynthia O'Neill Conger

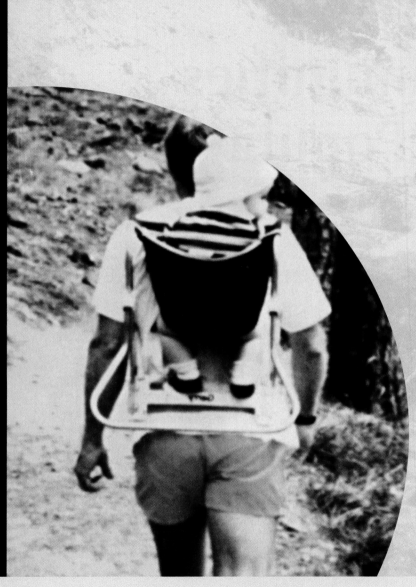

All of the information about exercise, eating right, and how my body works helped me change the physical me. The most important part is to understand that it's not as much about the weight as it is about making the connection. That means looking after yourself every day and putting forth your best effort to love yourself enough to do what's best for you. . . . The biggest change I've made is a spiritual one. It comes from the realization that taking care of my body and my health is really one of the greatest kinds of love I can give myself. . . . And there's no question I'm living a better life.

Oprah Winfrey (Greene & Winfrey, 1996, p. 32)

CHAPTER FOCUS

Basic Concepts of Health and Health Promotion
- Selected Definitions of Health Promotion and Wellness
- Community Health Promotion and Wellness

Factors Influencing Health Promotion and Wellness
- Changes in Societal Expectations
- Shifting Sands of the Health Care Delivery System

United States Government Initiatives
Public/Private Partnerships
Growing Consumerism and Emphasis on Self-Care

Models of Health Promotion and Wellness
- Holistic Wellness: Self-Inventory of Personal Wellness Using the Medicine Wheel
- The 4 + Model of Wellness

QUESTIONS TO CONSIDER

After reading this chapter, answer the following questions:
1. What is the difference between health promotion and wellness?
2. What are levels of prevention?
3. What do health promotion and wellness look like?
4. What factors influence health promotion and wellness?
5. What are the different models for health promotion?
6. How can community health nurses use these models in the promotion of health in their clients?
7. How can a nurse use these concepts to promote self-health?

KEY TERMS

Health-promoting behaviors	High-level wellness	Professional health promotion
Health promotion	Levels of prevention	Wellness
	Personal health promotion	

Health promotion and wellness are important concepts through-out nursing education and practice in all settings. Nurses promote good health and wellness for themselves, their loved ones, and clients. Generally, the major steps to health and wellness include healthy eating, proper exercise, adequate sleep, and time to un-wind and manage stress. Health promotion in this respect has al-ways been a nursing focus. As the health care delivery system moves further into managed care, however, health promotion and wellness become still more important. Health promotion and dis-ease prevention are the keys to managing health care costs. Pro-moting the health of individuals, families, populations, and com-munities is essential in nursing practice not only because it is the humane and ethical thing to do but also because of its practical and economic benefits.

It may be surprising to learn that there are several different definitions for the terms *health promotion* and *wellness*. There are definitions of health promotion and wellness for self, for other individuals, and even for populations and communities.

What do nurses really mean when they say they promote good health and wellness? There are many, many aspects of health promotion and wellness that will be important to know as a professional nurse. This chapter (1) briefly discusses basic con-cepts of health and health promotion as related to the concept of disease prevention, including definitions of *health promotion* and *wellness* as the terms are used in this chapter; (2) delineates fac-tors influencing health promotion and wellness; (3) demon-strates some ways of looking at health promotion and wellness by discussing some models of health promotion, risk evaluation, and analysis tools, plus wellness guides that might be useful to know about to promote health and wellness; and (4) introduces two recent models of wellness.

Basic Concepts of Health and Health Promotion

How people generally define health may influence how they de-fine health promotion (Baldwin, 1995; Green & Raeburn, 1990). For instance, if health is considered the absence of disease, the de-finition of health promotion would necessarily include the idea of disease prevention. However, if health is defined as a concept that expresses the positiveness of a full and joyful life, disease preven-tion is not a part of the definition. Edelman and Fain (1998) speak of this second characterization of health as "expanding con-sciousness, pattern or meaning recognition, personal transforma-tion, and tentatively, self-actualization" (p. 9). One example is a woman living with a chronic disease such as diabetes, who still considers herself a healthy person; she may see herself being as far along toward self-actualization as she can be.

In 1983, Brubaker conducted a linguistic analysis of the term *health promotion* in nursing literature and found that it was rarely defined specifically and often used as though it had the same meaning as disease prevention. There continues to be de-bate about the definition of health promotion and whether the definition must necessarily include disease prevention.

Historically, health promotion as a concept has been linked with disease prevention. Clark and Leavell (1965) depicted three levels of prevention—primary, secondary, and tertiary—in a model; primary prevention includes health promotion as part of the model. When primary prevention methods are used, the ba-sic premise of the model is that health-promotion activities "serve to further general health and well-being" (Clark & Leavell, 1965, p. 20). Because this is a model describing disease preven-tion factors, it leads one to connect health promotion with dis-ease prevention. In this particular model, primary prevention methods include health-promoting behaviors that are designed to improve general health and well-being, with the emphasis be-ing on preventing a disease in the first place. For instance, brush-ing teeth after meals is one step in preventing tooth decay, which would also be good for general health.

As early as 1965, Clark and Leavell noted that "health pro-motion is not applied for specific disease and as yet is not widely utilized" (p. 24). Identifying health-promoting strategies for sec-ondary and tertiary prevention still seems to be a bit difficult to-day, but health-promoting activities are important in these levels as well. *Secondary prevention* refers to the early detection of dis-ease and prevention of disease sequelae—"abnormal conditions resulting from a previous disease" (*Webster's Encyclopedic Dictio-nary*, 1996, p. 1747). A health-promotion action for a woman who has a diagnosis of fibrocystic breast disease would be to avoid caffeine. Poe and O'Neill (1997) determined that caffeine slows the process of the body's natural defenses, which normally results in the elimination of precancerous cells. Therefore, the potential for proliferation of abnormal cells is increased with caf-feine ingestion. Tertiary prevention focuses on the minimization of loss of function as a result of disease. Health-promotion activ-ities in tertiary prevention might include training for a competi-tion by a diabetic skier who has only one leg. Good and reason-able physical fitness promotes health.

Today there are also reasons for using health-promotion strategies, behaviors, or actions without necessarily having to consider prevention of disease. Someone may choose certain health-promotion actions just because the actions make the per-son feel good or healthy. For example, many people like to walk or run several times a week and comment that if they don't walk or run, they don't have as much energy during the day. In this ex-ample, these people are not specifically concerned about pre-venting disease, they just want to feel as good as they can.

Selected Definitions of Health Promotion and Wellness

For the purposes of this chapter, health promotion has two defi-nitions depending on if the nurse is applying health-promotion strategies to other people or if the nurse is promoting his or her own health. The definition of professional health promotion on behalf of others reflects the "organized actions or efforts that enhance, support, or promote the well-being or health of individuals, families, groups, communities, or societies" (Kulbok, Baldwin, Cox, & Duffy, 1997, p. 17). An example of this definition is when a school nurse teaches elementary school children the importance of washing hands to eliminate germs and dirt. The nurse first coats the children's hands with an invisible product that can be washed away with soap and water. After handwashing, a special light is shined on the children's hands; areas not carefully washed clean of the product glow green, demonstrating to the children that if hands are not carefully washed, "germs" may remain, much like the green, glowing product. Health education programs and physical education activities, to name two possibilities, are also examples of professional health promotion on behalf of others.

Personal health promotion reflects more emphasis on self-actualization and taking care of oneself. This definition identifies what motivates people "to attain and maintain their highest state of wellness, overall fitness, and self-actualization" (Baldwin, 1992, p. 10). For instance, the school nurse may recognize that walking daily for 30 minutes after work maintains physical fitness, dissipates work stress, and provides a sense of renewal and joy as she or he appreciates the spring flowers blooming.

What is the relationship between health promotion and wellness? As defined in this chapter, health promotion relates to behaviors or activities that result in wellness. Dunn (1959) describes **high-level wellness** as "an integrated method of functioning which is oriented toward maximizing the potential of which the individual is capable" (p. 447). The concept of high-level wellness is based on the assumption that every individual, regardless of personal challenges, has a potential for wellness within the limits placed by the challenge. In other words, high-level wellness is the highest level of well-being that a person can reach. To attain high-level wellness, there must be harmony in all aspects of a person's life. Box 13-1 lists two definitions of health promotion.

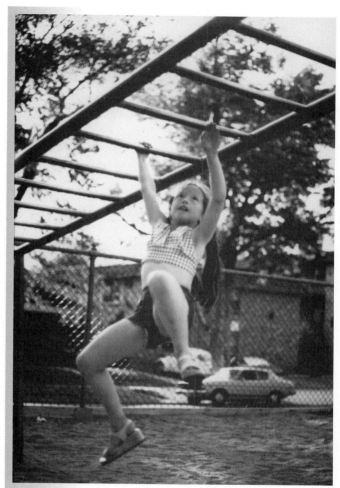

Children who are active earlier in life help decrease their risks for health problems as young adults.

BOX 13-1 KEY CONCEPTS: DEFINITIONS OF HEALTH PROMOTION

Health promotion by professionals on behalf of others is *"organized actions or efforts that enhance, support, or promote the well-being or health of individuals, families, groups, communities, or societies"* (Kulbok, Baldwin, Cox, & Duffy, 1997, p. 17).

Personal health promotion is *identification of what motivates people "to attain and maintain their highest state of wellness, overall fitness, and self-actualization"* (Baldwin, 1992, p. 10)

Health promotion and wellness, particularly when defined for one's own use, are closely related or even interrelated. In this chapter, *wellness* is a state of being; *health promotion* is how one gets there (Box 13-2). How one attains and maintains wellness is accomplished through various health-promoting behaviors. Examples of some health-promoting behaviors include (1) walking for at least 30 minutes 6 days a week, preferably with some intensity as though a bit late for an appointment (Bach, 1998); (2) eating foods that have omega-3 or monounsaturated fats, limiting daily total fat intake to less than 25% of total calories (Simopoulos, 1999); (3) adapting traditionally high-calorie or high-fat recipes to today's healthier levels (Jones, 1999); (4) meditating or visualizing to increase well-being (Cohen, 1998); and (5) learning how to relax (Cohen, 1998). Researchers today are emphasizing health-promoting activities such as these for individuals, families, populations, and communities to attain and

BOX 13-2 DEFINITIONS OF WELLNESS, HEALTH-PROMOTING BEHAVIORS, AND THE INTERRELATIONSHIP BETWEEN HEALTH PROMOTION AND WELLNESS

High-level wellness is *"an integrated method of functioning which is oriented toward maximizing the potential of which the individual is capable"* (Dunn, 1959, p. 447).

Health-promoting behaviors are *"any actions or behaviors taken by individuals to improve or promote well-being or health"* (Kulbok, Baldwin, Cox, & Duffy, 1997, p. 17). These *"behaviors [are those] that enhance, support, encourage and/or promote a healthy state"* (Kulbok, Carter, Baldwin, Gilmartin, & Kirkwood, 1999).

The interrelationship of health promotion and wellness *can be represented by the idea that wellness is a state of being, and health promotion is how one gets there.*

maintain states of wellness (Cohen, 1998; Mandle & Castle, 1998; McCarthy & Mandle, 1998a, 1998b; Sandhu, 1998).

A person can be sick and be moving toward wellness using health-promoting actions or behaviors or can have a chronic disease and actually be experiencing high-level wellness. Remember, high-level wellness means "maximizing the potential of which the individual is capable" (Dunn, 1959, p. 447). So, if the diabetic woman mentioned earlier in this chapter is maintaining a healthy lifestyle, has no difficulty managing her diabetes, is happy, and feels well-balanced in her life, it could be said that the woman is likely to be experiencing high-level wellness. The woman is maximizing the potential of which she is capable.

The woman with diabetes is the one most likely to know what her maximum potential can be and how close she is to reaching it in her life. What high-level wellness is, using Dunn's (1959) definition, for any particular person is defined by that person and may change over time.

How can a 22-year-old student nurse who is in a car accident and becomes a paraplegic reach high-level wellness? According to the aforementioned definitions, the student nurse has a potential to be more or less well within the boundaries of the limits set by the condition. "Wellness is a bridge that takes people into realms far beyond treatment or therapy—into a domain of self-responsibility and self-empowerment" (Ryan & Travis, 1991, p. 3). The student nurse has choices. Relating to personal life, the student nurse has the choice to (1) do nothing about overcoming the physical, emotional, mental, and spiritual challenges of being a paraplegic; (2) learn to use a wheelchair to go to classes and elsewhere; or (3) perhaps even go so far as to become a gold medalist in the

ParaOlympics. Professionally, the student nurse can bend to the pressure of the barriers and drop out of the nursing program or fight the system to remain, making adjustments as necessary. There is no reason that a full, satisfying, professional nursing career should be out of reach for this student.

It is important to note that nurses do not define high-level wellness for clients, but rather they assist clients in identifying what they are capable of reaching to maximize their potential for high-level wellness. Remember what was noted earlier in the chapter: high-level wellness is the highest level of well-being *that clients can reach.* An overweight, heavy-smoking, heavy-drinking person may think, and even state, the belief that he or she is healthy, but given Dunn's definition, it is unlikely that the person is experiencing high-level wellness and maximizing his or her potential to the best of his or her abilities. It is relatively easy to apply this concept to individuals, but how does high-level wellness translate to communities?

Community Health Promotion and Wellness

Communities have potential for high-level wellness as well. Communities can be defined within geographic boundaries or as population groups with special needs or interests (Baldwin, Conger, Abegglen, & Hill, 1998). Communities usually have systems in place, such as planning commissions or committees, to identify what is high-level wellness for that group. For example, one element of wellness identified in the motto for Sandy City, Utah, is support for family values. One way the community supports family values is by promoting healthy family activities. Toward this end, the community master plan establishes a network of neighborhood parks that will be developed as neighborhoods expand. This process maximizes the potential of the community to reach what it has defined as high-level wellness.

Some community interventions that support wellness are relatively easy to identify by community members. Others, especially related to population wellness, are more difficult for communities to pinpoint. Nurses often collaborate with community groups to identify these strengths, assets, problems, and needs.

People with chronic and even terminal diseases may live their lives in such a healthy and balanced manner that high-level wellness might be attained, at least for a time. A person can use health-promotion behaviors and activities even if ill or diseased "to become an active participant in the healing process instead of a passive recipient" (Ryan & Travis, 1991, p.3).

Factors Influencing Health Promotion and Wellness

It is important to recognize that health care in the United States is finally experiencing a shift in focus from a rather one-sided emphasis on present and potential disease to a more balanced focus that includes an equal emphasis on health promotion, wellness, risk reduction, and disease prevention (Baldwin, Conger, Abegglen, & Hill, 1998). Educating clients, defined as individuals, families, populations, or communities, regarding their health requires information about health-promotion activities that the clients consider relevant to them. It is because of this shift in focus that we now are more strongly accentuating the importance of understanding the "why's" and "how-to's" of health promotion and wellness. Some of the factors influencing health promotion and wellness are the changes in societal expectations, shifting sands of the health care delivery system, U.S. government initiatives, public/private partnerships, and growing consumerism and emphasis on self-care.

Changes in Societal Expectations

Over the years, people in the United States have vacillated as to what good health and wellness are all about. Some cultures had lifestyles that encompassed running and athletic feats, such as hunting, that sustained life; other groups were much more sedentary. Types of foods eaten varied, and little attention was paid to what foods were healthy or what foods were not; the important thing was being able to eat. Prior to the 1960s, the social system was such that the majority of people spent more time worrying

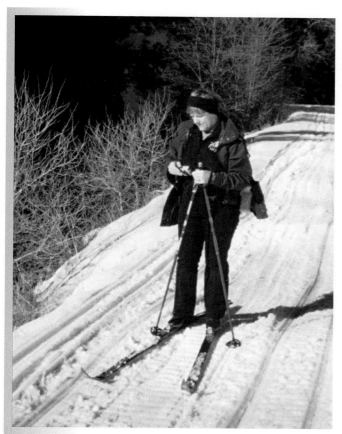

Vigorous exercise of large muscle groups lowers heart disease risks and promotes well-being in women.

about food, shelter, and safety (lower levels of Maslow's hierarchy) (Maslow, 1970) than self-actualization. The relationship of lifestyle and health had not been established scientifically. Health was primarily defined as the absence of disease, and health care delivery and research focused on controlling and trying to cure communicable diseases. The media played little or no role in sharing health-related information with the public other than reporting morbidity and mortality information.

Since the 1960s, societal expectations have changed. Increasing affluence has allowed the majority of society to move beyond a primary concern with food, shelter, and safety toward achieving self-esteem and self-actualization (Maslow, 1970). High-level wellness is a state of self-actualization, "maximizing the potential of which the individual is capable" (Dunn, 1959, p. 447). During the 1950s and 1960s, the leading causes of morbidity and mortality moved from communicable disease to chronic disease. With this shift, the health care profession had less success in controlling the causes of disease or in curing some of the diseases. Instead of cure, the focus became symptom management. It became more obvious that the method of control for chronic disease begins with health promotion and specific preventive measures. Since the mid-1960s, there has been a proliferation of research relating health promotion and wellness to lifestyle practices. This information has become so popular that the media has developed an interest in reporting health-promotion strategies. Today, experts on morning television programs regularly report the latest in health-related research and health-promotion strategies. With these societal changes in perception and the increasing costs of health care, pressure came to bear to look for the most cost-effective methods to deliver health care.

Shifting Sands of the Health Care Delivery System

The health care delivery system, as a fee-for-service system, focused on the treatment of illness rather than on health promotion and prevention of disease (Butterfield, 1993). However, research has demonstrated that the causes of most chronic illness are the practice of health-depleting behaviors *and* social and environmental barriers that limit the choices individuals, families, populations, and communities have relating to health-promoting activities. In addition, in a seminal article by McGinnis and Foege (1993), the chief preventable causes of death are translated to lifestyle choices and social influences. These causes include tobacco use; poor diet and activity patterns; alcohol consumption; exposure to environmental microbial or toxic agents; inappropriate use of firearms; promiscuous, unprotected sexual behaviors; motor vehicle accidents; illicit drug use; and socioeconomic barriers.

There are many social barriers that limit the choices clients have in relationship to health-promoting activities. Prime examples are those who live in inner cities or who live in rural or frontier areas. Food choices are limited by distance to full-service grocery stores and availability of transportation. The stores that are available tend to be small family-owned markets or gas station mini-marts. Both provide limited choice of foods at prices higher than full-service chain stores. In addition, gas station mini-marts may not sell produce but do sell high-fat, high-calorie convenience foods.

With the move to managed care and other community-based services for individuals and families and the realization that chronic illness and even death are grounded, for the most part, in lifestyle choices and social barriers, the focus of health care is changing. The principles of managed care require that health-promotion and disease-prevention activities be included in practice at both individual and population levels to prevent the costly occurrence of chronic disease and disability. For managed care organizations to realize profit, risk groups must be managed at both the individual and the aggregate levels (Baldwin, Conger, Abegglen, & Hill, 1998). Also, managed care organizations are becoming more involved in community activities such as community-based health centers, health fairs, Healthy Communities programs, and school-based clinics. Many managed care systems and other insurance companies encourage health-promotion education, activities, and behaviors for their members. In addition, industries have included wellness programs for employees, which may offer various types of reimbursement incentives, from lowering insurance premiums to giving bonuses to those members and employees who demonstrate health-promoting behaviors.

United States Government Initiatives

In the late 1970s, the Surgeon General of the United States, in a document titled *Healthy People,* reported to the nation about the expectations at that time regarding health promotion and disease prevention in this country (Baldwin, 1992, 1995; Kulbok & Baldwin, 1992; USPHS, 1979). The Surgeon General stated, "Let us make no mistake about the significance of this document, it represents an emerging consensus among scientists and the health community that the Nation's health strategy must be dramatically recast to emphasize the prevention of disease" (*Healthy People 2010*, 1998, p. 1).

In 1980, target outcomes, in the form of objectives for the year 1990, were given relating to the reduction of premature mortality in four age groups (*Laying the Foundation*, 1998). At that time, prevention of disease was the main thrust, with health-protection factors addressed and health promotion mentioned. Revised and updated objectives, written in 1990 for the year 2000 (*Healthy People 2000: National Health Promotion and Disease Prevention Objectives*), changed the order of health priorities. Health promotion became the first consideration in the list of three important factors: health promotion, health protection, and preventive services (Baldwin, 1992; Kulbok & Baldwin, 1992). In 1998, the document *Healthy People 2010 Objectives: Draft for Public Comment* (DHHS) was published to elicit public and professional input into the developed national objectives for the year 2010.

Nurses must be involved at all levels of policy development. They have been members of task forces developing the components of each *Healthy People* document, and with the availability of the Internet, nurses had opportunity to give input and feedback on the *Healthy People 2010* development.

The document provides a wonderful opportunity for nursing students to assess populations within their local regions related to progress toward one or more of the objectives. At Brigham Young University College of Nursing, beginning nursing students write a scholarly paper that is based on *Healthy People 2010* objectives. The students have 1 year, through several nursing courses, to complete the assignment. Students pick a topic such as immunizations or maternal-child issues, conduct a literature review, consider nursing implications, and assess what is being done in the local community for the population of interest. Recommendations are made as to additional approaches that might be taken, and these are shared with community agencies (personal communication, J. Abegglen, May 5, 1999).

Public/Private Partnerships

Through a cooperative agreement between the American Public Health Association (APHA) and the Centers for Disease Control and Prevention (CDC), a major collaborative process resulted in another document, *Healthy Communities 2000 Model Standards: Guidelines for Community Attainment of the Year 2000 National Health Objectives* (APHA, 1991). The approach and document are considered valuable resources for communities wanting to explore and develop local health-promotion standards (*Model Standards*, 1998). The APHA built on the *Healthy People 2000* objectives, developing step-by-step criteria for each objective. Each objective had a measurable "goal" attached to it. For instance, the objective to reduce coronary heart disease deaths might have a measurable goal to reduce *x* amount of these deaths per 100,000 people by some specific date. These guidelines for adapting measurable criteria to the national objectives have been adapted and used by leaders, including nurses and other health care professionals in many states, counties, regions, cities, and even some neighborhoods, who wish to facilitate more healthful lifestyles for the populations they serve.

The Healthy Cities program originated in 1985 with a presentation at an international meeting in Canada. The theme of the presentation was that health is the result of much more than medical care; people are healthy when they live in nurturing environments and are involved in the life of their community (Duhl, 1986). A recent publication, *Healthy People in Healthy Communities: A Guide for Community Leaders* (DHHS, 1998), links healthy cities with healthy people to create a healthy community in a guide to how other cities and communities developed and implemented their healthy community initiatives.

There have been numerous partnerships and group efforts in which nurses have collaborated with Healthy Cities and Communities projects throughout the country. Flynn and other community health nurses began "Healthy Indiana," which was an

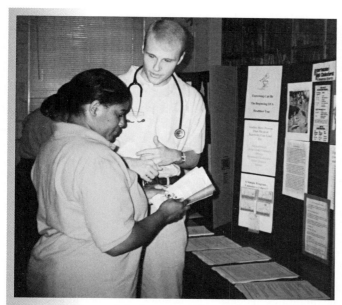

Education is a critical aspect of health promotion intervention. Health fairs are effective ways to share wellness information with large numbers of people.

early forerunner of ensuing Healthy Cities and Communities programs (Kellogg Foundation, 1988). Other examples include work with homeless populations (Greiner & Berry, 1992; Moore, Neff, Smith, & Weber, 1999) and nurse managed care centers (Drapo & Woods, 1992). The growth of community nursing organizations demonstrates how nurses believe our focus should be on partnering and collaborating with communities and special populations in health-promoting efforts. Nurse educators and local public health nursing directors continue to forge collaborative bonds with cities, communities, and target population groups in developing community/population health-promotion needs and assets assessments (Baldwin, 1995).

The following is an example of nursing student involvement with community-level health promotion interventions. The Brigham Young University College of Nursing in Provo, Utah, offers a community/population assessment elective course to both nursing undergraduate students and university honor students. Various city and county health departments and local communities have requested assistance in assessing the needs of key population groups. For example, the members of the Healthy Taylorsville Project requested the class's help in assessing the needs and viewpoints of the youth of the community. The college students collaborated with the school superintendent, principals, teachers, counselors, and junior and senior high school students. They produced a document outlining the needs of the youth and their suggestions and ideas about health-promotion strategies for the city of Taylorsville (Browning, Huls, Rather, & Stout, 1997). One example of the Taylorsville youths' suggestions was to place stoplights at two of the busiest streets in the growing city so that

students could safely cross those streets to get to and from school. The document will be a major guide toward anticipated changes for many of the needs stated by the youth (personal communication, J. I. Morgan, Director of Administrative Services, Taylorsville, Utah, March 1998).

Growing Consumerism and Emphasis on Self-Care

Since the late 1960s, consumers of health care have increasingly demanded information relating to their health care and to items that promote health. In the past, consumers almost complacently accepted what physicians and others in control of health care systems told them regarding their health care. Over the last 30 years, consumers have become better educated and more proactive in demanding their rights and insisting that health care professionals be accountable for their actions. Evidence can be seen in the proliferation of satisfaction surveys, opinion polls, and litigation, as well as in the nature of advertising. Information related to dietary management, such as lowering the fat content in recipes, and exercise activities that claim to be health promoting are seen throughout the media. People are requesting more information on labels in order to discern whether the item contains anything that might be non-health promoting, especially some-

RESEARCH BRIEF

Jette, A. M., Lachman, M., Giorgetti, M. M., Assmann, S. F., Harris, B. A., Levenson, C., Wernick, M., & Krebs, D. (1999). Exercise—It's never too late: The Strong-for-Life program. American Journal of Public Health, 89(1), 66–72.

The authors of a randomized controlled trial compared the outcomes of a home exercise program taught to 107 older persons (with a mean age of 75.4) with a control group of 108 people (with a mean age of 75.6) who did not receive the home exercise program training until after the study was completed. The Strong-for-Life program was based on a video of several exercise methods demonstrated by an exercise expert. Simple movements, those an older person might perform in daily functions, such as rotating wrist joints and reaching across the body, were incorporated into the exercises. Some exercises were done while sitting; others included short walking routines.

Striking results were noted regarding strength improvements. There is promise in using videos in home exercise programs designed for older people; the benefits of this type of health-promoting, cost-efficient exercise that can be done in the privacy of the home are appealing to the growing population of the elderly, as well as having health and cost benefits for the nation.

thing that might trigger an allergy or be too high in fat content. The health-promotion aspects of education have become a major focus for all age and ethnic groups.

Who is responsible for health? There is an expanding awareness that consumers must bear the responsibility for their own health. How can consumers do this? Self-care is the answer. Self-care is defined as those "activities initiated or performed by an individual, family, or community to achieve, maintain, or promote maximum health" (Steiger & Lipson, 1985, p. 12). Orem defines self-care as "the production of actions directed to self or to the environment in order to regulate one's functioning in the interest of one's life, integrated functioning, and well-being" (Orem, 1985, p. 31).

The impetus for the current interest in self-care began anew in the late 1970s and early 1980s. The U.S. Department of Health and Human Services (DHHS, 1982) published a document titled *Forward Plan for Health 1977-1981*. It seems remarkable to consider today, that for the first time ever, the authors of this report boldly suggested that lifestyle and psychosocial factors had a great impact on morbidity and mortality. A number of health-promotion elements such as nutrition, exercise, and fitness were mentioned.

In addition to the emphasis placed by government documents at that time, the popular press also supported the notion. In his book *Megatrends*, Naisbitt (1982, p. 131) forecast that self-care emphasizing health-promotion strategies would move health care out of the medical-institutional illness model into an era of self-responsibility for health and wellness.

The demand for self-care is currently coming from people themselves, private insurance carriers, managed care organizations, employers, and communities. In the past, individuals would never consider questioning the diagnoses or orders of their physicians. Insurance carriers now insist that there be at least two health care professionals' opinions before major surgery.

In addition, consumers are demanding information about complementary treatment options in addition to allopathic treatments suggested by physicians. Insurance and managed care companies are providing self-care books that assist subscribers to self-diagnose and self-treat simple illnesses and injuries, as well as provide tips on health-promoting activities for all members of the family. Incentives include managed care organizations paying bonuses to members for smoking cessation, weight loss, and other health-promoting activities that move the members toward high-level wellness. At the workplace, large companies implement organizational wellness programs that assist employees to maximize personal wellness. Research has shown that an employee experiencing high-level wellness uses fewer sick days and is more productive on the job (National Institute for Occupational Safety and Health, 1996; DHHS, 1998). At home or from a local library or other community establishment, clients can access numerous Internet sites on any subject relating to self-care.

Self-care and consumerism are processes that assist people to know about health-promoting items and activities. At the popu-lation and community levels, the Healthy Cities and Communities program depends heavily on people within communities to identify problems and assets and engage in problem solving and self-care to correct problems and promote maximal community wellness. The success of the *Healthy People 2010* objectives for the nation is equally dependent on client education in health-promotion and self-care strategies as well as policy changes to improve social conditions allowing for the context within which personal choices about health are made. To make informed health-promoting decisions, appropriate and correct health-promotion information must be available to clients, as well as to legislators who make the policies.

Models of Health Promotion and Wellness

Numerous models of health promotion and wellness might be useful guides to assessing and promoting health and wellness in communities, populations, families, and individuals. Many models have been constructed to explain, assess, plan, or evaluate health-promotion education programs, states of health, wellness, and illness, and preventive measures.

As early as 1952, researchers expressed the need for a model to help explain and predict why certain at-risk populations took preventive actions and others did not, even when there was very little or nothing being charged for the preventive services (Rosenstock, 1974). The first popular model developed was the health belief model (Becker, 1974; Hochbaum,1958; Padilla & Bulcavage, 1991; Rosentock,1974). In this model, "the individual's weighing of the positive and negative valences of the threats of illness was emphasized" (Baldwin, 1992, p. 27). How the individual perceived his or her susceptibility to an illness and what might be the perceived benefits and barriers to doing something about preventing the illness were important factors in the health belief model. Even when the individual decided it was in his or her best interest to take some action to prevent the illness, there needed to be a trigger or cue to action to motivate the person to carry out the action (Baldwin, 1992; Rosenstock, 1974).

Several other models have been developed that might be useful to the nurse of today. As researchers continue the quest to predict and explain what factors contributed to health-promoting and health-protecting behaviors, the multidimensionality of the process became clearer. Further developments of the predictors of preventive health behavior originating in the health belief model were instigated in later models. Cognitive factors such as clients' definitions of health and perceptions about health behaviors, including benefits, barriers, and control, were seen as important to clients' health-promoting behaviors. Modifying factors, ranging from demographic, biological, behavioral, and interpersonal to environmental, including access to care, as well as factors that might influence the initiating of health-promoting and health-protective behaviors, were explored. Many of these multidimensional factors can be seen in the health-promotion models constructed in the 1980s and early 1990s (Palank, 1991; Pender, 1987; Simmons, 1990) and in health hazard risk evaluation and appraisal tools and wellness guides, which began appearing in the early 1970s and 1980s.

Health hazard risk evaluation and appraisal tools are commonly designed in survey questionnaire form to provide quantitative data elicited from clients' responses regarding lifestyle and health habits. Questions regarding activities of daily living ranging from personal health habits, such as, "How often do you brush your teeth?" "In what way and how often do you exercise?" and "Are you sexually active?" to questions regarding seat belt use and consumption of caffeine products are often asked. Often, information is required regarding family and personal medical histories and various demographic data. The information from these questionnaires can then be compared with known national and local health statistics to make predictions and health-promotion recommendations regarding morbidity and mortality risks for the clients. Wellness guides are generally in a question and answer form, designed to appeal to consumers who may have a common health or wellness question or concern.

In the late 1980s, the *Guide to Clinical Preventive Services* (U.S. Preventive Services Task Force, 1989) was developed, and in 1995, a second edition was published to help guide primary care health professionals providing preventive services. These tools and guides are used by physicians' and nurse practitioners' offices, hospitals, health departments, managed care systems, and

other agencies to assist health care professionals counseling clients about reducing potential risks and increasing health-promoting behaviors. Models, tools, and guides continue to be designed to help explore factors involved in health promotion and wellness decision making for individuals, families, populations, and communities.

Two recent models are described to demonstrate how these techniques might be used to assess and facilitate wellness interventions: (1) holistic wellness: self-inventory of personal wellness using the medicine wheel (McDonald, 1997) and (2) the 4 + model of wellness (Baldwin & Baldwin, 1998). These models are similar in some respects to earlier models and tools in the assessment of multidimensional variables impacting health and wellness, but they differ somewhat in the approaches. Both of these models may be used with any ethnic population, as may several of the earlier models. The holistic wellness model allows clients to identify aspects that determine wellness and to define what well and unhealthy states are for them. The 4 + model of wellness also encourages client participation in the assessment of wellness and adds two other dimensions: the consideration of what might be the sources of nurture and depletion for a client and how the nurse might facilitate interventions with the client, focusing on those sources of nurture and depletion to promote health and wellness.

Holistic Wellness: Self-Inventory of Personal Wellness Using the Medicine Wheel

The medicine wheel is a sacred symbol that is common to almost all Native American tribes (Four Worlds Development Project, 1985, p. 9). Ivan McDonald, a member of the Blackfeet tribe and health educator for Indian Health Services in Browning, Montana, developed the holistic wellness model using the medicine wheel as a basis (see the figure on p. 296). Although the descriptors for this model are specific to the values and beliefs of the Blackfeet culture of Native Americans, the wheel can be used to assess wellness for any person of any culture. The descriptors of "healthy" states and "unhealthy" states for the spokes of the wheel should reflect the individuality of the person.

The holistic wellness model is grounded in the Native American understanding of existence. The medicine wheel, as a representation of this understanding, is depicted as a circle that comprises the four sacred directions. Each direction represents not only one of the basic elements necessary for survival, but also a human element.

The East is symbolic of the sun and fire and of one's own creative spirit. The South represents water and one's emotions. The West is the place of Mother Earth and one's intuition—the place of magic and dreams. The North represents air and minds filled with wisdom as one learns about the mystery of life.

Holistic wellness defines health in terms of the whole person, not only in terms of physical illness. The model represents how Native American people understand health as a balance within

RESEARCH BRIEF

Neuhauser, L., Schwab, M., Syme, S. L., Bieber, M., & Obarski, S. K. (1998). Community participation in health promotion: evaluation of the California Wellness Guide. Health Promotion International, 13(3), 211–222.

Short-term outcomes for participants using the California Wellness Guide were described and evaluated, using interviews from three population-based samples of women involved in the Women, Infants, and Children Supplemental Nutrition Program (WIC). From the pretesting stage to the end of the study at 8 months, the participants demonstrated significantly improved attitudes and knowledge regarding wellness information compared with the nonparticipants. Findings indicated that a wellness guide, such as the California Wellness Guide, which evolved from in-depth community involvement and contained many common health care topics, can raise the knowledge level and improve health-promotion and wellness behaviors of participants. This, in turn, could add immeasurably to the nation's health-promotion benefits.

RESEARCH BRIEF

Segal, L., Dalton, A. C., & Richardson, J. (1998). Cost-effectiveness of the primary prevention of non-insulin dependent diabetes mellitus. Health Promotion International, 13(1), 197–209.

A cost-effective analysis research study of intervention programs for the prevention of non–insulin-dependent diabetes mellitus (NIDDM) reported in international literature in recent years was undertaken. Epidemiological and clinical evidence pointed to weight loss, exercise, and fitness, plus appropriate nutrition, as health-promotion interventions leading to prevention of NIDDM. The research questions were aimed at whether preventing NIDDM was cost-effective in comparison with other potential resource use and if any NIDDM health-promotion programs were more cost-effective than other programs. Various media programs, such as the use of videos, and programs geared to overweight men compared most favorably in the study. NIDDM not only is a prevalent chronic disease today, but is also increasing in prevalence throughout the world, and many of the high-risk target populations are American Indian and Alaskan Native. Among the major risk factors for NIDDM is ethnicity.

HOLISTIC WELLNESS: SELF-INVENTORY OF PERSONAL WELLNESS USING THE MEDICINE WHEEL.

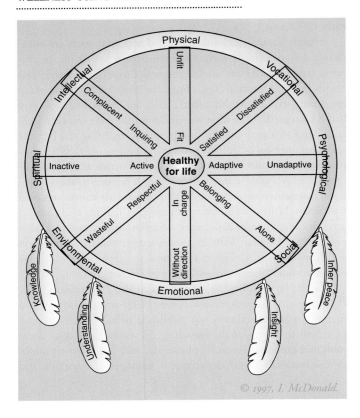

© 1997, I. McDonald.

the person and between the person and everything around him or her—physical, vocational, psychological, social, emotional, environmental, spiritual, and intellectual. It focuses on optimal health, prevention of disease, and positive mental and emotional states (personal communication, I. McDonald, April 1998).

The spokes of the medicine wheel radiate from a center circle that represents wellness or "Healthy for Life." The spokes contain dimensions of the specific wellness (as the Physical Wellness spoke has the dimensions of unfit and fit), with the more positive part of the dimension being closest to the center Healthy for Life circle in preceding figure. The spokes are defined as follows:

- Physical wellness: *maintenance of your body in good condition by eating right, exercising regularly, avoiding harmful habits, and making informed, responsible decisions about your health*

- Vocational wellness: *enjoyment of what you are doing to earn a living and/or to contribute to society*

- Psychological wellness: *maintenance of mental health or the ability to think reasonably clearly and to avoid wildly distorting reality*

- Social wellness: *ability to perform the expectations of social roles effectively, comfortably, and without harming others*

- Emotional wellness: *understanding emotions and knowing how to cope with problems that arise in everyday life; ability to endure stress*

- Environmental wellness: *personal and global risks to health, socioeconomic status, education, and various other environmental factors that affect health, such as noise pollution, radiation, air pollution, and water pollution*

- Spiritual wellness: *a state of balance and harmony with yourself and others; includes trust, integrity, principles, ethics, the purpose or drive in life, basic survival instincts, feelings of selflessness, degree of pleasure-seeking qualities, commitment to some higher process or being, and the ability to believe in concepts that are not subject to a "state of the art" explanation*

- Intellectual wellness: *having a mind open to new ideas; covers such activities as speaking, writing, analyzing, critical thinking, and judgment*

The eagle feathers at the bottom of the wheel represent the progression of personal development: knowledge, understanding, insight, and inner peace. Each element is a higher level than the one before. However, the element before must occur before one can aspire to the next level. The progression of the feathers is similar to the progression for each dimension reflected in the spokes of the wheel. As the client develops inwardly toward Healthy for Life, there is progress from knowledge to inner peace.

The holistic wellness model includes social and environmental aspects as they relate to a person's wellness. From the perspectives of many cultures, a person's wellness depends on social relationships and harmony with the environment. For example, for some societies in Australia and Mexico, physical illness can be caused by breaches of social norm. Although this is not necessarily a common idea in many Western societies, from the worldview of most cultures, personal illness or wellness may be a result of social and environmental interactions.

How to Use the Holistic Wellness Model

The nurse could use the holistic wellness model as an excellent visual depiction of a client's self-defined wellness state. The model can be used by health professionals to help clients in both assessing what the client's values are relating to the eight dimensions and determining how well he or she is functioning within each dimension. It is important to note, though, that if one dimension becomes the focus of changing behaviors, other dimensions may suffer from lack of attention. Therefore, facilitating interventions through the use of this model requires that the nurse and client together consider how to strengthen all of the dimensions as equally as possible. In addition, the holistic wellness model is handy for quick evaluations of progress. It is also important to understand that the balance may shift depending on circumstances and that as symbolized by the medicine wheel, there is constant motion.

Several examples of how to intervene and facilitate the client's considering a more healthful lifestyle using health-promoting behaviors include the following: (1) If the client considers himself or herself to be on the unfit dimension of the Physical spoke, discuss ways for the client to become more fit. What does the client like to do in the way of exercise, and what can the client physically and realistically do? If walking is difficult for an elderly person, perhaps suggest starting with moving every possible body joint two or three times during a television or radio commercial or a rest while reading. (2) If the client believes he or she is inactive on the Spiritual spoke, review what spirituality means to the client and see if he or she can discover ways to become more active in that realm. (3) If the client sees that he or she is without

direction on the Emotional spoke, address things that might be done by the client to make him or her feel more in charge of life. The major issue here is what does the client believe he or she can realistically do to develop health-promoting behaviors that will lead to the client being more healthy for life.

At a community level, the model could be applied by changing the names on the outer ring of the medicine wheel. For example, things such as public transportation, community pride, health care services, and so on could substitute for the physical, spiritual, and psychological elements. The spokes would translate similarly. For instance, public transportation might be present (meaning all possible modes of transportation are available) to absent (meaning there is no public transportation in the community). The feather could be redefined as knowledge to data, understanding to information, insight to creative solutions, and inner peace to harmony of factors.

The 4+ Model of Wellness

The 4+ model of wellness (Baldwin & Baldwin, 1998) is designed to assist critical thinking about things that might negatively deplete or positively nurture wellness in a client. There are two layers, much like transparent plastic overlays, to this model: (1) the four domains of inner self and (2) the outer systems. When layer 2 is placed over layer 1, the total 4+ model of wellness appears.

The 4+ model of wellness begins with the inner self layer, depicting a sphere containing the four domains of inner self (see the following figure) of the client. The client might be oneself, another individual, a family, population, or community. The

THE 4+ MODEL OF WELLNESS: THE FOUR DOMAINS OF INNER SELF.

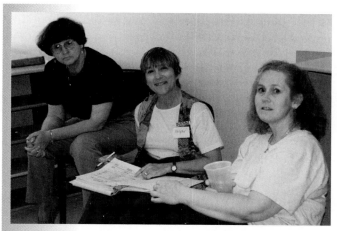

Dr. Joan H. Baldwin, chapter author (center), works with nurse practitioner students in a wellness program on Ute Indian reservation.

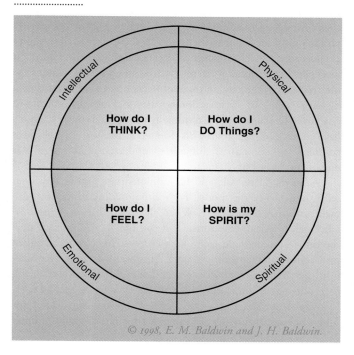

© 1998, E. M. Baldwin and J. H. Baldwin.

THE 4+ MODEL OF WELLNESS: THE OUTER SYSTEMS.

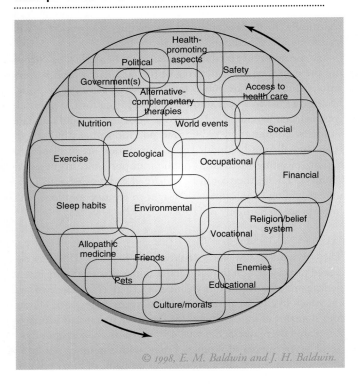

© 1998, E. M. Baldwin and J. H. Baldwin.

THE 4+ MODEL OF WELLNESS: THE FOUR DOMAINS OF INNER SELF PLUS THE OUTER SYSTEMS.

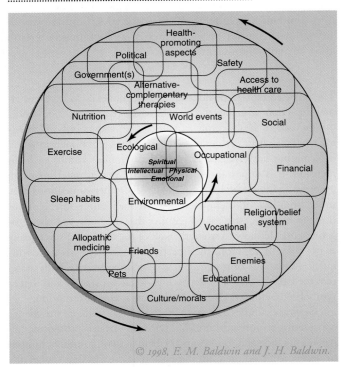

© 1998, E. M. Baldwin and J. H. Baldwin.

four domains of inner self are intellectual, physical, emotional, and spiritual (or spirit).

This portion of the 4+ model of wellness appears simple but is really quite complex. The intellectual component of the inner self relates to how the client thinks. The physical is how the client moves and senses things and includes all of the client's physiological (or inner workings, as in the case of a community as client) aspects. How a client feels anger, excitement, and so on is reflected in the emotional aspect, and the spiritual denotes the fire that drives the engine that connects one to others and to a higher power. The spiritual domain also includes the capacity to give love. Thus, the spiritual domain within each of us seems to have more than one role. This domain is likely to be the most complex and sometimes difficult to understand, although it is one of the most important to consider.

Achieving a holistic and harmonious state within the inner self is one part of the model. For example, think of the four domains of inner self as a tire. When all four of the domains—intellectual, physical, emotional, and spiritual—are "pumped up," the tire is rounded and rolls along evenly. This is what is meant by a holistic and harmonious state. This healthy state of harmony is further affected by interconnectedness and interaction with systems outside the inner self, which are depicted in the second overlay—the outer systems (see the figures above)—as facets of another sphere surrounding the sphere of the four domains of inner

self. The outer systems portion of this model is similar to the tool known as an *Ecomap,* which is discussed in chapter 2.

All of the elements of the outer systems sphere interact and interconnect with each other and all the four domains of inner self. Imagine the two spheres constantly rotating about each other so that all components of each sphere interact with other elements within their own sphere and with each other at some time. The preceding figure depicts the idea of layering the spheres—the 4+ model of wellness: the four domains of inner self plus the outer systems.

Think of the total model as a client system, one system with many moving components. Using the 4+ model of wellness, the nurse can look for things that might be depleting the elements of the inner self rather than nurturing the elements toward harmony. By working with the client to consider things that might deplete any one or all of the four domains and thinking of ways to strengthen those things that nurture the client, the nurse and client may be able to identify health-promoting actions for the client. Selected sources of nurture and depletion are listed in Box 13-3.

General observations

Strength in any domain, if not in excess, can nurture the other three domains. Also, depletion of any domain weakens and drains the other three domains.

BOX 13-3 THE 4+ MODEL OF WELLNESS: SELECTED SOURCES OF NURTURE AND DEPLETION

INTELLECTUAL

Sources of Nurture
- Books/intellectual media activities
- Observation/contemplation
- Experience/critical thinking
- Knowledge building more knowledge
- Practicing "brain work," that is, children's play and games; children learn this way and so do adults
- Planning for the future

Sources of Depletion
- Brainwashing—imposed conditioned responses
- Mind-numbing repetition
- Boredom
- Noise
- Interruption
- Stresses/stressors
- Codependent behavior encouraged by a perpetrator—can lead to posttraumatic stress syndrome

EMOTIONAL

Sources of Nurture
- Relief from stress
- Accomplishments
- Winning
- Physical well-being, exercise, diet
- Rest/relaxation
- Meditation/biofeedback, etc.
- Ability to "vent" appropriately

Sources of Depletion
- Physical illness
- Weak intelligence (inability to solve a problem)
- Isolation/noise/threats

PHYSICAL

Sources of Nurture
- Appropriate nutrition
- Outdoor/indoor activities/exercise
- Rest/relaxation
- Physical "work"
- Biofeedback/complementary health therapies, etc.
- Appropriate physiological workings
- Physical therapy

Sources of Depletion
- Disease/illness/prepathogenesis
- Toxins/environmental hazards
- Drug/substance abuse
- Poor nutrition/diet
- Lack of sleep
- Noise
- Stress/stressors/allergies
- Excessive exercise/exertion
- Trauma

SPIRITUAL

Sources of Nurture
- Giving love/connecting with others
- Being of service/loving animals
- Beauty/music/art
- Quiet/peace, meditation/prayer
- Physical exercise/cheering
- Being loved/hugs and pat-pats
- Intellectual stimulus/creating

Sources of Depletion
- Too much demand for support of others
- Failure to experience connectedness, love, belonging

Source: Baldwin & Baldwin, 1998.

Spiritual domain

On first consideration, the emotional and spiritual domains may appear similar, but in this model, these areas are quite different from each other. In this model, *spiritual* means the spirit or fire one has within. Excessive emotional highs may deplete the spirit.

Of importance in this model is that *spiritual* does not mean religion or religious. Religion is actually a piece of the outer system that impacts the inner self. Parts of a religion may indeed nurture the spirit, but sometimes, as in the case of overzealousness, depletion of the spirit may occur.

Observations about excesses

Excessive striving in any area can be destructive in all four domains. An illustration would be someone who exercises to an extreme, to the detriment of personal relationships with others.

Excessive pain can be a depleting factor. For example, it is hard to think when you are suffering severe pain. One kind of severe pain is depression. Severely depressed people become so immobilized in several of the domains that they cannot move themselves toward strength in any of the areas through simple exercise or nutrition or even interaction with loving people. Serious disease or weakness (which can cause excessive physiological and other problems) can deplete several domains and can be a major factor in the client suffering a downward spiral to total collapse and death.

Any excesses or "lacks" within any of the four domains throws the inner self sphere extremely "off balance or out of harmony." Think of the inner self sphere as being a tire; the difference in pressure on any portion of the tire will throw the tire off balance. People in various cultures speak of the tremendous importance of balance or harmony in a person's life.

Contemporary researchers and authors are proposing that changing and growing systems do not necessarily seek total equilibrium, that constant change alters the state of harmony or balance constantly (Coveney & Highfield, 1990; Prigogine & Stengers, 1984; Wheatley, 1994). This might explain how the assessment of a client on one day may be far different from a similar assessment another day or even later in the same day. This is why it is important to observe the client over time—to get a broader picture of what might be occurring within that client system. There does not have to be "equilibrium" to have balance or harmony; in fact, a well-functioning system is always in a state of nonequilibrium because it constantly and inevitably changes focus. A system that is flexible and open can constantly move, changing and adjusting to regain harmony or a state as close to harmony as possible (Wheatley, 1994).

How to Use the 4+ Model of Wellness with Individuals, Families, Populations, and Communities

The nurse should begin by assessing the four domains of inner self for oneself or a client. Then, the components of the outer systems, which encircle and move around the four domains of the inner self sphere, must be considered. By using the total 4+ model of wellness to assess the interactions and interconnectedness of the elements in the outer systems to all aspects of the inner self, the nurse will be able to critically assess and analyze much about himself or herself or others. The nurse and the client may be able to determine which factors to work on strengthening or nurturing and which factors might be diminished or deleted to "pump up" the client system's wellness. Remember that the client can be a family, group, population, or community, as well as an individual.

Individuals

Consider a grossly overweight, older man as an individual client. The client has been prescribed a diet that is nutritionally sound and, if followed, should help him lose weight. The client could be thinking he is trying to follow his prescribed diet, and he is perplexed about not being successful in losing weight. The nurse could explore with the client as many aspects as possible of his four domains of inner self, as well as the outer system components, to begin to figure out what interventions might facilitate health-promoting behaviors for this client. After working with the client to assess what might be sources of nurture and depletion for each of his four domains, the nurse (and, in some difficult cases, a team of health care professionals), along with the client, would develop a wellness plan. Ideally, finding ways to nurture the client's four domains and considering how the depleting sources could be diminished would constitute the initial part of the plan. For example, there might be work environment stressors (sources of depletion), such as the fact that donuts and other sweet, high-fat, and high-calorie foods are encouraged at break time at the workplace, which makes adhering to the prescribed diet difficult. Brainstorming with the client about how he might discuss his need to be on the prescribed diet with his supervisor and how difficult it has been to not eat the donuts when they are in full view could be one step in the process.

There will be some sources of nurture that the client could also strengthen. A source of nurture might be that the man has a dog as a pet. Possibly the man and his dog could work with children in a day-care center for developmentally disabled children. There have

RESEARCH BRIEF

Jorgenson, J. (1997). Therapeutic use of companion animals in health care. Image: The Journal of Nursing Scholarship, 29(3), 249–254.

An exploration of the research in several disciplines related to the use of animals for therapy in health care demonstrated applicability of the findings to enhance health-promoting nursing interventions for clients. A selective historical tour of the literature regarding the human-animal bond and its therapeutic effect in health care is a segue to more recent research on the subject. Considerations about the pros and cons of having animals interact with hospitalized clients are developed. The link between the benefits of stress reduction and positive psychoneuroimmunology changes in clients as a result of human-animal bonding therapies emerges as the strongest health promotion possibility for the use of this animal-assisted therapy.

CASE STUDY

How Everything Affects Everything— A Saga of One Man's Life and the Negative Influences on Him and the Families Involved

Sam had a difficult childhood. His mother left the family when Sam was about 3 or 4 years old. His father probably was devastated, but Sam was too young to understand all that had happened. Sam's paternal grandparents raised Sam, because Sam's father had to work long hours to even begin to make enough money to sustain himself, much less Sam. Sam's grandfather was strict and sometimes abusive to Sam's grandmother. No one in the family seemed to recognize that Sam believed that he was responsible in some way for his mother's leaving.

As Sam grew older, he became angry that his mother had left him, although he seemed to appreciate the fact that his grandparents took reasonable care of him. He was certain his father had no real love for him. Sam was a fairly bright young boy and did well in school. Sometime in the his teens, Sam began experimenting with marijuana. He managed to graduate from high school and began doing manual labor and odd jobs. He still lived with his grandparents.

Sam had several girlfriends over the next few years. The girls and many of his friends were younger than he was by several years. Sam was always the "leader" of the group. He and his friends abused alcohol and began taking many other kinds of "street drugs." Sam verbally abused his friends and girlfriends by telling them they were "stupid" and so on. Eventually, he married one of the young women. After a time, he was not only abusing her verbally, but also forcing her to start taking some of the drugs that he was taking.

Sam and his wife had a child. Amazingly, the child was healthy. As the child grew, Sam insisted on having the child by his side when Sam wanted the child to be there. Otherwise, Sam ignored the child. Sam said he "loved" the child, yet burdened the young child (then about 3 or 4 years of age) with Sam's concerns about money and Sam's belief that the child's mother was "no good." Sam also continued to have sexual liaisons

with other women. Sam's wife made several attempts to leave Sam, especially after some fairly severe beatings. The child often observed these situations. After several years of abuse, Sam's wife left him and took the child with her to live elsewhere. Sam threatened to find her and kill her if the child was not returned. After almost 2 years of legal interventions, Sam's wife won a divorce and legal physical custody of the child (meaning that the child would live with her, but that Sam might have some input into the raising of the child). Sam tolerated this process for a short time before he began verbally harassing and threatening his ex-wife on the phone.

There were several more months of harassment and the involvement of police and other legal interventions. When Sam was finally arrested for selling drugs and being intoxicated, among other things, the court agreed that Sam would be denied contact with his son.

1. Using the 4+ model of wellness, of Sam's four domains, how many were affected by his early life? by his high school adventures? by his adult life?

2. What additional information is needed in the scenario to assess Sam's wellness in the time before he went to jail? Consider what effect the outer systems components (e.g., social, vocational, environmental) may have had on Sam.

3. What sources of nurture and/or depletion are recognizable? Which of Sam's domains may have been affected, given the sources of nurture and/or depletion noted?

4. What health-promoting behaviors of Sam's family might have helped Sam during his early development? List Sam's family's possible sources of nurture and depletion.

5. While considering the 4+ model of wellness, what sources of nurture and/or depletion did the family of the ex-wife and child have? How might a nurse assist them to assess their own four quadrants individually and as a single-parent family?

6. How might a nurse help the ex-wife and child develop the health-promoting behaviors they might need individually and as a single-parent family?

7. Think about Sam's abuse of and involvement with substances. Consider his desire for drugs and Sam's early life and the life he was living as an adult. What view/attitudes might a nurse take as a logical and ethical approach toward Sam?

A Target Population Within a Community

The Teen Mothers' High School Program, which was located in one of the local high schools in the town of Urbansville, was used by more than 100 young, single women each year for 5 years. The City Council decided to participate in the formation of a community health-promotion program called "Healthy Urbansville." The council members wanted to improve the health-promoting aspects of their city. They called on leaders in the educational facilities in town, police/sheriff and fire departments, local business people, ecclesiastical representatives (e.g., of churches, temples, synagogues), and other local interested citizens, including representatives of the youth groups and senior citizens' centers, to be part of this community effort.

The city was fairly large and contained many community resource agencies and emergency funding processes to assist those in need. The city was located in an urban area of the western region of the country, with many parks and recreation areas. The city prided itself on the good relationships between its diverse populations, the cleanliness of the city, and the efforts toward appropriate city growth that had been in place for several years. There were several excellent libraries, theater and other media options, art and history museums, as well as restaurants of all kinds. Biomedical and complementary/integrative health therapies co-existed. There were churches of many different denominations readily accessible by most of the populations. Transportation opportunities were well distributed throughout the city, although there were continuing construction projects at various times throughout the dry seasons. There were, as in any large city, varying socioeconomic groups, including many homeless. Illicit drug dealing was being combated daily by the police and others, but it was

not out of hand. Violence was occasional, with robberies and burglaries being highest during the hotter months. Overall, the city considered itself a city with a future.

One of the major concerns of the Healthy Urbansville group that came forth after an in-depth community/population assessment process, which included the use of several surveys (plus the 4+ model of wellness), was that the rising numbers of teen pregnancies had a depleting effect on the community as a whole; families and resources within the community were hard hit. The age ranges of the teenage mothers was between 14 and 17; there were presently 1,000 young women in this age group, according to the most recent statistics. Statistically, teen pregnancies resulted in higher mortality rates than other age groupings. This concern became the main priority of the Healthy Urbansville group.

1. Using the 4+ model of wellness and given what this case study indicated, what assets (or sources of nurture) and what problems (sources of depletion) might exist in the community, Urbansville?

2. What might be the sources of nurture in the intellectual domain of the community? in the physical, emotional, and spiritual domains of the community?

3. Think of the teenage mothers in this community. What questions might you have regarding this target (at-risk) population? What are some of the sources of nurture (or assets) that might affect young women in the age group between 14 and 17 years of age? What are some of the potential sources of depletion (or problem areas) that might affect young women in this age group?

4. Given the sources of nurture (or assets) identified, what interventions might be made to strengthen these in the young women? What potential things might be done to diminish or delete the depleting sources (or problems)?

5. List several interventions for both the community and target population that could facilitate health-promoting behaviors for those client, either individually or by working to diminish a source of community depletion.

been many research articles relating the health-promoting aspects of the human-animal bond (Edney, 1992; National Institutes of Health, 1987). In addition, the process of connecting older people with younger people has many nurturing benefits (Piper, 1999). A service opportunity such as this could possibly nurture all four of

the client's domains, and certainly would nurture the children who are the recipients of this service (and maybe the dog, who might enjoy being with children).

Another important factor to remember when working with any client is that the client's goals or priorities in life may not be the same as what you might consider his, her, or its (in the case of a family, population, or community) goals or priorities "should" be. This is equally important to remember when establishing things that nurture or deplete a client. These also are factors in why clients do not always do what a health care professional tells the them to do. Too often, if clients choose not to do what the health care professional says, or cannot do something for some valid reason, health care professionals indicate that the clients are "noncompliant" or cannot figure out why clients do not do what is "good" for them. These episodes sometimes create ethical concerns, especially concerning whose needs are being met. Building trust, rapport, and respect with clients often encourages the clients, in due time, to follow health care professionals' suggestions for health-promoting behaviors.

Families

Using the 4+ model of wellness when assessing more than one individual becomes more complex than assessing an individual. Consider a family as a large client system comprised of several smaller systems, or individual family members. Look for sources of nurture for the family. These sources might include things such as being broad-minded, being creative, having good problem-solving skills, being flexible, having family members who are interconnected with each other and the outer systems of the family, sharing spirituality, and being appropriately nurturing of the family's spirit and the spirits of others. A family that has developed these characteristics and continues to derive nurture from them among others demonstrates a fair amount of harmony, health, and wellness. In the family Case Study that follows, look for potential sources of nurture and depletion in the various family clients.

Populations and Communities

Now, think about how the 4+ model of wellness might be used to examine a population or a community. If a family is a client system, then a population or a community can also be a client system; individuals within the population and individuals and target (or at-risk) populations within a community are the smaller systems within the larger client system of population or community. Remember that your own goals, values, and priorities are not necessarily those of populations or communities. These client systems also have their own goals, values, and priorities that can create ethical dilemmas for the nurse.

Sources of nurture for populations and communities may be similar to those for a family. As the client system becomes larger (as with more than one individual), the sources of nurture also become broader in many cases. Freedom from harassment, threats, or violence could be added to any level of client system sources of nurture but seems to be often pertinent to an at-risk or target population or community. Sources of depletion for a population could be the reverse of the sources of nurture. For instance, an at-risk population of unwed pregnant teenagers might be depleted by harassment, ridicule, or shunning by others with extreme moral views against unmarried young women being sexually active. The target population and community Case Study on p. 302 describes some of the things a nurse needs to consider when using the 4+ model of wellness.

• •

You have noticed that everything an Indian does is in a circle, and that is because the Power of the World always works in circles, and everything tries to be round. . . . The Sky is round, and I have heard that the earth is round like a ball, and so are all the stars. The wind, in its greatest power, whirls. Birds make their nests in circles, for theirs is the same religion as ours. . . . Even the seasons form a great circle in their changing, and always come back again to where they were. The life of a man is a circle from childhood, and so it is in everything where power moves.

Black Elk
Oglala Sioux Holy Man, 1863–1950

• •

CONCLUSION

This chapter contains a discussion of basic concepts of health and health promotion as related to disease prevention, including definitions of *health promotion* and *wellness* as the terms are used in this chapter; delineation of factors influencing health promotion and wellness; a brief summary of some ways of looking at health promotion and wellness by describing some models, guides, and tools involved in health protection, health promotion, wellness and risk evaluation, analysis, and reduction; and introduction of two recent models of wellness. Key concepts, case studies, research briefs, and critical thinking activities are presented to reinforce concepts and assist in "pushing the envelope" and expanding ideas for health-promotion interventions.

CRITICAL THINKING ACTIVITIES

1. Can a person who has been diagnosed with bipolar disorder and who is appropriately and successfully being managed with medications achieve high-level wellness?

2. Can a community experiencing a severe gang problem achieve high-level wellness? If so, how might this be done?

3. How might the Jedi Women (a community action group comprised of single, low-income mothers) define high-level wellness for their group? What activities might stimulate the group toward self-actualization?

4. What social barriers might keep clients from exploring health-promoting activities, including healthy eating, exercising, and so forth?

5. Why is it that lifestyle choices and social limitations and barriers exist? What situations might be lending themselves to building social barriers for clients?

6. Some population and community clients have noticeable limitations to their lifestyle choices, as noted in this chapter. Consider the populations that lived in major cities, as well as in rural and/or frontier areas, in the United States 50 years ago. Compare the positives and negatives of their lifestyle choices at that time to similar populations of today.

7. Discuss things a community or society could do to support an individual's self-care activities.

8. Describe how consumerism and self-care activities might encourage health-promotion and wellness behaviors.

9. Make a table with two columns. In the first, list self-care activities you engage in to nurture your wellness. In the second, list self-care activities you have not been doing but should. Plan interventions to include at least two new health-promoting behaviors in your daily life.

10. Identify two populations to which you belong. List five self-care practices these populations engage in for the benefit and nurture of their members.

11. How can communities engage in self-care?

12. Redefine the descriptors "unhealthy" and "well" for each of the spokes of the holistic wellness model as they fit from your or your client's cultural perspective.

13. Discuss the meaning of knowledge, understanding, insight, and inner peace, which are found on the eagle feathers on the bottom of the holistic wellness model, as they might fit your or your client's culture.

CRITICAL THINKING ACTIVITIES—CONT'D

14. With the client, evaluate the client's health at each spoke. Consider each spoke as having a weak or more negative dimension (e.g., on the physical spoke, unfit would be the weak dimension and fit would be the healthy dimension). Have the client place a dot on the spoke where the client thinks he or she is at the time on that spoke's dimension. The closer the client places the dot to the center of the wheel on any given spoke/dimension, the healthier the person considers himself or herself in regard to that dimension. Once a dot is placed on each spoke, the dots are connected to form a circle. The nurse and the client can visually evaluate whether the circle is balanced and where the weak dimensions are.

15. Discuss potential interventions and/or changes the client might decide to make to move himself or herself more toward the center of the holistic wellness wheel toward being "healthy for life."

16. For your own community, identify the system dimensions that would be important to assessing wellness.

17. Refer to Box 13-3. What other items could be added to the box to describe sources of nurture and sources of depletion for each of the four domains for an individual, a family, a population, or a community?

18. From Box 13-3, choose a source of nurture in one of the domains and describe how that source of nurture might affect another domain in a client.

19. How might an excess of any factor affect any (or all) of a client's domains?

20. If a person has a physical injury, which of the other domains besides the physical one might be affected? In what way(s)?

21. Consider a woman who is the sole support of several children and must also be the caregiver for an elderly, ill parent. What domains(s) in that person might be affected? How?

22. If that woman becomes totally depleted in several of her domains, how will the domains of the family she is caring for be affected? Describe.

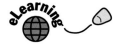

Explore Community Health Nursing on the web! To learn more about the topics in this chapter, use the passcode provided to access your exclusive web site: http://communitynursing.jbpub.com
If you do not have a passcode, you can obtain one at this site.

REFERENCES

American Public Health Association (APHA). (1991). *Healthy communities 2000 model standards: Guidelines for community attainment of the year 2000 national health objectives* (3rd ed.). Washington, DC: Author.

Bach, M. L. (1998). *ShapeWalking.* Los Angeles: Heel to Toe Fitness Walking.

Baldwin, E. M. & Baldwin, J. H. (1998). *4+ model of wellness.* Unpublished manuscript.

Baldwin, J. H. (1992). Moving towards harmony: Types and meanings of cues that prompt health-promoting decisions in women in the middle years. Doctoral dissertation, The Catholic University of America, Washington, DC. *UMI Dissertation Abstracts,* Order No. 9220772.

Baldwin, J. H. (1995). Are we implementing community health promotion in nursing? *Public Health Nursing, 12*(3), 159–164.

Baldwin, J. H., Conger, C. O., Abegglen, J. C., & Hill, E. M. (1998). Population-focused and community-based nursing—moving toward clarification of concepts. *Public Health Nursing, 15*(1), 12–18.

Becker, M. H. (Ed.). (1974). *The health belief model and personal health behavior.* Thorofare, NJ: Charles B. Slack.

Browning, B., Huls, J. Rather, R., & Stout, L. (1997). *Taylorsville youth assessment.* Unpublished manuscript. Provo, UT: Brigham Young University College of Nursing.

Brubaker, B. H. (1983, April). Health promotion: A linguistic analysis. *Advances in Nursing Science, 5,* 1–14.

Butterfield, P. G. (1993). Thinking upstream: Conceptualizing health from a population perspective. In J. M. Swanson & M. Albrecht (Eds.), *Community health nursing: Promoting the health of aggregates* (pp. 68–80). Philadelphia: W. B. Saunders.

Clark, E. G., & Leavell, H. R. (1953; 1965). Levels of application of preventive medicine. In H. R. Leavell & E. G. Clark (Eds.), *Preventive medicine for the doctor in his community: An epidemiologic approach* (3rd ed., pp. 14–38). New York: McGraw-Hill.

Cohen, J. (1998). Holistic health strategies. In C. L. Edelman & C. L. Mandle (Eds.), *Health promotion throughout the lifespan* (4th ed., pp. 333–356). St. Louis: Mosby.

Coveney, P., & Highfield, R. (1990). *The arrow of time: A voyage through science to solve time's greatest mystery.* New York: Fawcett Columbine.

Department of Health and Human Services (DHHS). (1982). *Forward plan for health 1977-1981.* Washington, DC: U.S. Government Printing Office.

Department of Health and Human Services (DHHS). (1998). *Healthy people in healthy communities: A guide for community leaders.* Washington, DC: Office of Disease Prevention and Health Promotion.

Department of Health and Human Services (DHHS). (1998). *Healthy people 2010 objectives: Draft for public comment.* Washington, DC: U.S. Government Printing Office.

Drapo, P. J., & Woods, E. (1992). Preparing community health nurses for the real world: Power, politics, and poverty. In *1991 Papers: State of the art in community health nursing education, research, and practice* (pp. 47–51). Lexington, KY: ACHNE.

Duhl L. J. (1986). *Health planning and social change.* New York: Human Sciences Press.

Dunn, H. L.(1959). High-level wellness for man and society. *American Journal of Public Health, 49,* 789.

Dunn, H. L.(1980). *High level wellness.* Thorofare, NJ: Charles B. Slack.

Edelman, C. L., & Fain, J. A. (1998). Health defined: Objectives for promotion & prevention. In C. L. Edleman & C. L. Mandle (Eds.), *Health promotion throughout the lifespan* (4th ed., pp. 3–24). St. Louis: Mosby.

Edney, A. T. B. (1992). Companion animals and human health. *Veterinary Record, 130*(4), 285–287.

Four Worlds Development Project. (1984). *The sacred tree.* Twin Lakes, WI: Lotus Light Publications.

Greene, B., & Winfrey, O. (1996). *Make the connection: Ten steps to a better body—and a better life.* New York: Hyperion.

Green, L. W., & Raeburn, J. (1990). Contemporary developments in health promotion: Definitions and challenges. In N. Bracht (Ed.), *Health promotion at the community level* (pp. 19–44). Newbury Park, CA: Sage Publications.

Greiner, P. A., & Berry, R. D. (1992). Student-faculty partnerships in a nurse-managed clinic for the homeless. In *1991 Papers: State of the art in community health nursing education, research, and practice* (pp. 67–69). Lexington, KY: ACHNE.

Healthy People 2010 (1998): http://web.health.gov/healthypeople/2010fctsht.html.

Hochbaum, G. M. (1958). *Public participation in medical screening programs: A socio-psychological study.* (Publication No. 572). Bethesda, MD: Public Health Service.

Jette, A. M., Lachman, M., Giorgetti, M. M., Assmann, S. F., Harris, B. A., Levenson, C., Wernick, M., & Krebs, D. (1999). Exercise—It's never too late: The strong-for-life program. *American Journal of Public Health, 89*(1), 66–72.

Jones, J. (1999). *Jeanne Jones' homestyle cooking made healthy.* Red Oak, IA: Rodale Press.

Kellogg foundation funds 3-year "healthy cities Indiana" project. (1988). *American Journal of Public Health, 78*(12), 5.

Laying the foundation for Healthy People 2010—The first year of consultation. (1998): http://web.health.gov/healthypeople/2010article.htm.

Kulbok, P. A, & Baldwin, J. H. (1992). From preventive health behavior to health promotion: Advancing a positive construct of health. *Advances in Nursing Science, 14*(4), 50–64.

Kulbok, P. A., Baldwin, J. H., Cox, C. L., & Duffy, R. (1997). Advancing discourse on health promotion: Beyond mainstream thinking. *Advances in Nursing Science, 20*(1), 13–21.

Kulbok, P. A., Carter, K. F., Baldwin, J. H., Gilmartin, M. J., & Kirkwood, B. (1999). The multidimensional health behavior inventory. *Journal of Nursing Measurement, 7*(2), 177–195.

Laffrey, S. C., & Kulbok, P. A. (1999). An integrative model for holistic community nursing. *Journal of Holistic Nursing, 17*(1), 88–103.

Mandle, C. L., & Castle, J. E. (1998). Health promotion & the individual. In C. L. Edleman and C. L. Mandle (Eds.), *Health promotion throughout the lifespan* (4th ed., pp. 119–143). St. Louis: Mosby.

Maslow, A. W. (1970). *Motivation and personality.* New York: Harper & Row.

McCarthy, N. C., & Mandle, C. L. (1998a). Health promotion & the family. In C. L. Edleman & C. L. Mandle (Eds.), *Health promotion throughout the lifespan* (4th ed., pp. 144–170). St. Louis: Mosby.

McCarthy, N. C., & Mandle, C. L. (1998b). Health promotion & the community. In C. L. Edleman & C. L. Mandle (Eds.), *Health promotion throughout the lifespan* (4th ed., pp. 171–192). St. Louis: Mosby.

McDonald, I. (1997). *Holistic wellness: self inventory of personal wellness utilizing the medicine wheel.* Unpublished manuscript.

McGinnis, J. M., & Foege, W. H. (1993). Actual causes of death in the United States. *Journal of the American Medical Association, 270*(18).

Model standards. (1998): www.apha.org/science/model/msmain.html.

Moore, V., Neff, D., Smith, G., & Weber, J. (1999). *The homeless in Utah County: Food & Care Coalition.* Unpublished manuscript. Provo, UT: Brigham Young University College of Nursing.

Naisbitt, J. (1982). *Megatrends.* New York: Warner Books.

National Institutes of Health. (1987). *The health benefits of pets.* (Publication No. 1988-216-107.) Washington, DC: U.S. Government Printing Office.

National Institute for Occupational Safety and Health (1996). *National Occupational Research Agenda.* (DHHS [NIOSH] Publication No. 96-115.) Washington, DC: U.S. Government Printing Office.

Neuhauser, L., Schwab, M., Syme, S. L., & Bieber, M. (1998). Community participation in health promotion: Evaluation of the California Wellness Guide. *Health Promotion International, 13*(3), 211–223.

Orem, D. E. (1985). *Nursing: Concepts of practice* (3rd ed.) New York: McGraw-Hill.

Padilla, G. V., & Bulcavage, L. M. (1991). Theories used in patient/health education. *Seminars in Oncological Nursing, 7*(2), 87–96.

Palank, C. L. (1991). Determinants of health-promotive behavior: a review of current research. *Nursing Clinics of North America, 26*(4), 815–832.

Pender, N. (1987). *Health promotion in nursing practice* (2nd ed.). East Norwalk, CT: Appleton & Lange.

Piper, M. (1999). *Another country: Navigating the emotional terrain of our elders.* Los Angeles: Riverhead Books.

Poe, B. S., & O'Neill, K. O. (1997). Caffeine modulates heat shock induced apoptosis in the human promyelocytic leukemia cell line HL-60. *Cancer Letters, 121,* 1–6.

Prigogine, I., & Stengers, I. (1984). *Order out of chaos.* New York: Bantam Books.

Rosenstock, I. M. (1974). Historical origins of the health belief model. In M. H. Becker (Ed.), *The health belief model and personal health behavior* (pp. 1–8). Thorofare, NJ: Charles B. Slack.

Ryan, R. S, & Travis, J. W. (1991). Introduction. In R. S. Ryan & J. W. Travis (Eds.), *Wellness: Small changes you can use to make a big difference* (p. 3). Berkeley, CA: Ten Speed Press.

Sandhu, G. K. (1998). Health promotion for the twenty-first century: Throughout the lifespan and throughout the world. In C. L. Edleman & C. L. Mandle (Eds.), *Health promotion throughout the lifespan* (4th ed., pp. 667–675). St. Louis: Mosby.

Segal, L., Dalton, A. C., & Richardson, J. (1998). Cost-effectiveness of the primary prevention of non-insulin dependent diabetes mellitus. *Health Promotion International, 13*(3), 197–211.

Simmons, S. J. (1990). The health-promoting self-care system model: Directions for nursing research and practice. *Journal of Advances in Nursing, 15*(10), 1162–1166.

Simopoulos, A. P. (1999). *The omega diet.* New York: HarperCollins.

Steiger, N. J., & Lipson, J. C. (1985). *Self-care nursing: Theory and practice.* Bowie, MD: Brady Communications.

United States Preventive Services Task Force. (1989). *A guide to clinical preventive services: An assessment of the effectiveness of 169 interventions.* Baltimore, MD: Williams & Wilkins.

United States Public Health Service (USPHS). (1979). *Healthy people: The surgeon general's report on health promotion and disease prevention.* (DHEW Publication No. 79-55071.) Washington, DC: U.S. Department of Health, Education, and Welfare.

United States Public Health Service (USPHS). (1980). *Promoting health/preventing disease: Objectives for the nation.* (DHHS Publication No. 0-349-256.) Washington, DC: Department of Health and Human Services.

United States Public Health Service (USPHS). (1989). *Promoting health/preventing disease: Year 2000 objectives for the nation.* Washington, DC: U.S. Department of Health and Human Services.

United States Public Health Service (USPHS). (1990). *Healthy people 2000: National health promotion and disease prevention objectives.* Washington, DC: U.S. Department of Health and Human Services.

Webster's Encyclopedic Unabridged Dictionary of the English Language. (1996). New York: Gramercy Books/Random House.

Wheatley, J. (1994). *Leadership and the new science: Learning about organization from an orderly universe.* San Francisco, CA: Berrett-Koehler.

Chapter 14

Nursing Informatics in Community Health Nursing Practice

Russell C. McGuire

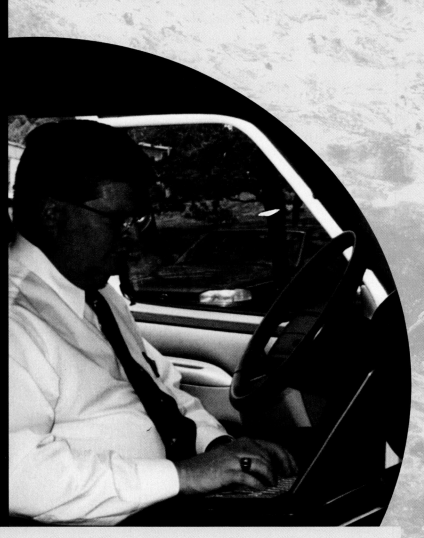

The worlds of health care, communication, and information tech-nologies are ever evolving, separately and together. As nurses in the community expand their practice definition to embrace new informa-tion technologies, opportunities for improved health care to popula-tions seem endless. This evolution is seen as a merger of health care technology with information and communications technology, foster-ing the design and implementation of health care management infor-mation systems in a variety of clinical practice settings.

QUESTIONS TO CONSIDER

After reading this chapter, answer the following questions:
1. What is nursing informatics?
2. How is the science of informatics used in nursing practice in the community?
3. What are the benefits of informatics?
4. How is client information managed using informatics?
5. What are some computer applications used in community health nursing?
6. How are management and network systems used in community health nursing practice?
7. What are the community health nursing benefits to using telehealth?

KEY TERMS

Database	Health management	Nursing classification	Nursing information
Distributed data	information systems	systems	systems
processing (DDP)	(HMIS)	Nursing data	Nursing knowledge
Electronic mail (e-mail)	Network client care	Nursing informatics	Telemedicine/telehealth
Electronic spreadsheets		Nursing information	

in data transmission, and increases in information systems' efficiency and data manipulation effectiveness.

Zielstorff, Hudgings, and Grobe (1993) describe characteristics related to nursing information systems. These characteristics apply to nursing information systems in any nursing clinical practice settings. Several assumptions that pertain to the information systems used in all nursing practice settings are discussed by Zielstorff and her colleagues. These assumptions are necessary for understanding how the profession of nursing can support development of effective nursing information systems. These assumptions are outlined in Box 14-1.

Community Health Nursing and Nursing Informatics

In community-based nursing practice, the implementation of nursing information systems must be integrated with data systems that collect client data for other disciplines. The profession of nursing leads the way in data collection, the use of standardized language classifications, and design support for automated systems that can assist in supporting the integration of other health care disciplines. This integration of nursing information is useful in community health nursing when multiple disciplines are responsible for the care of the client and his or her caregivers and when coordination of care is paramount in achieving expedient and successful outcomes.

Nursing informatics deals with the collection, manipulation, analysis, and interpretation of several levels of data, information, and knowledge. Community-based nursing deals with the same levels of data for which computer technology, nursing informatics, and communications technology are used to transform data into knowledge. The first level of data is related to clients and their caregivers. Data such as client sociodemographic status, medical history, physical examination results, integrated health care assessments, and treatment plans are examples of client-level

data or information. The second level of data is specific to the organization or agency. Examples of this level of data are an organization's productivity indicators, policies, and procedures, as well as the availability of community resources associated with a specific client's or caregiver's health care needs. The third level of data is domain specific. Domain-specific data are associated with care provided across the continuum of health care services delivery and are related to the client and caregiver responses (outcomes) to community health nursing interventions. Domain-specific data include the medical diagnosis and subsequent nursing diagnosis, the efficiency and applicability of specific nursing interventions and the subsequent client outcomes, and the data related to the specifics of providing care such as drug interactions with prescribed medications.

Benefits of Nursing Informatics for Community Health Nursing

The combination of nursing and information systems management produces several benefits for nurses practicing in the community. These benefits include (1) the management of client-level data; (2) the use of standardized nursing language to communicate what nurses do and how clients and their families respond to care; (3) provision of care in an efficient and productive manner; and (4) the use of information systems for research, health promotion, and illness prevention in the community.

Nursing Classification Systems

The different levels of data and subsequent levels of information and knowledge relevant to the practice of community-based nursing have been discussed thus far. To facilitate an understanding of how nursing languages are used to describe nursing practice and how standardized nursing languages are important in the context of automated nursing information systems, the discussion briefly turns to the evolution of **nursing classification systems.** It is important to remember that community health nurses use language as a medium for describing the client's clinical status, the appropriateness of the clinical care environment, the support systems available to the client, and the client's level of response to nursing intervention. To facilitate the use of language for communicating what nurses do, several professional nursing organizations have created initiatives to implement standardized nursing languages into clinical practice.

The American Nurses Association established the Steering Committee on Databases to Support Nursing Practice in 1990. The purpose of this committee was to develop policy to support the development of nursing classification systems, the uniformity of nursing data sets, and the implementation of a national data set. In 1992, the committee gave its support for the Unified Nursing Language System (UNLS). The UNLS is recognized by the National Library of Medicine for inclusion in the Unified Medical Language System. The Steering Committee on Databases to Support Nursing Practice currently recognizes five nurs-

TABLE 14-1   SUMMARY OF NURSING CLASSIFICATION SYSTEM FEATURES

NAME	MAJOR FEATURES
NANDA: North American Nursing Diagnosis Association (Warren & Hoskins, 1995)	Research-based nursing diagnosis system having nine different diagnosis patterns (exchanging, communicating, relating, valuing, choosing, moving, perceiving, knowing, and feeling).
Visiting Nurses Association of Omaha Community Health Problem and Intervention System (Martin & Scheet, 1995)	Three major components: (1) problems classification, (2) intervention scheme, (3) problem rating scale for outcomes. Developed for and researched in community-based nursing practice settings (home health, public health, school nursing, and clinic settings).
HHCC: Home Health Care Classification (Saba & McCormick, 1996)	Developed to provide a standardized language system for coding/categorizing the services provided by nurses in the home health practice setting. Coding scheme for nursing diagnosis, interventions, and outcomes that are easily coded for computer data collection and retrieval.
NIC: Iowa Intervention Project: Nursing Intervention Classification (McCloskey & Bulechek, 1996)	Large data set of research-based nursing interventions dealing with six domains (physiological basic and complex behavioral, safety, family, and health systems). Interventions have a specific label, are defined, and have a set of actions or activities performed by the nurse while providing client care.
NOC: Iowa Outcomes Project: Nursing Outcomes Classification (Johnson & Maas, 1997)	The classification contains 218 outcomes, which are listed in alphabetical order. Each NOC outcome has a specific definition, a list of indicators that are used in the evaluation of client status, scale of measurement, and a list of references used in development of the outcome. Five-point Likert type scales were developed for use with the outcomes to measure client status in relation to the outcome.

ing taxonomies: (1) the North American Nursing Diagnosis Association (NANDA), (2) the Visiting Nurses Association of Omaha Community Health Problem and Intervention System, (3) the Home Health Care Classification (HHCC), (4) the Iowa Intervention Project: Nursing Intervention Classification (NIC), and (5) Iowa Outcomes Project: Nursing Outcomes Classification (NOC). A brief summary of each classification system is provided in Table 14-1.

The use of standardized nursing classification systems as described in Table 14-1 provides community health nurses with a uniform description of problems, interventions, and related outcomes while providing care to clients and their caregivers. In the community health nursing practice setting, the use of standardized nursing languages can (1) facilitate the appropriate selection of nursing interventions for cost-effective and clinically effective health care delivery; (2) assist in predicting client and caregiver

outcomes; (3) foster transdisciplinary communications; (4) assist community health nursing managers in appropriate allocation of financial and personnel resources; (5) promote reimbursement for nursing services; and (6) articulate community health nursing's worth to health care policy planners at the state, federal, and international levels (Grier & McGuire, 1999).

Client Information Management

Health care is data intensive. Much of the collection of client-related clinical data takes a considerable amount of time and effort. The management of client-level data provides the community health nurse with an accurate assessment of clients' and their caregivers' situation for the purpose of planning, implementing, and evaluating care. Information systems allow for the organization of myriad data collected during an individual's admission to a community health care facility. This information can be stored for future retrieval, and the aggregation of this information can be analyzed for the benefit of the community.

Efficiency and Time Benefits

The use of nursing information systems can provide community health nurse managers and staff with efficiencies in productivity. The collection of client- and caregiver-centered information is often a time-consuming endeavor and uses financial and personnel resources. Savings in time are often demonstrated by the use of computer systems for communicating information over distance, over time, and to multiple users of the data. Clinical information can be shared with several users at the same time. An example is sharing laboratory results with a nurse practitioner at a remote community clinic at the same time the practitioner is consulting with a physician in a large tertiary center.

Information systems are used to manage health care information for population groups. Bargstadt (1998) described several benefits of information systems use in the community setting. These benefits include (1) collecting data to demonstrate clinical effectiveness of community health nursing care delivery to a specific population, (2) analyzing the collected clinical data for statistical comparison, (3) determining the cost-effectiveness of community health nursing programs on the care of clients and caregivers, and (4) using cost-effective data collection for outcome measurement.

Computer Applications in Community Health Nursing

Computer and communications technologies continue to grow rapidly in utilization with the community health care practice setting. This use will continue to grow in all segments of health care and will become more efficient and effective in meeting the goals of a community health care facility for information leading to sound clinical and financial decision making. Computer applications that support good communications and organization of clinically related data are available.

Electronic Mail

Computers have long been able to communicate with one another. In the past, communication between computer users had been an interactive endeavor; that is, both the sender and the receiver of the communication had to be at their respective terminals for the communication to take place. With today's elec-

tronic mail (e-mail) applications, the sender and receiver need not be at their respective computer terminals because the message can be sent in a "store and forward" manner. Depending on the type of operating system and e-mail software package, the typical e-mail system (e.g., Microsoft's Messaging) sets up a computerized mailbox that receives the incoming message and stores it for viewing by the receiving computer user when it is convenient. The received message can be read on the computer's monitor, saved for future reference, or printed. Messages can be configured with an "attached" or inserted file such as a word processing document, presentations, animation, sound bites, or electronic spreadsheets. In the community-based practice setting, messages of a critical nature (e.g., client status, critical laboratory reports, or case management information) can be sent to physicians or nurse practitioners from sources such as the laboratory, radiology department, health information systems departments, and remote sites such the public health department of home health agency.

Databases

Community-based health care delivery is data intensive. Client charts contain massive amounts of data that individually are just single pieces of unrelated information. When data are used in this unrelated manner, analysis is difficult to perform. But when data are combined in a structure that demonstrates relationships between data elements, powerful data analysis can begin. A **database** software package such as Microsoft's Access gives the com-

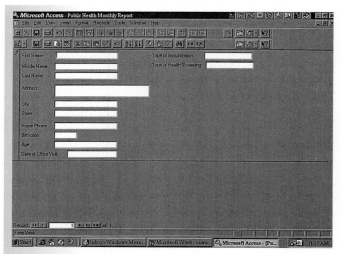

Example of database entry screen.

puter user the ability to generate records that have data elements grouped together for relational value. These individual records can be grouped, and further delineation of the data elements can be achieved. For example, a public health nurse might want to construct a monthly report of all clinic pediatric clients of a certain age or age group, data related to their visits, the immunization status of each client, and the type of health screenings that have been performed. If these data are first entered into a database program, age, dates of office visits, types of immunization, and types of health screening could be "queried" or selected by the nurse for the monthly report (see the figure on p. 314).

This type of database is known as *relational* because each data element in the database can be selected (or not selected) for report generation. Simple data analysis can then be performed on the individual and aggregate client care level.

Electronic Spreadsheets

Electronic spreadsheets assist the computer user with "crunching" or manipulating of large amounts of numerical data. The software displays a series of rows and columns in a gridlike depiction of a spreadsheet. This grid is displayed on the computer's monitor. Each box created by the intersection of a row and column is known as a *cell*. Individual numbers or formulas can be entered into the cell to calculate results for a given problem. For example, a home health nursing manager may want to know how many skilled nursing visits are a percentage of the total number of visits performed by all the professional staff in the agency. A column of cells is named "skilled nursing visits," and each of the registered nurses' monthly visits is entered in the cell next to their individual names. At the end of the column, the nurse manager designates one cell to enter a formula to (1) add all the cells that contain the registered nurses' monthly visits and (2) place the total number of professional visits for the agency into (3) a formula that would calculate a percentage (see the fig-

Example of electronic spreadsheet.

ure below). Sophisticated statistical analysis, supported by user-defined formulas that are a part of the spreadsheet software, can generate reports with graphs of a meaningful nature. Spreadsheet data can be "exported," that is, moved from one type of computer application to another.

For example, a nurse manager may want to perform some sophisticated statistical analysis that involves comparisons between two groups of clients. After collecting the desired data and entering these data into an electronic spreadsheet, the nurse manager can export the spreadsheet data file to a statistical package such as SPSS (Statistical Package for Social Sciences) for complex statistical comparisons.

Internet Applications in Community-Based Nursing Practice

As computer networks have become more established throughout the nation, and for that matter the world, additional opportunities for sharing data, information, and knowledge have presented themselves to health care providers. The establishment of the Internet has enabled many health care practitioners to communicate and thus share community health–related data. The Internet is the product of a communications network known as the *ARPAnet,* a network of American defense computers. This network was developed in the late 1960s to counter the detrimental effects of nuclear warfare on computer and communications technology. It was first used to link various major university academic computer centers where United States defense research was being conducted. As the academic centers proliferated and began to link to one another, the Internet became a conglomeration of academic, commercial, governmental, and personal web sites used for the exchange of information, services, and research. The Internet affords the computer user the luxury of communicating with health care professional from around the world. The Web has become a wonderful resource for communications, research, and education for community-based nurses and the clients and caregivers they serve. There are thousands of web sites easily accessed by computer users throughout the world.

Health Care Delivery System Management Software

Health care information systems software designers have developed many different financial and business solutions for various health care delivery settings. From the 1970s through the present, software developers focused most of their development on hospital software that dealt with financial issues such as cost, revenues, payer mix, and diagnosis-related group (DRG) identification and coding. Decision support systems were mostly aimed at answering business questions. Recently, an emphasis on clinical data collection and presentation has emerged in the development of software applications for health care. With the advent of managed care, prospective payment, managed care reimbursement, and increased competition in the health care industry, special health care application software has been and continues to be designed for the community-based practice setting.

Software applications and computer systems (as well as networks) are being developed from a clinical perspective. Outpatient clinics, public health departments, free-standing and hospital-based home health agencies, and schools are all excellent practice settings that have elements of information systems development. One example is the development of a home health information system by the Atlanta-based health information system vendor McKesson HBOC. The product, Pathways Homecare, which is based on a relational database, gives the home health nurse the opportunity to collect client care data at the point of care—the home setting. Sociodemographic data, client assessments, visit notes, clinical pathways used for specific disease states, generation of Medicare forms for billing purposes, and agency financial management have been incorporated into the application. The Windows-based Pathways Homecare has a user-friendly graphical interface that lends itself well to "point and click" data entry and manipulation within the software application.

Networked Client Care

Computers used in a stand-alone configuration are powerful, productive business, academic, and clinical tools. The power of computers is enhanced or increased when linked together. When linked together, computer users can share application software and files, communicate, and therefore increase productivity. Community-based health care delivery systems use networks (the linking of computer and communications technologies) to transfer data, images, and video (medical video and health care teleconferencing).

For this transmission of data, networks have been designed and implemented in many health care setting. Stallings and Van Slyke (1998) describe three types of networks that are used extensively in community-based health care practice: (1) wide area networks (WAN), (2) local area networks (LAN), and (3) wireless networks.

Wide area networks are used by health care facilities for data transmission and data communications over a long distance. For example, WANs are used for data transmission between several health care facilities and their central office. Local area networks connect computer users who are generally within the confines of an office complex or the same building. Wireless networks use radio frequency or infrared technology for data transmission. This type of network allows for greater mobility in hardware use within a facility. An outgrowth of network development is client-server computer architecture. As computer technology migrated from massive mainframe systems to smaller personal computers, the linkage of these personal computers to one another lead to client-server technology. The server, a computer (either a power-

ful minicomputer, a large-capacity personal computer, or a mainframe) is connected to several personal computer workstations. These "clients" can use application software that resides on the server. An example of this relationship can be demonstrated by the use of a database that resides on the server. A computer user at a remote workstation queries the relational database, asking the server for specific records. Instead of the server sending all the records to the computer user, the server sends only the records that are specified by the client workstation user.

Certain advantages are gained by using client-server technology in the community-based nursing practice setting. First, the system configuration is composed of several powerful machines that give the community health nurse a considerable amount of computer power at lower cost than traditional mainframe, centralized, "closed" computing systems. Second, the client-server computer architecture is considered to be open systems technology. Community health care program planners can choose from among several hardware and software vendors to configure their computer system based on specific organizational and clinical needs. Finally, the computer system can grow and be enhanced when the community health care organization's needs change. An example of this can be demonstrated in the community-based nursing practice setting.

Most community-based practice settings are influenced by external factors such as federal and state government health care reimbursement programs. As these programs change their reimbursement strategies and their regulations, different reporting and documentation requirements are generated for the service provider. When the community health care organization has an open systems architecture as a base for the computer system, new hardware (if needed) and software (for the new reporting requirements) can be installed easily with the existing system's configuration.

The advent of client-server technology has led to more use of a network concept known as **distributed data processing (DDP)**. In the DDP configuration, a community-based health care organization uses smaller computers as workstations at sites that can be situated within a single building or from off site, remote computing sites. These smaller competing sites are connected via telecommunications lines (POTS, T1 or T3, fiberoptic, or even satellite). The figure on p. 317 depicts a DDP configuration.

The advantages of developing and maintaining distributed data processing configuration are numerous. The remote sites (e.g., off-site health department offices) can respond more quickly to service demands if data processing capabilities are available at the remote sites. Backup systems are more often available to the entire community health care organization, minimizing downtime caused by equipment or software failure. As health care service demands change within a community (as a result of external factors such as changes in Medicare, Medicaid, or managed care penetration) a community-based organization can change the DDP configuration incrementally, often without

DISTRIBUTED DATA PROCESSING.

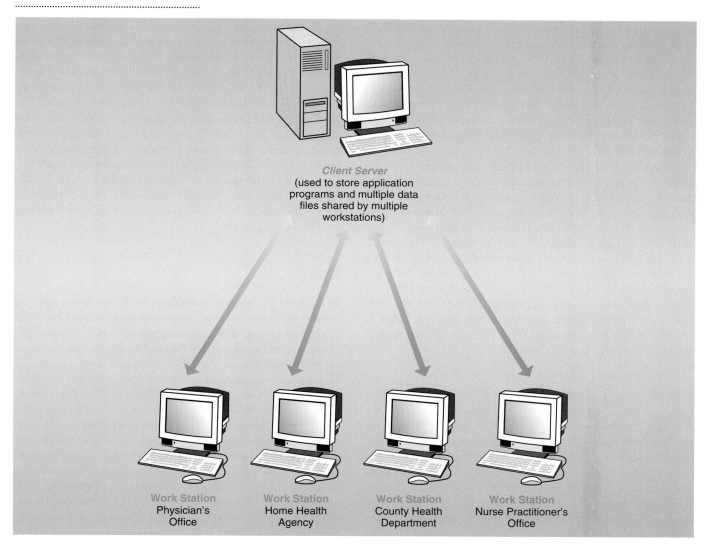

Client Server
(used to store application
programs and multiple data
files shared by multiple
workstations)

Work Station
Physician's
Office

Work Station
Home Health
Agency

Work Station
County Health
Department

Work Station
Nurse Practitioner's
Office

great expense to the organization. Finally, the computing needs of nurse executives, managers, and staff can be tailored easily within the DDP configuration. Analysis of client care data and more productivity at staff levels can be realized when a DDP system is developed, implemented, and maintained.

Communication Technology and Community Health Nursing

Much of the United States is considered rural in geography, and thus there are inherit challenges to providing access to health care services. Lack of access to health care facilities and to limited numbers of health care providers tends to decrease opportunities for service provision. Distance to health care facilities and access to skilled health care providers are but two challenges to individuals seeking health care services in both rural and inner-city environments. **Telemedicine/telehealth** is the delivery of medical services over telecommunications lines and is paving the way for providing specialized, skilled services in areas that would otherwise be without.

The following discussion demonstrates how current telehealth applications are being used in the community-based practice setting. As with all information and communications technology, these applications are evolving into faster, less expensive methods for delivering community-based health care services.

Telehealth Care Benefits

An example of the benefit that telehealth can provide can be demonstrated in home health care. Home health care is one of the fastest-growing industries in the United States. Along with this growth has come a certain amount of scrutiny with regard to reimbursement practices. In an effort to control cost, the federal government is in the process of converting from a cost-based reimbursement system to a prospective payment system based on the Balanced Budget Act of 1997. Managed care also is increasing in market penetration. As a response to the increased pressures to remain financially viable, home health care agencies are looking at many innovative technologies to supplement, enhance, and complement care. Crist, Kaufman, and Crampton (1996) discussed the advances of telemedicine and its application within home health agencies.

There are three basic types of data transmitted from the home setting to a central home health office via telecommunications. Data, which are generally client specific, can be sent from a remote site to the home health agency's central station. This can include data elements such as blood pressure, blood oxygen, pulse, temperature, blood glucose, weight, electrocardiograph results, and other measurements. The second type of data that can be collected and transmitted is audio (e.g., heart and lung sounds). Voice data can include anything from voice conversation to stethoscope sounds and messages. The third and final type of data transmitted through telecommunication is image. It can take the form of still image (i.e., still-frame photograph) or full-motion video.

Community Health Nursing Benefits of Telehealth Care

Crist and her colleagues describe a telemedicine system that has been evaluated in the Cincinnati area. This system was primarily developed for home use but could also be used in the hospital, physician's office, or nursing home. The device is a user-friendly computer-based device used to communicate daily with clients and their caregivers to support their health care needs. The system was designed using touch screen and audio to coach clients through treatment protocols. Other features available from the unit are vital signs devices, which include thermometer, pulse oximetry, blood pressure cuff, and electrocardiograph; digital stethoscope to record heart, lung, and gastrointestinal sounds; a medication reminder system to increase client compliance with medication administration; real-time telephone communication for scheduling activities; video transmission of client to nurse, nurse to client; and touch screens that allow for coaching to assist the client in routine medical procedures, which can include procedures such as dressing changes, medication administration, and the taking of vital signs.

The system provides for the hookup of future devices such as a blood glucose monitor, a scale for obtaining weight, an intravenous (IV) pump, and a ventilator. The system can be customized to meet the particular needs of the client during installation and also has an alarm function for changes in client status. This system allows for 24-hour response to client needs and care management with necessary skilled visits. The central nursing

station accumulates health care data such as vital signs, request for medication, communication events, and requests for assistance on each client for which a home-assisted nursing care (HANC) unit is installed. A unique feature of the system is the ability of the home health agency to change client protocols as client conditions change. The key factor to the successful application of the HANC network is the ability to customize the telecommunications systems for a particular clients needs.

Gains in staff productivity by using the HANC system were demonstrated in a cost-effectiveness study. Crist and her colleagues describe their research findings in a summary of retrospective chart review showing weekly savings for treatment therapy such as IV therapy ($2,207), wounds ($1,890), and diabetes ($1,807). They projected possible cost savings through the use of the telemedicine technology of approximately $255,000 per year for a total of 43 clients.

The Future of Informatics and Telehealth

The advent of telemedicine/telehealth brings a considerable amount of opportunity to community-based nursing practices. Client monitoring, client and caregiver education, transdisciplinary case conferences, and professional health care education are being achieved. Several researchers in telehealth see a future role for telecommunications in home care as an alternative to traditional in-home visits. Warner (1996) believes telehealth is a technological answer to proposed prospective payment systems being considered by Medicare. She bases this on the fact that agencies can be expected to be reimbursed at a fixed schedule rather than by the number of visits. Warner views the role of telecommunications as reducing unnecessary emergency room visits, reducing unnecessary/unscheduled physician office visits, providing early nursing intervention and prevention of repeat hospitalizations, and educating the client about early symptoms and managing these symptoms through a link to medical information (p. 792). The use of telehealth technology will enable the nurse to capture vital signs data (temperature, pulse, and blood pressure) at various times throughout the day without physically having to interact with the client. This collected data can then be used to revise the client's individualized care plan.

Warner envisions a nursing visit conducted through a telehealth system as encompassing the following: The nursing personnel places a call to the client's station using the client's home telephone number with two-way video communications and interactive audio; the nurse then interacts with the client, which consists of assessment, education, monitoring, and implementation of functions that would normally be made in person. Warner states that some telehealth systems allow the nurse to remotely control camera functions to get a closer view of wound sites and infusion sites as well as scanning the client's environment. Most systems will allow for an electronic capture of data elements necessary for a clinical record as well as still-frame photo and full-motion video. According to Warner, quality-of-care issues will also be met through enhanced productivity by replacing the travel time that nurses have in making their daily caseload assignments. Telehealth systems would also allow nurses to make visits in adverse weather conditions and in high-risk neighborhoods where safety is often threatened.

The use of telehealth systems can provide a telecommunications information system that is interactive between the nurse and the client, using text, video, audio, and/or graphics. Warner also advocates a telehealth utilization by diagnosis, with less severe acuities being matched with technologies that are also less technical. She places the complexity of client statuses on a continuum from less to more complex, more acute illnesses such as congestive heart failure, recovery after acute myocardial infarction, chronic obstructive pulmonary disease, and diabetes being on the higher end of the continuum and resulting in the need for more technical intervention. Warner discusses several factors that are related to determining when telehealth is appropriate for a particular client. A primary consideration should be the stability of the individual's disease processes. It is also necessary that the client possess sufficient cognitive ability, hearing, and vision to use the system or to have a caregiver to provide assistance In addition, consideration must be made for the client's and caregivers' feelings and beliefs with regard to allowing the system in their home (e.g., apprehension about technology, cost, or loss of privacy) (p. 794).

The future of nursing informatics will be based on supporting the individual practicing nurse's requirements for assessing, implementing, evaluating, and redefining care across all practice settings and teaching practicing clinicians how to use information and communication technologies. Gassert (1998), in her presentation to the American Medical Informatics Association, envisioned meeting these needs and those of clients and communities through a national nursing informatics agenda. Her two-part agenda includes (1) a strategic direction for preparing nurses in the use of information and communication technologies through the education of nursing students, practicing nurses, and nursing faculty and (2) strategies that impact client care, including preparing nurses for information and communication use at the undergraduate, graduate, and continuing education levels; developing funding and programs for teaching specialized nursing informatic skills and, with other health care providers, developing collaborative programs in telecommunications that "will enhance the quality of clinical practice for populations at risk and contribute to the education of health providers" (p. 266); increasing nursing faculty exposure to information and communication technology use in nursing individual clients, communities, and caregivers; and developing the use of public and private resources such as the Internet to increase accessibility of health care knowledge resources for health care providers and the public (p. 267).

RESEARCH BRIEF

Kinsella, A., & Warner, I. (1998). Telehealth and managing congestive heart failure. Caring, 17(6), 14–18.

In anticipation of delivering alternative visit services in a prospective payment environment, Kinsella and Warner (1998) describe how telehealth applications aid community-based nurses in extending their services to patients with congestive heart failure (CHF). Basic telehealth technology can assist the home health nurse with providing quality care services at the same time they reduce cost associated with an in-person visit. These basic tools induce the use of (1) blood pressure cuffs with telecommunication capability, (2) scales with scanning capabilities, (3) computer software packages that assist CHF patients and their caregivers with meal planning, and (4) telephonic reminder programs for medication compliance and supportive messaging. Other medical technologies with telecommunications capabilities include the use of vital signs monitoring equipment, electronic scales, patient education via multimedia, and automated critical pathways. Each of these technologies, when used appropriately by skilled nursing clinicians, are cost-effective, cost-efficient tools that provide care to patients and their caregivers.

CONCLUSION

The use of information and communications technology in support of community nursing functions will continue to increase and offer community health nursing leaders and staff care for the clients and family caregivers they serve. The specialty of nursing informatics offers strategies for using technologies such as those discussed in this chapter to (1) collect individual- and community-related data, (2) store and retrieve this data for clinical decision making (through the process of converting raw data into nursing information and ultimately into nursing knowledge), and (3) provide in-depth analysis of data for increasing productive service delivery while providing quality care.

Nursing informatics uses computer and communication technologies to collect information in a readily understandable format. To assist nurses in using computers to describe the care they render in a community-based practice setting, standardized nursing languages such as NANDA, NIC, NOC, HHCC, and Omaha were developed and continue to be added to through research efforts. Standardized languages in computer systems are used to assess clients and their communities, describe the care community health nurses perform, and are a basis for communications between community health nurses and other health care providers.

The use of computer applications such as e-mail, databases, and spreadsheets can provide community health nurses with tools to increase their productivity and knowledge. E-mail can be used to coordinate communications among health care providers in the community. Databases have been used to collect and organize massive amounts of client- and community-related data to be used in research and business analysis. Spreadsheets can be used to perform complicated mathematical or statistical calculations that support clinical decision making. Information and communication systems continue to offer exciting, new ways for community health nurses to maintain a cost-effective presence in the community even when distance is a challenge. The use of telemedicine/telehealth provides the community health nurse with several strategies for maintaining visual and/or audio contact with clients and family caregivers.

The future of nursing informatics and telehealth is bright and promising. Innovations in nursing science combined with advances in information and communication technologies will provide community health nurses and planners with tools that will increase their contact with the communities they serve.

CRITICAL THINKING ACTIVITIES

1. You have been chosen to introduce your public health nursing staff to e-mail and the Internet. Detail what you would do to develop a program for the staff, outlining the benefits and uses of this technology in community health.

2. Develop an e-mail message for new public health nurses who will be converting to an electronic client care system in 6 months. How will you evaluate the effectiveness of your communication?

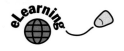

Explore Community Health Nursing on the web! To learn more about the topics in this chapter, use the passcode provided to access your exclusive web site:
http://communitynursing.jbpub.com
If you do not have a passcode, you can obtain one at this site.

REFERENCES

Bargstadt, G. (1998). Use of nursing information systems in the community setting. In S. Moorhead & C. Delaney (Eds.), *Information systems innovations for nursing* (pp. 213–226). Thousand Oaks, CA: Sage Publications.

Crist, T., Kaufman, S., & Crampton, K. (1996). Home telemedicine: A home health care agency's strategy for maximizing resources. *Home Health Care Management Practice, 8*(4), 1–9.

Gassert, C. (1998). The challenge of meeting patient's needs with a national nursing informatics agenda. *Journal of the American Medical Informatics Association, 5*(3), 263–286.

Graves, J., & Corcoran, S. (1989). The study of nursing informatics. *Image: The Journal of Nursing Scholarship, 21*, 227–231.

Grier, M., & McGuire, R. (1999). Nursing informatics: A means for change. In J. Lancaster (Ed.), *Nursing issues in leading and managing change* (pp. 533–553). St. Louis: Mosby.

Johnson, M., & Maas, M. (1997). *Iowa outcomes project: Nursing Outcomes Classification (NOC)* . St. Louis: Mosby.

Martin, K. S., & Scheet, N. J. (1995). The Omaha System: Nursing diagnosis, intervention, and client outcomes. *An emerging framework: Data systems advances for clinical nursing practice* (pp. 105–113). Washington, D.C.: American Nursing Association Publication, June. #NP-94.

McCloskey, J., & Bulechek, G. (1996). *Iowa intervention project: Nursing Intervention Classification (NIC)* (2nd ed.). St. Louis: Mosby.

Saba, V., & McCormick, K. (1996). *Essentials of computers for nurses* (2nd ed.). New York: McGraw-Hill.

Sebastian, J., & Stanhope, M. (1999). Managing resources. In J. Lancaster (Ed.), *Nursing issues in leading and managing change* (pp. 505–531). St. Louis: Mosby.

Stallings, W., & Van Slyke, R. (1998). *Business Data Communications* (3rd ed.). Upper Saddle River, NJ: Prentice Hall.

Warner, I. (1996). Telehealth home care. *Home Health Care Nurse, 14*(10), 791–796.

Warren, J. J., & Hoskins, L. M. (1995). NANDA's nursing diagnosis taxonomy: A nursing database. *An emerging framework: Data systems advances for clinical nursing practice* (pp. 49–59). Washington, D.C.: American Nurses Association Publication, June. #NP-94.

Zielstorff, R., Hudgings, C., & Grobe, S. (1993). *Next-generation nursing information systems: Essential characteristics for professional practice.* Washington DC: American Nurses Association.

Chapter 15
Health Education in the Community

Lucy Bradley-Springer

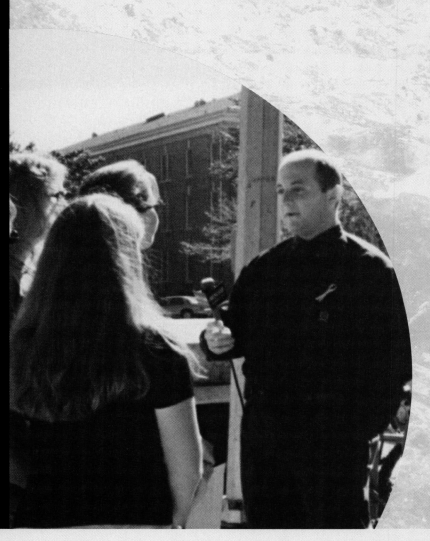

You may ask, "Why should I teach? Why would I want to change people's behaviors? I went to nursing school to give client care, not to teach. If I'd wanted to teach, I wouldn't have spent all this time learning to put catheters in and how to fill out care plans." The short answer is that **teaching** *is an essential part of nursing. Nurses teach because it is a part of client care. The longer answer is that teaching clients improves health care. Education positively influences health outcomes when clients experience fewer complications and faster recoveries; learn to care for themselves, increasing autonomy and self-confidence; and are better prepared to resume their usual lives.*

QUESTIONS TO CONSIDER

After reading this chapter, answer the following questions:

1. What is health education, and how does it differ in community settings?
2. What are behavior concepts and theories in education?
3. How are behavioral concepts and theories used to provide direction for health education programs?
4. What are principles of education, and how can they be integrated into health education practice?
5. What are the various situations in community health nursing in which education for behavior change can be incorporated into nursing care at the individual, group, and community levels?
6. What are the ethical issues in health education that have emerged from the current health care environment?

KEY TERMS

Absolutism	Behavior change	Discharge teaching	Learning theories
Adherence	Benefits	Domains of learning	Motivation
Advocacy	Cognitive dissonance	Empowerment	Paternalism
Autonomy	Community-based	Health education	Readiness
Barriers	teaching	Learning goals and	Self-efficacy
Behavior change theories	Compliance	objectives	Teaching

Wisdom is not a product of schooling, but the lifelong attempt to acquire it.

Albert Einstein

The purpose of health education is to change behaviors that put people at risk for injury, disease, disability, or death (Glanz, Lewis, & Rimer, 1990). This may sound blunt, but whether you call it modifying behavior or influencing behavior (Rankin & Stallings, 1996), it all boils down to the same thing: Nurses teach clients, families, groups, and communities with the primary goal of getting people to change behaviors in ways that focus on disease prevention, illness intervention, and health promotion. The mission of health education is to "reduce current and future suffering" by addressing "individual and social factors that contribute to health problems" (Guttman, Kegler, & McLeroy, 1996, p. i). This chapter explores the topic of health education: its theoretical bases, its application, the problems associated with it, and the community heath nurse's role in health education.

Health education can also increase the knowledge, skills, and confidence needed to make decisions. It improves continuity of care, decreases the risk of problem recurrence, and uses resources more efficiently. Educated clients and their families are better able to cope and more likely to recognize problems before they become severe. All of these benefits help nurses do their jobs because knowledgeable clients have fewer complications and present with fewer of the acute emergencies that require more complex care (Hunt, 1997).

Initially, health education concentrated on crisis management ("What do you need to know now that you've got a colostomy?"). However, the health care system in the United States is evolving. The emphasis is now on cost containment, health maintenance, and managed care (Damrosch, 1991). Over the past decade, health education has had to adjust to support client care in the midst of all these changes. Today health educa-

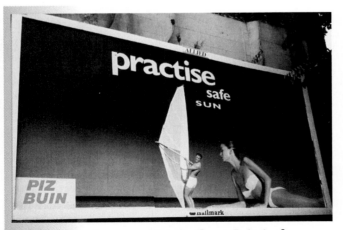

Public education campaign in Great Britain for prevention of skin cancer.

> **A CONVERSATION WITH . . .**
>
> *The fundamental conditions and resources for health are peace, shelter, education, food, income, a stable ecosystem, sustainable resources, social justice, and equity. Improvement in health requires a secure foundation in these basic prerequisites.*
>
> **—World Health Organization,** Ottawa Charter for Health Promotion, 1986.

tion includes disease prevention ("How do you keep from getting tuberculosis?" or "How can you decrease your risk of a stroke from hypertension?") and health promotion ("How can you change to a healthier diet?") as well as continuing to deal with acute care issues. In addition, whether the focus is on reducing the rates of childhood infections or the deaths from cancer, health education and community-based programs are essential components of attaining every goal in the *Healthy People 2010* agenda (DHHS, 2000). Selected *Healthy People 2010* objectives related to health education are included in a box at the end of this chapter (p. 343).

Although nurses are not the only health care professionals capable of teaching, their knowledge, skills, and access to clients, especially in the community, make them particularly well suited to this complex task (Spellbring, 1991).

Theoretical Bases

When dealing with complex issues, it is wise to work from a theoretical base. Theories describe, explain, and predict behaviors within a functional framework (Glanz, Lewis, & Rimer, 1990). Theories about health education and behavior change can help nurses understand behavior and thereby help them develop useful strategies that influence people's health.

Concepts

Theories are based on concepts that are used to form the propositions that give structure to a theory. Some important concepts that support client **autonomy** in health education are defined in Table 15-1. In addition, it would be helpful to discuss absolutism and paternalism, two concepts that have lost favor in health education not only because they tend to stifle autonomy, but also because they have not been found to be effective.

Absolutism is a tactic we have all used. When absolutism is used in health education, the teacher basically says, "This is what you must do." Absolutism requires absolute **adherence** to specific, prescribed strategies (Cates & Hinman, 1992), and we have all done it because, as nurses, we know that smoking is not healthy and eating broccoli is. Absolute health care messages are usually well intentioned. They are based on evidence that, if used consistently and correctly, the prescribed methods will make

TABLE 15-1	IMPORTANT CONCEPTS FOR HEALTH EDUCATION THEORY

CONCEPT	DEFINITION
Advocacy	Process in which clients are informed and supported so that they can make the best decisions possible (Spellbring, 1991); advocacy is a primary nursing function.
Barriers	Those individually determined things that associate cost with a particular behavior (Palank, 1991); costs can be thought of in terms of money, time inconvenience, difficulty, risk, or interpersonal effort. Not having child care, for example, is a barrier for a mother who needs to attend a Narcotics Anonymous meeting.
Benefits	Those individually determined things that reinforce or reward a particular behavior (Palank, 1991); in other words, one person may see weight loss as a main benefit of exercise, but another may see meeting friends at the gym as the primary benefit.
Cognitive dissonance	Tension or discomfort that accompanies actions that oppose personal beliefs (Rankin & Stallings, 1996); for example, a person who lectures co-workers about good nutrition eats chocolate cake and feels guilty about it.
Empowerment	Process of helping people develop the abilities to understand and control their personal situations; can be applied at individual, group, and community levels (Israel, Checkoway, Schulz, & Zimmerman, 1994).
Motivation	Complex concept that refers to those "forces acting on or within an organism that initiate, direct, and maintain behavior" (Redman, 1997, p. 7).
Readiness	Motivation to perform a particular action at a particular time (Redman, 1997).
Self-efficacy	Personal conviction of ability to carry out specific behaviors in order to achieve a desired end (Damrosch, 1991; Palank, 1991); the "I know I can do this" feeling.

people healthier. The problem is that complete **compliance** with any behavior is difficult. Think, for instance, about the last time you tried to lose weight or start exercising regularly. Were you always able to meet your goals? Did you always skip dessert? Did you show up at the gym every morning? Demanding absolute compliance with absolute behaviors is risky because most people cannot meet such high standards. When they fail to meet these standards, they can lose confidence in their abilities to change and give up (Strang, 1992). Maybe you have given up on some of your goals. Hopefully, you knew that missing a workout session or eating a piece of chocolate cake did not spell disaster. Hopefully, you chalked it up to experience and moved forward in your behavior change program. If you didn't, maybe it was because you believed an absolutist message: Do it right or don't do it at all. You can see how this would make health education and behavior change difficult.

Absolutism is perpetuated in an atmosphere of paternalism. **Paternalism** occurs when health care providers (or other "experts") decide what the client should do (Rankin & Stallings, 1996). Although this also is usually done with altruistic motives, it is counter to the concept of promoting client autonomy. Paternalism and absolutism demand compliance. Compliance carries the expectation that clients will do exactly what providers tell them to do. If they don't, they are labeled "noncompliant," a term that implies client responsibility for failure (Rankin & Stallings, 1996). The nursing philosophy of holistic client care

supports individuals in their efforts to make health decisions and behavior changes. Absolutism, paternalism, and demands for compliance are all counter to this philosophy.

Learning Theory

Much health education is based on **learning theories** that have been developed over the past several decades. These theories are usually familiar to nurses, but some of the more important learning theory contributions to health education are briefly discussed here. The behavioral theorists, including Pavlov, Thorndike, and Skinner, showed how teachers could connect a stimulus to a desired response. This leads to a conditioned change in behavior that occurs every time the stimulus is presented. A client could, for instance, learn that brushing her teeth in the morning is associated with taking her birth control pill. Developmental theories, on the other hand, state that individuals need to acquire competence at one level of a developmental process before moving to the next level. Piaget showed that children go through specific developmental stages in their intellectual abilities, Erikson defined the psychosocial stages of growth and development, and Maslow explained a hierarchy of human needs where basic needs (e.g., food and shelter) must to be met before working on higher level needs (e.g., social connections and self-actualization). In addition, Rogers contributed the concept of learner-centered care in which the client learns to make decisions and solve problems (Hunt, 1997; Spradley & Allender, 1996).

Adult learning theory provides important information for health education. This theory holds that motivation to learn is based on four assumptions (Knowles, 1973):

1. *Adults perceive themselves to be self-directed:* They want to have a say in what they learn.

2. *Adults have a variety of life experiences and are insulted if these experiences are ignored:* The wise teacher will build on these experiences.

3. *Adults learn better when they see an immediate need:* They are goal directed.

4. *Timing education to coincide with an immediate need is more effective because the learner will see the immediate goal and be ready to learn.*

Behavior Change Theory

Theories that specifically address behavior change and health education incorporate ideas from these learning theories. **Behavior change theories** provide direction for nurses who teach in a variety of situations. A brief overview of some of these theories is provided in Table 15-2.

TABLE 15-2   **OVERVIEW OF SELECTED THEORIES ABOUT HEALTH BEHAVIOR**

THEORY AND KEY COMPONENTS	CASE STUDY
Health belief model: Individuals are more likely to take action to improve health if: They perceive themselves to be at risk for a problem (susceptibility) The problem is seen as serious enough to warrant action (severity, perceived threat) The expected benefits of the action outweigh the anticipated costs (e.g., in terms of overcoming barriers related to time, effort, money) There is a personal sense of ability to perform the required actions (self-efficacy) (Mirotznik, Feldman, & Stein, 1995; Rosenstock, 1990)	Nina's mother and sister both died of breast cancer. Nina took care of her mother during the terminal phases of the disease, and she has told friends, "That was the most horrible thing I ever had to do." Nina was concerned about her own risk, so she talked to her nurse practitioner (NP). The NP gave Nina information about breast cancer, did a breast examination, scheduled Nina for a mammogram, and taught Nina how to do breast self-examination (BSE). **Follow-up:** Nina sees breast cancer as a terrible disease, and she feels that she may be at risk. She is motivated to protect her health but has trouble remembering to do BSE. Doing it actually frightens her: What if she should find a lump? At her next clinic visit, her NP provides Nina with a chart, watches her do BSE in the office, and discusses her concerns about finding a lump. The NP is able to assure Nina that she is doing everything right. Nina establishes a habit of BSE that works for her.
Harm reduction model: Health risks can be decreased by having clients ask, What is healthier, safer, or less risky than what I am doing now? and What steps am I willing and able to take in order to be healthier, safer, or less risky? Basic principles include the following: Most people are competent to make informed decisions about health behaviors; they are the only ones who know what will work for them in their specific situations. Needs are diverse and can be met in diverse ways; offering people a spectrum of potential behaviors is better than demanding that they adopt an absolute requirement. Incremental steps that provide chances for success work better than trying to make large, difficult changes where the risk of failure is high.	Bob, who smokes two packs of cigarettes a day, arrives at Occupational Health for his annual physical. He tells the nurse that he exercises regularly and feels "as healthy as a horse." He denies any smoking-related problems, saying, "Smoking is my only vice and I really like it. It relaxes me. I tried to stop smoking once and it was a disaster, so why bother? But I am worried about smoking around my kids—they've been sick a lot lately." The nurse asks, "What do you think would be healthier for your kids?" Bob lists ideas ranging from quitting smoking all together to not smoking in the house. The nurse then asks, "Which of these things do you think would work best for you?" Bob decides to try smoking only in his office at home where "the kids can't come anyway." **Follow-up:** The nurse helped Bob explore his options without taking over and telling him what to do. He was then able to choose a behavior that he thought would work in his situation. Bob sees the nurse several months later and says, "Hey, you know how we talked about smoking only in my office to protect my kids? Well it's working real well. The kids haven't been sick as often and I'm not smoking as much either. I'm down to a pack and a half a day." By helping Bob see his options and by not demanding that he quit smoking, the nurse gave

TABLE 15-2   **OVERVIEW OF SELECTED THEORIES ABOUT HEALTH BEHAVIOR—CONT'D**

THEORY AND KEY COMPONENTS	CASE STUDY
People may need social support, education, referrals, and assistance to make changes (Bradley-Springer, 1996; Caplan, 1995). **Goal-setting theory:** Setting goals can help people change health-related behaviors by focusing effort, persistence, and concentration on the goal. The following steps are used: Determine the client's commitment to change. Analyze the tasks required to make changes: Complex tasks need to be broken down into subgoals (strategic analysis); simple tasks can be motivated by a simple goal. Assess the client's self-efficacy for performing required behaviors and help with skill development as needed. Goals should be difficult enough to require significant effort; they should be optimistic as well as realistic. Provide feedback on progress (Strecher et al., 1995).	him the support he needed to make positive changes. Bob will now feel good about talking to the nurse if he wants to make further changes. At her last dental checkup, Ana's dentist pointed out that she had beginning gum disease and suggested that Ana start flossing. Ana said, "I know I should floss. I know how to do it. I floss for 2 or 3 days, but then I miss a day and I give up. I don't want to lose all my teeth like my mother did. I just can't keep it up." The dentist suggests that Ana set a goal of flossing every other day. **Follow-up:** Ana was committed to making a change and already possessed the required skills. By suggesting a specific, attainable goal, the dentist provided additional motivation. At her next checkup Ana says, "It worked! I'm flossing almost every day now. When I miss a day it's not that big a deal because I know I will be able to floss the next day." During her oral examination, the dentist is able to tell Ana that her gums look much better.
Theory of reasoned action: Behavioral intention to act is based on a combination of the following: Personal beliefs and evaluations about what will happen if the behavior is used (perceived chance of success) Personal attitudes and values about the behavior Feelings about what key people (family, friends, health care providers) in the person's life think about the behavior Motivation to change behavior (Carter, 1990) All things being equal, people are expected to act in accordance with their intentions (Miller, Wikoff, & Hiatt, 1992).	Sue, a nursing student, has been dating Jack for 2 years. They plan to get married after she graduates. They have discussed having a family and agree that they do not want children for several years. Sue and Jack want to become sexually active. They visit the Student Health Center, where a nurse explains birth control options. Jack encourages Sue to use birth control pills (BCPs). Sue is worried because some of her friends have told her that BCPs caused them to gain weight. **Follow-up:** Although Sue is worried about weight gain, she believes that BCPs are effective and easy to use. She is clear that she does not currently want a pregnancy. She has Jack's support. Sue rarely misses taking her vitamin pills, so she is sure that she can remember to take the pills every day. This model predicts that Sue is likely to use BCPs consistently and correctly.
Social learning theory: Individual behavior, personal factors, and the environment create a triad of components that interact to influence health behaviors: A change in one component of the triad has an effect on all components (reciprocal determinism). Personal factors include behavioral capability, self-control, self-efficacy, internal	Jose is a depressed 13-year-old who has just entered a new school. He hasn't made any friends at the new school, a problem he blames on being 20 pounds overweight. The people Jose admires most at school all seem to be thin. He also notices that they are active in after-school activities. Jose's mother reminds him that he is a good swimmer and encourages him to join the swim team. **Follow-up:** Jose's desire to lose weight is influenced by the rewards that he sees being given to slim people. His perception of his weight and his emotional response to it create a desire to change that is sup-

Continued

TABLE 15-2 **OVERVIEW OF SELECTED THEORIES ABOUT HEALTH BEHAVIOR—CONT'D**

THEORY AND KEY COMPONENTS	CASE STUDY
reinforcements, emotional coping response, and a belief that performing a behavior will lead to expected outcomes. The environment (everything external to the individual) and the situation (the individual's perception of the environment) provide opportunities to observe behaviors performed by others in the environment (vicarious learning) (Perry, Baranowski, & Parcel, 1990).	ported by his mother and his swimming ability. Jose knows that swimming can help. He tries out for the team and discovers that he can do the butterfly stroke better than anyone else. He joins the team, and in addition to exercising regularly and losing weight, Jose makes new friends and develops a more optimistic outlook.
Diffusion theory: New ideas, practices, or services (innovations) to improve health move from a resource (innovation developer) to the population (innovation users or adopters). Diffusion is more likely to occur if the innovation is cost-efficient, low risk, simple, flexible, and compatible with the social, economic, and value systems into which it is introduced. Innovations that are reversible (I can go back to where I was if I don't like it) and appear to be better than currently used methods have a better chance of being adopted. Diffusion can fail if the innovation does not work, if information about the innovation is not communicated well, if the potential user does not have the necessary resources for implementation, or if the innovation is in opposition to the user's value system. In addition, there may be a problem if components of the implementation process are abbreviated. An example of this would be when education about the innovation is omitted to save money. Maintenance of an innovation takes additional effort; without this, the adopted program can lose momentum and fade away (Orlandi, Landers, Weston, & Haley, 1990).	Injection drug users (IDUs) who do not share equipment to inject drugs are not at risk of infection with blood-borne diseases such as hepatitis B, hepatitis C, and human immunodeficiency virus (HIV). Activists in Metrotown, a community of 300,000, wanted to implement a needle and syringe exchange program (N/SEP) so that IDUs would have access to sterile injecting equipment. They gathered support from the city council, the health department, and law enforcement before setting up N/SEP sites around town. During the first week, only two IDUs brought in equipment to exchange. **Follow-up:** Activists (resource) did a good job in Metrotown of involving the established power systems. No doubt they convinced all of these entities that N/SEPs would be cost-effective, simple, reversible, and better than allowing used injecting equipment to accumulate on the streets of the city. The activists were less effective in communicating the benefits of N/SEPs to the intended users of the program. IDUs need to know that obtaining sterile equipment will decrease the risk of disease, will be easily accessible, and will not put them at risk for being targeted by the police. Although Metrotown has made a difficult public health decision, it will not be successful unless the innovation diffuses to the intended users.
Social marketing theory: Public acceptance of programs to improve health can be enhanced through marketing techniques. Marketing functions on a number of well-developed principles: Participants are offered benefits that are valued as being worth the cost (e.g., measured in effort, money, time). The consumer (client) is the central concern.	Everyone at Russell High School (RHS) is shocked when three students, all with blood alcohol levels over the legal limit, are killed in a car accident. The principal forms a committee of students, teachers, and administrators to develop a program to decrease drunk driving. After assessing the situation at RHS, the committee proposes a plan to encourage the use of designated drivers. The program is kicked off at an assembly where student leaders (athletes, class officers, cheerleaders) describe the program. They all wear t-shirts that say, "I care about my friends. I'm a designated driver." Students are regularly

TABLE 15-2	OVERVIEW OF SELECTED THEORIES ABOUT HEALTH BEHAVIOR—CONT'D
THEORY AND KEY COMPONENTS	**CASE STUDY**
Communication (in the form of advertising, public relations, direct marketing, promotion, and face-to-face encounters) is the key to getting information to the consumer. The marketing process has six stages that occur in a cycle: (1) analysis; (2) planning; (3) development, testing, and refinement of the plan; (4) implementation; (5) assessment of effectiveness; and (6) feedback to analysis (completing the cycle). Marketing strategies must be modified to function in situations in which social issues and health are the central concerns (Novelli, 1990).	reminded about the program in newspaper articles, intercom announcements, and student-lead discussions in homeroom classes. **Follow-up:** RHS used marketing strategies focused on consumers (students) to develop a program that would meet the objective to decrease drunk driving. Although the adults on the planning committee had some reservations about a program that seemed to condone drinking, they paid attention to the analysis provided by student representatives and approved the program. A survey done 3 months later showed that 40% of RHS students had been designated drivers, resulting in a significant decrease in drunk driving rates. An additional, unforeseen benefit was a decrease in the overall rate of drinking, a direct result of designated driving being seen as "cool."

The transtheoretical model, so called because it borrows from many other theories, provides new and helpful insights for health education. The central premise of the transtheoretical model is that people progress through a series of stages when they attempt to change behaviors. There are five stages of change: precontemplative, contemplative, preparation, action, and maintenance (Prochaska, Redding, Harlow, Rossi, & Velicer, 1994). Progression through the stages is rarely linear. People will change their minds, will hesitate, and may relapse several times before behavior change is permanent. Ten different processes are used to enhance progression through the stages of change:

1. *Consciousness raising (increasing the level of awareness)*
2. *Dramatic relief (experiencing and expressing feelings)*
3. *Environmental reevaluation (assessing how the environment affects the situation)*
4. *Self-reevaluation (assessing how a person thinks and feels about the situation)*
5. *Self-liberation (believing in the ability to change)*
6. *Helping relationships (caring and trusting relationships)*
7. *Social liberation (seeing social changes that support personal changes)*
8. *Counterconditioning (substituting more healthful behaviors for less healthful behaviors)*
9. *Stimulus control (restructuring the environment)*
10. *Reinforcement management (getting rewards)*

Table 15-3 gives an overview of the transtheoretical model, including examples of the 10 processes and interventions appropriate in each stage.

The Health Education Process

Health education is a process of planned teaching and support activities that help people learn (Spellbring, 1991). The education process follows the format of the nursing process, including assessment, planning, implementation, and evaluation (Rankin &

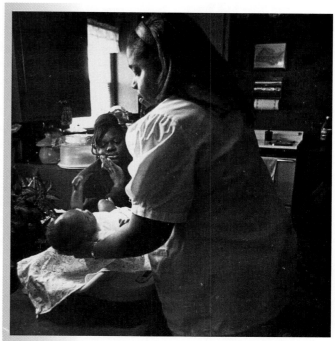

Nurse in the home setting educates new mother about newborn care.

TABLE 15-3	OVERVIEW OF THE TRANSTHEORETICAL MODEL (ALSO KNOWN AS THE STAGES OF CHANGE THEORY)

STAGE: CLIENT'S PERSPECTIVE	CASE STUDY AND INTERVENTIONS
Precontemplative: Unaware of or unwilling to consider the problem; defensive about the change issue, resistant to information about the behavior, and reluctant to initiate a behavior change program; not considering change within the next 6 months; has little confidence in ability to change; sees many reasons not to change	During a routine physical, Sam, a 26-year-old lawyer, says, "You know, I was listening to the radio on the way over here and a woman was talking about having AIDS (consciousness raising). This whole thing scares me (dramatic relief). It's not just gay guys anymore. I know that I've had some risks, but the things I do are a part of my life and the people I hang with (environmental reevaluation)." **Stage-specific interventions:** Raise awareness of the issue through community-appropriate public education and media programs. Provide information and feedback to increase individual awareness of physical, social, economic, and psychological problems related to the commission or omission of specific behaviors. Discuss the positive aspects of change. Do not spend time discussing details of specific change tactics or programs: You're wasting your time if it is clear that the client is not ready to think about changing.
Contemplative: Ambivalent; responds with "Yes, but . . . "; may see reasons to change as well as reasons to remain the same; indecisive, aware that a problem exists and more open to information, but still unsure of ability to change; intends to change behavior within next 6 months	Sam's nurse encourages him to continue talking about his concerns and those behaviors that make him think he has been at risk. He says, "Well, I have some crazy friends. I go out with them every Saturday. We compare notes on how much sex we get. We dare each other to do things like using a prostitute or having anal sex or coming on to a gay guy. I'm not proud of some of the things I've done. Maybe I'm getting too old for this (self-reevaluation)." **Stage-specific interventions:** Tip the balance in favor of change. It is important to see this stage as the time when the client will develop a commitment to change. It is still too early to look at strategies. The aim is to analyze risks and rewards of the behavior and to provide information. Clarify goals and discuss incentives to change. It is now time to emphasize negative aspects of not changing. A discussion of the risk for harm is appropriate.
Preparation: Expresses desire to do something to initiate change; some experimentation with new behaviors may already be occurring; thinks change may be possible; seriously planning change within next 30 days but has not set specific goals	When asked how this makes him feel, Sam responds by saying, with a sigh, "I guess I should think about being more careful. I don't want to get anything bad, especially AIDS. I need to change my act (self-liberation)." **Stage-specific interventions:** Now is the time to get down to details. Help the client find change strategies that are acceptable, accessible, appropriate, and effective. Encourage the client to experiment with a strategy: "Try it next time, see how you like it," or "Find out how your family/partner/friends react when you do it." Be available to the client to discuss issues related to moving into the action stage. Help the client establish specific objectives. In Sam's case, this could be limiting nights out with his friends to once a month.
Action: Engages in action to create desired change; feels developing confidence in personal self-efficacy; thinks reasons to change outweigh reasons not to; behavior modified to meet goal(s) for 6 months	Over the course of the next 6 months, Sam and the nurse meet several times to discuss his progress. During this time, Sam says, "I've talked about this with my friend Mia. She just listens and never acts like I'm a bad person even when I tell her bad things I've done (helping relationship). Since I've started talking about it, I've had people tell me that I'm right to be concerned and that I should be more careful—even some of my buddies agree (social liberation)." Sam begins to take specific actions to decrease his risks. He begins to use condoms and decides to have sex only when he wants to and not "on a dare" (counterconditioning). **Stage-specific interventions:** Be aware that this is not an easy process. Support change efforts. Clients will need continuing encouragement, help with problem solving, and a place to simply vent frustrations.

TABLE 15-3	OVERVIEW OF THE TRANSTHEORETICAL MODEL (ALSO KNOWN AS THE STAGES OF CHANGE THEORY)—CONT'D

STAGE: CLIENT'S PERSPECTIVE	CASE STUDY AND INTERVENTIONS
Maintenance: Challenged to continue change; feels expanding self-efficacy; continues behavior change for more than 6 months	As Sam becomes comfortable with his new behaviors, he reports that other things are changing. He says, "I realized that my problems were related to my friends. They didn't understand why I wanted to change. They called me a wimp. So I decided to quit hanging out with them (stimulus control). The good thing is that I feel better about myself. Mia even told me that she's noticed that I seem happier (reinforcement management)." **Stage-specific interventions:** Help the client maintain change. Problem solving and unconditional support for the client are extremely important during this stage. Relapse prevention efforts can include interactive discussions, role-playing, and "what if" sessions in which the client identifies risks for relapse and develops workable strategies.
Relapse (not a stage): An important event that can occur at any time in the change process; if relapse occurs, the client may express anger and question ability to maintain change; may be embarrassed or ashamed; may blame self or others (including health care providers) for relapse	Sam returns to clinic a year later. When asked about how he's doing, he blurts out, "I blew it. I ran into Jake a few weeks ago and we went for a drink. Before I knew it, we'd picked up a couple of women. I ended up in a strange apartment and no one ever thought about using condoms. I'm really embarrassed about this—especially after I made such a big deal out of being careful with my friends. Maybe I wasn't meant to be safe. Maybe I'm supposed to get the clap or HIV or something else that's just as bad. I can't even face Mia." **Stage-specific interventions:** Clients may get "stuck" in relapse if they resort to self-incrimination or self-blame. Help the client renew the change process at an earlier stage without getting demoralized. Explain that relapse is common and may occur many times before behavior change is permanent. Point out specific instances of success that show the client's abilities to change. Provide referral to needed services. Sam, for instance, may need a work up for sexually transmitted disease.

Source: Adapted from Bradley-Springer, 1996.

Stallings, 1996). While these steps are being taken, meticulous documentation should occur. The next section presents detailed information about each step in the education process, but before that, some important general points about education need to be made.

Education is client centered. An important question for the nurse to continually ask is, "How does *this* problem (e.g., diagnosis, stressor, need to change) affect *this* client?" To truly make the process client centered, nurses must remember that people live in complex social and culturally defined environments. Therefore, the involvement of family and significant others can help promote learning. In some cases, family involvement is essential, especially when health education is directed to children, clients with sensory deficits, or clients who are physically unable to perform the necessary skills. In general, involving others can provide social and emotional supports that help people make behavior changes (Rankin & Stallings, 1996). Unfortunately, clients do not always have healthy support structures, or they simply may not want others involved. In these cases, the nurse should not force the issue. Instead, referrals to community resources and support groups should be considered.

It does not do to leave a live dragon out of your calculations if you live near him.

J. R. R. Tolkien

Assessment

The task of assessment is to gather information. This can result in a huge amount of information that the nurse uses to determine needs and priorities. Obviously, educational needs cannot be determined without looking at the entire client. Learning needs evolve from a knowledge of the client's overall health problems (actual and potential). In most cases, some of the needs discovered through assessment will have a cognitive, skill, or attitudinal component that must be addressed through education (Rankin & Stallings, 1996).

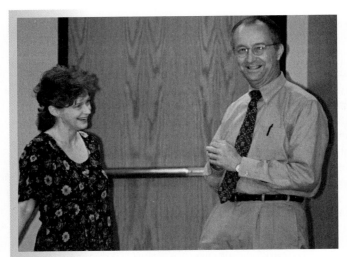

Chapter author Lucy Bradley-Springer and Kevin Morrisroe, RN, do a role play on Risk Assessment at a class in New Mexico.

Assessment requires active nurse-client interaction. This can be time-consuming, but the nurse can use assessment time to develop rapport with the client and significant others (Redman, 1997). Building a good working relationship during this phase will increase the amount of information the client reveals and will make the rest of the education process more enjoyable for both the client and the nurse. This is especially important in community health settings where nurses need to establish long-term relationships with individuals in the community. Table 15-4 lists some areas that need to be discussed during a health education assessment.

Data can be collected from a variety of sources, including direct observation, client records, other members of the health care team, and professional literature. The best way to get the client's point of view, however, is through an interactive interview. Client disclosure of information is enhanced by the following tactics (Rankin & Stallings, 1996):

- Establish an environment of trust. *This may require some time at the beginning of the conversation. Start by introducing yourself and telling who you are. ("Hi. I'm Faith Diaz, and I'm an RN from the home health agency.") Establish that you have experience in the area you will be addressing with the client. ("I've been working with people who've had your kind of surgery for 2 years.") Describe the intention of the interview and make it clear that questions are asked to help the client. As we all know, some of the questions that nurses need to ask can be embarrassing. Assure the client that there are health care reasons for asking each question and that all answers are confidential.*

- Choose the right time. *Be sure that you have time to adequately assess the client's needs. Ask if this is a good time for the client. Be sure the client is not in pain or anxious about*

an anticipated event. *If you know that your time is short, introduce the assessment session by saying, "I know you are anxious about your wound care. I only have 15 minutes to spend with you right now, and I need to ask you a few questions. Your answers will help me plan how I will teach you about your wound. I'll come back this afternoon, and we'll go over everything in detail. First, I'd like to know if you've ever had a wound like this before . . . "*

- Choose the right place. *The location of an interview should be comfortable and private. If it is not, the client (and the nurse) may concentrate more on the room temperature or the hard chairs or the constant interruptions than on the interview. If possible, do the interview on the client's "home turf." This can be in the client's home or a private room at the clinic. Asking questions in a known environment helps the client feel safe (Hunt, 1997).*

- Use open-ended questions. *Going through a list of "yes/no" questions does not provide the depth of information needed to develop effective, individualized teaching plans. Asking the client to describe her problems doing exercises after a mastectomy, for example, will get a lot of those "yes/no" questions answered without your even asking them. The client will also benefit from the experience of telling her story to an interested listener. Remember, clients (as adult learners) have unique perspectives that they need to share with you and that you should build into your teaching plan.*

- Use active listening skills. *Ask for clarification, summarize, and use open body language (nod, smile; do not act like you have to leave). These listening skills enhance interactions and ensure that you understand the client's meanings.*

When the interview is complete, summarize the main points and thank the client for spending time with you. Tell the client what you intend to do with the information and describe the next steps in the planning process. If you cannot continue the process at this time, tell the client when you will return.

Planning

During planning, the nurse and client discuss learning needs and potential goals. This is a negotiation process: The nurse provides input that the client uses to make decisions about specific interventions. The result of this process is a list of learning objectives. Hopefully, the list will not be too long, but some clients have many problems. In that case, it is best to prioritize the list by having the client choose those problems (1) that are most pressing (cause the most discomfort for the client) and (2) the client is most willing to work on (an estimate of readiness). Limiting the teaching session to one or two objectives is less intimidating than trying to make a large number of changes at the same time (Kreuter & Strecher, 1996).

Learning goals and objectives are established in the initial part of the planning phase. Goals and objectives provide an agreed-upon direction for implementation and a guide for eval-

TABLE 15-4   **ASSESSMENT VARIABLES**

WHAT TO ASSESS	ASSESSMENT QUESTIONS
Client understanding of the problem in question	What do you think is the cause of this problem?
	Why do you think it is happening now?
Client perception of need to change	How does the problem affect you?
	Has this problem limited your activities in any way?
Motivation to change: severity of problem and risks caused by the problem	How severe is the problem? Is it a short-term or a long-term problem? What harm could this problem cause you?
	What are the 2 to 3 main difficulties that you have because of this problem?
	What do you fear most about the problem?
	Why do you want to solve this problem?
Readiness to change	What would you like do to about the problem in the next few days (weeks)?
	What are the most important things that you would like to have happen?
Self-efficacy	How do you usually approach problems?
	How would you like to approach this problem?
	What do you think you can do about the problem?
	Have you tried to deal with this problem before? If so, what did you do and how did it turn out?
Perceived benefits to change	How would you feel if you solved this problem?
	If you didn't have the problem what would be better in your life?
Perceived barriers to change	What has kept you from dealing with this problem in the past?
	Do you see things that may prevent your dealing with this problem? If so, what are they?
Psychosocial issues	Who gives you the most support? Would you like her or him to be in on our teaching sessions?
	Also assess housing, economic status, educational background, community resources, cultural and religious contributions to health care, native language, and so on.
Learning skills	How do you learn best? Would you like reading materials or videotapes or group sessions or private counseling or . . . ?

Source: Adapted from Kreuter & Strecher, 1996; Palank, 1991; Rankin & Stallings, 1996; and Redman, 1997.

uation. Goals are broad statements of the desired outcome: Jason will manage insulin administration to control his blood sugar, for example. Objectives are specific, detailed statements. They describe behaviors that will help meet a goal. They describe what the client will do, define how it will be done, and prescribe time frames for task completion. Objectives for Jason could include the following:

1. *Before he is discharged in 3 days, Jason will be able to list the signs and symptoms of high and low blood sugar.*

2. *By tomorrow, Jason will be able to test his blood for glucose with the equipment he will use at home.*

3. *By the day before discharge, Jason will be able to use a prescribed sliding scale to accurately draw up and inject insulin in the ordered doses at the ordered times.*

4. *Within a week after discharge, Jason will describe the benefits of controlling his blood sugar.*

Notice that the objectives are specific and measurable. We will be able to tell when Jason accomplishes each objective (Rankin & Stallings, 1996).

Also notice that the objectives do not all look alike. That is because they address three different **domains of learning** (Redman, 1997). Some objectives refer to things that people need to know. These are called *cognitive objectives.* In Jason's case, the first objective asks him to know the signs of hyperglycemia and hypoglycemia. *Psychomotor objectives* refer to skills or behaviors. Jason will need to manipulate equipment (a skill) to meet the next two objectives. The final objective addresses an attitude: We want Jason to verbalize a positive outlook on his abilities. This objective occurs in the *affective* domain.

Knowing the type of objective helps the nurse and client decide on teaching and learning methods. Jason may be able to learn the symptoms of hyperglycemia from a brochure, for instance, but he will need to practice drawing up insulin and in-

TABLE 15-5   DOMAINS OF LEARNING

DOMAIN	GOALS AND OBJECTIVES	TEACHING METHODS	APPLICATION CASE: GOAL IS TO ENCOURAGE BREAST-FEEDING IN PREGNANT WOMEN WHO ATTEND A LOW-INCOME CLINIC.
COGNITIVE SUBDOMAINS			
Knowledge (to know)	To state, to list, to define, to recall, to name, to repeat	Lecture, one-on-one instruction, programmed instruction, videos or audio tapes, reading materials, questions and answers	Display breast-feeding posters in prominent places around the clinic. Run a continuous video on breast-feeding in the waiting room. Leave brochures and printed materials in examination rooms. Plan a series of lectures at a convenient time for clients.
Comprehension (to understand)	To explain, to label, to describe, to interpret	Lecture, one-on-one instruction, programmed instruction, video program, reading materials, learning guides, study questions	Arrange face-to-face sessions during prenatal visits; ask if client has questions or concerns. Follow up educational activities by asking, "What difference could breast-feeding make for your baby?"
Application (to use)	To illustrate, to apply, to give examples	Demonstration, group discussion, simulation exercises, games, role-play, clinical practice	Demonstrate breast care and the process of breast-feeding using a simulation model or a video. Encourage partner participation in education.
Analysis (to identify elements)	To compare, to contrast, to differentiate, to debate, to question	Group discussion, games, group interaction, simulation exercises, role-play, case studies	Arrange small group sessions where women can discuss concerns about breast-feeding. Role-play issues that emerge from group discussions.
Synthesis (to use in new ways)	To assemble, to prepare, to create, to design, to formulate	Group projects, group discussion, simulation exercises, games, role-play, case studies	Invite women from the community who are successfully breast-feeding to discuss the process in small groups of pregnant women. Support breast-feeding efforts after delivery.
Evaluation (to judge)	To assess, to justify, to measure, to choose	Group discussion, guided imagery, role-play, self-evaluation worksheet	Ask women to share success stories related to breast-feeding. Provide questionnaire that helps client assess values and fears about breast-feeding; follow up with a one-on-one discussion.
Psychomotor (to perform)	To assemble, to demonstrate, to control, to manipulate	Demonstration, practice with supervision, independent practice, return demonstration, role-play, simulation, clinical experience	Demonstrate breast care and the process of breast-feeding using a simulation model or a video. Provide guidance and positive reinforcement to women after delivery as they initiate breast-feeding with newborn.
Affective (to feel)	To tolerate, to accept, to defend, to adopt, to appreciate, to value	Group discussion, group project, simulation exercises, games, role-play, life experience	Encourage client involvement. Reinforce positive statements about breast-feeding. Encourage attendance at group sessions where breast-feeding is discussed.

jecting himself to really learn those skills. You cannot learn to give an injection by reading about it! Table 15-5 provides an in-depth overview of the domains of learning and teaching methods appropriate to each domain.

The planning stage is not complete until the client agrees to the goals, objectives, and teaching methods. Although Jason's plan looks good on the surface, he may have a morbid fear of sticking himself. In that case, the objectives and plan would need to be changed to have someone in his household learn the "sticking" skills (injections and finger sticks), but Jason should be able to meet the other objectives and may eventually overcome his fears and learn the "sticking" skills himself.

Implementation

During implementation, the nurse and client use information from the assessment and planning stages to make decisions about learning activities. Learning activities must focus on the established objectives. Interventions are tailored to the client's needs and abilities. Teaching plans are then put into action, but this is not a static process. The nurse continually observes and asks for feedback to track progress. The nurse should discuss any problems with the client, modifying the plan as needs change. This is called *formative evaluation*: It helps the teacher adjust the format of the education as the teaching progresses. Box 15-1 provides some general pointers to guide teaching.

BOX 15-1 POINTERS FOR HEALTH EDUCATION

- Design teaching based on assessments of individual clients: needs, ability, knowledge base, learning styles, expectations, culture, language, readiness to learn, and so on.
- Develop educational objectives with input from the learner. Validate that the objectives are relevant to the learner's needs. Objectives serve as the basis for instruction and evaluation.
- Create a learning environment. It should be comfortable and free of distractions.
- Keep things simple.
- Focus on one issue at a time. Keep learning sessions short. Concentrate on outcomes that will be immediately obvious (e.g., feeling and looking better because of exercise rather than the more distant issue of preventing heart disease).
- Be sure written materials are appropriate. Keep sentences short. Use words a layperson can understand. Define medical words in simple terms. Use a font style and size that are easy to read. Use pictures and diagrams to clarify concepts.
- Be specific. "Lose weight," for instance, is not as effective as, "Lose 2 pounds this week."
- Avoid threatening messages that generate fear. Mild anxiety enhances learning, but high fear levels can lead to denial, tuning out the message, or inability to concentrate.
- Explain what you will be teaching and why it is important. This provides an "advance organizer" to keep session centered on the topic.
- Provide for success. Divide learning tasks into sequential learning units that start with easier concepts and build to more difficult ones. Encourage success at each level before progressing to more difficult tasks. This enhances self-efficacy and personal satisfaction.

- Use a variety of teaching methods. People learn in different ways, and a combination of methods reinforces learning. Varying methods also keeps people involved.
- Provide visual learning materials. Seeing as well as hearing enhances retention.
- Show the client what is expected. Model behaviors to demonstrate how things are done.
- Skills (both verbal and physical) require practice. (Examples: role-play communication skills, use a plastic model to teach self-catheterization techniques, use syringes to practice drawing up insulin.)
- Involve all the senses in practice sessions. This reinforces learning on several levels.
- Provide immediate feedback that praises or corrects specific details during practice sessions. Highlight successes and express honest confidence in the learner's abilities to accomplish learning objectives. If you have doubts about the learner's abilities, do not give false praise. Instead, reassess with the learner and develop a new teaching plan.
- Develop mechanisms for support. Include family and friends in education as possible and as acceptable to the client. Support groups that focus on specific issues have been shown to enhance learning while encouraging positive change and maintenance of newly developed behaviors.
- Discuss resources for further information and/or practice.
- Review major points of each learning session. Discuss plans for follow-up, reinforcement, and expansion of learning experience.
- Keep learners involved: Ask for feedback and evaluation during teaching and learning.

Source: Adapted from Byham, 1992; Damrosch, 1991; and Spradley & Allender, 1996.

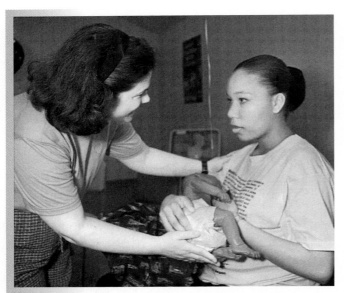

Nurse educating teen mom about breast-feeding.

Evaluation

Evaluation is a process of gathering information to assess the extent to which learning objectives have been met—or not met. There are a number of ways to evaluate learning, but all evaluation methods should be based on the learning objectives. Objectives that are written with appropriate action verbs will tell you how to evaluate outcomes. An objective that says the learner will be able to list the steps in cardiopulmonary resuscitation (CPR), for instance, can be evaluated by asking her to write those steps on a piece of paper. If the objective states that the learner will be able to perform CPR, however, you will need to watch the technique on a mannequin. Learning can be evaluated through quizzes, direct observation, physiological measures (is the client's blood pressure lower?), client self-report and self-monitoring, or input from other health care team members (Redman, 1997).

The outcome of evaluation is a list of learning that has been accomplished as well as a list of those learning objectives that have not been met. *Summative evaluation* is a summary of what has occurred and is usually used as a summary of client accomplishments when the nurse is closing out a case. More often, formative evaluation is used. As with the nursing process, information from formative evaluation feeds back to the assessment phase, and the teaching process repeats itself with new objectives, plans, and interventions until the client and the nurse are satisfied with the final result (Rankin & Stallings, 1997).

Health Education in Communities

All nurses, regardless of work site or specialty, are expected to teach individuals and their families about health-related matters. Nurses who work in the community have additional opportunities to help people change behaviors for the improved health of aggregate populations. The following section describes teaching efforts that can occur in community settings, including individual, group, and community education.

Individuals, Families, and Groups

People live in groups, and the family is the most basic social group. For purposes of this discussion, the *family* is what the client says it is. For some, family members are related by blood or marriage. For others, family members include close social (and sometimes sexual) ties with people who are not otherwise related. Families may be supportive or not supportive. They may be healthy or unhealthy. They may be large and extended or small and nuclear. Some people have rejected or cannot identify a family; others have been rejected by their families. Regardless of family process or content, the individual is greatly influenced by this first social unit (see chapters 30 and 31).

A *group,* on the other hand, is defined as people "with common goals interacting independently" (Rankin & Stallings, 1996, p. 202). Groups may come together for short periods to address one purpose (e.g., a bereavement support group) or may be more stable over time with larger purposes (e.g., a local unit of Alcoholics Anonymous) (see chapter 18). Families and groups are important entities for community health nurses to recognize. Families and groups may need direct education (e.g., the nurse teaches a parent group how to take an infant's temperature or how to recognize the signs of adolescent suicide), or they may need to be included as a support system for an individual client (e.g., the nurse includes family members in a discussion of safe food preparation for an immune-suppressed child). This chapter looks at two specific issues related to community education of individuals, families, and groups: discharge teaching and community-based teaching.

Discharge Teaching

Discharge teaching happens in formal inpatient and outpatient care settings, but it provides a basis for community care. Discharge teaching has become more complex in recent years because of changes in the way health care is provided. People are now discharged from acute care settings earlier, with less recuperation time. More procedures, including some that are quite complicated, are being done in outpatient settings. Hospitalization after delivery is usually less than 48 hours. All of these changes have led to people going home with more complex medications, treatments, pain, and anxiety. In addition, because the client spends less time in the formal care setting, there is less time for teaching. This is further complicated by the fact that teaching must often happen in the immediate aftermath of a procedure, a time when clients tend to be most anxious and least able to attend to educational messages (Hunt, 1997).

Nurses can overcome these barriers with careful assessment and planning. If possible, some teaching should take place in the clinic, home, or community before the acute event; preoperative education and prenatal classes are good examples of this. In addition, community resources need to be identified in advance: Is the family willing and able to provide care? Will home health services be required? Are there other options? Assessing these needs and establishing early contacts can ensure that the individual is well prepared. Bringing the needed supports (e.g., responsible family members or home care agencies) in early can decrease education time.

. . . .

To quit smoking is easy. I've done it hundreds of times.

Mark Twain

. . . .

. . . .

Learning is what happens when what you thought would work doesn't.

Unknown

. . . .

Education can then proceed through the teaching process as discussed earlier. Assessment should include a history of experiences that may influence this event, as well as individual and family coping mechanisms. Planning and implementation should be concise, clear, and supported by written information. Teaching should include demonstrations and return demonstrations for all treatments (e.g., dressing changes) and equipment (e.g., medication pumps). Follow-up telephone calls and referrals to community agencies for more intense follow-up should be scheduled (Hunt, 1997). The bottom line is that clients should not feel that they are on their own at the time of discharge. Ideally, they should feel secure in their own abilities to provide self-care. If this is not possible, clients should know how to arrange for the support they will need at home.

Community-Based Teaching

Discharge teaching provides information for clients who have been treated in a formal health care setting. More and more often, however, people need health education as a part of their daily lives. **Community-based teaching** can be complicated by a number of variables. The home setting itself can be difficult. The nurse will be on the client's "home turf," and there may be distractions from family members (especially if there are children in the house). In addition, teaching equipment will need to be brought into the house by the nurse, and the nurse may need to address learning needs for a wider range in individuals. Health education in the home must also be carefully coordinated among various care providers. To make matters even more difficult, all this must be done in a limited amount of time (Hunt, 1997). However, there are major advantages to teaching in the client's home:

- *The nurse can assess the client's environment and make changes in the teaching plan to compensate for problems and to take advantage of strengths.*

- *The family can be more easily involved.*
- *The client will usually be more comfortable in his or her own environment.*
- *The client will be learning in the environment in which he or she will be using new information to perform new skills and behaviors.*

Once again, application of the teaching process will help the nurse meet education goals. A most important step in community-based education is to keep the client and significant others involved in the entire process from assessment to evaluation. This helps the nurse address those issues of highest concern, establish trust within the family setting, and provide the basis for further education. Nurses serve as case managers in the community: They are the professionals who are responsible for coordinating information between the client and a variety of caregivers. In this process, nurses must cover objectives from each of the other care providers and integrate their orders with the needs of the client and family. To accomplish this complex task, nurses need to be aware of community resources so that they can make appropriate referrals. The result should be that community-based clients feel comfortable with their self-care (or family-care) status. Clients should move toward independent care or toward the knowledge that care will be maintained by trusted family members and/or professional providers (Hunt, 1997).

Community

Community health learning occurs when knowledge, attitudes, and/or behaviors change within an entire community. Over the past decade, major changes have been made in communities in areas such as seat belt use, limitations on smoking areas in public spaces, and decreased tolerance of drunk driving. All of these changes came about when individuals in communities stood up and demanded safer and more healthful environments. Changes such as these often require legislative action; at other times, a shift in the community norm is all that has to occur. Nurses have not often taken full advantage of their positions in communities to influence change, but they should. Education and political action are within the realm of what nurses should and can do to improve the health of communities and the individuals in those communities.

Communities consist of groups of people who identify membership in the community. These people share commonalties in language, tradition, ritual, and ceremony. They share values and norms and exert influence over each other. They have emotional connections, common needs, and a commitment to the community to meet those needs. Community may occur within a geographic location (as in a neighborhood or a town) or may be connected by something other than geography (as in ethnic or age-specific groups). Community is defined by all of these connections, so people who merely live in close proximity may not be a community (Israel, Checkoway, Schulz, & Zimmerman, 1994). An individual may have membership in more than one

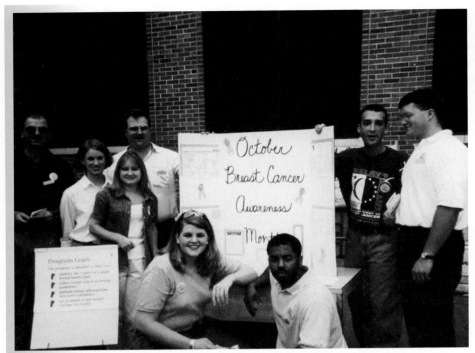

Breast cancer awareness education program for college students.

community and may have to deal with conflicting values from those communities. As you can see, a community has power that can affect **behavior change**. Although community support can be a powerful contribution to individual behavior change, lack of community support may doom an intervention to failure (Bigbee & Jansa, 1991). Table 15-6 gives a case study to illustrate the process of community education.

. . . .

There are some things you learn best in calm, and some in storm.
Willa Cather

. . . .

Community Assessment

As with individual health education, health education at the community level starts with community assessment, and as in individual education, the assessment needs to take into account the full spectrum of community variables. Individual behaviors take place within the context of community, and understanding this context can help nurses predict both barriers to and supports for behavior change (Israel, Checkoway, Schulz, & Zimmerman, 1994). The nurse needs a clear idea of what the community is: How do people in the community define *health* and *health care*? What is the norm for nutrition, elimination, exercise, sleep, sexuality, reproduction, and coping with stress? How is intellect supported? How does the community perceive itself? How are

roles and relationships established and supported? What does the community value? What ethnic and cultural identities exist in the community? What language(s) is(are) spoken? What ceremonies occur? What rituals are supported? How does the community share resources? Is there a sense of shared responsibility (Krozy, 1996)? Nurses can gather this information from community leaders, written histories and records, observations, consultations, and other community members.

Communities, like individuals, experience stressors. These stressors range from daily hassles (as in ongoing arguments from businesses that want to limit government controls) to chronic problems (e.g., homelessness or air pollution) to major events (e.g., the closing of an industry) to cataclysmic events (e.g., an earthquake or flood) (Israel, Checkoway, Schulz, & Zimmerman, 1994). Other community problems can include poverty, overpopulation, social injustice, lack of social organization, overcrowding (Krozy, 1996), a history of powerlessness, and tensions created by inequity and discrimination (Israel, Checkoway, Schulz, & Zimmerman, 1994). All of these contribute to community perceptions of powerlessness. Community empowerment, then, becomes a teaching strategy.

. . . .

The illiterate of the 21st century will not be those who cannot read and write, but those who cannot learn, unlearn, and relearn.
Alvin Toffler

. . . .

TABLE 15-6	COMMUNITY EDUCATION PROCESS CASE

Kris works as a school nurse at Center High School in a moderately sized Midwest city. At a weekly team meeting, she tells her friend Sam, "I am so frustrated—we have five pregnant girls already this semester." Sam, who works at two middle schools, says, "You think that's bad? I have a case of chlamydia in a sixth grader!" Others add their comments until one says, "We clearly have a problem. What should we do?" The nurses decide to "do something about the risks of teen sexual activity." Because they already know the community well, the nurses decide to assess the problem by listing positive and negative community factors related to the problem of teen sexual activity.

ASSESSMENT	PLANNING	IMPLEMENTATION	EVALUATION
Positive factors: The community has a number of agencies that could be involved, including Planned Parenthood, Big Brothers/Big Sisters, the YMCA, churches, etc. Community schools have good reputations; most students graduate and many go to college. The state department of education supports a sex education curriculum based on harm reduction. School nurses have a ratio of 1:2,000 students. **Negative factors:** The school board (SB) supports and enforces an abstinence-only sex education curriculum as a result of pressure from a few vocal parents and one of the churches in the community. There are limited programs for students who are not succeeding in school and/or extracurricular activities. Most student come from families with working parents, and the majority have several hours of unsupervised time after school. Kris has had a number of students at her school tell her, "I want to get pregnant, it'd be cool." A survey of the nurses reveals 25 known teen pregnancies and 42 known cases of sexually transmitted diseases (STDs) in students over the past 24 months.	The nurses struggle with the question of what to do with the assessment information. After a long brainstorming session, they develop a plan. Each nurse will do the following: • Meet with his or her principal(s) to inform and educate about the problem • Attend the next two meetings of the SB and ask to have the topic of teen sexuality placed on the agenda • Encourage the use of the state's harm reduction curriculum • Volunteer to teach sexuality classes in the 5th to 12th grades • Visit 2 to 3 community organizations (including churches) to discuss the problem, ask for support, and volunteer assistance to develop after-school programs.	The nurses complete their assigned visits to the principals, SB, and local organizations. Each nurse reviews the state sex education curriculum and volunteers to teach classes at his or her assigned school(s).	**Summative evaluation:** All assignments are completed. **Formative evaluation:** All of the principals support the nurses' efforts. One principal asks about sexual abuse in students' family and peer relationships. The SB refuses to add the issue to the agenda. All of the nurses will teach sex education classes, but several principals and health teachers refuse to allow a harm reduction curriculum until approval by the SB. Two churches and the YMCA are interested in setting up sports, games, and homework assistance programs after school. Planned Parenthood wants to develop a peer education program to address pressures to have sex in order to be "cool." **Follow up:** The nurses reassess the situation and plan for the next steps. The nurses will do the following: • Set up in-services for the nurses to learn about teaching a harm reduction curriculum • Set up nurse counseling services for any student who wants to discuss issues privately; available to all students, but especially for students in abusive relationships • Continue attending SB meetings; encourage principals, teachers, and parents to add their support at those meetings • Collaborate with agencies as new programs are developed and encourage other agencies to consider developing their own programs.

The good news is that communities also provide support for behavior change. The nurse should assess those things that enhance opportunities for education and change. These might include the emotional support given to community members who are trying to effect change. In addition, established agencies and services may already be available to support change. Information dissemination systems may be in place, and respected community members may be willing to sway opinion toward change (Israel, Checkoway, Schulz, & Zimmerman, 1994).

Planning for the Community

The main point that needs to be made about community planning should be obvious: Planning requires community involvement (Andrade & Doria-Ortiz, 1995). Shared decision making leads to better acceptance of change, support for the process, and commitment to programs that emerge from the process (Foran & Campanelli, 1995). Involving large portions of the community in planning can be difficult, but it is necessary. Representation should be sought from government, business, service, health care, and religious entities as well as from the individuals who will be targeted by the plan. Input can be gathered in community meetings, focus groups, and interviews with key informants. Opposing views must be sought, acknowledged, and considered in any planning activity (Krozy, 1996). Planning can then progress to setting educational goals and selecting an appropriate theory base, taking into account the strengths and weaknesses of the community.

Common broad-based goals for community health education are to (1) help people change unhealthy, unsafe, or risky behaviors; (2) equalize access to health and support services; and (3) decrease the incidence of preventable conditions that have a negative impact on the community (Krozy, 1996). Goals and more specific objectives need to be established and agreed upon during the planning process. Consider using *Healthy People 2010* in this process. It delineates national goals for specific health issues targeted to at-risk populations (DHHS, 2000).

....

You must learn from the mistakes of others. You can't possibly live long enough to make them all yourself.

Sam Levenson

....

Foran and Campanelli (1995) identified the components of successful community health programs: They are flexible, they use ongoing evaluation to identify design problems as soon as possible, they use evaluation to guide change, they are valued by the community, and they evolve by incorporating new ideas and technologies as change occurs. Planners should understand all of these elements. And remember: Planning should develop teaching interventions as well as evaluation tools.

Implementing Community Plans

Andrade and Doria-Ortiz (1995) encourage an implementation process that helps a community meet its own needs. This requires empowerment of community organizations, adequate resources and services to meet the needs of at-risk community members, and sufficient resources in the health care system. They recognize that programs and services (especially those targeted to underserved populations) must be available, accessible, acceptable, and accountable. Programs that do not meet these criteria will not be used.

It is important to remember that community education and change are long-term processes—they do not happen overnight. Even after programs are established, there must be commitment to a continuing process of assessment, planning, implementation, and evaluation. Implementation will be enhanced if the process is participatory (members of the community are involved), cooperative, collaborative, empowering, and balanced. Hopefully, the process will promote group identification, reinforcing the idea of a shared fate and the need to look at more global aspects of health (Israel, Checkoway, Schulz, & Zimmerman, 1994).

The assessment and planning process will help nurses identify appropriate sites for community education. Where are the natural community networks? Are they centered around employment, recreational, religious, or commercial functions? Will organizations that are not viewed as health care agencies (e.g., schools and churches) get involved? Can early health-promotion programs be established in neighborhood elementary and middle schools? Are community colleges open to health education efforts? Will the justice system support health education for people who live in prisons, jails, and halfway houses? Establishing programs specific to people who congregate in these sites can promote education in ways that target at-risk individuals (Andrade & Doria-Ortiz, 1995).

How health education is implemented also depends on assessment and planning. It helps to have a theoretical base (see Tables 15-2 and 15-3), knowing that some models are better for

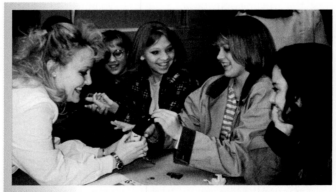

School nurse educating high school students about STDs.

> ## A Conversation With...
>
> **On education:**
> *Education is less and less a preparation for life and more and more a part of it.*
>
> *Our species thinks in metaphors and learns through stories.*
>
> *Relying on competition as a way of motivating learning eventually subverts not only cooperation but also the willingness to learn.*
> **—Mary Catherine Bates**

community intervention than others. Diffusion theory and social marketing theory, for example, were developed from community-focused research. The transtheoretical model also includes components of community action. Common teaching strategies for community intervention include lectures, small group work, facilitated discussions, demonstrations, printed and audiovisual materials, simulation exercises, guided imagery, and social marketing (Krozy, 1996). The important thing to remember is that the teaching strategy needs to match the learning objective (see Table 15-5) as well as the developmental level of the audience.

Evaluating Community Programs

As stated earlier, evaluation is an ongoing process in health education. Formal evaluation should be planned, and informal evaluation should be acknowledged and used in the process. Formative evaluation is used throughout the process. Summative evaluation occurs at a set point when goals are expected to have been met. Effective evaluation determines progress toward goals and identifies goals that have not yet been met. Data from evaluation are used to do the following:

* *Determine whether unmet goals are still a priority*
* *Plan interventions to address unmet goals*
* *Assess the impact of goals that have been achieved*
* *Assess evolving needs*
* *Establish new community goals and objectives*

The community health education process is much like the individual teaching process (it is cyclical and progressive in nature), but it is more complicated.

Beyond Community

Nurses who are involved in community education activities realize that some problems are too big to deal with on a community level. Sometimes, changes need to be made at the level of state and federal governments. Political advocacy then becomes a part of the health education agenda. Nurses can educate communities about the political process to encourage input into legislative ac-

tivities, knowing that communities with identified needs can often influence legislative outcomes. Some examples of community needs that have been addressed through legislative intent include drunk driving laws, water fluoridation bills, motorcycle helmet requirements, and funding for various initiatives from school-based health education programs to needle and syringe exchange programs. Andrade and Doria-Ortiz (1995) recommend the following legislative actions to support the health of the Mexican American community: provide national health insurance to cover the working poor, cooperate with Mexico to give health care in border communities, address high-risk diseases (e.g., diabetes and tuberculosis) and conditions (e.g., teen pregnancy and violence), increase Hispanic access to health professions schools, and ensure input from Hispanic communities into federal policy and legislative planning activities. Nurses can help communities achieve goals such as these.

....

Self-love is the only weight-loss aid that really works in the long run.

Jenny Craig
....

Ethical Issues in Health Education

Health education on the surface seems like an appropriate and ethical thing to do. After all, how ethical would it be to withhold information that could relieve suffering, prevent pain, and avert disease? But health education has its own controversies. Some of these are discussed next; others will become obvious to you as you educate individuals and communities.

A major problem occurs when there are unexpected, negative consequences because of health education. These can be the result of erroneous, poorly planned, or improperly implemented education efforts (Guttman, Kegler, & McLeroy, 1996). For instance, let's say that you want to teach a group of people who are newly diagnosed with cancer that there is hope. You ask four or five people with cancer to speak to your group. Unfortunately, several of the presenters are dealing with anger and depression because of their disease, and they take this opportunity to share their pain and frustration with the health care system. At the end of the session, your audience is likely to be confused (at the least) or to feel complete despair (at the worst). They may lose confidence in the ability to survive cancer treatment; they may even decide to forego therapy altogether and "get it over with." Although this example is quite blatant, problems can occur even under ideal circumstances.

One of the primary concerns that nurses have to address is the fact that, in many ways, health education manipulates clients to change behaviors. Granted, the changes we seek (based on our assessment of the latest scientific evidence) are for the client's benefit, but we are nevertheless clearly trying to influence change (Redman, 1997). This may be difficult for nurses to accept. We have, after all, been taught to respect individual autonomy. Manipulation, no matter how subtle, is hard to justify. This is not a reason to stop teaching or to stop advocating for policies such as motorcycle helmet laws. Instead, it is something that each nurse must weigh carefully before, during, and after health education programs. It also helps to differentiate manipulation from information dissemination. Giving a pregnant adolescent information on options, including the whole spectrum of choices involved in either continuing or terminating her pregnancy, for instance, is information dissemination that she can use to make an informed decision. Encouraging her to have an abortion, to give the infant up for adoption, or to have the baby and raise it herself is manipulation, especially if she makes her "informed" decision based on a lack of complete information that the nurse has failed to share.

Another issue is science itself and the rate at which knowledge expands (Redman, 1997). We have all heard clients say, "This is so confusing. How am I supposed to know what I should be doing? Last night there was a story on the news about how exercise can cause joint deterioration and here you are telling me that I need to exercise more!" Nurses have an obligation to keep up with advances in health care, but even nurses get confused. This all adds to the complex nature of education and reinforces the need to be able to read and critique research (see the following research briefs for examples of studies about health education).

One of the real social issues in client education has to do with the growing gap between the classes (Guttman, Kegler, & McLeroy, 1996). People who are financially secure are better equipped to act on advice to improve their health. Those without economic resources, however, often see health behaviors (e.g., exercise and eating well) as things they simply cannot afford. Poverty affects peoples' health, which further decreases the ability to earn a living or to get ahead. Nurses need to recognize that poor health practices may be related to social and economic barriers as much as they are related to a lack of knowledge, motivation, or positive attitudes. When this is the case, social and community solutions need to be explored rather than falling into the trap of victim blaming (Marantz, 1990). How appropriate,

RESEARCH BRIEF

Miller, P., Wikoff, R., & Hiatt, A. (1992). Fishbein's model of reasoned action and compliance behaviors of hypertensive patients. Nursing Research, 41, 104–109.

The authors of this study used the theory of reasoned action as a basis to examine medication compliance behaviors of 56 clients newly diagnosed as having hypertension. The purposes of the study were to (1) assess whether the constructs of reasoned action could be applied to clients with hypertension; (2) test whether intention was a sufficient predictor of behavior; and (3) test whether attitude, perceived beliefs of others, and motivation to comply were sufficient to determine intent. Demographic information and baseline physical data were collected during the first research visit. All subjects received extensive education about hypertension, medications, diet, smoking, exercise, and stress management. Six months later, subjects were asked to complete questionnaires that assessed attitude, perceived beliefs of others, motivation to comply, intention, and compliance behaviors related to diet, smoking, activity, stress, and medications.

Statistical analysis revealed that the model adequately predicted compliance to prescriptions for diet, smoking, activity, and stress, but not for medications. Compliance behavior was directly influenced by intention to comply. Intention, in turn, was influenced to varying degrees by attitude, motivation, and the perceived beliefs of others.

RESEARCH BRIEF

Swinburn, B. A., Walter, L. G., Arroll, B., Tilyard, M. W., & Russell, D. (1998). The green prescription study: A randomized controlled trial of written exercise advice provided by general practitioners. American Journal of Public Health, 88, 288–291.

The purpose of this study was to determine whether a written prescription for exercise in addition to verbal advice to exercise would increase physical activity more than verbal advice alone. Four hundred fifty-six sedentary adults (251 with at least one medical condition related to inactivity) were all given the same verbal information about increasing physical activity. Subjects were then randomly assigned to a control group (which received verbal information only) or an experimental group (which received a written prescription for exercise as well as verbal information). Activity levels were assessed 6 weeks later by a questionnaire that quantified time spent exercising over the previous 2 weeks.

There was an increase in physical activity for both groups, indicating that discussing the need had a beneficial effect. However, greater increases in the number of people who exercised and the amount of time spent exercising were seen for those who received both verbal and written information. The authors concluded that clients could be positively influenced to exercise and that this influence was enhanced by the use of written, goal-oriented prescriptions.

for instance, is it to blame an alcoholic for her liver disease? What if she was raised in a house where alcohol was used to deal with stress? What if her life has been filled with loss, abuse, and trauma? And what if her only solace is to sink into an alcoholic daze? Is this situation her fault? Maybe. Maybe not. Is she beyond help? No, but help is not easy to give if you blame the client for her disability. Repetitious, ineffective teaching will not help the situation either.

A final ethical issue that deserves attention has to do with community and cultural norms (Guttman, Kegler, & McLeroy, 1996; Redman, 1997). We each bring cultural biases into our social interactions. This is true of nurses as well as of clients. In addition to all of their other cultures, nurses bring the culture of health care and scientific bias into every encounter. This makes it difficult for nurses to deal with situations in which, for example, we know that fat infants grow up into fat adults, but the predominant culture believes that only fat babies are healthy. Nurses cannot ignore these conflicting values. They must instead use creative problem solving to develop acceptable solutions on a number of different levels. This can be a messy process with many trials and only a few successes. The alternative is to try to force the culture of science on people who are not going to accept it no matter how hard you try. So why not take some chances? The outcome could be that new messages or teaching methods or solutions emerge, and that could be the best possible conclusion to a difficult situation.

HEALTHY PEOPLE 2010

OBJECTIVES RELATED TO HEALTH EDUCATION

Educational and Community-Based Programs

School Setting

7.2 Increase the proportion of middle, junior high, and senior high schools that provide comprehensive school health education to prevent health problems in the following areas: unintentional injury; violence; suicide; tobacco use and addiction; alcohol and other drug use; unintended pregnancy; HIV/AIDS and STD infection; unhealthy dietary patterns; inadequate physical activity; and environmental health.

7.3 Increase the proportion of college and university students who receive information from their institution on each of the six priority health-risk behavior areas.

Health Care Setting

7.7 Increase the proportion of health care organizations that provide patient and family education.

7.8 Increase the proportion of patients who report that they are satisfied with the patient education they receive from their health care organization.

7.9 Increase the proportion of hospitals and managed care organizations that provide community disease prevention and health promotion activities that address the priority health needs identified by their community.

Source: DHHS, 2000.

CONCLUSION

Health education is an important intervention for nurses in all health care settings. The purpose of health education is to change behaviors and situations that put people at risk for injury, illness, disability, or death. It is a theory-based process that draws from learning theory as well as behavior change theory. The health education process is similar to the nursing process. It is appropriate in all clinical and community settings and can be applied to individuals, families, groups, and communities. Nurses may find that advocacy at the state and federal level is required to make personal and community behavior change possible. Nurses must also be aware that health education poses some important ethical issues.

CRITICAL THINKING ACTIVITIES

1. Develop teaching plans for each of the following situations. Identify and use a theory base that can help guide the process. Discuss assessment, planning, implementation, and evaluation as a part of your process.

- *Case 1:* Diane is a 48-year-old single mother who fractured her left wrist in a fall 3 weeks ago. The wrist was reduced in the hospital emergency room and set with a standard cast. Except for some pain and the need to modify a few of her activities, Diane has done well and feels that she will recover completely. Diane saw her nurse practitioner for a regular checkup 3 days ago. The nurse practitioner expressed concern about Diane's wrist and asked about the circumstances of the accident. When Diane described a situation that would not normally result in a fracture, the nurse practitioner ordered a scan to access bone density. The results show a 2.5% loss of bone mass. The nurse practitioner orders exercise and dietary changes. Diane and her provider agree to try these tactics for 6 months before considering medications. Diane's 14-year-old son lives with her. Her 20-year-old daughter recently married and moved out of state. The rest of Diane's family lives 350 miles away. She is the co-owner of a business that builds office complexes, and she typically works 10 to 12 hours a day. When you question her about her current diet and exercise routines, she shrugs and says, "To tell the truth, I'm way to busy to worry about those things. They just take up too much time."

- *Case 2:* Janet, the nurse at Allen Elementary School, has documented 12 cases of head lice during the past week. Most of the affected students are from one third grade class, but two cases came from a second grade class and one each came from a fifth grade class and another third grade class.

- *Case 3:* The nursing home in Sheridan County has a respite care center where families can leave elderly clients between the hours of 7 AM and 7 PM. The program provides meals, organized activities, and nap facilities for 22 clients with various physical and cognitive disabilities. Families who use the service give positive feedback about improvements in their abilities to cope with the stresses of caring for elderly relatives in the home. Sheila is an 86-year-old woman with confusion and delusions who is a regular client. Over the past week, Fred, the nurse manager, has noticed bruises around Sheila's wrists. Fred asks Sheila's daughter about the bruises, and she replies, "Oh, I guess she gets those from the restraints. She's started wandering around the house at night. I'm worried that she might fall and break a hip, so I talked to some of the other families at our last group meeting and several of them suggested that I tie Mama into bed at night."

- *Case 4:* Community Care Center is a comprehensive outpatient health care facility that serves injection drug users. In addition to methadone treatment, the center provides counseling services, case management, first aid, and routine annual physical assessments. The physician who does the physicals is only in the center 2 days a week. She approaches Anita, the clinic nurse, and expresses concern about the amount of chlamydia that she has diagnosed recently. She asks Anita, "What do you think we can do about this?" Although Anita agrees that the pattern the physician describes is an important concern, she worries about the ethical issues that could occur if the clinic takes any action. What ethical issues could develop? How can Anita address those issues for the clinic staff, clients, and surrounding community?

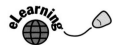

Explore Community Health Nursing on the web! To learn more about the topics in this chapter, use the passcode provided to access your exclusive web site:
http://communitynursing.jbpub.com
If you do not have a passcode, you can obtain one at this site.

REFERENCES

Andrade, S. J., & Doria-Ortiz, C. (1995). *Nuestro bienestar*: A Mexican-American community-based definition of health promotion in the southwestern United States. *Drugs: Education, Prevention, and Policy, 2,* 129–145.

Bigbee, J. L., & Jansa, N. (1991). Strategies for promoting health protection. *Nursing Clinics of North America, 26,* 895–913.

Bradley-Springer, L. (1996). Patient education for behavior change: Help from the transtheoretical and harm reduction models. *Journal of the Association of Nurses in AIDS Care, 7*(Suppl.), 23–33.

Byham, W. C. (with Cox, J., & Shomo, K. H.). (1992). *Zapp! in education: How empowerment can improve the quality of instruction and student and teacher satisfaction.* New York: Fawcett Columbine.

Caplan, D. (1995). Smoking: Issues and interventions for occupational health nurses. *AAOHN Journal, 43,* 633–643.

Carter, W. B. (1990). Health behavior as a rational process: Theory of reasoned action and multiattribute utility theory. In K. Glanz, F. M. Lewis, & B. K. Rimer (Eds.), *Health behavior and health education: Theory, research, and practice* (pp. 63–91). San Francisco: Jossey-Bass.

Cates, Jr., W., & Hinman, A. (1992). AIDS and absolutism: The demand for perfection in prevention. *New England Journal of Medicine, 327,* 492–494.

Damrosch, S. (1991). General strategies for motivating people to change their behavior. *Nursing Clinics of North America, 26,* 833–843.

Department of Health and Human Services (DHHS). (2000). *Healthy people 2010: Conference edition.* Washington, DC: United States Government Printing Office.

Foran, M., & Campanelli, L. C. (1995). Health promotion communications system: A model for a dispersed population. *AAOHN Journal, 43,* 564–569.

Glanz, K., Lewis, F. M., & Rimer, B. K. (Eds.). (1990). *Health behavior and health education: Theory, research, and practice.* San Francisco: Jossey-Bass.

Guttman, N., Kegler, M., & McLeroy, K. R. (1996). Health promotion paradoxes, antimonies and conundrums. *Health Education Research, 11*(1), i–xiii.

Hunt, R. (1997). Teaching. In R. Hunt & E. L. Zurek (Eds.), *Introduction to community based nursing* (pp. 182–225). Philadelphia: Lippincott.

Israel, B. A., Checkoway, B., Schulz, A., & Zimmerman, M. (1994). Health education and community empowerment: Conceptualizing and measuring perceptions of individual, organizational, and community control. *Health Education Quarterly, 21,* 140–170.

Knowles, M. S. (1973). *The adult learner: A neglected species.* Houston, TX: Gulf Publishing.

Kreuter, M. W., & Strecher, V. J. (1996). Do tailored behavior change messages enhance the effectiveness of health risk appraisal? Results from a randomized trial. *Health Education Research, 11,* 97–105.

Krozy, R. E. (1996). Community health promotion: Assessment and intervention. In S. H. Rankin & K. D. Stallings (Eds.), *Patient education: Issues, principles, practices* (3rd ed., pp. 245–271). Philadelphia: Lippincott.

Marantz, P. R. (1990). Blaming the victim: the negative consequence of preventive medicine. *American Journal of Public Health, 80*(18), 186–187.

Miller, P., Wikoff, R., & Hiatt, A. (1992). Fishbein's model of reasoned action and compliance behavior of hypertensive patients. *Nursing Research, 41,* 104–109.

Mirotznik, J., Feldman, L., & Stein, R. (1995). The health belief model and adherence with a community center-based, supervised coronary heart disease program. *Journal of Community Health, 20,* 233–247.

Novelli, W. D. (1990). Applying social marketing to health promotion and disease prevention. In K. Glanz, F. M. Lewis, & B. K. Rimer (Eds.), *Health behavior and health education: Theory, research, and practice* (pp. 342–369). San Francisco: Jossey-Bass.

Orlandi, M. A., Landers, C., Weston, R., & Haley, N. (1990). Diffusion of health promotion innovations. In K. Glanz, F. M. Lewis, & B. K. Rimer (Eds.), *Health behavior and health education: Theory, research, and practice* (pp. 288–313). San Francisco: Jossey-Bass.

Palank, C. L. (1991). Determinants of health-promotive behavior: A review of current research. *Nursing Clinics of North America, 26,* 815–832.

Perry, C. L., Baranowski, T., & Parcel, G. S. (1990). How individuals, environments and health behavior interact: Social learning theory. In K. Glanz, F. M. Lewis, & B. K. Rimer (Eds.), *Health behavior and health education: Theory, research, and practice* (pp. 161–186). San Francisco: Jossey-Bass.

Prochaska, J. O., Redding, C. A., Harlow, L. L., Rossi, J. S., & Velicer, W. F. (1994). The transtheoretical model of change and HIV prevention: A review. *Health Education Quarterly, 21*(4), 471–486.

Rankin, S. H., & Stallings, K. D. (1996). *Patient education: Issues, principles, practices* (3rd ed.). Philadelphia: Lippincott.

Redman, B. K. (1997). *The practice of patient education.* St. Louis: Mosby.

Rosenstock, I. M. (1990). The health belief model: Explaining health behavior through expectancies. In K. Glanz, F. M. Lewis, & B. K. Rimer (Eds.), *Health behavior and health education: Theory, research, and practice* (pp. 39–62). San Francisco: Jossey-Bass.

Spellbring, A. M. (1991). Nursing's role in health promotion: An overview. *Nursing Clinics of North America, 26,* 805–814.

Spradley, B. W., & Allender, J. A. (1996). *Community health nursing: Concepts and practice* (4th ed.). Philadelphia: Lippincott.

Strang, J. (1992). Harm reduction for drug users: Exploring the dimensions of harm, their measurement, and strategies for reductions. *AIDS and Public Policy Journal, 7,* 145–152.

Strecher, V. J., Seijts, G. H., Kok, G. J., Latham, G. P., Glascow, R., DeVellis, B., Meertens, R. M., & Bulger, D. W. (1995). Goal setting as a strategy for health behavior change. *Health Education Quarterly, 22,* 190–200.

Swinburn, B. A., Walter, L. G., Arroll, B., Tilyard, M. W., & Russell, D. (1998). The green prescription study: A randomized controlled trial of written exercise advice provided by general practitioners. *American Journal of Public Health, 88,* 288–291.

Chapter 16

Complementary and Holistic Health

Margaret A. Burkhardt

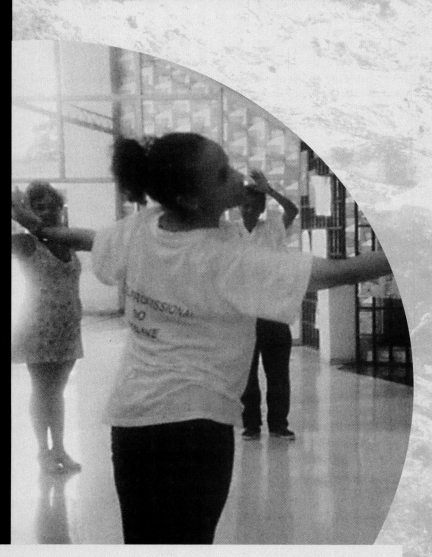

In recent years, health care professionals have become increasingly interested in therapies that lie outside the realm of conventional Western allopathic medicine. Many such therapies derive from folk wisdom, cultural perspectives, and healing practices of indigenous peoples and other ancient healing systems.

QUESTIONS TO CONSIDER

After reading this chapter, answer the following questions:

1. What is complementary health?
2. How does a nurse know when to choose a complementary intervention?
3. What are barriers to using complementary therapy?
4. What are some of the most common complementary therapies?
5. How does the community health nurse evaluate the effectiveness of complementary therapy?

KEY TERMS

Complementary health
Healing
Herbal therapies
Music therapy

Touch therapy
Office of Alternative
  Medicine (OAM)
Mind–body medicine

Health is wholeness, unfolding:
It is sharing, significantly, increasingly,
   in the varieties of human experience:
  physically, in the range of activities
   in which the human body can engage;
   not only aggression, but also conciliation,
   not only the proprieties, but also the singularities,
   not only to exhaustion, but also to the crest of vitality;
  sensually, in the possibilities of sensation;
   not confined to extremes:
    rage and excitement, passivity, suppression;
    not to pain:
    the pain of separation,
    the fear of aloneness;
   but knowing the quiet depths, the tenderness, the
    nuances flowing from tones, textures, odors,
    flavors;
    the joy of well-being, of union and reunion,
    the awesomeness of intimacy;
  culturally, socially, in the designs for living,
   across time and across the world:
   ways of talking, eating, dressing, pleasuring;
   ideas of beauty, of truth, of rightness.
It is growing in awareness:
  of sharing, significantly;
  of self;
  rising above existence, beyond time and space,
   the uniqueness of man.
And it is feeling good about it all, coming into Self-hood:
  expressing one's inner power,
  articulating one's reason-for-being,
  accepting one's sexuality,
   and interdependence:
   receiving and giving,
  holding on and letting go,
  following and guiding.
Toward wholeness:
  responding to the possibilities and limitations of human
   experience,
  reciprocating, resting, resurgent again;
  exploring, discovering
  opening, unfolding,
   from diffuseness toward coherence,
   simplicity toward complexity,
   disparity toward complementarity,
   vagueness toward decisiveness,
   confusion toward understanding,
   toward wholeness.

—Nancy Milio

More persons today are using alternative or unconventional therapies, either instead of allopathic modalities or combined with other nonallopathic approaches. These approaches are often termed complementary when they are used in addition to conventional therapies. In this chapter, *complementary therapy* is used regardless of the pattern of use, recognizing that health care providers need to be open to exploring various approaches to health and healing to support the best possible outcomes for clients.

RESEARCH BRIEF

Keegan, L. (1996). Use of alternative therapies among Mexican Americans in the Texas Rio Grande Valley. Journal of Holistic Nursing, 14(4), 277–294.

This descriptive study explored use of alternative health practices among Mexican Americans in the Texas Rio Grande Valley. A convenience sample of 213 subjects accessed through local clinics and hospitals were surveyed using a one-page bilingual written form designed to ascertain prevalence and use of alternative therapies, range of medical conditions for which subjects were currently seeking care, and demographic characteristics of subjects. Findings indicated that 44% of respondents had used an alternative practice one or more times in the past year, although 66% never reported the use of alternatives to their biomedical practitioner. The alternative practices used included herbal medicine, prayer/spiritual healing, massage, relaxation techniques, chiropractic, *curandero*, megavitamins, imagery, energy healing, acupuncture, biofeedback, hypnosis, and homeopathy. The most commonly used alternative therapies were herbal medicine, prayer/spiritual healing, massage, relaxation techniques, chiropractic, and visits to a Mexican folk healer (*curandero*).

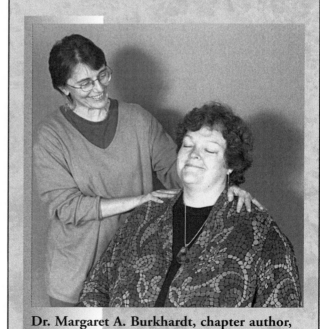

Dr. Margaret A. Burkhardt, chapter author, demonstrating healing touch with a client.

RESEARCH BRIEF

Olson, M., Sneed, N., LaVia, M., Virella, G., Bonadonna, R., & Michel, Y. (1997). Stress-induced immunosuppression and Therapeutic Touch. Alternative Therapies in Health and Medicine, 3(2), 68–74.

This experimental design pilot study focused on evaluating the effectiveness of therapeutic touch (TT) in reducing the adverse immunological effect of stress, as measured by changes in blood immunoglobulin levels, in a sample of highly stressed students. T-lymphocyte function (CD25) and immunoglobulin levels were the main outcome measures. Because this was a pilot study, there was a small sample size of 22 medical and nursing students who had scored one standard deviation above the mean on the SSTAI stress scale given during final examination periods 5 to 6 months before the national board examinations. Two weeks before the national examinations were given, the high stress students were randomly assigned to a TT or control group. Subjects in both groups completed the written stress scales, provided blood samples (1 week before, 1 day before, and 3 weeks after the board examination), and were given a standard dose of *Haemophilus* vaccine in the nondominant arm after the collection of the second set of data. In addition to this, the experimental group received three TT sessions approximately 24 hours apart during the week before the examination. Subjects receiving TT had significantly different levels of IgA and IgM from those in the control group, although there was no significant difference in IgG levels between the groups. There were no differences between the groups in the titers of antibodies to *H. influenzae*. Although the hypotheses were partially supported, the researchers acknowledge that, because of the small sample size, cautious interpretation of the results is indicated, and further research with larger sample sizes is needed to confirm findings.

Nurses within the community need to be familiar with various healing modalities used by their clients and aware of complementary modalities that may promote health, enhance healing, or contribute to unhealthy outcomes with clients. This chapter discusses a holistic framework for the integration of complementary therapies into care, understanding of complementary modalities, and assessment processes and ethical issues regarding **complementary health**. Selected complementary modalities are discussed that can be incorporated into community nursing care.

Care and love are the most universal, the most tremendous, and the most mysterious of cosmic forces; they comprise the primal and universal psychic energy.

Jean Watson

Holistic Framework

A holistic understanding of life that appreciates that each person is a bio-psycho-social-spiritual unity provides a framework for inclusion of complementary modalities into nursing care. Within a holistic framework, nurses are attentive to *healing* as well as to *curing* (Burkhardt, 1985; Quinn, 1989). Curing is a process that attends to disordered physical or psychological parts of a person, with a focus on disease processes and restoration of the integrity of a specific component (usually physiological) of a person. The allopathic approach focuses on curing by combating disease with techniques that produce effects different from those produced by the disease (Dossey & Guzzetta, 2000).

Healing, on the other hand, acknowledges that disharmony in a whole person may be manifesting as disease or illness and seeks to understand the totality of the lived experience for a person, taking into account the personal response to and meaning of the apparent disease or illness process (Burkhardt & Nagai-Jacobson, 1997b). Healing requires a relationship between the caregiver and care receiver that acknowledges common humanity and connectedness. Physical, emotional, and spiritual concerns are addressed within the healing relationship. Healing may manifest as cure in one or more of the bio-psycho-emotional realms but can be present without a cure. Quinn (1989) aptly notes that, although diseases may be cured, people need healing. The desire to promote health, or the need for healing or curing, which is not being addressed by conventional approaches, often leads people to complementary modalities. Complementary or alternative therapies generally focus on body-mind-spirit integration through healing by an individual, healing between two individuals, or healing at a distance (Dossey & Guzzetta, 2000).

It is particularly important for nurses who work within the community to practice holistic nursing. Dealing with clients and families within their home environments enables nurses to appreciate cultural considerations in healing and to assess clients' use of complementary modalities. Because holistic nursing has the healing of the whole person as its goal, nurses work in therapeutic partnership with clients and families to integrate those modalities that best facilitate the client's health and healing. Nurses also need to be aware of therapies that may be ineffective or cause potential harm when used alone or in combination with other modalities. The American Holistic Nurses' Association's description of holistic nursing presented in Box 16-1 provides a frame of reference for holistic nursing practice based on sound academic principles incorporating both the art and science of nursing.

BOX 16-1 AMERICAN HOLISTIC NURSES' ASSOCIATION DESCRIPTION OF HOLISTIC NURSING

Holistic nursing embraces all nursing practice that has healing the whole person as its goal. Holistic nursing recognizes that there are two views regarding holism: that holism involves studying and understanding the interrelationships of the bio-psycho-social-spiritual dimensions of the person, recognizing that the whole is greater than the sum of its parts; and that holism involves understanding the individual as an integrated whole interacting with and being acted on by both internal and external environments. Holistic nursing accepts both views, believing that the goals of nursing can be achieved within either framework.

Holistic practice draws on nursing knowledge, theories, expertise, and intuition to guide nurses in becoming therapeutic partners with clients in strengthening the clients' responses to facilitate the healing process and achieve wholeness.

Practicing holistic nursing requires nurses to integrate self-care in their own lives. Self-responsibility leads the nurse to a greater awareness of the interconnectedness of all individuals and their relationships to the human and global community, and permits nurses to use this awareness to facilitate healing.

Source: American Holistic Nurses' Association, 1994. Used with permission.

Historical Influences

Before discussing complementary health care modalities, let's take a brief look at the process through which allopathic or biomedical care became the accepted "conventional" approach to health care in the United States. The United States is often referred to as a "melting pot" of persons from many different cultures, educational and socioeconomic backgrounds, and experiences. Health care practices have evolved (and continue to do so) from the healing traditions of both native peoples and those who have immigrated to this country. Before the mid-1800s, practitioners from various health care systems, including allopathy, naturopathy, homeopathy, and botanics, were acknowledged as legitimate healers in the United States. Micozzi (1996) notes that the history of contemporary biomedicine as a scientific paradigm was as much influenced by social history as by scientific laws. Allopathic biomedicine began to predominate by the mid-1800s

and gained further prominence by the late 1800s through state licensing laws sponsored by and lobbied for by the American Medical Association.

Dossey and Swyers (1994) note that the prominence of biomedicine was shaped in part by two important developments. One development was in the realm of scientific discoveries, such as the identification of specific organisms as the cause of particular disease states and the identification of substances and vaccines that ward off the effect of pathogens, which greatly influenced the direction of biomedicine. The other was the 1910 release of Abraham Flexner's report titled *Medical Education in the United States and Canada*, which was influential in upgrading medical education programs, enabling medical schools with a stronger biomedical orientation to receive more financial backing from philanthropic foundations. This in turn prompted the stifling of medical schools teaching theories other than biomedical regarding the origin of illness and appropriate therapies. What was considered scientific was defined by biomedicine's "way of knowing," which emphasized that knowledge about the world requires empiricism (Micozzi, 1996). Other paradigms were either relegated to the "fringe" or subsumed into the biomedical paradigm. Although biomedicine gained power and prestige and became the gold standard for health care, small numbers of naturopathic, homeopathic, chiropractic, and practitioners of other healing systems continued to provide care.

Over the past several decades, however, health care consumers have become more active in seeking care outside the biomedical system. Some of the factors that may have contributed to this phenomenon include the following:

- *A shift away from infectious diseases as major causes of morbidity and mortality to health concerns that elude medical cure such as cancer, heart disease, hypertension, diabetes, and other chronic problems (Gordon, 1980)*

- *Increasingly depersonalized care and decreased personal control in health care decisions as a result of increased use of technology (Burkhardt & Nathaniel, 1998)*

- *A greater emphasis on self-care and personal responsibility for health*

- *A shrinking world that has allowed greater access to other cultures and their systems of healing*

- *Renewed appreciation that healing must address the whole body-mind-spirit person*

Although people have been using complementary therapies for years, the landmark study conducted by Eisenberg, Kessler, Foster, Norlock, Calkins, and Delbanco (1993) documented an unexpected frequency of use of these therapies and caused the medical establishment to take note. The results of this national telephone survey of 1,539 adults indicated that one in three Americans of all sociodemographic groups used complementary therapies, and of those who used these therapies, 72% did so without informing their conventional health care provider. This study also indicated that people tended to use complementary modalities for chronic rather than life-threatening conditions. To identify trends in alternative medicine use in the United States, Eisenberg, Rogers, Ettner, Appel, Wilkey, Van Rompay, and Kessler (1998) conducted another national telephone survey of 2,055 English-speaking adults in 1997 asking about their use of 16 therapies. The therapies included relaxation techniques, herbal medicine, massage, chiropractic, prayer or spiritual healing by others, megavitamins, self-help groups, imagery, commercial diet, folk remedies, lifestyle diet, energy healing, homeopathy, hypnosis, biofeedback, and acupuncture. Results of this survey indicated that alternative therapy use increased from 33.8% in 1990 to 42.1% in 1997. Use of herbal medicine, massage, megavitamins, self-help groups, folk remedies, energy healing, and homeopathy increased the most.

Keegan (1996) documented use of alternative therapies among Mexican Americans to be 44%, noting that 66% of this population never report the use of alternatives to conventional health care providers. Through a self-reporting survey of the use of complementary therapies among people in rural West Virginia, Burkhardt, Nathaniel, Nemeth-Pyles, and Boyd (1999) found that 83% of respondents (n = 545) used at least one of the 17 listed therapies within the past year. In this study, 41% of respondents reported that they never discuss these therapies with their health care provider and 34% only sometimes discuss these with their providers.

In response to growing awareness and use of complementary therapies, the National Institutes of Health (NIH) created the **Office of Alternative Medicine (OAM)** in 1992. The OAM was established to facilitate scientific and fair evaluation of complementary modalities that can contribute to the health and well-being of many people and reduce barriers to awareness and availability of promising complementary therapies. In 1998, the OAM was elevated to the National Center for Complementary and Alternative Medicine (NCCAM), one of the 25 institutes and centers of NIH. The NCCAM's mission is to conduct and support basic and applied research and training and to disseminate information on complementary and alternative medicine to practitioners and the public. The congressional mandate for the NCCAM provides for research training programs and a public information clearinghouse; however, the center is not a referral agency. The importance of research on and reliable information about complementary therapies is reflected in the increase in budget for the NCCAM from $2 million in 1993 to $50 million in 1999.

Complementary Modalities: What Are They?

Although the terms *alternative, complementary,* and *unconventional* are often used interchangeably in reference to nonbiomedical interventions, the term *complementary* best reflects the awareness that these therapies need to be considered adjuncts to, not replacements for, medical and surgical treatments. The definition of complementary modalities that was developed at the NIH/OAM Second Conference on Research Methodology in April 1995 notes that the broad domain of complementary and alternative medicine (CAM) encompasses all health systems, modalities, and practices other than those intrinsic to the politically dominant health system of a particular society or culture. CAM includes all practices and ideas self-defined by their users as preventing or treating illness or promoting health and well-being.

Each healing system (including biomedicine) has its own explanatory model that "summarizes the perceptions, assumptions, beliefs, theories, and facts that guide the logic of health care delivery" (Cassidy, 1996, p. 20). Some important distinctions between complementary and conventional medicine include differences in philosophical underpinnings, types of therapies offered, how therapies are administered, and interaction between practitioner and client (Cassidy, 1996; Dossey & Swyers, 1994). For example, in the biomedical model, the practitioner has traditionally been considered the authoritative expert who determines and designs care based on standardized treatments in which the client has variable involvement. With complementary systems, treatments are more often individualized and developed in collaboration with clients who are acknowledged as having responsibility for their own healing processes. Complementary systems generally appreciate that humans have natural built-in recuperative powers and often focus on therapies that enhance the client's natural healing processes. Unifying threads that are common to most complementary healing systems include emphasis on (1) one's relationships, sense of values, place in society, and sense of self; (2) the role of spiritual values and religion in health; (3) the impact on health of consciousness manifested through thoughts, feelings, attitudes, emotions, values, and perceived meanings; (4) diet, exercise, relaxation techniques, and modifications in lifestyle; and (5) utilization of whole foods and herbs rather than extracts (Dossey & Swyers, 1994). Many of these threads are common parts of nursing practice as well, and conventional medicine is beginning to pay more attention to them.

The NCCAM continues to use the seven fields of complementary and alternative health practice that were described in *Alternative Medicine: Expanding Medical Horizons* (National Institutes of Health, 1994) as the basis for the classification of alternative medical practices. The seven major categories of the classification each contain subcategories designated as *CAM*—practices that are not commonly used, accepted, or available in conventional medicine; *behavioral medicine*—practices that may fall within the domain of conventional medicine; or *overlapping*—practices that can be in either subcategory (NCCAM, 1999). The seven fields of practice with associated NCCAM classifications of alternative medicine practice are briefly summarized in the following section. Because the listing of specific modalities and therapies is updated and expanded on regularly, only a few selected examples are given for each category. The reader is encouraged to visit the NCCAM Web site for further information.

Diet, Nutrition, and Lifestyle Changes

This field focuses on the use of dietary and nutritional interventions in preventing illness, maintaining health, and reversing the effects of chronic disease. The rise in chronic illnesses related to diet has prompted a shift in nutritional research toward dealing with the effects of nutritional excess and away from eliminating nutritional deficiency. Evidence indicates that inadequate intake of some micronutrients may increase risks of problems such as coronary artery disease, cancers, and birth defects and that the required daily allowance for some minerals and vitamins may not be adequate to prevent chronic illnesses. Many alternative diets and dietary lifestyles that foster the inclusion of more fresh and freshly prepared fruits and vegetables, whole grains, and legumes may offer greater resistance to illness. For example, increased consumption of beans and lentils appears to decrease the risk of colon cancer (National Institutes of Health, 1994).

The NCCAM classifications *biologically based therapies* and *lifestyle and disease prevention* both relate to this field of practice. *Biologically based therapies*, which include naturally and biologically based products, may overlap with use of dietary supplements by conventional practitioners. The four subcategories are as follows:

1. Phytotherapy or herbalism: *plant-derived preparations used for therapeutic and preventative purposes, such as gingko biloba, echinacea, and green tea*

2. Special diet therapies: *dietary approaches used as alternative therapies for particular risk factors or for chronic disease in general, such as vegetarian, Pritikin, and macrobiotic*

3. Orthomolecular medicine: *products not covered in other categories that are used (usually in combinations and at high doses) as nutritional and food supplements for preventive or therapeutic purposes, such as ascorbic acid, co-enzyme Q10, and melatonin*

4. Pharmacological, biological, and instrumental interventions: *products and procedures applied in an unconventional manner, such as cartilage, enzyme therapies, iridology*

Lifestyle and disease prevention, which focuses on preventing illness, identifying and treating risk factors, and supporting healing, is concerned with integrative approaches for prevention and management of chronic conditions. The three subcategories are as follows:

1. Clinical preventive practices: *unconventional approaches, such as medical intuition and electrodermal diagnosis, used to screen for or prevent health-related concerns*

2. Lifestyle therapies: *changes or therapies based on unconventional systems of care or used in unconventional ways, such as dietary or behavioral changes, exercise, and addiction control*

3. Health promotion: *involves research on healing and the healing process, autoregulatory mechanisms, and factors affecting health promotion*

Mind-Body Control

This field focuses on the mind's capacity to affect the body and explores healing systems that make use of the interconnectedness of mind, body, and spirit. Most traditional healing systems acknowledge and incorporate the interconnectedness of mind-body-spirit, recognizing the power of each to affect the other. In the past 30 years, biomedicine has opened more to the awareness of the impact of the mind on the body, although exploring the role of spirituality in healing is still in its infancy. Mind-body-spirit interventions often enable clients to experience and express their illnesses in new and clearer ways and to explore the meaning aspects, which can have direct consequences on their health. Scientific exploration suggests that there is a complex interaction among the mind and neurological and immune systems (psychoneuroimmunology), which can be affected by interventions in this category.

The NCCAM classification of **mind-body medicine**, which involves psychological, social, behavioral, and spiritual approaches to health, relates to this field of practice. The four subcategories are as follows:

1. Mind-body systems: *whole systems that are used in combination with lifestyle or are part of traditional healing systems*

2. Mind-body methods: *specific modalities incorporating awareness of mind-body interaction in healing, such as yoga, t'ai chi, meditation, imagery,* **music therapy,** *and psychotherapy*

3. Religion and spirituality: *the nonbehavioral aspects of religion and spirituality that relate to biological function or clinical condition, such as nonlocality, confession, and spiritual healing*

4. Social and contextual factors: *interventions that are social, cultural, symbolic, or contextual in nature, such as caring-based approaches like holistic nursing, intuitive diagnosis, and community-based approaches like certain Native American rituals*

Alternative Systems of Practice

It is estimated that worldwide only 10% to 30% of human health care is delivered by conventional biomedically oriented practitioners. The remaining 70% to 90% of care varies from self-care according to folk principles to care sought within an organized health care system derived from traditions or practices that flow from paradigms of health and healing different from that of biomedicine. Some of these explanatory models have sound bases that have been developed, tested, and practiced over many more years than biomedicine. However, because they derive from a different worldview, the processes and modes of action of many of these modalities are not understood within the biomedical paradigm.

The NCCAM classification *alternative medical systems*, which addresses complete systems of theory and practice other than the Western biomedical approach, contains four categories:

1. Acupuncture and oriental medicine, *including herbal formulas, t'ai chi, and diet*

2. Traditional indigenous systems, *including Native American healing, Ayurvedic medicine, and traditional African healing*

3. Unconventional Western systems, *including homeopathy, environmental medicine, and Cayce-based systems*

4. Naturopathy, *including other natural systems and therapies*

Manual Healing

Touch or manipulation with the hands has been part of healing traditions as far back as one can explore. Although contemporary biomedical providers tend to be distanced from physical contact with clients because of attitudes of reliance on diagnostic equipment and tests, as well as legal and time constraints, at one time physicians' hands were considered their most important diagnostic and therapeutic tool. Manual healing methods derive from the understanding that dysfunction of one area of the body can affect the function of other discrete body parts. It is worth noting that osteopathic medicine was one of the earliest U.S. health care systems to use manual healing methods.

The NCCAM classification *manipulative and body-based systems* focuses on therapies and systems that are based on movement or manipulation of the body. The three subcategories are as follows:

1. Chiropractic medicine

2. Massage and body work, *including osteopathic manipulative therapy, Swedish massage, Chinese Tui Na massage and acupressure, and body psychotherapy*

3. Unconventional physical therapies, *including hydrotherapy, light and color therapies, and heat and electrotherapies*

Pharmacological/Biological Treatments

This includes any assortment of drugs, biological products, and vaccines not yet accepted by conventional medicine. Examples of some such products include cartilage products derived from sharks, chicken, and sheep, used for treating cancer; ethylene diamine tetraacetic acid (EDTA) chelation therapy, used for treating heart disease and preventing cancer; a liquid extract from mistletoe plants (iscador), used to treat tumors; and biologically guided chemotherapy.

The NCCAM classification *biologically based therapies*, which was discussed earlier, relates to this field of practice.

Bioelectromagnetic Applications

This is an emerging science studying how living organisms interact with electromagnetic fields. The understanding that electrical phenomena are found in all living organisms and that electrical currents in the body can produce magnetic fields extending outside the body is basic to this field of study. Exploration suggests that changes in the body's natural fields can produce physical and behavioral changes and that certain frequencies have specific effects on body tissues.

The NCCAM clarifications *biofield* and *bioelectromagnetics* relate to this field of practice. *Biofield* healing practices, which use subtle energy fields in and around the body for healing and health promotion, include healing touch, Reiki, therapeutic touch, and external Qi Gong. *Bioelectromagnetics* includes the unconventional use of electromagnetic fields for healing and health promotion.

Herbal Therapies

All cultures and healing traditions have included the use of plants and plant products. Many of today's drugs have herbal origins, and approximately 25% of drugs dispensed from pharmacies have at least one active ingredient derived from plants. According to the World Health Organization, an estimated 4 billion people (80% of the world's population) use **herbal therapies** for some aspect of primary care. Herbal therapies are a major component of indigenous healing traditions. Because of U.S. Food and Drug Administration regulations, herbal products can be marketed in the United States only as food supplements and can boast no specific health claims.

The NCCAM classification *biologically based therapies*, which was discussed earlier, relates to this field of practice. Aromatherapy is considered in this classification.

The national health goals of *Healthy People 2010: Increasing the Span of Healthy Life for Americans, Reducing Health Disparities among Americans, and Achieving Access to Preventive Services for all Americans* are designed to help bring the people of the United States to their full potential. The opportunities or objectives designated for achieving these goals relate to health promotion, health protection, and preventive services. Although the document does not address complementary modalities per se, many people use complementary therapies as part of their efforts to promote health and prevent illness. Most complementary modalities included in the classification system at the NCCAM relate to the goal of increasing the span of healthy life for people in this country. Appropriate use of complementary therapies and their practitioners may ultimately contribute to the goals of reducing health disparities. Because many complementary therapies focus on health promotion and illness prevention, appropriately integrating them into health care may promote access to preventive services for people in this country. Although research on the role of many complementary modalities in health promotion and prevention has expanded in recent years, more validation of the efficacy of these therapies is needed. Because health promotion strategies relate to individual lifestyle and choices, nurses need to be particularly aware of choices people make regarding the use of complementary therapies in dealing with health promotion and illness prevention.

Complementary Health and Community Nursing Practice

Community health nurses must remember that decisions about health care are based on more than scientific expertise. Health care choices are influenced by a person's values, culture, and spiritual and other beliefs; evaluation of risks, benefits, and economic considerations; and effects on lifestyle and role. All of these areas must be considered in deliberations about health care. Cassidy (1996) writes that "cultural relativity is pivotal to the study of alternative medicine, because each alternative system of medicine provides a different set of ideas about the body, disease, and medical reality" (p. 12). Community nurses need to be particularly attentive to the influence of culture because emotional, psychological, aesthetic, interpersonal, and other dimensions of health concerns differ across cultures and belief systems, impelling certain actions and constraining others (O'Connor, 1996). Our culture teaches us the meaning of health; how to be sick; and when, how, and from whom to seek care.

Community nurses must be aware of the values, goals, and beliefs of personal culture (their own and that of their clients), as well as the culture of the biomedical system and of other healing systems as they develop health care plans with clients. With this awareness, nurses can be more alert for potential conflicts and negative value judgments that may interfere with integrating complementary modalities into care. Consider, for example, a situation in which a nurse learns that her client with fibromyalgia is using herbs and vitamins recommended by a layperson who used kinesiology to determine what the client needed. Recognizing that the culture of the biomedical system would find this process unscientific alerts the nurse to potential negative value judgments from the client's biomedical practitioner regarding her choice and enables the nurse to consider ways to assist the client in integrating the different modalities. Clients are more likely to discuss their complementary health practices with nurses who approach them with an openness to exploring and including different modalities in care than they are with nurses who place judgments on such modalities.

The Right to Choose

Professional standards and codes of ethics direct nurses to respect each person and to value and support client autonomy. Basic to autonomy are the ability to determine personal goals, the ability to decide on a plan of action, and the freedom to act on one's choice. Consequently, the principle of client self-determination directs nurses to honor the right of persons to use modalities outside the realm of biomedicine in addressing their health care needs. When such choices are made, nurses may find it challenging to honor and respect the convictions derived from belief systems that underlie these choices, particularly when these beliefs are not understood or are contrary to their own. However, to deny such convictions in health care settings is "to deny the patient's very reality, sometimes risking serious psychological and emotional impact on patient and family alike, and always raising genuine ethical concerns about patient autonomy, provider beneficence, substituted judgment, and distributive justice" (O'Connor, 1996, p. 93). Attentiveness to client values and desires for treatment options requires nurses to take seriously the client's need for healing as well as curing, and the contributions to health offered by other explanatory models. When nurses do not understand the other modality or question the efficacy or safety of the choice, they must explore these considerations with the client. A nonjudgmental approach that is respectful of differing values and beliefs and alert for ethnocentric bias on the part of the nurse enhances joint exploration (Burkhardt & Nathaniel, 1996).

Nursing Assessment

To have a broad picture of the many factors affecting a client's health and healing, nurses need to be aware of the various therapies being considered or used by clients. Community nurses need to develop the ability to incorporate discussion of complementary therapies into their nursing assessment in an open way, because clients may be hesitant to bring up the subject. Discussion may be prompted through open-ended questions such as "What do you do to take care of your health on your own?" "What other things have you tried (or thought about trying) for this health concern?" and "Sometimes people with your condition want to try other remedies, and I wonder if this is something that you have considered?" Another approach to opening a discussion of complementary therapies is to explore the use of specific modalities commonly used in your area with questions such as "Have you ever seen a (chiropractor, acupuncturist, herbalist, etc.) for that problem?" "Have you considered seeing the (*curandera*, medicine person, spiritual healer, etc.)?" or "Have you been using (special vitamins, a macrobiotic diet, herbal remedies, etc.) for your illness?"

Nurses must be knowledgeable about various modalities and therapies to effectively discuss their use with clients. Nurses need not subscribe to particular complementary therapies to effectively assess how clients use these therapies. Nor do nurses need to be practitioners of other modalities to discuss them with clients, any more than they need to be able to do surgery to discuss it. However, community nurses must be able to create an atmosphere that encourages a nonjudgmental assessment of all modalities being considered or used, with a goal of using whatever is beneficial for and will meet the needs of the client and family.

Community nurses should become familiar with and develop at least a talking knowledge of complementary therapies that may be commonly used in their communities to be better able to discuss their use with their clients. Many therapies work as an adjunct to biomedical interventions, some may interact in unhealthy ways with particular biomedical treatments, and the efficacy of many modalities is not fully known. When discussing choices with clients, nurses should draw on studies with which they are familiar in offering relevant information regarding particular therapies, allowing clinical and personal experience into the conversation in judicious ways, yet recognizing that the nurse never has all the pertinent information and that uncertainty is inherent in health choices (Hufford, 1996b). Based on their assessment and knowledge regarding particular therapies, nurses may find it appropriate to support or recommend some complementary modalities while discouraging the use of others.

Hufford (1996b) suggests that the client has major responsibility for obtaining information regarding complementary therapies and making health choices in this regard. However, nurses need to have some knowledge about risks and benefits associated with these therapies. For example, although garlic may assist in lowering cholesterol, large doses can cause irritation to the digestive tract, which may result in some bleeding. Nurses should encourage clients to explore the validity of claims made about particular therapies and assist them in doing so, especially if the nurse perceives the therapy to be potentially harmful for the client. However, complementary modalities should not be discounted merely because they are not understood within the Western biomedical framework. When clients are interested in complementary therapies, nurses should help determine whether risks are involved. When the potential for significant risks exists and the client is committed to using the therapy, the nursing goal is to minimize risks while maximizing treatment. If the client does not have as strong commitment to the complementary modality, nurses should encourage ongoing discussion of known risks and benefits related to various options (Hufford, 1996a). As part of their assessments, nurses need to determine the congruency between client and nursing goals regarding healing and curing; they also should review options considered viable by each as a means of meeting these goals. Maintaining an openness to working with traditional systems and their healers facilitates more effective and culturally congruent nursing and health care.

Potential Barriers to Use of Complementary Therapies

Professional integrity requires nurses to take an honest look at potential barriers that may limit availability of and access to complementary therapies for clients and that may hinder the research of complementary therapies. Dossey and Swyers (1994) suggest that barriers to use of complementary therapies can be structural in nature or can relate to regulatory, economic, and belief systems. Structural barriers include problems caused by a lack of common classification systems and definitions between biomedicine and complementary modalities, difficulty in obtaining original research on complementary therapies because they are not published in English in scientifically reviewed literature, and lack of understanding of culturally based explanatory models. For example, a family may wish to obtain more information about the efficacy of an herbal preparation that they heard may help with their mother's chronic illness, but the major research is

published in Chinese. Regulatory and economic barriers include current federal mechanisms for regulating medical research, which do not favor the evaluation of many forms of complementary treatments; the cost of conducting the necessary laboratory and clinical trials of a product or procedure; and the existence of state medical practice acts that limit the practice of healing arts to holders of medical licenses. An example of this barrier is the limited access to naturopathic physicians because they are not licensed in most states.

Belief barriers include ideological skepticism flowing from comfort with the status quo, belief that high technology interventions are more effective, and attitudes that any modality other than biomedicine is unscientific. These barriers include attitudes of conventional practitioners that consider use of herbal preparations rather than as medical intervention a waste of money because they have not been "scientifically" studied, even when the client is experiencing benefit from the preparations. Although the work of the NCCAM and other organizations is helping reduce these barriers, nurses need to be alert for situations in which clients experience limited access to or availability of complementary modalities.

Power relationship between the nurse and client can present barriers to the client's use of complementary therapies. The nurse is in a role of power and authority derived from professional knowledge and skills. Persisting paternalistic attitudes within health care settings, which foster the dependent role for clients, may manifest as attitudes indicating that approaches to managing health concerns other than those proposed by the nurse are unacceptable and without sound basis. Consider, for example, a nurse who is very willing to support the physician's recommendation of surgery or strong narcotics for the management of severe pain but who is unwilling to discuss the client's interest in trying acupuncture, declaring that such approaches are unreliable. When nurses assume that a client's values and thought processes are the same as their own, they may believe that the only reasonable courses of action are those that they would choose. Such attitudes may prompt nurses to question the decision-making capacity of clients who choose complementary therapies in lieu of or in addition to conventional therapies or label them as noncompliant, both of which can present barriers to the client's use of therapies that may enhance the healing process.

Integrating Complementary Therapies into Community Nursing Care

As noted previously, holistic care should be the goal of all nursing practice. Although holistic care presumes attention to physical, mental, emotional, and spiritual concerns, many look upon spirituality as complementary therapy. The tendency to view body and spirit as separate and unrelated entities (which persists within contemporary health care settings) supports the view that physical concerns are the prime focus of biomedicine and that spirituality has little or no place in biomedical care. However, body-mind-spirit are inextricably intertwined, and spirituality cannot be separated from physical and emotional health.

This section briefly discusses ways of integrating spirituality and selected complementary modalities into nursing care. When considering integrating any modality into practice, nurses need to address two fundamental concerns: (1) safety—the potential side effects and risks for harm when the therapy is used alone or in combination with other therapies, and (2) efficacy—the therapy produces the effect that it is intended to produce. The examples of complementary modalities presented here are chosen because they can be particularly valuable nursing interventions that clearly fall within nursing's domain of practice. Educational programs are available through which nurses can become certified practitioners of many of these therapies. Although it is within nursing's domain of practice to address diet, nutrition, and lifestyle changes, nurses must recognize that when such modalities are considered complementary or alternative, they are based on nonorthodox systems of healing or are applied in unconventional ways. Nurses need to be aware that their clients are using these modalities, their reasons for using them, and potential risks and benefits.

The nursing role includes supporting that which promotes health and healing, advising caution where risks are involved, facilitating open communication about various options, and honoring the client's right to choose. Nurses can become knowledgeable about, and through training become, practitioners of alternative healing modalities such as acupuncture, oriental medicine, homeopathy, and Ayurvedic medicine. Some aspects of other healing systems may be easily integrated into nursing care, such as use of particular acupressure points for relief of headaches or nausea. However, nurses need to be aware of the scope of practice stated in their state's nurse practice act and incorporate only those modalities that are within their scope of nursing practice.

Spirituality

Spirituality is the essence of who one is, a unifying or animating force that permeates all of one's life and being. This essence is expressed in and through connectedness with one's self, with others, with nature, and with a God or a Life Force. Although one's spirituality and relationship with God or Life Force is often nurtured and expressed through one's religious beliefs and practices, for many, spirituality transcends the boundaries of religion. Spirituality is connected to values and is vital to the process of discovering meaning and purpose in life. Spiritual issues are core life issues that are often related to mystery, suffering, forgiveness, grace, hope, and love (Burkhardt & Nagai-Jacobson, 1997a, 2000).

The nursing assessment of spirituality requires attentive listening, the ability to be fully present with the client in this moment, and good communication skills. Assessment of spiritual concerns with clients includes exploration of issues of meaning and purpose; important values, beliefs, and practices; prayer or meditation styles; important relationships and their influence on the present circumstances; and desires for connection with religious groups or rituals. The process of assessment often is part of the intervention because merely providing the opportunity for clients to talk of their spiritual concerns enables them to become more aware of their spiritual journey and its impact on present life experiences. Because people often use story and metaphor in expressing their spirituality and spiritual concerns, nurses can approach spirituality by encouraging people to tell their stories. In this process, nurses can gain insight into those connections that support and inspire a client, relationships in need of healing, sources of strength, experiences that have given life meaning, and ways in which the person questions the meaning of life. Nurses can help clients attune to their spirituality by exploring and incorporating meaningful rituals into care such as sacred readings, drumming, and music; facilitating processes focused on mindfulness such as relaxation exercises, imagery, and paying attention to physical sensations; and fostering consideration of the place and meaning of prayer for clients and the ways they do or do not experience God or Life Force in their lives. Nurses need to be aware of their own spiritual perspectives to honor their own values and beliefs without imposing them on clients.

Prayer

The experience of prayer or some form of connecting to the "beyond" is fundamental to human life and experience. Dossey (1993, 1996, 1997, 1998) discusses the extensive evidence indicating that prayer and religious devotion are associated with health outcomes. He notes that research on intercessory prayer and distant intentionality indicate that open-ended, nondirective prayer such as "Thy will be done" or "Whatever is best for all concerned" is more efficacious than prayers for particular outcomes. He also reminds us that prayer does not require scientific evidence for validation. Prayer is an appropriate nursing intervention, whether the nurse prays for or with clients or arranges for clients to have the quiet and privacy needed for prayer or meditation. Nurses who include prayer as part of their client care need to remember that prayer has many forms and expressions and is culturally conditioned.

When nurses incorporate prayer for clients into their personal spiritual practices, they should not presume to know what the client needs; rather, they should express prayer in terms such as, "Whatever is for the client's highest good." Nurses who wish to pray with clients should do so with the client's permission and encourage clients to use their own forms and expressions of prayer. Very often, clients in health care institutions need nurses to help them make sacred space within daily routines in order to attend to their own prayer, either alone or with others.

Music Therapy

Music has been a vital part of all cultures and societies and has been linked with healing throughout history. Guzzetta (1997,

2000) notes that music therapy complements conventional therapies by providing clients with integrated body-mind experiences and by facilitating relaxation, self-healing, and active participation in health and recovery. Music can promote relaxation and can produce changes in emotions, behavior, and physiology. Music can be used alone or in conjunction with prayer, meditation, relaxation exercises, and guided imagery. Musical vibrations can help restore or maintain the body's regulatory function; can help reduce pain, anxiety, isolation, and psychophysiological stress; can enhance the immune system; and can facilitate development of self-awareness and help improve memory (Guzzetta, 1997, 2000).

Guzzetta reminds us that, when considering using music therapy with clients, nurses need to assess clients' music preferences, the importance of music in their lives, and the types of music that make them happy, sad, relaxed, tense, and so forth. Nurses must be aware that no one selection or type of music is best for all people or in all situations and that the client's mood and preferences determine the types of music used and the goals of each session. Nurses can introduce clients to music therapy, initially guide them through the process, and help them develop their own healing scripts and music libraries. Guzzetta (1997, 2000) offers guidelines for incorporating music therapy into clinical settings and provides a script that nurses can use with clients during a music therapy session. Research conducted through the music therapy program at the University of Miami indicated that music contributed to an increase in levels of melatonin and human growth hormone (leading to better sleep patterns and fewer aches and pains) in Alzheimer's clients and that the combined use of music and guided imagery in clinical trials contributed to lower liver enzymes in clients with chronic hepatitis B and lower levels of stress hormones in healthy persons (Simonton, Cohen, Kumar, McKinney, & Tims, 1997).

Imagery

Imagery is a way of using the imagination and connecting with the more subtle aspects of inner experiences that may involve all senses—vision, taste, smell, touch, and hearing. Images, which can be considered a bridge between conscious processing of information and physiological change, can be produced by conscious as well as subconscious acts and may precede or follow physiological change (Dossey, 1997; Schaub, 2000). Imagery enables access to our emotions and to our spiritual or higher self. Dossey (1997) describes several types of imagery: receptive, active, symbolic, process, correct biological, end-state, general healing, packaged, customized, and interactive guided imagery. Although nurses can use any type with clients to enhance their healing processes, they need to appreciate individual variations of images, colors, shapes, symbols, and meanings related to cultural diversity. Nurses can use imagery to help promote a sense of well-being with clients; encourage healthy behaviors; and help them modify their perceptions about their diseases, strengths, treatments, and healing capacities. Relaxation exercises are a form of imagery. An example of a situation in which imagery can be incorporated into nursing care is with bone or wound healing. Before the session, in terms the client can understand, the nurse describes the basic biological process involved in the healing. The imagery process begins with a relaxation exercise. While the client is in a relaxed state, the nurse instructs the client to imagine the natural process of healing that is occurring, helping the client by quietly describing the elements of the healing process, and ultimately imagining oneself as fully healed and back to normal activities. Many resources are available for nurses who wish to develop skills in integrating imagery into nursing care (Achterberg, Dossey, & Kolkmeier, 1994; Dossey, 1997; Schaub, 2000), including a nurses' certification program in interactive imagery sponsored by the American Holistic Nurses' Association and the Academy for Guided Imagery.

Herbal Therapies

Herbal and natural therapies, which have been used for healing in all cultures from before the time of written history, are becoming more common and are available in grocery stores and regular pharmacies. Although many natural and herbal preparations can enhance health and contribute to the prevention of disease, they are not necessarily safe just because they are natural (Duke, 1997; Murray, 1995). Because plants cannot be patented, little research has been done in the United States on plants as a medicinal agents and there is a lack of standardization regarding the amount of the active ingredient of the plant that is in any particular herbal preparation (Murray, 1995). Although research on plants as medicinal agents is only in its infancy in this country, there is research to support the efficacy of many herbal and natural preparations (e.g., St. John's Wort and gingko biloba) that has been done in other countries (Murray & Pizzorno, 1998). Because many clients use herbs and other natural preparations, nurses need to become knowledgeable about common herbs, their uses, and potential interaction with pharmaceutical drugs. Nurses need to ask about use of herbal and natural preparations in the same way they include discussion of other medications. Of particular importance is advising clients who take herbal preparations to read labels and buy only those that have standardized extracts of the active herb. Students are encouraged to explore the many good references available that discuss the healing benefits, side effects, and interactions of various herbal and natural preparations.

Aromatherapy

Aromatherapy refers to the therapeutic use of the essential (concentrated) oils extracted from different parts of aromatic plants. The oils, which are widely available, may be applied to the body through massage, inhaled as mists, used as a compress, or mixed into an ointment. Although research on the health benefits of aromatherapy is in its infancy, use of this therapy shows promise in promoting relaxation; relieving stress, anxiety, pain, discomfort, insomnia, and restlessness; promoting wound healing; enhancing self-esteem; and stimulating immune function (Stevensen, 1995). Although aromatic oils have been used for varied purposes for centuries, recent years have seen a resurgence in the use of aromatherapy among lay people as well as nurses. Robins (1999) notes that aromatherapy is a safe therapy, with few adverse reactions reported in the literature, although its mechanisms of action and efficacy need further research. Robins suggests that nurses who wish to consider using aromatherapy as an adjunct in nursing practice should have some formal training, use caution when using these oils with people with very sensitive skin or severe respiratory disorders, and be aware that most of these oils should not be ingested.

Touch Therapy

Touch is essential for human survival and development. **Touch therapy** includes a broad range of hand techniques that a nurse can use on or near the body to support the client's movement toward balance, wholeness, and optimal functioning (Shames, 1997, 2000). Touch interventions used by nurses include both physical and energetic healing modalities such as therapeutic massage, therapeutic touch, healing touch, acupressure, shiatsu, and reflexology. Massage (particularly of the back) has long been considered an important nursing intervention used to promote relaxation, relieve muscle discomfort, and stimulate circulation. Many books and educational programs are available for nurses who want to expand their skills with therapeutic massage.

Therapeutic touch (TT), a noninvasive healing technique developed by a nurse, Dr. Delores Krieger (1979), involves touching with conscious intent to heal. In TT, the nurse works from a centered state using the natural sensitivity of the hands to assess the client's energy fields and treat imbalances. Healing touch (HT) (Hover-Kramer, Mentgen, & Scandrett-Hibdon, 1996) is a collection of energy-based healing techniques, which, like TT, are noninvasive. The HT practitioner also works from a centered state to assist in making energy available to clients through application of systemic and localized techniques. In addition to promoting relaxation, decreasing anxiety, and balancing energy, research sug-

gests that these therapies can enhance immune functioning (Olson, Sneed, LaVia, Virella, Bonadonna, & Michel, 1997) and promote wound healing (Wirth, 1992). Continuing education workshops, academic courses, and certification programs are available for nurses who wish to develop skills in these modalities. Acupressure, shiatsu, and reflexology are systems that use the application of pressure (with fingers, thumbs, or a blunt instrument) to specific points along energy pathways (meridians) of the body (acupressure and shiatsu) or in the feet or hands (reflexology). Continuing education workshops and certification programs are also available for nurses who wish to study these modalities.

> ## " A CONVERSATION WITH... "
>
> *In considering, re-considering Caring in the Community, perhaps a case can be made for Pure Caring, in that it is non-institutional, real-living situations, in the community where the most authentic, and yet demanding aspects of personal-professional caring become manifest. What the nurse offers first, by way of establishing relationship-centered care, is Self: by this I mean bring one's whole self into the present. It is from this professional and philosophical orientation that authentic caring can be witnessed and experienced at its finest.*
>
> **—Jean Watson, PhD, RN, FAAN, HNC**
> **Distinguished Professor of Nursing,**
> **Endowed Chair in Caring Science,**
> **University of Colorado Health Sciences Center,**
> **Denver, Colorado 80262 USA**
> **September 29, 2000**

CONCLUSION

This chapter has discussed the use of complementary therapies within a holistic nursing frame of reference. Nurses must be aware that many people use complementary therapies in addition to biomedical interventions but often do not disclose this to their biomedical practitioners. Complementary modalities encompass all health systems, modalities, and practices other than those intrinsic to the politically dominant health system of a particular society or culture and include all practices and ideas self-defined by their users as preventing or treating illness or promoting health and well-being. Many complementary modalities are based in cultural healing practices, which derive from different explanatory models than that of biomedicine.

Nurses need to be attentive to client values and desires for treatment options, taking seriously the client's need for heal-ing as well as curing and the contributions to health offered by other explanatory models. If nurses do not understand the other modality or question the efficacy or safety of the choice, they should explore these considerations with the client. Nurses need to be aware of the various therapies being considered or used by clients so that they are aware of the many factors affecting a client's health and healing. Community nurses need to develop the ability to incorporate discussion of complementary therapies into assessment in an open way and work toward integration of complementary therapies with conventional interventions. Holistic nursing care implies attentiveness to spiritual concerns as well as to physical and emotional concerns. Prayer, imagery, music therapy, and touch therapy are examples of complementary modalities that can be incorporated into health care with clients in the community.

CRITICAL THINKING ACTIVITIES

1. Explore the history and current practice of a healing system other than biomedicine and interview a practitioner of that modality. Compare and contrast that healing system with biomedicine relative to explanatory model, preparation of practitioners, treatment modalities, and interaction with clients. Discuss the extent to which each system focuses on healing and curing.

2. Shauna is an outpatient oncology nurse who has cared for 53-year-old Marita during her 4 years of living with breast cancer. Marita has endured surgery and radiation and is currently undergoing another course of chemotherapy for recently discovered metastasis. Marita tells Shauna that she thinks the medical therapies are only making her sicker and that she has been doing a lot of reading about other ways of dealing with cancer. Marita says she is seriously considering discontinuing chemotherapy treatments and seeking healing through prayer and herbal remedies. She also indicates that she knows God can heal, but that if she is to die, she would rather die with dignity than be stuck in a hospital attached to machines. It is clear from what Marita says that she has thoughtfully considered the various options with their risks and benefits. Shauna tells the physician about Marita's plans; the physician exclaims that Marita is "out of her mind" and suggests that family members be enlisted to persuade Marita to continue with conventional interventions. What do you think of Marita's plan? What personal values are evident in Marita's decision? How do you think you would respond if you were in Marita's situation?

3. How can Shauna respond to Marita in a way that demonstrates respect for persons and supports her autonomy?

4. What perspective is reflected in the physician's response? How might the suggestion to enlist family assistance be considered coercion?

5. How do you think a holistic nurse would approach Marita and her care?

6. Talk with someone who uses as complementary health modality on as regular basis and discuss why they use the modality, the benefits of the modality, whether they discuss the therapy with biomedical practitioners, the cost, and how they pay for the modality.

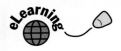

Explore Community Health Nursing on the web! To learn more about the topics in this chapter, use the passcode provided to access your exclusive web site: http://communitynursing.jbpub.com
If you do not have a passcode, you can obtain one at this site.

REFERENCES

Achterberg, J., Dossey, B. M., & Kolkmeier, L. (1994). *Rituals of healing*. New York: Bantam Books.

American Holistic Nurses' Association. (1994). P.O. Box 2130, Flagstaff, AZ 86003-2130. http://www.ahna.org.

Burkhardt, M. A. (1985). Nursing, health and wholeness. *Journal of Holistic Nursing, 3*(1), 35–36.

Burkhardt, M. A., & Nagai-Jacobson, M. G. (1997a). Psychospiritual care: A shared journey embracing life and wholeness. *Bioethics Forum, 13*(4), 34–41.

Burkhardt, M. A., & Nagai-Jacobson, M. G. (1997b). Spirituality and healing. In B. M. Dossey (Ed.), *Core curriculum for holistic nursing* (pp. 42–51). Gaithersburg, MD: Aspen.

Burkhardt, M. A., & Nagai-Jacobson, M. G. (2000). Spirituality and health. In B. M. Dossey, L. Keegan, & C. E. Guzzetta (Eds.), *Holistic nursing practice* (3rd ed., pp. 89–119). Gaithersburg, MD: Aspen.

Burkhardt, M. A., & Nathaniel, A. K. (1996). Patient self-determination and complementary care. *Bioethics Forum, 12*, 24–30.

Burkhardt, M. A., & Nathaniel, A. K. (1998). *Ethics & issues in contemporary nursing*. Albany, NY: Delmar.

Burkhardt, M. A., Nathaniel, A. K., Nemeth-Pyles, M., & Boyd, J. (1999). *Utilization of complementary health practices among people in southern West Virginia*. Presentation at the 18th Annual American Holistic Nurses' Association Conference: Holistic Nursing, Heritage to Vision. Phoenix, AZ, June 16–20, 1999.

Cassidy, C. M. (1996). Cultural context of complementary and alternative medicine systems. In M. S. Micozzi (Ed.), *Fundamentals of complementary and alternative medicine*. New York: Churchill Livingstone.

Dossey, B. M. (1997). Imagery. In B. M. Dossey (Ed.), *Core curriculum for holistic nursing* (pp. 188–195). Gaithersburg, MD: Aspen.

Dossey, B. M., & Guzzetta, C. E. (2000). Holistic nursing practice. In B. M. Dossey, L. Keegan, & C. E. Guzzetta (Eds.), *Holistic nursing: A handbook for practice* (3rd ed.). Gaithersburg, MD: Aspen.

Dossey, L. (1993). *Healing words*. New York: HarperCollins.

Dossey, L. (1996). *Prayer is good medicine*. San Francisco: HarperCollins.

Dossey, L. (1997). The return of prayer. *Alternative Therapies in Health and Medicine, 3*, 10–17, 113–120.

Dossey, L. (1998). *Be careful what you pray for . . . you just might get it*. San Francisco: HarperCollins.

Dossey, L. & Swyers, J. P. (1994). Introduction. In National Institutes of Health, *Alternative medicine: Expanding medical horizons* (NIH Publication No. 94-066). Washington, DC: U.S. Government Printing Office.

Duke, J. A. (1997). *The green pharmacy*. Emmaus, PA: Rodale Press.

Eisenberg, D. M., Kessler, R. C., Foster, C., Norlock, F. E., Calkins, D. R., & Delbanco, T. L. (1993). Unconventional medicine in the United States. *New England Journal of Medicine, 328*, 246–252.

Eisenberg, D. M., Rogers, B. D., Ettner, S., Appel, S., Wilkey, S., Van Rompay, M., & Kessler, R. C. (1998). Trends in alternative medicine use in the United States, 1990-1997. *Journal of the American Medical Association, 280*(18), 1569–1575.

Gordon, J. S. (1980). The paradigm of holistic medicine. In A. Hastings (Ed.), *Health for the whole person*. Boulder, CO: Westview Press.

Guzzetta, C. E. (1997). Music therapy. In B. M. Dossey (Ed.), *Core curriculum for holistic nursing* (pp. 196–204). Gaithersburg, MD: Aspen.

Guzzetta, C. E. (2000). Music therapy. In B. M. Dossey, L. Keegan, & C. E. Guzzetta (Eds.), *Holistic nursing: A handbook for practice* (pp. 585–610). Gaithersburg, MD: Aspen.

Hover-Kramer, D., Mentgen, J., & Scandrett-Hibdon, S. (1996). *Healing touch: a resource for health care professionals.*

Hufford, D. J. (1996a). *Ethical dimensions of alternative medicine*. Presentation at the First Annual Alternative Therapies Symposium: Creating Integrated Healthcare. San Diego, January 18–21, 1996.

Hufford, D. J. (1996b). Informed consent and alternative medicine. *Alternative Therapies in Health and Medicine, 2*, 76–78.

Krieger, D. (1979). *The therapeutic touch*. Englewood Cliffs, NJ: Prentice Hall.

Micozzi, M. S. (1996). *Fundamentals of alternative and complementary medicine*. New York: Churchill Livingstone.

Murray, M. (1995). *The healing power of herbs* (2nd ed.). Rocklin, CA: Prima Publishing.

Murray, M. & Pizzorno, J. (1998). *The encyclopedia of natural medicine* (2nd ed.). Rocklin, CA: Prima Publishing.

National Institutes of Health. (1994). *Alternative medicine: Expanding medical horizons* (NIH Publication No. 94-066). Washington, DC: U.S. Government Printing Office.

O'Connor, B. B. (1996). Medical ethics and patient belief systems. *Alternative Therapies in Health and Medicine, 2*, 92–93.

Olson, M., Sneed, N., LaVia, M., Virella, G., Bonadonna, R., & Michel, Y. (1997). Stress-induced immunosuppression and therapeutic touch. *Alternative Therapies in Health and Medicine, 3*(2), 68–74.

Quinn, J. F. (1989). On healing, wholeness, and the haelan effect. *Nursing and Health Care, 10*, 553–556.

Robbins, J. L. W. (1999). The science and art of aromatherapy. *Journal of Holistic Nursing, 17*(1), 5–17.

Schaub, B. G. (2000). Imagery. In B. M. Dossey, L. Keegan, & C. E. Guzzetta (Eds.), *Holistic nursing: A handbook for practice* (pp. 539–584). Gaithersburg, MD: Aspen.

Shames, K. H. (1997). Touch. In B. M. Dossey (Ed.), *Core curriculum for holistic nursing* (pp. 205–210). Gaithersburg, MD: Aspen.

Shames, K. H. (2000). Touch. In B. M. Dossey, L. Keegan, & C. E. Guzzetta (Eds.), *Holistic nursing: A handbook for practice* (pp. 613–638). Gaithersburg, MD: Aspen.

Simonton, O. C., Cohen, D. Kumar, M., McKinney, C., & Tims, F. (1997). *Music as a healing force*. Presented at Second Annual Alternative Therapies Symposium: Creating Integrated Healthcare, Orlando, April 16–19, 1997.

Stevensen, C. J. (1996). Aromatherapy. In M. S. Micozzi (Ed.), *Fundamentals of alternative and complementary medicine* (pp. 137–148). New York: Churchill Livingstone.

Wirth, D. (1992). The effect of non-contact therapeutic touch on the healing rate of full thickness dermal wounds. *Subtle Energies, 1*, 1–20.

Chapter 17
Global Health

Janet Gottschalk, Susan Scoville Baker, and Sharyn Janes

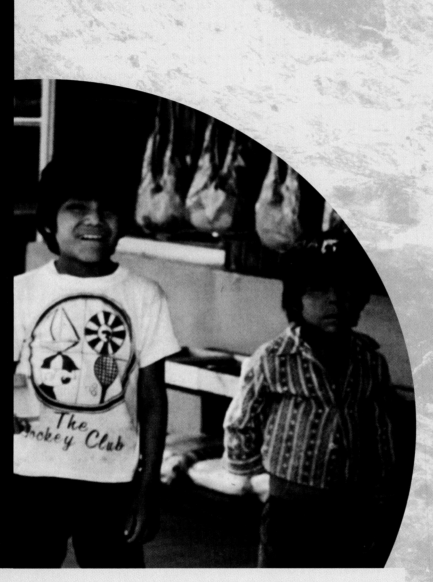

In a world connected by supersonic transports and cyberspace, nurses need to be alert to developments in the changing world. Nurses need to continually update and modify their nursing practices in accordance with changing global political, social, economic, and cultural realities.

Chapter Focus

Questions to Consider

After reading this chapter, answer the following questions:

1. How has globalization affected international health?
2. What roles do international agencies play in world health efforts?
3. How is world health influenced by international economics and trade?
4. What roles do nurses play in international health?
5. How do nongovernmental agencies contribute to global health efforts?
6. How does the International Council of Nurses collaborate with other organizations to improve health care and nursing worldwide?

Key Terms

Alma Ata
"Health for All"
International health
International Monetary
  Fund

Nongovernmental
  organizations
North American Free
  Trade Agreement
Poverty

Primary health care
Privatization
The Carter Center
United Nations (UN)
United Nations Children's
  Fund (UNICEF)

World Bank
World Health
  Organization (WHO)
World Trade Organization

Most professional nurses have a working knowledge of local and state realities that directly influence their nursing practice. Many nurses are also aware of the links between federal legislation, financing mechanisms, and the daily practice of nursing. An increasing number are also actively engaged in health policy at the national level. But this is not enough for nurses living and working in the 21st century. Nurses also need to be knowledgeable about global issues and their impact on health care and people's health statuses throughout the world.

A relatively small number of U.S. nurses have had the valuable experience of working in countries outside the United States, especially in the most resource-poor countries of Africa, Asia, and Latin America. They have been privileged to share, firsthand, people's struggles for water, food, health care, and freedom from violence of all kinds. More importantly, they have often shared in people's struggles for acknowledgment of their own personal dignity and for their right and the right of their countries to social and economic development. As nurses become key players in the global health community, their focus must shift from the specific issues related to international nursing to the broader issues of **international health** (Wright, Godue, Manfredi, & Korniewicz, 1998).

Unfortunately, as one West African leader expressed it, most poor peoples and countries seem to be trying to climb up an escalator that is going down. In other words, the gaps between rich and poor are getting larger, both between countries and within countries, and statistically most of the poor of this world are getting poorer. The sick are also getting sicker, and the numbers of maternal deaths per year (approximately 750,000 worldwide) and the numbers of children who suffer from severe malnutrition remain unacceptably high. See Table 17-1 for a description of disparities.

Globalization and International Health

The world today is radically different from the one in which most of today's nursing leaders were educated. In the 1970s and 1980s, the United States began the painful recovery from its involvement in the controversial Vietnam War. People looked at the world according to the rigid divisions and categorizations of the Cold War. It was common practice at that time to divide the world into the "First," or Western, capitalist World; the "Second," or Eastern, communist World; and the "Third," or neutral World. Generally speaking, the Third World was also considered to include the poorest nations of the world.

During those Cold War days, the battles for supremacy between the First World and Second World were fought on the soils of Africa, Asia, and Latin America. One way the superpowers (primarily the United States and the Soviet Union) competed for acceptance of their respective economic and political systems was through foreign aid and assistance programs to friendly countries among the underdeveloped or developing nations. Foreign aid was primarily intended to be used for economic development, which included education and health care. Immunization and family planning programs were financed and training programs were developed for nurses, midwives, and medical assistants in many of the countries served. Unfortunately, many of these programs failed because of corrupt government officials or political dissension within many of the developing countries.

In 1989, however, the competition for allies among developing nations ended with the economic collapse of the Soviet Union. The United States is the only real superpower left, and so we have a world in which the terms *First World, Second World,* and *Third World* have little meaning. Instead, we have a world in which nations are divided into two categories: the rich, industrialized nations of the North and the poorer, developing nations of the South. The terms *North* and *South* are somewhat confusing, however, because some of the richer nations, such as Australia, are actually geographically located in the southern hemisphere, while some of the poorer nations, such as India, are located in the northern hemisphere. Pockets of the "North" and the "South" are also found within cities and nations throughout our world.

TABLE 17-1   **DISPARITIES BETWEEN INDUSTRIALIZED AND DEVELOPING NATIONS OF THE WORLD**

AVERAGE STATISTICS FOR **1990s**	INDUSTRIALIZED WORLD	DEVELOPING WORLD
Percentage of world population	23	77
Percentage of global gross national product (GNP)	85	15
GNP per person	$12,510 ($19,840 in U.S.)	$710
Percentage of population growth rate	0.8	2.3
Number of people living in poverty	0.3 billion	1.2 billion
Life expectancy	74.5 years	62.8 years
Maternal mortality (per 100,000)	24	290
Child younger than 5 years old mortality (per 100,000)	18	116
Percent of population below the poverty level	2	32

Source: Adapted from Benetar, 1998.

Unfortunately, after spending millions of dollars on unsuccessful, poorly designed, and often corrupt health and education programs to assist the poor of the world, the industrialized nations of the North now seem to be suffering from "compassion fatigue," and most have generally lost interest in what happens to the developing nations of the South, preferring instead to concentrate on their own economic growth. With the exception of the Scandinavian countries, most nations, including the United States and Canada, have drastically reduced their budgets for foreign aid or overseas development programs. For example, the United States Agency for International Development's funding for international family planning programs followed an upward trend for 30 years until 1996, when the U.S. Congress reduced funds for international family planning by 35% (USAID, 1998). Arms, of course, are still being sold to poorer countries, but this appears to be for purely economic reasons or to maintain the North's technological capacity and military preparedness.

Role of International Agencies

The United Nations

The **United Nations (UN)** was established on October 24, 1945, when its permanent charter was ratified by 50 nations. In 1999, there were 188 member countries of the United Nations. The idea for the establishment of the UN grew from the discussions conducted at the 1943 Allied conferences held by the nations opposed to the fascist (Axis) nations of World War II (Germany, Italy, and Japan). The mission of the UN is to maintain international peace and security; to foster international cooperation in solving economic, social, cultural, and humanitarian problems and in promoting respect for human rights and fundamental freedoms; and to be a center for harmonizing the actions of nations in attaining these common ends (U.S. Department of State, 1999a).

At the time it was established and throughout the Cold War era, the UN was a relatively influential international organization and was respected by most of the nations of the world for its fairly successful health care, education, and peacekeeping efforts. Today, although the global need is greater than ever, the UN has lost much of the strength it once mobilized to confront the world's most intractable problems. Today it is an organization badly weakened by some of its founding members, including the United States, who had for several years refused to pay its assigned dues. Concerns voiced in the U.S. Congress related to some UN operations (primarily international family planning programs) in the mid-1990s resulted in nonpayment of dues. However, in recent years, the United States has been paying its UN dues in full annually, although back dues are still owed. In 1997, the U.S. Congress drafted legislation that would have enabled the United States to pay $926 million of the more than $1 billion in back dues owed to the UN if certain reforms were made within the UN and its agencies. However, the president was forced to veto the legislation because of the ongoing dispute over the U.S. support for international family planning programs. Debate still continues over the issue, although most American citizens support payment of the dues owed (U.S. Department of State, 1999b). In the meantime, the UN specialized agencies and commissions such as the World Health Organization, the United Nations Fund for Population Activities (UNFPA), the United Nations High Commission for Refugees (UNHCR), and the United Nations Children's Fund have difficulty mobilizing adequate resources and expert personnel. In fact, at times the UN does not have paper for its copiers, nor money to pay its translators or peacekeeping forces.

Over the years, the UN has created special bodies, such as the United Nations Children's Fund, to respond to economic and social challenges. There are also 18 independent intergovernmental organizations that are related to the UN by special agreements but are not under UN authority. They have their own memberships, charters, budgets, and staffs. These include such organizations as the World Health Organization, the World Bank, and the International Monetary Fund. See Box 17-1 for a list of addresses for health-related UN agencies.

BOX 17-1 SELECTED UN ADDRESSES

United Nations Public Inquiries Unit	United Nations, GA-57 New York, NY 10017 www.unsystem.org	Tel: (212)963-4475 Fax: (212)963-0071 E-mail: inquiries@un.org
World Health Organization Distribution and Sales	20 Avenue Appia 1211 Geneva 27 Switzerland	Tel: (22)791-22-76 Fax: (22)291-48-57 E-mail: publications@who.ch
UNICEF Division of Communication	3 United Nations Plaza New York, NY 10017 www.unicef.org	Tel: (212) 326-7000 Fax: (212) 887-7465 E-mail: pubdoc@unicef.org
United Nations High Commission for Refugees	P.O. Box 2500 1211 Geneva 2 Switzerland www.unhcr.ch	Refugees 1775 K St. NW, #300 Washington, DC 20006

The World Health Organization

Organized efforts at providing a global health network date back to the 1830s, when an international alliance was formed to combat the cholera epidemic that was sweeping Europe. Sporadic efforts continued throughout the next century until the **World Health Organization (WHO)** was founded in 1948 through a special agreement with the UN. The accomplishments of the WHO in the 20th century are outlined in Box 17-2. The primary objective of the WHO is for all people to attain the highest possible level of health. According to the WHO, health is a state of complete physical, mental, and social well-being and not merely the absence of disease or infirmity. In support of its objective, the four major functions of the WHO are as follows:

1. To give worldwide guidance in the field of health
2. To set global standards for health
3. To cooperate with governments in strengthening national health programs
4. To develop and transfer appropriate health technology, information, and standards (WHO, 1999)

BOX 17-2 OVERVIEW OF THE WORLD HEALTH ORGANIZATION ACTIVITIES IN THE 20TH CENTURY

1945   The United Nations Conference on International Organization in San Francisco unanimously approved a proposal by Brazil and China to establish a new, autonomous, international health organization.

1946   The International Health Conference in New York approved the WHO constitution.

1947   The World Health Organization (WHO) interim commission organized assistance to Egypt to combat the cholera epidemic.

1948   The WHO constitution was ratified on April 7 (now celebrated as World Health Day each year), when the 61 member nations signed it. Later, the First World Health Assembly was held in Geneva, Switzerland, with delegations from 53 member nations in attendance.

1951   The text of the International Sanitary Regulations was adopted by the Fourth World Health Assembly.

1969   The International Sanitary Regulations were renamed the International Health Regulations.

1973   The WHO executive board reported widespread dissatisfaction with health services. Radical changes were needed. The Twenty-Sixth World Health Assembly decided that WHO should collaborate with, rather than assist, its member nations in developing practical guidelines for their national health care systems.

1974   The WHO launched the Expanded Programme on Immunization to protect children from poliomyelitis, measles, diphtheria, whooping cough, tetanus, and tuberculosis.

1977   The Thirtieth World Health Assembly set a goal of "Health for All by the Year 2000."

1978   The joint WHO/UNICEF International Conference at Alma Ata adopted a declaration on primary health care as the key to obtaining the goal of "Health for All by the Year 2000."

1979   The United Nations General Assembly, along with the Thirty-second World Health Assembly, reaffirmed that health is a powerful tool for socioeconomic development and world peace. A global commission certified that smallpox had been eradicated worldwide.

1981   The global strategy for "Health for All by the Year 2000" was adopted. The United Nations General Assembly endorsed the global strategy and encouraged other international organizations to collaborate with the WHO.

1987   The United Nations General Assembly expressed concern about the expanding AIDS epidemic. The WHO launched the Global Programme on AIDS.

1988   The Forty-First World Health Assembly set a goal to eradicate poliomyelitis by the year 2000.

1993   The Children's Vaccine Initiative was launched by the WHO in collaboration with other international health organizations.

1996   The WHO Centre for Health Development opened in Kobe, Japan.

1998   Fiftieth anniversary of the signing of the WHO constitution.

Source: WHO, 1999.

Infectious disease has long been a major focus of the WHO. Efforts have been successful in the control, elimination, and eradication of diseases throughout the world. (These terms are defined in Box 17-3.) One of the major accomplishments of the WHO was the worldwide eradication of smallpox. Smallpox was endemic in 31 countries and claimed nearly 2 million lives a year. A systematic effort to vaccinate entire populations in endemic countries began in 1967. By 1972, the incidence of the disease had significantly decreased, with cases occurring in only eight countries. The last case of smallpox occurred in Somalia in 1977. Today, the WHO is making great progress toward eradicating two diseases in the world (dracunculiasis and poliomyelitis) and eliminating four more (leprosy, neonatal tetanus, Chagas' disease, and iodine deficiency disorders) (WHO, 1999).

In 1977, the World Health Assembly set a goal to be reached by the end of the 20th century that all people would obtain a level of health that would permit them to lead socially and economically productive lives. This led to the development of "Health for All by the Year 2000." It is important to realize that "**Health for All**" does not mean that there will be an end to all disease and disability. It means that health resources are evenly distributed and that basic health care is available to everyone. The focus is on health care in community settings such as homes, schools, and workplaces (WHO, 1999).

In 1978, delegates from 134 nations and representatives from WHO nongovernmental organizations met in **Alma Ata**, in the former Soviet Union (now Almatay, Kazakhstan) and committed themselves and their resources to the achievement of "Health for All by the Year 2000" through primary health care (PHC). PHC emphasizes the needs and involvement of the community and uses health strategies that are accessible, acceptable, affordable, and appropriate (Barnes, Eribes, Juarbe, Nelson, Proctor, Sawyer, Shaul, & Meleis, 1995; Gottschalk, 1996).

The concept of **primary health care** is based on health education in the community, an adequate food supply for good nutrition, an adequate supply of safe water, basic sanitation efforts, maternal and child care, family planning programs, immunization against the major infectious diseases, prevention and control of local endemic diseases, appropriate treatment of common diseases and injuries, and the provision of essential drugs (WHO, 1999).

• •

Our success—WHO's and yours—will depend on shaping public opinion and stimulating public action through elected representatives and civil society—at local, national, regional, and global levels. The fundamental message we send is that health is a fundamental human right, enshrined in the Universal Declaration of Human Rights. This means more than universal access to health care. It depends on the assurance of many other rights in the Declaration: access to education and information, the right to food in sufficient quantity and of good quality, the right to decent housing, and the right to live and work in an environment where known health risks are controlled.
Gro Harlem Brundtland, Director General,
World Health Organization United Nations,
Geneva, Switzerland, November 23, 1999

• •

United Nation's Children's Fund

The **United Nation's Children's Fund** (**UNICEF**) was founded in 1946 to assist millions of sick and hungry children in war-torn Europe. It soon became apparent that children all over the world needed help. Today UNICEF's primary objective is to provide support for the world's most disadvantaged children without discrimination. The children in the countries with the greatest need receive the highest priority. UNICEF is in the forefront of organizations working to help the more than 1 billion people in the world who live in extreme **poverty**. Through programs and services aimed at ending hunger, helping refugees, controlling disease, saving the environment, and securing human rights, UNICEF strives to improve the lives of all the world's children (UNICEF, 1999a).

A major focus of UNICEF is the worldwide problem of malnutrition. Malnutrition is implicated in half of all child deaths worldwide, yet this global crisis has stirred little public alarm. Malnutrition is a silent and invisible emergency. In addition to death, the results of malnutrition extend to the millions of survivors who are left physically and mentally disabled and chronically vulnerable to illness. Good nutrition not only is the key to the healthy development of individuals, families, and communities, but may contribute to overcoming some of the global burden of chronic and degenerative diseases, maternal mortality, and infectious diseases such as malaria and acquired immunodeficiency syndrome (AIDS). UNICEF has had much success in recent years with its nutrition programs. For example, 12 million children a year are having their diets supplemented with iodized salt to prevent irreversible mental impairment, and more than 60% of the world's children are receiving vitamin A supplements. Vitamin A deficiency impairs a child's resistance to disease and contributes to nearly 25% of all deaths among children younger than 5 (UNICEF, 1998, 1999b).

BOX 17-3 DEFINITIONS OF TERMS RELATED TO WHO INFECTIOUS DISEASE EFFORTS

Control: *the ongoing operations or programs aimed at reducing the incidence and/or prevalence of a specific disease*

Elimination: *the reduction of disease transmission to a predetermined, very low level*

Eradication: *no new disease cases occur anywhere in the world, and continued control efforts are unnecessary*

Source: WHO, 1999.

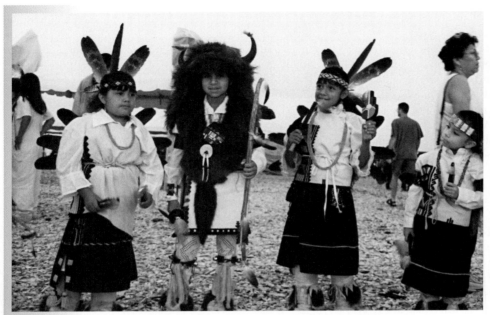

The health care needs of indigenous people in all countries must be addressed within the context of their culture.

During this final year of the 20th century, a child will be born, bringing the world's population to 6 billion. What lies ahead for this 6 billionth baby, no one can say. But for the majority of the world's poor are children. Early death from preventable disease, illiteracy, or traumatic conflict often awaits them. For the 6 billionth child and for all children, the odds can and should be better.

Carol Bellamy, Executive Director of UNICEF,
Progress of Nations, 1999

The Carter Center

The Carter Center, a nonprofit organization located in Atlanta, was founded by Jimmy and Rosalynn Carter in 1982. The Carter Center is a private, nonpartisan organization associated with Emory University and governed by an independent board of trustees, chaired by former U.S. President Jimmy Carter. Activities, directed by resident experts and scholars, are designed and implemented in cooperation with Jimmy and Rosalynn Carter, networks of world leaders, other nongovernmental organizations (NGOs), and partners in the United States and the rest of the world. The Carter Center has been instrumental in alleviating global health problems through its assistance in reducing Guinea worm disease (dracunculiasis) by 97% in Africa, India, Pakistan, and Yemen and its launching of a program to prevent river blindness (onchocerciasis) among people in Africa, Latin America, and Yemen (Carter Center, 1997).

The World Bank and International Monetary Fund

Since the fall of communism and the general acceptance of capitalism as the world's preferred economic system, two financial institutions associated with the UN—the **World Bank** (WB) and the **International Monetary Fund** (IMF)—have attempted to meet the needs of a changing world economy. Founded in 1944, the World Bank is a development institution whose goal is to reduce poverty by promoting sustainable economic growth in its client countries. The World Bank provides nearly $30 billion annually to assist developing countries. The money comes from tapping the world's capital markets and through contributions from wealthier member nations. The World Bank consists of five closely associated institutions (described in Table 17-2). Over the past few decades, the World Bank has been instrumental in reducing poverty and raising the standard of living in many developing countries. For example, the average life expectancy has increased by nearly 10 years, per capita incomes have doubled, the proportion of children attending school has risen from less than half to more than three-quarters, and the infant mortality rate has been reduced by 50%. Although these successes are noteworthy, more rapid progress is desperately needed. Of the 4.7 billion people who live in the 100 countries served by the World Bank, 3 billion live on less than $2 a day and more than 1 billion live on less than $1 a day (U.S. dollars), 40,000 are dying of preventable diseases each day, 130 million do not attend school, and more than 1 billion do not have safe drinking water (World Bank Group, 1999).

TABLE 17-2   **WORLD BANK INSTITUTIONS**

INSTITUTION	FUNCTION
The International Bank for Reconstruction and Development (IBRD)	The IBRD provides loans and development assistance to middle-income countries and poor countries with good credit. Voting power is linked to the member country's relative economic strength. Most of the funds come from the sale of bonds in the international capital markets.
The International Development Association (IDA)	The IDA is important in the poverty reduction mission of the World Bank. The focus is on interest-free loans and other services to the poorest countries. Contributions from wealthier member countries provide most of the financial resources.
The International Finance Corporation (IFC)	The IFC finances private sector investments and provides technical assistance and advice to governments and businesses in the developing world. In partnership with private investors, loan and equity finance for business ventures is also provided.
The Multilateral Investment Guarantee Agency (MIGA)	MIGA encourages foreign investment in developing countries by insuring against loss caused by noncommercial risks. Technical assistance is given to help countries distribute information about investment opportunities.
The International Centre for Settlement of Investment Disputes (ICSID)	ICSID assists with conciliation or arbitration of investment disputes between foreign investors and their host countries.

Source: World Bank Group, 1999

The International Monetary Fund, established in 1946, is a cooperative institution with 182 voluntary member nations whose purpose is to do the following:

- *Promote international monetary cooperation*
- *Facilitate the expansion and balanced growth of international trade*
- *Promote exchange stability*
- *Foster economic growth and high levels of employment*
- *Provide temporary financial assistance under adequate safeguards to its member nations having payment balance difficulties (IMF, 1999)*

Operating globally, these powerful financial institutions routinely impose structural adjustment programs (SAPs) on nations seeking loans for domestic development purposes or to strengthen their weak, unstable currencies and economic systems. As a consequence, poor nations seeking funds from the WB or IMF are asked to "adjust" their behaviors according to accepted market principles. For example, the IMF lends money to member nations who are having trouble meeting financial obligations to other member nations, but only if economic reforms are undertaken to eliminate their repayment difficulties for their own good and the good of the other member nations (IMF, 1998). These required economic reforms often include in-

creasing exports despite falling world commodity prices, which then leads to further economic difficulty for the struggling nation. Nations that already have limited social services for their needy populations are required to decrease their government spending even further (Kolko, 1999).

It is often difficult to identify direct causal links between the IMF-imposed SAPs and a country's increased poverty levels, decreased access to health services, and increased morbidity and mortality rates. However, researchers and concerned health professionals are gathering these data to support efforts to change the requirements for IMF or WB loans to poor countries.

In 1996, the WB and the IMF spearheaded the highly indebted poor country initiative (HIPC). The goal of HIPC is to assist severely impoverished countries with unsustainable debt burdens to become solvent. HIPC was established to assist 41 poor countries, 33 of them in Africa. The targeted countries have infant mortality rates one-third higher and maternal mortality rates nearly three times greater than other developing countries. More than a third of the children in these countries have not been immunized, and half the population is illiterate. Progress has been slow and painful. By the end of 1999, only two countries—Uganda and Bolivia—had received economic relief, and commitments for HIPC support had been made to only five additional countries. Countries targeted for aid must pass rigid, and often inappropriate, criteria to be eligible for HIPC. For ex-

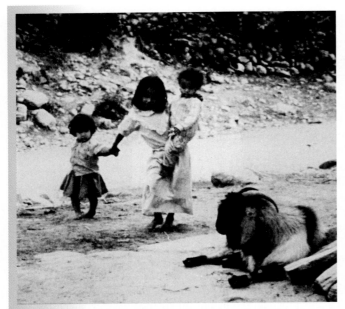

Female children as young as 8 must take primary responsibility for younger children in many underdeveloped countries.

ample, 3 to 6 years of draining structural adjustment programs that increase poverty are required to qualify for assistance (UNICEF, 1999b).

In 1999, Canada, Germany, the United Kingdom, and the United States called for reforms to speed up the HIPC process and debt cancellation for the poorest countries. International groups also have started campaigns to cancel the debts of the poorest countries. In a recent study, 27 developing countries were surveyed with only 9 reporting spending more on basic social services than on debt repayment. Six African countries surveyed spend more than twice as much on debt services than on services such as nutrition, safe water sanitation, health care, and education (UNICEF, 1999b). (Contact information for the IMF and other world financial institutions can be found in Box 17-4.)

The debt bondage that ensnares hundreds of millions of the world's poorest people, particularly in Africa, provides clear evidence. As though bound to feudal lords, their lives and labour have been mortgaged to rich country banks and governments, often by leaders they did not choose, to finance projects that did not benefit them. Debt, like an oppressive political system, strips them of their rights. And its tyranny is particularly painful now, with sub-Saharan Africa in the grip of an unprecedented calamity as AIDS spreads remorselessly.
Sir Shridath Ramphal, Co-Chairman of the Commission on Global Governance, *The Progress of Nations 1999*, UNICEF

The Effects of International Corporations

Other problems have resulted from the formation of regional trading blocks and common markets, such as the North American Free Trade Association and other regional free trade areas. Concurrent with the development of such trading blocks has been the development of the **World Trade Organization** (WTO) in 1995, an organization that many political analysts say is ultimately more powerful than the UN. Much of the WTO's power comes from transnational corporations or multinational corporations, which are powerful companies and industries that can force unwilling nations to open their markets and shores to foreign investors and industries. Policies that impose any conditions on foreign investment are prohibited for all 134 member nations, regardless of how foreign investments conduct business in their countries. These companies may exploit the natural resources of these relatively defenseless countries, logging their forests to the point of extinction and destroying their local farmers and small industries. When a member nation challenges the practices or laws of another member nation, the case is brought before a WTO tribunal. Once a WTO final ruling is made, the losing country can change their law to conform to WTO requirements, pay permanent compensation to the winning country, or face trade sanctions. Any law that may pose a barrier to free trade is

BOX 17-4 RELEVANT FINANCIAL INSTITUTIONS AND ORGANIZATIONS

World Bank	*1818 H Street NW* *Washington, DC 20433*	*Tel: (202) 477-1234* *Fax: (202) 477-6391*
International Monetary Fund	*700 19th St. NW* *Washington, DC 2043*	
Women's Eyes on the World Bank—U.S.	*c/o Oxfam America DC Office* *1511 K St. NW* *Washington, DC 20005*	*Tel: (202) 783-7305* *Fax: (202) 783-8739*
50 Years Is Enough: U.S. Network *for Global Economic Justice*	*1025 Vermont Ave. NW, Suite 300* *Washington, DC 20005*	*Tel: (202) 463-2265* *Fax: (202) 879-3186*

ruled against, regardless of its effect on labor rights or environmental or public health protection (Global Trade Watch, 1999a).

The **North American Free Trade Agreement** (NAFTA) was signed into U.S. law in 1994. Economists and major business interests point to some of NAFTA's positive consequences, including an increased market share and decreased production costs for certain industries. However, some of its negative consequences are clearly visible in communities that have suffered from lowered wages, environmental pollution, and human rights violations on all sides of the Canadian, U.S., and Mexican borders. Away from the borders, other less desirable consequences of NAFTA can be seen in towns with vacant factories and increased unemployment. For example, in the United States, Guess, Inc., cut the percentage of its clothes made in Los Angeles from 97% before NAFTA to 35% in 1997, when work was sent to sewing factories in Mexico, Peru, and Chile. More than 1,000 Los Angeles workers lost their jobs (Global Trade Watch, 1999b).

Canada and Mexico have also suffered at the hands of NAFTA. The Canadian unemployment rate was high before NAFTA as a result of massive layoffs and plant closings in the late 1980s and early 1990s. The addition of NAFTA has added significantly to the problem by contributing to increased unemployment and the undermining of Canada's strong social programs, particularly unemployment insurance and national health care (UNITE, 1999).

In Mexico, NAFTA has failed to protect the rights of the workers. Although NAFTA contains a provision that requires

FYI

Of the 4.4 billion people in developing countries, nearly three-fifths lack access to safe sewers, a third have no access to clean water, a quarter do not have adequate housing, and a fifth have no access to modern health services of any kind.

More than 110 million active land mines are scattered in 68 countries, with an equal number stockpiled around the world. Every month more than 2,000 people are killed or maimed by mine explosions.

The three richest people in the world have assets that exceed the combined gross domestic product of the 48 least developed countries.

It is estimated that the additional cost of achieving and maintaining universal access to basic education for all, basic health care for all, reproductive health care for all women, adequate food for all, and clean water and safe sewers for all is roughly $40 billion a year—or less than 4% of the combined wealth of the 225 richest people in the world.

Source: UNDP, 1998a.

RESEARCH BRIEF

Little, R. E., Monaghan, S. S., Gladen, B. C., Shkyryak-Nyzhnyk, Z., & Wilcox, A. J. (1999). Outcomes of 17,137 pregnancies in 2 urban areas of Ukraine. American Journal of Public Health, 89(12), 1832–1836.

To explore the state of reproductive health in Central and Eastern Europe since the dissolution of the Soviet Union, a study was conducted in two urban areas of the Ukraine. During a 19-month period between 1992 and 1994, 17,137 pregnancy outcomes were recorded. Sixty percent of the pregnancies were voluntarily terminated, generally before the 13th week. In pregnancies delivered after 20 weeks' gestation, fetal mortality was 29 per 1,000, nearly five times the rate among Caucasians in the United States. Perinatal mortality was estimated to be 35 per 1,000, about three times the U.S. rate. The data documented elevated reproductive risks in a former Soviet state. This study is believed to be the first to count and report pregnancy outcomes in the former Eastern block using World Health Organization definitions and research procedures.

Mexico to protect the rights of businesses, there is no such provision for the protection of Mexico's labor laws. Current trade agreements protect investors, multinational corporations, patent and copyright holders, and speculators. The only group not protected are the workers. So when Mexico fails to enforce its labor laws, resulting in Mexican workers' wages being kept low and their rights denied, there is nothing that can be done (UNITE, 1999).

* *

Individual nurses, national nurses' associations, and ICN have a responsibility to monitor the development and impact of international trade agreements that affect nursing, health and social policy, including access to health services, employment opportunities of health workers, and profession regulation.

Judith Oulten, Chief Executive Officer,
International Council of Nurses
Geneva, Switzerland, November 18, 1999

* *

Hope for the Future
UN Conferences

Uncertain as the future may appear for many peoples and nations in our world today, there is also considerable reason for optimism. During the 1990s, the UN sponsored a series of mega-conferences dealing with the major social and environmental

> **BOX 17-5 MAJOR UNITED NATIONS CONFERENCES IN THE 1990S**
>
> - Children's Summit, New York, New York, USA
> - UN Conference on Environment and Development (Earth Summit), Rio de Janeiro, Brazil
> - World Conference on Human Rights, Vienna, Austria
> - UN Conference on Population and Development, Cairo, Egypt
> - World Summit on Social Development, Copenhagen, Denmark
> - Fourth World Conference on Women, Beijing, China
> - UN Conference on Human Settlements, Istanbul, Turkey

" A CONVERSATION WITH... "

This is the time to declare as we approach the great millennium that women must be made free. We cannot be free as long as our human rights are violated, as long as we don't have economic equality and as long as we are not participating in gender-balanced political bodies.

In all of our countries women have been in the forefront of the struggle for freedom and liberation, not only for themselves but for others, as well as themselves, to create democracies instead of hypocrisies which seek to deny them equality.

... A war still continues against the women of this world. And we must use the strength of this women's commission and the strength of the UN to end that war, to end the war against the civil rights of women and the human rights of women, and our children and people everywhere.

—**Bella Abzug,**
United Nations, March 31, 1998

issues of our times and the foreseeable future. The titles of these conferences read like a litany of our world's challenges and included issues related to children, the environment, population and development, human rights, social development, women, and urbanization (Box 17-5).

At these conferences, a new phenomenon became increasingly evident: the rise, power, and sophistication of peoples' organizations, called **nongovernmental organizations** (NGOs) or civil society organizations (CSOs). Because so many of the world's health problems are a result of the status of women and children, women from the barrios, favelas, farms, and neighborhoods of the world are leading many of the most effective and astute of these organizations. Many of these women continue to monitor their governments' efforts to improve living conditions in their countries. For example, in Turkey, nongovernmental organizations are proactively supporting girls' education programs. The Turkish NGOs recognize that education will provide young women with the skills necessary to have a voice in the political, economic, and social elements of their society (Global Issues, 1998). In Sri Lanka, work is being done to significantly reduce maternal mortality by increasing educational opportunities for women and providing reproductive and health services programs (Senanayake, 1998). In 1996, the Uganda Women's Network established a women's governance task force to promote women's access to power and decision making (Mobilizing Beyond Beijing, 1999). One mechanism, the annual meeting of the UN's Commission on the Status of Women (CSW), has become a focal point for concerned and committed women. During the CSW's 1998 meeting, the late Bella Abzug, co-founder of the New York-based Women's Environment and Development Organization, pleaded for social justice for women throughout the world.

American Women Activists

Operating against the same backdrop of tremendous change that is occurring worldwide, women in the United States developed a "Women's National Action Agenda." Like other women throughout the world, American women are concerned about the growing gap between rich and poor, the epidemics of violence and racial and ethnic tensions in their communities, the breakdown of social structures from the family to government, the threats to their and their children's environments, and the threats to their future that come from a rapidly globalizing economy.

American women are mobilizing for action. Whether they meet in small groups or use modern electronic communications, women all over the United States are organizing and networking with other women throughout the world to ensure that governments and international organizations faithfully carry out the commitments they made at the many UN conferences. In the United States, several steps have been taken to honor the commitments made at the UN Fourth World Conference on Women held in Beijing, China, in 1995. Some examples are listed in Box 17-6.

These women's groups reflect on the changes and dangers in the world around them and demand access and influence in the decisions being made at policy levels. Believing strongly in their abilities and insights, such women want to be involved at the times decisions are made and not after the fact. They sense great opportunities and possibilities for changes. Even more, they are filled with hope for the future.

BOX 17-6 U.S. COMMITMENTS TO THE UN FOURTH WORLD CONFERENCE ON WOMEN

- The President's Interagency Council on Women was created for implementation of the Beijing Platform of Action.
- The Women's Bureau at the Department of Labor initiated a year-long campaign to make changes in workplace policies and practices to improve conditions for women and their families.
- The Office of Violence against Women at the Department of Justice led a comprehensive campaign to fight violence against women through new legislation and assistance to states and communities.

Source: Mezvinsky, 1996.

Nurses' Global Vision

Economic and foreign trade issues, UN conference agendas, and women's activist groups may not at first appear of immediate concern to most nurses. However, nurses living and working in the 21st century need to expand their vision of nursing practice from one that concentrates principally on individual client care in local or regional settings to one that encompasses the entire world in all its complexities. Nurses need to sharpen their awareness of changing global, social, political, and economic realities. More importantly, nurses need to study the consequences of these global realities on their local individual and community practices.

International Council of Nurses

The International Council of Nurses (ICN), with headquarters in Geneva, Switzerland, is the world's first and widest reaching international organization for health professionals. Founded in 1899, ICN is a federation of the national nurses' associations in more than 120 countries. Its goals are to do the following:

- *Bring nursing together worldwide*
- *Advance nurses and nursing worldwide*
- *Influence health policy (Brush, Lynaugh, Boschma, Rafferty, Stuart, & Tomes, 1999; ICN, 1999)*

The core values of ICN are visionary leadership, inclusiveness, flexibility, partnership, and achievement. ICN standards and guidelines for education, practice, and research are accepted globally as the basis of nursing policy. Some of the areas that ICN is particularly active in are listed in Box 17-7. ICN continually strives to ensure quality nursing care for all the world's people through the presence of a well-respected nursing profession and a competent nursing workforce (Brush et al., 1999; ICN, 1999).

BOX 17-7 EXAMPLES OF INTERNATIONAL COUNCIL OF NURSING ACTIVITIES

International classification of nursing practice (ICNP)

Advanced nursing practice and entrepreneurship

HIV/AIDS

Women's health

Primary health care

Nursing regulation

Continuing education

Ethics and human rights

Credentialing

Socioeconomic welfare for nurses

Occupational health and safety

Pay for services

Human resources planning

Career development

Source: ICN, 1999.

Nursing's New Blueprint

Nurses need only look to the WHO's "Health for All" strategy to find a blueprint for future activities. The Global Advisory Group on Nursing and Midwifery was established in 1992 in response to resolution WHA45.5, "Strengthening nursing and midwifery in support of strategies for health for all," adopted by the World Health Assembly in May 1992. The major role of the Global Advisory Group on Nursing and Midwifery is to advise the director general of the WHO on all nursing and midwifery services, particularly regarding assessing nursing and midwifery service needs, assisting countries to develop national action plans for nursing and midwifery, and monitoring progress in strengthening nursing and midwifery in relation to health for all. One of the important collaborating partners of nursing and midwifery at the WHO is the International Council of Nurses (WHO, 1998).

Still, in many countries, especially where women hold culturally subservient roles, much work needs to be done to elevate the professional status of nursing. In these countries, nursing is viewed as a low-status and menial occupation, whereas medicine is considered a high-status and prestigious career, often resulting in an overabundance of physicians. These physicians often continue focusing on curative interventions rather than fostering preventive care, which is essential for primary health care to be successful (Orchard & Karmaliani, 1999). However, the World Health Assembly has recognized that, given the opportunity, nurses can address many primary health care needs in their communities. Nurses, for example, can mobilize communities to take control of their health by serving as an advocate for the community's health needs and ensuring that community leaders have a voice. They can help clients learn to understand and manage chronic diseases such as diabetes, asthma, and hypertension. They can provide technologically sophisticated home care, enabling clients to remain at home with loved ones. They can provide compassionate treatment and support to the aged, the homeless, the marginalized, refugees, immigrants, and others who would not otherwise have access to care (WHO, 1998).

Health Care and Nursing Around the World

Czech Republic
Sharon L. Oswald and Elizabeth A. Simnons

The Czech Republic is a small Eastern European country bordered by Germany, Poland, Austria, and Slovakia. Until 1989, the Czech Republic was part of the Soviet state of Czechoslovakia. The current population of the Czech Republic is greater than 10 million, with an average life expectancy of 74 years of age and an infant mortality rate of 6.67 per 1,000 live births.

With the dismantling of the Soviet Union in 1989, the Czech Republic embarked on a rapid path of change from a socialist to a capitalist society. The Czech Republic went from the private sector representing less than 1% of the gross domestic product in 1989 to accounting for more than 56% in 1994 (Lastovicka, Marcincin, & Mejstrik, 1995). The **privatization** of industry contributed greatly to a sense of social cohesion throughout the country.

However, even with the general success of privatization, reform of the health care system has been met with criticism and resistance. Few have questioned the need for reforms; however, many have questioned the suitability of the methods used to change the system. Under the previous communist regime, the Czech health care system was characterized by universal coverage, national control, absence of competition, and inefficiencies. From World War II until 1992, health care was free to all citizens. The system, based on the national health service model, was hierarchical in nature and controlled by the government. The Czech Republic was split into regional health authorities, which in turn were further divided into district authorities. Although all health policies were established by the central government, committees headed by medical doctors controlled the regional and district authorities (Rubas, 1995; Zarkovic, Mielck, John, & Beckmann, 1994). The amount of money physicians and nurses received under this system depended on the type of health care institution, the hospital's capabilities, and the number of employees (Vyborna, 1994).

Just before privatization, the Czech health care system developed extensively and the number of nurses and physicians grew to approximately 4.7% of the Czech labor force. At the same time, hospital efficiency and equipment quality and reliability substantially deteriorated (Deppe & Oreskovic, 1996). The oversupply of health professionals, coupled with the lack of any concrete incentive to work, created a workforce overflowing with unmotivated, unproductive workers. In a country where medical personnel were paid barely livable wages, efficiency and customer service were not strong points. Furthermore, until 1993, hospitals were funded according to occupancy. Therefore, the incentive existed for administrators and doctors to keep the beds occupied (Earl-Slater, 1996), adding to the inefficiency of the system.

The transformation of the health system began in 1990, when the Czech parliament adopted a new health care system that was to guarantee access to health for all, privatization of health care providers, and community participation. In 1992, fundamental reform was initiated, beginning with a tax on wages to fund the new health care system and the introduction of compulsory health insurance. Health insurance was made mandatory for all citizens; however, the state theoretically assumed responsibility for those who were unable to pay. By design, the system was supposed to support the belief that health was not dependent on wealth and the wealthy were not responsible for the poor.

The Czech government established an insurance-based system that is administered by the newly formed General Health Care Insurance Office (GHIO), an independent insurance body. The GHIO was funded by a 13.5% tax on gross income, of which employers were required to pay two-thirds while their employees paid one-third. Working closely with the government, the GHIO was charged with redistributing the money collected from the mandatory tax. The GHIO holds approximately 84% of the insured market and is required by law to accept anyone who applies for insurance (Earl-Slater, 1996; Vyborna, 1994). Employer-backed private insurance companies were permitted for employee groups of 20,000 or more (Vyborna, 1994). Hospitals (state, municipal, and private) may contract with whichever insurance companies they choose.

An initial step toward health care reform was the decentralization of state-owned institutions (Vyborna, 1994). Community health centers (physician practices) were also privatized; however, restrictions were placed on the range of services that could be provided. In many cases, ownership of community health centers (physician practices) was transferred by the state to local town halls and leased back to individual physicians. In these cases, the state was responsible for the upkeep of the facilities. The other alternative was the sale of a health center to a private owner, a religious entity, or a nonprofit organization. In these situations, the owners were responsible for upkeep and equipment.

Since privatization, employment levels in companies throughout the Czech Republic have remained constant, including the health care industry. As a result, the overemployment of health care professionals in the 1980s continues to put a strain on hospital budgets. In addition, pricing for health services places some unpredicted pressures on hospital operating budgets. A point system has been developed to control escalation of health care costs. This system does not impose cost controls on the hospitals, but instead places budget controls on all health care facilities. If hospitals or other facilities are unable to stay within their budgets, government officials reduce funding as a form of punishment, rather than attempt to renegotiate the budget or examine problem areas. With hospital employment levels hovering well above American standards and reimbursement for services established at the whim of the government, hospitals have found it difficult to stay in business. This problem is compounded by the prorated system of reimbursement. Reimbursement decreases with each corresponding day a client remains in the hospital.

In addition, although nurses and physicians were the most vocal groups in support of health care reform, they were the first to stage a public protest against the direction that the reform efforts were taking. Nurses and physicians have played a positive role in changing the public's attitude toward health care. Three physician/nurse strikes resulted initially from requests for higher salaries. As a result, nurses' salaries have been increased by an average of 30%. The Ministry of Health created the post of director of nursing in 1991, primarily to facilitate changes in nursing education and to define the role of nurses in the changing health care system (Misconiova, 1992).

Although in theory the privatization effort seemed logical and consistent with the changing economic conditions, in practice it has proven problematic. Both economic and social problems have surfaced. As government officials and management concentrated on the operational problems, they limited their focus on economic issues, disregarding the social concerns. However, privatizing a social system is considerably more complex than privatizing business. Health care is a physiological need—any threat to that need will automatically lead to some form of resistance. In the Czech Republic, health care is considered an inalienable right. By 1996, there was a public cry for the end of privatization. What has resulted is a stagnated transformation. As of the summer of 1998, privatization remained at a standstill—but progress toward health care access and quality remains a primary goal of the new government.

Cuba

Juana Daisy Berdayes Martínez, Anayda Fernández Naranjo, and Alavara Leonard Castillo

Cuba, a Caribbean island nation with a population of 11 million, is located between the Caribbean Sea and the Atlantic Ocean approximately 90 miles off the coast of the United States. After the Cuban revolution in 1959, Cuba experienced many economic and social transformations, which led to the development of its current health care policy. The belief in the right to health care for all citizens and the duty of the state to guarantee it brought about the provision of free health services for all Cuban citizens. A process of reorganization and expansion of the national health system was initiated based on the primary care model. Several

measures were taken to guarantee accessibility of health services for all. For example, new hospitals in rural zones and in mountains were constructed, greatly increasing the number of hospital beds nationwide. Health professionals no longer worked in private practices, but instead became part of the government's primary care system (Jardnes, Ouviña, & Aneiro Riba, 1991).

From its beginnings, the Cuban public health system has included the participation of the community in its historic evolution. In 1964, the first polyclinic was created to deliver comprehensive health care to communities. Community participation in health care was reinforced in 1975 with the creation of health advisory committees in each community. The health advisory committees are made up of people in the community who participate in analyzing the health of the community and facilitating collaboration between the health care system and community residents. In 1984, the new Cuban primary care model was introduced, with family physicians and nurses as essential components. Family practice physician offices, staffed by a physician and one or two nurses, began to spring up in every neighborhood. The principles of primary care proclaimed in Alma Ata in 1978 were applied in creative ways and adjusted to the economic and social conditions of Cuba. In this way, the truly humanistic dimensions of medicine and health care were applied to the care of people in their own communities, where they live, work, study, or play. As a result, Cuba met the WHO's "Health for All" 2000 objectives in 1985. Although Cuba is considered a developing country, its health indices are comparable to those of developed countries such as the United States. The life expectancy for Cubans is 75 years of age, and the leading causes of death are heart disease, malignant tumors, accidents, and cerebrovascular diseases.

Since 1989, with the economic collapse of the Soviet Union, with whom Cuba conducted 85% of its commercial trade, the living conditions of the population have deteriorated. In addition, the 40-year-old economic embargo of Cuba by the United States has contributed significantly to the economic depression. The health services that have been affected most are organ transplant and other technology programs, surgical activity, the availability of medications, and the acquisition and maintenance of medical equipment. Despite these resource limitations, the goals of the Ministry of Public Health are focused on maintaining free and accessible health care for all citizens and continuing the progress attained in the years since the revolution. Some of the future goals include expanding home care with medical and nursing surveillance for clients with acute conditions, increasing outpatient surgery services, and increasing emphasis on secondary and tertiary prevention.

The infant mortality rate, considered one of the best indicators of the health status of a population, has steadily decreased. Despite adverse economic conditions, the infant mortality rate was 7.8 per 1,000 in 1999, placing Cuba among the top 25 countries in the world with the lowest infant mortality rates. More than 99% of Cuba's children are born in hospitals or other health institutions. Vaccine-preventable diseases such as poliomyelitis, diphtheria, pertussis, measles, and tetanus have been controlled or virtually eliminated. In 1998, 98.5% of all children younger than 2 years of age were immunized.

At present, Cuba has 64,000 physicians (1 for every 170 inhabitants) and 82,527 nurses (17,568 of whom have baccalaureate degrees). More than 30,000 physicians and 32,000 nurses work in family practice settings in the community, with an emphasis on health promotion and illness prevention.

Nurses working in communities are in privileged situations to identify and satisfy the needs or problems of families. By interacting with individuals and families in the community daily, the nurse is able to develop a holistic view of the health status of the community and its members. The work of the community health nurse corresponds to the needs of the population of the community where the family physician's office is located. The nurse works with the physician in a synchronized relationship. Together they provide health care for between 120 and 140 families, through office appointments and community visits to homes, day-care centers, schools, cafeterias, and so on (Eisen, 1996) During office visits, the nurse performs treatment procedures, immunizations, and physical examinations. Other activities include case management, health teaching, and research (Jardnes, Ouviña, & Aneiro Riba, 1991).

The physician-nurse team devotes half of each day to community visits, primarily home visits. The physical contact with the family environment allows the team to assess the environmental conditions in which the family lives, as well as the family's health practices, lifestyle, customs, and family relationships (Eisen, 1996).

Despite the difficulties encountered during recent years, Cuba offers a health system that is highly developed and effective. Because of the focus on primary care in the community, Cuba's main health indicators, such as an average life expectancy of 75 years of age, are comparable to those of industrialized countries, placing Cuba far ahead of the rest of Latin America and other developing countries around the world.

Iran
Marjaneh Fooladi

Iran, a country with a population of 60 million, is located in East Asia, bordered by the Gulf of Oman, the Persian Gulf, the Caspian Sea, Azerbaijan, Armenia, Turkmenistan, Pakistan, Afghanistan, Turkey, and Iraq. The average life expectancy in Iran is 70 years of age, and the infant mortality rate is 30 per 1,000 live births. Iran is a religious state known as the Islamic Republic of Iran. Shiite Islam is the official religion.

Since the Iranian Revolution of 1979, the health status of Iran has changed a great deal. Iran lost many of its devoted medical doctors, nurses, and medical technicians during the Eight Years War with Iraq because hospitals were one of the major war targets of Iraq.

The medical schools continue training doctors despite their losses in the war and those who fled to the United States. At the end of 1993, 73% of Iranians had access to health care, compared with 50% at the end of 1980 (the end of the revolution), and childhood immunizations for children younger than 12 years old reached 92% by the end of 1995.

The greatest success in the health care system during the postrevolution era has taken place in the rural and urban poor sections of the country. These sections were the most underserved areas during the prerevolution period. Today, these two sections have been so prosperous and well served in Iran that the WB brought a group of African officials to see it.

Another striking factor since the revolution is that women are encouraged to seek higher education, especially in medical schools. Today, 90% of women receive higher education, compared with 38% before the revolution (Friedman, 1996). Another noteworthy factor in the health care system is gender segregation. Gender segregation requires hospitals to segregate care given to men and women. In the present health care system, female nurses care for female clients and male nurses care for male clients. By the same token, female physicians care for female clients and male physicians care for male clients in most levels of health care, including primary, secondary, and tertiary (Iran gender segregation, 1998).

In villages, life, death, health, and sickness are often attributed to God's will, and they are accepted in a spirit of fatalism. Accordingly, poor health is accepted, and medical aid is sought only when the illness interferes with one's daily work routine. A large number of Iranians believe in natural herbs, folk medicine, and the Holy Koran as curative means for illnesses. For instance, many Iranians use the *Book of Healing,* written by Avicenna (Abu Ali Cina, 980–1037 AD). This book contains descriptions of herbal medicine, dosages, and exercises, as well as general health rules. Because many medical problems are regarded as part of the supernatural, they are handled by religious leaders, whose services have been solicited in areas such as gaining someone's affection and love or ensuring the birth of a male child for couples who desire a son (Carter, 1978).

For serious illnesses, the family may consult a village herbalist or a medical doctor. Historically, in villages where there was not a medical doctor or health clinic, barbers were called to perform circumcisions and tooth extractions. Occult powers were given to midwives, who were viewed as specialists in the diseases of women and children (Carter, 1978).

In Iranian society, mothers carry a heavy load of responsibility on their shoulders as health care providers. The members of the family depend on mothers to handle their health problems and administer their everyday remedies. In return, mothers train their daughters in traditional medical lore, using magical formulas and herbs and preparing foods based on particular rules for certain illnesses.

Some of the most common terms for illness and their meaning as expressed by an Iranian client include the following:

- Chashm e bad *(evil eye)—believed to be a malicious spell cast on individuals through the eyes of another person or beast. Peo-*

ple who believe their illness has resulted from evil eyes seek cure through praying and reading from the Holy Koran.

- Ghalbam gerefteh *(distress of the heart)*—indicates a feeling that the heart is being squeezed; it denotes severity from mild excitation of the heart or palpitation to fainting and heart attack. It also can be an expression that the individual is feeling blue or sad *(Good, 1980)*.

- Saram seda meekoneh *(pounding in one's head)*—expresses a general feeling that something is wrong; it may mean a feeling of anxiety *(Good & Good, 1982)*.

- Balancing "hot" and "cold" foods—normally hot and cold categories are based on the Galenic-Islamic medical tradition *(Good, 1980)*. These are not related to food temperature. Iranians put a great deal of emphasis on their diet. They include lots of fruits and vegetables in their diets, and they avoid excess fat. Culturally, they avoid processed foods, preferring to cook only with fresh ingredients. They refuse to eat incompatible foods at the same time. For example, fish and yogurt are incompatible. Honey and walnuts are considered hot, whereas cucumbers, watermelon, and yogurt are deemed to be cold.

The following are a few home remedies commonly used by Iranians to prevent and treat symptoms of minor ailments:

- *Teas or herbs such as* gole gohv zaboon *are used for treatment of nervousness*

- *Nabbot (recrystallized sugar) is used to treat stomach upset and offset the cold foods*

- *Mint tea and cilantro seeds are used to induce relaxation and sleep*

- *Sucking quince seeds is used to relieve a sore throat*

- *Getting enough rest and exercise*

- *Keeping warm or dressing adequately (Hafizi, 1996; Lipson, 1992)*

Nepal

Debendra Manandhar

Nepal is a small country, with a population of 24 million, bordered by China and India. As a result of poverty and very limited access to health services, its health statistics are among the worst in Asia. The infant mortality rate is estimated to be 74 per 1,000 live births; the mortality rate of those younger than 5 is 189 per 1,000 live births; the maternal mortality rate is 8.5 per 1,000 women aged 15 to 49. The average life expectancy at birth is estimated to be 58 years.

The major causes of ill health lie primarily in widespread and extreme poverty and in an associated lack of basic infrastructures. This can be illustrated by the existing ratio of health personnel, hospitals, and hospital beds to population. There is just 1 doctor per 16,800 population, and even more important is the limited nursing staff, 1 nurse per 4,700 population. Similarly, there is 1 hospital per 161,948 population and 0.3 hospital beds per

1,000. These ratios are very low compared with the other South Asian countries (UNDP, 1998b).

Four health systems co-exist simultaneously in Nepal. These systems are divided into four broad categories: the home-based system, the traditional faith healing system, the Ayurvedic (traditional Hindu) system, and the allopathic (modern Western) system.

Limited access to health services and the relatively low quality of public health institutions, along with the prohibitive costs of allopathic medicine and modern health services, force most households to rely on home remedies. The most common home remedies include folk remedies passed down from generation to generation and local herbs. Over-the-counter Western medicines, which are almost completely unregulated, are being used in increased numbers.

The failure of many home remedies invites intervention from community-level faith healers. Such healers base their treatment on an intimate knowledge of the sick person, divine invocation of ancestors, and herbal remedies. Healers often specialize in particular techniques, and specific healers are consulted according to the nature of the illness. The number of such healers is very large, indicating the legitimacy of the system. One study estimated the number of local faith healers at 400,000 to 800,000, which roughly translates to one faith healer for every six households. The significant role of local healers has been widely noted. The majority of sick persons in the rural areas who eventually visit the allopathic health clinic had first consulted a tradition faith healer. The majority of the women in rural areas use the services of faith healers for childbirth, partly because women prefer to deliver a baby at home.

The Ayurvedic (traditional Hindu) system of healing has been practiced in South Asia since ancient times. It is based on the physiological characteristics of the sick person, the symptoms

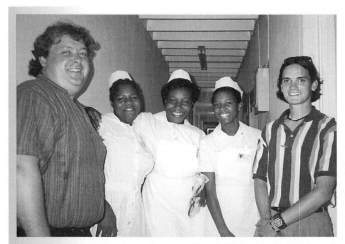

American nursing students talk about nursing school experiences with nursing students in Jamaica.

of the illness, and a detailed pharmacological knowledge of herbs. The herbal treatments that households and local faith healers use are often borrowed from the Ayurvedic system. Most Ayurvedic healers work within the private domain, although there is some public support. Ayurvedic healing in the public sector is performed through one central Ayurvedic hospital with 50 beds, one 15-bed zonal hospital, 172 dispensaries in 55 districts, and a central drug-manufacturing unit (UNDP, 1998b).

Nepal began using a modern allopathic public health system at the end of 19th century. By 1955, there were 34 small-scale hospitals with a total of 623 beds and 24 dispensaries. An organized national public effort to spur the development of modern health services started in the mid-1950s. A large-scale malaria control program was launched in 1955; the leprosy and tuberculosis control projects were initiated in 1966; the smallpox eradication program was launched in 1968; and a family planning and maternal and child health board was established in 1968. In 1971, the Division of Basic Health Service was formed within the Department of Health to provide basic health to a maximum number of people. Small-scale public hospitals were established at various regional and district centers. In 1977, the successful smallpox eradication project was converted to the expanded program for immunization. Other health programs such as nutrition support and diarrhea control were integrated in 1980. Private and international nongovernmental organization initiatives also led to the establishment of rural health posts, clinics, hospitals, and drug retail outlets. One teaching hospital was also established within the public sector. Public health offices were established in all districts.

Significant steps were taken by the Nepalese government to expand the public health network in the mid-1980s and early 1990s. A national policy decision led to the formation of a unified group of volunteer community-based female health workers to provide basic health services, including health education and basic first aid treatment. At present, they number more than 42,000. Although their educational level is low, their achievements in terms of community sensitization to health-related issues and referrals to health care clinics are significant. Another national policy decision created an integrated institutional structure of public health at the local and regional levels. Implementation of this policy is leading to the establishment of community-level health posts in all parts of the country.

These governmental policies, together with expanding private initiatives, have led to a gradual rise in trained health personnel and health facilities at various levels. As of 1997, local clinics had been established in 3,187 of the 3,912 villages. A total of 75 public hospitals are functioning today in different regions. Approximately 40 hospitals and nursing homes have been established under private initiative. In addition, larger numbers of health clinics and laboratories have been set up under private sector as well. In addition, there has been a significant increase in the number of health personnel and hospital beds per unit of population (UNDP, 1998b).

The formal health sector is organized through the Ministry of Health (MOH), with central offices of the various programs based in Kathmandu. The MOH is by far the largest single provider of formal health services. The MOH expenditure comprises nearly 50% of total expenditure on health care. Since its inception in the 1950s, the MOH has undergone almost continuous restructuring to become an integrated public health system with emphasis on preventive care (UNDP, 1998b).

In every district, there is a District Health Office (DHO). Beside planning, management, and organization of health activities, the DHO is also made responsible for mobilizing all health and health-related institutions and supervising and monitoring the activities of these institutions regularly. At present, there are 1,196 physicians, 2,986 nurses, 240 Ayurved physicians, 130 Ayurved assistants, 1,186 health assistants, 4,015 village health workers, and 42,000 female community health volunteers (UNDP, 1998b).

Private providers of health services in Nepal include private nonprofit providers, modern private for-profit providers, and traditional providers. The nonprofit providers are composed of nongovernmental organizations and international NGOs (INGOs). NGOs include small, local grassroots organizations as well as the national NGOs, such as Family Planning Association of Nepal, Nepal Red Cross Society, and so on. There are approximately 20 nonprofit hospitals with more than 1,000 beds. In most cases, the hospitals are run on a partial cost recovery basis. NGOs and INGOs provide support for governmental health services or parallel private health services.

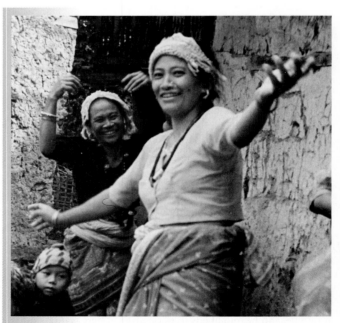

Although maternal mortality is still a significant problem for Nepalese women, it is being addressed by increases in postpartum care technology as Nepal struggles to improve the health status of women.

The Nepal Social Welfare Council (SWC) estimates that NGOs operate about 235 primary health centers and that about 24% of all local rural health facilities are managed by NGOs. Forty percent of the budgets of NGOs that are registered with SWC are spent on health services, although health activities differ in scope and quality. The quality of health care services provided by NGOs is perceived to be better than those provided by the public sector. The strengths of NGOs include close contacts with local communities, nonbureaucratic structures, management flexibility, and higher staff motivation. Many of the NGOs have been experimenting with different methods of community financing schemes, which include sale and supply of drugs to retail outlets and community-based prepayment schemes.

Besides large local and international NGOs, many community-based organizations (CBOs) are involved in providing health care to communities. However, there is little documentation of the efforts of smaller grassroots level health CBOs.

Another kind of private sector providers are for-profit organizations. There has been significant growth in private nursing homes and clinics, especially in the urban areas. There are currently about 15 private for-profit hospitals and nursing homes with more than 200 beds.

Traditional healers are considered important private providers. Payment to the traditional healers is made both in cash and in kind. Many studies found the role of the traditional healers in the rural communities to be of great importance. In Nepal, there are still many remote places where it is almost impossible for the government to provide appropriate health care because of the mountainous terrain and local sociocultural beliefs. In such cases, traditional healers are the only source of health care.

Sadly, despite the growth in the health infrastructure in recent years, nearly 80% of the population are still not receiving health care services. Although the number of local clinics has increased, they are still ill equipped. The annual drug rations allocated to local clinics are adequate for only 3 to 6 months. Physicians and nurses often are absent from the rural-based clinics and regional and district hospitals. A major reason for this inadequate access to health care is related to poverty. The per capita health expenditure in Nepal is very low ($7) compared with other South Asian neighbors such as India ($21), Pakistan ($12), and Sri Lanka ($18).

South Africa
Ntombodidi Muzzen-Sherra (Zodidi) Tshotsho

South Africa, a country with a population of more than 40 million, is located in the most southern apex of the African continent. The average life expectancy in South Africa is 57 years of age, and the infant mortality rate is 52 per 1,000 live births. Before 1994, when the present government of South Africa was democratically elected, the majority of the population had limited or no access to health care services because of the legacy of apartheid. The laws and policies of the apartheid regime discriminated against the majority of South Africans on the basis of race and skin color. Between 35% and 55% of the South African population lived in poverty, with 53% of them living in rural areas. Poverty was rampant primarily because of the country's poor infrastructure and lack of resources in the rural areas, including poor transportation facilities.

Since the new government has been in place, many major changes have taken place in South Africa to ensure that health care services are accessible, affordable, and rendered in an equitable manner to the majority of the people. The National Department of Health published a *White Paper for the Transformation of the Health System in South Africa* on April 16, 1997, outlining a set of policy objectives and principles for the transformation of the health care system (Government Gazette No. 17910, 1997). The goals outlined in the white paper included the following:

- *Unifying the previously fragmented services at all levels into a comprehensive and integrated national health system (NHS)*
- *Improving equity, accessibility, and utilization of health services*
- *Extending the availability and ensuring the appropriateness of health services*
- *Developing health promotion activities*
- *Improving health sector planning and monitoring of health status and services*

The health services have been reorganized with emphasis on planning and implementing health care services in accordance with primary health care principles. The responsibilities of health care services have been passed down from the national level to the provincial and district levels. The country is divided into nine provinces, with each one having its own department of health. A district health system for the delivery of services at the district level has been established in each province. Separate functions for all three levels of the health care system have been designated to avoid duplication of services and to ensure a well-coordinated comprehensive health care system.

Some of the roles of the National Department of Health include providing leadership for the formulation of legislation and health policy, building the capacity of the provincial health departments to provide effective health services, ensuring equity in the allocation of resources to the provinces and municipalities, developing a coordinated health information system, and forming partnerships with other national health departments and international agencies.

The mission of the provincial health departments is to promote and monitor the health of the people in the provinces and develop and support a caring and effective primary health care system. Some of the roles and functions of the provincial health departments include developing the capacity to deliver the full range of health services within the provinces, distributing resources (personnel, equipment, and facilities) to achieve accessible and cost-effective delivery of services, decentralizing all aspects of administration and management for services to allow local democratic participation in the control of health services, and achieving strategic, functional, and managerial integration of health services of both provincial and district health services.

Each province is divided into a number of functional districts. The main purpose of the district health system in South Africa is to decentralize responsibility for health care delivery and place it at the local level. This level of the health care system is responsible for the overall management and control of its own budget and the provision and purchase of a full range of comprehensive primary health care services within its area of jurisdiction. All services are rendered in collaboration with other governmental, nongovernmental, and private structures. In some provinces, district management teams are already in place and functioning well.

Equitable, accessible, and affordable comprehensive primary health care services in South Africa are slowly becoming a reality, as evidenced by a substantial increase in the number of clinics built since the inception of the new health care system; free health care services for children younger than 5 years of age and pregnant women; changes in the education and training of health care workers; meals provided at schools to reduce the prevalence of malnutrition among children; compulsory community service for newly qualified medical practitioners; control measures for alcohol, illicit drugs, and tobacco; HIV/AIDS prevention measures and services to reduce the personal and social impact of HIV/AIDS; and the Expanded Program on Immunization (EPI) to control the seven vaccine-preventable diseases common in children—childhood tuberculosis, diphtheria, pertussis, tetanus, polio, measles, and hepatitis B (Masakhane, 1998).

The transformation of health services in South Africa is not without problems, however, as some sectors of the community are critical of these changes and seem not to appreciate the principles on which the present health care system is based. High unemployment rates, poverty, and the upsurge of violence are only a few of the factors contributing to the limited successes of health care services. One of the biggest problems is the limited successes in controlling HIV/AIDS and tuberculosis. Despite the many problems, appreciable strides have been made in improving the health of the people in the rural areas. The rural areas are being provided with electricity, running water, telephones, and adequate housing (Sefularo, 1998).

CASE STUDY

A Nursing Student's Story

Border issues affect everyone. During a clinical experience at a level 1 trauma center, another student and I were assigned to a room in the emergency room. A 16-year-old boy was brought in by the triage nurse. He was in obvious respiratory distress. He had renal failure, a Hickmann to right anterior chest wall, soiled dressings, bilateral rales, and +3 pitting edema. After assessment by the first-year resident, the chief resident was called and determined that this boy was not a candidate for emergency dialysis. An interpreter was called, and it was learned that the boy was from Honduras and had no medical coverage. He was admitted for observation. Following up on the client's status the next day, we found the notation "illegal" recorded again and again in his medical record. Social Services could not help this young man. While we vis-ited the client, the chief nephrologist came to see him. He wanted us to translate for him as he gave discharge instructions. There would be no dialysis, and the Hickmann would not be removed. He said, "Marry a U.S. citizen or go back to your country. You will be discharged today."

We told the client we were sorry and asked for his phone number. We told him we would try to do something. We knew that there is no hemodialysis in Honduras and that Social Services could have attempted to make referrals. We did some research and found a hospital willing to treat our client and referred our client there. In this cultural experience, we were able to integrate respect for human rights, client advocacy, and ethics with critical care skills to assist this client. We hope that we empowered this client to use available community resources to care for himself despite cultural differences.

Jamy Josey, 1998.

CONCLUSION

From its very beginning in Alma Ata, Russia, in 1978, the "Health for All" era was based on the defining principles of social justice and equity. Two decades later, with injustice and inequity still rampant in the world, the WHO has recommitted itself to the use of primary health care as the principal means of achieving health for all. The WHO has called for a new global health policy and strategy to address some of the old and new obstacles confronting people in their search for health: poverty, debt, environmental deterioration, and increases in violence of all kinds. This renewed global health effort will address the determinants and trends in health status, inequalities in that status, and access to health services. The focus is to be on equity, solidarity, and social justice.

• •

It is important to recognize that the development of nursing and its status as a profession is very much related to its social contract. This contract varies around the world, but the overall theme is fairly consistent. Nursing is looked to for committed service to all peoples in need. Nursing is seen as responding to need, regardless of class, race, ethnicity, gender, or political affiliation. What this means is that nursing is fundamentally important to the pursuit of equity and social justice. It also means that nursing has a far-reaching impact that goes well beyond those individuals and families that nurses touch each day.
Marla Salmon, ScD, RN, FAAN,
Dean, Emory School of Nursing,
Atlanta, 1998

• •

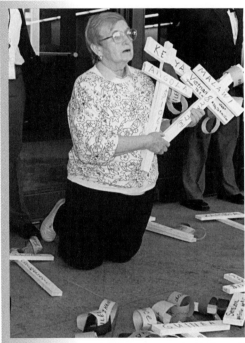

Chapter author Janet Gottschalk kneels in the doorway of the International Monetary Fund, Washington, DC, in April 1999 in an appeal for the cancellation of debt for poor nations.

If these last years have taught globally conscious nurses anything, it is that we all share one world and an increasingly fragile ecosystem. Whatever the color of our skin—whatever language we speak or religion we profess—we are united in dreaming the same dreams for ourselves and families.

Unfortunately, the same negative global forces affect each of us and have the same deadly consequences wherever we live and work. As nurses we will be challenged to step aside from the ordinary and known and venture out into the complex worlds of international economics and politics, areas previously unknown to many nurses.

Years ago there was a popular saying: "Thinking globally . . . act locally." Today that saying is insufficient. To meet the challenges on the horizon, you will need to think and act globally as well as locally.

The challenges facing nurses and others with whom we share our world are enormous. The consequences of inaction, locally and globally, are also enormous. We nurses need the courage individually and as groups to analyze, strategize, act—in true partnership with others—to build a world of peace based on justice for all.

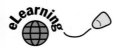

CRITICAL THINKING ACTIVITIES

1. Which groups or organizations in your community are working locally to improve people's lives?

2. Are nurses actively involved with any of these groups? If so, in what capacity?

Explore Community Health Nursing on the web! To learn more about the topics in this chapter, use the passcode provided to access your exclusive web site: http://communitynursing.jbpub.com
If you do not have a passcode, you can obtain one at this site.

REFERENCES

Abzug, B. (1998, March 31). *Address to United Nations*. New York: United Nations.

Barnes, D., Eribes, C., Juarbe, T., Nelson, M., Proctor, S., Sawyer, L., Shaul, M., & Meleis, A. I. (1995). Primary health care and primary care: A confusion of philosophies. *Nursing Outlook, 43*, 7–16.

Benetar, S. R. (1998). Global disparities in health and human rights: A critical commentary. *American Journal of Public Health, 88*(2), 295–300.

Brush, B. L., Lynaugh, J. E., Boschma, G., Rafferty, A. M., Stuart, M., & Tomes, N. J. (1999). *Nurses of all nations. A history of the International Council of Nurses, 1899–1999*. Philadelphia: J. B. Lippincott.

Carter Center. (1997). *At a glance. The Carter Center*. Atlanta: Author.

Carter, N. L. (1978). Social systems. In H. H. Smith (Ed.), *Iran: A country study*. Washington, DC: American University.

Deppe, H-U., Oreskovic, S. (1996). Back to Europe: Back to Bismarck? *International Journal of Health Services, 26*(4), 777–802.

Earl-Slater, A. (1996). Health care reforms in the Czech Republic. *Journal of Management in Medicine, 10*(2), 13–22.

Eisen, G. (1996). The primary attention in Cuba. The physician's team, the family nurse and the polyclinic. *Public Health Cuban Magazine, 22*(2), 117–124.

Friedman, T. L. (1996). The talk of Tehran. *The New York Times, 145*(50542), p. 27.

Global Issues. (1998). U.S. backs "well-being" programs for women. *USIA Electronic Journal, 3*(2): www.usia.gov/journals/.

Global Trade Watch. (1999a). *The MAI shell game. The World Trade Organization*: www.tradewatch.org.

Global Trade Watch. (1999b). *A sampling of NAFTA related job loss . . . NAFTA trade adjustment assistance*: www.citizen.org.

Good, B. J., & Good, M. D. (1982). Toward a meaning: Centered analysis of popular illness categories: "Flight illness" and "heart distress" in Iran. In A. J. Marsella & G. M. White (Eds), *Cultural conceptions of mental health and therapy*. Dordrecht: Reidel.

Good, M. D. (1980). Of blood and babies: The relationship of popular Islamic physiology to fertility. *Social Science and Medicine, 146*, 147–156.

Gottschalk, J. (1996). Primary health care: The foundation. In *Community as partner: Theory and practice in nursing* (pp. 7–9). Philadelphia: J. B. Lippincott.

Government Gazette No. 17910. (1997, April). *White paper for the transformation of the health system in South Africa*. Pretoria: South African Government Printing Office.

Hafizi, H. (1996). Iranians. In J. G. Lipson, S. L. Dibble, & P. A. Minarik (Eds), *Culture and nursing care* (pp. 169–179). San Francisco: UCSF Nursing Press.

International Council of Nurses (ICN). (1999). *About the International Council of Nurses*: www.icn.ch/abouticn.htm.

International Monetary Fund (IMF). (1998). *What is the International Monetary Fund?* www.imf.org/.

International Monetary Fund (IMF). (1999). *About the IMF*: ww.imf.org/.

Iran gender segregation. (1998). *Off Our Backs, 28*(6), 3.

Jardnes J. B., Ouviña J., & Aneiro Riba, R. (1991). Education in the science of health in Cuba. *Public Health Cuban Magazine, 25*(4), 387–407.

Josey, J. (1998). *National League for Nursing Education Summit*. Chicago, IL. [DAY/MONTH?]

Kolko, G. (1999). Ravaging the poor: The International Monetary Fund indicted by its own data. *International Journal of Health Services*, *29*(1), 51–57.

Lastovicka, R., Marcincin, A., & Mejstrik, M. (1995). Corporate governance and share prices in voucher privatized companies. In J. Svejnar (Ed.), *Czech Republic and economic transition in Eastern Europe*. San Diego: Academic Press.

Lipson, G. J. (1992). The health and adjustment of Iranian immigrants. *Western Journal of Nursing Research*, *14*(1), 10–29.

Little, R. E., Monaghan, S. S., Gladen, B. C., Shkyryak-Nyzhnyk, Z., & Wilcox, A. J. (1999). Outcomes of 17,137 pregnancies in 2 urban areas of Ukraine. *American Journal of Public Health*, *89*(12), 1832–1836.

Masakhane, J. (1998, October 29). List of healthy results. *Pretoria News*, p. 20.

Mezvinsky, M. M. (1996). *Beyond Beijing: U.S. Commitments*: www.feminist.com/beijing.htm.

Misconiova, B. (1992, September/October). Healing a sick society. *World Health*, 4–5.

Mobilizing Beyond Beijing. (1999). *Country and regional news on follow-up to Beijing*: www.interaction.org/pub.

Orchard, C. A., & Karmaliani, R. (1999). Community development specialists in nursing for developing countries. *Image: The Journal of Nursing Scholarship*, *31*(3), 295–299.

Rubas, L. (1995, May 30). The intended reforms in health care Ministry of Health of the Czech Republic. Ministry of Health, Czech Republic Parliament, Prague.

Salmon, M. E. (1998). Nursing equity and social justice. *Reflections*, *24*(2), 8–11.

Sefularo, M. (1998). Health and development of social welfare—North West Province. *Pretoria News*, p. 8.

Senanayake, P. (1998). Safe motherhood: A success story in Sri Lanka. *World Health*, *51*(1), 28-29.

UNDP (1998a). *Human development report*. New York: Author.

UNDP. (1998b). *Nepal: Human development report*. Kathmandu: Author.

UNICEF. (1998). *The state of the world's children*: http://unicef.org/sowc98/silent.htm.

UNICEF. (1999a). *Action Against Poverty. NetAid: Ending extreme poverty*: www.unicef.org/netaidright.htm.

UNICEF. (1999b). *Progress of nations*: www.unicef.org/pon99/legcom2.htm.

UNITE. (1999). *The NAFTA scam*: www.uniteunion.org.

U.S. Department of State. (1999a, April 27). *The United Nations*: www.un.int/missions/usa/iofact8.htm.

U.S. Department of State. (1999b). *U.S. financial commitment to the U.N.*: www.un.int/missions/usa/iofact2.htm.

USAID. (1998). *Making a world of difference one family at a time*: www.usia.gov/ journals/itgic/0998/ijge/gj-14.htm.

Vyborna, O. (1994). *The reform of the Czech health care system*. Working paper. Co-sponsored by the Ford Foundation, in conjunction with Center for Economic Research and Graduate Education Charles University and Economics Institute of the Academy of Sciences of the Czech Republic.

World Health Organization (WHO). (1998). *Nursing and midwifery at WHO (HDP/NUR)*: www.who.int/hdp/nur/index.htm.

World Health Organization (WHO). (1999). *About WHO*: www.who.int/aboutwho/.

World Bank Group. (1999). *Why do we need a World Bank?* www.worldbank.org.

Wright, M. G. M., Godue, C., Manfredi, M., & Korniewicz, D. M. (1998). Nursing education and international health in the United States, Latin America, and the Caribbean. *Image: The Journal of Nursing Scholarship*, *30*(1), 31–36.

Zarkovic, G., Mielck, A., John, J. J., & Beckmann, M. (1994). *Reform of the health care systems in former socialist countries: Problems, options, scenarios*. Germany: GSF-Forschungszentrum, Oberschleissheim.

Chapter 18
Groups in the Community

Peggy "Margaret" Hickman and Marilyn Givens King

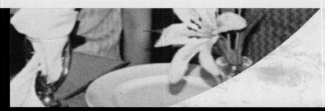

Humans are social beings and, as such, tend to congregate in groups. **Groups** *consist of two or more people who have a collective identity, communicate with each other regularly, and share a common purpose or goal.*

CHAPTER FOCUS

Characteristics of Effective Groups
Collective Identity
Shared Purpose
Communication
Group Norms
Participation
Shared Leadership
Cohesion
Shared Decision Making
Conflict Management
Problem Solving

Stages of Group Development
Group Formation
Group Maintenance: Cohesion, Norms, and
   Conflict Resolution
Group Dissolution

Group Functions
Group Tasks
Roles of Group Members
Groups as Change Agents
Concepts Related to Change

Types of Groups

Working with Groups
Group Leadership
Ethical Considerations
Evaluating Groups

QUESTIONS TO CONSIDER

After reading this chapter, answer the following questions:
1. What are group characteristics?
2. What are the stages of group development?
3. What kinds of functions do groups exhibit?
4. What are the different types of groups that community health nurses might be involved in?
5. How is group process evaluated?
6. What is group leadership? How does it apply in community health nursing?

KEY TERMS

Change	Force field analysis	Internal maintenance	Outcome evaluation
Coalitions	Goal attainment tasks	tasks	Participation
Cohesion	Groups	Leadership	Partnership
Decision making	Impact evaluation	Norms	Process evaluation
Empowerment			

In the course of their professional activities, nurses work with a wide variety of groups to achieve population health promotion and restoration goals. In addition, nurses are members of work-related groups focused on continuous improvement of health care, the health care system, and the nursing profession.

Working with groups in community settings is an essential component of public health and community health nursing practice. *Healthy People 2000, Healthy People 2010, and Healthy Communities 2000* indicate that national health objectives cannot be met effectively unless health professionals work in **partnership** with community and professional groups (APHA, 1991; DHHS, 1991, 2000) (Box 18-1). In a similar vein, professional nursing standards include repeated statements that the nurse is to practice *in partnership* with others to achieve desired health outcomes that are collectively held (ANA, 1986, 1991, 1996).

In many situations, nurses are able to work more effectively and efficiently when they work in groups than when they work individually. Some advantages of groups are as follows:

- *Can accomplish tasks that may not be achievable by individuals*
- *Bring a wider range of resources, skills, and talents to bear on complex health issues*
- *Provide a means of decision making that allows for multiple and sometimes conflicting views to be evaluated and synthesized*
- *Have a synergy that surpasses the capacity of individuals to attain health goals*

The Case Study on p. 389 is an example of a clinical situation in which nurses working together form a community coalition to implement a teen health program that is much more comprehensive and effective than the services the nurses provided separately.

Working with groups requires a knowledge of group characteristics and dynamics, as well as a set of basic group facilitation

BOX 18-1 NATIONAL HEALTH STANDARDS AND OBJECTIVES

COLLECTIVE RESPONSIBILITY FOR CHANGE

Healthy People 2000: *"While the responsibility for change lies with each of us, it also lies with all of us, and individuals cannot be expected to act alone"* (DHHS, 1991, p. 85).

Healthy People 2010: *"Community health is profoundly affected by the collective behaviors, attitudes, and beliefs of everyone who lives in the community"* (DHHS, 2000, p. 3).

Healthy Communities 2000: *"Improvements in public health require active community ownership and commitment"* (APHA, 1991, p. xxiv).

PRACTICE PARTNERSHIPS AMONG HEALTH CARE PROVIDERS AND OTHERS

Healthy People 2000: *"Practice can take the form of partnerships with nonprofessionals in the pursuit of individual, family, and community health care. The effectiveness and efficiency of preventive services . . . will be enhanced by such partnerships"* (DHHS, 1991, p. 87).

Healthy Communities 2000: *"Disease prevention is a shared partnership . . . Cooperation among major community groups and organizations creates the foundation for communities to establish and achieve [health] goals and objectives"* (APHA, 1991, p. xviii).

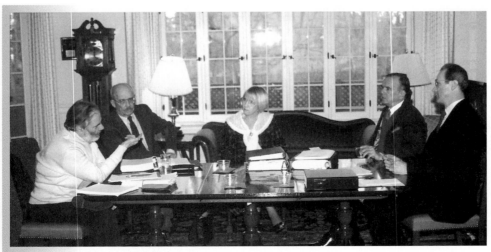

Formal group with agenda.

CASE STUDY

Working with Groups to Plan a Teen Health Clinic

J. C. Roberts, a school health nurse in an urban high school, runs a school-based education center targeting health problems affecting the student population. Lee Sorrel, a nurse in a nearby public health center, runs an after-school teen clinic to provide care for the same set of health problems. Although both nurses spent much time and energy implementing their respective programs, local teens are not using the services of either. After discussing their mutual frustration at a district nursing meeting, J. C. and Lee decide to work together. They form an advisory group made up of local teens to help them evaluate the two programs. The group learns the following:

- Students fear negative repercussions if teachers see them going into the health education center at school.

- Desired educational topics, such as safe sex and pregnancy prevention, cannot be offered by the health education center under existing school policy.

- Using a "problem-oriented" clinic has a negative social stigma among their peers.

- Many teens who might attend the health department clinic are working after school.

The group recommends a community-based program that includes social activities, health and education services, and job skills training. The nurses and advisory committee members initiate a coalition of community leaders and organizations that mobilizes resources for a comprehensive teen program at the local community center. The program is highly successful. Local teens are using a broader range of services than the school or health department were able to offer separately.*

On a sheet of paper, list all the individuals (e.g., the two nurses, the teens), agencies, organizations, and community officials or representatives that should be part of the community coalition. Next to each, list examples of the knowledge, skills, and resources that each can potentially contribute to the pool of information that will be used as the basis for informed decision making.

1. Take a pencil and cover each entry, one at a time. What would be lost each time?

2. Look at each entry. What are the potential sources of power and influence for each?

3. Brainstorm a list of ground rules that would support shared leadership and decision making.

Look at the individuals, agencies, organizations, and community officials or representatives that you identified in the previous questions. Make a list of the potential sources and topics of conflict within this group.

1. What detrimental effects to individuals and the group might result from these conflicts?

2. What strengths might the group derive from these potential conflicts?

3. Brainstorm a list of ground rules that would support positive conflict management.

---

skills. Our understanding of groups and group behavior is based on a body of interdisciplinary research from the fields such as sociology, anthropology, business, and health (Bracht, 1990). A variety of nursing theories, such as *Parse's Theory in Practice*, also help guide nursing practice with groups (Kelley, 1995). This chapter introduces the basic concepts, leadership skills, and ethical considerations needed for effective group development, maintenance, and evaluation.

Characteristics of Effective Groups

A *group* is defined as two or more people who have a collective identity, communicate with each other regularly, and share a common purpose or goal. Although collective identity, shared goals, and open communication are defining characteristics of groups, additional characteristics associated with groups that can function effectively include group norms, cohesion, active participation, shared leadership, shared decision making, problem solving, and conflict resolution.

Collective Identity

Although groups are made up of unique individuals, effective groups develop a sense of collective identity. The group identity may be explicit and related to a shared characteristic of the group members. For example, "Bosom Buddies" groups are made up primarily of breast cancer survivors, and the "West End Neighborhood Association" denotes a group of people who define their collective identity based on shared geographic-political boundaries.

Shared Purpose

In addition to having a common identity, groups have a shared purpose or goal that transcends the individual goals of group members. Group goals must be clearly understood and relevant to all members of the group. Within effective groups, goals are determined cooperatively and clarified or modified to fit as closely as possible with individual goals (Berdahl & Craig, 1996).

Communication

Stable mechanisms of open communication in which each member of the group gives and receives information is a characteristic of effective groups. Mutual acceptance, trust, and understanding are basic to open communication patterns in which group members can freely share thoughts and feelings. Traditionally, a component of communication patterns in effective groups included regular face-to-face interaction. However, current health practice uses electronic means quite effectively to facilitate group communication. Electronic tools for collaboration developed in the 1980s have evolved into highly sophisticated Internet-based methods of communication and decision making in groups whose members are geographically dispersed (Dennis & Valacich, 1994; Laudon & Laudon, 1988; Lebie, Rhoades, & McGrath, 1996; Preboth & Wright, 1999; Reagan-Cirincione, 1994; Sharf, 1997).

Health information clearinghouses provide extensive lists of health-related groups that meet and communicate online. Research about online groups that focus on illnesses such as cancer, diabetes, and alcoholism has found that the Internet actually strengthens group communication because there are no signs of age, gender, race, social status, dress, weight, disabilities, and other distinctions (Madara, 1997). However, a challenge for nurses and others using the Internet for group work is to develop ways of communicating thoughts and feelings in the absence of traditional visual cues.

Group Norms

Norms are the spoken and unspoken rules and politics that govern group behavior (Loomis, 1979). Because groups often bring together people with a variety of assumptions about acceptable group behavior, effective groups make implicit norms explicit by discussing and developing written rules for group conduct. If starting a new group, one may want to begin the first meeting by having the group identify some ground rules about which they agree and post this list where everyone can see it. The group may add additional rules as needed at subsequent meetings.

Participation

Groups are more effective when all members are active participants. **Participation** means that all group members listen and are listened to, share in decision making, and contribute to the achievement of group tasks and objectives. Ground rules such as "Everyone will be given a chance to talk," "Only one person talks at a time," "No interrupting," "Everyone's ideas are important," and "Everyone has a vote" can help promote active participation in groups. Community development and organizational behavior research indicates that participation by all group members increases group motivation, leads to greater involvement in group activities, is associated with higher levels of commitment to group plans and objectives, and contributes to greater success in achievement of group goals (Cooke & Szumal, 1994; Minkler, 1997).

Shared Leadership

Although individuals within a group may exhibit a variety of **leadership** styles, effective groups distribute leadership among their members. As the need for formal leadership arises, various members of the group take turns in assuming leadership roles. As with participation, shared leadership is associated with higher levels of group motivation, involvement, commitment, and goal attainment (Hirokawa & Keyton, 1995; Schitterkate, 1996). One way to promote shared leadership is to end each meeting with the development of the agenda for the next meeting and have different group members volunteer to be discussion leaders for each item on the agenda.

Cohesion

Group **cohesion** refers to the ability of the group to "stick together," that is, retain members who can work together over a sufficient period of time to achieve group goals. Group cohesion is related to factors such as the following (Sampson & Marthas, 1981):

- *Positive interpersonal relations among group members*
- *The desire of members to continue as part of the group*
- *The degree to which members like and are satisfied with the group's composition*
- *The level of acceptance, trust, and support among group members*

Cohesive groups put effort into team building and maintenance as well as task achievement. Setting ground rules that show respect for diversity and for the dignity and worth of each member of the group is an important part of ensuring group cohesion.

Shared Decision Making

In effective groups, power and influence within the group are shared relatively equally. All members are involved in setting goals, gathering information, identifying alternative ways to achieve goals, and deciding on the plan of action. An assumption underlying shared **decision making** is that each group member has information of value that will contribute to informed decision making. Input is based on a group member's knowledge, skills, and access to needed resources, rather than on the member's formal title or position in the organization or community. For shared decision making to be effective, all group members should understand the following (Ramey, 1993):

- *The nature of the goal and task being undertaken*
- *Alternative approaches and strategies for achieving the goal or accomplishing the task*
- *Potential consequences (positive and negative) of each alternative being considered*
- *The social, economic, and environmental costs of each alternative to individuals, families, and organizations in the community, as well as to the community as a whole*

A goal of groups should be to expand the knowledge and skills of its members in ways that will empower the group to make efficacious, informed decisions (Minkler, 1997; Ramey, 1993).

Conflict Management

One of the strengths of a group lies in its ability to bring together individuals and organizations that have diverse views about an issue or problem. With diversity, the potential for conflict is high, so conflict management is critical. Conflict that is not managed effectively can be harmful to individuals and can destroy group cohesion and productivity; however, conflict also has a high potential for promoting involvement in a group and increasing the creativity and quality of decision making. Therefore, effective groups view conflict as a source of potential strength and develop productive ways of managing and resolving conflict.

Problem Solving

Finally, groups must have the ability to solve problems collectively in ways that are long lasting and require minimal energy. Effective groups develop ways to identify problems early, provide opportunities for anticipatory problem solving, and develop mechanisms for evaluating the effect and quality of solutions.

Stages of Group Development

Like individuals and families, groups go through several stages of growth and development. Many classic theories of group development (Table 18-1) reflect the belief that groups move by stages from a collection of unique, diverse individuals with conflicts to a cohesive group that maintains itself and achieves ongoing tasks and goals (Bion, 1961; Tuckman, 1965; Yalom, 1985). Others, including more recent theories, believe that the life cycle of a group includes several stages of group formation, maintenance, and dissolution (Berman-Rossi, 1992; Feinberg, 1980).

Group Formation

Group formation may take place in two phases: group initiation and group expansion. *Group initiation* is the phase in which the nurse and other members of a small planning body define the preliminary goal of the group and take care of arranging the first group meeting. *Group expansion* occurs as the larger group verifies and clarifies its purpose and begins the process of goal achievement.

Group formation begins with the planning group asking a series of critical questions: What is the purpose of the group? Why form a new group? What will this group do that is not already being done by other groups? How large should the group be? Who should be invited to join? How long should this group exist?

The answers to these questions will vary according to the type of group being developed. In general, groups should be kept small enough for all members of the group to interact with each other. Group membership and anticipated longevity will be closely related to the purpose of the group. For example, educational groups may be formed for a specified period of time and be open to all interested persons, whereas a support group may be ongoing and be open primarily to people affected by a specific health problem.

After the initial decisions about group membership and purpose have been made, someone must take responsibility for arranging a place and time for the initial group meeting, inviting prospective members to attend, and conducting the first meeting. The initial meeting is very important because it sets the stage for how well the group will develop and perform. At the initial meeting, invited participants should be involved in clarifying the group's purpose and goals and determining whether additional members are needed for the group to achieve its goals effectively and efficiently.

TABLE 18-1 STAGES OF GROUP GROWTH AND DEVELOPMENT: A COMPARISON OF THEORIES

| | STAGES OF GROUP DEVELOPMENT | | | | |
THEORISTS	INITIATION	MAINTENANCE			DISSOLUTION
Bion (1961)	Flight	Fight		Unite	
Tuckman (1965)	Forming	Storming	Norming	Performing	
Yalom (1985)	Orientation	Conflict	Harmony	Maturity	
Feinberg (1980) Berman-Rossi (1992)	Formation	Conflict resolution	Norms	Cohesion	Dissolution

CASE STUDY

Health Needs of the Rural Elderly Population

Darla Parker, RN, BSN, works with a small home health agency that is located in a rural Appalachian community. Population in the county is estimated to be 13,798, with 2,578 people between the ages of 55 and 64. Another 3,459 people are older than 65. Demographic data indicate that the elderly population will continue to grow, with the "graying of America" and young adults leaving the area to find work. Chronic health problems among the older population of this county include high rates of cancer, especially late-stage diagnosed uterine and breast cancers, chronic lung diseases that includes a high rate of black lung disease, and high rates of cardiovascular diseases. The incidence of cigarette smoking, sedentary lifestyles, and obesity are also high for this community.

In consultation with Shirley Janeff, director of the regional office on aging, Darla learned that a recent assessment of the community had found that a number of elderly citizens with chronic health problems were having difficulty getting access to needed health care resources. Results of this survey also showed needs for transportation, for home caregivers, and for help with the purchase of medications. Janeff said, "I think the problem is complex, but some of the problems we are encountering are related to changes in Medicare reimbursement policies that limit access to home health and also that people are simply not informed about the many resources available to them in the community." Darla responded, "I know we can't solve the problems with reimbursement at this time,

but maybe we can do something to inform people about resources." When Darla returned to her office she talked with her supervisor about setting up a task force to investigate some possible solutions to these issues. Her supervisor, Mary Jane, agreed with the need to work on this issue and suggested that Darla proceed.

Two weeks later, Darla met with representatives of a variety of service agencies to develop some approaches to the documented needs of the elderly citizens of the community. After much discussion of the assessment data, the group decided to put on a health fair as one strategy to inform the community of the many resources in the area. At this first meeting, the group selected a date to coincide with Older Americans Month. They decided to hold it outdoors at the local county park, but they also identified another site in case of rain on the chosen date. The task force met two more times to complete planning for the event.

1. What are some factors Darla needs to consider when putting together a task force to plan this project? As you answer this question, think about the advantages and disadvantages of inviting various community and organizational representatives.

2. Once she has established the task force, what is Darla's role with the group? What are expected behaviors of the different possible roles she could assume?

3. At the first meeting, Darla is elected by the group to be the chairperson. What does it mean to be a leader? Describe leadership behaviors you would expect to see Darla exhibit.

4. Whenever a group of people come together to work on an issue or a project, conflict is a possibility. How could Darla intervene with the group to control conflict and keep them moving toward their goal?

Stakeholder analysis is a technique often used to identify potential group members. In the example (planning teen health services) in the Case Study on p. 389, two nurses initiated group development by inviting some teens from the local high school to come together to form an advisory group. At the first meeting, the nurses may have used the technique of stakeholder analysis to identify other teens who might represent segments of the student population not included in the first meeting. Similarly, when the group expanded and formed a community coalition, stakeholder analysis would have been a useful way to identify potential coalition members (Box 18-2).

Group Maintenance: Cohesion, Norms, and Conflict Resolution

As the expanded group moves into an active working phase, it must establish its rules of behavior (norms) and begin the process of developing group cohesion and conflict resolution. The success of this stage is related to sharing of leadership and participa-

BOX 18-2 HOW TO CONDUCT STAKEHOLDER ANALYSIS

1. Identify the specific issue, health topic, or problem that is the intended focus of the group.

2. List all agencies, organizations, and/or individuals who affect or are affected by the issue, health topic, or problem that is the intended focus of the group.

3. Narrow the list to a workable size by asking two questions about each potential participant:

   • What can this person, agency, or organization contribute to achieving this group's goal?

   • What will be lost if this person, agency, or organization does not participate in the group?

4. Refine the initial list, based on the answers in step 2, adding names and addresses of each person, agency, or organization who will be invited.

5. Invite each stakeholder to participate in the next group meeting.

tion and to the degree that goal achievement and group maintenance roles are fulfilled by group members.

Group Dissolution

When a group has achieved its stated purpose and goals, it is faced with the decision of whether to dissolve or continue with new goals and objectives (Keyton, 1993). The dissolution stage can be tricky if the group has developed tangible assets. In some cases, a group may decide to merge with another group having similar purposes. Consensus building and conflict resolution are essential if group dissolution is to be achieved in a positive manner.

Group Functions

Group functions may be divided into two categories: the activities that group members must perform if the group is to function effectively and efficiently and the role of groups themselves in creating the conditions that improved the health and quality of life of individuals and families in the community (change agent role).

Group Tasks

Groups must carry out two sets of tasks—internal maintenance tasks and goal attainment tasks—to function effectively. **Internal maintenance tasks** are the activities of group members that help

the group move smoothly through the stages of development, such as formation and maintenance of a teen advisory board and community coalition. **Goal attainment tasks** are the activities that must be performed by members of the group so that the group can define and achieve its collective purposes and desired outcomes, such as establishment of comprehensive teen health services that are acceptable and accessible.

Roles of Group Members

Although the entire group shares responsibility for these tasks, there are many different roles that individual members can play in carrying out these tasks (Charns & Schaefer, 1983; Clark, 1994a, 1994b; Cole, 1998; Maznevski, 1994).

Group Maintenance Roles

Behaviors that ensure good relationships among group members are needed for groups to survive, grow, and function effectively. The roles related to group maintenance help the group spend its time and energy on goal achievement rather than on meeting the needs of the membership. While reading about each role, think about what you would do to carry out each role if you were one of the nurses involved in one of the groups planning teen health services.

Gatekeeper: The role of the gatekeeper is to ensure that everyone who wants to make a contribution to the group has an opportunity to do so. This includes finding ways of allowing and encouraging quieter group members to voice their opinions, as well as helping more vocal group members express themselves in ways that do not dominate others. In recent years, some groups have been exploring the use of computers and decision science technology to facilitate gatekeeping.

Encourager: The encourager complements the work of the gatekeeper by creating a climate of acceptance within the group so that members feel free to express themselves.

Conflict manager: As noted earlier, conflict is an inherent part of effective group functioning. The role of the conflict manager is to facilitate a tone of harmony and compromise in which individuals with strongly held beliefs and opinions can modify their personal views in favor of the greater good of the group. A strategy that is often effective in reducing tension is the appropriate use of humor.

Standard setter/tester: When group relationships have broken down, the standard setter helps the group diagnose the situation and develop and implement standards of group behavior that will help correct the problem.

Goal Attainment Roles

The roles of group members related to achievement of shared goals and objectives reflect behaviors that move the group through a process of planning and decision making. Continue to think about what you would do if you were one of the nurses in the teen health services project as you read about group attainment roles.

Initiator: The initiator is responsible for stating and clarifying the group's goals, defining or specifying the problem (if any) being addressed, and proposing how the group should proceed. At first, the initiating behaviors may come from the formal group leader, but as the group matures, the initiating role is shared. For example, one of the nurses may have been the initiator during the first teen advisory board meeting, but teen members of the group also would fulfill initiator roles in later meetings.

Opinion and information seeker/giver: For a group to move forward with developing activities and interventions, it is critical that a member of the group facilitate honest and open sharing of diverse opinions and a wide array of information.

Clarification/elaboration builder: A group member who accepts this role is responsible for clarifying ideas and proposals presented to the group and for helping the group develop the communication and synergy to combine and build on individual ideas.

Summarizer: Periodically, someone in the group needs to summarize what is taking place so that important ideas and decisions are not lost. In some groups, the person who takes minutes may perform this role.

Decision-making facilitator: The decision-making facilitator checks group progress toward decision making and readiness for closure. Premature closure tends to result in decisions that are made with insufficient information or that lack member "buy in." On the other hand, group members become bored and restless when closure is delayed too long. Both extremes have a negative impact on group cohesion.

Consensus builder: The consensus builder helps the group frame diverse ideas and opinions into proposals or decisions that reflect the corporate wishes of the group.

As a student nurse, you have learned communication skills that will help you perform group maintenance and goal attainment roles when working with face-to-face groups. If your nursing care involves working with groups, your care plan should include strategies for helping group members develop the skills and knowledge needed for shared leadership and task-related roles.

Researchers from a variety of disciplines are examining the tasks and roles needed for successful computer-mediated groups. Although the task-related roles and communication skills are similar to those of face-to-face groups, there is an additional set of technology-related skills and knowledge that must be developed (Hollingshead & McGrath, 1995; Sosik, 1997).

Groups as Change Agents

Much of the current knowledge about group dynamics and groups as agents of **change** originates in the social psychology research conducted by Kurt Lewin in the 1930s and 1940s. Lewin found that the traditional methods of education, such as lecturing and individual instruction, were effective in transmitting units of information but did not result in learning and behavior change. Instead, he found that people learn best in a social con-

text through group discussion and decision-making approaches. Think about the various teaching/learning strategies you have encountered during your nursing education. Although you may have encountered copious amounts of information in lecture-based courses, it is likely that the courses using problem-based learning or group discussion focused on decision making have been more effective in helping you acquire the knowledge and skills that you use in the clinical setting.

Lewin also found that learning and behavior change were much greater in groups with democratic (participatory) leadership than in groups with autocratic (top-down) leadership (Lewin, 1949). Subsequent educational and health-related research not only has affirmed Lewin's findings but has contributed to the development of the highly effective **empowerment** approaches to health promotion and restoration (Minkler, 1997; Moreland & Hogg, 1993; Sampson & Marthas, 1981). The shared leadership and shared decision making approaches discussed earlier in this chapter are examples of how participatory leadership may be used in nursing practice with groups.

Concepts Related to Change

Lewin's subsequent research on motivation, behavior change, and group dynamics led to the development of two concepts of change that serve as the foundation for many contemporary health promotion and disease prevention models. The first concept, known as **force field analysis,** states that behavior is strongly influenced by the forces in the social fields surrounding people. Forces that promote or support change are considered *driving forces.* Forces that oppose or inhibit change are *restraining forces.* To bring about individual or collective change, the practitioner must analyze the strength and direction of the forces that are preserving the status quo and develop action steps to strengthen the driving forces, while diminishing or changing the direction of the restraining forces (see the following three figures on p. 395). The analysis and action steps are group activities in which all members participate. For example, during the planning process, community coalition members may have identified individuals, groups, and social norms that were supportive of or opposed to each of the health services proposed for the teen health center. If the forces opposing the service outweighed support for the service, the group might ask, "Are there ways we help people feel more positive about this service? If not, is the opposition so strong that we should not offer this service at the teen center?" It is especially useful to conduct force field analysis on controversial areas, such as contraception education or services for teens.

Lewin's second concept is that change occurs in stages. During the first stage, unfreezing, the forces that preserve the status quo are analyzed and strategies targeting specific driving and restraining forces are developed. In the second stage, moving, the strategies are implemented. The modified forces (e.g., new behaviors, policies, organizational structures) are tested and evaluated. In the third stage, refreezing, the changes that are to be

LEWIN'S CHANGE PROCESS.
STAGE 1: UNFREEZING. ANALYZE THE STRENGTH
AND DIRECTION OF FORCES PRESERVING STATUS QUO.

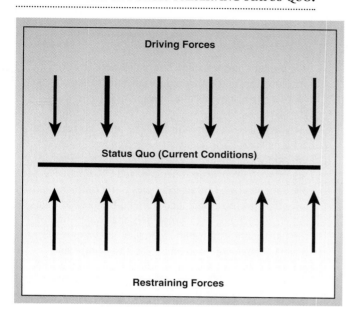

STAGE 3: REFREEZING. REINFORCE AND PRESERVE CHANGES.

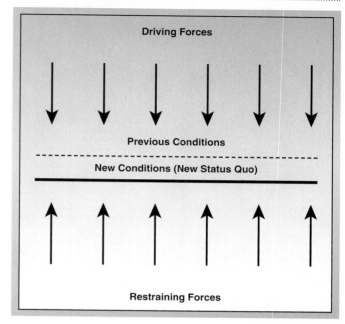

adopted are reinforced by repetition, policy change, and other long-term change approaches (Lewin, 1951).

For example, nurses may be involved in groups that have a goal of reducing health problems related to tobacco use. During

STAGE 2: MOVING. CHANGE THE STRENGTH
OR DIRECTION OF FORCES.

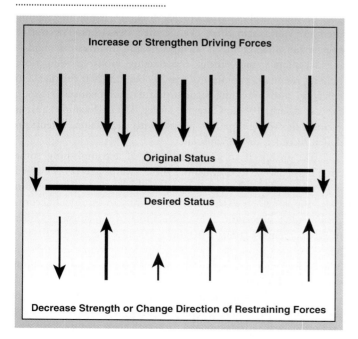

the unfreezing stage, group members would analyze a variety of physical, social, cultural, economic, educational, political, and environmental factors that provide positive or negative support for tobacco use by community members. One strategy might be to reduce the harmful effects of secondhand smoke in public places such as restaurants. The group might work with local restaurant owners to develop trial smoke-free nights and evaluate the impact of voluntary no-smoking policies on business (moving). If the trial period shows that business remains the same or increases, restaurant owners may adopt long-term smoke-free policies (refreezing). Furthermore, if restaurant owners develop positive opinions about smoke-free environments, they may be less of a restraining force (or may even become a driving force) if the group expands its strategies to include a local no-smoking ordinance.

Types of Groups

So far the main type of group discussed has been a health planning coalition. In reality, groups have diverse goals and purposes. Groups that nurses may find themselves working with to achieve health goals include educational or learning groups, support groups, self-help groups, therapy groups, task groups, focus groups, and coalitions (Aspen Reference Group, 1997). A nurse's role within a group depends on the type of group with whom she or he is working.

Educational or *learning* groups are designed to provide members with knowledge and understanding regarding a specific issue

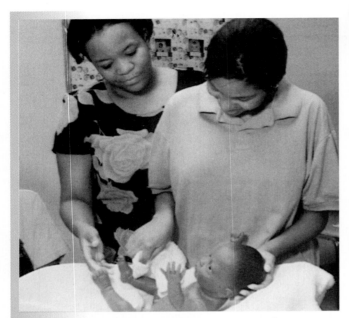

Parenting groups are an effective strategy for improving teen parenting skills.

RESEARCH BRIEF

Dumka, L. E., Garza, C. A., Roosa, M. W., & Stoerzinger, H. D. (1997). Recruitment and retention of high-risk families into a preventive parent training intervention. The Journal of Primary Prevention, 18(1), 25–39.

Recruitment and retention strategies were developed, implemented, and evaluated for an eight-session preventive parenting education program. This program was designed for high-risk minority parents from low-income inner-city communities. The program recruited 142 one- and two-parent families. Demographics of the sample were 78% Mexican immigrant or Mexican American, 15% African American, and 9% Anglo, Native American, and other. Examples of recruitment and retention strategies included framing the goal as helping children, having staff members that were fluent in the participants' preferred languages, showing respect, having convenient class schedules, providing transportation, and initiating mentoring and referral procedures. Implementation of recruitment and retention strategies resulted in a rate of 70% participation from the families recruited; 48% of the families attended five to eight sessions. Another 22% of families attended one to four sessions. Married and cohabiting mothers had a higher attendance rate than single mothers, as did Spanish-speaking mothers compared with English-speaking Hispanic mothers.

or area of need. The nurse's role in these groups is to provide structure and focus for group learning. The nurse may also be the educational provider (Toseland, 1995). Examples of educational groups include Lamaze childbirth classes and diabetes education programs.

Support groups help members cope with situational crises, life transitions, and a variety of chronic health problems through the provision of emotional support, information, and guidance. The nurse's role with support groups is to facilitate group interaction and process and to serve as a role model of acceptance (Schopler & Galinsky, 1993; Sharf, 1997; Yates, 1995). Examples of support groups are Alzheimer's caregiver groups, hospice bereavement groups, and breast cancer support groups.

Self-help groups are defined by self-governance and a common concern or problem. Group members provide each other with emotional support, information, education, social advocacy, and sometimes material aid. High value is placed on experiential knowledge as a form of special understanding of a group member's experiences. Although nurses and other health professionals generally do not have a formal role in these groups, health professionals often make referrals to these groups (Humphreys, 1997; Ogborne, 1996; Schubert & Borkman, 1991; Social Policy Corporation, 1997; Stewart, 1990). Examples of self-help groups are Alcoholics Anonymous and Overeaters Anonymous.

Therapy groups provide treatment, most often professional, for people experiencing an emotional disturbance. The primary goal of these groups is to provide members with insight into themselves and help them change their behaviors. The nurse's role within these groups is therapeutic and involves role modeling acceptance and caring, encouraging group participation, helping members explore the reasons behind their feelings and behavior, and providing structure and maintenance of group process (Clark, 1994a; Corey & Corey, 1992). Examples might include therapy groups for people with depression, attention-deficit disorder, or schizophrenia.

Task groups have a primary goal of accomplishing some specified activity. Consequently, these groups are time limited and disband when the task is completed. The nurse's role within task groups, which is to facilitate progress toward goal accomplishment, is determined by the membership position of leader or group member (Bracht, 1990; Skvoretz & Fararo, 1996). Examples of task groups include a community group to establish a recreation center or a group of teachers, parents, and the school nurse planning a health fair.

Focus groups provide a forum for obtaining data through group interviews about a variety of issues of concern to nurses and other health professionals. Although these groups have pri-

RESEARCH BRIEF

Houseman, C., Butterfoss, F. D., Morrow, A. L., & Rosenthal,
J. (1997). Focus groups among public, military, and private
sector mothers: Insights to improve the immunization process.
Public Health Nursing, 14(4), 235–243.

Six focus groups were conducted with 41 mothers (25
African Americans and 16 Caucasians) to gather information regarding immunizations and services received
in the public health (n = 27), military (n = 4), and
private (n = 10) sectors. Results indicated that these
women were positive about immunizations but identified many barriers to obtaining immunizations for
their children. Strategies for improving the immunization process included enhancing information dissemination, improving appointment and reminder systems,
decreasing waiting time, developing and/or improving
transportation systems, improving the clinic environment, and making immunizations less traumatic.

marily been used in the business arena for marketing purposes, nurses and other health professionals are now using the approach to obtain information from clients about health services and needs. The nurse's role within a focus group is to establish a non-threatening and positive environment and to facilitate group process (Aspen Reference Group, 1997; Butterfoss, Houseman, Morrow, & Rosenthal, 1997; Quible, 1998).

Coalitions bring together people, organizations, community groups, factions, and constituencies in a working group to influence outcomes on a specific issue or problem to achieve a common goal. Advantages of coalitions include conservation of resources, potential to reach more people, greater credibility in numbers, enhanced information exchange, and cooperation among participating groups (Aspen Reference Group, 1997; Wandersman, Goodman, & Butterfoss, 1997). The nurse's role may include chairperson, facilitator, or group member.

Working with Groups

This section is focused on general information about group leadership that can be adapted to a variety of settings. When working with specific types of groups, such as therapeutic or support groups, you should supplement the theory base you are using to guide your nursing care of groups with the research and theories specific to the specialty area linked to that type of group.

Group Leadership

Two leadership styles—democratic and autocratic—were identified earlier in the chapter as part of the discussion about change. Although the democratic leadership style is most closely associ-

ated with long-term learning and change, both styles have utility (Hickman, 1990; VanOostrum & Rabbie, 1995).

Democratic leadership, more commonly known as *participatory leadership*, refers to the approach that involves group members in all levels of information gathering, discussion, analysis, decision making, and evaluation. In a more restrictive form of democratic leadership, group members are presented with information as a basis for informed decision making. Participatory leadership builds group cohesion and contributes to individual and collective empowerment. A strength of participatory/shared leadership is that it builds a broad base of support for long-term change. A corresponding reality is that the decision-making and change process will take longer to achieve.

Autocratic leadership, also known as *authoritarian leadership*, is the "top-down" style of leadership found in many health care settings. The authoritarian leadership style also is reflected in the approach to teaching, planning, and behavior change used by many educators in the health professions. Two advantages of this approach are the volume of information that can be transmitted in a short time and the speed with which change can be made. On the negative side, knowledge does not necessarily lead to learning and growth, and changes made in this manner tend to be short-lived unless supported by major "selling" campaigns. Table 18-2 offers a comparison of different leadership styles.

America would be a better place if leaders would do more long-term thinking. In Iroquois society, leaders are encouraged to remember seven generations in the past and consider seven generations in the future when making decisions that affect people.
Wilma Mankiller, Principal Chief, Cherokee Nation

Both styles of leadership have some usefulness. When a decision must be made quickly or rapid change is essential, then a shift toward a more authoritarian leadership style may be indicated. For example, an infection control nurse might be working with a group of day-care center operators. During an outbreak of a communicable disease, the infection control nurse might *tell* the day-care operators what control measures they *must* adopt immediately to stop the outbreak (autocratic approach). However, in most group settings, the participatory leadership style is the preferred approach. For example, the infection control nurse might work with the group on a long-term basis to help the day-care operators develop and test the efficacy of a variety of strategies for preventing communicable diseases in their businesses (democratic approach). Furthermore, leadership style may be modified to fit with the capacities of group members. Factors such as age, physical or mental impairment, and physical disability may affect a group member's ability to engage in participatory or shared leadership (Cole, 1998; Seers & Woodruff, 1997; Toseland, 1995).

TABLE 18-2   **A COMPARISON OF LEADERSHIP STYLES**

	PARTICIPATORY LEADERSHIP	AUTHORITARIAN LEADERSHIP
Nurse's roles	Facilitator Partner with expertise	Director Expert information provider
Group members' roles	Co-leaders Partners with expertise Decision makers	Recipients of information Providers of feedback Targets of change
Leadership actions	Ask questions Stimulate/guide discussion Link to resource providers	Tell/lecture Lead discussion Arrange for resources
Outcomes	Learning Empowerment Sustained change	Short-term change Knowledge expansion

Ethical Considerations

Group leadership brings with it some ethical considerations. Group leaders potentially have great power. Many of the world's belief systems warn of the corrupting effects of power that is not grounded in a set of higher moral values and a sense of responsibility. Furthermore, a skillful leader may be tempted to guide the group in the direction he or she believes is best for the group. Another consideration is that shared leadership, empowerment, and change will likely shift the existing balance of power. You also may face the dilemma of realizing that a group's actions or decisions may adversely affect individuals within the group or others in the community. Different approaches to ethical decision making will generate questions to guide reflective thinking. Some of these questions may include "How is my leadership style affecting the lives of the members of the group?" "Whose goals are being pursued?" "How is the balance of power being shifted?" "Who potentially benefits from this group's decisions and actions?" and "Who is potentially harmed?"

Evaluating Groups

Groups may be evaluated for process, impact, and outcome. **Process evaluation** often is focused on group dynamics and interactions. A useful tool for process evaluation is the *group interaction diagram.* The evaluator draws a circle that includes the initials of each member of the group. For each interaction, the evaluator draws an arrow from the person talking to the person being addressed. The direction and number of the arrows will show communication patterns within the group. In authoritarian groups, most of the interaction will be between the leaders and individual members of the group. In participatory groups, the direction of the arrows should be more evenly distributed. The diagram will also identify both nonparticipants and discussion dominators. It may be helpful to begin a new diagram when a new topic is introduced or after a major decision is made. Each diagram should be labeled clearly. (The following figures show examples of group interaction diagrams.)

Impact evaluation focuses on intermediate behavior changes among group members or by those whose behavior the group is attempting to change. **Outcome evaluation** is based on the degree to which the group's goal and objectives have been met.

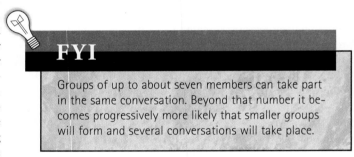

FYI

Groups of up to about seven members can take part in the same conversation. Beyond that number it becomes progressively more likely that smaller groups will form and several conversations will take place.

BEGINNING A PROCESS RECORDING DIAGRAM.

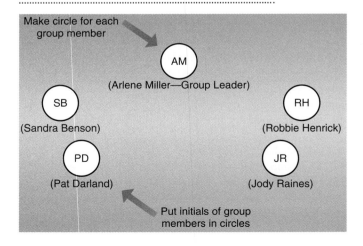

PROCESS RECORDING PATTERN ASSOCIATED WITH AUTHORITARIAN LEADERSHIP.

....

Discussion primarily between leader and individual group members.

PROCESS RECORDING PATTERN ASSOCIATED WITH DEMOCRATIC LEADERSHIP.

....

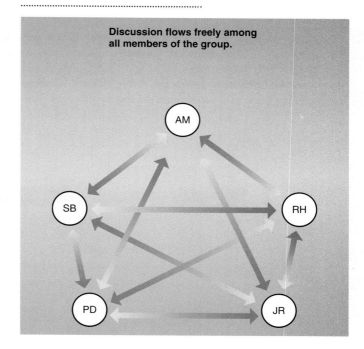

Discussion flows freely among all members of the group.

FYI

Groups of more than 10 or 12 people have difficulty taking part in the same conversation unless one member assumes a leader role and regulates interaction so that everyone has a chance to contribute. Conversations directed to the group tend to become more formal at this size. Group members "address" the group rather than talk.

FYI

Group think is a sociological phenomenon characterized by decision-making processes that are driven by consensus. The group tends to reject information or alternatives that do not fit with group's original plan.

CONCLUSION

In this chapter, several types of groups encountered in nursing practice have been described. Concepts, research, and strategies for effective nursing care of and with groups have been discussed. Although the focus of this chapter has been on working with small face-to-face groups, many of the concepts and skills are applicable to work with groups of all sizes, including community populations. For example, participatory leadership at the group level corresponds with the community development approach at the community level, and authoritarian leadership fits within the social planning model of community organization.

CRITICAL THINKING ACTIVITIES

1. As a student nurse, you are probably involved in a variety of on-campus and clinical groups. Observe the next meeting of one of these groups and answer the following questions:

   • Does everyone participate in discussions and decision making? What is happening in the group that fosters active participation? What are some of the barriers to active participation? Is leadership shared among various members of the group? What do you think about these observations?

   • In your community health nursing clinical group, brainstorm a list of ground rules for participation. Decide which ones you will adopt as a group. Post them and try them out at your next clinical group meeting. What are the outcomes of using these ground rules?

   • As a group, develop and implement some strategies for shared leadership. What are the outcomes?

   • What are the sources of conflict within the group? Is conflict viewed as a potential strength or as something to be avoided? How is conflict managed? In your clinical group, brainstorm some ground rules for positive conflict management. Try them out. Do they work? Why or why not?

2. Observe the different roles played by members of groups in which you are participating as a student nurse.

   • What are the goal achievement and group maintenance roles played by each person in the group? Does one person play more than one role? Do more two or more people play the same role?

   • What are the different strategies that you might use to assist a group in goal achievement and group maintenance?

3. In your community health nursing clinical group, take turns fulfilling each of the goal achievement and task maintenance roles.

   • Discuss your reactions and feelings related to each role. Evaluate each other's role performance. Which roles are most comfortable for you? Which roles do your classmates observe you performing most in other group settings?

   • Develop a list of facilitating questions for each role.

4. Interview a nurse who is facilitating a group over the Internet. (*Hint:* Some of the members of the nursing faculty may be conducting classes and groups using the Internet.)

   • How does this person facilitate group maintenance and goal attainment using the Internet?

- With your classmates, brainstorm how you would modify your behavior and questions for each group role if you were using the Internet.

5. Observe the various learning situations (formal and informal settings) that you have been in. Think about the various teaching/learning approaches and activities that you have encountered.

- Which approach(es) have involved you in reflection and critical thinking?
- What is the relation between knowledge and behavior?
- List 10 things that you know about health promotion but do not personally practice. Select one that you would like to target for change.
  - What are the driving and restraining forces that preserve your current behavior?
  - How can you change these forces? Develop an action plan that includes the stages of unfreezing, moving, and refreezing.
  - How would a group approach fit with your proposed change?
- List the groups in your community that fall into the category of groups that create or support change. How can you use these groups in nursing practice?
- Make a list of health-related groups in your community. What is the purpose of each group? How does each group contribute to the health of individuals, families, or populations in your community?
- Visit three of these groups. If possible, visit three different types of groups. Observe the behavior of group leaders. What leadership styles are being used? How well do these leadership styles fit with the group's type and purpose? What leadership style would you use with each group? Why?

6. There are many practical activities that must take place to ensure effective group meetings. Some of these activities may include arranging the time and place for the meeting, arranging the meeting room (e.g., lights, sound, seating, food, other resources, clean-up), inviting people to attend, setting the agenda, leading the meeting, taking minutes or notes (if appropriate), and evaluating outcomes. Select one of the types of group that might be found in one of your clinical settings. Make a table that has three columns. Label the first column "Practical Considerations." List all the specific activities that you can identify that would need to take place if your meeting is to be a success. Label the second and third columns "Participatory Leadership" and "Authoritarian Leadership." In the columns under each of these leadership styles, describe how you would ensure that the activities listed in the first column are carried out.

- What are the similarities between the second and third columns? the differences?
- What are the sets of skills needed for each of these leadership styles? Which of these skills do you already possess? What self-directed learning activities will help you expand your skills and knowledge base for effective group leadership?
- Which of these leadership styles are most comfortable for you? Why? What do you think about this?

7. You have been asked to develop an educational program about asthma for parents of elementary schoolchildren. One step you plan to use in developing the program is to bring together a focus group of parents to identify what they need to know.

- Describe and explain the selection process you will use to identify participants for the focus group.

CRITICAL THINKING ACTIVITIES—CONT'D

- What is your role as the group leader (before, during, and after the meeting)?
- How will you fulfill this role? What theories, concepts, and strategies will you use to guide your group leadership activities?

8. Observe the different ways that nurses work with groups in your community health clinical setting. Select one of these nurses and interview him or her.

- What types of groups does he or she work with?
- What is his or her role with each group?
- What skills does he or she think are needed to work with these groups effectively?
- What are the greatest challenges encountered when working with groups?
- What advice would he or she give to student nurses who will be working with groups in the community?
- Write a self-evaluation focused on working with groups. How effectively do you work in groups? What group-related skills, knowledge, and experience do you already possess? How can you strengthen these during your remaining nursing education? after graduation?
- What additional group-related skills, knowledge, and experience do you need to develop as part of your nursing education to increase your group work? after graduation?

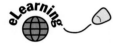

Explore Community Health Nursing on the web! To learn more about the topics in this chapter, use the passcode provided to access your exclusive web site:
http://communitynursing.jbpub.com
If you do not have a passcode, you can obtain one at this site.

REFERENCES

American Nurses Association (ANA). (1986). *Standards of community health nursing practice*. Washington, DC: Author.

American Nurses Association (ANA). (1991). *Standards of clinical nursing practice*. Washington, DC: Author.

American Nurses Association (ANA). (1996). *Scope and standards of advanced practice nursing practice*. Washington, DC: Author.

American Public Health Association (APHA). (1991). *Healthy communities 2000: Model standard* (3rd ed.). Washington, DC: APHA.

Aspen Reference Group. (1997). *Community health education and promotion: A guide to program design and evaluation*. Gaithersburg, MD: Aspen.

Berdahl, J., & Craig, K. (1996). Equality of participation and influence in groups: The effects of communication medium and sex composition. *Computer Supported Cooperative Work, 4*, 179–201.

Berman-Rossi, T. (1992). Empowering groups through understanding stages of group development. *Social Work with Groups, Special Issue, 5*(2–3), 239–255.

Bion, W. (1961). *Experiences in groups and other papers*. New York: Basic Books.

Bracht, N. (1990). *Health promotion at the community level*. Newbury Park, CA: Sage Publications.

Burnside, I. (1994). *Working with older adults: Group process and techniques*. Boston: Jones and Bartlett.

Butterfoss, F., Houseman, C., Morrow, A., & Rosenthal, J. (1997). Use of focus group data for strategic planning by a community-based immunization coalition. *Family and Community Health, 20*(3), 49–59.

Charns, M., & Schaefer, M. (1983). *Health care organizations: A model for management*. Englewood Cliffs, NJ: Prentice Hall.

Clark, N. (1994a). *The nurse as group leader*. New York: Springer.

Clark, N. (1994b). *Team building: A practical guide for trainers*. New York: McGraw-Hill.

Cole, M. (1998). *Group dynamics in occupational therapy*. Thorofare, NJ: Slack.

Cooke, R., & Szumal, J. (1994). The impact of group interaction styles on problem-solving effectiveness. *Journal of Applied Behavioral Science, 30*(4), 415–437.

Corey, M., & Corey, G. (1992). *Groups: Process and practice*. Pacific Grove, CA: Brooks-Cole.

Department of Health and Human Services (DHHS). (1991). *Healthy people 2000: National health promotion and disease prevention objectives. Full report with commentary*. Washington, DC: U.S. Government Printing Office.

Department of Health and Human Services (DHHS). (2000). *Healthy people 2010: Conference edition*. Washington, DC: U.S. Government Printing Office.

Dennis, A., & Valacich, J. (1994). Group, sub-group, and nominal group idea generation: New rules for a new media? *Journal of Management, 20*(4), 723–736.

Dumka, L. E., Garza, C. A., Roosa, M. W., & Stoerzinger, H. D. (1997). Recruitment and retention of high-risk families into a preventive parent training intervention. *The Journal of Primary Prevention, 18*(1), 25–39.

Feinberg, N. (1980). A study of group stages in a self-help setting. *Social Work with Groups, 3*(1), 41–50.

Hersey, P., & Blanchard, K. (1982). *Management of Organizational Behavior*. Englewood Cliffs, NJ: Prentice Hall.

Hickman, P. (1990). Community health and development: Applying sociological concepts to practice. *Sociological Practice, 8*, 125–132.

Hirokawa, R., & Keyton, J. (1995). Perceived facilitators and inhibitors of effectiveness in organizational work teams. *Management Communication Quarterly, 8*(4), 424–446.

Hollingshead, A., & McGrath, J. (1995). Computer-assisted groups: A critical review of the empirical research. In R. Guzzo, E. Salas, & Associates (Eds), *Team effectiveness and decision making in organizations*. San Francisco: Jossey-Bass.

Houseman, C., Butterfoss, F. D., Morrow, A. L., & Rosenthal, J. (1997). Focus groups among public, military, and private sector mothers: Insights to improve the immunization process. *Public Health Nursing, 14*(4), 235–243.

Humphreys, K. (1997). Individual and social benefits of self-help groups. *Social Policy, 27*(3), 12–19.

Kelley, L. (1995). Parse's theory in practice with a group in the community. *Nursing Science Quarterly, 8*(3), 127–132.

Keyton, J. (1993). Group termination: Completing the study of group development. *Small Groups Research, 24*(1), 84–100.

Laudon, K., & Laudon, J. (1988). *Management information systems: A contemporary perspective*. New York: Macmillan.

Lewin, K. (1949). Frontiers in group dynamics: Concept, method and reality in social science, social equilibrium, and social change. *Human Relations, 1*, 5–41.

Lewin, K. (1951). *Field theory in social science*. New York: Harper.

Loomis, M. E. (1979). *Group process for nurses*. St. Louis: Mosby.

Madara, E. (1997). The mutual-aid self-help online revolution. *Social Policy, 27*(3), 20–27.

Maznevski, M. (1994). Understanding our differences: Performance in decision-making groups with diverse members. *Human Relations, 47*(5), 531–550.

Minkler, M. (1997). *Community organizing & community building for health*. New Brunswick, NJ: Rutgers University Press.

Moreland, R., & Hogg, M. (1993). Theoretical perspectives on social processes in small groups. *British Journal of Social Psychology, 32*, 1–4.

Ogborne, A. (1996). Professional opinions and practices concerning Alcoholics Anonymous: A review of the literature and a research agenda. *Contemporary Drug Problems, 23*(1), 93–105.

Quible, Z. (1998). A focus on focus groups. *Business Communication Quarterly, 61*(2), 28–36.

Preboth, M., & Wright, S. (1999). Online support groups. *American Family Physician, 57*(6), 1379.

Ramey, J. (1993). Group empowerment through learning formal decision making processes. *Social Work with Groups, 16*(1–2), 171–185.

Reagan-Cirincione, P. (1994). Improving the accuracy of small group judgement: A process intervention combining group facilitation, social judgement analysis, and information technology. *Organizational Behavior and Human Decision Process, 58*(2), 246–270.

Sampson, E. E., & Marthas, M. (1981). *Group process for the health professions* (2nd ed.). New York: John Wiley and Sons.

Schitterkatte, M. (1996). Facilitating information exchange in small group decision-making groups. *European Journal of Social Psychology, 26*(4), 537–556.

Schopler, J. H., & Galinsky, M. J. (1993). Support groups as open systems: A model for practice and research. *Health and Social Work, 18*(3), 195–207.

Schubert, M. A., & Borkman, T. J. (1991). An organizational typology for self-help groups. *American Journal of Community Psychology, 19*(5), 769–787.

Seers, A., & Woodruff, S. (1997). Temporal pacing in task forces: Group development or deadline pressure? *The Journal of Management, 23*(2), 169–186.

Sharf, B. (1997). Communicating breast cancer on-line: Support and empowerment on the Internet. *Women & Health, 26*(1), 65–84.

Skvoretz, J., & Fararo, T. (1996). Status and participation in task groups: A dynamic network model. *American Journal of Sociology, 101*(5), 1366–1414.

Social Policy Corporation. (1997). The future of self-help. *Social Policy, 27*(3), 2–3.

Sosik, J. (1997). Effects of transformational leadership and anonymity on idea generation in computer-mediated groups. *Group and Organization Management, 22*(4), 460–487.

Stewart, M. J. (1990). Professional interface with mutual-aid self-help groups: A review. *Social Science and Medicine, 31*(10), 1143–1158.

Toseland, R. (1995). *Group work with the elderly and family caregivers*. New York: Springer.

Tuckman, B. (1965). Developmental sequence in small groups. *Psychological Bulletin, 63*(6), 384–399.

VanOostrum, J., & Rabbie, J. (1995). Intergroup competition and cooperation within autocratic and democratic management regimes. *Small Group Research, 26*(2), 269–195.

Veninga, R. (1982). *The human side of health administration: A guide for hospital nursing and local public health administrators*. Englewood Cliffs, NJ: Prentice Hall.

Wandersman, A., Goodman, R. M., & Butterfoss, F. D. (1997). Understanding coalitions and how they operate: An "open systems" organizational framework. In Minkler, M. (Ed.), *Community organizing & community building for health*. New Brunswick, NJ: Rutgers University Press.

Yalom, I. (1985). *The theory and practice of group psychotherapy*. New York: Basic Books.

Yates, R. (1995). *Developing support groups for individuals with early-stage Alzheimer's disease*. Baltimore: Health Professions Press.

Unit IV

Common Community Health Problems

Chapter 19

Communicable Disease

Sharyn Janes and Gale A. Spencer

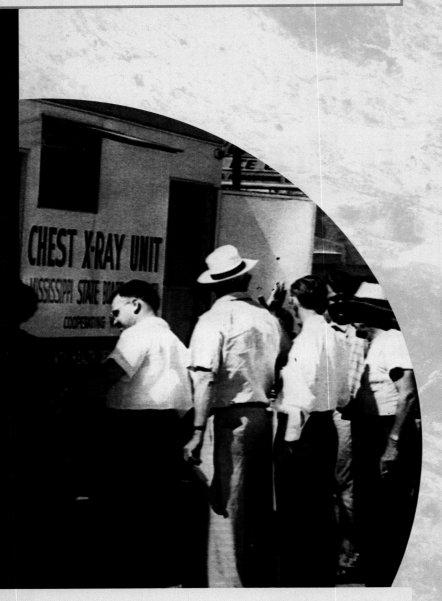

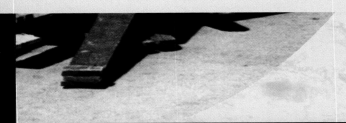

Some 1,500 people, mostly children and working age adults, will die in the next hour from infectious diseases, many that could be prevented for less than the cost of a few bottles of aspirin.

World Health Organization, June 17, 1999

QUESTIONS TO CONSIDER

After reading this chapter, answer the following questions:

1. What is the current infectious disease threat both in the United States and worldwide?
2. What are the reasons for the emergence of new diseases and the reemergence of diseases previously under control?
3. What are the factors that make up the chain of infection?
4. What are the different types of immunity?
5. How do vaccines aid in the prevention of communicable disease?
6. What is the role of the community health nurse in the prevention and treatment of infectious disease?

KEY TERMS

Acquired immunity	Immunity	Period of infectivity	Vector
Active humoral immunity	Incubation period	Personal surveillance	Virulence
Agent	Isolation	Quarantine	Zoonoses
Fomites	Passive immunity	Reservoir	
Herd immunity	Pathogenicity	Segregation	

The Problem of Communicable Disease

Communicable disease, or infectious disease, has always been a focus of community health nursing practice. In fact, at the end of the 19th century, when public health nursing emerged as a nursing specialty, communicable diseases were the leading cause of illness and death. During the early years of the 20th century, nurses continued to care for large numbers of adults and children who were sick or dying from a wide variety of infectious diseases. The typhoid epidemic in the early 1900s and the great influenza

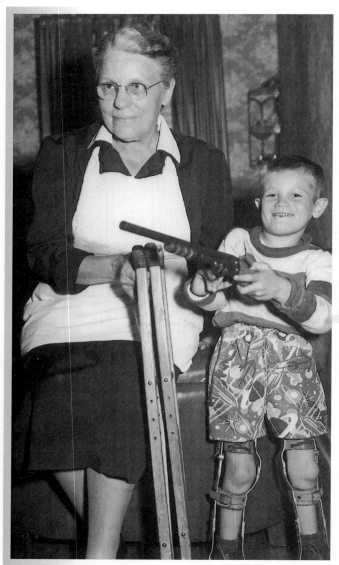

A home visit provided the public health nurse with an opportunity to assess a child with polio in familiar surroundings (circa 1951).

pandemic of 1918, which killed 20 million people worldwide (CDC, 1998a), are just two examples of infectious diseases that caused enormous suffering and death. Tuberculosis (TB) was a leading killer until well into the 1930s and 1940s, when TB sanitariums were overflowing. Nursing students in hospital schools in bigger cities were routinely tested for antibodies against TB, and most of them who came from rural areas tested positive. After a year in the urban hospital wards of the 1930s and 1940s, it was almost a certainty that nursing students would test positive for TB (Garrett, 1994).

The development of antibiotics, particularly penicillin, in the mid-1940s curbed the spread of bacterial infections and significantly decreased the number of deaths from infectious diseases like TB and typhoid fever. Vaccinations against diseases such as polio, whooping cough, and diphtheria, along with urban sanitation efforts and improved water quality, dramatically lowered the incidence of infectious diseases (CDC, 1998a). So although infectious disease still took an enormous toll in the rest of the world, a shift in leading causes of morbidity and mortality from infectious diseases to chronic diseases in industrialized nations like the United States caused attention to be focused on chronic conditions such as heart disease, cancer, and diabetes. Antibiotics became the "wonder drugs" of the latter half of the 20th century, and modern medicine triumphed. Or so we thought.

As early as the 1950s, penicillin began to lose its effectiveness against infections caused by *Staphylococcus aureus*. In 1957, and again in 1968, new strains of influenza originating in China rapidly spread throughout the world. During the 1970s, several new diseases were identified in the United States and elsewhere, including Legionnaires' disease, Lyme disease, toxic shock syndrome, and Ebola hemorrhagic fever. The 1980s brought human immunodeficiency virus/acquired immunodeficiency syndrome (HIV/AIDS) and a resurgence of TB, which rapidly spread throughout the world. By the 1990s, it was apparent that the threat of infectious disease was again a global reality (CDC, 1998a).

Now that we have entered the 21st century, we are again faced with infectious diseases that challenge medical and nursing practice. Some are old and familiar, like TB and influenza, and others are new and unfamiliar, like Ebola and hantavirus. Many of the new challenges are viral in origin, but the overuse and misuse of antibiotics over the last half century have also caused drug-resistant and often fatal strands of bacterial infections to emerge (Box 19-1). In fact, in much of the world, the most dangerous emerging diseases are not viral but bacterial or parasitic (Garrett, 1994).

The entire world is becoming much more vulnerable to the eruption and spread of both new and old infectious diseases. Infectious disease is a global problem brought about by recent dramatic increases in the worldwide movement of people, goods, and ideas. Not only are people traveling more, but they

BOX 19-1 FACTS ABOUT ANTIBIOTICS AND ANTIBIOTIC RESISTANCE

- Alexander Fleming, a Scottish scientist, discovered the first antibiotic in 1928.
- Antibiotics became widely available in the 1940s.
- Two million pounds of antibiotics were produced in the United States in 1954. Today, more than 50 million pounds are produced.
- Antibiotics work by either killing bacteria or inhibiting their growth. They do not work on viral infections.
- People consume more than 235 million doses of antibiotics yearly. The Centers for Disease Control and Prevention estimates that 20% to 50% of that use is unnecessary.
- Antibiotic resistance occurs when bacteria causing a specific infection are not destroyed by the antibiotics taken to halt the infection. Unnecessary and improper use of antibiotics promotes the spread of antibiotic-resistant bacteria.

Source: Data from CDC, 1999a.

States. Some of the contributing factors are the emergence of new diseases, poverty, environmental changes, mass population shifts, and economic and social globalization. It is interesting to note that five of the six communicable diseases included on the list of the 10 deadliest diseases in the world were previously thought to have been contained, according to the World Health Organization's 1997 World Health Report (*Drug resistance,* 1998) (Table 19-1).

• •

The single biggest threat to man's continued dominance on the planet is the virus.

Joshua Lederberg, Nobel Laureate

• •

To address the increasing threat of infectious diseases, nurses must understand the problem from global and historical perspectives. There are many roles for nurses in the battle against infectious diseases. From a community health nursing perspective, primary and secondary prevention concepts must guide nursing practice. A holistic approach that includes health education, environmental health, political action, human rights, and cultural competency is the key. Communicable disease is, after all, not a new concept. Microbes have been an enemy of humans since ancient times. They did not disappear just because science developed drugs and vaccines or because Europeans and Americans cleaned up their cities and towns, and they certainly will not go away when humans choose to ignore or downplay their existence (Garrett, 1994). This chapter describes the present-day threat of infectious diseases and explores the role of community health nurses. Selected *Healthy People 2010* objectives related to communicable diseases are listed on the following page.

are traveling more rapidly and going to more places than ever before (Mann, 1994). Currently, one of every three people throughout the world dies from infectious diseases each year. Infectious diseases are the number one cause of death worldwide and are the sixth leading cause of death in the United

TABLE 19-1   TEN MOST DEADLY DISEASES

NAME OF DISEASE	COMMUNICABLE OR NONCOMMUNICABLE	DEATHS (IN MILLIONS)
1. Coronary heart disease	Noncommunicable	7.2
2. Cancer (all types)	Noncommunicable	6.3
3. Cerebrovascular accident	Noncommunicable	4.6
4. Acute lower respiratory infection	Communicable	3.9
5. Tuberculosis	Communicable	3.0
6. Chronic obstructive pulmonary disease	Noncommunicable	2.9
7. Diarrheal diseases	Communicable	2.5
8. Malaria	Communicable	2.1
9. HIV/AIDS	Communicable	1.5
10. Hepatitis B	Communicable	1.2

[1]Diseases in bold color represent reemerging infectious diseases.

Source: American Association for World Health, 1998c.

HEALTHY PEOPLE 2010

OBJECTIVES RELATED TO COMMUNICABLE DISEASES

Food Safety

10.1   Reduce infections caused by food-borne pathogens.

10.2   Prevent an increase in the proportion of isolates of *Salmonella* species from humans and from animals at slaughter that are resistant to antimicrobial drugs.

10.6   Improve food employee behaviors and food preparation practices that directly relate to food-borne illnesses in retail food establishments.

Immunization and Infectious Diseases

Diseases Preventable Through Universal Vaccination

14.1   Reduce or eliminate indigenous cases of vaccine-preventable disease.

14.2   Reduce hepatitis B.

14.5   Reduce invasive pneumococcal infections.

Diseases Preventable Through Targeted Vaccination

14.6   Reduce hepatitis A.

14.7   Reduce Lyme disease.

Infectious Diseases and Emerging Antimicrobial Resistance

14.9   Reduce hepatitis C.

14.11   Reduce tuberculosis.

14.15   Increase the proportion of international travelers who receive recommended preventive services when traveling in areas of risk for select infectious diseases: hepatitis A, malaria, typhoid.

Vaccination Coverage and Strategies

14.27   Increase routine vaccination coverage levels of adolescents.

14.29   Increase the proportion of adults who are vaccinated annually against influenza and ever vaccinated against pneumococcal disease.

14.30   Reduce vaccine-associated adverse events.

Source: DHHS, 2000.

Transmission of Infectious Agents

The role of nurses in the control of infectious disease prevention and treatment is based on an understanding of ways in which diseases are transmitted from one person to another. *Transmission* is "any mechanism by which an infectious agent is spread from a source or reservoir to a person" (Benenson, 1995, p. 544). There are three general modes of transmission: direct, indirect, and airborne.

Chain of Infection

The chain of infection is defined as the minimum requirements for an infectious or communicable disease to occur. Six factors make up the chain of infection: (1) an etiological agent or pathogen, (2) a source or reservoir of infection, (3) a means of escape from the source or reservoir (portal of exit), (4) a mode of transmission, (5) a portal of entry into the new host, and (6) a susceptible host.

The causative **agent** or pathogen is any substance or factor that can cause disease. Agents may be bacteria, virus particles, chemicals, or any other plant or animal substance that can cause illness, disease, disability, or death. Causative agents differ both in their ability to cause disease and in their ability to cause serious illness. **Pathogenicity** refers to the agent's capacity to cause disease in an infected host, whereas **virulence** defines the ability of the agent to produce serious illness. For example, both botulism and salmonella are highly pathogenic agents (they can easily cause disease), but botulism is much more virulent (it causes more severe disease).

The source of infection, or **reservoir**, is the habitat or medium in which the agent lives and/or multiplies. Reservoirs can be living things (e.g., humans, animals, insects) or inanimate objects (e.g., food, intravenous [IV] fluids, feces, surgical instruments, stuffed animals) that are conducive to the maintenance or growth of the agent. Reservoirs of infection are human beings, animals, and environmental sources. Humans become reservoirs of infection when the infectious agent has entered the body and established itself. There are three levels of infection in humans: (1) colonization, (2) inapparent infection, and (3) clinically overt disease.

Colonization occurs when the agent is present on the surface of the body or in the nasopharynx and multiplies at a rate sufficient to maintain its numbers without producing any identifiable evidence of a reaction in the person. Inapparent infection (subclinical infection) occurs when the agent is not only present but multiplies in the human reservoir. In an inapparent infection, the agent causes a measurable reaction; however, it does not cause the human to have symptoms of illness. Inapparent infections are usually identified only through laboratory testing (Benenson, 1995). Finally, clinical disease occurs when the agent is present in the human and causes physical symptoms. The time interval between initial contact with an infectious agent and the first appearance of disease symptoms is the **incubation period** (Benenson, 1995). The communicable period, or **period of infectivity,** is the time during which an infectious agent may be transferred directly or indirectly from an infected person to another person, from an infected animal to humans, or from an infected person to animals. All infected persons, including those with colonization, are reservoirs for the agent. Animal reservoirs are mainly domestic animals and rodents.

Zoonoses are animal diseases that are transmissible to humans under natural conditions. Animals transmit the disease directly to humans, but these diseases usually are not transmitted from human to human. Examples of zoonoses are bovine TB, rabies (although theoretically it can be transmitted by humans), and anthrax. Environmental reservoirs also transmit directly to humans. An example of an environmental reservoir is hookworm in soil. Inanimate objects such as food, surgical instruments, and human feces can also be reservoirs for diseases.

The agent leaves the reservoir through a portal of exit. Portals of exit and portals of entrance are similar. They include the following, listed in order, starting with the more common portals: respiratory, oral, gastrointestinal, reproductive, IV, urinary, skin, cardiovascular, conjunctival, and transplacental.

The last factor in the chain of infection is a susceptible host. The agent must enter a human host who is vulnerable to the specific disease agent. Susceptibility can be related to factors such as age, immunological status, lifestyle habits, or the presence of other infectious diseases or chronic illnesses.

Routes of Infection

The agent then must be transmitted to the next susceptible host through a mode of transmission. Transmission can be direct, indirect, or airborne.

Direct transmission consists of the direct and immediate transfer of an infectious agent from one infected host or reservoir to a portal of entry in the new host. This may be through direct contact that occurs through biting, kissing, or sexual intercourse or by direct projection of droplet spray into the conjunctiva of the eye or mucous membranes of the eye, nose, or mouth. The projection of droplet spray occurs with sneezing, coughing, talking, singing, or spitting and is usually limited to a distance of approximately 1 meter (Benenson, 1995).

Indirect transmission usually occurs through a vector or by a vehicle. A **vector** is some form of living organism, usually an animal or an arthropod. Arthropods are insects such as flies and mosquitoes. Flies often carry organisms that are picked up on their feet or proboscis and transferred to food or water. When the organism is carried in this manner, it is called *mechanical vector-borne transmission* because the organism (or agent) does not multiply in the carrier. Mosquitoes, however, are often carriers of biological vector-borne transmission as multiplication and development of the organism occurs in the mosquito before the organism is transmitted to the new host through a bite (or inoculation). An example of this type of vector-borne disease is the transmission of malaria by the bite of a mosquito.

Vehicle-borne transmission is defined as contaminated inanimate objects, called **fomites,** which serve as an intermediate means by which an infectious agent is transported and introduced into a susceptible host through an appropriate portal of entry (Benenson, 1995). Examples of fomites are toys, bedding, soiled clothes, surgical instruments, and contaminated IV fluids. An example of a vehicle-borne disease is salmonella, which can be transmitted from a kitchen countertop contaminated while thawing raw chicken for dinner.

Airborne transmission occurs through droplet nuclei and dust, which are particles suspended in the air in which microorganisms may be present. Droplet nuclei result from the evaporation of fluid from droplets disseminated by coughing, talking, or sneezing between one infected person and another host. Droplet nuclei can remain suspended in the air for long periods in a dry state. During this time, some droplet nuclei retain their infectivity, while others lose their infectivity or virulence. The particles are very small and are easily breathed into the lungs, where they are retained. When these particles reach the terminal air passages, they begin to multiply and an infection begins in the new host (Benenson, 1995). Pulmonary TB and legionellosis (Legionnaires' disease) are two illnesses that are transmitted by droplet nuclei.

Dust particles in which microorganisms may be present can also become airborne and thus can be breathed into the lungs and cause infection. Contaminated bedding and clothes are examples of objects that can create dust that may carry infectious microorganisms from one infected person to another host. Dust particles contaminated with deer mouse feces may be one way to transmit hantavirus to human hosts.

The cycle of transmission can be broken by breaking the chain of infection—by eliminating the agent, eliminating the reservoir of infection, eliminating transmission at the portal of exit or the portal of entry, or eliminating susceptible hosts.

Susceptibility Versus Immunity

For a disease to be transmitted, the new host must be susceptible to that disease. The concept of immunity forms the basis of understanding host resistance to disease. **Immunity** is the increased resistance on the part of the host to a specific infectious agent (Valanis, 1999). There are two types of acquired immunity found in humans: active and passive.

Acquired immunity can occur after having had the disease or through vaccination. If a person is infected with the disease

BOX 19-2   VACCINE-PREVENTABLE DISEASES

Adenovirus	Meningococcal
Anthrax	infections
Cholera	Mumps
Chickenpox (varicella)	Pertussis
Diphtheria	Plague
Hepatitis A	Pneumococcal
Hepatitis B	pneumonia
Haemophilus	Polio
influenzae	Rabies
Influenza	Tetanus
Japanese encephalitis	Typhoid
Measles	Yellow fever

Source: CDC, 1994.

Communicable Disease Prevention

One of the foundations of public health is the prevention and control of communicable disease. Timmreck (1998) states that the three key factors in the control of communicable disease are as follows:

1. *The removal, elimination, or containment of the cause or source of infection*

2. *The disruption and blockage of the chain of disease transmission*

3. *The protection of the susceptible population from infection and disease*

Approaches to the control of communicable disease should be based on the levels of prevention—primary, secondary, and tertiary.

Primary Prevention

Primary prevention activities are targeted at intervening before the agent enters the host and causes pathological changes. This level of prevention attempts to increase the host's resistance, inactivate the agent (source of infection), or interrupt the chain of infection.

A major focus of primary prevention is on increasing the resistance of the host. This can be accomplished through health education and/or immunization. Health education can target many subjects to increase the resistance of the host. It can identify a variety of activities that will improve the host's resistance, such as frequent handwashing, proper nutrition, adequate rest, and proper attire. Immunization is another method of primary prevention that increases the host's resistance. Immunization uses vaccines that are obtained either from the agent in a killed, modified, or variant form or from fractions or products of the agent (Valanis, 1999). Vaccines are available for many common infectious diseases. See Box 19-2 for a list of vaccine-preventable diseases.

Inactivating the agent involves stopping the agent by chemical or physical means. The protection of food has become particularly important in the last few years, with frequent foodborne illness outbreaks occurring as a result of improper storage, preparation, and handling. Proper temperatures must be maintained to inactivate the agent when storing, preparing, and cooking food. Proper food handling, which includes handwashing during preparation, is also important. Many bacterial agents (e.g., staphylococci, salmonellae, and *Escherichia coli*) can contaminate food and make the consumers of the food extremely sick. Irradiation of food (particularly beef and vegetables) has been suggested as a method of control, but this continues to be vigorously debated. Chemical methods are also used to inactivate agents. Chemical methods are used to chlorinate water supplies and to treat sewage, as well as to disinfect infectious or potentially infectious materials.

A common method of breaking the chain of infection is environmental control. Environmental control is aimed at providing clean and safe air, food, milk, and water; managing solid

(with or without clinical signs and symptoms), the disease agent stimulates the body's natural immune system. However, if the person is inoculated with the agent (in a killed, modified, or variant form), the vaccination artificially stimulates the immune system (see Box 19-2 for a list of vaccine-preventable diseases). Both methods of acquired immunity result in active humoral immunity because the human body produces its own antibodies when the immune system is stimulated. **Active humoral immunity** is based on a B-lymphocyte response, which results in immunity that lasts for several years with diseases such as tetanus or a lifetime with diseases such as measles or mumps (Benenson, 1995). **Passive immunity** can be acquired either through the transplacental transfer of the mother's immunity to a disease to her unborn child or from the transfer of already-produced antibodies into a susceptible person (such as the use of immune serum globulin for persons exposed to hepatitis A). Passive immunity is based on a cellular, T-lymphocyte sensitization. Passive immunity is of short duration, lasting from days to months (Benenson, 1995).

Herd immunity is the resistance of a population or group to the invasion and spread of an infectious agent (Benenson, 1995). Herd immunity is based on the level of resistance a population has to a communicable disease because of the high proportion of group members in the population who cannot get the disease because they have been previously vaccinated or have previously had the disease. Jonas Salk, one of the developers of the polio vaccine, suggested that if 85% of the population were immunized against polio (the herd immunity level), a polio epidemic would not occur (Timmreck, 1998). Herd immunity provides barriers to the direct transmission of infection through a group or population because the lack of susceptible individuals in the population stops the spread of infection.

waste (garbage) and liquid waste (sewage); and controlling vectors (insects and rodents). Environmental control may target the reservoir, such as chlorination of a water supply. Environmental control may also be aimed at destroying the vector that transports the agent. One way a community may target the vector is to spray swamp areas (known to serve as reservoirs) with an insecticide to prevent mosquito-borne viral encephalitis. However, when this method is used, care must be taken to preserve the ecosystem as much as possible. Another method of breaking the chain of transmission is to encourage good personal hygiene and use of protective clothing. Methicillin-resistant *S. aureus* (MRSA) is an increasingly difficult nosocomial infection seen on medical and surgical floors in hospitals and in nursing homes. Health care providers must protect themselves and their clients by using proper hygiene and standard precautions when caring for all clients.

Primary prevention also includes restricting the spread of infection to human reservoirs and preventing the spread to other susceptible human hosts (Valanis, 1999). The four most commonly used methods are isolation, quarantine, segregation, and personal surveillance.

Isolation is the separation of infected persons during the period of communicability (Benenson, 1995; Valanis, 1999). These infected persons may be under one of several different types of isolation (strict isolation, contact isolation, respiratory isolation, tuberculosis isolation, enteric precautions, and drainage/secretion precautions). See Valanis's *Epidemiology in Health Care* (1999) or Harkness's *Epidemiology in Nursing Practice* (1995) for identification of types of isolation and diseases requiring precautions.

Quarantine is the restriction of healthy persons who have been exposed to a person with a communicable disease during the period of communicability. These persons are considered contacts of the infected human host. Quarantine prevents further transmission of the disease during the incubation period if the healthy contacts should become infected. Quarantine usually occurs for the longest usual incubation period of the disease. Quarantine is rarely if ever used today; however, before vaccination for diphtheria, it was often used in the United States.

Segregation is another method to control the spread of communicable disease. It is used to separate and observe a group of people who are infected with a specific disease. Segregation has been used in some countries to separate HIV-infected individuals from the general public in order to control the spread of AIDS. The United States still has public health laws that allow the segregation of persons with TB; however, those laws are rarely enforced, although in the early part of the 20th century, persons with TB were segregated from the general public in hospitals known as *sanitariums*. With the advent of new drug therapies and treatment, these sanitariums are no longer necessary.

Personal surveillance is close medical or other supervision of contacts and identified carriers of a specific disease without restricting their personal movement (Benenson, 1995). For example,

public health officials continue to require personal surveillance of persons known to have had TB and to be carriers of typhoid.

As distinct from personal surveillance, disease surveillance is the continuing investigation of all incidence and spread of a disease that are relevant to effective control (Benenson, 1995). Public health surveillance is the systematic collection, analysis, interpretation, dissemination, and use of health information. Surveillance and data systems provide information on morbidity, mortality, and disability. Surveillance information is used to plan, implement, and evaluate public health programs to control communicable disease. To provide maximum benefits, surveillance data must be accurate, timely, and available in useful form (DHHS, 1991).

Although successful disease surveillance involves collaboration among federal, state, and local agencies, the U.S. Public Health Service (PHS) takes a leading role. PHS activities include collecting and analyzing health information at the national, regional, and when possible, state and local levels; providing data to federal, state, and local agencies for further analysis or use; assisting states and local agencies in conducting public health surveillance and evaluating data; and coordinating a network of federal, state, and local public health surveillance for diseases of public health importance (DHHS, 1991).

Secondary Prevention

Secondary prevention activities are targeted at detecting disease at the earliest possible time to begin treatment, stop progression, and initiate primary prevention activities to protect others in the community. Secondary prevention in infectious disease contributes to primary prevention because it restricts the infection to the human reservoir and prevents its spread to other susceptible individuals. Case finding and health screening are common activities used to accomplish this task. An example of case finding is following up on food handlers who may be infected during an outbreak of hepatitis. Screening for new cases of diseases can significantly decrease the spread of infection. Examples include screening for TB, through tuberculin testing, to detect and treat cases of TB among new immigrants; screening for herpes simplex virus type 2 in pregnant women to prevent infection to the infant during the birth process; screening for venereal diseases as a requirement for marriage licenses in some states; and administering gamma-globulin or immune serum after exposure to hepatitis.

Health education also plays a significant role in secondary prevention because it provides education about signs and symptoms, which enables individuals to identify illness and seek care early. Knowledge of health risk behaviors that contribute to the spread of disease may influence infected individuals to modify their behavior and thus assist in the prevention of the spread of disease.

Tertiary Prevention

Tertiary prevention limits the progression of disability (Timmreck, 1998). Hearing impairment from frequent ear infections, paralyzed limbs from polio, impaired vision from severe con-

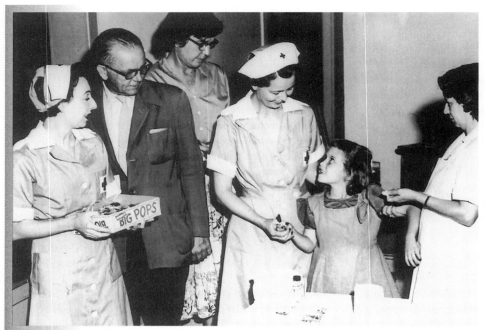

Nurses and physician administering Salk polio vaccine to a child (circa 1955).

junctivitis, and shingles are just a few of the possible disabilities resulting from infectious disease. Treatment of symptoms and rehabilitation vary with each specific disease.

Control of Diseases

Vaccine-Preventable Diseases

Immunization is one of the most accepted and cost-effective preventive health practices in the United States. In the last 50 years, vaccines have prevented countless days of illness and hundreds of thousands of deaths. Most health care providers take for granted the rarity of vaccine-preventable diseases; many health care providers will never see a child with diphtheria, measles, or polio. Childhood immunization needs and practices are discussed in chapter 34. Therefore, this chapter focuses on the vaccine-preventable diseases of adults and the need for adults to be immunized against them.

Adult immunization is extremely important. Approximately 70,000 adults in the United States die each year from vaccine-preventable diseases or their complications, compared with approximately 500 people (children and adults) who die of childhood vaccine-preventable diseases (Gardner & Schaffner, 1993; Thurm, 1998). Between 1980 and 1992, the number of deaths from infectious diseases rose 58% in the United States. Even when HIV-associated diagnoses are removed, deaths from infectious diseases still increased 22% during this period (DHHS, 2000). In fact, each year in the United States alone, at least 45,000 adults die

SABIN ORAL SUNDAY

POLIO PREVENTION PROGRAM

This Certifies That

Ruth Sancier

(NAME)

HAS RECEIVED SABIN ORAL POLIO VACCINE TYPE:

(1)   (3)   (2)

BRING THIS CARD FOR NEXT IMMUNIZATION. AFTER THIRD IMMUNIZATION, GIVE CARD TO YOUR FAMILY DOCTOR.

SABIN ORAL SUNDAY

POLIO PREVENTION PROGRAM

This Certifies That

Marshall Sancier

(NAME)

HAS RECEIVED SABIN ORAL POLIO VACCINE TYPE:

(1)   (3)   (2)

BRING THIS CARD FOR NEXT IMMUNIZATION. AFTER THIRD IMMUNIZATION, GIVE CARD TO YOUR FAMILY DOCTOR.

Vaccination cards from polio prevention program (circa 1956).

As informed providers, nurses are in a unique position to educate health planners, legislators, and community leaders about immunizations and preventive care. Nurses can serve as advocates for immunizations personally and through professional organizations.

At a time when costs are skyrocketing, it is encouraging to know how much can be accomplished with relatively low cost prevention. Nurses need to be in the forefront to inform our citizens about health promotion and prevention activities as important aspects of personal health care.

—Hillary Rodham Clinton
Source: Clinton, 1993.

from complications resulting from influenza, pneumonia, or hepatitis B, despite the availability of safe and effective vaccines to prevent these diseases. Approximately 90% of flu-related deaths occur in people age 65 and older (Thurm, 1998).

Hepatitis

Viral hepatitis encompasses several distinct infections. All are hepatatrophic and have similar clinical presentations. However, they differ in their cause and in some clinical, pathological, immunological, and epidemiological characteristics. Their prevention and control also vary (Benenson, 1995).

Hepatitis A

Hepatitis A is a highly contagious viral infection of the liver. In 1995, 31,582 cases were reported in the United States (CDC, 1995a). However, it is the most common vaccine-preventable disease in travelers (*Fact about hepatitis A for adults,* 1996). The hepatitis A virus (HAV) is found in the stool of infected people. The mode of transmission is person to person by the fecal-oral route. The infection is passed on by infected persons who do not wash their hands after having a bowel movement and contaminate everything they touch. Outbreaks have been related to contaminated water and to food prepared by food handlers who are infected with the hepatitis A virus. People are also infected with hepatitis A by eating contaminated raw shellfish, fruits, or vegetables.

People at risk for being infected with hepatitis A include the following (*Hepatitis learning guide,* 1998):

* *Those who share a household with someone who is infected with hepatitis A*
* *Individuals in a day-care center (adult employees or children) where a child or employee is infected with hepatitis A*

* *Those who travel to countries such as Africa, Asia (other than Japan), the Caribbean, Central and South America, Eastern Europe, the Mediterranean basin, and the Middle East*
* *Residents or staff of custodial institutions*
* *Homosexual men*

The symptoms of hepatitis A differ from person to person. Although many people infected with hepatitis A have no symptoms (particularly children), those with symptoms usually have an identifiable pattern. These symptoms include fever, nausea, vomiting, jaundice, diarrhea, fatigue, abdominal pain, dark urine, and loss of appetite. Respiratory symptoms, joint pain, and rash occasionally occur (*Facts about hepatitis A for adults,* 1996).

The incubation period is from 15 to 50 days, with the average time being approximately 28 days. The period of infectivity is during the last half of the incubation period, up to and including a few days after the onset of jaundice (Benenson, 1995).

Hepatitis A is prevented through the following means (Benenson, 1995):

* *Vaccination with the hepatitis A vaccine (with an initial injection providing protection for up to 1 year, with a booster dose [6 to 12 months after the first dose] providing prolonged protection)*
* *Education of the public about good sanitation and proper hygiene, with careful emphasis on handwashing*
* *Proper water and sewage treatment*
* *Education of employees in child day-care centers about the need for thorough handwashing after every diaper change and before feeding children or eating*
* *Immunization of child day-care employees*
* *Cooking shellfish to the proper temperature (85 to 90° C, or 185 to 190° F)*
* *Immunization with the hepatitis A vaccine of all travelers going to developing countries*

Hepatitis B

Hepatitis B is also a highly contagious virus that infects the liver. It is caused by the hepatitis B virus (HBV), which infects approximately 300,000 Americans annually. In the United States, more than 1 million people are chronically infected with HBV. Globally, there are an estimated 300 million HBV carriers (*Hepatitis learning guide,* 1998). The virus is found in the blood and body fluids of infected people. All persons who test positive for the hepatitis B antigen are potentially infectious. The mode of transmission can be person to person through sexual contact as well as through direct contact with blood or blood products resulting from sharing of needles or razors and from infected mother to infant during the birthing process. Hepatitis B is often described as a silent disease because it often infects people without making them feel ill. Infants are usually asymptomatic, and small children usually have a milder case of the disease. When symptoms do occur, the infected person will often complain of flulike symptoms, with loss of appetite, nausea and vomiting, stomach cramps, and extreme fatigue, which may progress to jaundice. Hepatitis B can progress to fulminating hepatic necrosis and death. Each year, 4,000 to 5,000 Americans die from hepatitis B (Benenson, 1995). Antiviral therapies are being used to treat active HBV with limited success.

The incubation period for hepatitis B is 45 to 180 days, with an average of 60 to 90 days. Hepatitis B occurs worldwide with little seasonal variation. Hepatitis B is prevented by the hepatitis B vaccine, which consists of a series of three intramuscular (IM) injections of the hepatitis B vaccine over 6 months. This vaccine is used to protect everyone, from newborn infants to older adults (*Facts about hepatitis B for adults,* 1997).

Hepatitis C

Hepatitis C is also a viral infection of the liver. It has been referred to as *parenterally transmitted hepatitis,* and before blood donor screening, it was the most common cause of posttransfusion hepatitis worldwide. Ninety percent of hepatitis C occurrence in Japan, the United States, and Western Europe is as a result of blood transfusions (*Hepatitis C,* 1997).

Hepatitis C virus (HCV) is found worldwide. The World Health Organization (WHO) estimates that up to 3% of the world's population is infected with HCV (*Hepatitis learning guide,* 1998). In the United States, hepatitis C currently accounts for 20% of acute viral hepatitis cases. Its occurrence is highest in IV drug users and hemophilia clients; moderate in hemodialysis clients; low in heterosexuals with multiple partners, homosexual men, health care workers, and family members of HCV clients; and lowest in volunteer blood donors (Benenson, 1995). The reservoir for the virus is in humans. The mode of transmission is indirect, spread through contaminated needles and syringes; however, this accounts for fewer than 50% of the infected cases in the United States. Transmission rates through household contact and sexual activity appear to be low, and perinatal transmission is uncommon. The route of transmission cannot be identified in more than 40% of infected clients (Benenson, 1995).

The incubation period of hepatitis C is from 2 weeks to 6 months, with most cases occurring within 6 to 9 weeks after infection. Most infected individuals with hepatitis C are asymptomatic (up to 90%); this includes even those with chronic disease (*Hepatitis C,* 1997). The most common symptoms are fatigue, nausea, vague abdominal discomfort, and jaundice. Severity ranges from inapparent cases (approximately 75%) to rare fulminating, fatal cases (Benenson, 1995). Although the disease appears to be less severe than hepatitis A or B in the acute stage, clients with chronic HCV infection develop chronic liver disease (occurring in more than 60% of adult clients). Of those developing chronic liver disease, 30% to 60% will develop chronic ac-

tive hepatitis, and 5% to 20% will develop cirrhosis. There also appears to be an association between HCV infection and hepatocellular carcinoma (Benenson, 1995). Treatment with interferon is effective in approximately 20% of clients, and ribavirin has been shown to be somewhat effective as an antiviral agent against hepatitis C when used in combination with interferon (*Hepatitis C,* 1997).

Prevention measures for hepatitis C include the following (*Hepatitis C,* 1997; *Hepatitis learning guide,* 1998):

- *Universal screening of blood and blood products*
- *Effective use of standard precautions and barrier techniques*
- *Sterilization of reusable equipment and destruction of disposable equipment*
- *Public health education regarding the risks of using unsterilized equipment*

Because there is no vaccine against hepatitis C, prevention is the primary strategy against the virus.

Hepatitis D

Hepatitis D virus (HDV) is a defective, single-stranded RNA virus that requires the helper function of HBV to replicate. HDV is found worldwide, but its prevalence varies. Because it requires the HBV to replicate and to infect cells, it occurs either epidemically or endemically in populations with high rates of HBV infection. (Benenson, 1995). Places where HDV is found to be endemic are Africa, southern Italy, Romania, parts of Russia, and South America. Populations that have high rates of hepatitis D are hemophiliacs, drug addicts, people with frequent blood exposures, residents in homes for the developmentally disabled, and male homosexuals. Humans serve as the reservoir for hepatitis D. The modes of transmission are similar to those of hepatitis B, with direct contact with blood or blood products the most efficient. Sexual transmission is less efficient than that of hepatitis B, and perinatal transmission is rare. The onset of hepatitis D is usually abrupt, with signs and symptoms similar to those of hepatitis B. Hepatitis D varies from being self-limiting to progressing to chronic hepatitis. Hepatitis D can be acquired either as a co-infection with hepatitis B or as a superinfection in persons with chronic HBV infection. When it is acquired as a co-infection, the person has a greater risk of severe acute disease, with a 2% to 20% chance of fulminant hepatitis. Chronic HBV carriers who acquire hepatitis D as a superinfection have a greater chance of developing chronic HDV infection. The superinfection with HDV has been found to increase the development of chronic liver disease with cirrhosis 70% to 80% compared with 15% to 30% of clients with HBV alone (*Hepatitis learning guide,* 1998).

The incubation period is approximately 2 to 8 weeks. Peak infectivity is thought to occur just before the onset of the illness. Symptoms are similar to those of hepatitis B and are identified as joint pain, abdominal pain, loss of appetite, nausea and vomiting, fatigue, and jaundice. No vaccine exists for HDV. The method of control is immunization with the hepatitis B vaccine; however, this is effective only in persons who are not already infected with HBV. For those infected with HBV, avoidance of any possible exposure to HDV is the only preventive measure (*Hepatitis learning guide*, 1998).

Hepatitis E

Hepatitis E is similar to hepatitis A in that there is no evidence of a chronic form. The fatality rate for hepatitis E is also similar to that of hepatitis A, except in pregnant women during the third trimester, when the fatality rate may reach 20%. Hepatitis E virus (HEV) is transmitted by the fecal-oral route. Contaminated water from feces of infected humans is the most commonly documented vehicle of transmission. Person-to-person transmission (seen in hepatitis A) does not appear to be a mode of transmission in hepatitis E, because secondary household cases are not common during outbreaks. The attack rate is highest in young adults; cases are uncommon in children and the elderly (Benenson, 1995).

The reservoir is unknown at this time, and an animal reservoir is possible. In the United States, as well as in most other industrialized countries, hepatitis E cases have been documented only among travelers returning from HEV-endemic areas (Benenson, 1995). HEV is endemic in Mexico, Central America, Asia, North Africa, the Middle East, and a few sub-Saharan African countries along the western coast (*Hepatitis learning guide*, 1998).

The incubation period is 15 to 64 days, with the mean incubation period ranging between 26 to 42 days (Benenson, 1995). Symptoms for hepatitis E are loss of appetite, nausea and vomiting, fever, fatigue, and abdominal pain. Many people who contract HEV have no symptoms. Prevention of hepatitis E relies primarily on the provision of clean water. Hygiene practice must be strict among travelers to prevent contracting hepatitis E when traveling in developing countries, such as avoiding drinking water and beverages with ice, uncooked shellfish, and uncooked fruits and vegetables (*Hepatitis learning guide*, 1998). There is no vaccine and no identified treatment at this time; thus, prevention is very important.

Influenza

Influenza is another vaccine-preventable disease important in adults. Influenza is often called "the flu." It is an extremely contagious viral infection of the nose, throat, and lungs. In temperate zones, epidemics occur in the winter season, and in tropical zones, they occur during the rainy season. Influenza derives its importance from the rapidity with which epidemics occur, the high morbidity rate, and the severity of the complications that result from the infection. During major epidemics, the most severe illnesses and deaths occur in the elderly population and in those with debilitating diseases. In 1997, the flu vaccination rate for adults 65 and older was only 65.5% ("Immunizations lag," 1999).

CASE STUDY

You are a nurse in a neighborhood-based clinic. In October, Mrs. Clark, a 75-year-old woman, comes into the clinic for her regular yearly physical examination. Mrs. Clark is in good health overall, with relatively few minor complaints. Last year, as part of her yearly visit, Mrs. Clark had been given an influenza vaccination. During this visit, however, Mrs. Clark tells you that she does not need to be vaccinated against influenza because she had gotten her "flu shot" last year. She also said, "I don't want the flu shot this year because I know somebody who got sick from it. I don't want to get sick."

1. Should you convince Mrs. Clark to get the influenza vaccination this year? Why or why not?

2. What other vaccines should you consider offering to Mrs. Clark?

3. What are the client education considerations for Mrs. Clark?

There are three types of influenza viruses: A, B, and C. Type A is associated with widespread epidemics and pandemics, type B is associated with regional or widespread epidemics, and type C is associated with sporadic and minor localized outbreaks (Benenson, 1995). Occurrence is worldwide. The United States has an epidemic almost every year with type A, type B, or sometimes with both A and B.

Influenza symptoms are fever, myalgia, headache, sore throat, dry cough, and some gastrointestinal symptoms, such as nausea, vomiting, and diarrhea. Humans are the primary reservoir, with swine and avian reservoirs as likely breeding grounds for new strains. The mode of transmission is airborne, which is aerosolized or droplet material from the respiratory tract. The incubation period is very short, ranging from 1 to 3 days. People are infectious from 1 to 2 days before onset of symptoms to 4 to 5 days after onset (CDC, 1995b).

Most cases of influenza are preventable through a vaccine. Because the virus changes from year to year, it is necessary to be vaccinated yearly. The following people should receive a yearly vaccine: people 65 years and older, people with chronic disease (cardiac and/or respiratory), people who are immunocompromised, pregnant women who will be in their second or third trimester during the flu season, residents in long-term care facilities, health care workers, and adolescents receiving long-term aspirin therapy (who are at risk for Reye's syndrome) (*Facts about influenza for adults*, 1997; National Institute of Allergy and Infectious Diseases, 1997a).

Pneumococcal Disease

Pneumococcal disease is an acute bacterial infection. It is characterized by a rapid onset with shaking chills, fever, pleural pain, a productive cough, dyspnea, tachycardia, anorexia, malaise, and extreme weakness. Its onset is not as rapid in the elderly, and the first evidence is usually by x-ray examination. In infants and young children, the onset may be characterized by fever, vomiting, and convulsions. Pneumococcal disease is most severe in infants and elders, with higher death rates in both groups. The mortality rate is 5% to 10% with antibiotic therapy but can be as high as 60% for infants in developing countries where antibiotics are unavailable. The infectious agent is *Streptococcus pneumoniae* (pneumococcus). Its occurrence is worldwide, with peaks in the winter and early spring in temperate zones. However, it occurs in all climates and in all seasons (Benenson, 1995).

The reservoir for pneumococcal disease is in humans, and pneumoncocci are often found in the lungs of healthy people worldwide. The mode of transmission is airborne through droplets spread either by direct transfer or by indirect transfer when droplets have recently contaminated articles of clothes or bedding with discharge from the respiratory track. Person-to-person transmission is common. The incubation period is approximately 1 to 3 days.

Pneumococcal disease can be prevented through vaccination with polyvalent vaccine. Although this vaccine is not effective in children younger than 2 years of age (Benenson, 1995), it is safe in all others, and one immunization lasts most adults a lifetime against almost all the bacteria that cause pneumococcal disease. The following adults should be vaccinated: people 65 and older, people with chronic diseases, people who are immunosuppressed, residents of long-term care facilities, Alaska Natives, and American Indian populations (*Facts about pneumococcal disease for adults,* 1997). In 1997, the vaccination rate for adults 65 or older was only 45.5% ("Immunizations lag," 1999).

Routine Vaccines Indicated for Adults

All adults should be protected against many of the same diseases as adolescents and children. The tetanus and diphtheria (Td) vaccine should be given to all adults (Table 19-2). It is important for adults to be immunized against diphtheria and tetanus because 1 of every 10 people who get diphtheria will die from it, and 40 to 60 cases of tetanus occur each year, resulting in at least 10 deaths. Approximately 50% of Americans 50 years and older are inadequately immunized against tetanus and diphtheria (*Facts about adult immunization,* 1997).

TABLE 19-2   **ADULT IMMUNIZATION SCHEDULE**

VACCINE	TIMING OF IMMUNIZATIONS
Hepatitis A virus (HAV) for those at risk*	Two doses are needed to ensure long-term protection. Travelers to countries where the disease is common should get the first dose at least 4 weeks before departure.
Hepatitis B virus (HBV) for those at risk*	First dose; second dose 1 month later; third dose 5 months after second dose.
Influenza (flu)	Given yearly in the fall to people age 65 and older. Also recommended for people younger than 65 who have heart disease, lung disease, diabetes, and other chronic conditions, as well as for others who work or live with high-risk persons.*
Measles, mumps, rubella (MMR)	Two doses 1 month apart are recommended for adults born in 1957 or later if immunity cannot be proved.†
Pneumococcal	Usually given to those age 65 and older. Also recommended for people younger than 65 who have chronic illnesses such as those listed for influenza, and also for those with kidney disorders and sickle cell anemia.* A repeat dose 5 years later may be given for those at highest risk.*
Tetanus, diphtheria (Td) if initial series was not given in childhood	First dose; second dose 4 to 6 weeks later; third dose 6 to 12 months after the second dose; booster shot every 10 years.
Chickenpox (varicella)	Two doses are recommended for persons 13 and older who have not had chickenpox.‡

*Consult health care provider to determine level of risk.
†Should not be given to pregnant women or those considering pregnancy within 3 months of vaccination.
‡Should not be given to pregnant women or those considering pregnancy within 1 month of vaccination.

Based on the recommendations of the Advisory Committee on Immunization Practices, National Coalition for Adult Immunizations, CDC, 1997.

Adults born before 1957 do not usually require the measles, mumps, and rubella vaccine because most of these adults have acquired immunity as a result of having the diseases during childhood. However, all adults born after 1957 should be immunized (see Table 19-2). Women of childbearing age should be given the rubella vaccine unless they have documentation of immunization after their first birthday. Currently, approximately 12 million women of childbearing age are susceptible to rubella. If rubella occurs during pregnancy, severe birth defects, miscarriages, and stillbirths can result (*Facts about adult immunization,* 1997). Although laboratory evidence of rubella immunity is acceptable, a stated previous history of rubella is unreliable and should not be accepted as proof of immunity. Before giving rubella immunization, the nurse should determine the likelihood of pregnancy during the next 3 months. The nurse should discuss with the woman her plans for reliable birth control during the following 3 months. Although there is no evidence that the rubella vaccine or other live viruses cause birth defects, the possibility exists. Thus, health care providers should not give any live vaccine to women known to be pregnant.

All adults without a reliable history of varicella disease (chickenpox) should receive the varicella vaccine. Adults who are either at highest risk for susceptibility or at high risk for exposing people to varicella should be targeted for varicella immunization (see Table 19-2). These adults include teachers, college students, military personnel, health care workers, and family members of immunocompromised persons. Although varicella is not considered a serious disease of childhood, adults are 25 times more likely to die from the disease. Adolescents and adults who develop varicella are 10 times more likely to require hospitalization and/or develop pneumonia, bacterial infections, and encephalitis (*Facts about adult immunizations,* 1997).

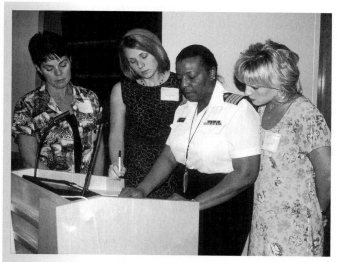

Mississippi nurses discuss immunization rates in their state with Captain Joyce Goff, RN (U.S. Public Health Service), Nurse Epidemiologist, at the Centers for Disease Control and Prevention, Atlanta.

Emerging and Reemerging Infectious Diseases

Infectious diseases continue to be a problem for all people, regardless of age, gender, lifestyle, ethnicity, or socioeconomic status. New and mutated infectious diseases that have the potential to cause suffering and death and impose an enormous financial burden on individuals and society are always emerging. Two examples occurred in 1997, when a new strain of influenza that had never been seen in humans began to kill previously healthy people in Hong Kong and strains of *S. aureus* with diminished susceptibility to vancomycin were reported in both Japan and the United States. If scientists cannot replace antibiotics that are losing their effectiveness, some diseases may become untreatable, as they were in the preantibiotic era (CDC, 1998a).

* *

Everybody knows that pestilences have a way of recurring in the world; yet somehow we find it hard to believe in ones that crash down on our heads from a blue sky.
Albert Camus, 1948, *The Plague*

* *

Emerging infectious diseases are diseases that have appeared for the first time or that have occurred before but are appearing in populations where they had not previously been reported. Reemerging infectious diseases are familiar diseases caused by well-understood organisms that were once under control or declining but are now resistant to common antimicrobial drugs or are gaining new footholds in the population and increasing in incidence (AAWH, 1997; Dzenowagis, 1997).

Concern about emerging and reemerging infectious diseases prompted a 1992 report issued by the Institute of Medicine (IOM) of the National Academy of Sciences. The report, "Emerging Infections: Microbial Threats to Health in the United States," concluded that emerging and reemerging infectious diseases are a major threat to the health of Americans and challenged the U.S. government to take action. The IOM report (1992) defines emerging or reemerging infectious diseases as those diseases whose incidence has increased within the last two decades of the 20th century or threatens to increase in the near future. Modern conditions that favor the spread of disease are listed in Box 19-3.

* *

I think the weakest point in the United States is our false security that there will be no problems . . . we still have this feeling in the United States that we don't need to worry, that it's someone else's problem . . . but these diseases don't respect barriers. They don't respect borders.
Dr. David Heymann, Director of the Office of Emerging Infectious Diseases at the World Health Organization, 1997

* *

BOX 19-3 MODERN DEMOGRAPHIC AND ENVIRONMENTAL CONDITIONS THAT FAVOR THE SPREAD OF INFECTIOUS DISEASES

- Global travel
- Globalization of the food supply and centralized processing of food
- Population growth and increased urbanization and overcrowding
- Migration due to wars, famines, and other artificial or natural disasters
- Irrigation, deforestation, and reforestation projects that alter the habitats of disease-carrying insects and animals
- Human behaviors, such as intravenous drug use and risky sexual behavior
- Increased use of antimicrobial agents and pesticides, hastening the development of resistance
- Increased human contact with tropical rain forests and other wilderness habitats that are reservoirs for insects and animals that harbor unknown infectious agents

Source: CDC, 1998a.

BOX 19-4 SOME EXAMPLES OF THE IMPACT OF PREVENTION ACTIVITIES TO REDUCE MORBIDITY AND MORTALITY FROM EMERGING INFECTIOUS DISEASES FROM 1994 TO 1998

Decreased number of nosocomial outbreaks of multidrug-resistant tuberculosis from 9 between 1990 and 1993 to none in 1996 and 1997 as a result of the implementation of control measures in hospitals

Decreased incidence of hepatitis B by more than 60% from 1985 to 1996 primarily as a result of changes in high-risk behaviors and increased immunizations

Decreased incidence of hepatitis C by more than 80% from 1989 to 1996, primarily as a result of changes in high-risk behaviors and improved screening of the blood supply

Source: CDC, 1998a.

As a result of the IOM report, in 1994 the Centers for Disease Control and Prevention (CDC) and other health care groups launched a national effort to support public health efforts to control the negative impact of infectious diseases. As funds became available the CDC, in partnership with the IOM, state and local health departments, medical and public health professional associations, and international organizations implemented a plan titled "Addressing Emerging Infectious Disease Threats: A Prevention Strategy for the United States." The four major goals of the plan and the implications for nursing are described in Table 19-3.

Box 19-4 outlines some of the outcomes of the CDC's national effort to control the negative impact of infectious diseases 4 years later.

Food-Borne Disease

Infections caused by food-borne parasites or viruses are common. Each year in the United States, millions of people get sick from food-borne diseases and thousands die. In recent years, food-borne illness has become one of the fastest growing threats to community health in the United States (Foodborne illness, 1998; Mahon, Slutsker, Hutwagner, Drenzek, Maloney, Toomey, & Griffin, 1999). Much of the reason for this is that enormous quantities of food are being produced in central locations and then being widely distributed to all parts of the country (Mahon et al., 1999) (Table 19-4). There have also been sharp increases in the number and types of food being imported from other countries. In response to these factors, the National Food Safety Initiative was created in 1997 to improve the safety of the nation's food supply (CDC, 1998a; Foodborne illness, 1998). The health care for people with food-borne illnesses can be very expensive. The yearly cost for food-borne illnesses in the United

A CONVERSATION WITH . . .

With all our experience, we have not gone far on the road to eradicating disease. This knowledge keeps us humble. We have trouble outthinking a virus. Even smallpox humbled us until the very end. That virus seemed to have a better understanding of nature, human behavior, and ways to achieve immortality than the entire smallpox eradication team. The emergence and reemergence of infections must be approached with humility.

—**William Foege, MD**
former director of the CDC
and the Carter Center, Emory University, Atlanta
Source: Foege, 1998.

| TABLE 19-3 | GOALS OF CDC PLAN OUTLINED IN *ADDRESSING EMERGING INFECTIOUS DISEASE THREATS: A PREVENTION STRATEGY OF THE UNITED STATES* |

GOALS OF CDC PLAN (CDC, 1994)	ROLE OF NURSES IN CDC PLAN (COHEN & LARSON, 1996)
GOAL I SURVEILLANCE Detect, promptly investigate, and monitor emerging pathogens, the diseases they cause, and the factors influencing their emergence.	**GOAL I SURVEILLANCE** Support, explain, and circulate to the nursing community any recommendations made by CDC and their partner agencies focusing on the implications for nursing.
GOAL II APPLIED RESEARCH Integrate laboratory science and epidemiology to optimize public health practice.	**GOAL II APPLIED RESEARCH** Promote a population-based, epidemiological, systems approach for nursing practice and research.
GOAL III PREVENTION AND CONTROL Enhance communication of public health information about emerging diseases and ensure prompt implementation of prevention strategies.	**GOAL III PREVENTION AND CONTROL** 1. Collaborate with other professions and policy-making groups to support, endorse, and evaluate global strategies to prevent or reduce the threat of emerging infectious diseases. 2. Communicate with other nursing groups and recommend that they develop and disseminate policies and standards to prevent the spread of emerging infections. 3. Identify mechanisms to promote the appropriate prescription and use of antibiotics. 4. Address strategies to enhance host resistance and immunity. 5. Take a leadership role in initiatives to promote preventive strategies. 6. Take an active role in promoting science education for students in grades K through 12.
GOAL IV INFRASTRUCTURE Strengthen local, state, and federal public health infrastructures to support surveillance and implement prevention and control programs.	**GOAL IV INFRASTRUCTURE** Serve as a clear voice to policy makers for support of public health, public education, public health infrastructure, and policies that protect the environment and promote ecological balance.

States is $5 to $6 billion in medical costs and lost productivity (National Institute of Allergy and Infectious Diseases, 1998a).

Foods can serve as a medium for growing bacterial pathogens or as a passive vehicle for transferring parasitic or viral pathogens. Most food-borne infections are directly related to foods of animal origin such as meat, fish, shellfish, poultry, eggs, and dairy products (Kaferstein & Meslin, 1998). Many food-borne bacterial diseases have emerged or increased during the last two decades. Some of the factors that bring about the multiplication and distribution of these bacteria in food are poor hygienic practices at the animal husbandry, slaughterhouse, and food processing levels as well as poor food preparation practices.

Prevention

There are three measures of protection against food-borne pathogens (Kaferstein & Meslin, 1998):

1. Prevention of contamination of food

2. Prevention of growth of pathogens

3. Prevention of the spread and survival of pathogens

First, the quality of food at the production level must be improved. The environmental conditions under which food animals are raised and the use of fertilizers and pesticides for food plants must be monitored and controlled.

Second, food processing technology must be improved and used to prevent the survival and spread of food pathogens. Pas-

TABLE 19-4   EXAMPLES OF MULTISTATE FOOD-BORNE OUTBREAKS IN THE UNITED STATES, 1994–1999

Year	Organism	Number of States	Food Source
1994	Shigella flexneri	2	Green onion, probably contaminated in Mexico
1994	Listeria monocytogenes	3	Milk, contaminated after pasteurization and shipped interstate
1995	Salmonella enteritiditis	41	Ice cream premix hauled in trucks that had previously carried raw eggs
1996	Cyclospora cayetanensis	20	Raspberries from Guatemala, mode of contamination unclear; cases also reported in the District of Columbia and two Canadian provinces
1996	Escherichia coli O157:H7	3	Unpasteurized apple juice, probably contaminated during harvest
1996	Norwalk virus	5	Oysters contaminated before harvest
1997	Salmonella infantis	2	Alfalfa sprouts, probably contaminated during sprouting
1997	Cyclospora cayetanensis	18	Raspberries imported from Guatemala, mesclun lettuce, and products containing basil; cases also reported in the District of Columbia and two Canadian provinces
1997	Hepatitis A	4	Strawberries from Mexico distributed through the USDA Commodity Program for use in school lunches
1998–1999	Listeria monocytogenes	22	Hot dogs and deli meats, probably contaminated while packaging

Source: CDC, 1998a, 1999d.

teurization, sterilization, and irradiation contribute significantly to food safety by reducing or eliminating disease-causing organisms.

Third, all food handlers must be educated in the principles of safe food preparation. This is probably the most critical line of defense, because most food-borne diseases are a result of one or more of the following (Kaferstein & Meslin, 1998):

- *Insufficient cooking of food*
- *Preparation of food too many hours before it is eaten, along with improper storage*
- *Use of contaminated raw food*
- *Cross-contamination where food is prepared*
- *Food preparation by infected persons*

Nurses' Roles in Prevention

Because many cases of food-borne diseases are a result of mishandling food in the home, community health nurses who visit families in their homes are in an excellent position to provide education for the persons in a family who are responsible for food handling and preparation (Kaferstein & Meslin, 1998). Female caregivers should be specifically targeted because they often prepare the food for infants and young children, elders, and others who are unable to cook for themselves.

School nurses can be successful in reducing the incidence of food-borne infections by educating children in the schools about the concepts of food safety. Educating children is not only an effective way to communicate safe food handling procedures to parents but is also a way to implant the principles of safe food preparation in the minds of future adults (Kaferstein & Meslin, 1998). School nurses should monitor school food programs and educate school food services personnel about proper handling and storage of foods. Educational programs should also be provided for teachers because of the amount of "food treats" that are served in the classrooms, especially in elementary schools.

Common Food-Borne Diseases in the United States
Campylobacteriosis

Campylobacteriosis, caused by bacteria of the genus *Campylobacter*, is one of the most common diarrheal diseases in the United States. The symptoms (diarrhea, abdominal pain, fever, nausea, and vomiting) usually develop within 2 to 5 days after exposure and typically last 1 week. Most people infected with *Campylobacter* will recover with no treatment except for drinking plenty of fluids for the diarrhea. However, in more severe cases, an antibiotic such as erythromycin can be used. Most cases of campylobacteriosis are a result of handling or eating raw or undercooked poultry. Most cases occur as isolated, sporadic events, although small outbreaks have been reported. More than 10,000 cases are reported to the CDC each year. However, because many cases are undiagnosed or unreported, campylobacteriosis is estimated to affect more than 2 million people every year, approximately 1% of the population (CDC, 1998b).

Listeriosis

Listeriosis, caused by the bacterium *Listeria monocytogenes,* has been recognized as a serious public health problem in the United States. The symptoms are fever, muscle aches, and sometimes nausea or diarrhea. If the infection spreads to the nervous system, headache, stiff neck, confusion, loss of balance, or seizures can occur. *L. monocytogenes* is found in a variety of raw food, such as uncooked meats and vegetables, as well as in processed foods that become contaminated after processing. The disease primarily affects pregnant women, newborns, and adults with weakened immune systems. An estimated 1,100 people become ill from listeriosis each year, and 250 of them die. Most deaths occur among immunocompromised and elderly clients. Infected persons are treated with antibiotics (CDC, 1999b).

Salmonellosis

Salmonellosis, caused by many different kinds of *Salmonella* bacteria, is a diarrheal disease that has been known for more than 100 years. The symptoms (diarrhea, fever, and abdominal cramps) usually develop within 12 to 72 hours after exposure and usually last 4 to 7 days. Salmonellosis usually does not require any treatment, but if the client becomes severely dehydrated or the infection spreads from the intestines to other body parts, rehydration with IV fluids and antibiotic therapy may be necessary. *Salmonella* can be transmitted to humans by eating foods contaminated with animal feces. Many raw foods of animal origin are frequently contaminated, but fortunately, thorough cooking kills *Salmonella.* Foods may also be contaminated by the unwashed hands of an infected food handler. Approximately 40,000 cases of salmonellosis are reported in the United States each year, but the actual number of cases may be 20 or more times greater (CDC, 1998c).

Escherichia coli O157:H7

Escherichia coli O157:H7 is an emerging cause of food-borne illness. *E. coli* O157:H7 is one of the hundreds of strains of the bacterium *E. coli.* Most strains of *E. coli* are harmless and live in the intestines of healthy humans and animals, but *E. coli* O157:H7 produces a powerful toxin that can cause severe illness. The combination of letters and numbers in the name refers to specific markers on the surface of the bacterium that distinguishes it from other types of *E. coli.* The symptoms of *E. coli* O157:H7 are bloody diarrhea and abdominal cramps, although sometimes there are no symptoms. Most people recover in 5 to 10 days without antibiotics or other specific treatment. In about 2% to 7% of infections, particularly among young children and elders, hemolytic uremic syndrome develops. This complication causes destruction of the red blood cells and kidney failure. Hemolytic uremic syndrome is a life-threatening condition usually treated with blood transfusions and kidney dialysis. With intensive care treatment, the death rate for hemolytic uremic syndrome is 3% to 5%. About one-third of persons with hemolytic uremic syndrome have permanent abnormal kidney function

and may require long-term dialysis. Most cases of *E. coli* O157:H7 are associated with eating undercooked, contaminated ground beef; drinking raw milk; or swimming in or drinking sewage-contaminated water (CDC, 1999c).

Vector-Borne Diseases

A *vector* is an "animal, particularly an insect, that transmits a disease-producing organism from a host to a non-infected animal" (Neufeldt, 1996, p. 1478). Vector-borne diseases were responsible for more human disease and death from the 17th century through the early 20th century than all other causes combined (Gubler, 1998). In the late 1800s, mosquitoes were discovered to transmit such diseases as malaria, yellow fever, and dengue from human to human. By 1910, other major vector-borne diseases, such as African sleeping sickness, plague, Rocky Mountain spotted fever, Chagas' disease, sandfly fever, and louse-borne typhus, all had been shown to be transmitted by blood-sucking arthropods (Gubler, 1998).

Most prevention programs have centered on vector control. Through a global effort during the 20th century, most of the vector-borne diseases in the world had been effectively controlled, primarily by the elimination of arthropod breeding sites and limited use of chemical insecticides (Table 19-5). However, the benefits of vector-borne disease control programs were short-lived. Vector-borne diseases such as Lyme disease and malaria began to emerge and reemerge in different parts of the world during the 1970s, and the numbers have greatly increased over the last three decades. Although the reasons for the resurgence are complex and poorly understood, two factors have been identified: (1) the diversion of financial support and subsequent loss of public health infrastructure and (2) reliance on quick fix solutions such as insecticides and drugs (Gubler, 1998).

Lyme Disease

In the 1990s, Lyme disease was listed as the most important emerging infection in the United States, accounting for 90% of vector-borne illness (Herrington, Campbell, Bailey, Cartter, Adams, Frazier, Damrow, & Gensheimer, 1997). First identified in 1975, when unusually high numbers of children living in Lyme, Connecticut, were diagnosed with juvenile arthritis, the annual number of reported cases of Lyme disease increased 25-fold between 1982 and 1998, with a total of 103,000 reported cases. The disease has steadily been moving into many different geographic regions in the United States (Pinger, 1998). In 1996, 45 states reported cases of Lyme disease to the CDC (Herrington et al., 1997). More than 16,000 cases were reported in the United States in 1996, and in 1997, there were more than 12,500 cases reported (CDC, 1999e).

The disease is caused by infection with the spirochete *Borrelia burgdorferi,* transmitted by infected *Ixodes scapularis* ticks in the northeastern, mid-western, and southern states and *I. pacificus* on the west coast (Herrington et al., 1997; National Institute of Allergy and Infectious Diseases, 1998b). These ticks generally

TABLE 19-5   SUCCESSFUL GLOBAL VECTOR-BORNE DISEASE CONTROL/ELIMINATION PROGRAMS

DISEASE	LOCATION	YEAR(S)
Yellow fever *(Aedes aegypti)*	Cuba	1900–1901
Yellow fever	Panama	1904
Yellow fever	Brazil	1932
Anopheles gambiae infestation	Brazil	1938
A. gambiae infestation	Egypt	1942
Louse-borne typhus	Italy	1942
Malaria	Sardinia	1946
Yellow fever	Americas	1947–1970
Malaria	Americas	1954–1975
Malaria	Global	1955–1975
Yellow fever	West Africa	1950–1970
Onchocerciasis	West Africa	1974–Present
Bancroft's filariasis	South Pacific	1970s
Chagas' disease	South America	1991–Present

Source: Gubler, 1998.

feed on white-tailed deer and the white-footed mouse. The recent increase of the white-tailed deer population in the northeast and the influx of humans living in rural areas have probably contributed to the increased incidence of Lyme disease (National Institute of Allergy and Infectious Diseases, 1998b).

The symptoms of Lyme disease are multistage and multisystem. Early disease symptoms include a red rash resembling a bull's-eye forming over the tick bite and systemic flulike symptoms such as headache, muscular aches and pains, and fatigue. If untreated, symptoms can progress to include heart problems such as an irregular heart rate, shortness of breath, or dizziness; neurological problems such as meningitis, Bell's palsy, numbness, pain, or weakness in the limbs, or poor muscle coordination; and arthritis that shifts from joint to joint, with the knee being most commonly affected. About 10% to 20% of untreated clients develop chronic arthritis (National Institute of Allergy and Infectious Diseases, 1998b; Pinger, 1998).

Most cases of Lyme disease can be treated with antibiotic therapy. The earlier the treatment is begun, the more successful the treatment will be. However, early diagnosis is difficult because many of the disease symptoms mimic those of other disorders, and the distinctive bull's-eye rash is absent in more than 25% of those infected (National Institute of Allergy and Infectious Diseases, 1998b). It is important for the nurse to interview clients presenting with flu symptoms thoroughly to determine whether possible exposure to deer ticks could have occurred, particularly in warm weather months.

Malaria

Malaria is one of the oldest known diseases, with the first recorded case appearing in 1700 BC in China. In ancient Chinese, it was called "the mother of fevers" (The mother of fevers, 1998). Malaria is the most important of all vector-borne diseases because of its global distribution, the numbers of people affected, and the large numbers of deaths (Gubler, 1998). Worldwide, 10% to 30% of all hospital admissions and 15% to 25% of all deaths of children younger than 5 years of age are attributed to malaria. Each year, approximately 300 million people are infected by it, and as many as 2.7 million die, most of them residing in developing countries. The death toll includes more than 1 million children younger than 5 years of age (Liese, 1998; The mother of fevers, 1998).

Today, cases of malaria are reported in more than 100 counties throughout the world. Although more than 90% of cases occur in sub-Saharan Africa, the disease is also found in parts of Asia, the western Pacific, and Central and South America (Box 19-5). About 40% of the world's population, totaling more than 2 billion people, are currently at risk (The mother of fevers, 1998). Air travel has brought the disease to the doorsteps of industrialized countries, resulting in increased illness and death among travelers to areas with endemic disease (Nchinda, 1998). Although malaria is not endemic to the United States, it is the most common imported disease in the United States, with approximately 1,000 suspected cases being imported each year (Gubler, 1998). In recent years, clusters of malaria have occurred in California, New Jersey, New York, Texas, and Michigan, and 1,200 cases were reported to the CDC in 1995 (Pinkowish, 1998). Although malaria is not a widespread problem in the United States, nurses should be alert for imported malaria infection in their clients who travel abroad.

Malaria in humans is caused by a protozoon of the genus *Plasmodium* and the four subspecies, *falciparum, vivax, malariae,* and *ovale* (Nchinda, 1998). *P. falciparum* causes the most severe

RESEARCH BRIEF

Shankar, A. H., Genton, B., Semba, R. D., Baisor, M., Paino, J., Tamja, S., Adiguma, T., Wu, L., Rare, L., Tielsch, J. M., Alpers, M. P., & West, K. P., Jr. (1999, July 17). Effect of vitamin A supplementation on morbidity due to Plasmodium falciparum in young children in Papua, New Guinea: A randomised trial. Lancet, 354, 203–208.

A team of researchers in New Guinea followed 480 children between the ages of 6 and 60 months for 1 year. In the part of New Guinea where the study was done, 55% of preschool children carry *Plasmodium falciparum*, the parasite that causes malaria. The children were randomly assigned to groups that received high-dose vitamin A or a placebo every 3 months. By the end of the study, children who had received vitamin A had a 30% reduction in clinical episodes of malaria sickness and a 36% reduction of *P. falciparum* levels in the blood. In the age group normally experiencing the highest malaria sickness rate (12 to 36 months old), there were 35% fewer malaria attacks, 68% lower levels of *P. falciparum* in the blood, and 26% fewer enlarged spleens (a common result of malaria) in the children receiving the vitamin A. Although vitamin A reduced the number of acute clinical episodes of malaria, no statistical differences were found between the percentage of children in both groups who became infected with the malaria parasite. The researchers concluded that vitamin A supplements could be a cost-effective nonpharmacological treatment for malaria but would not be an effective method of primary prevention.

---

form of the disease in humans (Molyneux, 1998). The disease is transmitted through the bite of *Anopheles* mosquitoes (Marsh & Waruiru, 1998; Nchinda, 1998). Once inside the human host, the malaria organism enters the bloodstream and travels directly to the liver, where it hides and multiplies. After about 2 weeks, the newly produced organisms burst out of the liver into the bloodstream, where they attack red blood cells. These new malaria organisms rapidly reproduce in the bloodstream over the next few days until there are tens of millions of them. It is at this point that the human host begins to feel symptoms of illness (Marsh & Waruiru, 1998).

The first signs of illness are usually fever and malaise, often accompanied by a severe headache. At this stage of the illness, many people think they are experiencing the flu. Other malaria symptoms, such as vomiting, diarrhea, or coughing, might lead nurses or other health care providers to suspect gastric upset or respiratory infection. Malaria is a great imitator, making it important for nurses to suspect any fever as a potential case of malaria for clients who have recently traveled to a country where

BOX 19-5 FACTORS CONTRIBUTING TO THE RESURGENCE OF MALARIA

- Increased resistance of malaria organisms to drugs currently used for treatment
- Civil wars in many countries, forcing large populations to relocate to different geographic regions
- Changing rainfall patterns and water development projects (e.g., dams, irrigation systems), which create new mosquito breeding places
- Poor economic conditions resulting in reduced health budgets and inadequate funding for drugs
- Changes in mosquito biting patterns, from indoor to outdoor biters

Source: Nchinda, 1998.

the disease is known to exist. Early diagnosis and rapid treatment are the keys to the secondary prevention efforts necessary to keep the disease from progressing to a complicated or severe state (Marsh & Waruiru, 1998).

Zoonoses

Many of the infectious diseases that have emerged or reemerged in the past few years have been zoonotic. Zoonoses are diseases that are caused by infectious agents that can jump from species to species—jumping from vertebrate animals to humans (Murphy, 1998; Neufeldt, 1996). Throughout time, humans have interacted with the other animals that share this earth. Whether domesticated work animals, animals raised or hunted for food, family pets, or unwanted household pests, animals and their products are an integral part of our daily lives (Meslin & Stohr, 1998). A variety of both domestic and wild animals carry viruses, bacteria, or parasites that can be transferred to humans either through direct contact with the animals and their waste products or through food products of animal origin (Heymann, 1998). Zoonotic diseases seem to be increasing at rapid pace for several reasons: Global human populations are increasingly bringing people into closer contact with animal populations; modern air travel has made it possible to travel to the other side of the world in a matter of hours; enormous environmental changes have been brought about by human activity; and bioterroristic activities are increasing, and the infectious agents of choice are usually zoonotic (Murphy, 1998).

Hantavirus

Hantavirus pulmonary syndrome was first recognized in the southwestern United States in 1993 when several deaths occurred from acute respiratory distress syndrome (Hantavirus infection, 1993; Toro, Vega, Khan, Mills, Padula, Terry, Yadon,

Valderrama, Ellis, Pavletic, Cerda, Zaki, Wun-Ju, Meyer, Tapia, Mansilla, Baro, Vergara, Concha, Calderon, Enria, Peters, & Ksiazek, 1998). Initial symptoms include fever, muscle aches and pains, gastrointestinal upset, and headache. Cardiac dysfunction follows, with a 40% to 60% mortality rate (Toro et al., 1998).

Deer mice are the primary reservoir hosts for the southwestern U.S. hantavirus. Infection can occur when saliva or feces particles are inhaled in aerosol form during direct contact with the mice or when dried materials contaminated by mouse excreta are loosened, directly introduced into open wounds or eyes, or ingested in contaminated food or water. Humans can also become infected through deer mouse bites (Hantavirus infection, 1993). Avoidance of contact with the deer mouse population is the best way to prevent infection and control disease. Risks can be controlled through environmental hygiene practices that deter deer mice from inhabiting home and work environments (Hantavirus infection, 1993).

Pet Diseases

Pets, especially cats and dogs, are considered members of the family by many people worldwide. People give their pets names, share their food, and sometimes even share their beds with them, all in exchange for unconditional love (De Menezes Brandao & Anselmo Viana da Silva Berzins, 1998). Unfortunately, pets can be a source for zoonotic diseases. However, if pets are well nourished, properly vaccinated, and regularly examined by a veterinarian, there is little to fear (Chomel, 1998).

Cat-scratch fever, caused by *Bartonella henselae*, is generally a benign local inflammation of the lymph nodes transmitted through a break in the skin caused by a cat scratch. However, in people with weakened immune systems, it causes bacillary angiomatosis, a life-threatening vascular disease in which tumors are formed from blood cells. The organism is transmitted from cat to cats primarily by fleas (Chomel, 1998).

In countries where plague is endemic, cats can become infected or carry fleas from infected rodents they may have killed. Several cases of bubonic and pneumonic plague in humans in the United States have been associated with pet cats (Chomel, 1998).

Pets can carry infectious agents such as *Campylobacter* or *Salmonella*, which can cause diarrheal and gastrointestinal illness. Puppies and kittens with diarrhea pose the greatest risk. Reptiles are also carriers of a wide variety of *Salmonella* species. Pet turtles and iguanas have been linked to several severe, and even fatal, cases of *Salmonella* among young children worldwide. It is easy to see why handwashing is extremely important after handling pets and before eating (Chomel, 1998).

Rabies

Rabies is probably the best known and most feared of the zoonoses because the disease is almost always fatal in humans once symptoms occur. The WHO estimates that more than 50,000 deaths from rabies occur a year, but the figure may actually be higher because of the large number of deaths worldwide that go unreported. In the United States, the number of rabies-related deaths has declined from more than 100 annually in 1900 to only one or two per year in the 1990s. Modern prevention efforts have proven almost 100% effective, with U.S. deaths occurring only in people who do not recognize their risk and fail to seek medical treatment (CDC, 1999f).

The virus is usually transmitted through bites from infected animals, but in rare cases, it can also be transmitted through infected licks on mucous membranes, inhaled infected bat secretions, and corneal transplants from undiagnosed human donors. Reservoirs for infection are domestic dogs and cats as well as many wild animals such as skunks, raccoons, foxes, wolves, and bats (Wilde & Mitmoonpitak, 1998). Before 1960, most rabies cases were in domestic animals, but now, more than 90% of cases occur in wild animals (CDC, 1999f). Efforts by U.S. wildlife agencies have helped control rabies in wild animal populations in recent years.

After entering the host, the rabies virus multiplies slowly at the portal of entry. It then invades the surrounding nerve tissue and slowly migrates to the spinal cord and brain. Once there, it multiplies, causing a rapid death. The incubation period can range from a few days to many years (Wilde & Mitmoonpitak, 1998). Rabies in humans is preventable by immediately cleans-

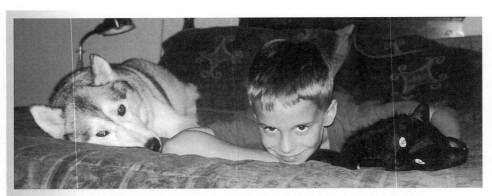

In American households, pets are members of the family. Children are especially vulnerable for exposure to infectious agents carried by pets.

ing all animal bites with soap and water and using rabies immune globulin and vaccine as indicated (Benenson, 1995; Wilde & Mitmoonpitak, 1998). Current rabies vaccinations are the best protection for pets and other domestic animals, thus significantly reducing the risk of exposure for humans.

Parasitic Diseases

Parasitic diseases, although more common in developing countries, have been on the rise in recent years in the United States. According to *Webster's Dictionary* (Neufeldt, 1996, p. 981), a *parasite* is an animal that lives on or in an organism of another species, from which it derives sustenance or protection without benefit to, and usually with harmful effects on, the host. The most common parasites are helminths (worms and flukes) and one-celled protozoans.

Helminths

Pinworm infection (enterobiasis) occurs worldwide and is the most common helminth intestinal infection in the United States, with the highest prevalence in school-aged children, followed by preschoolers. The prevalence is low in adults except for mothers of infected children. Pinworm infection often results in no symptoms, but in some persons, there may be perianal itching and disturbed sleep. Diagnosis can be made by applying cellophane tape to the perianal region early in the morning before bathing or defecating. Transmission occurs by direct transfer of infective eggs from the anus to the mouth or indirect transfer through contaminated clothing, bedding, food, or other fomites. Treatment with oral vermicides and disinfection of clothing and bedding is usually effective (Benenson, 1995).

Roundworm infection (ascariasis) occurs worldwide, with the highest prevalence in children between 3 and 8 years of age living in moist, tropical countries. Typically, no symptoms occur. Live worms, passed in stools or occasionally through the mouth or nose, are often the first sign of roundworm infection. Transmission occurs by ingestion of infective eggs from soil contaminated with human feces or from uncooked produce contaminated with soil containing infective eggs; it is not transmitted directly from person to person. Treatment with oral vermicides is usually effective (Benenson, 1995).

Hookworm infection (ancylostomiasis) is widely endemic in tropical and subtropical climates but can also occur in temperate climates. Approximately 1 billion people (about one-fifth of the world's population) are estimated to be infected with hookworms. In persons with heavy infections, there is severe iron deficiency, which leads to severe anemia. Children with heavy, long-term infection may have hypoproteinemia and may be delayed in physical and mental development. Light hookworm infections generally produce no clinical symptoms. Diagnosis is made by finding hookworm eggs in feces. Transmission occurs by larvae in the soil penetrating the skin, usually of the foot. The larvae then enter the bloodstream and travel to the lungs, where they enter the alveoli and migrate up the trachea to the pharynx. They are swallowed and reach the small intestine, where they develop into mature half-inch worms in 6 to 7 weeks. They attach to the intestinal wall and suck blood. Treatment with vermicides is usually effective (Benenson, 1995; CDC, 1998d).

Protozoans

Giardiasis

Giardiasis is a disease caused by *Giardia lamblia,* a microscopic, one-celled parasite that lives in the intestines of humans and animals. This parasite is found in every part of the United States and every region of the world. In recent years, giardiasis has become one of the most common water-borne diseases in the United States. Transmission is through the fecal-oral route or through ingestion of contaminated food or water from swimming pools, lakes, rivers, springs, ponds, or streams. The most common symptoms of giardiasis are diarrhea, abdominal cramps, nausea, fatigue, and weight loss. Symptoms usually appear within 1 to 2 weeks after exposure and generally last 4 to 6 weeks, but they can last longer (CDC, 1998e).

Persons at risk for giardiasis are child care workers, children in diapers who attend day-care centers, international travelers, hikers, campers, or anyone who drinks untreated water from a contaminated source. Because chlorine does not kill *G. lamblia,* several community outbreaks have been linked to contaminated community water supplies (CDC, 1998e).

Giardiasis is difficult to diagnose and may require examination of several stool specimens over several days. The pharmacological treatment for giardiasis is metronidazole (Flagyl). Nurses can help prevent giardiasis outbreaks in their communities by teaching clients in community settings to wash their hands after using the bathroom and before handling food, to wash and peel all raw vegetables and fruits, and to avoid drinking water from any source unless it has been filtered or chemically treated (Benenson, 1995; CDC, 1998e).

Cryptosporidiosis

Cryptosporidiosis, often called *crypto,* is a disease caused by *Cryptosporidium parvum,* a microscopic, one-celled parasite. Although not a new disease in the developing world, cryptosporidiosis made its first major appearance in the United States in 1993, when 400,000 people became ill with diarrhea after drinking contaminated water. Today, crypto has become a major threat to the U.S. water supply. Transmission is through the fecal-oral route or through ingestion of food or water contaminated with stool, including water in recreational parks or swimming pools (CDC, 1998f, 1998g).

Immunocompromised persons are most at risk for crypto infection, particularly HIV-positive persons or persons receiving chemotherapy for cancer treatment. Other persons at risk for infection are child care workers, children in diapers who attend day-care centers, persons exposed to human feces by sexual contact, and caregivers of persons infected with crypto. The most common symptoms are watery diarrhea and cramps, which in some cases can be severe. Weight loss, nausea, vomiting, and fever may also occur (CDC, 1998g, 1998h; Guerrant, 1997).

Currently, no cure exists for crypto, but some drugs (e.g., paromomycin) may reduce the severity of the symptoms. Oral rehydration powders and sports drinks can help prevent dehydration. Nurses can help at-risk populations reduce their risk by teaching them to wash their hands often with soap and water; to avoid sex that involves contact with stool; to avoid touching farm animals; to avoid touching the stool of pets; to wash and/or cook food; to be careful when swimming in lakes, rivers, pools, or hot tubs; to drink safe water; and to take extra precautions when traveling, particularly to developing countries (CDC, 1998f, 1998g, 1998h).

HIV/AIDS

The most significant emerging disease in the world during the last 20 years is HIV/AIDS (see chapter 20). AIDS is the life-threatening, late clinical stage of infection with HIV. The disease was first recognized as a distinct syndrome in 1981, and the virus was first isolated in 1983 (Benenson, 1995).

If I were going to imagine a real terror it would be a deadly virus that kills 100% of its victims, but incubates so slowly, say a decade, that millions of people are infected before they know it. It would be a virus that is transmitted sexually, attacking young adults while it takes advantage of our social inhibitions and bigotry about sex.

Dr. Joe McCormick, Chairman,
Community Health Sciences Department,
Aga Khan University, Pakistan

As of December 31, 1998, the cumulative number of reported AIDS cases in the United States was 688,200. Total deaths from AIDS in the United States was 410,800 (CDC, 1999g). Worldwide, 1,393,784 AIDS cases were reported (Pan American Health Organization, 1999). Estimated HIV cases were between 650,000 and 900,000 and 30.6 million worldwide (AAWH, 1998a; Pan American Health Organization, 1999).

HIV can be transmitted from person to person through unprotected sexual contact, through direct contact with blood or blood products through sharing needles or razors, and from mother to baby during gestation or the birthing process (Benenson, 1995). HIV/AIDS is addressed further in chapter 20.

Tuberculosis

TB is the leading cause of death worldwide from an infectious agent. Approximately 2 billion people, one-third of the world's population, are infected with TB, with about 3 million deaths

TUBERCULOSIS CASE RATES, UNITED STATES, 1997.

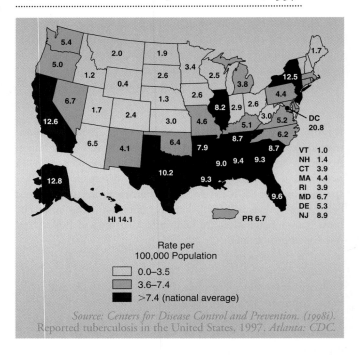

Rate per 100,000 Population	
□	0.0–3.5
▨	3.6–7.4
■	>7.4 (national average)

Source: Centers for Disease Control and Prevention. (1998i). Reported tuberculosis in the United States, 1997. Atlanta: CDC.

occurring annually (AAWH, 1998b; National Institute of Allergy and Infectious Disease, 1997b; Torres, 1998).

Historically, TB has been one of the great scourges of humankind. It was a leading killer in the United States until the advent of antibiotics in the 1950s. For the next 30 years, TB was on a steady decline, at least in the developed countries (AAWH, 1998b; Grimes & Grimes, 1995). The 1980s, however, saw a sharp increase in TB cases, which has been primarily the result of the development of multidrug-resistant strains of the disease (AAWH, 1998b; Grimes & Grimes, 1995). Other reasons for the upsurge include the spread of TB in institutional living facilities such as shelters and correctional facilities, a declining public health infrastructure, increased immigration from regions where TB is endemic, and the HIV/AIDS pandemic (Clark, Cegielski, & Hassell, 1997).

TB continues to be a major health problem in the United States, where an estimated 10 to 15 million people are infected, with about 10% of these people expected to develop active disease (Torres, 1998). Although the number of reported TB cases in the United States has shown a steady decline again in the past few years, cases are still high among high-risk groups such as the incarcerated, the homeless, elders, and HIV-infected persons, as well as underrepresented racial and ethnic groups and immigrants from countries with high TB rates and inadequate control measures (AAWH, 1998b; National Institute of Allergy and Infectious Diseases, 1997b; Torres, 1998).

REPORTED TUBERCULOSIS CASES BY RACE/ETHNICITY, UNITED STATES, 1997.

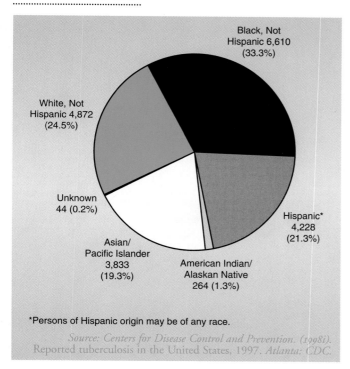

*Persons of Hispanic origin may be of any race.

Source: Centers for Disease Control and Prevention. (1998i). Reported tuberculosis in the United States, 1997. Atlanta: CDC.

TB is caused by *Mycobacterium tuberculosis* and is transmitted by droplets in the air. It usually affects the lungs (pulmonary), which accounts for 75% of all cases, although other body organs may be involved (extrapulmonary) about 25% of the time (National Institute of Allergy and Infectious Diseases, 1997; Torres, 1998). TB can live in an infected person's body and not cause illness. This is called *inactive* TB or TB infection. Approximately 5% of people with inactive TB develop active TB or TB disease later in life. Only about 10% of all persons infected with TB actually develop active TB. Symptoms of active TB include fatigue, weight loss, fever, chills, and night sweats. Symptoms of pulmonary TB also include a persistent cough, chest pain, and bloody sputum (Torres, 1998).

TB is both preventable and curable. Prevention is focused on treating persons with inactive TB infection prophylactically with anti-TB medications such as isoniazid (INH) for 6 to 12 months. It is extremely important for infected persons to complete the preventive therapy treatment both to prevent progression to active disease and to prevent the development of drug-resistant organisms (Torres, 1998).

Treatment for persons with active TB disease commonly includes such drugs as INH, rifampin, pyrazinamide, ethambutol, and streptomycin. These drugs are usually prescribed in various combinations. It is important that persons with active TB take the medication therapy prescribed for at least 6 months (Torres, 1998).

Multidrug-resistant TB disease (MDR-TB) may occur when medications are not taken consistently for the 6 to 12 months necessary to completely destroy the *M. tuberculosis* organism. In some U.S. cities, more than 50% of TB clients fail to complete their prescribed course of therapy. Many of these clients are homeless persons, drug addicts, or other persons living in poverty, who may not be reliable about taking their medications. Many individuals with TB may feel better after only a few weeks of therapy and stop taking their medications because of unpleasant side effects. MDR-TB is difficult to treat. Even with treatment, the death rate for MDR-TB clients is 40% to 60%, the same as for clients who receive no treatment (National Institute of Allergy and Infectious Diseases, 1997b; Torres, 1998).

The best method of treatment for persons in high-risk circumstances is direct observed therapy (DOT). DOT is a community-based prevention program in which a nurse or other health care provider is paired with a person infected with TB to ensure that the client follows the prescribed treatment plan. DOT programs have been successful in curing 95% of clients with pulmonary TB (Torres, 1998) and have the potential to save millions of lives worldwide over the next few years (DOTS: A breakthrough, 1998).

The HIV/TB Connection

The WHO estimates that 4.4 million people worldwide are co-infected with HIV and TB, with an estimated 80,000 to 100,000 of them living in the United States. Worldwide, TB is the leading killer among people infected with HIV. TB is listed as an AIDS-defining opportunistic infection for people who are infected with HIV. TB often occurs early in the course of HIV infection and may be the first indication that a person has HIV (HIV-related conditions, 1999; National Institute of Allergy and Infectious Diseases, 1997b). In the United States, approximately 8% of people co-infected with HIV and TB develop active disease each year. In comparison, otherwise healthy people infected with *M. tuberculosis* have approximately a 10% lifetime risk of developing active TB (National Institute of Allergy and Infectious Diseases, 1997b).

Early diagnosis and treatment of TB are critical for HIV-infected clients because the risk for drug-resistant TB is higher among people with HIV infection compared with other groups (MMWR, 1998; Moore, McCray, & Onorato, 1999). For people with HIV infection, the death rate for MDR-TB is as high as 80%. Because TB symptoms are the same as the symptoms for many other HIV-related opportunistic infections, TB is easy to overlook initially. HIV-infected clients may not react to tuberculin skin testing because their immune systems are suppressed (HIV-related conditions, 1999; National Institute of Allergy and Infectious Diseases, 1997b). A comprehensive health history is an essential tool for assisting nurses and other health care providers to identify TB exposure risks in HIV-infected clients.

Global Disease Eradication Efforts

Despite the emergence and reemergence of infectious diseases in recent years, significant advancements in the elimination or eradication of some diseases that have existed for centuries have occurred through a united global effort. The eradication of smallpox by 1979 is thought to be the greatest triumph of modern public health (Garrett, 1994). The WHO, in collaboration with other international public and private health organizations, has targeted seven other communicable diseases for eradication in the beginning of the 21st century. These diseases are polio, measles, leprosy, river blindness, Chagas' disease, guinea worm disease, and lymphatic filariasis. According to the WHO, these crippling and sometimes deadly diseases can be eliminated in parts of the world and even completely eradicated worldwide within a generation. The methods being used to accomplish this goal are immunization and vaccination, drug therapy, community training, health education, and national disease surveillance efforts (Wittenberg, 1998).

CONCLUSION

Community health nurses have played a significant role in the prevention, control, and treatment of communicable diseases throughout recent history. Nurses' skills and knowledge will continue to be a vital part of global eradication efforts well into the 21st century.

CRITICAL THINKING ACTIVITIES

1. As a nurse working with the WHO, what actions would you take to eliminate the reservoir for a vector-borne diseases such as malaria? What kind of actions would you take to eliminate the reservoir for an airborne disease such as legionellosis?

2. Discuss the differences between active immunity and passive immunity. Give two examples of each kind of immunity. How long does immunity last for each example?

3. Identify one infectious disease and discuss primary, secondary, and tertiary prevention methods appropriate for that disease on the community level.

4. Compare and contrast the five viral types of hepatitis. Identify similarities and differences regarding the following:

   - Occurrence in the world
   - Infectious agent
   - Reservoir
   - Incubation period
   - Methods of control

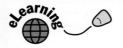

Explore Community Health Nursing on the web! To learn more about the topics in this chapter, use the passcode provided to access your exclusive web site: http://communitynursing.jbpub.com
If you do not have a passcode, you can obtain one at this site.

REFERENCES

Adult Immunization Schedule. (1997). *National coalition for adult immunization:* www.medscape.com/NCAI/.

American Association for World Health (AAWH). (1997). *Emerging infectious diseases: Reduce the risk.* Washington, DC: Author

American Association for World Health (AAWH). (1998a). *Be a force for change.* Washington, DC: Author.

American Association for World Health (AAWH). (1998b). *TB alert.* Washington, DC: Author.

American Association for World Health (AAWH). (1998c). Drug resistance opens new door for old threats. *AAWH Quarterly, 12*(1), 4–5.

Benenson, A. S. (Ed.). (1995). *Control of communicable diseases in manual* (15th ed.). Washington, DC: American Public Health Association.

Centers for Disease Control and Prevention (CDC). (1994). *Addressing emerging disease threats: A prevention strategy for the United States.* Atlanta: U.S. Department of Health and Human Services.

Centers for Disease Control and Prevention (CDC). (1995a). Summary of notifiable diseases, United States 1995. *Morbidity and Mortality Weekly Report, 44*(53), 3.

Centers for Disease Control and Prevention (CDC). (1995b). *Epidemiology and prevention of vaccine-preventable diseases.* Atlanta: U.S. Department of Health and Human Services.

Centers for Disease Control and Prevention (CDC). (1998a). *Preventing infectious diseases: A strategy for the twenty-first century.* Atlanta: U.S. Department of Health and Human Services.

Centers for Disease Control and Prevention (CDC). (1998b). *Campylobacter.* Atlanta: U.S. Department of Health and Human Services: www.cdc.gov/ncidod/diseases/bacter/campyfaq.html.

Centers for Disease Control and Prevention (CDC). (1998c). *Salmonellosis.* Atlanta: U.S. Department of Health and Human Services: www.cdc.gov/ncidod/diseases/foodborn/salmon.html.

Centers for Disease Control and Prevention (CDC). (1998d). *Hookworm infection.* Atlanta: U.S. Department of Health and Human Services: www.cdc.gov/ncidod/dpd/hookworm.html.

Centers for Disease Control and Prevention (CDC). (1998e). *Giardiasis.* Atlanta: U.S. Department of Health and Human Services: www.cdc.gov/ncidod/dpd/giardias.html.

Centers for Disease Control and Prevention (CDC). (1998f). *Cryptosporidiosis: A guide for persons with HIV/AIDS.* Atlanta: U.S. Department of Health and Human Services: www.cdc.gov/ncidod/diseases/crypto/hivaids.html.

Centers for Disease Control and Prevention (CDC). (1998g). *Cryptosporidiosis.* Atlanta: U.S. Department of Health and Human Services: www.cdc.gov/ncidod/dpd/crypto.html.

Centers for Disease Control and Prevention. (1998h). *Cryptosporidiosis: Control and prevention.* Atlanta: U.S. Department of Health and Human Services: www.cdc.gov/ncidod/dpd/control.html.

Centers for Disease Control and Prevention (CDC). (1998i). *Reported tuberculosis in the United States, 1997.* Atlanta: U.S. Department of Health and Human Services.

Centers for Disease Control and Prevention (CDC). (1999a). *Antibiotic resistance. A new threat to your and your family's health.* Atlanta: U.S. Department of Health and Human Services: www.cdc.gov/ncidod/dbmd/antibioticresistance/default.html.

Centers for Disease Control and Prevention (CDC). (1999b). *Listeriosis.* Atlanta: U.S. Department of Health and Human Services: www.cdc.gov/ncidod/diseases/foodborn/lister.html.

Centers for Disease Control and Prevention (CDC). (1999c). *Escherichia coli O157:H7.* Atlanta: U.S. Department of Health and Human Services: www.cdc.gov/ncidod/diseases /foodborn /e_coli.html.

Centers for Disease Control and Prevention (CDC). (1999d). *Update: Multistate outbreak of Listeriosis.* Atlanta: U.S. Department of Health and Human Services: www.cdc.gov/od/oc/media/pressrel/r990114.html.

Centers for Disease Control and Prevention (CDC). (1999e). *Lyme disease: Introduction.* Atlanta: U.S. Department of Health and Human Services: www.cdc.gov/ncidod/dvbid/lymeinfo.html.

Centers for Disease Control and Prevention (CDC). (1999f). *Rabies: Introduction.* Atlanta: U.S. Department of Health and Human Services: www.cdc.gov/ncidod/dvrd/rabies/introduction/intro.html.

Centers for Disease Control and Prevention (CDC). (1999g). *HIV/AIDS prevention.* Atlanta: U.S. Department of Health and Human Services: www.cdc.gov/nchstp/hiv_aids/stats/cumulati.html.

Chomel, B. B. (1998). Diseases transmitted by pets. *World Health, 51*(4), 24–25.

Clark. P. A., Cegielski. J. P., & Hassell, W. (1997). TB or not TB? Increasing door-to-door response to screening. *Public Health Nursing, 14*(5), 268–271.

Clinton, H. R. (1993). Nurses in the front lines. *Nursing & Health Care, 14*(6), 286–288.

Cohen, F. L., & Larson, E. (1996). Emerging infectious diseases: Nursing responses. *Nursing Outlook, 44*(4), 164–168.

De Menezes Brandao, M., & Anselmo Viana da Silva Berzins, M. (1998). When does a pet become a health hazard? *World Health, 51*(4), 20–21.

Department of Health and Human Services (DHHS). (1991). *Healthy People 2000: National health program and disease prevention objectives.* Washington, DC: U.S. Government Printing Office.

Department of Health and Human Services (DHHS). (2000). *Healthy People 2010: Conference edition.* Washington, DC: U.S. Government Printing Office.

DOTS: A breakthrough in TB control. (1998). *World Health, 51*(2), 14–15.

Drug resistance opens new door for old threats. (1998). *American Association for World Health Quarterly, 12*(1), 4.

Dzenowagis, J. (1997). Using electronic links for monitoring diseases. *World Health, 50*(6), 8–9.

Facts about adult immunization. (1997). Bethesda, MD: National Coalition for Adult Immunization: www.nfid.org/factsheets/adultfact.html.

Facts about hepatitis A for adults. (1996). Bethesda, MD: National Coalition for Adult Immunization: www.nfid.org/factsheets/hepaadult.html.

Facts about hepatitis B for adults. (1997). Bethesda, MD: National Coalition for Adult Immunization: www.nfid.org/factsheets/hepbadult.html.

Facts about influenza for adults. (1997). Bethesda, MD: National Coalition for Adult Immunization: www.nfid.org/factsheets/influadult.html.

Facts about pneumococcal disease for adults. (1997). Bethesda, MD: National Coalition for Adult Immunization: www.nfid.org/factsheets/pneuadult.html.

Foege, W. H. (1998). Controlling emerging infections: Lessons from the smallpox eradication campaign. *Emerging Infectious Diseases, 4*(3), 412–413.

Foodborne illness. (1998, July/December). *AAWH Quarterly, 12*(3–4), 8.

Gardner, P., & Schaffner, W. (1993). Immunization of adults. *New England Journal of Medicine, 328,* 1252–1258.

Garrett, L. (1994). *The coming plague. Newly emerging diseases in a world out of balance.* New York: Farrar, Straus, and Giroux.

Grimes, D. E., & Grimes, R. M. (1995). Tuberculosis: What nurses need to know to help control the epidemic. *Nursing Outlook, 43*(4), 164–173.

Gubler, D. J. (1998). Resurgent vector-borne diseases as a global health problem. *Emerging Infectious Diseases, 4*(3), 442–449.

Guerrant, R. L. (1997). Cryptosporidiosis: An emerging, highly infectious threat. *Emerging Infectious Diseases, 3*(1).

Hantavirus infection—Southwestern United States: Interim recommendations for risk reduction. (1993, July 30). *Morbidity and Mortality Weekly Report, 42,* 1–13.

Harkness, G. A. (1995). *Epidemiology in nursing practice.* St. Louis: Mosby.

Hepatitis C. (1997). Geneva: World Health Organization.

Hepatitis learning guide. (1998). Abbott Park, IL: Abbott Diagnostics.

Herrington, J. E., Campbell, G. L., Bailey, R. E., Cartter, M. L., Adams, M., Frazier, E. L., Damrow, T. A., & Gensheimer, K. F. (1997). Predisposing factors for individuals' Lyme disease prevention practices: Connecticut, Maine, and Montana. *American Journal of Public health, 87*(12), 2035–2038.

Heymann, D. L. (1998). Zoonoses—disease passed from animals to humans. *World Health, 51* (4), 4.

HIV-related conditions. Focus on: Tuberculosis (1999, June/July). *HIV Frontline. A Newsletter for Professionals Who Counsel People Living with HIV, 37,* 6.

Immunizations lag among older adults. (1999, April). *The Nation's Health. The Official Newspaper of the American Public Health Association, 29*(3), 24.

Institute of Medicine. (1992). *Emerging infections: Microbial threats to health in the United States*. Washington, DC: National Academy Press.

IntelliHealth news. (1998, September 21). Rabies may explain the vampire legend. *The PointCast Network.*

Kaferstein, F. K., & Meslin, F. X. (1998, July/August). Keeping foods of animal origin safe. *World Health, 51*(4), 28–29.

Liese, B. H. (1998, May/June). A brake on economic development. *World Health, 51*(3), 16–17.

Mahon, B. E., Slutsker, L., Hutwagner, L., Drenzek, C., Maloney, K., Toomey, K., & Griffin, P. M. (1999). Consequences in Georgia of a nationwide outbreak of salmonella infections: What you don't know might hurt you. *American Journal of Public Health, 89*(1), 31–35.

Mann, J. M. (1994). Preface. In *The coming plague. Newly emerging diseases in a world out of balance*. New York: Farrar, Straus, and Giroux.

Marsh, K., & Waruiru, C. (1998). What is malaria? *World Health, 51*(3), 6–7.

Meslin, F. X., & Stohr, K. (1998). Animals that infect humans. *World Health, 51*(4), 5.

MMWR. (1998, October 30). Prevention and treatment of tuberculosis among patients infected with human immunodeficiency virus: Principles of therapy and revised recommendations. *Morbidity and Mortality Weekly Report, 47*(RR-20), 5.

Molyneux, M. (1998). Severe malaria. *World Health, 51*(3), 8–9.

Moore, M., McCray, E., & Onorato, I. M. (1999). Cross-matching TB and AIDS registries: TB patients with HIV co-infection, United States, 1993–1994. *Public Health Reports, 114*, 269–277.

Murphy, F. A. (1998). Emerging zoonoses. *Emerging Infectious Diseases, 4*(3), 429–435.

National Institute of Allergy and Infectious Diseases. (1997a, December). *Flu*. Washington, DC: Department of Health and Human Services.

National Institute of Allergy and Infectious Diseases. (1997b, March). *Tuberculosis*. Washington, DC: Department of Health and Human Services.

National Institute of Allergy and Infectious Diseases. (1998a, January). *Foodborne diseases*. Washington, DC: Department of Health and Human Services.

National Institute of Allergy and Infectious Diseases. (1998b). *Lyme disease. The facts, the challenge*. Washington, DC: Department of Health and Human Services.

Nchinda, T. C. (1998). Malaria: A reemerging disease in Africa. *Emerging Infectious Diseases, 4*(3), 398–403.

Neufeldt, V. (Ed.). (1996). *Webster's new world college dictionary* (3rd ed.). New York: Macmillan.

Pan American Health Organization. (1999). *AIDS/sexually transmitted diseases.* Washington, DC: www.paho.org/english/aid/aidstd.html.

Pinger, R. L. (1998). Lyme disease: An emerging health threat. *The Community. The Official Jones and Bartlett Community Health Newsletter, 1,* 1–2.

Pinkowish, M. D. (1998, August 15). Infectious diseases: Still emerging in 1998. *Patient Care, 32–35, 39–40, 42, 47, 51–52.*

Shankar, A. H., Genton, B., Semba, R. D., Baisor, M., Paino, J., Tamja, S., Adiguma, T., Wu, L., Rare, L., Tielsch, J. M., Alpers, M. P., & West, K. P., Jr. (1999, July 17). Effect of vitamin A supplementation on morbidity due to Plasmodium falciparum in young children in Papua New Guinea: a randomised trial. *Lancet, 354,* 203–208.

Shute, N. (1998). Hepatitis C: A silent killer. *U.S. News & World Report, 124*(24), 60–66.

The mother of fevers. (1998, March/April). *World Health, 51*(2), 12–13.

Thurm, K. (1998, November). Adult immunizations save lives. *Closing the Gap. A Newsletter of the Office of Minority Health.* Washington, DC: Department of Health and Human Services.

Timmreck, T. C. (1998). *An introduction to epidemiology.* (2nd ed.). Boston: Jones and Bartlett.

Toro, J., Vega, J. D., Khan, A. S., Mills, J. N., Padula, P. Terry, W., Yadon, Z., Valderrama, R., Ellis, B. A., Pavletic, C., Cerda, R., Zaki, S., Wun-Ju, S., Meyer, R., Tapia, M., Mansilla, C., Baro, M., Vergara, J. A., Concha, M., Calderon, G., Enria, D., Peters, C. J., & Ksiazek, T. G. (1998). An outbreak of hantavirus pulmonary syndrome, Chile, 1997. *Emerging Infectious Diseases, 4*(4), 687–694.

Torres, M. (1998, July). Tuberculosis update. *National Council of La Raza Center for Health Promotion Fact Sheet.*

Valanis, B. (1999). *Epidemiology in health care.* (3rd ed.). Stamford, CT: Appleton & Lange.

Wilde, H., & Mitmoonpitak, C. (1998). Canine rabies in Thailand. *World Health, 51*(4), 10–11.

Wittenberg, R. L. (1998). From the president. Efforts toward eliminating seven diseases from the globe. *American Association for World Health Quarterly, 12,*(2), 2.

Chapter 20

Sexually Transmitted Diseases and HIV/AIDS

Sharyn Janes, Janet St. Lawrence, Julia B. St. Lawrence, and Barbara Aranda-Naranjo

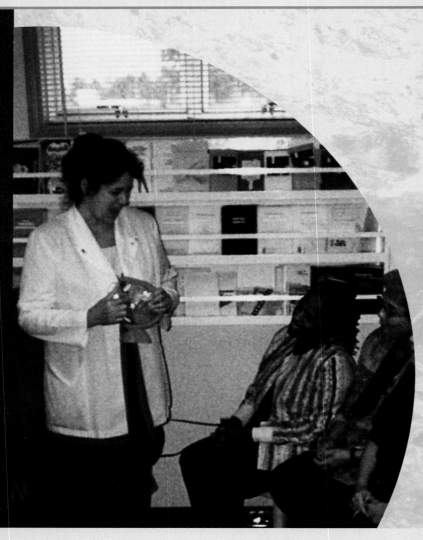

Sexual activity is a way to express intimacy and positive emotions, enable reproduction, and provide physical pleasure, but it also can be associated with potentially harmful consequences. The undesired outcomes from sexual activity include unintended pregnancies and sexually transmitted diseases (STDs), including infection with the human immunodeficiency virus (HIV), which can lead to acquired immunodeficiency syndrome (AIDS). STDs have been described as America's "hidden epidemic" because the rates of some STDs are now higher than they were three decades ago and the United States has the highest rates of STDs in the industrialized world.

QUESTIONS TO CONSIDER

After reading this chapter, answer the following questions:
1. How are STDs affecting global health?
2. What are some of the most common STDs in the United States?
3. What are some of the major health consequences of STDs?
4. How is the HIV/AIDS pandemic affecting global health?
5. What are some of the populations at risk for HIV in the United States and why?
6. How is the U.S. health care system handling the overload of sexually transmitted diseases and HIV/AIDS?
7. What is the role of the nurse in the diagnosis and treatment of STDs and HIV/AIDS?
8. What are some of the prevention efforts being done by communities?
9. What is the role of the community health nurse in prevention efforts?

KEY TERMS

Chlamydia
Gonorrhea
Herpes simplex
Human immunodeficiency
  virus (HIV)

Acquired
  immunodeficiency
  syndrome (AIDS)

Human papillomavirus
Ryan White CARE Act
Sexually transmitted
  diseases

Syphilis
Transtheoretical model of
  behavior change

Scope of the Problem

Rates of some **sexually transmitted diseases (STDs)** are higher in the United States than in some developing countries (Aral & Holmes, 1991). In 1996, the reported incidence of gonorrhea in the United States was 124 cases per 100,000 persons, 26 times greater than the rate in Germany and 50 times greater than the rate in Sweden (CDC, 1997a). Similar disproportions exist for all of the curable STDs, such as gonorrhea and syphilis, all of which are substantially higher in the United States than in other developed countries. For viral STDs, the discrepancy is not as great between the United States and other countries in the developed world, but the overall disease burden in this country is staggering. For example, the herpes simplex virus type 2 (HSV-2) infection, a persistent, incurable viral infection, is present in more than 20% of American adults, an estimated 45 million infected individuals (CDC, 1997a).

More than 12 million Americans become infected with STDs every year (Institute of Medicine, 1997) and 5 of the 10 most frequently reported diseases in this country are STDs: gonorrhea, chlamydia, **acquired immunodeficiency syndrome (AIDS)**, primary and secondary syphilis, and hepatitis B. In fact, 87% of cases of the top 10 reportable diseases are STDs (CDC, 1996). The actual rate is probably more than double the number of reported cases, because STDs are widely underreported in this country. See Box 20-1 for clinical presentations of STDs.

The number of identified STDs continues to grow as newly emerging infections are identified. Since 1980, eight new STDs have appeared in the United States. Many of these, such as human papillomavirus (HPV), HIV, and hepatitis B, are viral diseases that are incurable at present. Bacterial STDs such as gonorrhea, syphilis, and chlamydia are curable in most cases but are still present at unacceptably high levels in the United States.

There is no such thing as a "typical" STD client. STDs affect people of all socioeconomic levels, races, ethnicities, genders, ages, and religions. STDs are almost always transmitted from one person to another during sexual intercourse. They are transmitted most efficiently during anal or vaginal intercourse and less efficiently during oral intercourse. Some STDs, such as hepatitis B and HIV, can also be transmitted parenterally and are particularly problematic among intravenous drug user who share injection equipment. In some cases, a pregnant woman can transmit an STD to her infant prenatally, during birth, or postnatally during breast-feeding, as happens with HIV, for example.

Against this backdrop of high STD rates, some subpopulations have higher STD incidences than average. In most parts of the United States, sexually active adolescents, regardless of their race or socioeconomic status, have a 5% to 10% prevalence of chlamydial infection (CDC, 1993). In addition, men who have sex with other men, especially young men, generally have higher rates of STDs (Lafferty, Hughes, & Handsfield, 1997). STDs are also common among persons who use illicit drugs, including both injection drug users (IDUs) and non-IDUs. There is also geographic variability, with bacterial STD rates sharply higher in the southeastern United States and in many urban areas than for the country as a whole (Nakashima, Rolfs, Flock, Kilmarx, & Greenspan, 1996).

The presence of an STD greatly increases the risk of HIV transmission during sexual activity (Wasserheit, 1992). A recent study of syphilis conducted in several large U.S. cities found that 18% of clients with early syphilis also were infected with HIV (Rolfs, Joesoef, Hendershot, Rompalo, Augebraun, Chiu, Bolan, Johnson, French, Steen, Radolf, & Larsen, 1997). Ulcerative STDs such as syphilis bleed easily and come into contact with vaginal, cervical, oral, urethral, or rectal mucosa during sexual activity. This is of concern because HIV is routinely found in the exudate of genital ulcers of both men and women with HIV infection (Schacker, Ryncarz, Goddard, Diem, Shaughnessy, & Corey, 1997). In both men and women, inflammatory STDs such as gonorrhea and chlamydia increase both the prevalence of HIV shedding and the "viral load" of HIV present in genital secretions (Atkins, Carlin, Emery, Griffiths, & Boag, 1996), both of which probably lead to increased infectiousness. Among HIV-infected men with gonorrhea, for example, HIV shedding in semen is 10-fold higher, but when the gonorrhea is treated, the HIV shedding decreases significantly (Cohen, Hoffman, Royce, Kazembe, Dyer, Daly, Zimba, Vernazza, Maida, Fiscus, & Eron, 1997). In addition, both ulcerative STDs (e.g., herpes, syphilis, chancroid) and nonulcerative STDs (e.g., gonorrhea, chlamydia) disrupt normal epithelial and mucosal barriers to infection, increasing an infected person's susceptibility to HIV infection (Levine, Pope, Bhoomkar, Tambe, Lewis, Zaidi, Farshy, Mithcell,

---

BOX 20-1   CLINICAL PRESENTATIONS OF SEXUALLY TRANSMITTED DISEASES

In the case of sexually transmitted diseases (STDs), one organism does not cause one identifiable syndrome. Instead, similar presentations can be caused by different STDs. For example, pelvic inflammatory disease (PID) can be caused by gonorrhea, chlamydia, or other bacteria. Genital ulcers can be caused by herpes, chancroid, or syphilis, as well as by other infections. Some STDs, such as syphilis or HIV/AIDS, have many different clinical presentations and mimic many other health problems. Some diseases that were at one time not perceived as being particularly serious now are known to lead to very serious outcomes. For example, human papillomavirus infection (HPV) was widely associated with genital warts but not regarded as a serious condition until after it was discovered that HPV also causes several types of cancers.

& Talkington, 1998; Spinola, Orazi, Arno, Fortney, Kotylo, Chen, Capagnari, & Hood, 1996). If individuals at risk for HIV infection could be more effectively accessed and treated for other STDs, it could have a substantial impact on lowering HIV transmission (Garnett & Anderson, 1995; Robinson, Mulder, Auvert, & Hayes, 1997). See Box 20-2 for a list of basic facts about STDs.

Common STDs

The term *STD* refers to more than 25 infectious organisms that can be transmitted during sexual contact; they cause dozens of different clinical presentations. Five of the most common STDs are described briefly in the following sections. Table 20-1 lists the 25 STDs that are currently known and their associated health conditions. HIV/AIDS is discussed separately in a later section.

Syphilis

Syphilis is a systemic disease caused by *Treponema pallidum.* The disease progresses through three stages, with different clinical presentations at each stage:

1. Primary infection: *ulcer or chancre at the infection site*

2. Secondary infection: *rash, mucocutaneous lesions, and adenopathy*

3. Tertiary infection: *cardiac, neurological, ophthalmic, auditory, or gummatous lesions*

Latent syphilis is defined as the periods when patients are seropositive but have no signs or symptoms. Treatment of latent syphilis is important to halt the progression of the disease. Although most associated with tertiary infection, central nervous system disease can occur at any stage of syphilis. Persons diag-

nosed with syphilis showing any neurological symptoms such as ophthalmic or auditory symptoms, cranial nerve palsies, and signs and symptoms of meningitis should have a cerebrospinal fluid examination. Severe dementia can occur if syphilis infection is left untreated (CDC, 1998a).

Pregnant women should be screened for syphilis in the early stages of pregnancy because early treatment of the mother's syphilis infection has a high success rate in preventing the baby from acquiring congenital syphilis. In communities in which the prevalence of syphilis is high or for patients at high risk, serological testing should also be done at 28 weeks' gestation and at delivery. No infant should leave the hospital or birthing center without the mother having been screened for syphilis at least once during pregnancy. Children born with congenital syphilis can have birth defects affecting all systems, including severe neurological abnormalities (CDC, 1998a).

Penicillin G, given intramuscularly, has been an effective treatment for syphilis for many years. It is a cure in the early stages of syphilis and helps slow disease progression and prevent complications in later stages. Dosage and duration of treatment depend on the stage and severity of the disease. For patients with penicillin allergies, doxycycline or tetracycline can be used. However, patients with poor treatment compliance histories or those who are pregnant should be desensitized and treated with penicillin. All sexual partners should be identified and treated (CDC, 1998a).

After remaining at a steady level through the 1970s and into the 1980s, syphilis increased substantially from 1987 to 1990, then began to decrease once again (CDC, 1997a). This waxing and waning illustrates how syphilis and other STDs can reemerge with alarming intensity. The most recent increase was associated with new patterns of behavior related to illicit drug use, particularly crack cocaine users and their sex partners. Unfortunately, traditional public health strategies proved to be less effective in curtailing syphilis when it emerged in this new context because illicit drug users tend not to seek treatment for a variety of reasons, including fear of legal prosecution (Andrus, Fleming, Harger, Chin, Bennet, Horan, Oxman, Olson, & Foster, 1990; Farley, Hadler, & Gunn, 1990).

Chlamydia

Chlamydia, caused by *Chlamydia trachomatis,* is the most common bacterial STD in the United States, with more than 4 million cases reported annually (CDC, 1995a; NIAID, 1998). The highest rates of chlamydia occur in those who are 15 to 19 years of age. As many as 85% of the infections in women and 40% of the infections in men are asymptomatic and will not be detected or treated without widespread screening programs. Although chlamydia is easily treated with antibiotics, more than 1 million women every year develop pelvic inflammatory disease (PID) as a result of unrecognized and untreated cervical chlamydia infections (Rolfs, Galaid, & Zaidi, 1992).

If symptoms occur, they usually appear within 1 to 3 weeks after exposure. Early signs of chlamydia include abnormal genital

TABLE 20-1   SEXUALLY TRANSMITTED DISEASES

PATHOGEN	ASSOCIATED INFECTIONS AND CONDITIONS
BACTERIAL	
Neisseria gonorrhoeae	Urethritis, epididymitis, proctitis, cervicitis, endometritis, salpingitis, perihepatitis, bartholinitis, pharyngitis, conjunctivitis, vaginitis, disseminated gonococcal infection, chorioamnionitis, premature rupture of membranes, premature delivery, amniotic infection syndrome
Chlamydia trachomatis	All of the above except disseminated gonococcal infection, plus otitis media, rhinitis, pneumonia in infants, and Reiter's syndrome
Mycoplasma hominis	Postpartum fever
Ureaplasma urealyticum	Nongonococcal urethritis
Treponema pallidum	Syphilis
Gardnerella vaginalis	Bacterial vaginosis
Haemophilus ducreyi	Chancroid
Calymmatobacterium granulomatis	Donovanosis (granuloma inguinale)
Shigella spp.	Shigellosis in homosexual men
Campylobacter spp.	Enteritis, proctocolitis
VIRAL	
Human immunodeficiency virus (HIV)	Acquired immunodeficiency syndrome (AIDS)
Herpes simplex virus	Initial and recurrent genital herpes, aseptic meningitis, neonatal herpes
Human papillomavirus (more than 70 types have been identified)	Condyloma acuminata, laryngeal papilloma, cervical intraepithelial neoplasia and carcinoma, vaginal carcinoma, anal carcinoma, vulvar carcinoma, penile carcinoma
Hepatitis B virus	Acute hepatitis B infection, chronic active hepatitis, polyarteritis nodosa, chronic membranous glomerulonephritis, hepatocellular carcinoma
Hepatitis A	Acute hepatitis A
Cytomegalovirus (CMV)	Heterophil-negative infectious mononucleosis, congenital CMV infection with gross birth defects and infant mortality, cognitive impairment (mental retardation, sensorineural deafness), and protean manifestations in an immunosuppressed host
Molluscum contagiosum virus	Genital molluscum contagiosum
Human T-cell lymphotrophic virus, types I and II	Human T-cell leukemia or lymphoma
Human herpesvirus type 8	Kaposi's sarcoma (uncertain), body cavity lymphoma
PROTOZOA	
Trichomonas vaginalis	Trichomonal vaginitis
Entamoeba histolytica	Amebiasis in men who have sex with men
Giardia lamblia	Giardiasis in men who have sex with men
FUNGI	
Candida albicans	Vulvovaginitis, balanitis
ECTOPARASITES	
Phthirus pubic	Pubic lice infestation
Sarcoptes scabiei	Scabies

Source: Institute of Medicine, 1997.

discharge or painful urination. However, these symptoms often are ignored because they are so mild. Chlamydia can be transmitted during vaginal, anal, or oral sex with an infected partner. Pregnant women may pass the infection to their newborns during delivery, leading to neonatal eye infections or pneumonia (NIAID, 1998).

Chlamydia is completely curable if diagnosed before complications occur. The antibiotics most commonly used are a 1-day course of azithromycin or a 7-day course of doxycycline. Other antibiotics such as erythromycin or ofloxacin are also effective. Pregnant women are treated with azithromycin, erythromycin, or amoxicillin. Sexual partners should be identified and treated to prevent reinfection (CDC, 1998a; NIAID, 1998).

Gonorrhea

Gonorrhea, a bacterial infection caused by *Neisseria gonorrhoeae*, is spread through vaginal, anal, or oral sexual activity with an infected partner. Pregnant women can pass the infection to their newborns during delivery, leading to eye infections in their babies. The early symptoms are often mild, and many women never develop symptoms. This can be problematic because untreated gonorrhea can lead to serious complications such as PID. If symptoms occur, they usually appear within 2 to 10 days after exposure. Initial symptoms in women include pain or burning with urination and yellow or bloody vaginal discharge. More advanced symptoms, such as abdominal pain, bleeding between menstrual periods, vomiting, or fever, usually indicate progression to PID. Men usually experience a penile discharge and burning with urination that may be severe. Symptoms of rectal infection include anal itching, discharge, or painful bowel movements (CDC, 1998a; NIAID, 1998).

Gonorrhea is becoming increasingly resistant to antibiotics, resulting in more expensive treatment because the usual options are no longer effective. As recently as 1976, almost all gonorrhea infections could be cured with penicillin (Aral & Holmes, 1991). Since that time, resistant strains steadily increased from 2% of the gonorrhea infections in 1987 to 30% in 1994 (CDC, 1995a). One of the most effective treatments for gonorrhea is ceftriaxone, which can be given in a single dose. Other effective antibiotics include cefixime, ciprofloxacin, or ofloxacin. Because gonorrhea often occurs simultaneously with a chlamydial infection, combination therapy with ceftriaxone and doxycycline or azithromycin is often effective. Since dual therapy for gonorrhea and chlamydia was initiated, the incidence of chlamydia has decreased significantly in some populations (CDC, 1998a; NIAID, 1998).

Herpes Simplex Virus

Sexually transmitted **herpes simplex** virus (HSV) infection is widespread and produces intermittent painful ulcers. Although the ulcers can be treated, the underlying infection persists and ulcers recur (Quinn & Cates, 1992). This is of concern because HSV can be transmitted to a sex partner even in the absence of a genital ulcer and can also be passed from an infected mother to her newborn during childbirth. Approximately 200,000 to 500,000 new cases of HSV occur each year in the United States, and it is estimated that 45 million individuals are currently infected. This prevalence estimate means that one of every four women and one of every five men in the United States will become infected with HSV during their lifetimes (CDC, 1997a, 1998a; NIAID, 1998).

There are two types of HSV, both of which can cause genital herpes. HSV type 1 most often causes fever blisters and cold sores around the mouth area, but it can cause genital herpes also. HSV type 2 generally causes genital lesions, but it can also cause sores around the mouth. Eighty percent of people with genital herpes never develop symptoms or do not recognize them. If symptoms do occur, they will usually appear within 2 to 10 days after exposure. The first episode of ulcers usually lasts 2 to 3 weeks. Early symptoms include genital itching or burning; pain in the legs, buttocks, or genital area; and vaginal discharge. Later symptoms include lesions inside the vagina or in the urinary tract. Small red bumps occur first, followed by blisters, and then painful sores (CDC, 1998a; NIAID, 1998).

Genital herpes cannot be cured, but it can be controlled with acyclovir. Treatment with acyclovir also reduces the risk of transmission to sexual partners. A baby born with herpes can develop encephalitis, severe rashes, and eye problems. Early treatment with acyclovir greatly reduces serious complications in infants. Delivery by cesarean section also greatly reduces the risk of newborn infection (CDC, 1998a; NIAID, 1998).

Human Papillomavirus

Human papillomavirus (HPV) is one of the most common STDs in the world, occurring across all socioeconomic levels. An estimated 24 million Americans are infected with HPV, and as many as 1 million new infections occur every year. Of the more than 60 known types of HPV, 20 are spread through sexual contact. Low-risk types of HPV cause genital warts (condylomata acuminata). Other high-risk types of HPV can cause vaginal, cervical, and anal cancers (CDC, 1998a; NIAID, 1998).

Genital warts are very contagious. Approximately two-thirds of people who have sexual contact with a person with genital warts will develop warts, usually within 3 months of exposure. In women, warts can occur inside and outside the vagina, on the cervix, or around the anus. In men, warts can occur on the tip or shaft of the penis, on the scrotum, or around the anus. Left untreated, genital warts may disappear or may grow into a raised fleshy growth with a cauliflower-like appearance. Because there is no way to predict whether warts will disappear or grow, people who suspect that they have genital warts should seek treatment (CDC, 1998a; NIAID, 1998).

The primary goal of treatment is removal of the warts. Although there is no cure for HPV, treatment can induce wart-free periods. Treatment varies with each individual case and is guided by the preference of the client, the experience of the health care provider, and the available resources. Available treatment include client-applied therapies (e.g., podofilox, imiquimod) and provider-applied therapies (e.g., cryotherapy, podophyllin resin, trichloroacetic acid, bichloracetic acid, interferon, surgery). Like many other STDs, HPV often has no visible symptoms. It is estimated that nearly 50% of people infected with HPV are unaware of their infection and the risk of transmission to others.

Examination of sex partners is not necessary because chance of reinfection is minimal, and in the absence of a cure, treatment to reduce transmission is not realistic. However, sex partners should be counseled about the implications of having a partner who has HPV. Because there is no cure for HPV, clients and sex partners should be aware that the client might remain infectious after the warts are gone. Condom use may decrease the risk of infection but does not eliminate it (CDC, 1998a; NIAID, 1998).

Health Consequences of STDs

Most people are not aware of the long-term health consequences of STDs other than HIV/AIDS. There are several reasons why STDs rarely command attention or concern. Many STDs are without symptoms and go undetected until years after infection, when serious sequelae appear. Many of the major adverse outcomes that do occur from STD infections arise years after the initial infection, so the connection is not made between the original infection and the later consequence, except for the awareness that HIV-infection leads to AIDS. Viral STDs, in particular, often result in lifelong infection for which there is no cure at present. Public discourse is also hampered by the stigma of STDs. Finally, many people—including health providers—find it difficult to discuss sexual behavior openly and comfortably. This can make it difficult for a health provider to take a client's sexual history or to counsel a client effectively about his or her sexual health.

Cancers

Several STDs are associated with cancers, although this relationship goes largely unrecognized among the general public. These include HPV, hepatitis B virus, human T-cell lymphotrophic virus type 1, human herpesvirus type 8, and Epstein-Barr virus. Studies find that cervical infection with HPV is associated with 80% of cases of invasive cervical cancer (NIH, 1996), and women with HPV cervical infections are more than 10 times more likely to later develop invasive cervical cancer (Schiffman, 1992). In the United States, approximately 16,000 new cases of cervical cancer are diagnosed each year (American Cancer Society, 1996). This number alone does not begin to convey the physical or emotional anguish experienced by literally hundreds of thousands of women who develop precancerous cervical lesions.

Although cancers of the vulva, vagina, anus, and penis are less common than cervical carcinoma, they equal nearly 50% of the total numbers of cervical cancer cases. Each of these is associated with HPV infection, and when HIV is also present, the likelihood that HPV will progress to cancer is increased.

Reproductive Health Problems

Many reproductive health problems are the consequence of unrecognized or untreated STD infections. Such reproductive health problems may be short term, as is the case for PID, pregnancy complications, or epididymitis, or long term, such as infertility.

Pelvic Inflammatory Disease

PID is one of the most serious threats to women's reproductive health. Most cases result from chlamydial or gonorrheal infection that initially involves the cervix but later migrates into the uterus and through the fallopian tubes into the pelvic or abdominal cavity (Jossens, Schachter, & Sweet, 1994). Each year, more than 1 million women in the United States experience an episode of PID (Rolfs, Galaid, & Zaidi, 1992). At least one-fourth of these women will have serious long-term outcomes, the most common of which are ectopic pregnancy and infertility. Other complications include chronic pelvic pain and painful intercourse caused by the scarring in the pelvis that can result from PID.

Ectopic Pregnancy

Ectopic pregnancies can result from partial blockage of the fallopian tubes as a result of PID. Women who have had an episode of PID are 6 to 10 times more likely to have an ectopic pregnancy. Ectopic pregnancies are a leading cause of first-trimester fetal deaths and one of the leading causes of maternal death during pregnancy (Marchbanks, Annegers, Coulam, Strathy, & Kurland, 1988).

Infertility

When the fallopian tubes are blocked or damaged as the result of an STD infection, infertility can result. It is estimated that 15% of women's infertility is a consequence of tubal damage caused by PID (Institute of Medicine, 1997). Many of these women experienced PID symptoms that were so mild that they went unrecognized and untreated until a fertility workup identified PID.

Health Consequences for Pregnant Women and Infants

STDs create many complications for pregnant women and their infants (Brunham, Holmes, & Embree, 1990). Pregnant women with STDs can transmit the infections prenatally, during birth, or after birth. Common STDs that are known to create adverse outcomes in pregnant women and their babies include chlamydia, gonorrhea, syphilis, cytomegalovirus, genital herpes, and HIV. Some STDs, such as HPV, hepatitis B, and human T-cell lymphotrophic virus type 1, produce sequelae years and even decades after the initial infection (Institute of Medicine, 1997). STDs can cause even more severe and potentially life-threatening conditions in fetuses or newborns because of their immature nervous system. Brain damage, spinal cord abnormalities, and sensory impairments are of particular concern. Newborns infected with hepatitis B have a 90% chance of being lifelong carriers of the disease.

HEALTHY PEOPLE 2010

OBJECTIVES RELATED TO SEXUALLY TRANSMITTED DISEASES

Bacterial STD Illness and Disability

25.1   Reduce the proportion of adolescents and young adults with *Chlamydia trachomatis* infections.

25.2   Reduce gonorrhea.

25.3   Eliminate sustained domestic transmission of primary and secondary syphilis.

Viral STD Illness and Disability

25.4   Reduce the proportion of adults with genital herpes infection.

25.5   Reduce the proportion of persons with human papillomavirus.

STD Complications Affecting Females

25.6   Reduce the proportion of females who have ever required treatment for pelvic inflammatory disease.

25.7   Reduce the proportion of childless females with fertility problems who have had a sexually transmitted disease or who have required treatment for pelvic inflammatory disease.

25.8   Reduce HIV infections in adolescent and young females aged 13 to 24 years that are associated with heterosexual contact.

STD Complications Affecting the Fetus and Newborn

25.9   Reduce congenital syphilis.

25.10   Reduce neonatal consequences from maternal sexually transmitted diseases, including chlamydial pneumonia, gonococcal and chlamydial ophthalmia neonatorum, laryngeal papillomatosis (from human papillomavirus infection), neonatal herpes, and preterm birth and low birth weight associated with bacterial vaginosis.

Personal Behaviors

25.11   Increase the proportion of adolescents who abstain from sexual intercourse or use condoms if currently sexually active.

25.12   Increase the number of positive messages related to responsible sexual behavior during weekday and nightly prime-time television programming.

Community Protection Infrastructure

25.13   Increase the proportion of tribal, state, and local sexually transmitted disease programs that routinely offer hepatitis B vaccines to all STD clients.

25.14   Increase the proportion of youth detention facilities and adult city or county jails that screen for common bacterial sexually transmitted diseases within 24 hours of admission and treat STDs (when necessary) before persons are released.

25.15   Increase the proportion of all local health departments that have contracts with managed care providers for the treatment of nonplan partners of clients with bacterial sexually transmitted diseases (gonorrhea, syphilis, and chlamydia).

Personal Health Services

25.16   Increase the proportion of sexually active females aged 25 years and younger who are screened annually for genital chlamydia infections.

25.17   Increase the proportion of pregnant females screened for sexually transmitted diseases (including HIV infection and

Continued

HEALTHY PEOPLE 2010—cont'd

bacterial vaginosis) during prenatal health care visits, according to recognized standards.

25.18 Increase the proportion of primary care providers who treat clients with sexually transmitted diseases and who manage cases according to recognized standards.

25.19 Increase the proportion of all sexually transmitted disease clinic clients who are being treated for bacterial STDs (chlamydia, gonorrhea, and syphilis) and who are offered provider referral services for their sex partners.

Source: DHHS, 2000.

Health Consequences for Men

The consequences of some STDs are similar in both men and women. HPV, for example, is associated with penile and anal cancers in men, although both are less common than cervical cancer among women. Most people are not aware that STDs produce long-term sequelae such as infertility for men, but Over and Piot (1993) found that the health burden of chancroid, chlamydia, gonorrhea, HIV, and syphilis was high among men as well as among women.

Mortality of STDs

Most STD-related deaths are associated with AIDS, which has received considerable attention from the media. However, many other STDs cause fatal complications in adults and in fetuses and infants. A recent study concluded that the three leading causes of STD-related deaths in women are due to cervical cancer (57% of deaths), AIDS (29%), and hepatitis B and C (10%), all of which are related to viral STDs.

HIV/AIDS

By impairing and eventually destroying the immune system, HIV progressively eliminates the body's ability to fight infections and certain cancers. A badly weakened immune system is unable to fight off microbes that would not cause illness in a healthy person. These life-threatening diseases are called *opportunistic infections* and are generally the first sign that an HIV-infected person has progressed to AIDS. AIDS is the end stage of HIV disease, which includes the whole spectrum of HIV infection, from initial infection with the virus to clinical AIDS and eventual death. HIV is found in semen, vaginal secretions, blood, and breast milk. HIV does not live outside the body and can be transmitted only through unprotected anal, vaginal, or oral sex; contaminated needles for injection drug use; contaminated blood products; or from an infected mother to her infant during pregnancy or delivery or through breast-feeding. The most common route of transmission is sexual contact (AAWH, 1997, 1998; NIAID, 1999a).

In 1993, the criteria for an AIDS diagnosis were amended to include three additional opportunistic infections (invasive cervical cancer, tuberculosis, and recurrent pneumonia) with a positive HIV antibody test and/or a CD4 blood cell count of 200 cells/mm^3. Before 1993, a positive HIV antibody test and a diagnosis of 1 of 23 specific opportunistic infections were the only criteria for an AIDS diagnosis. As a result, AIDS cases were undercounted before 1993.

Scope of the Problem

Since its discovery in 1981, HIV/AIDS has had a devastating effect in many regions of the United States and the world. Through June 30, 1999, a total of 711,344 AIDS cases were reported in the United States, with a total of 420,201 deaths. The figure on p. 445 lists the total AIDS cases by state or territory through December 1998. AIDS is the fifth leading cause of death in the United States for people 25 to 44 years old, after unintentional injuries, cancer, heart disease, and suicide (NIAID, 1999b). However, these figures are just the tip of the iceberg, because only AIDS cases are reportable in many states, not cases of HIV infection that have not progressed to AIDS. In 1999, only 34 states reported HIV cases to the CDC. Also, the reports did not include people tested at anonymous sites or those unaware of their HIV status. Therefore, the total number of people thought to be living with HIV infection in the United States is between 650,000 and 900,000, with 40,000 new cases occurring each year (AAWH, 1999; NIAID, 1999b).

An overview of HIV/AIDS in other parts of the world is even more serious. It is estimated that there were more than 34.3 million people worldwide living with HIV by the end of 1999. More than 95% of them live in developing countries, where social, economic, cultural, and political conditions that contribute to the spread of the virus are more prevalent (see the following figure). In 1998 alone, more than 5.8 million new HIV infections occurred around the world, approximately 16,000 new infections each day. In fact, it is estimated that every minute, 11 people in the world are infected with HIV. The most frightening concern for worldwide prevention and treatment efforts is the

HIV/AIDS IN THE UNITED STATES. TOTAL **AIDS** CASES REPORTED THROUGH DECEMBER 1998.

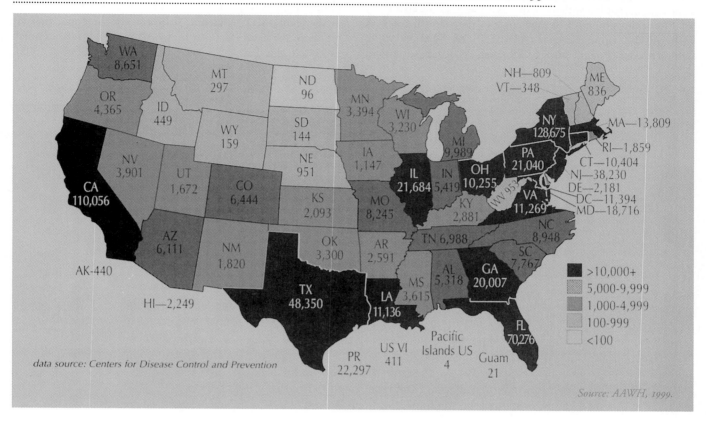

WA 8,651
OR 4,365
ID 449
MT 297
ND 96
MN 3,394
WI 3,230
NY 128,675
NH—809
VT—348
ME 836
MA—13,809
NV 3,901
UT 1,672
WY 159
SD 144
NE 951
IA 1,147
MI 9,989
OH 10,255
PA 21,040
RI—1,859
CT—10,404
NJ—38,230
CA 110,056
CO 6,444
KS 2,093
IL 21,684
IN 5,419
KY 2,881
WV 953
VA 11,269
DE—2,181
DC—11,394
MD—18,716
AZ 6,111
NM 1,820
OK 3,300
MO 8,245
AR 2,591
TN 6,988
NC 8,948
SC 7,767
AK—440
TX 48,350
LA 11,136
MS 3,615
AL 5,318
GA 20,007
HI—2,249
PR 22,297
US VI 411
Pacific Islands US 4
Guam 21
FL 70,276

data source: Centers for Disease Control and Prevention

Legend:
- >10,000+
- 5,000-9,999
- 1,000-4,999
- 100-999
- <100

Source: AAWH, 1999.

ADULTS AND CHILDREN ESTIMATED TO BE LIVING WITH **HIV/AIDS** IN 1999.
TOTAL CASES OF **HIV/AIDS** WORLDWIDE: 34.3 MILLION.

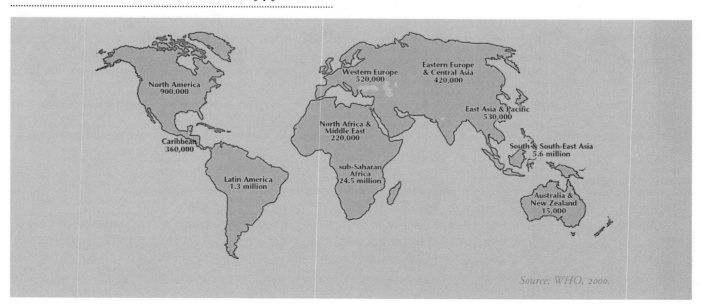

North America 900,000
Western Europe 520,000
Eastern Europe & Central Asia 420,000
East Asia & Pacific 530,000
Caribbean 360,000
North Africa & Middle East 220,000
South & South-East Asia 5.6 million
Latin America 1.3 million
sub-Saharan Africa 24.5 million
Australia & New Zealand 15,000

Source: WHO, 2000.

fact that 90% of HIV-infected people, especially in developing countries, do not know they are infected. Sadly, in the absence of an affordable cure, most of the people in the world living with HIV will die within a decade (AAWH, 1999; NIAID, 1999b; Schwartlander, Pisani, Walker, Monasch, & Gerbase, 1998).

United Nations estimates of the world population for 2050 have been recently downgraded from 9.4 billion to 8.9 billion because of the global AIDS epidemic. Estimates for the population increases in the nations hardest hit by AIDS are down by as much as 23% (Cook, Lavelle, Shapiro, Brownlee, & Robinson, 1998).

BOX 20-3 CHRONOLOGY OF THE BATTLE AGAINST AIDS

June 1981:	The U.S. Centers for Disease Control and Prevention (CDC) published the first report of a rare type of pneumonia, Pneumocystis carinii, in five gay men in Los Angeles.
July 1982:	U. S. health officials coined the term AIDS (acquired immunodeficiency syndrome) to describe the new disease.
December 1982:	The U.S. government issued a warning that the blood supply might be contaminated.
January 1983:	Heterosexuals were identified to be at risk for AIDS.
May 1983:	Dr. Luc Montagnier's team at the Pasteur Institute in Paris reported their discovery of the retrovirus believed to cause AIDS.
April 1984:	Dr. Robert Gallo at the National Cancer Institute announced that his laboratory had also isolated the AIDS retrovirus.
January 1985:	Montagnier and Gallo published the genetic sequence of the AIDS viruses they had identified. A lawsuit resulting from their competing claims was settled in March 1987, with the United States agreeing to share patent royalties.
March 1985:	The U.S. Food and Drug Administration (FDA) approved the first AIDS antibody test, which was immediately used to screen the nation's blood supply.
April 1985:	The first International Conference on AIDS began in Atlanta.
July 1985:	Journalists reported that actor Rock Hudson had AIDS, which brought the epidemic into the public limelight.
October 1986:	U.S. Surgeon General C. Everett Koop issued a landmark report on the AIDS epidemic that called for public health measures and sex education.
March 1987:	The FDA approved the antiretroviral compound zidovudine (AZT), the first AIDS drug.
May 1987:	President Ronald Reagan, who took office in 1981, made his first speech on the AIDS epidemic.
June 1987:	Citing public health concerns, the United States barred HIV-infected immigrants and travelers from entering the country.
October 1987:	U.S. scientists began preliminary tests of the first experimental AIDS vaccine.
October 1987:	Randy Shilts published his definitive chronicle of the AIDS epidemic, And the Band Played On.
June 1989:	The FDA approved aerosolized pentamidine for the prevention of P. carinii pneumonia, one of the biggest killers of AIDS patients.
April 1990:	Ryan White died after contracting AIDS from the blood supply 5 years earlier. He was an 18-year-old hemophiliac whose ostracism from his hometown in Indiana became a symbol of AIDS intolerance.
August 1990:	The Ryan White CARE Act was signed into law by the U. S. Congress.
November 1991:	All-star basketball player Magic Johnson announced that he had HIV disease.
July 1992:	The first reports of a combination drug treatment for AIDS were published.
December 1995:	The FDA approved saquinavir (Invirase), the first protease inhibitor.
July 1996:	At the 11th International Conference on AIDS in Vancouver, Canada, reports on newly infected patients on multidrug therapy whose viral loads dropped to undetectable levels suggested that the virus could possibly be held in check.

Source: Gorman, 1996.

....

And that was the day that we knew, oh! In the world there is a new disease called AIDS. I thought surely this will be the greatest war we ever fought. Surely many will die. And surely we will be frustrated, unable to help. But I also thought the Americans will find a treatment soon. This will not be forever.
                Dr. Jayo Kidenya, Bukoba, Tanzania, 1985

....

The introduction of the "triple-drug cocktails" (various combinations of two antiretroviral drugs and a protease inhibitor) in 1996 caused a significant drop in new AIDS cases and AIDS deaths in the United States. The new drug therapies, often referred to as *highly active antiretroviral therapies* (HAART), have enabled persons infected with HIV to live longer, more healthful lives by slowing the progression of HIV infection into AIDS and lowering the death rate from AIDS complications. The estimated number of new AIDS cases decreased 18% from 1996 to 1997 and 11% from 1997 to 1998. At the end of 1998, an estimated 297,137 people in the United States were living with AIDS, a 10% increase from 1997 (NIAID, 1999a). Unfortunately, the "drug cocktails" effective in controlling the HIV disease progression in the United States are not available to most of the people infected with HIV in the rest of the world. The high cost of the drugs (approximately $10,000 a year per client) exceeds the health care budgets of developing countries, where 95% of HIV-infected persons live (AAWH, 1998, 1999). Box 20-3 details a timeline of the fight against the AIDS epidemic.

....

The advance of antiretroviral drugs in industrialized countries has left some with the illusion that the worst of the AIDS epidemic has passed. Nothing could be further from reality in the developing world where the silent, voracious epidemic is wiping out the historic gains of the public health and economic development efforts of the last 20 years.
                Her Excellency Janat Mukwaya,
                Minister of Gender, Labour,
                and Social Development, Uganda
                UNICEF, *Progress of Nations,* 1999

....

Treatment is problematic in the United States as well. Drug resistance and side effects are beginning to develop in clients who

FYI

In some African countries, such as Zimbabwe and South Africa, life expectancy is expected to decrease by 20 years during the next few years as a direct result of the AIDS epidemic (Miramontes, 2000).

are long-term "drug cocktail" therapy recipients. The cost is also prohibitive for many uninsured and underinsured patients. **Ryan White CARE Act** funding (Box 20-4) is providing the necessary drugs for some, but the number of clients needing treatment is increasing while funding is not. Also, while progression to clinical AIDS and eventual death has been slowed, the number of people with HIV remains high and continues to rise in certain populations (AAWH, 1998).

Populations at Risk for HIV/AIDS

The HIV/AIDS pandemic has affected different populations in different ways around the world. In the United States and Europe, HIV/AIDS has been primarily a male disease, with high rates of infection among homosexual and bisexual men, IDUs, and their sexual partners. In the early years of the U.S. epidemic, hemophiliacs were also infected at high rates because of contaminated blood products used in the production of factor VIII. However, after April 1985, when testing of the blood supply for HIV antibodies was initiated, the incidence of HIV in this population greatly declined and has remained low. In the rest of the world, however, the male/female HIV infection ratio has always been nearly equal, with transmission primarily through heterosexual contact (Vuylsteke, Sunkutu, & Laga, 1996). In recent years, we have seen new trends in HIV/AIDS infection in industrialized nations like the United States. Although infection rates remain high among homosexual and bisexual men, IDUs, and their sexual partners, the numbers of women, adolescents, and members of underrepresented ethnic groups, particularly African Americans and Latinos, have risen at alarming rates (AAWH, 1998).

Men Who Have Sex with Men

The fact that AIDS was first identified in 1981 in the American homosexual, Caucasian, male population, and was in fact called *gay-related immune deficiency syndrome* (GRID) for a short time, greatly affected the way it was perceived worldwide (Coxon, 1996; Shilts, 1987).

Because homosexual behavior is stigmatized in most societies, efforts aimed at prevention or treatment were limited early in the pandemic. However, gay organizations such as the Gay Men's Health Crisis Center in New York City and ACT UP (AIDS Coalition to Unleash Power) were formed at the beginning of the U.S. epidemic and continue to be instrumental in providing information and influencing HIV/AIDS policy.

The efforts of the gay population to spread the prevention message have resulted in reported behavioral changes among gay, white males, with a subsequent drop from 53% of all reported AIDS cases in 1995 to 50% in 1996. However, men who have sex with men (MSM) still continue to account for the largest number of people living with AIDS by risk group (AAWH, 1997; NIAID, 1999b). It would be a mistake to think that high-risk behaviors are no longer a problem in the gay community. Young gay men who have never lived in a world without AIDS

BOX 20-4 RYAN WHITE CARE (COMPREHENSIVE AIDS RESOURCES EMERGENCY) ACT

Signed into law by the U.S. Congress on August 18, 1990, to improve the quality and availability of care for people with HIV/AIDS and their families.

Managed by the Health Resources and Services Administration (HRSA), an agency of the U.S. Department of Health and Human Services.

HRSA's HIV/AIDS Bureau administers the programs under four titles and Part F.

- Title I provides grants to metropolitan areas that are disproportionately affected by the HIV epidemic. Grants are awarded to the chief elected official and are used to fund services such as outpatient health care; support services like case management, home health and hospice care, housing and transportation assistance, nutrition services, and day care and respite care; and inpatient case management services that expedite discharge and prevent unnecessary hospitalization.

- Title II provides grants to the states and territories to provide services for people living with HIV/AIDS. Some of these services include home and community-based health care and support services; continuation of health insurance coverage; pharmaceutical treatments through an AIDS drug assistance program; local organizations that assess needs and organize and deliver HIV ser-

vices in collaboration with health care providers; and direct health services.

- Title III supports outpatient HIV early intervention services for low-income, medically under-served people in existing primary care systems. Educational, clinical, and psychological services are provided for prevention, treatment, and support through community and migrant health centers, homeless programs, local health departments, family planning centers, and so on.

- Title IV provides comprehensive, community-based, family-centered services for women, children, adolescents, and families. Eighty-two percent of the people served are from poor, minority families with limited access to housing and transportation.

- Part F provides funding for special programs and services related to HIV/AIDS. Examples include the following:

  - *Special Projects of National Significance (SPNS) Program*—supports the development of innovative models of HIV/AIDS care designed to address minority and hard to reach populations

  - *AIDS Education and Training Center Program*—national network of 15 centers that provide HIV/AIDS education and training for health care professionals

Source: AAWH, 1997, 1998.

and who are possibly motivated by a sense of hopelessness, fatigue, or frustration with safer sex practices are engaging in unprotected intercourse with greater frequency. This may be partly due to their misguided perceptions that HIV/AIDS is a disease of older gay men or that their peers are not practicing safer sex (AAWH, 1998). As a result, in 1999, the CDC estimated that 60% of new HIV infections among men were through homosexual sex (NIAID, 1999b). Research data suggest that gay men of color are engaging in high-risk sexual behavior, which may be influenced by poverty, greater reliance on heterosexual activity, and invisibility to researchers and policy makers (Coxon, 1996).

Community prevention programs must continue to address the needs of MSM, particularly young gay and bisexual men and gay and bisexual men of color. The involvement of social and political leaders in the community is important to be able to overcome cultural barriers related to homophobia and stigmatization. Prevention efforts must be geared to both uninfected and infected MSM, because research shows that HIV-infected MSM are continuing to practice high-risk sexual behavior. Treatment and prevention of other STDs are critical for this population be-

cause studies of MSM who are treated in STD clinics have shown consistently high rates of HIV infection. Because HIV transmission is two to five times more likely to occur in people with STDs, aggressively treating STDs can help reduce the rate of new HIV infections (CDC, 1999a).

Ethnic Minority Populations

In recent years, HIV/AIDS has disproportionately affected the African American and Hispanic/Latino communities in the United States. In fact, AIDS is the number one killer of African Americans between the ages of 25 and 44. In 1998, racial and ethnic minorities accounted for more than 50% of reported AIDS cases in the United States. This is particularly significant considering that racial and ethnic minorities make up only 25% of the total population. Table 20-2 describes rates of new AIDS cases in the United States in 1998 by race and ethnicity. It is important to note that although AIDS death rates dropped by 28% for Caucasians from 1995 to 1996, the decrease in AIDS death rates was only 10% for African Americans and 16% for Latinos during that same period (AAWH, 1997, 1999; CDC, 1995b).

TABLE 20-2   RATE OF NEW AIDS CASES REPORTED IN THE UNITED STATES IN 1998 BY RACE AND ETHNICITY

RACE OR ETHNICITY	RATE OF REPORTED AIDS CASES PER 100,000
Caucasian (not Hispanic/Latino)	8.4
African American (not Hispanic/Latino)	81.9
Hispanic/Latino	34.7
Asian/Pacific Islander	4.1
Native American/Alaska Native	9.4

Source: NIAID, 1999b.

Table 20-3 describes AIDS death rates in the United States in 1998 by race and ethnicity.

Although the statistics in Tables 20-2 and 20-3 reflect the fact that African American and Hispanic/Latino populations are disproportionately affected by HIV/AIDS, they are not meant to suggest that individuals are at high risk for HIV/AIDS just because they are members of ethnic minority groups. Community prevention efforts for HIV/AIDS must consider not only the multicultural nature of our U. S. society, but also social and economic factors such as poverty, unemployment, and poor access to health care that disproportionately affect ethnic minority populations.

Ethnic minority groups, especially African American and Hispanic women and MSM, are at high risk for HIV infection as a result of the following:

- *Disparities between socioeconomic classes in access to quality health care*
- *The link between HIV and tuberculosis, and HIV and STDs*
- *Unsuccessful efforts to address illicit drug use in the United States*
- *Lack of culturally relevant HIV prevention programs and messages*

Social barriers also play a significant role in blocking HIV/AIDS education efforts in ethnic communities, especially in African American and Hispanic communities, where HIV/AIDS is still identified with homosexuality and drug use. Until HIV/AIDS prevention and treatment efforts gain support from the community, including churches and political leaders, HIV/AIDS will continue to affect ethnic minority groups in disproportionate numbers (AAWH, 1998).

Injection Drug Users

There are between 1.1 and 1.5 million IDUs in the United States, costing society an estimated $58.3 billion each year. Sharing used needles has been a well-known route of transmission for many years, yet injection drug use continues to contribute to the spread of HIV disease in significant proportions. The impact of injection drug use on HIV transmission goes far beyond the circle of those who inject drugs. Sexual partners of IDUs are at high risk for HIV infection, as well as babies born to mothers who are IDUs or who have had sex with IDUs. Injection drug use has directly or indirectly accounted for more than one-third (36%) of all AIDS cases in the United States since the beginning of the epidemic. In 1998, injection drug use was associated with 31% of all new AIDS cases. From the beginning of the epidemic, women have been disproportionately infected, with 59% of all AIDS cases among women associated with being IDUs or having sex with IDUs, compared with 31% of cases among men (AAWH, 1998; CDC, 1999b).

Substance abuse prevention is strongly related to HIV prevention, so comprehensive community-based programs must

TABLE 20-3   AIDS-RELATED DEATH RATES IN THE UNITED STATES IN 1998 BY RACE AND ETHNICITY

RACE OR ETHNICITY	AIDS-RELATED DEATH RATE PER 100,000
Caucasian (not Hispanic/Latino)	3.3
African American (not Hispanic/Latino)	32.5
Hispanic/Latino	12.2
Asian/Pacific Islander	1.3
Native American/Alaska Native	4.2

Source: NIAID, 1999b.

provide information, skills, and support for reducing risks for both. Community HIV/AIDS prevention programs require a wide range of approaches, including the following (CDC, 1999b):

- *Initial drug use prevention*
- *Street outreach programs*
- *Access to high-quality substance abuse treatment programs*
- *HIV prevention programs in correctional facilities*
- *Comprehensive health care for HIV-infected IDUs*
- *HIV risk-reduction counseling for IDUs and their sex partners*

Effective substance abuse treatment programs that assist people to eliminate drug use not only eliminate the risk of HIV transmission through contaminated needles, but also reduce the risk of engaging in behaviors that contribute to the risk for sexual transmission. Unfortunately, the need for substance abuse treatment in the United States greatly outweighs the ability to provide it. There is a long waiting list for admission to available drug treatment programs and U.S. laws exist that restrict the possession, distribution, or sale of any drug injection equipment. The U.S. government bans the use of federal funds for needle exchange programs that allow IDUs to exchange dirty needles for clean ones to reduce the transmission of HIV. This policy remains in effect despite the fact that scientific studies have provided sufficient evidence that needle exchange programs, when combined with a comprehensive prevention program, reduce HIV transmission without increasing drug use. Therefore, IDUs across the country continue to inject drugs and share needles despite the risk of HIV (AAWH, 1998).

The absence of needle exchange programs and insufficient numbers of substance abuse treatment programs make efforts aimed at HIV prevention for IDUs even more critical. IDUs should be taught to use sterile needles and to never reuse needles. But if using sterile needles is not always possible, IDUs should be taught to clean their needles with a chlorine bleach and water solution between uses. However, it should be noted that cleaning needles with bleach is not as safe as using sterile needles (AAWH, 1998; CDC, 1999b).

Adolescents

Worldwide, greater and greater numbers of adolescents are infected with HIV. More than half of new infections in 1998 occurred in those 15 to 24 years of age, with approximately 7,000 young people becoming infected each day. Adolescents in developing countries are most affected, but the risk is growing for teens in industrialized countries too. In the United States and Canada, HIV is spreading at an alarming rate, with 25% of all new infections in the United States occurring in young people between the ages of 13 and 21. AIDS-related illnesses are the sixth leading cause of death among people between the ages of 15 and 24 in the United States. For all AIDS cases among males in the 13 to 24 age group in 1998, 51% were MSM, 10% were IDUs, and 9% were infected heterosexually. In 1998, among young women in the same age group, 47% were infected heterosexually and 14% were IDUs (AAWH, 1998; CDC, 1999c; NIAID, 1996b; UNICEF, 1999).

Sexual exposure accounts for the majority of adolescent HIV infections. For young men, the biggest sexual risk is homosexual contact, and for young women, it is heterosexual contact. Adolescents engage in multiple high-risk behaviors, often associated with drug and alcohol use. One in 50 high school students reports having injected an illegal drug, and alcohol and other drug use is common, often leading to high-risk sexual behavior (Staton, Leukefeld, Logan, Zimmerman, Lynam, Milich, Martin, McClanahan, & Clayton, 1999). The CDC Youth Risk Behavioral Surveys consistently show that approximately 50% of all high school students have had sexual intercourse. By the time teens reach 12th grade, almost 70% have had sexual intercourse. Nearly one in four sexually active 12th graders have had four or more sex partners, yet less than half of them report consistent condom use (AAWH, 1998, 1999; Woods, 1998).

....

A review of over 50 studies revealed that sexual health education programs do not encourage sexual experimentation. When quality criteria are met, such programs actually help to delay the age of first intercourse. They also reduce sexually transmitted diseases and unwanted pregnancy in adolescents who are sexually active.

UNAIDS, 1999
(Joint United Nations Programme on HIV/AIDS)

....

Adolescents are difficult to engage in the care needed for the diagnosis and treatment of HIV disease. Adolescents believe they are invincible and tend to deny they are at risk. This belief may cause them to engage in high-risk behavior, delay HIV testing, or delay or refuse treatment when they have tested positive for HIV. When adolescents are treated by health care providers for other reasons, HIV risk is seldom discussed. Recent studies show that fewer than half of adolescents with histories of "survival sex" (sex to earn money to live on the street), injection drug use, same-gender sexual behavior, or prior STD infection seek treatment or help for these HIV-related issues. Thus, prevention is the key weapon in reducing the incidence of adolescent HIV/AIDS (Woods, 1998). Behavioral science has shown that young people respond best to a balance of different approaches to prevention. To be effective, a wide range of activities must be implemented in communities. For example, school-based programs must include kindergarten through 12th grade education programs that address not only HIV prevention but also prevention for STDs, unintended pregnancy, and tobacco and drug use and pro-

RESEARCH BRIEF

Jemmott, J. B., Jemmott, L. S., & Fong, G. T. (1998). Abstinence and safer sex: HIV risk-reduction interventions for African American adolescents. Journal of the American Medical Association Online, 279(18), 1529.

Randomized control studies with 659 African American adolescents in Philadelphia were conducted to evaluate the effectiveness of sexual abstinence and safe sex intervention programs. The average age of the participants was 11.8 years. Saturday programs were held in which adolescents participated in one of three different intervention programs consisting of eight 1-hour modules each. One intervention program focused on delaying sexual intercourse or delaying its frequency. Another intervention program focused on safe sex education with an emphasis on condom use. The control intervention program focused on health matters unrelated to sex. Analyzing self-reported data within the cohort, the researchers found that the abstinence intervention had an effect after the first 3 months, as compared with the control group, but not after 6 or 12 months. The safe sex group participants reported increased rates of condom use at all follow-ups. This group also reported less sexual intercourse at the 6- and 12-month follow-ups than either the abstinence group or the control group.

grams that encourage healthy eating and physical exercise. School programs should address social norms that regulate gender roles, develop good decision-making skills, and increase self-esteem and self-efficacy. Other community-based programs to reach teens not in school are needed for homeless and runaway youth, juvenile offenders, or school dropouts (CDC, 1999c).

Women

Women are one of the fastest growing groups of people living with HIV/AIDS (AAWH, 1999; Nyamathi, Bennett, & Leake, 1995). Women account for 43% of cumulative AIDS cases worldwide. In a little more than a decade, the proportion of all AIDS cases reported in the United States among adult and adolescent women more than tripled, from 7% in 1985 to 23% in 1998 (CDC, 1999d). AIDS is now the third leading cause of death in women age 25 to 44 and is the leading cause of death for African American women in that age group. For most of these women, heterosexual sex and injection drug use are the primary means of HIV transmission (AAWH, 1998; Lawless, Kippax, & Crawford, 1996). HIV infection rates are highest among poor ethnic minority women. In fact, the rate of HIV/AIDS among African American women is 18 times higher

than among Caucasian women. The rate of HIV/AIDS among Hispanic women is eight times higher than among Caucasian women (AAWH, 1998).

Cultural, legal, religious, and economic factors often limit the amount of control many women have over their own bodies, thus putting them at increased risk for HIV infection (AAWH, 1997). For example, condom requests by women are often misinterpreted by male partners as an indication of mistrust or infidelity, leading to loss of the male partner or domestic violence. Women with minimal education and job skills are often unable to negotiate safer sex practices because of economic dependence on their partners for both themselves and their children. Many poor women may exchange sex for money, gifts, or other favors, and exchange of sex for addictive drugs is common (O'Leary & Jemmott, 1995).

Cultural and economic factors also account for many women not having access to preventive care and early treatment, resulting in later diagnosis and earlier death. Research, prevention, and care activities for women have been slow to develop (Mann & Tarantola, 1996), even though the numbers of women infected in the developing world has been equal to men since the beginning of the pandemic. Much of this may be related to the unequal role and status of women worldwide (Mann & Tarantola, 1996). Another factor may be that, until recently, the proportion of cases of AIDS in women in the industrialized world, where most of the research is conducted, were much lower than for men.

Because most of women with HIV/AIDS are of childbearing age, most of the research involving women with HIV has centered on reproduction, with an emphasis on the fetus or infant (Lawless, Kippax, & Crawford, 1996). In the United States, approximately 6,500 women with HIV become pregnant and give birth each year. As a result of the ACTG 076 study of drug treatment in perinatal AIDS transmission, treatment of HIV-infected pregnant women with AZT (zidovudine) has become the standard of care, thereby reducing perinatal HIV infection to approximately 8%. Perinatal infection rates before AZT therapy during pregnancy ranged from 25% to 30%. Although it is a positive breakthrough that fewer children are becoming infected with HIV, the negative side is that, by the year 2000, as many as 80,000 children in the United States had been orphaned by HIV. Parents with HIV/AIDS, particularly mothers because they are often single parents, are confronted with the difficult decisions about what and how to tell their children about their illness and

FYI

In the African country of Zambia, 1 in 3 children are AIDS orphans living on the streets (Miramontes, 2000).

who will care for their children if they die (Rotheram-Borus, Draimin, Reid, & Murphy, 1997).

As a result of the emphasis on the maternal role, many women living with HIV have been stigmatized as a potential source of infection instead of being regarded as people with their own health care needs. HIV/AIDS is often associated with guilt or blame because becoming infected with HIV implies failure in the traditional and expected role of women as caregivers and moral guardians who are responsible for the next generation (Lawless, Kippax, & Crawford, 1996).

Community efforts at HIV prevention need to put more emphasis on interventions aimed at women. Conventional education programs that address male and female condom negotiation and use, routine HIV testing, and drug abuse still need to be implemented, but programs that address domestic abuse, self-esteem, and self-efficacy also need to be developed and implemented. In addition, community-supported domestic crisis centers, day-care facilities, educational and job training programs, and support groups specifically for women at risk need to be established.

Children

The first cases of children with AIDS were reported in the United States in 1983, 2 years after the syndrome was described in adults. By 1997, the CDC had reported 8,086 cumulative cases of AIDS in the United States for children younger than 13 years of age (AAWH, 1998). Because children have immature immune and nervous systems, HIV infection produces a wide range of developmental problems and negatively affects almost every vital organ of the body (AAWH, 1997).

More than 90% of children are infected with HIV through vertical transmission (mother to child). Vertical transmission can take place in several ways, including transmission while the fetus is still in the uterus; during the birth process, when the baby comes into direct contact with large quantities of the mother's blood and vaginal fluids; and during breast-feeding. However, the chance of transmission during breast-feeding is minimal (AAWH, 1997). Although HIV infection in newborns in the United States has decreased dramatically since the introduction of AZT therapy during pregnancy, the rest of the world has not been as fortunate. The prohibitive cost of AZT therapy has made it impossible for countries in the developing world, where 90% of HIV infections occur, to obtain it. However, there is hope. In 1998, studies in Thailand showed a much shorter and less expensive course of AZT therapy may be effective in reducing vertical HIV transmission by as much as 50%. This shorter course of therapy may be a realistic option for developing countries (CDC, 1998b).

HIV infection can be definitively diagnosed in virtually all infected infants by 6 months of age, and in nearly all by 1 month of age, using viral diagnostic assays. A positive virological test indicates presumptive HIV infection. Diagnostic testing should be performed between birth and 48 hours of age, and again at 1 to 2 months and 3 to 6 months of age for a definitive diagnosis.

AIDS is the most publicized disease in the world, but its impact on children has received an inadequate response. Adults can and must do their part to ease the suffering of children infected with HIV, help children in HIV-affected homes and communities, and enable all children living in the shadow of HIV risk to grow up uninfected. But it may be that the epidemic's future course will be shaped by the actions of those it is increasingly affecting: the children who live in a world with AIDS.

UNAIDS, 1997
(Joint United Nations Programme on HIV/AIDS)

Nursing Care of Families with HIV

Nursing care for families with HIV-infected children requires an in-depth assessment of the needs of all members of the family. The nurse should initially ask the primary caregiver, usually the mother, but sometimes the father or grandparent, who is considered to be family and who in the family knows about the HIV status.

This analysis should include the physical, psychological, social, and spiritual needs of every member of the family. It is also helpful to draw a family genogram to determine the relationships and lines of communication in the family. The assessment cannot be done in one visit, and the nurse should be sensitive to the emotional stress of the primary caregiver and plan accordingly for a series of visits to complete the assessment.

A multidisciplinary family care plan may be developed based on the initial assessment and the input of team members such as the psychologist, physician, or social worker. The primary caregiver can give input into the care plan and may be provided with a copy. The care plan should be updated at least quarterly, especially for families with three or more infected members.

Educational sessions for every member of the family may be established based on the initial and subsequent assessments and recorded as goals and objectives on the care plan (e.g., "Mrs. Jones will be able to give her baby John the accurate doses of AZT as evidenced by drawing up the AZT dose and giving it to John at the specified time"). Educational sessions may also include addressing social, emotional, or spiritual issues (e.g., "Mrs. Jones will identify three ways to decrease stress in her life as evidenced by walking three times a day, placing the children in respite care three days a week, and so on"). The nurse must consider that there will be episodic failures for the caregiver in achieving objectives and must be prepared to help the family through these normal episodes (Crespo-Fierro, 1997).

The entire plan of care and the coordination for meeting the multiple needs of any family must take place using a sensitive and compassionate approach. Many women and children feel isolated, depressed, and overwhelmed by their HIV infection. The nurse and the multidisciplinary staff can give anticipatory guidance and thereby increase the quality of life for the entire family.

CASE STUDY

Providence Home and Family Services, Inc.

In 1989, the University of Texas Health Science Center in San Antonio, Texas, established the South Texas AIDS Center for Children and Families, a Ryan White Title IV-funded demonstration project, with John Mangos, MD, as director and Barbara Aranda-Naranjo, RN, as assistant director. The mission of the project was to provide comprehensive health services to children and their families infected and affected by HIV disease.

During the first year of the project, many children experienced the death and/or debilitation of one or both parents. Many of the children were being left orphans or needed a safe place to stay while their parents were hospitalized. After observing this phenomena, nurse Barbara Aranda-Naranjo saw a need for a residential/respite care for children. After discussion with Dr. Mangos and other community leaders, she approached another nurse colleague, Sr. Barbara Hyzak, RN, and began exploring the idea of a respite center. Sr. Barbara Hyzak was a member of the Sisters of Divine Providence, a Catholic order of nuns, and the director of the Stella Maris Clinic. The clinic, located in the west side of San Antonio, served the poor and migrants that had worked in the area for more than 30 years. As a result of changes in migrant employment and the establishment of other for-profit and non-profit clinics, the sisters were looking for a new mission for the clinic.

After discussion about the needs of the children and families living with HIV infection, a proposal was developed to present to the clinic board of directors. The proposal included the description of the needs of the population and the link with the South Texas AIDS Center. In addition, the primary goal of the proposal was to set up a residential care center and day care in place of the Stella Maris clinic. The development of the proposal was a joint effort with the University of Texas Health Science Center, the Sisters of Divine Providence, and other community-based organizations such as Project ABC.

Providence Home was established in 1990 as a non-profit agency to serve the needs of women, children, and their families infected and affected by AIDS. The Texas Department of Health granted Providence Home a license as a special care facility. The home offers services to infants and children from birth to 13 years of age. The services included residential as well as respite care for children. The first director was Sister Barbara Hyzak, RN.

In 1993, the home opened the Providence Home Learning Center as a therapeutic day-care center. The learning center is open five days a week from 9 AM to 3 PM. The capacity of the learning center is 30 children.

Providence Home is staffed with full-time and part-time employees. The University of Texas Health Science Center, the South Texas AIDS Center, and the University of the Incarnate Word Nursing School provide nursing, medical, and psychological support. A vast number of volunteers and nursing students also make contributions to Providence Home's quality of health services. The current director of Providence Home is Carol Bova-Rice; the Sisters of Divine Providence continue to sponsor the home.

Applying the nursing assessment of the environment, two nurses in this case study were able to observe a need in the community, develop a proposal, and create a home from an existing health center. The collaboration by these two nurses assisted in the creation of both a residential and respite center that has met the needs of many families living with HIV infection in South Texas. More than 100 families have benefited from the services of Providence Home, which continues to serve the changing needs of families living with HIV infection.

STDs and the U.S. Health Care System

Problems of Access

Most of the disease burden produced by sexually transmitted infections, including HIV/AIDS, could be prevented or treated with increased access to services, expanded screening and treatment, and behavior changes that lower STD risk. Clearly, a widespread availability of high-quality STD care is necessary to ensure that infections are detected and treated in a timely and appropriate manner. If this were the case now, both STD and HIV transmission would be diminished (Institute of Medicine, 1997). Instead, Americans have limited awareness of their need for STD care, compounded by limited access to STD services. Misinformation is also a problem

•••••••••••••••••••••••••••••••••

Yes, it's true life can be scary, but life can also be exciting, thrilling, and fabulous. And to be honest with you, I would much rather have life than the alternative. I don't regret this disease. It's taught me some valuable lessons—helped me face some exciting and new challenges and introduced me to some charming people. All of which never would have happened had it not been for this disease. It's true I may die tomorrow. But if I

do die, I'm going to die happy, without regrets. If I had to live my life all over again, I wouldn't change a thing. I'd take it all—AIDS included. I don't have HIV, I have AIDS and I am proud of who I am. And I am proud of the person I am going to become. My name is Rob Lanier and I have AIDS and I am alive. I am alive! I am alive!

Rob Lanier died in 1995, at the age of 28

•••••••••••••••••••••••••••••••••

" A CONVERSATION WITH . . . "

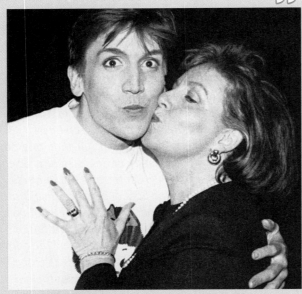

Dr. Ann Lanier congratulates her son, Rob, on his one-man stage play. New York City, 1994.

On Saturday, February 18, 1995, we held a memorial for Rob at the Ridiculous Theater in New York City—among his friends and family—among stage props and red gels and sound equipment and fading velvet curtains—among wigs and green eyeliner—among photographs of him in a multitude of silly costumes—with him in his laughing face and somber mood. Among 200 daffodils and hundreds of daffodil bulbs tied up in yellow tulle and small green ribbons, we ate his favorite food and listened to his collection of music. We shared a moment of love with friends and family who played tribute to him by playing the flute, dancing, reading poetry, and performing dramatic readings. We told stories of his generosity, his silliness, his love of living—and among all the daffodils and all the promises of spring and life, we said good-bye to his physical presence on earth.

Such a strong and loving spirit will stay with us. As his mother, I will always see the boy who organized a production of "Candide" using the children who lived on his mountainside in Colorado. The little boy in Texas who talked his rough and tumble cousins into putting on a musical production for all the relatives in his grandfather's barn among the bales of hay. The young man trying out for the role of the older "young prince" in the summer production of "Richard III" in Boulder. When called back for the fourth time, the director said, "I'd love to cast you as the young prince, but you're three inches taller than the lead." The young man who lied about his age so he could go to work to help his single mother. The young man, who in his free time, spent long hours directing the senior citizens group in their production of "Blithe Spirit." The young man who played the role of the father in "What's the Matter with Father?" because it had a special meaning to him that he never explained. The young man who walked 4 miles in the Colorado winter to take his SATs. The young man who tried out for NYU's Tisch School of the Arts by performing a piece he wrote, "Gorilla Warfare in Texas." The young college student who worked double shifts and tried to pawn his watch to get the money to go to Paris for all the love and adventure it promised.

We, as his family, will always see the man who lived and worked among people he loved, in all the tears and laughter of the theater. We will see the man with our family on the Chesapeake Bay that he loved, with the red and gold of fall leaves, the dogs, and the boats. And with the family that came much later in life than it should have, with whom he felt loved and accepted for being "Rob" and was always chosen first for a game of Trivial Pursuit. Above all we remember his last play, "Mortality Waltz," that taught us about coming of age, about life, and about living with AIDS.

Until his last breath, Rob did just as he promised in his play. He lived every moment of his life. He said, "I will not

A CONVERSATION WITH... cont'd

discuss dying. I will only talk of living." He did just that. He never spoke of dying again. His energy—his sense of love and life—stayed with him, as it will always stay with each of us who loved him. Family and friends were with him and held his hands long after that beautiful spirit left his body and wrapped around us like a cloak. We cry now because we must reach back into our memories to pull out his laughter—to see his smile—to hear him tell us stories—to feel his arms around us—or to see him wink. We desperately miss the touch, feel, and smell of that wonderful person, and the world will miss so many more gifts he had to offer.

—Dr. Ann Lanier,
Mother of Rob Lanier

HEALTHY PEOPLE 2010

OBJECTIVES RELATED TO HIV

13.1   Reduce AIDS among adolescents and adults.

13.2   Reduce the number of new AIDS cases among adolescent and adult men who have sex with men.

13.3   Reduce the number of new AIDS cases among females and males who inject drugs.

13.4   Reduce the number of new AIDS cases among adolescent and adult men who have sex with men and inject drugs.

13.5   Reduce the number of cases of HIV infection among adolescents and adults.

13.6   Increase the proportion of sexually active persons who use condoms.

13.7   Increase the number of HIV-positive persons who know their serostatus.

13.8   Increase the proportion of substance abuse treatment facilities that offer HIV/AIDS education, counseling, and support.

13.9   Increase the number of state prison systems that provide comprehensive HIV/AIDS, sexually transmitted diseases, and tuberculosis (TB) education.

13.10   Increase the proportion of inmates in state prison systems who receive voluntary HIV counseling and testing during incarceration.

13.11   Increase the proportion of adults with tuberculosis (TB) who have been tested for HIV.

13.12   Increase the proportion of adults in publicly funded HIV counseling and testing sites who are screened for common bacterial sexually transmitted diseases (STDs) (chlamydia, gonorrhea, and syphilis) and are immunized against hepatitis B virus.

13.13   Increase the proportion of HIV-infected adolescents and adults who receive testing, treatment, and prophylaxis consistent with current Public Health Service guidelines.

13.14   Reduce deaths from HIV infection.

13.15   Extend the interval of time between an initial diagnosis of HIV infection and AIDS diagnosis in order to increase years of life of an individual infected with HIV.

13.16   Increase years of life of an HIV-infected person by extending the interval of time between an AIDS diagnosis and death.

13.17   Reduce new cases of perinatally acquired HIV infection.

Source: DHHS, 2000.

because the public is generally unaware of the seriousness of STDs. Almost one in five Americans believe that all STDs are curable, and more than half are not aware that having an STD facilitates HIV transmission. STDs that cause genital lesions can create a portal of entry for HIV. Even without lesions, STDs increase the number of CD4 target cells in cervical secretions, thereby increasing HIV susceptibility in women. In fact, people who are already infected with an STD are two to five times more likely to become infected with HIV. Yet only half the public health departments in this country provide STD services, compared with 97% that provide immunizations (AAWH, 1999; Landry & Forrest, 1996).

Public Health Services

Even where public STD services are available, access to those services is often restricted by limited hours of operation. Almost 40% of health departments do not see clients the same day they seek care, despite the fact that they may be both infected and infectious. Most health care providers do not routinely take a sexual history or screen for STDs in primary care settings (CDC, 1997b). Thus, the harsh reality is that in many areas of the country, people actively seeking STD care are unable to receive timely services. A recent survey in states with high rates of syphilis demonstrated the magnitude of this problem, finding substantial numbers of clients who were turned away by STD clinics because the clinics' schedules were full, which sometimes occurred by early to midmorning (Gibson, 1996).

Private and Other Health Services

STD care is often lacking outside of dedicated STD clinics. Community outreach for STD prevention is especially limited, although this can be an important role for community nurses, who will encounter persons at high risk for STD or HIV infection in community settings. Innovative approaches to delivering STD care outside the traditional categorical STD clinics are increasingly being explored. When family planning services and STD care are integrated under a broader rubric of reproductive health services, the burden of chlamydial infections was reduced substantially (DeLisle, 1997). Prenatal and obstetrical care settings are additional venues where STD/HIV screening, treatment, and prevention counseling can be provided, at the same time enhancing the prevention of perinatal infections and other STD-related adverse outcomes of pregnancy (Goldenberg, Andrews, Yuan, MacKay, & St. Louis, 1997; Goldenberg, Vermund, Goepfert, & Andrews, 1998). Traditional public health clinics will not reach all of the people who need STD care, and greater effort is needed to stimulate and encourage private providers to take sexual histories, screen for asymptomatic infections, and provide a range of STD services in their practices. More recently, managed care organizations have emerged as a dominant organizational framework for medical care across much of the United States, particularly for the more disadvantaged segments of the population, and could serve many individuals at risk

for STDs. However, a recent survey of managed care organizations that primarily serve clients at risk for STDs revealed that none had any plans for STD prevention programs, although most had plans for offering courses on diabetes, nutrition, and smoking cessation (American Social Health Association, 1998).

Increasing STD clinical services and prevention counseling in community settings may have substantial benefits because services could be extended to persons at high risk of infection but who do not seek health care from within familiar surroundings. New technologies for STD diagnosis using urine, self-collected swabs, and other noninvasive specimens now enable outreach screening for people who may not use formal health care in nontraditional settings (Rietmeijer, Yamaguchi, Ortiz, Montstream, LeRoux, Ehret, Judson, & Dougis, 1997).

Screening and Prevention

People often do not know they are infected with STDs because they do not have or do not recognize symptoms. Because most studies of STDs are conducted in health care settings where people have sought care because they did experience symptoms, the proportion of infectious persons who are symptomatic has usually been overestimated. More recent studies of STD screening outside of health care settings (e.g., in jails, workplaces, and other community-based settings) reveal that a large number of

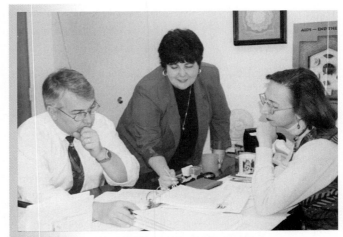

Chapter author Dr. Sharyn Janes (center) plans a statewide HIV education program for health care providers with Craig Thompson (left), Director of the STD/HIV Division of the Mississippi State Department of Health, and Cheryl Hamill, RN, Director of the Resource Center of the Delta Region AIDS Education and Training Center at the University of Mississippi Medical Center.

persons with gonorrhea and chlamydia have no symptoms or signs of infection (Grosskurth, Mayaud, Mosha, Todd, Senkoro, Newell, Gabone, Changalucha, West, & Hayes, 1996).

The fact that gonorrhea and chlamydia so often do not produce any symptoms has many implications for community health nursing because no matter how effectively access to health care is enhanced, many of these silent infections will go undetected and untreated unless screening and treatment are provided in nontraditional settings. Even though asymptomatic individuals will not access health care specifically for STD testing or treatment, they do visit a variety of health care settings for other purposes. There are many opportunities to identify and treat asymptomatic but infected persons in health care settings when they present for other unrelated problems (e.g., in emergency rooms, in family planning clinics, during routine or sports physicals, during immunization visits) and in non–health care settings such as schools and jails.

The Role of Community Health Nurses

To prevent the spread of STDs, it is not enough to screen for and treat infections; community nurses also need to be able to help individuals change their behavior by counseling about how to prevent infections and reinfections. It is not who one is but what one does that determines whether a person becomes infected or reinfected with an STD. Screening and treating infection are effective for a current infection, but unless individuals can be helped to change their behavior, they may continue to behave in ways that put them at risk for further infections.

A number of different behaviors can be targeted to reduce infections: increasing the seeking of appropriate health care, improving clients' adherence to medication and cooperation with efforts to notify their partners of possible infection, reducing the rate of partner change, and lowering the number of sex partners. Increasing consistent and correct condom use can prevent some infections, such as gonorrhea and HIV, but is less effective with other STDs such as HPV. The most effective counseling interventions are those that are directed at a specific behavior. Perhaps the most difficult task facing community health nurses is identifying the behaviors that warrant change for specific clients and matching their intervention to the clients' readiness to change behavior.

Decisions about the behaviors in need of change should be based on a careful assessment of the client's sexual and drug-use history. Although many nurses are uncomfortable taking such histories, most clients view sexual and drug histories as an expected part of a medical examination (Croft & Asmussen, 1993; Warner, Rowe, & Whipple, 1999). At the very least, information should be gathered about the number and type of sexual partners (regular and occasional partners), types of sex practiced, condom use (with regular and occasional partners), use of both injected

and noninjected drugs, and in the case of IDUs, information about their use of sterile syringes and disinfection of shared injection paraphernalia. It is only by taking such histories that behaviors that are placing the client at risk can be identified. These behaviors should then be the target of the nursing intervention.

All too often, however, the goals of an intervention are vague (e.g., staying healthy, losing weight, preventing an STD), rather than focusing on a specific changeable behavior (e.g., always using a condom with every partner, telling one's partner to always use a condom). It is the latter type of intervention that is most likely to produce successful behavior changes. The distinction between overly broad goals and specific behaviors is not always obvious. For example, "using condoms" is not a specific behavior but a broad goal. Condoms are used for specific sexual activities with specific partners, and the factors that influence condom use for vaginal sex with a spouse are different from those that can influence condom use with an occasional partner. Furthermore,

RESEARCH BRIEF

Lauby, J. L., Smith, P. J., Stark, M., Person, B., & Adams, J. (2000). A community-level HIV prevention intervention for inner-city women: Results of the women and infants demonstration projects. American Journal of Public Health, 90(2), 216–222.

This study examined the effects of an HIV prevention intervention on women's condom-use behaviors. The community-level intervention targeted sexually active women of child-bearing age in four different inner-city communities. At the beginning of the study, nearly 70% of the participants did not intend to use condoms with their sexual partners. After two years of theory-based and culturally specific intervention activities, increases in talking with partners about condoms and attempting to use condoms with partners were significantly larger in the intervention communities than in comparison communities. The results of this study show that (1) large-scale community interventions can be implemented successfully in low-income, inner-city neighborhoods; (2) many women were still not using condoms, which confirms the necessity for relevant, effective prevention interventions that target women; and (3) a community-level intervention can affect women's condom-use behavior. To be successful in low-income neighborhoods, interventions must address social, economic, and cultural issues that affect the target population's access to information and its ability to focus on health-related behaviors.

while using a male condom is a behavior for men, for women, the goal may be a behavior that influences the partner's behavior.

People also differ in their readiness for change. The type of counseling a nurse provides is more effective when it is matched to the individual's readiness to make changes. The transtheoretical model of behavior change is a helpful framework for understanding individual differences and for identifying appropriate interventions (Prochaska, Redding, Harlow, Rossi, & Velicer, 1994). Some individuals who are engaging in risky behaviors will have no intention of changing their behavior or adopting more healthful behaviors (precontemplative stage). Any one of several strategies (e.g., recognizing that the behavior is putting them at risk) may help those individuals to consider change, whether immediately or in the future (contemplative stage). After deciding to change the behavior, initial attempts to adopt new behaviors may follow (preparation or ready for action stage). Eventually, a new behavior is adopted (action stage) and will become a routine part of the person's life (maintenance stage). Movement through these stages may be sequential, or the person may skip some stages or relapse back to an earlier stage, and then cycle back through the stages several times before he or she successfully reaches long-term maintenance of a new behavior.

To help people change behavior, the nurse should first determine where each person is on this continuum of behavior change and then develop an intervention to help him or her move toward the next stage. Generally speaking, if the person has decided to make a change, has the skills to be able to perform the new behavior, and does not face environmental barriers that will prevent him or her from making the change, it is almost certain that the new behavior will be performed.

Once the risk assessment has been completed and a decision reached about what behavior needs to be the first target of an intervention, the next step is to assess the person's readiness and capability to perform that behavior. This can easily be evaluated by asking the client if he or she plans on starting (or continuing) to practice the risk-reducing behavior. For example, "Do you plan to use condoms every time you have sex with your boyfriend? How sure are you about this?" If the person wants to perform the behavior but has not been able to do so, it is important to determine whether this is because he or she does not have the skills to act on the good intentions or whether environmental constraints are preventing him or her from doing so. Depending on which of these is operating, the intervention can be directed at increasing the person's skill or at helping the individual to overcome the perceived barriers. If, on the other hand, the person has no intention of performing the safer behavior, the intervention can be directed at helping to motivate the person to make a change. This may involve helping the person to change his or her attitudes about the behavior, addressing social pressures to perform or not perform the behavior, or reinforcing beliefs that the client can do so successfully (self-efficacy).

For example, let's assume that a sexual history indicated that a client was at risk for acquiring an STD because she had no intention whatsoever of using a condom for vaginal sex with her boyfriend. The following questions provide an example of how to elicit information that would help guide counseling for this client:

- *Do you feel mostly positive or mostly negative about always using a condom for vaginal sex with your boyfriend?*

- *Do people who are important to you think you should or should not always use a condom when you have vaginal sex with your boyfriend?*

- *Considering all of the things that can make it difficult to always use a condom, how certain are you that you could always use a condom for vaginal sex with your boyfriend?*

If the first question reveals that the person has negative attitudes toward using condoms, the next step is to try to understand the person's beliefs about using condoms. For example, the client can be asked to describe what she thinks will happen if condoms are always used for vaginal sex with her boyfriend. More specifically, the client can be asked to describe what she thinks are the advantages and the disadvantages. Counseling can then be directed at disputing counterproductive beliefs that lead to negative outcomes and at increasing or strengthening beliefs that will lead to positive outcomes.

If the client's answers to the second question indicate that important others are opposed to consistent condom use, then it becomes important to understand which of the people in the client's social network support and oppose condom use. The client can be asked about specific individuals in her social network who would oppose consistent condom use and to describe who would think consistent condom use for vaginal sex with her boyfriend was a good thing to do. The interaction can then be directed at clarifying misperceptions or pointing out others in the client's life who would be supportive.

Finally, if the client was positively predisposed to using condoms and had supportive social relationships but little sense of self-efficacy with respect to condom use, then a more careful examination of the reasons for the client's low self-efficacy need to be examined. The client can be asked to describe the things that make it hard to consistently use condoms with her boyfriend (barriers) and to describe things that would make it easier to consistently use condoms (facilitators). The intervention can then be directed at helping the client overcome barriers or find ways to facilitate condom use. It is also essential to pay attention to whether the person has the skills to be able to carry out the behavior. This may involve demonstrating how to use a condom correctly and having the client practice the behavior several times using a model to gain both comfort and familiarity with using a condom. It may involve helping her practice how to negotiate with her boyfriend for condom use.

When nurses understand their clients' behavioral skills, beliefs, and attitudes, it becomes possible to tailor an appropriate, brief, and practical intervention strategy for each client, helping them move along the continuum of change described earlier. Changing behavior can be difficult, and it is a good idea to check with the client at the next visit to see if any difficulties arose. If so, the nurse can help with problem solving to overcome these impediments.

At the community level, successful population interventions often take the form of media campaigns, peer counseling, diverse educational strategies, and partnerships with community-based organizations. Community health nurses should be directly involved with policy development as related to the prevention and treatment of STDs and HIV/AIDS.

A Conversation With...

I am on the road to AIDS. I knew it first in 1991. I had just survived a bitter divorce. I was not ready to have a three and a one year old, no husband, and AIDS. If I offered a prayer those days, it might have been, "Why me, O Lord? Why me?" Over time, whatever my complaints had been gave way to something better and more useful. I began to see AIDS as less than a curse in my life, and more as a call to speak out, to show courage to my children, and to ask others to consider healing instead of indifference and compassion instead of judgment. I was not a victim, I was a pilgrim, called by God to walk humbly and obediently with other pilgrims on the road to AIDS. I didn't know what I could do that might make a difference. But I decided to speak out. For gay men who had been rejected by their families, I spoke out. For women who were isolated, and frightened, and powerless, I spoke out. From the echoing halls of the United States Senate to the whisper-quiet corridors of hospitals, I spoke out—believing that by speaking out, I could make a difference.

And then I looked around to see what difference I had made. I was still a pilgrim walking down the road to AIDS. Those who had lined the pilgrims' road still called out judgments, still rejected those who were sick and dying, still hurled insults and discrimination at pilgrims as we marched by. That had not changed. The only change I saw was that the pilgrim band grew larger every year. The number of women first doubled, then tripled, then went beyond counting. And the pilgrims were increasingly drawn from communities of color. The hard, plain truth was that I couldn't change it. Only God could do that. And so with Carvin Winans and a few friends, the idea of Gospel Against AIDS was born, conceived in the belief that we need to reach into our neighborhoods—into the apartments and the alleyways, the gas stations and the beauty shops.

And that's why we're here. To tell the nation's policy makers that our children are growing sick and dying, to insist that power and money support compassion and hope. To remind the nation that we need forgiveness. To remember when AIDS was a "gay disease," we did not care, as if those who were gay were less than God's children; and to confess that now as our women and children become infected, we do care—that's why we seek forgiveness. Once we were a part of the crowd that said, "They do not matter. Let them go...." But we are here to say that they do matter, that they are not less than God's other children.

Because AIDS is creating orphans who need parents, who need community, who need love and comfort that only flows from God's children—that's why we're here. We are here for the "good news" of the gospel. It is a gospel of oneness. Jews and Gentiles, blacks and whites, gays and straights, men and women—all are God's children, all are welcome in God's house.

I am now a veteran pilgrim on the road to AIDS. I've learned that pilgrims sometimes lose hope. The virus wears us down. The medications wear us out. The sleeplessness, the lesions, and the cancers—like a faucet dripping in the dark, they take away our hope drop by drop. We read happy headlines about promised cures, but it isn't a cure that we experience—it's fever, sores, and family members who grow angry at our anger and hopeless at our hopelessness. Some of us have given up hope that even God could love us.

God's family needs to show others that the gospel is not about judgment, but about grace. It is a gospel not of death, but of life—a hopeful gospel, a healing gospel. What science cannot heal, God's family can embrace. And what life itself cannot sustain, the gospel can heal. That is why we're here and that is why there is a Gospel Against AIDS.

—Mary Fisher,
Gospel Against AIDS, December 6, 1997

CONCLUSION

STDs are a hidden epidemic with enormous health and economic consequences in this country. They remain hidden because so many Americans are unable to address sexual health issues openly and because of the biological and social characteristics of these diseases.

All Americans have a vested interest in STD prevention because every community is affected by STDs and everyone directly or indirectly pays for the costs of these diseases. STDs are public health problems that lack easy solutions because they are rooted in fundamental human behavioral and social problems. Despite the barriers to open discussion of sexuality, there are prevention programs that are effective and that can be implemented on a local level.

Ultimately, multifaceted approaches are needed at both the individual and community levels to produce the best results. Although no intervention is perfect, together they can have a synergistic and positive impact on lowering the disease burden in this country. Subpopulations such as adolescents and disenfranchised adults will need special attention and outreach efforts.

To develop more effective STD treatment and prevention in the United States will require full participation by the public and private sectors. Community health nurses can be key stakeholders in modifying how STD services are provided and by accepting new responsibilities to ensure that the hidden epidemic of STDs in this country is addressed.

CRITICAL THINKING ACTIVITIES

1. What are some of the reasons the United States has vastly higher rates of STDs compared with other developed countries?

2. How can you, as a community health nurse, play an important role in changing the STD burden in the United States?

3. How comfortable are you in talking about sexual health and sexual behavior with your family? with your friends? with your clients?

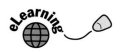

Explore Community Health Nursing on the web! To learn more about the topics in this chapter, use the passcode provided to access your exclusive web site: http://communitynursing.jbpub.com
If you do not have a passcode, you can obtain one at this site.

REFERENCES

Alter, M. J., & Mast, E. E. (1994). The epidemiology of viral hepatitis in the United States. *Gastroenterology Clinics of North America, 23*, 437–455.

American Cancer Society (1996). *Cancer facts and figures—1996.* Atlanta: Author.

American Association of World Health (AAWH). (1997). *Give children hope in a world with AIDS.* Washington, DC: Author.

American Association of World Health (AAWH). (1998). *Be a force for change.* Washington, DC: Author.

American Association of World Health (AAWH). (1999). *AIDS—end the silence.* Washington, DC: Author.

American Social Health Association (ASHA). (1998). Managed care and STDs: Can the promise be fulfilled? *STD News. A quarterly newsletter of the American Social Health Association, 6*(1), 1, 9.

Andrus, J. K., Fleming, D. W., Harger, R. D. R., Chin, M. Y., Bennet, D. V., Horan, J. M., Oxman, G., Olson, B., & Foster, L. R. (1990). Partner notification: Can it control epidemic syphilis? *Annals of Internal Medicine, 112*, 539–543.

Aral, S. O., & Holmes, K. K. (1991). Sexually transmitted diseases in the AIDS era. *Scientific American, 264*, 62–69.

Atkins, M. C., Carlin, E. M., Emery, V. C., Griffiths, P. D., & Boag, F. (1996). Fluctuations of HIV load in semen of HIV positive patients with newly acquired sexually transmitted diseases. *British Medical Journal, 313*, 341–342.

Brunham, R. C., Holmes, K. K., Embree, J. E. (1990). Sexually transmitted diseases in pregnancy. In Holmes, K. K., Mardh, P. W., Sparling, P. F., Weisner, P. I., Cates, W., Lemon, S. M., & Stamm, W. E. (Eds.), *Sexually transmitted diseases* (2nd ed., pp. 771–801). New York: McGraw-Hill.

Centers for Disease Control and Prevention (CDC). (1993). Recommendations for the prevention and management of *Chlamydia trachomatis* infections. *Morbidity and Mortality Weekly Report, 42*, 1–39.

Centers for Disease Control and Prevention (CDC). (1995a). *Annual report 1994. US Department of Health and Human Services, Public Health Service.* Atlanta: Author.

Centers for Disease Control and Prevention (CDC). (1995b). Facts about HIV/AIDS and Race/Ethnicity. In *HIV/AIDS Prevention.* Rockville, MD: CDC National AIDS Clearinghouse.

Centers for Disease Control and Prevention (CDC). (1996). *Sexually transmitted disease surveillance 1995. US Department of Health and Human Services Public Health Service.* Atlanta: Author.

Centers for Disease Control and Prevention (CDC). (1997a). *Sexually transmitted disease surveillance 1996. US Department of Health and Human Services Public Health Service.* Atlanta: Author.

Center for Disease Control and Prevention (CDC). (1997b). Gonorrhea among men who have sex with men—Selected sexually transmitted disease clinics, 1993–1996. *Morbidity and Mortality Weekly Report, 46*, 889–892.

Center for Disease Control and Prevention (CDC). (1998a). 1998 Guidelines for treatment of sexually transmitted diseases. *Morbidity and Mortality Weekly Report, 47*(RR-1). Atlanta: U.S. Government Printing Office.

Centers for Disease Control and Prevention (CDC) (1998b). *Status of perinatal HIV prevention. U.S. declines continue: Hope for extending success to developing world.* [Online]. Available: www.cdc.gov/nchstp/hiv_aids/pubs/facts/perinatl.htm.

Centers for Disease Control and Prevention (CDC) (1999a). *Need for sustained HIV prevention among men who have sex with men.* [Online]. Available: www.cdc.gov/nchstp/hiv_aids/pubs/facts/msm.htm.

Centers for Disease Control and Prevention (CDC) (1999b). *Drug associated HIV transmission continues in the United States.* [Online]. Available: www.cdc.gov/nchstp/hiv_aids/pubs/facts/idu.htm.

Centers for Disease Control and Prevention (CDC) (1999c). *Young people at risk: HIV/AIDS among America's youth.* [Online]. Available: www.cdc.gov/nchstp/hiv_aids/pubs/facts/youth.htm.

Centers for Disease Control and Prevention (CDC) (1999d). *HIV/AIDS among U.S. women: Minority and young women at continuing risk.* [Online]. Available: www.cdc.gov/nchstp/hiv_aids/pubs/facts/women.htm.

Cohen, M. S., Hoffman, I. F., Royce, R. A. Kazembe, P., Dyer, J. R., Daly, C. C., Zimba, D., Vernazza, P. L., Maida, M., Fiscus, S. A., & Eron, J. J., Jr. (1997). Reduction of concentration of HIV-A in semen after treatment of urethritis: Implications for prevention of sexual transmission of HIV-1. *Lancet, 349*, 1868–1873.

Cook, W. J., Lavelle, M., Shapiro, J. P., Brownlee, S., & Robinson, L. (1998). AIDS spread cuts population odds. *U.S. News & World Report, 125*(18), 15.

Coxon, A. P. M. (1996). Male homosexuality and HIV. Section I: Behavior changes among homosexual men. In J. Mann & D. Tarantola (Eds.). *AIDS in the World II*. New York: Oxford University Press, 252–254.

Crespo-Fierro, M. (1997). Compliance/adherence and care management in HIV disease. *Journal of the Association of Nurses in AIDS Care, 8*(4), 43–54.

Croft, C. A., & Asmussen, L. (1993). A developmental approach to sexuality education: Implications for medical practice. *Journal of Adolescent Health, 14*, 109–114.

Department of Health and Human Services (DHHS). (2000). *Healthy People 2010: Conference edition*. Washington, DC: U.S. Government Printing Office.

DeLisle, S. (1997). Preserving reproductive choice: Preventing STD-related infertility in women. *SIECUS Report, 23*, 18–21.

Farley, T. A., Hadler, J. L., & Gunn, R. A. (1990). The syphilis epidemic in Connecticut: Relationship to drug use and prostitution. *Sexually Transmitted Diseases, 17*, 163–168.

Garnett, G. P., & Anderson, R. M. (1995). Strategies for limiting the spread of HIV in developing countries: Conclusions based on studies of the transmission dynamics of the virus. *Journal of Acquired Immune Deficiency Syndrome and Human Retrovirology, 9*, 500–513.

Gibson, J. (1996). Providers of syphilis care in the southeastern United States. *Sexually Transmitted Diseases, 23*, 40–44.

Goldenberg, R. L., Andrews, W. W., Yuan, A. C., MacKay, H. T., & St. Louis, M. E. (1997). Sexually transmitted diseases and adverse outcomes of pregnancy. *Clinical Perinatology, 24*(1), 23–41.

Goldenberg, R. L., Vermund, S. H., Goepfert, A. R., & Andrews, W. W. (1998). Choriodecidual inflammation: A potentially preventable cause of perinatal HIV-1 transmission? *Lancet, 352*(9144), 1927–1930.

Grosskurth, H., Mayaud, P., Mosha, F., Todd, J., Senkoro, K., Newell, J., Gabone, R., Changalucha, J., West, B., & Hayes, R. (1996). Asymptomatic gonorrhoea and chlamydial infection in rural Tanzanian men. *BMJ, 312*(7026), 277–280.

Institute of Medicine. (1997). *The hidden epidemic: Confronting sexual transmitted diseases*. Washington, DC: National Academy Press.

Jossens, M. O., Schacter, J., & Sweet, R. L. (1994). Risk factors associated with pelvic inflammatory disease of differing microbial etiologies. *Obstetrics and Gynecology, 83*, 989–997.

Lafferty, W. E., Hughes, J. P., & Handsfield, H. H. (1997). Sexually transmitted diseases in men who have sex with men: Acquisition of gonorrhea and nongonococcal urethritis by fellatio and implications for STD/HIV prevention. *Sexually Transmitted Diseases, 24*, 272–278.

Landry & Forrest (1996). Public health departments providing STD services. *Family Planning Perspectives, 25*, 261–266.

Lawless, S., Kippax, S., & Crawford, J. (1996). Dirty, diseased and undeserving: the positioning of HIV positive women. *Social Science and Medicine, 43*(9), 1371–1377.

Levine, W. C., Pope, V., Bhoomkar, A., Tambe, P., Lewis, J. S., Zaidi, A. A., Farshy, C. E., Mithcell, S., & Talkington, D. F. (1998). Increase in endocervical CD4 lymphocytes among women with non-ulcerative sexually transmitted diseases. *Journal of Infectious Diseases, 177*, 164–174.

Mann, J., & Tarantola, D. (Eds.). (1996). *AIDS in the world II*. New York: Oxford Press.

Marchbanks, P. A., Annegers, J. F., Coulam, C. B., Strathy, J. H., & Kurland, L. T. (1988). Risk factors for ectopic pregnancy: A population-based study. *Journal of the American Medical Association, 259*, 1823–1827.

Miramontes, H. (2000). The global challenges of the HIV/AIDS pandemic. *Journal of the Association of Nurses in AIDS Care, 11*(4), 11–12.

Nakashima, A. K., Rolfs, R. T., Flock, M. L., Kilmarx, P., & Greenspan, J. R. (1996). Epidemiology of syphilis in the United States, 1941–1993. *Sexually Transmitted Diseases, 23*, 16–23.

National Institutes of Allergy and Infectious Diseases (NIAID). (1998). *Sexually transmitted diseases*. Bethesda, MD: National Institutes of Health.

National Institutes of Allergy and Infectious Diseases (NIAID). (1999a). *HIV infection and AIDS*. Bethesda, MD: National Institutes of Health.

National Institutes of Allergy and Infectious Diseases (NIAID). (1999b). *HIV/AIDS statistics*. Bethesda, MD: National Institutes of Health.

National Institutes of Health (NIH). (1996). *Consensus Development Conference statement on cervical cancer*. National Institutes of Health, Bethesda MD, April 1–3, 1996.

Nyamathi, A. M., Bennett, C., & Leake, B. (1995). Predictors of maintained high risk behaviors among impoverished women. *Public Health Reports, 110*(5), 600–606.

O'Leary, A., & Jemmott, L. S. (Eds.). (1995). *Women at risk. Issues in the primary prevention of AIDS.* New York: Plenum Press.

Over, M., & Piot, P. (1993). HIV infection and sexually transmitted disease. In Hamison, D. T., Mosley, W. H., Measham, A. R., & Bohadilla, J. L. (Eds.), *Disease control priorities in developing countries* (pp. 455–472). New York: Oxford University Press.

Prochaska, J. O., Redding, C. A., Harlow, L. L., Rossi, J. S., & Velicer, W. F. (1994). The transtheoretical model of change and HIV prevention: A review. *Health Education Quarterly,* 481–486.

Quinn, T. C., & Cates W. R. (1992). Epidemiology of sexually transmitted diseases in the 1990s. *Advances in Host Defense Mechanisms, 8,* 1–37.

Rietmeijer, C. A., Yamaguchi, K. J., Ortiz, C. G., Montstream, S. A., LeRoux, T., Ehret, J. M., Judson, F. N., & Dougis, J. M. (1997). Feasibility and yield of screening urine for *Chlamydia trachomatis* by polymerase chain reaction among high-risk male youth in field-based and other nonclinic settings. A new strategy for sexually transmitted disease control. *Sexually Transmitted Diseases, 24,* 429–435.

Robinson, N. J., Mulder, D. W., Auvert, B., & Hayes, R. J. (1997). Proportion of HIV infections attributable to other sexually transmitted diseases in a rural Ugandan population: simulation model estimates. *International Journal of Epidemiology, 26*(1), 180–189.

Rolfs, R. T., Galaid, E. I., & Zaidi, A. A. (1992). Pelvic inflammatory disease: Trends in hospitalization and office visits: 1979 through 1988. *American Journal of Obstetrics and Gynecology, 166,* 983–990.

Rolfs, R. T., Joesoef, M. R., Hendershot, E. F., Rompalo, A. M., Augebraun, M. H., Chiu, M., Bolan, G., Johnson, S. C., French, P., Steen, E., Radolf, J. D., & Larsen, S. (1997). A randomized trial of enhanced therapy for early syphilis in patients with and without human immunodeficiency virus infection. *New England Journal of Medicine, 337,* 307–314.

Rotheram-Borus, M. J., Draiman, H., Reid, H. M., & Murphy, D. A. (1997). The impact of illness disclosure and custody plans on adolescents whose parents live with AIDS. *AIDS, 11*(9), 1159–1164.

Schacker, T., Ryncarz, A., Goddard, J., Diem, K., Shaughnessy, M., & Corey, L. (1997). *Frequent recovery of replication competent HIV from genital herpes simplex virus lesions in HIV-infected persons.* Paper presented to the National STD Conference, Tampa, FL.

Schiffman, M. D. (1992). Recent progress in defining the epidemiology of human papillomavirus infection and cervical neoplasia. *Journal of the National Cancer Institute, 84,* 394–398.

Schwartlander, B., Pisani, E., Walker, N., Monasch, R., & Gerbase, A. (1998). AIDS strengthens its grip on the world. *World Health, 51*(6), 20–21.

Shilts, R. (1987). *And the band played on. Politics, people, and the AIDS epidemic.* New York: Penguin Books.

Spinola, S. M., Orazi. A., Arno, J. N., Fortney, K., Kotylo, P., Chen, C. Y., Capagnari, A. A., & Hood, A. F. (1996). *Haemophilus ducreyi* elicits a cutaneous infiltrate of CD4 cells during experimental human infection. *Journal of Infectious Diseases, 173,* 394–402.

Staton, M., Leukefeld, C., Logan, T. K., Zimmerman, R., Lynam, D., Milich, R., Martin, C., McClanahan, K., & Clayton, R. (1999). Risky sex behavior and substance use among young adults. *Health & Social Work, 24*(2), 147–154.

UNICEF (1999). *The Progress of Nations 1999.* [Online]. Available: www.unicef.org/pon99/aidsdat3.htm.

Vuylsteke, B., Sunkutu, R., & Laga, M. (1996). Epidemiology of HIV and sexually transmitted infections in women. In J. Mann & D. Tarantola (Eds.). *AIDS in the world II.* New York: Oxford Press, 97–109.

Warner, P. H., Rowe, T., & Whipple, B. (1999). Shedding light on the sexual history. *American Journal of Nursing, 99*(6), 34–41.

Wasserheit, J. N. (1992) Epidemiologic synergy: Interrelationships between human immunodeficiency virus infection and other sexually transmitted diseases. *Sexually Transmitted Diseases, 9,* 61–77.

Woods, E. R. (1998). Overview of the Special Projects of National Significance Program's 10 models of adolescent HIV care. *Journal of Adolescent Health, 23*(2), 5–10.

World Health Organization (WHO). (2000). *WHO report on global surveillance of epidemic-prone infectious disasters.* [Online]. www.WHO.int.

Chapter 21

Substance Abuse as a Community Health Problem

Jean Haspeslagh and Judith A. Barton

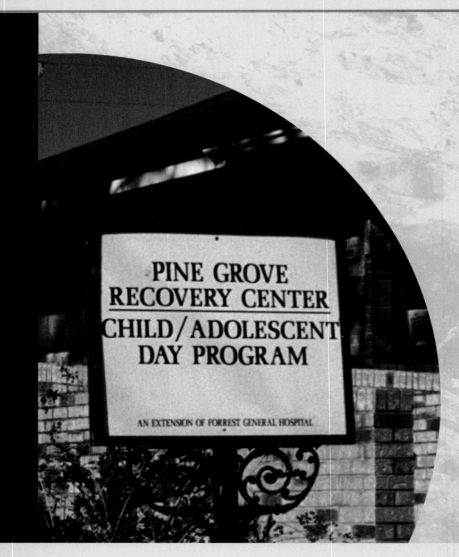

Macduff: What three things does drink especially provoke?
Porter: Marry, sir, nose-painting, sleep and urine. Lechery, sir; it provokes and unprovokes. It provokes the desire, but it takes away the performance; therefore, much drink may be said to be an equivocator with lechery; it makes him and it mars him; it sets him on, and it takes him off, it persuades him, and disheartens him; makes him stand to and not stand to, in conclusion, equivocates him in a sleep, and, giving him the lie, leaves him.
—Macbeth, Act 2, Scene 3

CHAPTER FOCUS

QUESTIONS TO CONSIDER

After reading this chapter, answer the following questions:

1. What is the scope of substance abuse in the community?
2. What are the most commonly abused drugs?
3. What are the community health consequences of substance abuse?
4. What are the risk factors associated with substance abuse?
5. How does a nurse's self-awareness relate to addressing the problem of substance abuse in the community?
6. How are primary, secondary, and tertiary prevention strategies implemented in the community?
7. What are specific intervention strategies for various age groups in the prevention of substance abuse?
8. What specific population groups are most at risk for substance abuse?
9. What is the role of the community health nurse in substance abuse prevention in schools and in the workplace?

KEY TERMS

Addiction	Dependence	Project STAR	Social modeling theory
Alcoholism	Family functioning	Return to work contract	Substance abuse
Comprehensive school health	Interdiction	Secondary prevention	Supply
	Primary prevention	Social control	Tertiary prevention

Substance abuse is a familiar topic that we find much focus on in society today. The president has a drug policy director working on political responses to drug use and abuse; the media always includes articles or news items speaking to the magnitude of the problem as it affects society. Often, community health nurses find they are directly involved in working with clients who are living with the effects of substance abuse on themselves and their families. These effects range from major health problems such as liver disease to major social problems such as drug dealing. It is the community health nurse's role to be ready to provide intervention at the primary, secondary, and tertiary levels when addressing substance abuse. This chapter provides insight into ways that you, as a community health nurse, can prepare yourself to work with substance abuse as a community health problem.

The Nature of Substance Abuse as a Community Health Problem

Definitions of Substance Abuse

When speaking of substance abuse, one finds a number of terms used in the literature, including *substance abuse, chemical dependence,* and *addiction.* In this chapter, *substance abuse* is used to cover the broad spectrum of abuse of alcohol and other drugs, including dependence and addiction. **Substance abuse** is the use of any drug (alcohol, street drugs, or prescription medications) that results in a loss of control over the amount taken and when it is taken. It also includes continuation of drug use regardless of the consequences (physical, social, and psychological). Misuse of prescription drugs is a form of substance abuse often encountered in the community. Box 21-1 lists the major classes of abused drugs.

. . . .

There was a time when all I cared about was the next game, the next party, the next tee time. I've come to a crossroads. I can't think of one thing that drinking has done that's been good for me or my family. I'm not saying everyone in the world should quit drinking, but I wasn't the best drinker in the world, so I'm quitting it.

Brett Favre, Green Bay Packers Quarterback, 1999

. . . .

Dependence or **addiction** is present when there are physiological symptoms that occur with withdrawal of the substance. However, the important thing to remember is that, whether or not the individual is experiencing dependence or is "merely" overusing or misusing drugs, the effects on the person and the community are similar.

Scope of Substance Abuse

The use and abuse of alcohol and other drugs contribute to one of the major public health problems facing society today. The use and abuse of alcohol and other drugs are widespread across all

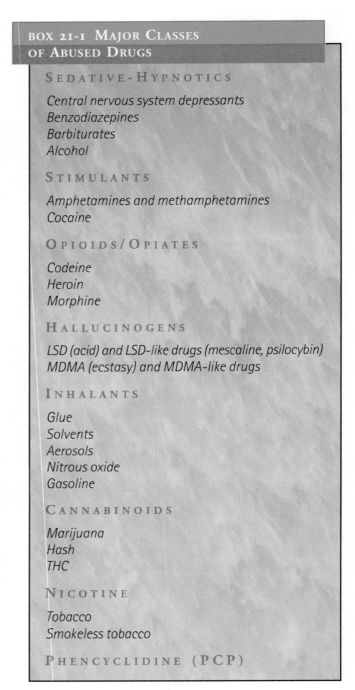

BOX 21-1 MAJOR CLASSES OF ABUSED DRUGS

SEDATIVE-HYPNOTICS

Central nervous system depressants
Benzodiazepines
Barbiturates
Alcohol

STIMULANTS

Amphetamines and methamphetamines
Cocaine

OPIOIDS/OPIATES

Codeine
Heroin
Morphine

HALLUCINOGENS

LSD (acid) and LSD-like drugs (mescaline, psilocybin)
MDMA (ecstasy) and MDMA-like drugs

INHALANTS

Glue
Solvents
Aerosols
Nitrous oxide
Gasoline

CANNABINOIDS

Marijuana
Hash
THC

NICOTINE

Tobacco
Smokeless tobacco

PHENCYCLIDINE (PCP)

races and ethnic groups in society; furthermore, someone you know at work could be using drugs (Box 21-2). A 1997 survey conducted by the Harvard School of Public Health indicated that 56% of the people surveyed considered drugs the most serious problem facing young people in the United States today. Alcohol use and abuse are occurring at a younger age, making the need for prevention programs in schools essential. For young people going off to college, the military, or first jobs, their newly

BOX 21-2 MOST DRUG USERS ARE
IN THE WORKFORCE

*"The typical drug user is not poor and unem-
ployed," Barry McCaffrey, the White House drug
policy director, said in a statement. "He or she can
be a co-worker, a husband or wife, a parent."*

*A report issued by the U.S. Department of
Health and Human Services (DHHS) found that
7.7% of workers ages 18 to 49 had used illegal
drugs in the past month. (The report was based on
research conducted by the Substance Abuse and
Mental Health Services Administration). Nationwide, 7 in 10 drug users were full-time workers in
1997.*

*The report also found that 19% of restaurant
workers, 14% of construction workers, and 10% of
transportation and material-moving workers used
illegal drugs.*

*DHHS officials are using the report's findings
to encourage medium-sized businesses to establish treatment programs that will increase workplace safety and productivity and lower substance
abuse and its human and economic effects.*

Source: Associated Press, 1999.

found independence also includes new peer pressures to drink, smoke, or use recreational drugs. In addition, as persons live longer and experience more chronic health problems, they are faced with an existence that includes the use of multiple drugs. Along with the benefits associated with improved pharmacological management of chronic conditions, it is necessary to acknowledge the problems associated with the misuse of these same agents.

Illicit Drug Users

An estimated 13.6 million Americans used some form of illicit drugs in 1998. This number indicates that 6.2% of the population 12 years and older used an illicit drug in the month prior to the survey, titled the National Household Survey on Drug Abuse (NHSDA), as conducted by the Substance Abuse and Mental Health Service Administration (SAMHSA, 1998). Although this number is slightly less than the 13.9 million illicit drug users in 1997, the difference is not statistically significant. However, by comparison, the number is greatly reduced from its highest level, in 1979, when the estimate was that 25 million or 14.1% of Americans used illicit drugs.

Marijuana continues to be the most commonly used illicit drug, used by 81% of current illicit drug users. Approximately

60% of current illicit drug users use only marijuana. Therefore, approximately 40% of current illicit drug users in 1998 (an estimated 5.4 million Americans) were current users of illicit drugs other than marijuana. The rates of use of cocaine, heroin, hallucinogens, and inhalants in the total population age 12 and older did not significantly change between 1997 and 1998. However, reports of increasing heroin and methamphetamine abuse have been prominent over the past few years, based on emergency departments' and drug treatment facilities' reports. The 1998 NHSDA did show an increasing rate of past-month heroin use from 1993 to 1997, and an increasing rate of lifetime heroin smoking, snorting, or sniffing between 1994 and 1997. Furthermore, most new heroin users in recent years were younger than 26.

In 1998, about a third of illicit drug users were 35 and older. In 1979, the peak year for drug use prevalence, only 10.3% of drug users were age 35 and older. An analysis of this statistic indicates that the high users of drugs in 1979 are the middle-aged drug users of today.

In the 1998 NHSDA, illicit drug use for African Americans (8.2%) remained somewhat higher than for whites (6.1%) and Hispanics (6.1%). As in prior years, men continue to have higher rates of current illicit drug use than women (8.1% versus 4.5%). In terms of regional illicit drug use, 7.3% of users resided in the Western region, 6.7% in the North Central region, 5.8% in the Northeast, and 5.5% in the South. The rates of illicit drug use in metropolitan areas are higher than in nonmetropolitan areas.

Illicit drug use rates remain highly correlated with educational status. Among young adults 26 to 34 years old, those who had not completed high school had the highest rates of current use (9.8%), whereas college graduates had the lowest rate (4.8%).

Use of Alcohol

In 1998, approximately 113 million persons 12 and older, or about 52% of the total population, were current alcohol users. The alcohol use rate did not change between 1997 and 1998. This was true for both binge drinking and heavy drinking (Box 21-3). It is also important to note that the level of alcohol use is strongly associated with illicit drug use.

Rates for current alcohol use were greater than 60% for those ages 21 to 44 in 1998; for younger and older age groups, the rates were lower. Binge drinking was a particular problem

BOX 21-3 WHAT CONSTITUTES BINGE
AND HEAVY DRINKING?

Binge drinking: 5 or more drinks on the same occasion in the past month.

Heavy drinking: 5 or more drinks on the same occasion at least 5 different days in the past
month.

among 18- to 25-year-olds (college-age individuals). Alcohol use tends to be more moderate among African Americans than among other racial/ethnic groups. Men's use of alcohol (59% in the past month) was greater than women's use (45% in the past month). Although the overall rate of alcohol use is lower in rural areas than in metropolitan areas, the rates of binge drinking and heavy alcohol use in rural areas were similar to the rates in non-rural areas. In contrast to the pattern for illicit drugs, the higher the level of education, the more likely the current use of alcohol. In 1998, 65.5% of adults with college degrees were current drinkers, compared with only 40.4% of those having less than a high school education (SAMHSA, 1998).

Use of Tobacco

Tobacco use continues to be a major public health concern, with 60 million current smokers in the United States (SAMHSA, 1998). This actual number of tobacco smokers represents a smoking rate of 27.7% for those 12 and older. The rate did decrease from 29.6%, and this drop was statistically significant. Current smokers were more likely than nonsmokers to be heavy drinkers and illicit drug users. The use of cigars rose significantly from 1997 (5.9%) to 1998 (6.9%). In addition, an estimated 3.1% of the population are current users of smokeless tobacco. This rate has remained steady since 1991.

The current smoking rate among young adults ages 18 to 25 continues to move upward from 34.6% in 1994 to 41.6% in 1998. The smoking rate among 12- to 17-year-olds was 18.2%, with no change in use from recent years. Smoking rates are similar among different races and ethnic groups. Males had higher rates of smoking than females (29.7% versus 25.7%). Lower educational attainment was correlated with higher tobacco use (SAMHSA, 1998).

Youthful Illicit Drug Users

The Monitoring the Future study (National Institute on Drug Abuse, 1998) concluded that illicit drug use by 8th, 10th, and 12th graders is finally heading down after 6 years of steady increases. However, the authors of this study, Johnston, O'Malley, and Bachman (1998), point out that the improvement is still very modest.

Marijuana is still the most widely used illicit drug, even though its use is decreasing. In 1998, nearly half (49%) of all 12th graders said they had used marijuana. Although there was evidence of some decline in alcohol use at all three grade levels, fully one-third (33%) of all high school seniors reported being drunk at least once in the 30-day interval preceding the survey.

Stimulant (amphetamine) use showed a noticeable turnaround. Use of stimulants has declined for 2 years. The annual prevalence rates in 1998 for stimulants were 7.2% for 8th graders, 10.7% for 10th graders, and 10.1% for 12th graders.

Inhalant use also showed a downward trend; however, the 1998 rate of use was higher in younger children (8th graders) at 11.1% compared with 10th graders at 8% and seniors at 6.2%. Hallucinogen use was down slightly, with 9% of seniors, 6.9% of sophomores, and 3.4% of 8th graders reporting some use of this illicit drug during 1998.

················

If we hear somebody's sniffing something, we're not shocked—It's an everyday occurrence.
Sophomore high school student, Newark, Delaware

················

Some categories of illicit drugs did not show an improvement in 1998 over the 1997 survey data. Heroin use remained the same in 1998 as compared with 1997, but cocaine and tranquilizers continued to show a gradual increase in use by youth.

Overall, the conclusions of the 1998 survey of illicit drug use among youth was promising. The study points out that behaviors change very slowly, and often only after there has been some reassessment by young people about the dangers of drugs and how acceptable they are in the peer group. Perhaps the seniors of 1998 saw the negative consequences happening to past seniors as they moved into substance dependence. Other effects could include more attention being paid to drug issues by community groups, parents, government, and the media. The 1998 Monitoring the Future study also points out that fewer music industry performers are singing the praises of drugs than in the early 1990s. The analysis of this shift is that it could made a real difference for teenagers.

Impact of Substance Abuse on Society

An August 1999 report issued by the Department of Health and Human Services reported that drug- and alcohol-related abuse kills approximately 35,549 Americans each year and that drugs and alcohol cost taxpayers nearly $246 million in unnecessary health care costs, extra law enforcement, auto crashes, crime, and lost productivity. The annual financial losses to victims of alcohol-related violence (approximately 500,000 persons annually) total more than $400 million, while the average victim of such violence paid $1,500 out of pocket for related medical expenses. According to the National Treatment Improvement Study (1997), the cost of treatment for substance abuse ranges from a low of $1,800 to a high of approximately $6,800 per person, while the cost of incarceration (prison) has been estimated at $18,330 annually.

The U.S. Department of Transportation (1999) reported that alcohol was involved in 15,935 traffic fatalities, or 38.4% of all 1998 fatalities. The Drug Enforcement Administration of the U.S. Department of Justice (1997) reported that alcohol abuse was a factor in 4 in 10 violent crimes and that approximately 4 in 10 criminal offenders reported using alcohol at the time they committed their offense. The National Justice Institute asserts that abuse of alcohol and other drugs by criminal offenders, parolees, and probationers contributes to 80% of crime in the

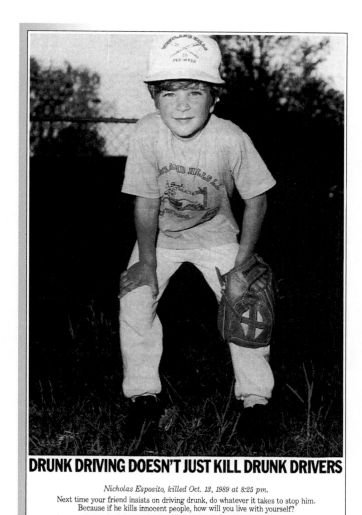

DRUNK DRIVING DOESN'T JUST KILL DRUNK DRIVERS

Nicholas Esposito, killed Oct. 13, 1989 at 8:25 pm.
Next time your friend insists on driving drunk, do whatever it takes to stop him.
Because if he kills innocent people, how will you live with yourself?

FRIENDS DON'T LET FRIENDS DRIVE DRUNK.

U.S. Department of Transportation

The tragic outcomes of drunk driving due to alcohol abuse.

United States. In incidents of spouse abuse, alcohol use by the offender was documented in 75% of reported cases.

Impact of Substance Abuse on the Individual

The effects of substance abuse on the individual are many and range from loss of a job and loss of relationships to major health problems. Substance abusers find themselves at greater risk for death as a result of auto accidents and violence (suicide and homicide), cirrhosis, and hemorrhagic cerebrovascular disease (Stein, 1997). They are also more likely to develop chronic health problems such as central nervous system neuropathy, impaired cognition, cardiovascular disease, hypertension, and chronic gastrointestinal problems, including gastritis. Acute and chronic pancreatitis and liver disease are often associated with alcohol abuse. Nutritional deficiencies and anemia are often identified and are a result of not only poor dietary habits but more importantly the physiological changes that result from abuse of alcohol and other drugs.

Although low self-esteem is a common characteristic exhibited by the person who abuses substances, no personality factors or other behaviors have reliably differentiated substance abusers from other individuals. It would appear that low self-esteem appears to be more a result of the substance abuse rather than a causative factor (West & Kinney, 1996, p. 28). After reviewing psychological theories related to substance abuse, Goldsmith (1997, p. 6) concluded that the idea that there is an addictive personality is a myth. It appears that the depression, anxiety, and lack of self-esteem are as much a result of the substance use as they are causative factors.

Participation in high-risk behaviors such as intravenous drug use and promiscuous sexual activity put the substance abuser at greater risk for acquiring sexually transmitted diseases. Kimball, Beckley, and Ngugi (1998) indicated that there are increasingly high rates of positive tests for human immunodeficiency virus (HIV) in high-risk groups, which include intravenous drug users, "sex workers" (i.e., prostitutes), and those who have multiple sex partners. Individuals who are using illicit drugs and need to find ways to pay for their drugs often turn to prostitution to help support their habit, placing them in this high-risk group.

Risk Factors for Substance Abuse
Society's Influence
Media Influences

Societal factors that influence the use and abuse of alcohol and other drugs are all around us. Television and movies present the use of alcohol and tobacco as glamorous, a rite of passage, something the sophisticated person does. The Research Briefs on p. 470 highlight recent studies on the potential influence of the media on substance use in our society.

Advertisements tell us we need a break, we need to relax and unwind, and what better way then by having a drink or smoking? We live in a fast-paced world where people are encouraged not to feel. Ads remind us that if it hurts, take something; if you are stressed, have a drink, take a pill, smoke another cigarette.

Societal Attitudes

Attitudes toward legal and illegal substances, abuse of substances, and interventions and treatment for drug-addicted individuals vary according to society, community, ethnicity, social status, gender, and time. In other words, substance abuse is a socially constructed concept. Sometimes drug use is considered okay, and other times it is not okay. For example, the use of amphetamines or tranquilizers by a businessperson might be considered a

RESEARCH BRIEF

Kelly, K., & Donohew, L. (1999). Media and primary socialization theory. Substance Use and Misuse, 34(7), 1033–1045.

Portrayal of Substance Use in the Media

This study examined the frequency and nature of substance use in the most popular movie rentals and songs of 1996 and 1997. The intent was to determine the accuracy of public perceptions about extensive substance use in media popular among youth. Because teenagers are major consumers of movies and music, there is concern about the potential for media depictions of tobacco, alcohol, and illicit drugs to encourage use.

The study examined the 200 most popular movie rentals and 1,000 of the most popular songs from 1996 and 1997. Substances included in the study were illicit drugs, alcohol, tobacco, and over-the-counter and prescription medicines. The researchers examined what was used, by whom, how often, under what circumstances, and with what consequences.

Findings revealed that 98% of the movies studied depicted illicit drugs, alcohol, tobacco, or over-the-counter and prescription medicines. Fewer than half (49%) the movies portrayed short-term consequences of substance use, and only 12% depicted long-term consequences.

The major finding from the song analysis was the dramatic difference among music categories (country, alternative rock, hot 100, rap, and heavy metal), with substance references being most common in rap. Illicit drugs were mentioned in 63% of rap songs versus about 10% of the lyrics in all other categories.

RESEARCH BRIEF

Robinson, T. N., Chen, H. L., & Killen, J. D. (1998). Television and music video exposure and risk of adolescent alcohol use. Pediatrics, 102(5), 1202–1209.

Study Links Television Viewing Time with High School Student Drinking

A Stanford University study of 1,533 9th graders found that high school students who watch lots of television and music videos are more likely to start drinking than other youngsters. Youngsters who rented movies were less likely to start drinking, while playing video and computer games had no effect. Watching TV and music videos made no difference in the drinking habits of those who had already begun to drink alcohol.

RESEARCH BRIEF

Amaro, H. (1999). An expensive policy: The impact of inadequate funding for substance abuse treatment. American Journal of Public Health, 89(5), 657–659.

Substance Abuse Policies Related to Societal Attitudes

Although public health policies and practices are making slow but sure progress toward improving the health of particular groups of Americans (e.g., children with infectious diseases, cancer patients) through insurance coverage, screening, and treatment, the prevention and treatment of substance use has not kept up.

The federal government's continued policy of spending nearly double the amount on supply reduction (interdiction) as on demand reduction (prevention and treatment) is considered perplexing by public health professionals because of the large treatment gap for substance abuse.

It is estimated that although more than 5.3 million persons in the United States are in severe need of substance abuse treatment, only 37% receive such treatment. It is estimated that providing treatment to all in need could save more than $150 billion over the next 15 years, at a price tag of just $21 billion. In other words, funding treatment for persons addicted to drugs is good fiscal policy because every dollar invested in drug treatment generates $7 in savings of future costs!

matter of personal judgment, but the use of the same drugs by a young person who wishes to experience their effects produces much more emotion. Society's influence can again be seen when one looks at alcohol, which was actually prohibited in the United States through a constitutional amendment—the Eighteenth Amendment, passed by the U.S. Congress in 1920. After 13 years of unsuccessful efforts to enforce the law, prohibition was repealed. Currently, tobacco use is increasingly being viewed as deviant, and those individuals and groups who use tobacco are experiencing stigmatization and subsequent discrimination.

Substance abuse as a criminal activity or as a disease

Alcoholism in American culture has been defined as a chronic disease manifested by repeated drinking causing injury to the drinker's health and/or social or economic functioning. Alcohol for individuals 21 years of age and older is legal in the United States, and being defined as a chronic disease has shifted alcohol-related problems from the category of sin or crime to the category of sickness. Nevertheless, many in our society tend to stereotype the alcoholic as a skid row derelict. Consequently, many persons who regularly drink to excess do not seek treatment because they do not see themselves as fitting that stereotype. Although excessive use of alcohol has been viewed as a disease, the excessive use of other psychoactive drugs in our society has not (Carroll, 1996). Currently, however, there is some movement toward defining alcohol and drug addiction as meeting the criteria for a disability under the Americans with Disabilities Act (ADA). The medical community is taking leadership in this movement. The American Medical Association (AMA) and the American Society of Addiction Medicine (ASAM) are particularly concerned about managed care denials for individuals with drug addictions. Although it appears that our society is far from decriminalization of illicit drug use or the legalization of drugs, there is a growing concern about the prevention and treatment of drug addiction. For example, in spring of 1998, General Barry McCaffery, current director of the Office of National Drug Control Policy, announced that the administration will ask Congress for an increase of $491 million for both prevention and treatment programs (ASAM, 1998). The Research Brief on p. 470 discusses current substance abuse treatment policy, which is based on the attitude that substance abuse is a criminal activity to deter rather than a disease to treat. The conversation with Betty Ford, former President Ford's wife (below), contributed especially for this nursing textbook, discusses addictions and the need for more emphasis on treatment of addictions as a disease.

A CONVERSATION WITH...

Alcoholism and other drug addiction is an equal opportunity disease—women and men, young and old, all walks of life are affected. It is a complex disease of mind, body, and soul.

The chronic nature of alcoholism and other drug addiction is often what gets in the way of understanding and awareness. There continues to be many myths about this illness and much stigma attached to alcoholics and addicts.

The Betty Ford Center, in addition to having over 38,000 women, men, and their families participate in our treatment programs, offers unique training opportunities. Licensed professionals and students take part in the Professional in Residence Program, which is an experiential, hands-on-program. Nurses, in particular, who are often on the frontline of intervention and treatment, have been eager participants in this training experience.

There is no question that our national drug policy is failing. I believe that is because the majority of emphasis continues on interdiction rather than treatment and prevention. This failure has even led to calls of legalization. Legalization would be an invitation to young people to use drugs. This would be a disaster. We need to change the emphasis of our national programs.

—Betty Ford,
Founder of the Betty Ford Center
Source: Betty Ford, personal communication,
October 25, 1999.

Cultural Influences

Research has demonstrated that peer pressure, particularly for youth, is highly correlated to the use of illicit substances. If peer pressure to use substances is joined with other cultural influences, the risk of use becomes even stronger. For example, Goldsmith (1997) found that first use of alcohol and drugs often occurs in a social setting, suggesting that peer pressure and positive social/group attitudes about using substances, availability of the drugs, and pro-use norms in the community contribute to substance abuse.

Think about the many cultural influences for and against the use and potential abuse of drugs in the United States. Will the restriction of billboards promoting the glamour of cigarette smoking reduce the use of tobacco? Are the current movement by the National Organization for the Reform of Marijuana Laws and the resurgence of the use of marijuana in Hollywood movies going to have an influence on the use of marijuana in our society?

The Family's Influence

Although in modern society many of the socialization functions of the family have been taken over by other institutions such as schools, churches, or the media, the family remains a significant agent of socialization. Parents normally take care to monitor their offspring's behavior and pass on the language, values, norms, and beliefs of their culture. Research in the area of adolescent substance abuse has demonstrated that the family can have a positive effect in reducing the risk of initiation into alcohol, tobacco, and other drug use among children and youth (Hahn, 1993; Hahn & Rado, 1996; Hahn, Simpson, & Kidd, 1996). For example, a young man who is raised in a family where all the male role models drink heavily will most often follow their lead. The opposite is also true—the person who is raised in a family or culture where there are strong prohibitions against drinking may be more inclined to experiment with alcohol at a later time, hopefully when he or she is more mature and will not end up abusing alcohol.

The family can play a role in either maintaining a family member's escalation into substance abuse or their recovery from substance abuse. Non–substance-abusing family members initially experience emotions such as anger, fear, resentment, guilt, and shame when they first recognize that a spouse or child is a substance abuser. Because many people in our society view substance abuse as a character weakness, non-substance-abusing family members often share in the stigma (i.e., discrediting and discrimination) imposed on the substance abuser. Literature indicates spouses and parents most likely have inaccurate knowledge about the extent of their spouse's or child's substance abuse activities and therefore are inclined to show a great deal of tolerance of untoward behavior among family members, often taking a long time to acknowledge that a problem exists. In most cases, families attempt to cope with the abuser's problem; however, in some cases, the problem is dealt with by means of divorce or ejection of the adolescent (Barton, 1991; Weinberg & Vogel, 1990).

A family history of alcoholism or addiction as well as biochemical and genetic factors also make certain family members more sensitive to the effects of substances. Research in this area, although not totally confirming, is becoming more definitive as to the correlation between familial alcoholism and offspring alcoholism (Hill, 1998). In addition, the problem of drug dependence during pregnancy is known to lead to babies who show withdrawal symptoms (Schneider, Fischer, Diamant, Hauk, Pezawas, Lenzinger, & Kasper, 1996) and the concern could be that these children will exhibit tendencies toward substance abuse in their youthful and adult lives.

The Workplace's Influence

Substance abuse in the workplace is a concern for both employers and consumers of products and services. The cost in lost work time alone accounts for $10 billion a year (Naegle, 1993). This does not include such things as the cost of intervention, treatment, and reduced productivity. How substance abuse is viewed in the workplace is important. Does management send a message that drinking and using drugs in the workplace is unacceptable? Does management simply avoid confronting the issue of substance abuse with the stand that "We don't have anyone on our staff who does that"? Failure to acknowledge that substance abuse can be a problem in the work environment is itself a problem that can lead to further risk for employees. Acknowledgment that substance abuse can be a problem for many workers, creation of health promotion and prevention programs, and policies related to treatment for workers will put all workers on alert that the demands of work require workers to deal with their substance abuse problem.

Personal Factors

Substance abuse affects people of all ages, socioeconomic groups, and occupations. Box 21-4 lists populations vulnerable to substance abuse. Young people remain the most vulnerable to substance abuse, with the highest rate of illicit drug use occurring in those younger than 20 years of age (35.6%), while only 1% of illicit drug use occurs in the over-50 group. There appears to be little difference between whether the individual lives in an urban or rural setting (SAMHSA, 1997).

According to the 1996 household survey (SAMHSA, 1997), the use of illicit drugs appears to be higher in young people who have dropped out of high school and lowest in college graduates. Similarly, although 60% of individuals use alcohol, the group most likely to binge or fall into the heavy drinking category tends to be individuals between 18 and 35 years of age who have not completed high school. Alcohol use is also strongly associated with illicit drug use, with 31% of drinkers using illicit drugs.

When looking at risk factors for alcoholism and addiction, it is essential to consider such things as the biochemical and genetic factors that make one individual more sensitive to the effects of drugs, prenatal exposure to drugs, and preexisting or co-existing psychiatric disorders. Box 21-5 provides a list of individual risk factors nurses should be alert to during any assessment.

Research has indicated that there is no one clear-cut cause for substance abuse disorders. However, for some persons, one or more factors may predominate (Clark, Kanas, Smith, & Landry, 1995). It has been found that for many people, a family history of alcoholism or addiction is a red flag indicating that the risk of becoming addicted or dependent on alcohol and/or other drugs is greater. It would stand to reason then that babies who were born addicted because of maternal drug abuse will be at a higher risk for developing substance abuse problems should they experiment with alcohol or other drugs when they are older.

BOX 21-4 VULNERABLE POPULATIONS

- Children and adolescents
- High school dropouts
- People with duel diagnoses
- People with family history of alcoholism/addiction
- Unemployed individuals
- College students

BOX 21-5 INDIVIDUAL RISK FACTORS

- Family history of substance abuse
- Genetic/biochemical factors
- Prenatal exposure
- Psychiatric disorders

The existence of preexisting or co-existing psychiatric disorders may also contribute to substance abuse. Anthenelli (1997) and Waller (1997) found evidence that persons with both a psychiatric diagnosis and a substance abuse problem are not uncommon. Persons with antisocial personality disorders, schizophrenia, and bipolar disorders are at greater risk for developing a substance abuse disorder. Goldsmith (1997) emphasized that "alcohol exaggerates both mood disorders and anxiety and that alcohol and drugs cause organic mood and organic anxiety disorders" (p. 6).

In an age when families are often scattered and talking with a neighbor appears to be a lost art, the sharing and receiving of emotional support is difficult for many people in our society. The image of rugged individualism, self-reliance, and high achievement often discourages people from allowing others to see their vulnerability and leads them to seek other ways of dealing with emotional pain. For some individuals, using alcohol or other drugs becomes their way of coping with their emotional pain. What results is a vicious cycle in which the person experiences emotional pain, uses alcohol or drugs to relieve that pain, experiences emotional pain related to consequences of substance abuse, and turns back to the substance to dull the emotional pain.

Nursing Assessment

Nurses' Attitude Self-Assessment

For community health nurses to work effectively with substance abusers, it is important that they develop an awareness of their own issues and attitudes about substance abuse. The nurse's attitudes regarding use of legal and illicit drugs, about those people who use or abuse drugs, and past experiences with substance abuse/abusers need to be assessed.

One of the first areas of self-awareness that needs to be addressed is what feeling the nurse has about the use of alcohol, tobacco, and recreational drugs. Questions to ask oneself include the following:

- *What do I believe about the use of alcohol, tobacco, and recreational drugs? Is it morally wrong?*

- *Is it okay to use alcohol and tobacco but not marijuana or other recreational drugs? marijuana but not any other illegal drugs?*

- *Is the use of any mind-altering substance up to the individual's freedom of choice?*

The second area that one needs to examine is one's attitude about the substance abuser.

- *How do I feel about the person who uses and abuses alcohol, tobacco, or other drugs?*

- *Is that person just weak-willed, immoral, or undisciplined or ill and in need of treatment?*

- *Is the answer to the substance abuse problem punishment and incarceration?*

Third, the community health nurse must look carefully at how past experiences with substance abuse/abusers may have influenced attitudes toward those individuals who abuse substances. Nurses should ask themselves the following questions:

- *Who have I known who abused alcohol or other drugs? How did their substance abuse affect me and my relationship with them?*

- *Was I raised in an alcoholic or addicted family? What did this mean to me? Have I received any assistance in dealing with my own issues?*

- *Have I ever lost someone who was important to me as a result of substance use?*

- *Have I ever been physically, sexually, or emotionally abused by someone who was abusing alcohol or other drugs?*

For some people, asking and answering these questions may bring up uncomfortable, painful feelings. If this occurs, it is important that available resources be used to work through those feelings. For those individuals who have never shared their experiences, working with substance abusers may be difficult unless those unresolved issues are addressed. Failure to do so may result in the nurse's unconsciously avoiding interactions, being judgmental, and failing to be therapeutic when working with this population.

Drug History

One of the nurse's critical tasks when substance abuse is suspected is to conduct a drug history, taking note of the drugs of choice, the route of administration, the amount used, the frequency of use, and polysubstance use. Box 21-6 summarizes key elements to address in a drug history. Information regarding the initiation of drug use, including the age and drugs first used, is important. Drug histories may need to be repeated to get a more accurate picture of what drugs have been used and how often. The substance abuser may give inaccurate information initially for a number of reasons: confu-

---

BOX 21-6 KEY ELEMENTS IN A DRUG HISTORY

- What drug/drugs have been taken? In what combination?
- What route was used to administer the drug (e.g., injection, intravenous, oral, sniffed, smoked)?
- How much of the drug was taken?
- What is the frequency of drug use?
- When was the drug last taken?
- At what age did drug use begin?

Recognizing the Signs of Substance Abuse

To address substance abuse issues, it is essential that the nurse recognize that abuse of drugs is multifaceted, with a variety of substances being used either singularly or in combination (see Box 21-1 for a listing of major classes of abused drugs). The community health nurse needs to be aware of those major drug groups that are subject to abuse. In addition, for community health nurses, knowledge regarding the signs of substance abuse is essential if they are to recognize such abuse early so that intervention can be planned. Efforts must be made to detect the problem as soon as possible. Common signs indicative that an individual may be abusing one or more substances are found in Boxes 21-7 and 21-8. Becoming familiar with the indicators of potential substance abuse is important for nurses, particularly those who work in primary care or community settings because it is at these nonstigmatizing medical settings (as opposed to drug abuse treatment centers) that the substance abuser may first make contact with health care professionals. The assessment process, however, is not always straightforward. The early stages can be difficult to recognize. The psychological, social, and physical manifestations vary widely, depending on the particular sub-

sion because of drugs, fear, lack of trust, and uncertainty regarding what drugs were taken. The latter is often a problem with street drugs because the purity of these substances is often questionable.

stance or substances used, the amount used or the frequency of use, and factors such as age and the physical health of the user (Grant & Hodgson, 1991).

Interventions
Society's Response

Society today is increasingly responding to the problems associated with substance abuse in a two-pronged approach: politically and as a health care issue. In the past, the political response to substance abuse was focused on punishment for the use or supplying of illicit drugs. Indeed, the acquisition and sales of illicit drugs continues to be the focus, with emphasis on law enforcement and punishment. However, the 1998 National Drug Control Strategy (NCADI, 1998) now speaks to the importance of prevention. It indicates the need for a "balanced" program that addresses not only the **supply** (i.e., support to developing countries to put an end to their drug market) and **interdiction** (i.e., to stop drug trafficking at U.S. borders) issues, but also prevention, education, and treatment. The 1998 strategies recognize substance abuse problems as being international and long term, and as such they must be addressed with realistic programs that support families, schools, and communities and that include the international aspects of drug control. The following are the five goals of the 1998 strategy (NCADI, 1998):

Goal 1: *Educate and enable America's youth to reject illegal drugs as well as alcohol and tobacco.*

Goal 2: *Increase the safety of America's citizens by substantially reducing drug-related crime and violence.*

Goal 3: *Reduce health and social costs to the public as a result of illegal drug use.*

Goal 4: *Shield America's air, land, and sea frontiers from the drug threat.*

Goal 5: *Break foreign and domestic drug sources of supply.*

These strategies do recognize that persons who are addicted need assistance. The strategies hold individuals accountable for their negative behaviors but offer treatment that can help change those self-defeating destructive behaviors.

Healthy People 2010 has recognized the seriousness of substance abuse and has identified 25 objectives related to alcohol and other drugs and 21 specifically focused on tobacco. Much of the emphasis in the objectives is placed on youth and decreasing the use and abuse of alcohol, tobacco, and other drugs within this group. One of the biggest needs identified in *Healthy People 2010* is access to culturally, linguistically, and age-appropriate service, education, and research necessary to meet the objectives. In addition, it is recognized that ongoing research must be undertaken to identify changes, evaluate the effectiveness of interventions and programs, and determine where further emphasis is needed. See the box on pp. 476 and 477 for selected *Healthy People 2010* objectives.

Primary Prevention

Primary prevention involves the *prevention* of diseases or conditions through protective factors, as well as through health-*promotion* activities. In the case of substance abuse, the first level of intervention pertains to activities that are begun before drug abuse occurs (Carroll, 1996). Typical primary prevention techniques include education for responsible decision making, knowledge of risk factors, legislation and law enforcement, interdiction activities, and programs to strengthen resistance to substance abuse.

One example of a primary prevention program conducted on a community level is the Kansas City comprehensive community program for drug abuse prevention with high- and low-risk adolescents. The program targeted early adolescent children within the community because research has demonstrated that this is the first risk period for onset of drug use. The program targeted multiple agencies within the community—schools, parents, community leaders, and mass media. Drug use resistance skills training took place for adolescents in grades six or seven, parent-school organizations set agendas to review school prevention policies, and parents were trained in positive parent-child communication; community leaders were organized into a drug abuse prevention task force; and considerable media coverage was given to the program. Research on the outcomes of the program indicate that the community-based prevention program

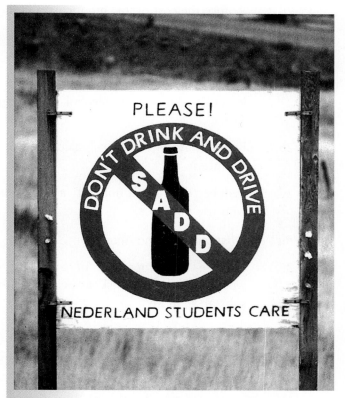

Public education involves the entire community.

HEALTHY PEOPLE 2010

OBJECTIVES RELATED TO SUBSTANCE ABUSE AND TOBACCO USE

Substance Abuse

Adverse Consequences of Substance Use and Abuse

26.1   Reduce deaths and injuries caused by alcohol- and drug-related motor vehicle crashes.

26.3   Reduce drug-induced deaths.

26.4   Reduce drug-related hospital emergency department visits.

26.5   Reduce alcohol-related hospital emergency department visits.

26.7   Reduce intentional injuries resulting from alcohol- and illicit drug–related violence.

26.8   Reduce the cost of lost productivity in the workplace due to alcohol and drug use.

Substance Use and Abuse

26.9   Increase the age and proportion of adolescents who remain alcohol and drug free.

26.12   Reduce average annual alcohol consumption.

26.15   Reduce the proportion of adolescents who use inhalants.

Risk of Substance Use and Abuse

26.17   Increase the proportion of adolescents who perceive great risk associated with substance abuse.

Treatment for Substance Abuse

26.18   Reduce the treatment gap for illicit drugs in the general population.

26.20   Increase the number of admissions to substance abuse treatment for injection drug use.

26.21   Reduce the treatment gap for alcohol problems.

State and Local Efforts

26.23   Increase the number of communities using partnerships or coalition models to conduct comprehensive substance abuse prevention efforts.

26.24   Extend administrative license revocation laws, or programs of equal effectiveness, for persons who drive under the influence of intoxicants.

26.25   Extend legal requirements for maximum blood alcohol concentration levels of 0.08% for motor vehicle drivers aged 21 years and older.

Tobacco Use

Tobacco Use in Population Groups

27.1   Reduced tobacco use by adults.

27.2   Reduced tobacco use by adolescents.

27.3   Reduce initiation of tobacco use among children and adolescents.

Cessation and Treatment

27.5   Increase smoking cessation attempts by adult smokers.

27.6   Increase smoking cessation during pregnancy.

27.7   Increase tobacco use cessation attempts by adolescent smokers.

HEALTHY PEOPLE 2010—cont'd

Exposure to Secondhand Smoke

27.9   Reduce the proportion of children who are regularly exposed to tobacco smoke at home.

27.11 Increase smoke-free and tobacco-free environments in schools, including all school facilities, property, vehicles, and school events.

27.12 Increase the proportion of worksites with formal smoking policies that prohibit smoking or limit it to separately ventilated areas.

Social and Environmental Changes

27.14 Reduce the illegal buy rate among minors through enforcement of laws prohibiting the sale of tobacco products to minors.

27.16 Eliminate tobacco advertising and promotions that influence adolescents and young adults.

27.18 Increase the number of tribes, territories, and states and the District of Columbia with comprehensive, evidence-based tobacco control programs.

Source: DHHS, 2000.

CASE STUDY

A nurse at a university health services clinic has noticed a high number of females from sororities coming into the clinic complaining of "hangover" symptoms during the rush season. She begins to compare the numbers with the year before and finds a 200% increase in the number of females who have presented with alcohol-related symptoms. The nurse would like to do a population assessment of the sororities at the university and plan educational programs and interventions related to responsible and safe alcohol use.

1. Who should the nurse contact first to begin the assessment process?

2. What kind of demographic information would the nurse need to know in the planning of appropriate interventions?

3. Are there other professionals and laypersons who need to be involved in educational interventions for this population group?

4. How should the sororities be involved with the assessment, planning, and intervention related to safe alcohol use?

5. What kinds of evaluation measures could the nurse use to determine intervention effectiveness?

was effective in reducing cigarette smoking and marijuana use at the 9th and 10th grade levels (3 full years after delivery of the school-based program). The program did not demonstrate a significant reduction in the use of alcohol by 9th and 10th graders who had participated in the program. However, the program was equally effective with both high- and low-risk adolescents. Overall, the program suggests that social/behavioral approaches to prevention that are addressed to whole populations can be effective and that prevention effects can be enduring (Johnson, Pentz, Weber, Dwyer, Baer, MacKinnon, & Hansen, 1990).

Programs that involve students in the design of a prevention campaign have two advantages. One is that students are mobilized to become involved in the prevention of substance abuse among peers; second, the messages in health educational materials will be relevant to the population. For example, at the University of Colorado at Boulder, students in journalism classes had a unique assignment: Create an ad campaign aimed at college students that emphasizes responsible drinking. Students in the class knew that their peers would not respond to fear tactics because college-age youth still have a tendency to think that nothing tragic will happen to

A FOCUS ON PREVENTION: AN ADVERTISEMENT CAMPAIGN DESIGNED BY UNIVERSITY OF COLORADO COLLEGE STUDENTS FOR COLLEGE STUDENTS.

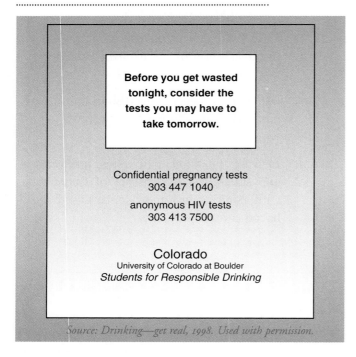

Before you get wasted tonight, consider the tests you may have to take tomorrow.

Confidential pregnancy tests
303 447 1040

anonymous HIV tests
303 413 7500

Colorado
University of Colorado at Boulder
Students for Responsible Drinking

Source: Drinking—get real, 1998. Used with permission.

them. The class decided it would be best to focus on social issues like sexually transmitted diseases and poor sexual performance. The students created six print and voice ads that appeared in newspapers, buses, and movie theaters as well as on a local radio station (Drinking—get real, 1998). See the figure above for an example of a relevant health education message developed by students themselves.

Community health nurses can and will be more and more involved in participating in population-focused intervention such as the previously mentioned programs. In addition, preventing the initial use of illicit substances or intervening to prevent further escalation of illicit substance use by our nation's youth before they move into adulthood should be a goal for all community health nurses who work with youth and their families. This goal is especially true for school health nurses, public health nurses, and nurses working in community-based primary care settings. Efforts to prevent a public health problem before it begins or arresting it quickly in the early stages is far more effective than waiting until a substance abuse problem is firmly established. Remember, always include prevention strategies and keep substance abuse assessment criteria in mind whenever you are working with youth.

Secondary Prevention

Secondary prevention efforts are focused on the early stages of substance abuse. The goal of secondary prevention is *to detect and arrest substance abuse* before the individual becomes physically addicted and the problem becomes a chronic condition.

Efforts are made to detect the problem as soon as possible and to begin treatment so that the condition does not progress. Health professionals need training in substance abuse as a significant health problem. Nurses and other health professionals need knowledge of high-risk populations and indicators of possible substance abuse, skills in assessment for the problem, and knowledge of interventions at the individual, family, and community levels. Common signs that an individual may be abusing one or more substances are listed in Box 21-8. Becoming familiar with the indicators of potential substance abuse is important for nurses, particularly those nurses working in community-based primary care settings, because it is at these nonstigmatizing medical settings (as opposed to a drug abuse treatment center) that the substance abuser may first make contact with health professionals. The assessment process, however, is not always straightforward. The early stages can be difficult to recognize. The psychological, social, and physical manifestations vary widely, depending on the particular substance or substances used, the amounts used or frequency of use, and other factors such as age and physical health of the user (Grant & Hodgson, 1991). The primary aims of the assessment are outlined in Box 21-9.

After early detection and a beginning willingness on the part of the individual and his or her family to break the silence of denial, the next task involves getting the substance abuser into treatment to prevent physiological addiction. Perhaps the entire family is in a crisis state. The nurse would be involved, along with a health care team, in crisis intervention with the family. It is no longer wise or necessary to assume that the individual needs to "hit bottom" before he or she can be helped. Indeed it is detrimental for the individual and the family to receive help only after the loss of physical and mental health, family and friends, job, and self-respect. The substance-abusing individual needs to initiate treatment. Persuading the individual to do so at an early stage in substance abuse is difficult but can be accomplished. If possible, intervention is best implemented

BOX 21-9 SECONDARY PREVENTION: PRIMARY AIMS OF SUBSTANCE ABUSE ASSESSMENT

- To meet the goal of secondary prevention with early detection and referral
- To obtain as much accurate information as possible about the individual's substance(s) use (frequency, amounts)
- To identify the factors associated with substance abuse, such as physical illnesses and social and psychological problems
- To identify the strengths and weaknesses of the individual and his or her family and ability to cope with and assist in the management of the problem

Source: Adapted from Grant & Hodgson, 1991.

through a coalition of a health care team and family members of the substance abuser. Planning for an actual confrontation is often the best way to "shock" the individual into seeking treatment. Depending on the circumstances, the best time for confrontation is when the substance abuser's defenses are low, for example, shortly after the loss of a job, a drunk-driving arrest, a warning from a physician about a health problem, or the threat of a divorce (Carroll, 1996).

In addition to an intervention such as confrontation, nurses can be involved in a generalized intervention developed by the World Health Organization (WHO) titled SCRAP. **SCRAP** stands for a focus on the substance abusers' (1) social relationships, (2) confidence in ability to change, (3) reasons to change, and (4) alternative activities, as well as on (5) preventing relapse. WHO

promotes this approach to intervening with substance abusers because it is easily taught to nonprofessional community workers, family, and friends of the substance abuser. See Box 21-10 for further explanation of the SCRAP approach to working with substance abusers (Grant & Hodgson, 1991).

Tertiary Prevention

The third level of prevention, **tertiary prevention**, is initiated during later or advanced stages of substance abuse. Tertiary interventions include physical, mental, and social treatment procedures; detoxification; institutionalization; or outpatient drug-maintenance programs. You will find community health nurses working in all aspects of tertiary care. Many hospitals have drug treatment units. County mental health services sponsor detoxification centers where nurses are needed to do medical assessments, counseling, and referral. A major role for community health nurses in tertiary care is case or care management involving ongoing assessment and care coordination among the various services a chronic substance abuser may need in order to slowly move toward a potential recovery.

The primary goal of tertiary prevention is *to prevent reactivation* of substance-abusing behaviors (Carroll, 1996). Many health authorities now view dependence on alcohol or other drugs as a chronic relapsing disease. As such, drug dependence is often marked by a return of the substance abuse problem. Some professionals believe that it is more reasonable to think in terms of remissions (a lessening or reduction of the problem and its associative symptoms) rather than a cure (NIDA, 1998). Box 21-11 is a partial listing of potential tertiary treatment programs.

BOX 21-10 SECONDARY PREVENTION: SCRAP INTERVENTIONS

- *Social supports and relationships:* Help the family with better communication to include increasing communication to solve problems more efficiently, increase the amount of praise and positive comments within the family, and reduce the frequency of conversations about past negative incidents.

- *Confidence in ability to change:* Provide encouragement that every person who is suffering from substance abuse tries to stop many times before succeeding; pointing out small or large successes; when a relapse occurs, point out that this is bound to happen and that preventing relapse is a skill that has to be learned.

- *Reasons for changing:* Help the client identify two or three main reasons to stop drug or alcohol abuse (e.g., to save marriage, improve health); identify an activity client does regularly every day (e.g., commute to work, drink coffee throughout day); have client think about reasons for stopping substance abuse problem and bring up positive images of what could happen if a change occurs; ask client to bring these images to mind every time he or she is involved in routine activity in order to reinforce these images.

- *Alternatives to drug use:* Help the client (particularly if he or she does not have a job) devise a list of possible pleasurable activities; obtain the client's commitment to become involved in one or more of these activities; and take a keen interest in your client's achievements.

- *Preventing relapse:* Help the client identify high-risk situations (e.g., family fights, weekends without planned activities); think of ways to cope with or avoid these situations.

Source: Adapted from Grant & Hodgson, 1991.

BOX 21-11 TERTIARY PREVENTION: PARTIAL LISTING OF SUBSTANCE ABUSE TREATMENT OPTIONS

DRUG-FREE TREATMENTS

- Therapeutic community
- Self-help groups such as Alcoholic Anonymous and Narcotics Anonymous
- Psychotherapy, including cognitive, behavioral, supportive-expressive, and family therapy
- Behavioral therapy specifically aimed at prevention of relapse

DRUG-BASED TREATMENTS

- Methadone maintenance for heroin addicts
- Naltrexone (nonaddicting narcotic antagonist, also used in treating alcoholism)
- Antabuse (blocks alcohol metabolism)
- Psychoactive medication when indicated

Source: Carroll, C. (1996). Drugs in modern society (4th ed.). Dubuque, Iowa: Brown and Benchmark.

Although treatment is the focus of tertiary prevention, it is essential that common barriers to treatment be removed or reduced. Emotional support must be available. This is a primary intervention area for community health nurses because all nurses receive education and experience in interpersonal interaction with caring as a philosophical base. Financial support must be ensured through social policies that promote workplace drug assistance programs or through job counseling, job training, and a return to employment. Child care may also be an important treatment enhancer (Carroll, 1996).

Interventions with Special Populations
Children and Adolescents
Youthful deaths and substance abuse

Seventy-two percent of all deaths among school-age youth and young adults in the United States result from four causes: auto accidents, other unintentional injuries, homicide, and suicide (Kann, Warren, Harris, Collins, Williams, Ross, & Kolbe, 1996). Research has also shown that Native Americans, African Americans, males, and those youths with the least education and income are at greater risk of both overall and injury-specific youth mortality (Singh & Yu, 1996). Furthermore, many of these unintentional injury deaths are associated with substance abuse (Mezzich, Giancola, Tarter, Lu, Parks, & Barrett, 1997; U.S. Department of Transportation, 1995). It is particularly disturbing that U.S. suicide rates are highest among persons 15 to 24 years of age and in those older than 65 years of age. The association between suicide and the abuse of alcohol and other drugs is also a significant problem as highlighted in data gathered from the Drug Abuse Warning Network (DAWN), a large-scale drug abuse data collection system sponsored by the National Institute on Drug Abuse. DAWN records substances linked with emergency department admissions in various metropolitan areas of the United States. According to the 1996 DAWN report on annual trends in total drug-related episodes in emergency departments (SAMHSA, 1996), the most commonly reported motive for taking a substance (37%) was suicide.

Specific prevention programs for children and adolescents

The type of substance abuse prevention program most often used in schools has been either the presentation of factual information about the dangers of substance use (fear-arousal) or "affective" education to enhance self-esteem, responsible decision making, and social development. One program that is very popular in school districts and communities is the Drug Abuse Resistance Education (DARE) program. The DARE curriculum is organized into 17 classroom sessions conducted by a police officer, coupled with activities taught by the regular classroom teacher. DARE combines the fear-arousal approach with the affective educational approached just described (Carroll, 1996). Despite the long tradition of these two approaches to prevention of substance abuse among youth, it is abundantly clear from scientific research that these approaches are not effective, or have

only a short-term effect (Botvin & Botvin, 1992; Resnicow & Botvin, 1993). Why do these approaches fail to prevent substance abuse among youth? First, they fail to address the psychosocial factors promoting substance use, particularly peer pressure. Second, although the affective programs attempt to reduce the intrapsychic motivations to engage in substance use, the methods used are inadequate in that they do not place enough emphasis on skills training using behavior-change techniques (Botvin & Botvin, 1992).

One program that is demonstrating effective prevention results is Project STAR (Students Taught Awareness and Resistance). **Project STAR** is a comprehensive, community-based drug and alcohol prevention program that is primarily based in a community's schools. The school-based program encompasses teaching drug use resistance skills and enhancement of individual competence. The program also includes parents, the media, community development, and health policy interventions. Project STAR begins by getting the whole community motivated and involved in the issue of youthful substance use. Teachers are given extensive standardized training. The 10-session, school-based curriculum includes a correction on normative expectations regarding drug use (i.e., the actual number of similar-age peers who use drugs); recognition and counteraction of adult, media, and peer influences on drug use; peer and environmental resistance training; assertiveness training; problem solving for difficult situations; and a public statement of commitment to avoid drug use. Teaching methods used in the program include role-playing; group feedback; the use of teacher and peer leaders; homework assignments requiring students to interview family members regarding family drug use rules; techniques to avoid using drugs; and methods to counteract media, peer, and family influences to use drugs (MacKinnon, Johnson, Pentz, Dwyer, Hansen, Flay, & Wang, 1991).

Literature in the area of substance abuse prevention is abundant. Project STAR is but one program. However, there is a consensus in the literature that substance use prevention must begin early and that drug use resistance programs (in particular programs that use peer influences) are far superior to programs that focus on information and general affective programs involving self-esteem enhancement and problem-solving skills (Bukoski, 1997; U.S. Department of Transportation, 1995).

Families

Many of the studies on families and illicit substance use by youths within the family are based on **social modeling theory.** Using this perspective, Fleming, Brewer, Gainey, Haggerty, and Catalano (1997) examined the relationship among parental drug use, bonding to parents, and child substance use. The families in this study were headed by substance abusers in methadone treatment for opiate addiction. The results of this study support the social development model and suggest that family interventions for preventing substance use in children of substance abusers should focus on reducing parental drug use and promoting bonding to parents who are abstinent.

Social control through parental involvement with youth is a second area of research that has been conducted on families as a risk factor in substance abuse in youth. In a study of male narcotic addicts, Nurco and Lerner (1996) found that intact family structure and parental disapproval of misbehavior by subjects was identified as significant deterrents to later addiction. Aseltine (1995) studied the reciprocal associations of family and peer relations and adolescent drug use over time. In this study, parental social control (e.g., being alert, having rules) was found to be stronger at the initiation stages of drug use but less than peers at maintenance. Parents may also indirectly help in the prevention of adolescent drug use by acting as friendship "gatekeepers," thus preventing youths from associating with other youths who are using drugs.

A third area of research on family and risk factors for substance abuse is the influence of family functioning and drug use. Researchers at Arizona State University followed 179 adolescents, ages 11 to 15, over a 3-year measurement period. All youth entered into the study as nonusers of illicit drugs. Over the 3-year measurement period, 88 initial abstainers began to use substances. Results showed that older adolescents and adolescents from disorganized home environments were more likely to initiate substance use than younger adolescents and those from homes high in family organization that exhibited good communication and good problem solving (Hussong & Chassin, 1996). The Research Brief above highlights the importance of having fathers involved in family functioning.

Family-focused interventions

The family has been viewed as a target of nursing care since the time of Florence Nightingale. The practice of nursing in the United States began in family homes. There is a return to the im-

RESEARCH BRIEF

Center on Addiction and Substance Abuse. (1999). CASA survey: Many dads AWOL in the battle against teen substance abuse: *www.casacolumbia.org.*

In an analysis of family structure and substance abuse risk, the Center on Addiction and Substance Abuse found that children living in two-parent families who have a fair or poor relationship with their father are at 68% higher risk of smoking, drinking, and using drugs compared with all teens living in two-parent households. The average teen living in a household headed by a single mother is at 30% higher risk compared with all teens in two-parent households. The results of this survey emphasized that "parent power" is the key to preventing drug use by children and youth.

portance of family nursing in the 21st century as health care finance reform is moving health care back into community settings. How do nurses intervene with families in which one or more members of the family has a substance abuse problem? Craft and Willadsen's (1992) investigation into nursing interventions related to family provides a taxonomy of general nursing interventions that are appropriate to use with substance-abusing families. Table 21-1 provides a list of generalized family-focused interventions to use when caring for a family in which one or more members has a substance abuse problem. It is important to note that these interventions fall within the practice domain of nursing. Often, nurses feel that they do not have the practice skills to deal with a family in which one or more

---

TABLE 21-1   FAMILY NURSING INTERVENTIONS AND THEIR DEFINING ACTIVITIES

NURSING INTERVENTION	DEFINING ACTIVITIES
Family support	Promotion of family interest and goals
Family process maintenance	Minimization of disruption in family environment
Family integrity promotion	Promotion of family cohesion and unity
Family involvement	Promoting all family members in problem solving their situation of having one or more family members with a substance abuse problem
Family mobilization	Utilization of family strengths to influence substance abusing member(s) in positive direction
Caregiver support	Provision of necessary information, advocacy, and emotional support
Family therapy	Interaction with the family as a change agent to move family toward a more productive way of living
Sibling support	Helping family understand the need to provide support (and attention) to nonabusing sibling when another sibling is the substance-abusing family member
Parent education	Assistance to parents to understand effects of different substances and theories on causes of substance abuse

Source: Adapted from Craft & Willadsen, 1992.

members has a substance abuse problem. Nurses do have skills in family support, education, facilitation of problem solving, and so on, which should be and are effective nursing interventions to be used when a family needs nursing care for a substance abuse problem.

Schools

Although there has been a downward trend in adolescent substance use since 1996, schools are definitely a target for substance abuse prevention; the 1998 Monitoring the Future survey indicated that the lifetime prevalence use of any illicit drug was 29% for 8th graders, 44.9% for 10th graders, and 54.1% for 12th graders. Indeed, the critical period for initial experimentation with one or more drugs and the subsequent development of regular patterns of use typically spans the beginning to middle adolescent years (NIDA, 1996).

The movement known as **comprehensive school health** is a broad strategy for improving student health. This movement views education and health as highly integrated. The movement proposes that healthy children learn better and cautions that no curriculum can compensate for deficiencies in student health status (Kann, Collins, Pateman, Small, Ross, & Kolbe, 1995). The goal of the movement is to improve student risk behaviors in the areas of alcohol and other drugs, unintentional injuries, tobacco, diet, physical activity, and sexual intercourse (Symons, Cinelli, James, & Groff, 1997). Despite growing support for the movement among parents, communities, and the federal government, local school leaders, who are under tremendous pressure to improve academic achievement, and other political stakeholders often remain unconvinced that improving student health represents a means to achieve improved academic outcomes. Instead, the current primary approach toward students with substance abuse behaviors is to discipline the offenders—suspending or expelling students, thus putting the youth at more risk for academic failure and future life difficulties.

Workplace

Substance abuse in the workplace is a concern for both employers and consumers of products and services. In communities without occupational health nurses, the community health nurse is sometimes called on to provide employers with assistance in the development of programs to address workplace substance abuse problems. In addition to the signs of substance abuse found in Boxes 21-7 and 21-8, signs specifically found in the workplace are listed in Box 21-12.

To deal effectively with substance-abusing employees, it is necessary to take some proactive measures. For this to occur, it is important to consider not only the needs of the company but also the legal issues, equal employment opportunity laws, the National Labor Relations Act, drug-free workforce rules and regulations, the ADA, Department of Transportation drug testing rules and regulations, and just cause dismissal regulations (Naegle, 1993).

> ### BOX 21-12 WORKPLACE SIGNS OF POTENTIAL SUBSTANCE ABUSE
>
> - Decreased productivity or work fall off
> - Decreased quality of job performance
> - Increased work-related injuries, accidents, or illness
> - Increased absenteeism, especially just before or after days off (e.g., holidays or vacations)
> - Increasingly longer breaks and meal times

It is important to develop policies and processes for dealing with substance use and abuse in the workplace. Many times, nurses will be asked to participate in committees that develop these policies, particularly policies that are being developed by their own employers. These policies should be provided to new employees and periodically reviewed with all employees to ensure that they fully understand the policies and how the policies affect them. Any substance abuse policy needs to include a statement regarding drug testing. This statement needs to include when drug testing will be done (e.g., on employment, randomly). It should also include how the testing will take place, who will do it, how the security of the specimen will be maintained, who will pay for the testing, and how confidentiality of results will be handled.

For any drug policy to be effective, the employers, management personnel, and supervisory personnel should become familiar with what alcoholism, addiction, and substance abuse are; how to recognize them; and the appropriate way to handle an employee experiencing such problems. Often, it is the community health nurse who is called on to assist in providing educational programs regarding substance abuse.

Many employers turn to community-based employee assistance programs (EAPs) to address the issue of substance-abusing employees. For EAPs to be effective, it is essential that any service, counseling, or intervention be kept separate from supervision of employees, with maintenance of confidentiality critical. The nurse working in a community-based EAP needs to be sure that policies and procedures regarding follow-up with supervisors who refer employees for assistance are handled in such a way that the employee's confidentiality is maintained. Reviewing policies and procedures regularly and being sure that they are in compliance with governmental rules and regulations is essential, and the nurse will often be actively involved in this process.

Rural

Approximately 27% of all Americans and 26% of the total elderly population live in rural areas (Bull, 1998). Farm foreclosures and the declining farm economy are stressors faced by those living in rural communities. In addition, rural communities are aging, with all of the health concerns associated with getting older.

> BOX 21-13 FACTORS TO CONSIDER WHEN PLANNING RURAL SUBSTANCE ABUSE INTERVENTION PROGRAMS
>
> - Geographic distance
> - Transportation
> - Rural economy
> - Shortage of health care providers
> - Shrinking tax base
> - Isolation
> - Access
> - Issues of stigmatization

Limited income, unemployment, and poverty are added stressors for rural families. Although illicit drug use does not appear to be as much of a problem in rural communities, high alcohol consumption and tobacco use, especially smokeless tobacco, are concerns. Attempts at establishing and carrying out prevention programs in rural communities are directly related to the rural nature of these communities. Key factors that the community health nurse needs to consider in planning for this population include the following: a shortage of health care providers, geographic distance, isolation, transportation, access, rural economy, a shrinking tax base, and issues of stigmatization (Box 21-13).

For substance abuse prevention programs to be effective in rural communities, they must be accessible and at neutral sites such as schools, churches, and community centers. Prevention efforts need to target those groups at greatest risk. Smoking and the use of smokeless tobacco are of particular concern in rural communities. Information about the health effects of smokeless tobacco should be made available and included in any drug prevention program. Potential users need to be made aware of not only the addictive nature of smokeless tobacco but also the long-term health effects (AHCPR, 1996). Box 21-14 is a summary of the health effects of dipping and chewing smokeless tobacco, which is a particular problem in rural communities.

Because depression and alcohol abuse can be co-existing conditions in rural communities, programs that provide for self-esteem building, decreased negative self-talk, building of support

> BOX 21-14 HEALTH EFFECTS OF SMOKELESS TOBACCO
>
> - Oral cancer
> - Gum problems
> - Loss of teeth
> - Heart problems

networks, and identification of accessible resources are needed. The community health nurse is often the person who is called on to plan, develop, and sometimes conduct these programs. The nurse may also become involved in planning and implementing groups for rural women conducted through the church, planning and implementing men's groups at the volunteer fire department hall, or arranging support groups for all substance abuse prevention efforts.

Neighborhoods

The communities and neighborhoods where people live, work, play, and raise their families are important areas for addressing the problems associated with substance abuse. Interventions that are focused on the substances (drugs) are often aimed at eliminating the accessibility of drugs, limiting the sale of alcohol and tobacco, and providing education regarding the health effects of tobacco and drug use. Efforts to discourage and prevent substance abuse in neighborhoods have been found to be effective means of providing intervention to people where they live. For many individuals, the idea of using official agencies (e.g., hospitals, clinics, health departments, social welfare agencies) is unpleasant. Fears of authority and prior experiences that might have been embarrassing or upsetting often discourage the use of such agencies, making it difficult to accept intervention and treatment. People prefer contacts with community health nurses in their own neighborhoods. Neighborhood programs that actively involve residents have been shown to be highly effective in drug prevention efforts. The community health nurse is often asked to assist in the development of such a program. The first step the nurse needs to take is to assess the neighborhood. Six questions need to be asked (Office of Substance Abuse Prevention, 1989):

1. *Do convenience stores, liquor stores, and gas station mini-marts in your neighborhood check identification of people purchasing alcohol and tobacco? Do they sell beer in six-packs, not singles?*

2. *Do bars and restaurants in the neighborhood refuse service to intoxicated patrons? make sure intoxicated patrons get rides home? promote nonalcoholic drinks during happy hours?*

3. *Do employers in your neighborhood have a policy on alcohol use? Do they require nonalcoholic beverages to be served at social events they sponsor? Do they refuse to pay for alcoholic drinks at business meals? Do they provide for transportation, if needed, after social events where alcohol is served?*

4. *Can you find health messages about alcohol and tobacco use on local radio and TV stations?*

5. *Is there a communitywide policy that prevents alcohol- and drug-related problems at sporting events, rock concerts, and other large community gatherings?*

6. *Do local schools, universities, and sports centers accept advertising for alcoholic beverages or tobacco that is displayed at the sports arenas or in program?*

It is important that community health nurses not only assume a role in promoting neighborhood involvement, but also become actively involved themselves. The community health nurse can assist with as well as encourage others to take the following six steps (Office of Substance Abuse Prevention, 1989):

1. *Write letters to support legislation on alcohol and drug policy.*

2. *Join a coalition of organizations involved with alcohol and drug policy.*

3. *Organize educational programs about alcohol- and drug-related programs.*

4. *Work with the media on developing health messages regarding alcohol, tobacco, and drug use.*

5. *Work with community organizations to implement alcohol-safe policies for large community events.*

6. *Set up programs to monitor the granting of new alcohol licenses.*

The community health nurse is seen as a leader and role model within the community. As a role model, it is important that residents see nurses taking proactive roles in drug prevention efforts. When issues related to substance abuse arise, nurses should take the lead in informing elected officials about the need to support legislation and programs for prevention and treatment. Write and call your political leaders urging action. Ask others to also contact their elected officials. It is also important to activate supporters of prevention programs regarding legislation about substance abuse prevention, especially if there is a threat to such programs. Meet with elected officials and speak about your concerns. If necessary, mobilize the community to take action regarding substance abuse through letter writing, petitions, and other positive actions to make the neighborhood needs known.

Women

The 1996 household survey indicated that 4.1 million women between the ages of 15 and 44 are drug users. Use of drugs and alcohol by women is not a new phenomenon, but the response to women who are substance abusers is often different than it is for their male counterparts. In the 1980s, it was reported that women who were alcoholic were considered sicker, wives of alcoholics were considered enablers, and husbands of alcoholic wives were looked at with respect for putting up with their wives' problem (Sandelowski, 1981). Things are beginning to change, but some issues still need to be addressed when working with the problems associated with substance abuse in women. Women's drug use differs from men's in that they often use prescription drugs in combination, are less likely to have a stable relationship/marriage, and most often have children living with them (Morgan & Kinney, 1996). How these women view themselves is an important factor in addressing issues of their substance abuse. The Research Brief above addresses the issue of pregnant women and substance abuse.

RESEARCH BRIEF

Kearney, M., Murphy, S., Irwin, K., & Rosenbaum, M. (1996). Salvaging self: A grounded theory of pregnancy on crack cocaine. Nursing Research, 44(4), 208–213.

In-depth interviews were conducted with 60 pregnant or postpartum women who were crack cocaine users in order to better understand the issues and problems these women face. Findings suggested fears about bearing a drug-dependent baby and/or concerns about losing custody were very real. Guilt, fear, and pressure to take action were common feelings. The women initially dealt with the threats to their self-esteem by delaying acknowledging the pregnancy and seeking care. However, once they did acknowledge the pregnancy, they attempted to make the best of the situation by decreasing drug use, trying to improve their diet, and trying to avoid conflict and worry. When health care providers were perceived as threatening custody of the child, they tried to avoid the health care system and "relied on their own self-care to optimize pregnancy outcomes" (p. 212).

For the community health nurse, it is essential that the nurse recognize the fears and concerns of the substance abusing pregnant woman and provide avenues for entry into care that support the mother to be and foster trust and safety rather than fear and distrust.

Most treatment programs use a model that was developed when the majority of persons receiving treatment were men. Women tend to be hesitant about entering treatment programs that use confrontation and mixed-sex groups. For substance abusing women, who often have experienced abuse (physical and verbal) from men, verbalizing their vulnerability in a mixed group is difficult if not impossible. Low self-esteem is an issue for this population. Providing same-sex groups where the women feel safe and supported and are received in a nonjudgmental manner is helpful in facilitating the treatment process. The same-sex groups also provide the opportunity for women to openly discuss relationship issues.

Treatment issues related to the pregnant woman and to women with children need to be addressed. The 1996 household survey reported that of the women who used drugs, 3.2% were pregnant and 6.2% had one or more children younger than 2 years of age. The highest incidence of substance abuse in pregnant women is found in women younger than 25 years of age, with a large percentage of these women being unmarried. A major problem is the lack of treatment programs geared to caring for women who are pregnant and using drugs or for women with children who are using drugs.

Community health nurses need to focus their attention on two areas when addressing the problems associated with substance abuse in women: education and advocacy. Educating women about the effects of alcohol and drug use is essential, especially with young women who are of childbearing age. Knowledge about the effects of drug use on the unborn child is essential for young women to make informed decisions (Kinney, 1996). Second, it is essential that the community health nurse take an advocacy position and lobby for treatment programs that adequately provide for women with young children, addressing such issues as child care, treatment for the pregnant woman, and physical and sexual abuse. Currently, treatment outcome studies have been funded by SAMHSA in 13 states to monitor the effectiveness of programs developed to address these needs of women who are pregnant or have young children. The results of these studies will provide useful information in planning programs designed to help women with their substance abuse. Community health nurses have an obligation to keep informed about which programs are most effective in treatment and prevention of substance abuse and its associated problems if they are to meet the needs of this special population.

Elders

Substance abuse in the elderly population is often a hidden problem. It has been estimated that by the year 2030, the fastest growing segment of the population will be persons older than 85 years of age. Fewer than 50% of elders live in institutions, and at least half of older people have some health problems. According to the 1996 National Household Survey, this group has the lowest rate of illicit drug use and the highest use of over-the-counter drugs. Prescription medication use is also a reality for 60% to 78% of the older population. Nelson (1998) indicated that one of the major concerns with this population results from the adverse effects of drug-drug and drug-alcohol interaction, leading to an increased risk for illness, injury, and death (Table 21-2).

Adams and Kinney (1996) suggest that even minimal alcohol use/abuse can be a problem for the older person. The problem in

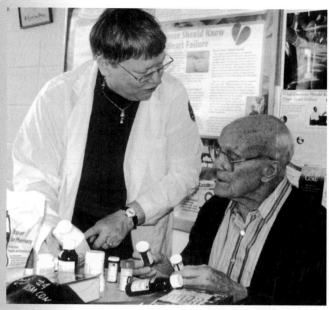

Chapter author, Dr. Jean Haspeslagh, assists an elder client with understanding multiple drug interactions.

part is due to alcohol interaction with other prescription drugs, as well as the physiological changes that are associated with aging, such as impaired absorption and excretion of those substance (Meiner, 1997). For example, alcohol use by an older person who is taking a nonsteroidal antiinflammatory agent increases the likelihood of gastrointestinal bleeding. Problems such as these are further complicated by the movement of former prescription medications into the over-the-counter category (Kinney, 1996).

It is essential that the community health nurse recognize the potential for problems because it is often the nurse who must sort out the elder's shoebox of prescription and over-the counter-medications and make sense of what that individual is really tak-

TABLE 21-2	COMMON ALCOHOL-DRUG INTERACTIONS TO LOOK FOR IN THE ELDERLY

DRUG CATEGORY	INTERACTION/EFFECT
Antibiotics	Nausea, vomiting, headache, possible seizures, reduced effectiveness of the medication
Anticoagulants	Acute alcohol consumption = increased risk of hemorrhage
	Chronic alcohol consumption = reduced blood thinning effect and potential for blood disorder
Antidepressants	Increased sedative effects, elevated blood pressure
Antidiabetic medications	Nausea, headache
	Acute alcohol consumption = prolonged effect
	Chronic alcohol consumption = decreased effect
Cardiovascular medications	Dizziness, fainting, reduced effectiveness of some antihypertensives

ing. Therefore, it is important that the nurse recognize the possibility that alcohol use/abuse could be a complicating factor.

For the elderly population with multiple chronic health problems, additional factors that may contribute to alcohol and drug abuse are limited income, inadequate instructions regarding their medications and alcohol interaction, and poor follow-up. Community health nurses must carefully assess the older person's medication regimen and determine how well it is being followed.

When attempting to determine whether there is a substance abuse problem, the family and friends of the elder are often the first to identify the potential problem. Nelson (1998) reported that the elderly most at risk for a substance abuse problem are those who are "widowed, single, living in disadvantaged areas, blue-collar workers, and those with criminal records" (p. 28). Nelson also indicated that older women have the potential to develop drinking problems later in life as a result of such factors as outliving their spouses and having a higher poverty rate. Community health nurses, especially those who work with the elderly in their homes, need to be aware of the potential for a substance abuse problem and provide necessary referral should the problem be identified. An effective treatment program must take into consideration the health problems and necessary medications to treat those problems when planning care. When working with the elder who has a substance abuse problem, it is important for the community health nurse to recognize that this person is a survivor and to build on that strength when planning care. Any intervention planned by the community health nurse must include contact for the elder with other people and assistance in identifying ways to provide meaningful activity for the elder.

Primary prevention efforts should focus on teaching about age-specific dangers of alcohol use, particularly in relation to medications that are being taken. The Council on Scientific Affairs of the AMA indicated that there are no safe guidelines for drinking for older adults. Prevention programs need to include content that reviews medications and their appropriate use, problems associated with mixing medications and alcohol, mixing prescription and over-the-counter medications, and proper disposal of medications. The Office of Substance Abuse Prevention suggests that programs encouraging responsible use of medications be implemented. They encourage having "dumping contests" (i.e., a contest for throwing away outdated and no longer used medications). We need to remember that prevention efforts are not just for the young and that our elderly also need our assistance if they are to avoid problems with substance misuse and abuse.

Nurses and Other Health Care Professionals

Nurses and other health care professionals are another group at risk for substance abuse problems. Accurate reports of substance abuse in the general population of nurses and health care providers is difficult to determine because denial is a key component of alcoholism and substance abuse, thus lessening the likelihood of accurate self-reporting in surveys. The American Nurses Association has estimated that approximately 6% to 8% of nurses have a substance abuse problem (Kinney, 1996).

Because substance abuse in nurses affects not only the nurse but also those who receive health care and those who work with the nurse, it is important that community health nurses recognize the issues associated with nurses who abuse substances. Community health nurses will encounter substance-abusing nurses and other health care professionals in the community both as clients and as colleagues. Factors influencing how you may respond can be found in Box 21-15.

As with any chronic condition, recognition that the condition exists is the first step toward rehabilitation. Signs of substance abuse in nurses range from mood swings to blackouts. Box 21-16 presents a list of indicators of substance that may be noticed in a nurse's job performance. Deteriorating work performance is often one of the later signs of the problem. One recovering nurse reported that even at the peak of her active drug use, she continued to receive good performance evaluations from her supervisor. During that time, she was never confronted about her performance even though she was experiencing blackouts (periods when she was unable to recall what happened).

A number of programs have been developed to address the needs of substance-abusing nurses. In addition to community treatment programs and employee assistance programs, programs specially designed for the recovering nurse have been developed to assist the nurse toward recovery and to monitor the nurse's progress. There are two types of programs: those sponsored by state nurses associations and those associated with state boards of nursing. The latter programs have legal power, provide oversight to the nurse, and have power to grant permission to work with certain stipulations (requirements) that must be met to retain a nursing license. Such programs ensure that the substance-abusing nurse is meeting those requirements placed on the license to practice.

BOX 21-15 FACTORS INFLUENCING RESPONSES TO SUBSTANCE-ABUSING NURSES

- Prior experience with someone else who is a substance abuser
- Hold a view that a nurse is a "superhuman being" who should be able to avoid such behavior
- Hold a strong moralistic view of substance abuse as being morally wrong
- Feel anger at anyone who would "steal" medication from clients
- Feel fear and anxiety that this could easily happen to themselves

BOX 21-16 INDICATORS OF POSSIBLE SUBSTANCE ABUSE IN NURSES

ANY SUBSTANCE

- Frequent medication errors
- Poor documentation—illogical, sloppy, illegible
- Client complaints
- Withdrawal, isolation—removing self from professional committees and organizations
- Signs out more controlled substances than others
- Volunteers to work extra hours or assignments that provide access to drugs

NARCOTICS

- Incorrect counts of controlled substances
- Large amounts of drugs wasted
- Significant variation in quantity of drugs required on the unit when that nurse is working
- Discrepancies between client's and nurse's reports of pain
- Client reports of ineffective pain medication only when suspected nurse gives the medication
- Client complaints of pain or restlessness only when the suspected nurse is working

Sources: Crosby & Bissell, 1989; Sullivan, Bissell, & Williams, 1988.

BOX 21-17 RESOURCES FOR RETURN TO WORK CONTRACT REQUIREMENTS

Crosby, L., & Bissell, L. (1989). *To care enough* (pp. 255–260). Minneapolis: Johnson Institute.

Durburg, S., & Werner, J. (1989). Re-entering the professional practice environment. In M. R. Haack & T. L. Hughs (Eds.), *Addiction in the nursing profession* (pp. 119–171). New York: Springer.

Naegle, M. (1993). *Substance abuse education in nursing* (vol. 3, pp. 231–235). New York: National League for Nursing.

counseling sessions, and written reports. Box 21-17 is a list of resources that provide information on return to work contract requirements.

Haspeslagh (1990) found that returning to work was a process during which the recovering nurse could either cope successfully or relapse. The time when nurses are most vulnerable for relapse is between 3 months and 1 year after treatment. There are three factors that put recovering nurses at risk for relapse: not working their aftercare program, not going to aftercare/support groups, and only doing what is required for their license or family, not for themselves. She also found that nurses who had the support of colleagues and supervisors who were knowledgeable about substance abuse and relapse were more likely to not relapse. For community health nurses, it is important to be able to recognize issues associated with substance abuse in nurses and other health care professionals. It is essential for the nurse to understand the importance of confronting substance abuse in nurses and to provide support for the returning recovering nurse. It is imperative that the community health nurse be cognizant of the signs of relapse and the proper steps to take if a co-worker begins to take that walk down the path to relapse.

Nurses returning to active nursing must have a **return to work contract.** This contract protects the nurse and the agency employing the nurse, and ultimately the clients. This contract should include the stipulations for returning to work, the length of time for the stipulations, frequency of random drug screens, restrictions on license, required group and individual

FYI

In a study by Trinkoff and Storr (1998), nurses who smoke vary by specialty group. The researchers defined cigarettes use as smoking more than 10 per day. Psychiatric nurses had the highest prevalence (23%), followed by emergency nurses and gerontological nurses (both at 18%). The lowest incidence of smoking was reported by pediatric critical care nurses.

Source: Trinkoff, A. M., & Storr, C. L. (1998). Substance use among nurses: differences between specialties. American Journal of Public Health, 88(4), 581–585.

CONCLUSION

Substance abuse is a major public health concern. Community health nurses have a responsibility to address this problem as both health care professionals and private citizens. Looking at yourself and identifying your own issues and biases regarding the substance abuser is the first step to developing and providing appropriate care for those populations affected by substance abuse. The nurse must take an active role in assessment and early identification of persons at risk for substance abuse. Planning and implementing prevention programs is a primary role for community health nursing practice. Working with community leaders in the planning and implementation of programs that address the issues of drugs and youth, programs for women and children, drug-related crime, and community-focused prevention programs must be addressed if the *Healthy People 2010* objectives are to be achieved.

CRITICAL THINKING ACTIVITIES

1. In the 1998 legislative session, the state legislature passed three bills related to alcoholic beverages. One bill set a zero tolerance level (when tested, no level of alcohol can be present) for intoxicated adolescents picked up by authorities. The second bill raised the alcohol level allowed in beer sold in the state, thus allowing for a stronger beverage. The third bill permitted the establishment of microbreweries in the state.

   - What kind of message do these three bills send?
   - If you were a resident of this state, how would you react?
   - What do you see as the major issue(s) related to the passage of these three bills?
   - What moral and ethical dilemmas can you identify?
   - What options are available to address these issues?

2. You are a community health nurse working in home health. One day the client's daughter tells you the following about one of the agency's home health aides:

   I really like Mrs. Green, she is a good person and has so many responsibilities, but I need to tell you she does tend to fall asleep when she is staying with dad. Last week he said that he thought he smelled alcohol on her breath but couldn't be sure. I've noticed she has been late coming to work more and more. Monday, when she came, she had a number of bruises and looked like she might have fallen down. I hate to complain, but I'm concerned about dad's safety. I also like Mrs. Green and am concerned about her.

   - How would you respond to the daughter?
   - What should the agency do about Mrs. Green? Why?
   - What is your responsibility?
   - How would you feel in this situation?

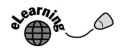

Explore Community Health Nursing on the web! To learn more about the topics in this chapter, use the passcode provided to access your exclusive web site:
http://communitynursing.jbpub.com
If you do not have a passcode, you can obtain one at this site.

REFERENCES

Adams, W., & Kinney, J. (1996). The elders. In J. Kinney (Ed.), *Clinical manual of substance abuse* (2nd ed.). St. Louis: Mosby.

Agency for Health Care Policy and Research (AHCPR). (1996). *Clinical practice guidelines on smoking cessation.* Washington, DC: Department of Health and Human Services.

Amaro, H. (1999). An expensive policy: The impact of inadequate funding for substance abuse treatment. *American Journal of Public Health, 89*(5), 657–659.

American Society of Addiction Medicine (ASAM). (1998). *Addiction medicine news*: www.asam.org.

Anthenelli, R. (1997). A basic clinical approach to diagnosis in patients with comorbid psychiatric and substance use disorders. In N. Miller (Ed.), *The principles and practice of addictions in psychiatry* (pp. 119–126). Philadelphia: W. B. Saunders.

Aseltine, R. H. (1995). A reconsideration of parental and peer influences on adolescent deviance. *Journal of Health Social Behavior 36*(2), 103–121.

Associated Press. (1999, September 8). Seven in ten drug users work full time, report says. *Hattisburg American*, p. 4A.

Baldwin, L, & Smith, V. (1997). Relapse in chemically dependent nurses: Prevalence and contributing factors. *Issues, 15*(1): www.ncsbn.org/documents/issues.

Barton, J. A. (1991). Parental adaptation to adolescent drug abuse: An ethnographic study of role formulation in response to courtesy stigma. *Public Health Nursing, 8*(1), 39–45.

Botvin, G. J., & Botvin, E. M. (1992). Adolescent tobacco, alcohol, and drug abuse: Prevention strategies, empirical findings, and assessment issues. *Developmental and Behavioral Pediatrics, 13*(4), 290–301.

Bukoski, W. J. (Ed.) (1997). Meta-analysis of drug abuse prevention programs. NIDA *Research Monograph, 170.*

Bull, C. (1998). Aging in rural communities. *National Forum, 18*(2), 34–41.

Carroll, C. (1996). *Drugs in modern society* (4th ed.). Dubuque, IA: Brown and Benchmark.

Center on Addiction and Substance Abuse. (1999). *CASA survey: Many dads AWOL in the battle against teen substance abuse*: www.casacolumbia.org.

Chen, K., & Kandel, D. (1995). The natural history of drug use from adolescence to mid-thirties in a general population sample. *American Journal of Public Health, 85*(1), 41–47.

Clark, H. W., Kanas, N., Smith, D., & Landry, M. (1995). Substance-related disorders: Alcohol and drugs. In Goldman, H. (Ed.), *Review of general psychiatry* (4th ed., pp. 190–213). Norwalk, CT: Appleton & Lange.

Craft, M. J., & Willadsen, J. A. (1992). Interventions related to family. *Nursing Clinics of North America, 27*(2), 517–531.

Crosby, L., & Bissell, L. (1989). To care enough. Minneapolis: Johnson Institute.

Department of Health and Human Services (DHHS). (1997). *Drug use survey shows mixed results for nation's youth*: www.health.org/mtf/pressre.

Department of Health and Human Services (DHHS). (1999). *Substance abuse: A national challenge*: www.dhhs.gov.

Department of Health and Human Services (DHHS). (2000). *Healthy People 2010: Conference edition.* Washington, DC: U.S. Government Printing Office.

Drinking—get real. (1998, December). *The Coloradan* (p. 2).

Durburg, S., & Werner, J. (1989). Re-entering the professional practice arena. In M. Haack & T. Hughs (Eds.), *Addiction in the nursing profession* (pp. 119–171). New York: Springer.

Fleming, C. B., Brewer, D. D., Gainey, R. R., Haggerty, K. P., & Catalano, R. F. (1997). Parent drug use and bonding to parents as predictors of substance use in children of substance abusers. *Journal of Child and Adolescent Substance Abuse, 6*(4), 75–86.

Goldsmith, R. J. (1997) The integrated psychology for addiction psychiatry. In N. Miller (Ed.), *The principles and practice of addictions in psychiatry* (pp. 3–10). Philadelphia: W. B. Saunders.

Grant, M., & Hodgson, R. (Eds.). (1991). *Responding to drug and alcohol problems in the community.* Geneva: World Health Organization.

Haack, M. R., & Hughes, T. L. (Eds.). (1989). *Addiction in the nursing profession.* New York: Springer.

Hahn, E. J. (1993). Parental alcohol and other drug (AOD) use and health beliefs about parent involvement in AOD prevention. *Issues in Mental Health Nursing, 14*, 237–247.

Hahn, E. J., & Rado, M. (1996). African American head start parent involvement in drug prevention. *American Journal of Health Behavior, 20*(1), 41–51.

Hahn, E. J., Simpson, M. R., & Kidd, P. (1996). Cues to parent involvement in drug prevention and school activities. *Journal of School Health, 66*(5), 165–170.

Haspeslagh, J. (1990). Recovering nurses' perceptions of job re-entry. Unpublished PhD dissertation. Louisiana State University Medical Center, New Orleans.

Hill, S. Y. (1998). Alternative strategies for uncovering genes contributing to alcoholism risk: Unpredictable findings in a genetic wonderland. *Alcohol, 16*(1), 53–59.

Hussong, A., & Chassin, L. (1996). Substance use initiation among adolescent children of alcoholics: Testing protective factors. *Journal of Studies on Alcohol, 58*(3), 272–279.

Johnson, C. A., Pentz, M., Weber, M., Dwyer, J., Baer, N., MacKinnon, D., & Hanson, W. (1990). Relative effectiveness of comprehensive community programming for drug abuse prevention with high-risk and low-risk adolescents. *Journal of Consulting and Clinical Psychology, 58*(4), 447–456.

Johnston, L. D., O'Malley, P. M., & Bachman, J. G. (1998). *Drug use by American young people begins to turn downward:* www.isr.umich.edu.

Kann, L., Collins, J. L., Pateman, B. C., Small, M. L., Ross, J. G., & Kolbe, L. J. (1995). The School Health Policies and Programs Study (SHPPS): Rationale for a nationwide status report on school health programs. *Journal of School Health 65*(8):291–294.

Kann, L., Warren, C. W., Harris, W. A., Collins, J. L., Williams, B. I., Ross, J. G., & Kolbe, L. J. (1996). Youth risk behavior surveillance-United States 1995. *Mortality and Morbidity Weekly Report CDC Surveillance Summary, 45*(4), 1–84.

Kearney, M. H., Murphy, S., Irwin, K., & Rosenbaum, M. (1995). Salvaging self: A grounded theory of pregnancy on crack cocaine. *Nursing Research, 44*(4), 208–213.

Kelly, K., & Donohew, L. (1999). Media and primary socialization theory. *Substance Use and Misuse, 34*(7), 1033–1045.

Kimball, A., Beckley, S., & Ngugi, E. (1998). International aspects of the AIDS/HIV epidemic. In P. Lee & C. Estes (Eds.), *The nation's health* (5th ed., pp. 114–136). Sudbury, MA: Jones and Bartlett.

Kinney, J. (1996). *Clinical manual of substance abuse* (2nd ed.). St. Louis: Mosby.

Kelly, K., & Donohew, L. (1999). Media and primary socialization theory. *Substance Use and Misuse, 34*(7), 1033–1045.

MacKinnon, D. P., Johnson, C. A., Pentz, M. A., Dwyer, J. H., Hansen, W. B., Flay, B. R., &Wang, E. Y. (1991). Mediating mechanisms in a school-based drug prevention program: first-year effects of the Midwestern Prevention Project. *Health Psychology 10*(3), 164–172.

Manning, G. (1995). Surviving disciplinary hearings: A new board members primer. *Issues, 16*(2): www.ncsbn.org/documents//accufacts/issues.

Meiner, S. (1997, July). Polypharmacy in the elderly. *Advance for Nurse Practitioners*, 29–33.

Mezzich, A. C., Giancola, P. R., Tarter, R. E., Lu, S., Parks, S. M., & Barrett, C. M. (1997). Violence, suicidality, and alcohol/drug involvement in adolescent females with a psychoactive substance use disorder and controls. *Alcoholism Clinical and Experimental Research, 21*(7), 1300–1307.

Morgan, S., & Kinney, J. (1996). Women. In J. Kinney (Ed.), *Clinical manual of substance abuse* (2nd ed., pp. 318–332). St. Louis: Mosby.

Naegle, M. (1993). *Substance abuse education in nursing.* (vol 3). New York: National League for Nursing.

National Clearinghouse for Alcohol and Drug Information (NCADI). (1997). *Substance abuse resource guide older Americans:* www.health.org/pubs/elderly/doceld.htm.

National Clearinghouse for Alcohol and Drug Information (NCADI). (1998). *Drug control strategy: An overview:* www.health.org/ndcs98/ivc.html.

National Council of State Boards of Nursing (NCSBN). (1999). National council compares two regulatory approaches to the management of chemically impaired nurses: An interim report. *Issues, 18*(1): www.ncsbn.org/documents/accufacts/issues.

National Institute on Drug Abuse (NIDA). (1996). *Facts about teenagers and drug abuse:* www.nida.nih.gov/NIDACpsules/NCTeenagers.

National Institute on Drug Abuse (NIDA). (1998). *Monitoring the future—1998.* Rockville, MD: Department of Health and Human Services.

National treatment improvement study. (1997): www.health.org/nties 97/employ.htm.

Nelson, M. (1998). Alcohol use in the older adult. *The American Journal for Nurse Practitioners*, *2*(6), 24–32.

Nurco, D., & Lerner, M (1996). Vulnerability to narcotic addiction: Family structure and functioning. *Journal of Drug Issues*, *26*(4), 1007–1025.

Office of Substance Abuse Prevention. (1989). *Prevention Plus II: Tools for creating and sustaining drug-free communities.* Rockville, MD: Department of Health and Human Services.

Office of Substance Abuse Prevention. (1991). *Prevention Plus III: Assessing alcohol and other drug prevention programs at the school and community level.* Rockville, MD: Department of Health and Human Services.

Resnicow, K., & Botvin, G. (1993) School based substance use prevention programs: Why do effects decay? *Preventive Medicine*, *22*, 484–490.

Robinson, T. N., Chen, H. L., & Killen, J. D. (1998). Television and music video exposure and risk of adolescent alcohol use. *Pediatrics*, *102*(5), 1201–1209.

Sandelowski, M. (1981). *Women, health, & choice.* Englewood, NJ: Prentice Hall.

Schneider, C., Fischer, G., Diamant, K., Hauk, R., Pezawas, L., Lenzinger, E., & Kasper, S. (1996). Pregnancy and drug dependence. *Wiener Klinisch Wochenschrift*, *108*(19), 611–614.

Singh, G. K., & Yu, S. M. (1996). Trends and differentials in adolescent and young mortality in the United States, 1950–1993. *American Journal of Public Health*, *86*(4), 560–564.

Stein, M. (1997) Medical disorders in addicted patients. In N. Miller (Ed.), *Principles and practice of addictions in psychiatry* (pp. 144–154). Philadelphia: W. B. Saunders.

Substance abuse among women. (1998). *Public Health Reports*, *113*, 13.

Substance Abuse and Mental Health Services Administration (SAMHSA). (1996a). *Discussion of results of 1996 household survey*: www.health.org/pubs/95hhs/discuss.

Substance Abuse and Mental Health Services Administration (SAMHSA). (1996b). *Annual trends in annual drug-related episodes*: www.health.org/ppubs/dwn96.

Substance Abuse and Mental Health Services Administration (SAMHSA). (1997). *Preliminary results from the 1996 national household survey on drug abuse*: www.health.org/pubs/nhsda/96hhs.

Substance Abuse and Mental Health Services Administration (SAMHSA). (1998). *Discussion of results from the 1997 national household survey on drug abuse*: www.health.org/pubs/nhsda/98hhs/findings/12results.htm.

Sullivan, E., Bissell, L., & Williams, E. (1988). *Chemical dependency in nursing.* Menlo Park, CA: Addison-Wesley.

Symons, C., Cinelli, B., James, T. C., & Groff, P. (1997). Bridging student health risks and academic achievement through comprehensive school health programs. *Journal of School Health*, *67*(6), 220–227.

U.S. Department of Justice, Drug Enforcement Administration (DEA). (1997). *Drugs of abuse*: www.usdog.gov/dea/pubs/abuse.

U.S. Department of Labor (DOL). (1998). *An employer's guide to dealing with substance abuse*: www.gov/dol/asp/public/programs/drugs/employers.htm#An.

U.S. Department of Transportation, National Highway Traffic Safety Administration. (1995). *Understanding youthful risk taking and driving: Interim report*: www.nhtsa.dot.gov/.

U.S. Department of Transportation, National Highway Traffic Safety Administration. (1999, September 15). *Press release*: www.dot.gov/affairs/nhtsa4499.htm.

Waller, M. (1997). Addictions and psychiatric settings. In N. Miller (Ed), *Principles and practice of addictions in psychiatry* (pp. 135–143). Philadelphia: W. B. Saunders.

Weinberg, T. S., & Vogel, C. (1990). Wives of alcoholics: Stigma management and adjustments to husband-wife interaction. *Deviant Behavior*, *11*, 331–343.

West, D., & Kinney, J. (1996). Overview of substance use and abuse. In J. Kinney (Ed.), *Clinical manual of substance abuse* (pp. 17–39). St. Louis: Mosby.

Chapter 22
Violence and Nursing's Response

Sherry Hartman and Debrynda B. Davey

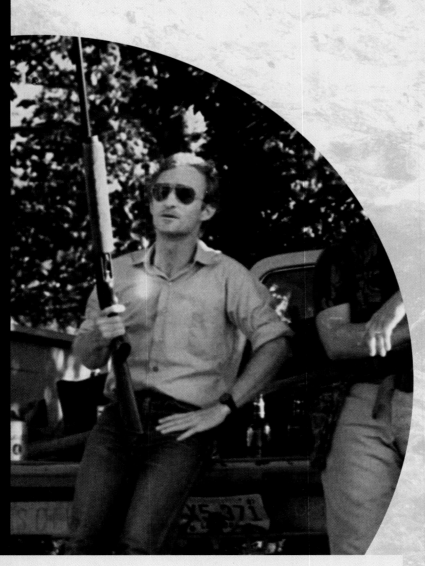

When there is light in the soul, there is beauty in the person
When there is beauty in the person, there is harmony within the home
When there is harmony within the home, there is order in the nation
When there is order in the nation, there is peace in the world.

—Lau Tzu

CHAPTER FOCUS

From Criminal Justice to Public Health

Defining and Explaining Violence

Types of Violence in U.S. Society
- Violence in the Family
- Youth Violence
- Workplace Violence
- Mass Violence and War

Interventions to Prevent Violence
- Microlevel Interventions with Individuals and Families
- Mesolevel Interventions: Community Structures
- Macrolevel Interventions: Society and Culture

 Healthy People 2010: Objectives Related to Injury and Violence Prevention

QUESTIONS TO CONSIDER

After reading this chapter, answer the following questions:
1. How does a public health approach to violence differ from a criminal justice approach?
2. What are the forms of behavioral violence?
3. What are the forms of structural violence?
4. What are the factors that contribute to violent behavior?
5. What populations are at greater risk for violence?
6. What is the typical pattern of abuse episodes in family violence?
7. What are the forms of violence among youths?
8. What factors contribute to youth violence?
9. What roles do nurses have in relation to the global issue of the violence of war?
10. What primary, secondary, and tertiary interventions contribute to the prevention of violence?

KEY TERMS

Abuse	Behavioral violence	Learned helplessness	Structural violence
Batterer	Domestic violence	Learned hopefulness	

Americans have been living with increasing violence for decades. Citizens express concern for their personal safety, and cities have created multidisciplinary crime task forces to address the problem. These initiatives are often heavily focused on protection and ensuring safety against what seems to be an overwhelming problem with no certain solution (City of Hattiesburg, 1995).

• •

Real success for new health agendas will depend on researchers involving themselves in finding ways to help reduce community violence.

Sr. Rosemary Donley, past president of
Sigma Theta Tau International,
Reflections, Fall 1996

• •

From Criminal Justice to Public Health

Violence has been a part of humankind's world at least since recorded history. Our oldest texts are rife with tales of violence at individual and collective levels. In more recent history, violent behavior has been regarded as a social problem having moral overtones, with prevention efforts focused on tertiary prevention through imprisonment, capital punishment, and sometimes, psychosocial rehabilitation. Violence had remained primarily a criminal justice issue of deviant and antisocial behavior until just over a decade ago. In discussing interpersonal violence, Hawkins (1999) commented that "one of the widely noted developments of the past decade is the trend toward viewing interpersonal aggression and violence as a public health concern rather than as a matter to be handled exclusively by the criminal justice system" (p. 87). It was in the 1980s that the Centers for Disease Control and Prevention (CDC) initiated efforts to prevent injuries from violence by using a public health approach. Both a rapid rise in homicide rates in the United States and a growing acceptance by public health workers of the importance of behavioral factors in the etiology of disease and injury encouraged the efforts. Violence was becoming a "behavior-based epidemic that kills and injures as certainly as a disease of the flesh" (Jones, 1993, p. 9). It became accepted that the nation needed to have more than a criminal justice approach to violence.

Criminal justice approaches, however, continue to attend to violence with secondary and tertiary interventions after violence has occurred. A public health approach does not imply that violence is only or mainly a problem of health or that responsibility for solutions lies with health professionals. It provides a multidisciplinary, scientific approach that brings the methods of epidemiology to study how primary prevention strategies can reduce violence (Mercy, Rosenberg, Powell, Broome, & Roper, 1993). A public health approach implies the belief that violence is a learned behavior and therefore can be changed and prevented. Describing the scope of the problem, identifying risk and protective factors, evaluating interventions, and implementing promising community programs are the components of the CDC approach to prevention.

Nurses have long played a role in addressing the trauma of violence and its health consequences and continue to be highly involved. In 1991, the American Nurses Association (ANA) issued a statement about physical violence against women that reflected the important nursing research that had been done in the area. In recognition of the magnitude of the health problems related to violence, several other nursing organizations have since issued position statements on violence. These organizations include the National Black Nurses Association (1994), the American College of Nurse-Midwives (1995), the Association of Emergency Room Nurses (1996), and the National Nursing Summit on Violence against Women (1997). Most recently, the American Association of Colleges of Nursing (AACN) issued a position statement on violence as a public health problem (1999). Violence against women, children, and elders in familial or intimate relationships was given special emphasis as a form of violence with high incidence and prevalence resulting in morbidity and mortality and requiring health care interventions. As part of the overall epidemic of violence, domestic violence has been described as a dilemma in disguise or a silent epidemic (Markin, 1996).

This chapter provides a public health approach to violence and examines many varieties of its expression. Some forms will be more common and will be familiar from courses focusing on women's health, children's health, and mental health. The emphasis here is on populations at risk and interventions directed to communities and populations. The broader context within which violence occurs and the complex interplay of individuals with their larger community and with society need to be understood in order to take on the task of reducing harm from violence.

Defining and Explaining Violence

Depending on the discipline and purposes of inquiry, conceptualizations and explanations of violence vary. The most common and narrow definition of violence is of physical harm at an interpersonal level. Barash (1991) defines the more traditional meaning, which suggests that violence is physical and readily apparent through direct injury or the infliction of pain. Gilligan (1997) distinguishes one form of violence as **behavioral violence,** which refers to "the non-natural deaths and injuries caused by individuals against individuals, such as the deaths we attribute to homicide, suicide, soldiers in warfare, capital punishment, and so on" (p. 192). Such violence is related to interpersonal interactions. There is little known about what leads individuals to use violence as a relational tool.

Proposed explanations of individual behavioral violence include biological causes such as instinct, heredity, race, lesions of the brain, drugs and alcohol, and various neurochemical causes such as increased testosterone or lowered serotonin. In psychological theories, violent behavior is sometimes further distinguished as "emotive" aggression, as seen in crimes of passion, and "instrumental" aggression governed by rewards and punishments stimulated by a number of personal or material gains such as power, status, money, and sex. Developmental approaches look to early life experiences and parental relationships that develop violence potential. Related to this is the belief that violence is learned in the family from the social role models, which may sanction physical punishment and the privacy of family interactions.

Personality or character disorders in which the person is inadequate in coping and communications is another perspective. In the cases of child and elder abuse, stress, inadequacy, and frustration from the dependency of the child or elder explain the abuser's violence.

There are multiple ways in which health can be compromised as a result of violence, especially when psychological and social health are included. The preceding definitions and explanations of violence focus on the individual. However, scientific study of violence is in its infancy, and there appear to be many forms of violence and multiple etiologies (Potter, 1999). Barash (1991) expands the traditional definition by describing "another form of violence, one that is more indirect and insidious. This structural violence is typically built into the very structure of social and cultural institutions." **Structural violence** is defined by Gilligan (1997) as "the increased rates of death and disability suffered by those who occupy the bottom rungs of society, as contrasted with the relatively lower rates experienced by those above them. . . . These excess deaths . . . are a function of class structure; and that structure is itself a product of society's collective human choices, concerning how to distribute the collective wealth of the society" (p. 192).

Such definitions move beyond behavioral science perspectives and recognize destructive actions that do not necessarily involve a direct relationship between the victim and the institution or person responsible for the harm. Such a perspective includes actions causing nonphysical harm, subtle or covert forms of violence, actions with long-term consequences, and socially sanctioned violence (e.g., capital punishment, spanking). It broadens the field to any avoidable action that violates a human right or prevents fulfillment of a basic human need (Salmi, 1993).

Broader definitions are congruent with both the public health approach and nursing's holistic approach to individuals, which recognizes the need to view the individual as part of a greater whole. Systems theory, multivariate theories, and ecological theories applied to violence recognize this need for a comprehensive approach to explanation (O'Neil & Harway, 1997; Potter, 1999; Van Soest, 1997).

The figure on the right shows the relationship of behavioral and structural violence. There are several implications of the model for understanding violence. First, there are reciprocal effects of the micro, meso, and macro system levels on each other. Individual behavior is affected by all levels: personal characteristics and the environment of institutions and culture. The top level is the most obvious overt form of violence that we can see

and assess. The second two levels refer to the unseen covert forces that guide thoughts, words, and actions. These can be forces or situations that in subtle ways hinder health, growth, and development of individuals or certain groups of individuals. For example, at the institutional or mesosystem level, the policies for reporting domestic violence have the potential to put the victim at greater harm from retaliation by the abuser. Because there are no required assessment training or screening policies, women often remain undiagnosed for domestic violence. Until quite recently, in many states, it was legal for a husband to rape his wife. Many of the barriers to access to health care described in chapter 7 are the result of bureaucracy and oppressive social policy and are examples of structural violence at the institutional level.

Like the young fish who asks the wise, old fish, "So what is this 'ocean' I hear others talking about?" individuals live their lives surrounded and affected by the forces represented by the macrosystem. This is shown in unconscious acceptance of inequalities and deprivations such as differential infant mortality rates, premature death, or lack of political representation. These indicate the excess suffering of some groups over others. Seldom, however, are the forces leading to this type of suffering referred to as *violence*. Whitlock (1996) delineates a long list of instances

RELATIONSHIP OF BEHAVIORAL AND STRUCTURAL VIOLENCE.

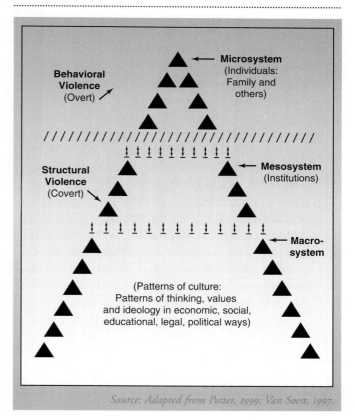

Source: Adapted from Potter, 1999; Van Soest, 1997.

of past and sometimes current structural violence. He is focused on African American suffering, but the examples apply to many groups: erasure of ethnic languages, names, and religions; depiction of certain ethnic groups and their culture in dehumanizing terms and images; segregation laws, welfare agencies, and government interventions that disrupt family units; intensive marketing of harmful substances such as tobacco and alcohol to certain groups; educational denial of admission, restrictive entrance requirements, underfunding, and lowered expectations of educational performance; and inaccessibility to loans, mortgages, real estate, or other property. Some of these are recognized, and laws have been put in effect to remedy the potential harmful effects to peoples' lives and well-being. However, much structural violence continues unacknowledged and unrecognized by the majority.

According to Van Soest (1997), the pattern of thinking that is most revealing is the continued easy acceptance of threat or use of violence as a method of social control and an appropriate method of problem solving. In the United States particularly, our history uncovers the pattern and cultural values:

> The American culture of violence is reflected in the history, attitudes, belief systems, and coping styles of the population in dealing with conflicts, frustrations, and the quest for wealth and power. Historically, violent traditions have made a clear imprint. Recall the genocidal wars against Native Americans by the early settlers; the lawlessness of the American frontier; the violence of slavery; the fratricidal Civil War; the massacres of early union organizers; the long history of violence against racial, ethnic, and political minorities; the violence against women; the romanticizing of the gangsters of the Roaring Twenties; and the imperialistic wars against Third World countries. . . . In addition, manifestations of violence on television and film have grown. Violence sells. . . . Furthermore, the United States was also the first country to use atomic weapons on populated areas and has maintained an enormous stockpile of nuclear weapons for more than four decades (Schachter & Seinfeld, 1994, p. 347).

One example of the cultural propensity to use force and attack to solve problems is the frequent characterization of health and social problems as an enemy that becomes an opponent to engage in battle, as "war" is waged against drugs and violence. Just as the child who experiences violence is thought to learn to respond with violence, some believe that meeting violence with violence at the structural and cultural levels also breeds a cycle of violence. Gilligan (1997) explains how the horrific violence committed by the prisoners he worked with may seem senseless if studied in isolation. Combining the insights of psychiatry with a public health approach to violence, he believes their violent acts have a logic when seen as a response to structural violence of social conditions that stimulate shame and guilt. He details how these emotions lead to violent acts that are counterviolence to the social conditions of structural violence. He lists poverty, race, age discrimination, and gender asymmetry as the most important of these. Related others can be added to his list.

Box 22-1 summarizes and adds to the work of Potter (1999), who reviewed the research on violence and classified influences based on an ecological model. In public health terms, these can be viewed as factors associated with the risk of violent behaviors. From this perspective, the presence or absence of certain factors or circumstances determines the likelihood of instigating violence. This compilation is not exhaustive of the various influences that have been studied related to violence, nor do the influences always lead to violence. They are also interrelated, as described earlier. A complex interaction between individuals, their varied environments, and existing social ills combine to lead to violence.

Types of Violence in U.S. Society
Violence in the Family

In the AACN (1999) position paper on violence, domestic violence was the only type of violence addressed, suggesting the importance of this area to nursing. Community health nurses en-

A Conversation With . . .

No matter where we are from or what our philosophy of life, to a greater or lesser extent, we are all sorry to hear of other's suffering . . . .Wars, crime, violence of every sort, corruption, poverty, deception, fraud, and social, political, and economic injustice are each the consequence of negative human behavior. And who is responsible for such behavior? We are. . . . There is not a single class or sector of society which does not contribute to our daily diet of unhappy news.

. . . These human problems, because they are all essentially ethical problems, can be overcome. The fact that there are so many people, again from every sector and level of society, working to do so is a reflection of this intuition: There are those who join political parties to fight for a fairer constitution; those who become lawyers to fight for justice; those who care, both on a professional and on a voluntary basis, for the victims of harm. Indeed, we are all, according to our own understanding and in our own way, trying to make the world—or at least our bit of it—a better place for us to live in.

—His Holiness the Dalai Lama
Source: His Holiness the Dalai Lama. (1999). *Ethics for the new millennium* (pp. 24-25). New York: Riverhead Books.

BOX 22-1 INFLUENCES RELATED TO VIOLENT BEHAVIOR

MICROSYSTEM

Individual

- Genetics related to personality traits or cognitive styles associated with aggression
- Neurobiology, diet, hormones, neurochemistry
- Prenatal and perinatal factors
- Antisocial personality disorder
- Alcohol and/or drug use
- High stress level
- Younger than 30 years of age
- Lack of understanding of partner's differing gender role socialization
- Low self-esteem
- Access to firearms and willingness to use firearms

Family, Peers, School

- Poor parenting skills
- Poor supervision
- Separated from family at early age
- Physical and/or sexual abuse or neglect
- Witness of violence in home
- Unstable or unsafe home
- Rejection by peers
- Witness peers fighting
- Knowing peers carry weapons
- Schools in disrepair

MESOSYSTEM

- Collective powerlessness in neighborhood/community
- Collective sense of confusion in transient neighborhoods
- Poor economy with joblessness
- Schools (especially urban) with high stress and frustration
- Group or gang membership or rivalry
- Oppressive work environment

MACROSYSTEM

- Poverty
- Income inequality
- Low socioeconomic status
- Community instability
- Racial and ethnic mix of community
- Housing and population density
- Exposure to dramatic violence in media (TV, music, film)
- Economic activities supporting violence such as gun and drug trafficking
- Declining public assistance programs
- Denigration of minorities, gays, ethnic groups, refugees, people with disabilities, and so on
- Organizational structures that maintain and tacitly support aggression toward women
- Changes in gender roles that produce fears of power loss in males
- Tacit acceptance of violence to resolve conflict: war and weapons, child punishment
- Pornography of women is legal and considered erotica

counter individuals in family settings and work closely with families; thus, they have frequent opportunities to intervene.

....

War, to sane men at the present day, begins to look like an epidemic insanity, breaking out here and there like the cholera or influenza, infecting men's brains instead of their bowels.
Ralph Waldo Emerson, *Miscellanies,* 1884

....

Family violence is a pervasive and often lethal problem of epidemic proportions, with far-reaching challenges and conse-quences for all members of society. Family violence is often silent and hidden from view—a family secret. It physically, emotionally, financially, and spiritually devastates victims and their children. It threatens the stability of the family and violates communities' safety and economies by costing billions of dollars annually in medical expenses, sick leave, absenteeism, and nonproductivity (Davey & Davey, 1998; Kent-Wilkerson, 1996).

There is growing recognition that family violence is a major health problem for women and children in the United States as well as around the world. Family violence presents unique challenges and opportunities for health care providers. Because victims of family violence and their children are found across health care services, as are nurses, nurses are in unique positions to assess and identify those affected by family violence. As such, nurses, and especially community health nurses, have the opportunity to be leaders in the prevention of family violence. Nursing approaches to domestic violence have an advocacy orientation that can be absent from other health care professionals. Research has shown that health care professionals can contribute to further subjugation of domestic violence victims. In many cases, those victimized by violence are viewed as a deviant group. Those victimized are most often members of disenfranchised groups, minority or ethnic groups, and/or women and children. Professionals may try to distance themselves from such groups and their problems by holding the belief that it is the problem of an "other" or deviant group. Many nurses who work and research in this area are believed by some to have avoided the victim blaming that is characteristic of some disciplines. Their research has grown out of clinical, grassroots concerns that have developed an activist agenda and a recognition of survivors' needs for empowerment (Campbell, Harris, & Lee, 1995).

Throughout history, the leading causes of premature death have been infectious diseases and violence. For two centuries, the world has made gains against infectious diseases and despite the problems of emerging infections, as well as the development of resistance to antibiotics and insecticides, the world is a much safer place when it comes to microorganisms than ever before in history. The same is not true of violence. The age of science has provided more efficient means of inflicting violence, and it has changed the ethic of violence. People can now kill and maim without confronting the effects of their actions due to the distance, time and filters placed between them and the victims. Many forces in society have made it possible for arms to be acquired by almost anyone, regardless of age, wealth, or propensity for violence. What is the cost of this situation and is there real hope for changing the equation?

Foege, 1997

According to Campbell, Harris, and Lee (1995), there are three main theories to explain family violence. The first emphasizes the abuser and the possible behavioral or psychopathological causes, such as mental illness, developmental disability, or substance abuse. In the family violence model, "the cycle of violence," with its use of force, is created when violence is learned in childhood and transmitted across generations. The third theory speculates that stressful situations precipitate violence. For example, violence arises when adults are unable to cope appropriately with the stress of unemployment or caring for a dependent elder. Children with special needs can increase stress and potential abuse (Wallach & Lister, 1995). Other researchers have looked to the many conflicts in roles and expectations between males and females and suggest that a pattern of male control over females explains male violence toward women (O'Neil & Harway, 1997).

The invention of nuclear weapons has changed everything—except the way we think . . . .We shall require a substantially new manner of thinking if mankind is to survive.

Albert Einstein

Domestic Violence Against Women

Domestic violence is known by many names: *spouse abuse, wife abuse, wife beating, battering, marital assault, woman battery,* and *intimate partner abuse.* These terms are sometimes used interchangeably, and occasionally, a term is used to refer to a specific problem (e.g., *family violence* to indicate wife and children are being battered). There are also many behavioral and legal definitions of domestic violence, which sometimes makes it unclear what is meant by the term. This lack of clarity can lead to inconsistencies in health care providers' identification and interventions as well as differences in research terminology. Author Dr. Anne L. Ganley, in *Improving the Health Care Response to Domestic Violence: A Resource Manual for Health Care Providers* (1996), offers the following definition of domestic violence: "Domestic Violence is a pattern of assaultive and coercive behaviors, including physical, sexual, and psychological attacks, as well as economic coercion, that adults or adolescents use against their intimate partners" (p. 16).

In 1995, the Fourth World Conference on Women, held in Beijing, developed a platform for action on violence against

A CONVERSATION WITH . . .

Nurses historically have been in a key position to assess and prevent domestic violence. We typically spend more time with patients and their families than any other health care professional. We are with people at all the important times in their lives and can see how patients and families interact with each other. National surveys also have shown that patients trust nurses and are likely to confide in us.

. . . We cannot let another year go by without having a strong, nationwide educational and assessment program to educate health care professionals to assess for domestic violence and work with women to promote their health and safety.

After all, asking the right questions won't hurt women. Not asking those questions, certainly will.

—Patricia Underwood, PhD, RN,
Secretary of the American
Nurses Association, 1999

women and defined it as follows: "Violence against women: any act of gender-based violence that results in, or is likely to result in, physical, sexual or psychological harm or suffering to women, including threats of such acts, coercion or arbitrary deprivation of liberty, whether occurring in public or private life" (United Nations Division for the Advancement of Women, 1995).

Most abusive relationships are male batterers of female victims; however, the reverse may be true. Domestic violence also occurs in gay and lesbian relationships. It cuts across all of society, all ethnic and cultural groups, and all educational and socioeconomic levels. Three types of batterers have been described based on the severity of their violence, who they direct violence toward, and their degree of personality disorder. Some batter with less severity and only within the family; others use more violence, mostly in the family, and show some signs of distress and emotional instability; and the most severe batterers are violent outside the family, often have criminal activity, alcohol and drug abuse, and antisocial personality disorder (Hotzworth-Monroe & Stuart, 1994). More attention has been given to the characteristics of male batterers than to abused women because these characteristics have been found to be more helpful in assessing risk of partner violence. Batterers are not a homogenous group and vary greatly in their profiles. However, there are some generalities (Hampton, Vandergriff-Avery, & Kim, 1999). Batterers often suffer from low self-esteem and have a need to use power and control tactics over victims. They usually minimize their own behavior and blame the victim for the violence. They tend to be more jealous, abusive to children, and sexually aggressive toward partners. After battering episodes, batterers manipulate by offering remorse, loving words, and promises to change—anything to gain control over the partner. Alcohol often is involved in partner violence.

Characteristics of victims of abuse have been described more from the viewpoint of their reactions and the consequences of the abuse. Three viewpoints describe the consequences for the victim. Walker (1984) suggested that the syndrome of woman battering leads to **learned helplessness.** Women are viewed as helpless, passive victims who restrict their behaviors because they lose the ability to predict whether their actions will be effective. Others have seen battered women as **survivors** who unsuccessfully seek help from the abuse (Gondolf & Fisher, 1988). What is viewed as helplessness is just the reality of a situation in which resources to enable escape are inadequate. Women logically try to protect themselves and their children, but police response, child care, shelter, education and employment opportunities, and community support are lacking or are already overwhelmed. A third approach that counters learned helplessness in women draws on the societal expectation that women must be responsible for maintaining relationships. Relationship hope is present in women in general and **learned hopefulness** in battered women is their belief that the perpetrator will change behavior or personality (Barnett & LaViolette, 1993). The concept explains why women stay with or return to abusers, especially if the abusers

enroll in treatment programs. Box 22-2 outlines the signs that may indicate a women is the victim of domestic violence.

The prevalence statistics found in Box 22-3 have been obtained from numerous studies. There are few national sources of epidemiological data on domestic violence; the National Family Violence Surveys (Straus & Gelles, 1990) and the National Crime Victimization Survey are the largest. Most states collect data from law enforcement agencies. Although these sources provide information on trends, it is generally believed that domestic violence is seriously underreported and severely underdiagnosed by health care providers.

Child Maltreatment

Child abuse may be defined within the legal sphere as the commission of acts resulting in physical or mental harm (i.e., injury) to a child younger than 18 years of age. Neglect implies acts of omission that lead to such results. **Abuse** can be sexual, physical, psychological, and emotional. Broad definitions include any in-

---

BOX 22-2 INDICATORS OF OCCURRENCE OF DOMESTIC VIOLENCE

- Recurrent trauma history
- Proximal injuries, such as to head, neck, torso, breast, abdomen, or genitals
- Patterned, multiple, or bilateral injury
- Poor explanations or no explanations for injuries
- Concealing or acting ashamed of injuries
- Delay in seeking treatment for injury with wounds in various stages of healing
- Physical injury during pregnancy, especially to abdomen or breasts
- Signs of depression: flat affect, failure to make eye contact, mood swings, poor hygiene
- Other psychological cues such as suicidal thoughts, anxiety, difficulty sleeping, panic attacks
- Alcohol or substance abuse symptoms
- Chronic pain with no known cause
- Seeking medical care for minor problems to maintain contact with professional
- Missing scheduled appointments or only coming for acute care
- Overly protective, controlling partner who visits professionals with client and refuses to leave his or her side

Sources: Cassidy, 1999; Scott-Tilley, 1999.

BOX 22-3 FACTS ABOUT DOMESTIC VIOLENCE

- In 1998, two out of five women surveyed experienced at least one type of violence in their lifetime (The Commonwealth Fund, 1999).

- It was also estimated that 31% of women experience domestic violence by a spouse or intimate partner, 3% within the last year (The Commonwealth Fund, 1999).

- Rates of domestic violence are 116 per 1,000 for a violent act and 34 per 1,000 for severe violence, with rates the highest for the following groups (Straus & Gelles, 1990):
  - Young adults ages 18–24
  - African American males
  - Families with income less than $20,000 per year
  - Women in central cities
  - Couples who have been together for the shortest time

- Pregnancy makes women particularly vulnerable, with 4% to 14% of all pregnant women and 20% of pregnant adolescents experiencing physical violence from an intimate partner (Campbell, 1999).

- Attempts to terminate the relationship may precipitate the abuse; 75% of victims are divorced, separated, or single (Campbell, 1992).

- Male to female violence represents a more serious public health concern than female to male violence (Schafer, Caetano, & Clark, 1998):
  - Women are eight times more likely to be victims of intimate partner homicide.
  - Women are seven times more likely to be assaulted by an armed intimate.
  - One in three women will be assaulted by an intimate male partner in her lifetime.
  - Women experiencing violence are more likely to have it be repeated.

- Of women murdered in the United States, 42% are killed by their intimate male partners (Family Violence Prevention Fund, 1997).

- Of very-low-income mothers, 83% have experienced severe physical violence and/or sexual abuse during their lives (Family Violence Prevention Fund, 1997).

- Violence by an intimate is more lethal, with 52% involving injury (41% needing medical care) compared with 20% when victimized by a stranger (Bachman & Saltzman, 1995).

---

terference with the child's development. Child sexual abuse is any sexual activity with a child in which consent is not or cannot be given, including use of force or threat of force. It is all sexual contact between an adult and child, regardless of deception or the child's knowledge of the sexual nature of the acts (Berliner & Elliot, 1996).

Incidence of child abuse

Child protective agencies in 1995 investigated a total of nearly 2 million reports of child maltreatment involving an estimated 3 million children, a rate of 43 incidents per 1,000 children. This was an increase of 49% since 1986. Thirty-six percent of the reports were substantiated, an incidence rate of 15 per 100 for children younger than 18. Fifty-two percent of these were for neglect, 25% for physical abuse, and 13% for sexual abuse. The majority were 7 years of age or younger, and 21% were teenagers. More than 1,100 died as a result of the abuse (Kotch, Muller, & Blakely, 1999). In one survey, parents admitted a rate of physical abuse 16 times the official reported rate and sexual abuse 10 times greater (Frietag, Lazoritz, & Kini, 1998). Although poverty and single parent families are at increased risk, all socioeconomic levels and family patterns experience child mal-

treatment. Box 22-4 shows some of the risk factors associated with child abuse.

Estimates are that three children a day die from maltreatment. This is an underestimate, however, because studies have indicated that approximately 85% of deaths from maltreatment were coded as some other cause on death certificates (McClain, Sacks, Froehlke, & Ewigman, 1993). Younger children are at highest risk. Child abuse ranks as the second leading cause of death, after accidents, for children from 1 to 5 years of age. From 1993 to 1995, of the fatalities that occurred, 85% were children younger than 5 years of age, and 45% were children younger than 1 year of age. Thirty-seven percent of fatalities were from neglect, 48% from abuse, and 15% from both; 49% who died had previous contact with Child Protective Services (Prevent Child Abuse America, 1996b).

Consequences of abuse for survivors vary depending on the nature of the act, the child's age, and the general environment. Physical harm can include deformity or disfigurement, sexually transmitted disease, and pregnancy. Emotional scars of shame, vulnerability, anger, and betrayal can persist through adulthood (Prevent Child Abuse America, 1996a). Other long-term effects are depression, sexual disturbances, and substance abuse. Emo-

BOX 22-4 KEY FACTS ABOUT CHILD PHYSICAL AND SEXUAL ABUSE

- Girls are sexually abused 3 times more often than boys.

- Surveys show at least 20% of women and 5% to 16% of men experienced sexual abuse as children.

- Two percent of all forms of confirmed abuse occurred in day-care or foster care settings.

- The most vulnerable age for sexual abuse is 7 to 13 years.

- Children are mostly abused by adult related to them or known to their families; however, up to 30% may be by strangers.

- Children are more likely to be physically abused by their fathers than by their mothers, and more severe abuse is committed by men.

- Mothers who are victims of domestic violence are more likely to abuse their children.

- There is a dramatic increase in adolescents who commit sexual aggression against other children.

- Single-parent families and families in poverty are at increased risk of abuse.

- Younger and less educated parents are at greater risk to abuse their children than older or more educated parents.

- Families in which prenatal care was absent or inadequate or in which the mother is depressed are at greater risk.

Source: Aron & Olsen, 1997; Frietag et al., 1998; Prevent Child Abuse America, 1996a.

tional maltreatment can lead to later social dysfunction and poor academic functioning. Abused and neglected children are at increased risk for delinquency and have higher rates of arrest for violent crime (Kotch, Muller, & Blakely, 1999). Just as abused women are thought to develop a learned helplessness, children are likewise susceptible. They are hindered in developing a strong sense of self-sufficiency and control and have difficulty experiencing a sense of initiative (Davies & Flannery, 1998). Health prob-

CASE STUDY

The School Nurse and "Routine Checks"

As the school nurse for Ridgewood High School, you are seeing students this morning for checkups required after absences because of illnesses. Two students in particular cause you to suspect that further intervention might be needed.

Sam Parker is returning after 2 days out with the "flu." He arrives with his newest best friend, and they both look haggard and tired and smell faintly of what might be alcohol. Sam has a new tattoo in the form of a pyramid and is wearing clothes that look a lot like his friend Elliot's. They both are wearing similar bands of jewelry around their arms. Sam has an expensive, shiny, new-looking watch. You ask about his mother, whom you have met before at a social club, but Sam says he hasn't seen her much lately. Sam is angry about having to report to the clinic and has been hit-

ting the door jam repeatedly with his fist. Before releasing Sam, you ask him if everything is going okay for him. He replies, "Yeah, no problem!" As he leaves your office you contemplate what you observed.

Jilly Tucker, 17 years old, comes in next and gingerly moves to sit down. She has fresh red marks on her neck. She is beginning to show her pregnancy, which is about 5 months along. Jilly's boyfriend waits in the hall. You ask Jilly how she and Scott are getting along. She looks away and answers that all is going well. Your next question is about how long she and Scott have been dating. "About a little over 4 months now," she replies. "Jilly, is Scott the father of your baby?" you ask. "No" is the reply. When you do an unplanned prenatal check, Jilly has bruises on her abdomen.

1. What further assessment would be needed for both young people?

2. What interventions might result and with who if your suspicions are correct?

| TABLE 22-1 | PHYSICAL AND BEHAVIORAL INDICATORS OF CHILD MALTREATMENT |

PHYSICAL INDICATORS		BEHAVIORAL INDICATORS
Physical abuse	Unexplained bruises (in various stages of healing) Unexplained burns, especially cigarette burns or immersion burns Unexplained fractures, lacerations, or abrasions Swollen areas Evidence of delayed or inappropriate treatment for injuries	Self-destructive Withdrawn and/or aggressive, behavioral extremes Arrives at school early or stays late as if afraid to be at home Chronic runaway (adolescents) Complains of soreness or moves uncomfortably Wears clothing inappropriate to weather to cover body Bizarre explanation of injuries Apprehensive when other children cry
Physical neglect	Abandonment Unattended medical needs Consistent lack of supervision Consistent hunger, inappropriate dress, poor hygiene Lice, distended stomach, emaciated Inadequate nutrition	Regularly displays fatigue or listlessness, falls asleep in class Steals food, begs from classmates Reports that no caretaker is at home Frequently absent or tardy Self-destructive School dropout (adolescents) Extreme loneliness and need for affection
Sexual abuse	Sexual abuse may be *nontouching*: obscene language, pornography, exposure; or *touching*: fondling, molesting, oral sex, intercourse Torn, stained or bloody underclothing Pain, swelling, or itching in genital area Difficulty walking or sitting Bruises or bleeding in genital area Venereal disease Frequent urinary or yeast infections	Withdrawn, chronic depression Excessive seductiveness Role reversal, overly concerned for siblings Poor self-esteem, self-devaluation, lack of confidence Peer problems, lack of involvement Massive weight change Suicide attempts (especially adolescents) Hysteria, lack of emotional control Inappropriate sex play or premature understanding of sex Threatened by physical contact, closeness Unwilling to change clothes in front of anyone Exhibits fantasy or babylike behavior Frequent nightmares High level of unexplained anxiety
Emotional abuse	Emotional abuse may be name-calling, insults, put-downs, etc., or may be terrorization, isolation, humiliation, rejection, corruption, ignoring Speech disorders Delayed physical development Substance abuse Ulcers, asthma, severe allergies	Habit disorder (sucking, rocking, biting) Antisocial, destructive Neurotic traits (sleep disorders, inhibition of play) Passive and aggressive, behavioral extremes Delinquent behavior (especially adolescents) Developmentally delayed

Source: National Children's Advocacy Center (1998): www.ncac-hsv.org/indicate.html.

lems in later life are also strongly linked to childhood abuse. Abused children exhibit behaviors that are viewed as public health problems—smoking, heavy alcohol use, overeating, physical inactivity, promiscuity, and drug use—as a way of coping with damaging experiences in early life. These coping mechanisms lead to the chronic diseases that are the common causes of mortality and morbidity (Felitti, Anda, Nordenberg, Williamson, Spitz, Edwards, Koss, & Marks, 1998).

Know everything you can about your children's activities and friends. Monitor children's activities and participate with them. Do not allow children to play alone in fields, on playgrounds, or in other dangerous or isolated areas.

Teach your children about strangers.

Teach your children to refuse anything from strangers, including money, gifts, and rides. Know where new items come from.

Teach your children how to safely enter home alone. Teach them how to pretend you are home and how to answer the phone if they are alone.

Teach your children to keep a safe distance from strangers and not to give strangers directions for help. Adults need to get help from other adults.

Use secret codes with your children (for use when may need to positively identify each other or ask for help).

Do not let your children go to public places, especially restrooms, alone. Develop a family plan stressing where to meet if lost, when you are away from home. Do not have children meet you in the parking lot.

Do not place your children's names on their clothing or on the outside of their possessions.

Teach your children to say NO to "touches" on the part(s) of their bodies covered by a swimming suit.

Teach your children to say NO, to TELL SOMEONE, and to GET AWAY if someone bothers them.

Join with other concerned parents to set up safety systems for your neighborhood.

Teach your children about secrets and that some "secrets" have to be told if children and their parents are to be kept safe.

Source: Project SAFE, HISD, and the Child Abuse Prevention Network, Houston, TX.

Table 22-1 lists both behavioral and physical signs of child maltreatment. Box 22-5 provides information for educating parents on protecting their children from abuse.

Elder Maltreatment

Elder maltreatment can be compared with child maltreatment regarding the dependent situation of the victim. Elders who are abused are frail and often mentally or physically impaired. They have a special relationship with and are dependent on a family member or caregiver. Federal definitions of elder abuse, neglect, and exploitation were first used in the 1987 amendments to the Older Americans Act. Categories of abuse include domestic abuse, institutional abuse, self-abuse, and neglect. State statutes define these with various degrees of specificity. As with children, abuse takes the forms of physical, sexual, and emotional abuse; neglect; and abandonment. Elders are also at risk for financial or material exploitation.

Caring for frail elders can be difficult and stressful. Elders who are mentally or physically impaired are especially needy of special care that the family or caregiver is ill equipped to provide. Both skills and resources in the form of family or financial support may be lacking. Increased stress and poor coping combine to lead to stress. The more impaired and dependent the elder, the greater the likelihood of maltreatment. Adult children who abuse are often dependent on the parent themselves because of their own mental, social, emotional, or financial problems. Abuse signals their response to their own inadequacies. As with other forms of abuse, the learned behavior is passed through the generations as children who were abused learn and reciprocate when a parent becomes vulnerable. Often, caregivers are themselves elderly and are unable to care for another.

There are no federal laws providing protective services and shelters for elderly victims, but all 50 states have such legislation. These laws establish guidelines for reporting and investigating suspected abuse and vary widely in terms of age and circumstances for eligibility. In many states, separate laws exist to cover long-term care and other institutions. All states have laws authorizing a long-term care ombudsman program, which is a requirement for receiving federal funds. They are advocates for those residing in long-term care.

Demographics of elder abuse

The following statistics are from the National Elder Abuse Incidence Study, reported in 1998 and drawn from 1996 data.

> This first-ever National Elder Abuse Incidence Study brings a severely under-reported problem out of the shadows. This study estimates that at least one-half million older persons in domestic settings were abused and/or neglected, or experienced self neglect during 1996, and that for every reported incident of elder abuse, neglect or self neglect, approximately five go unreported (Tatara, Kuzemskus, Duckhorn, & Bivens, 1998, p. 1).

Box 22-6 shows the types of maltreatment experienced by elders. Neglect is most common and abandonment least common. For all types of abuse, as age increases abuse increases. For those who are physically abused, 43% are older than 80 and only 5.5% are 60 to 64 years of age. Income affects abuse, with those who are poorer being more likely to be neglected and abandoned. In all categories of abuse except abandonment, more than 75% of

Neglect: 49%   *Financial abuse: 30%*
Emotional abuse: 35% *Abandonment: 3%*
Physical abuse: 26%

BOX 22-7 INDICATORS OF ELDER MALTREATMENT

PHYSICAL ABUSE

- Bruises, black eyes, welts, lacerations, and rope marks
- Bone fractures, broken bones, and skull fractures
- Open wounds, cuts, punctures, untreated injuries in various stages of healing
- Sprains, dislocations, and internal injuries/bleeding
- Broken eyeglasses/frames
- Physical signs of being subjected to punishment
- Signs of being restrained
- Laboratory findings of medication overdose or underutilization of prescribed drugs
- An elder's report of being hit, slapped, kicked, or mistreated
- An elder's sudden change in behavior
- Caregiver's refusal to allow visitors to see an elder alone

SEXUAL ABUSE

- Bruises around the breasts or genital area
- Unexplained venereal disease or genital infections
- Unexplained vaginal or anal bleeding
- Torn, stained, or bloody underclothing
- An elder's report of being sexually assaulted or raped

EMOTIONAL/PSYCHOLOGICAL ABUSE

- Being emotionally upset or agitated
- Being extremely withdrawn and uncommunicative or nonresponsive
- Unusual behavior usually attributed to dementia (e.g., sucking, biting, rocking)
- An elder's report of being verbally or emotionally mistreated

NEGLECT

- Dehydration, malnutrition, untreated bed sores, or poor personal hygiene

- Unattended or untreated health problems
- Hazardous or unsafe living condition/arrangements (e.g., improper wiring, no heat, or no running water)
- Unsanitary and unclean living conditions (e.g., dirt, fleas, lice on person, soiled bedding, fecal/urine smell, inadequate clothing)
- An elder's report of being mistreated

ABANDONMENT

- The desertion of an elder at a hospital, nursing facility, or other similar institution
- The desertion of an elder at a shopping center or other public location
- An elder's report of being abandoned

FINANCIAL OR MATERIAL EXPLOITATION

- Sudden changes in bank account or banking practice, including an unexplained withdrawal of large sums of money by a person accompanying the elder
- The inclusion of additional names on an elder's bank signature card
- Unauthorized withdrawal of the elder's funds using the elder's ATM card
- Abrupt changes in a will or other financial documents
- Unexplained disappearance of funds or valuable possessions
- Substandard care being provided or bills unpaid despite the availability of adequate financial resources
- Discovery of an elder's signature being forged for financial transactions or for the titles of his/her possessions
- Sudden appearance of previously uninvolved relatives claiming their rights to an elder's affairs and possessions
- Unexplained sudden transfer of assets to a family member or someone outside the family
- The provision of services that are not necessary
- An elder's report of financial exploitation

Source: National Center for Elder Abuse (1999, June): www.gw-japan.com/NCEA.

the abused are female. Whites are abandoned less than other groups. Only 23% can care for themselves; 47% cannot care for themselves at all. The majority of those maltreated are confused and 43% are depressed. Females experience more of all forms of abuse except for abandonment.

Perpetrators of elder mistreatment are only slightly more likely to be male (52.5%), but males are much more likely to

abandon (83%). Those who abuse are mostly younger than 60, but those older than 80 are the next most likely to abuse. Children of the elderly are the largest group of abusers (47%), with spouses next (19%). Those who abuse are overwhelming white (77%), except for those who abandon, who are more likely to be African American. Those elders who neglect themselves are most likely to be white females older than 75 with confusion who are only somewhat able to care for themselves. Box 22-7 outlines the indicators of the various forms of elder maltreatment.

Patterns of Behavior in Family Violence

Many individuals who use violence in their intimate relationships grew up in homes where they saw violence between adults and were abused themselves. Many saw frequent drug abuse by adults. They themselves often abuse alcohol and other drugs. They have little experience with men and women dealing successfully with each other to solve problems nonviolently. They tend to have rigid ideas about men's and women's roles. Many do not use violence outside of the home, and some have no criminal record before a family violence incident. They find approval for their behavior in daily life through media, entertainment, and sports events, as well as from peers.

For batterers, family violence is often a pattern of behaviors directed at a victim. It is not an isolated event. It is a pattern of multiple episodes of a variety of abusive acts, which occur over the course of the familial relationship. In each episode, there is often a build up of tension, followed by a violent episode, followed by remorse, gifts, and attention. Each episode builds on the last and sets the stage for future events. Some perpetrators use a particular set of abusive behaviors repeatedly, whereas others use a wide variety of behaviors randomly. These abusive and coercive behaviors take several different forms, including physical, sexual, psychological, and economic. Box 22-8 gives examples of family violence, which

---

BOX 22-8 EXAMPLES OF ABUSIVE BEHAVIORS OCCURRING IN FAMILIES

PHYSICAL ABUSE: INFLICTING INJURY OR ILLNESS, WITHHOLDING NECESSITIES OF HEALTH

- Spitting
- Scratching
- Biting
- Grabbing
- Shaking
- Choking
- Twisting
- Slapping
- Pushing
- Restraining
- Burning
- Punching
- Using weapons
- Inappropriate use of drugs
- Inappropriate use of physical restraint
- Force feeding
- Withholding food, medications, assistive devices

SEXUAL ABUSE: COERCING ANY SEXUAL CONTACT WITHOUT CONSENT, UNDERMINING SEXUAL IDENTITY

- Coerced sex
- Unwanted touching
- Sexual assault or battery
- Rape
- Sodomy
- Coerced nudity

- Sexually explicit photographing
- Forced prostitution
- Undermining sexuality by critizing desirability

PSYCHOLOGICAL ABUSE: INSTILLING FEAR, ISOLATING, UNDERMINING SENSE OF SELF-WORTH

- Verbal assaults
- Insults
- Threats
- Destruction of pets or property
- Intimidation
- Humiliation
- Harassment
- Isolation from family or friends
- Withholding transportation and/or phone access
- Isolation from regular activities
- Silent treatment
- Forced social isolation
- Ongoing accompaniment
- Constant "checking up"

ECONOMIC ABUSE: TAKING FUNDS, MAKING FINANCIALLY DEPENDENT

- Cashing checks without authorization
- Forging signature on checks
- Stealing money or possessions
- Deceiving into signing any financial documents
- Improper conservatorship, guardianship, or power of attorney
- Controlling financial resources
- Accumulating bills for which victim is responsible

includes domestic violence, intimate partner violence, spouse abuse, child abuse, elder abuse, battering, and wife beating.

Youth Violence
Scope of the Problem

For public health care providers, there is growing concern over the victimization and violent behavior of children and youth. Despite a decrease in overall violent crime rates and indications that there are declines in fighting and weapon carrying among U.S. adolescents (Brener, Simon, Krug, & Lowery, 1999), violent injury and death disproportionately affect youth in the United States. Hennes (1998) presents evidence that violence rates, homicides, firearm-related mortality, and homicide-related arrests among children and adolescents are rapidly rising. The at-risk group of perpetrators has shifted to younger ages, and females appear to be more involved in violent behavior (Office of Juvenile Justice and Delinquency Prevention, 1999). Young African American males ages 14 to 17 have the greatest and most rapidly growing homicide arrest rates. Homicide and suicide are the third and fourth leading causes of death among children, adolescents, and young adults ages 5 to 24. For those younger than 15, homicide and suicide rates are higher in the United States than in the rest of the industrialized world. Box 22-9 presents further evidence of the problem of youth violence.

School Violence

Although less than 1% of all homicides among school-age children (5 to 19 years of age) occur in or around school grounds or on the way to and from school, violent events against youths at school are an increasing health concern. Whether children turn their aggression against others or toward themselves, the increasing climate of violence is evident. As the baseline of violence rises, the chance of deadly incidents increases. Society demands that our schools be safe for our

---

BOX 22-9 FACTS ABOUT YOUTH VIOLENCE

- Teenagers are two and a half times more likely than adults to be victims of violence.

- In 1996, 6,548 young people 15 to 24 years old were homicide victims, an average of 18 youth homicides per day.

- Homicide is the second leading cause of death for 15- to 24-year-olds and the leading cause of death for African Americans and Hispanics in this age group.

- In each year since 1900, more than 80% of homicide victims 15 to 19 years old were killed with a firearm. In 1996, the rate was 85%.

- Arrest rates for weapons offenses among youths 10 to 17 years old doubled between 1987 and 1993, then dropped by 15% in 1995.

- The majority of homicides committed by juveniles involve handguns.

- More teenagers in the United States die from firearm injuries than from all natural (noninjury) causes combined.

- A national survey reported that one-fourth of serious violent crimes and one-third of property crimes were committed by teenagers.

Sources: CDC, 1999a; Wakefield, Gardner, & Guillett, 1998.

BOX 22-10 FACTS ABOUT SCHOOL VIOLENCE

- Of school-associated violent deaths, 65% were students; 11% were teachers or other staff members; and 23% were community members who were killed on school property.

- Of school homicide or suicide victims, 83% were males.

- Of the fatal injuries, 28% happened inside the school building; 36% occurred outdoors on school property; and 35% occurred off campus.

- The deaths occurred in 25 states across the country and happened in both primary and secondary schools and in communities of all sizes.

- Approximately one-third (32.9%) of students nationwide had had property (car, clothing, or books) stolen or deliberately damaged on school property one or more times within a 12-month period.

- Of students, 14.8% had been in a physical fight on school property one or more times within a 12-month period, with male students (20%) significantly more likely than female students (8.6%) to have been in a physical fight on school property.

WEAPONS AT SCHOOL

- Of high school students, 18.3% carried a weapon (e.g., gun, knife, club) within a 30-day period; 5.9% carried a gun within a 30-day period.

- Of high school students, 8.5% carried a weapon on school property within a 30-day period, with males (12.5%) significantly more likely than female students (3.7%) to have carried a weapon on school property.

- Within a 12-month period, 7.4% of high school students were threatened or injured with a weapon on school property, with male students (10.2%) significantly more likely than female students (4%) to have been threatened or injured.

Source: CDC, 1999a.

children, yet as Box 22-10 shows, schools are not always safe places. School violence has received more attention with the increase in multiple victim events, most notably at Columbine High School in Littleton, Colorado, in 1999, where two stu-

dents on a shooting and bombing rampage killed 12 fellow students, a teacher, and themselves, and wounded many others. See Box 22-11 for additional information regarding hate crimes.

BOX 22-11 HATE CRIMES: CAN COMMUNITY HEALTH NURSES REALLY DO ANYTHING TO PREVENT THE DAMAGE?

The effects of hate crime on any particular community are not limited to bleeding victims in the emergency department of the hospital or scenes from Columbine High School. Why hate crimes? Why now? And what can nurses possibly do to prevent it from occurring?

The significance of hate crimes to the community goes beyond the physical injuries of the victims. If you do not believe that hate crimes affect you and your community, consider the following questions: Did your perception of safety in your school change after the first time you heard about shootings at school? Did it the second? What about the third and all the times after that? Have you ever changed your behavior in an effort to avoid potential harm that might come to you based on some personal characteristic of yours? Is there anywhere in your community that you avoid because you do not "belong there" and fear that harm would come to you if you went there? These are just a few of the ways that hate crime shapes our perceptions of safety, the ways in which we interact, and our actions toward each other.

Is there anything about you that someone else might not like? Anything about your physical nature: the color of your skin, your gender, any disability? What about your sexual orientation or practices, your ethnic or national origin or that of your family, or your religious practices? Remember, this is not asking about your tolerance of others; this is asking about the potential tolerance of others toward you.

In short, the answer is that there are always people out there who will react negatively toward you based on some personal characteristic of yours. It does not have to be logical, it does not have to be justified, and it does not have to be out in the open.

It is human nature to reject what makes us uncomfortable or what we do not understand and seek the company of others like ourselves. The more positive expression of this tendency is demonstrated within social circles: With common interests or shared charac-

teristics, more can be accomplished as a group. People of the same religious faith gather together to practice that faith and celebrate its tenets; those who share fondness for a sport find others to play with or observe with; and those who share characteristics such as being parents of small children or having the same disability find support and advice in each other's company. Nurses are always being reminded that there is strength in numbers; by joining together, nurses can influence legislation and make changes in the way things are done. People are more powerful in groups.

Neutrality is also possible. An individual may "agree to disagree" with someone else on some point of difference, if there are other points they share. An example of this would be friendship between people of different religious faiths. Neither person is expected to relinquish his or her beliefs; neither one is "right" or "wrong." If they are willing to seek out points of sharing and commonality rather than focus on differences, people from widely differing groups can also share strength and enrich each others' experience. This is a true expression of tolerance: acceptance of others based not on their similarity to oneself, but on the merits of their own characteristics.

The dark side of this aspect of human nature emerges when the characteristics of one's own group are considered the only correct ones. It is not enough to associate with others like oneself. Those who are different are less trustworthy, dangerous, less human. The discomfort felt when in the presence of someone different from this "norm" leads to action against that individual. Those who are different must be kept out, moved away, eliminated. There are untold millions of examples of this intolerance in human history; all people, of all cultures, share in this inheritance.

This is the origin of hate crimes. One of the aphorisms of Hippocrates is, "Of two pains existing at the same time, but not in the same place, the stronger obscures the other." Hatred in this case is the stronger pain, drawing attention from its quieter companions, fear of the other, fear of the unknown, fear of what is different.

Continued

This fear is intolerable, and the reaction of the individual is hatred for the thing that has caused this discomfort. The hatred is louder, obscuring the existence of the fear, but the fear is there.

At present, the federal statute regarding hate crimes is 18 U.S.C. §245, which covers the threat, attempt to use, or use of force to injure, intimidate, or interfere with "any person because of his race, color, religion, or national origin" who is participating in one of six federally protected activities. These are (1) enrolling in or attending a public school or public college; (2) participating in or enjoying a service, program, facility, or activity provided or administered by any state or local government; (3) applying for or enjoying employment; (4) serving in a state court as a grand or petit juror; (5) traveling in or using a facility of interstate commerce; and (6) enjoying the goods or services of certain places of public accommodation.

The Hate Crimes Prevention Act of 1999 (S. 622 and H. R. 1082) seeks to eliminate the "federally protected activities" requirement because some cases that have satisfied juries as to bias motivation had to be dismissed because the victims were not involved in one of the six protected activities. This act also seeks to add gender, perceived or actual sexual orientation, and disability to the list of bias motivations. Other attempts at legislation with similar intent were the Violent Crime Control and Law Enforcement Act of 1994 and the Bias Crimes Compensation Act of 1993, neither of which made it into law.

Are you surprised? Many members of the public assume that any crime motivated by bias can be prosecuted as a hate crime; with a vague sense that there are "hate crime laws," they believe the issue to be closed. There are also misperceptions of the purpose of hate crimes legislation.

If bias against a certain religion is the motivation for killing someone, is the victim any less dead than if the action had taken place during a robbery? Aren't they both murder, which is against laws that already exist? Is it less heinous if the victim was at home rather than participating in one of the six federally protected activities? Is it more wrong to kill someone who is in one group than someone who is in an-

other? Why should the motivation for the act or the identity of the victim make any difference in the prosecution? Then answers are: no, yes, no, no, and please pay attention, because that comes next.

Burt Neuborne, the John Norton Pomeroy Professor of Law at the New York University School of Law, testified before the Senate on May 11, 1999, in support of the Hate Crimes Prevention Act of 1999 (S. 622). He stated, "The First Amendment does not protect violence merely because it is motivated by hatred. No principle of First Amendment law shields a violent offender against increased punishment because the crime was motivated by group hatred." The two things to note here are "increased punishment" and "group hatred." Remember the nature of prejudice: Another group of people is perceived as a threat. Neuborne contended that the heavier penalties for hate crimes would act as a deterrent against activities of hate and that hate crimes legislation would have "educational value" because it singles out the unacceptability of organized bias crimes. Murder is a crime; the perpetrator should be punished. But if the murder is part of the program of a hate group, should that group not also be punished? What if the murderer is not a member of a hate group but singles out victims with certain characteristics?

The victims of random crime are no less valuable than the victims of hate crime; that is not the reason different penalties are sought. The reason that hate crimes are different from other crimes: Existing laws punish random actions, while hate crime laws seek to punish organized activities of hate, whether they are the actions of hate groups or of individuals.

Nurses can have an effect on hate crimes and the communities they damage. The politics of difference can have a chilling effect on the pursuit of justice; by authoring or monitoring legislation, nurses can promote politics of equity. The 104th Congress asked the Library of Congress to make federal legislative information available via the Internet. Beginning in January 1995, this information has been available through Thomas, a service of the Library of Congress. This is one online source that should remain current for many years to come; the URL is http://thomas.loc.gov. By using this resource, nurses can follow the progress of federal legislation.

BOX 22-11 HATE CRIMES: CAN COMMUNITY HEALTH NURSES REALLY DO ANYTHING TO PREVENT THE DAMAGE?—cont'd

Nurses can also work to promote tolerance in their communities. If fear is the basis for prejudice, then understanding and information are the countermeasures. This is not something that can be imposed from outside. Peace comes from partnering with the community. It is important to respect the concerns of the members of the community and help them to move toward their own acceptance and tolerance of others. To that end, I offer this quotation from C. S. Lewis:

For every one pupil who needs to be guarded from a weak excess of sensibility there are three who need to be awakened from the slumber of cold vulgarity. The task of the modern educator is not to cut down jungles but to irrigate deserts. The right defence [*sic*] against false sentiments is to inculcate just sentiments. By starving the sensibility of our pupils we only make them easier prey to the propagandist when he comes. For famished nature will be avenged and a hard heart is no infallible protection against a soft head (p. 27, *The Abolition of Man*).

Written for educators in 1944, this is relevant for nurses working with the community now; fear and mistrust have created deserts that separate people from each other, and the apathy that grips the population must be akin to the slumber of which Lewis wrote. Promoting tolerance of diversity and providing learning opportunities form the best protection against hard hearts; the "soft heads" will never be any less soft until efforts are made to improve the situation.

Regina Hood Posey, RN, MSN

Gangs

Gang membership has been found to be closely associated with carrying weapons and being involved in physical fights. Having family and friends who are gang members also was related to increased violence (Powell, 1997). Although the majority of youth, even those in high-risk neighborhoods, are not involved with gangs, in one survey, 36% of the youth in high risk areas reported pressure to join gangs. Those who had been gang members most often became full members at age 13. Gangs are not confined to urban areas. In municipal and county jurisdictions with a population less than 25,000, as many as 68% reported gang activity. More than 7,000 different gang sets have been identified in the United States. Many of these are engaged in drug trafficking. For a better understanding of the dynamics associated with gangs, gang members, and their contribution to violence see Box 22-12.

Gun Control

According to one expert on youth violence, the proportion of youths committing violent acts has not altered, but the lethality of those acts is greater. Dr. Delbert Elliot, Director of the Center for the Prevention and Study of Violence at the University of Colorado at Boulder, states, "The same event 10 or 15 years ago would result in a bloody nose or a black eye, but now both guys have guns and somebody dies" (Blackmer, 1994). In addition to smoking and drinking, owning and using firearms has become a part of youthful experimentation. Ease of access has contributed to the situation, and interest in public health policy on gun control has become more intense. In 1996, 34,234 deaths resulted from firearms. Government statistics reveal that 44% of deaths from firearms were homicides, 51% suicides, and only 3.4% accidental (National Center for Health Statistics, 1998).

When a gun is present in the home, the risk of suicide by those residing there is three times greater and the risk of homicide is five times greater (MMWR, 1994). Some studies indicate that increased concentration of firearms (indicated by permits issues, new sales, or surveys of ownership) is associated with increased firearm robbery, assault, and homicide. Likewise, other studies indicate that those who have violent tendencies are more likely to seek and use guns (DiGuiseppi, 1995). Both the ANA and the American Public Health Association have been advocates for policy proposals to decrease access to guns. In 1999, U.S. Representative Carolyn McCarthy, a nurse, gained support from the ANA for the Children's Gun Violence Prevention Act of 1999 (H.R. 1342). The box on p. 513 demonstrates two nurses' opposing positions on gun control.

Dating Violence

The Youth Violence and Suicide Prevention Program (1999) of the CDC provides the following information about dating violence. Much of the information has been obtained from young people in high school and college within the context of dating and courtship relationships. Depending on the definition of violence, reported nonsexual courtship violence rates range from 5% to 65%, with higher rates found when threats and verbal abuse are included in the definition.

On average, the prevalence of nonsexual dating violence is 22% among male and female high school students and 32% among college students. Females experience slightly more violence than males. Among female college students, 27% experienced at least one episode of rape or attempted rape since the age of 14, of which only 5% were reported to police. Sexual assaults often go unreported to police. From 80% to 95% of rapes on

BOX 22-12 VIOLENCE IN THE COMMUNITY SETTING: UNDERSTANDING GANGS, CULTS, AND OTHER DEVIANT GROUPS

Gangs and cults are about power, fear, intimidation, crime, and very often extreme forms of violence, including murder. Gang and cult activities cut across all socioeconomic, racial/ethnic, and gender boundaries and exist in rural, inner-city, suburban, and other community configurations where an opportunity for power, revenge, and rewards associated with crime (especially drug sales) exists. Preadolescence and adolescence are times in which youngsters experiment, rebel, and often feel very insecure (a feeling that is commonly generated by their own subculture) during this critical transition period. Thus, youngsters are susceptible to gang/cult activity and the trappings associated with this subculture.

Gang and cult are terms referring to specific types of groups but here are used to also represent similar deviant groups that may operate within a community setting. The term gang or cult is defined as a group composed of three or more individuals who have a common identity and who have committed at least one crime, whether the crime is a felony or misdemeanor. There are other groups of individuals who have created ganglike organizations with a central focus of providing for their membership and/or immediate community needs; however, they have not (nor do they intend to) committed any crimes.

Within the "street setting," gangs will generally refer to themselves as an "organization." In fact, many gangs will admit to being an organization but will vehemently deny being a gang. Gangs will even go as far as to say they do not "jump in" their members, but "bless" or "invite" them into the organization. "Jumping in" is when gang members beat a new recruit; if the new member happens to be a female, she is "sexed in" (has sex with male members of the gang) as part of her initiation into the gang. These activities prove a new member's worth, loyalty, and desirability for membership. When female members choose to be beat in to a gang rather than to be sexed in they are generally more respected by the membership.

There are differences between gangs and cults. A gang tends to focus more on economic and personal or interpersonal needs of its membership, whereas a cult tends to focus on some religious or spiritual belief system, along with an individual's need to belong

and identify with a group. Although there are gangs that almost totally focus on economics, which are most often associated with the drug trade, there are gangs that thrive on racial and/or ethnic hate. Within this context, the difference between an occult and a cult warrants a brief discussion. An occult is a nontraditional religious belief system in which a group tends to believe; however, there is no emphasis on manipulating and controlling its members (or others) for deviant means. On the other hand, cults will often have almost the same beliefs as an occult, but their focus will be to control and manipulate their membership and others for deviant and criminal purposes. In addition, the typical cult tends to focus more on its leader's desire for power, whims, and fantasies rather than improving the lives of its members. Last, there is a gang/cult category called a "hybrid" that tends to be a combination of belief systems that may include traditional or nontraditional religious beliefs in combination with ethnic/racial hate, along with various criminal activities.

The question often asked is, "Why would an individual join a deviant group?" Well, affiliations with deviant groups tend to focus around a person's real or perceived needs and/or wants, which are often associated with concepts such as identity, low self-esteem, recognition, protection, drug habit, revenge, reward, power, desire for structure and discipline, respect, sex, understanding, excitement, hate, acceptance, and love; however, the bottom line for joining deviant groups is most often focused around economics, and the economics of gang activity is correlated with crime and violence.

WARNING SIGNS OF GANG/CULT MEMBERSHIP

- Unexplained wealth in the form of large amounts of cash
- Unexplained change in types and designs of jewelry
- Lack of participation in typical family activities such as church, school, family outings, and attention to chores
- Unexplained and atypical music being honored
- Habitual lying or distorting the truth
- Aggressive or violent behavior toward family or former friends
- Drug/alcohol use

BOX 22-12 VIOLENCE IN THE COMMUNITY SETTING: UNDERSTANDING GANGS, CULTS, AND OTHER DEVIANT GROUPS—cont'd

- Defiance of authority
- Blaming others for his/her troubles and concerns
- Unexplained tattoos
- Denial of a problem
- Refurbishing or reorganizing his/her room and fixtures
- Expressing feelings of rejection
- Association with youngsters of similar styles of dress, grooming, writing, and language

Although some items may not necessarily be gang related, a combination of items may point to an association.

CRIMES AND VIOLENT BEHAVIOR ASSOCIATED WITH GANGS/CULTS

- Criminal exploits associated with joining
- Criminal adventures connected with moving up in rank or position within the gang/cult structure
- Protecting turf
- Saving face or protecting one's honor
- Drug sales
- Drug deals that go bad because of someone being ripped off or cutting the quality of drugs
- Use of weapons, especially firearms and knives
- Stealing and robbery
- Home invasions
- Extortion
- Intimidation, harassment
- Sexual offenses, both heterosexual and homosexual
- Animal abuse and mutilation
- Drive-by shootings
- Homicides
- Vandalism
- Graffiti
- Maiming to prove a point or intimidate
- Abduction of both children and adults
- Ritual abuse

Levels of gang involvement in membership roles will often vary according to the type of gang and peculiarities associated with individual gangs. These in- clude (1) wannabes—potential members who are trying to prove themselves and are very often the most dangerous of all membership levels; (2) peripheral—those youngsters that are not in, but not out, and at times participate in gang-related activities; (3) regulars—youngsters who are members and participate regularly in gang-affiliated activities; (4) leaders—hard-core members who direct gang-affiliated endeavors and who are in contact with upper level leadership within a geographical region; and (5) imitators—those individuals who are not (and most likely would never be) gang members but "talk the talk" and "walk the walk," wear the clothing, and try to impress others through being "cool." Any of these five levels of gang involvement or affiliation can be dangerous for both participants and those that come into contact with them in the community setting.

GANG-ASSOCIATED SIGNS AND SYMBOLS

Blood/People and Vice Lord Gangs
- Left orientation
- Color red
- Five-point star
- Pyramid
- Cane

White Supremacists
- Skull and crossbones
- Rebel flag
- Swastika
- Anarchy symbol

Folks/Crips and Gangsters Gangs
- Right orientation
- Color blue
- Six-point star
- Pitchfork
- Three-point crown

Cults
- Pentagrams
- Inverted pentagrams

Continued

> **BOX 22-12 VIOLENCE IN THE COMMUNITY SETTING: UNDERSTANDING GANGS, CULTS, AND OTHER DEVIANT GROUPS—cont'd**
>
> - Circles
> - Candles (red, white, black)
> - Celtic crosses
> - Ankhs
>
> **RESPONSE TO GANG/CULT ACTIVITY**
>
> *The response to gang and cult activity should focus on strategies associated with prevention, intervention, and suppression. Prevention tactics are those strategies that the home/school/community select to prevent gangs/cults from forming and/or exploiting others. Intervention focuses on those techniques that are employed in the home/school/community setting that respond to youngsters who are on the fringes of gang/cult involvement or are actually participants. Suppression is more associated with enforcement, prosecution, and incarceration of members who have*
>
> *committed a crime within the community and/or suspension/expulsion for violating school district policy. To adequately combat gang/cult activities the home/school/community has to work together and employ all three strategies or the youngsters will manipulate the system and take advantage of the structural void that is created. The two most important issues that must be overcome before an effective gang/cult response is possible are for all entities within a community to admit that a problem exists and to overcome agency and individual jurisdictional issues (turf issues). There is no single solution to cult- or gang-related violence within our communities; however, there is hope especially when a community is aware of what is happening around them, admits that a problem exists, and collectively responds through strategies associated with prevention, intervention, and suppression.*
>
> **Johnny R. Purvis, PhD**

campus are committed by acquaintances. In one study, more than half of 1,000 female students studied had experienced a form of unwanted sex, predominately by steady dating partners. In addition to being at risk for sexual violence from known assailants, other factors attributed to perpetrators include early sexual experiences (forced or voluntary), sex role stereotyping, negative attitudes toward women, alcohol use, and rape myths held by men.

Suicide

Although suicide occurs in all age groups and is the ninth leading cause of death for all Americans, it is the third leading cause of death for young people 15 to 24 years of age. More than 90% of suicides in the United States are among whites, with males committing suicide almost four times more often than females. More than half the suicides among Native Americans were young males ages 15 to 24. Suicide rates have increased in the last 20 years for those between 10 and 19 years of age, among young African American males, and among elderly males. The problem has grown especially among African American youth, with an increase of 157% from 1980 to 1995 (CDC, 1998a). Firearms were used in 60% of suicides. Suicides among young people are often seen in clusters, with a number of youth committing suicide in the same community.

Increasing suicide rates for all groups of youth are explained by family disintegration and ease of access to alcohol, drugs, and lethal methods of suicide. Increased suicide among young African

American populations may be due to the growing African American middle class and the adoption of the coping methods of the larger society. It may also be due to reporting differences (CDC, 1998a). Of the 16,262 students in grades 9 to 12 who participated in the CDC's Youth Risk Surveillance Survey in 1997, 21% had seriously considered suicide, 16% had made a specific plan for suicide, 8% had actually attempted suicide, and 3% had made a suicide attempt that resulted in injury, poisoning, or overdose that had been treated by a doctor or nurse (CDC, 1998b).

In addition to prevention efforts to screen and counsel youth who are having difficulties coping, nurses will also be involved with the survivors of suicide. An average of five family members and many friends and acquaintances remain after a suicide (Praeger & Bernhardt, 1985). Survivors often have anger and guilt over an event that many would prefer not to discuss. Nurses intervene during the immediate shock and the eventual integration of the event into the survivors' lives.

Causes of Youth Violence

The theories on causation of youth violence are similar to those cited earlier for violence in general and to family violence. The focus with youth is on the early development of aggressive behavior and the tendencies for it to exhibit at earlier ages. The escalation of violence may, as proposed earlier, be due to societal factors that have made youth aggression more destructive than in the past. Easy access to handguns is one factor. A second strong

FYI

Gun Control

Nurses Debate the Question: Are Tighter Gun Control Restrictions the Answer to the Epidemic of Violence in Schools, Workplaces, and Communities?

Yes

There is some truth in the slogan "Guns don't kill people, people kill people"; nevertheless, people without access to guns are more often than not stymied in their murderous impulses, whether those impulses arise from a distorted perception of reality or from evil. Of course, a substantive cure for the epidemic of violence in our country includes meaningful employment for all, better mental health programs, warm and welcoming families for all children, improved educational systems, increased serenity, and the uprooting of all forms of bigotry. But while we as people are struggling to bring all these about, ought we not, at the very least, do what is within our immediate grasp? It is within our current legislative and enforcement power to: (1) make illegal the sale and possession of those particular guns for which the purpose is to kill lots of people quickly; (2) make the ownership of all guns as traceable as that of the automobile; (3) disqualify for gun ownership persons who have committed felonies or given evidence of potential harm to themselves or to others. For reasons of public health and the common good we restrict entry into school for children who have not been immunized. It seems only common sense that we also restrict the possession of firearms in an effort to control the public health menace of easy killing.

—Mary Margaret Mooney, DNSc, ARNP, FAAN
Dubuque, Iowa

No

I do not believe that tighter gun control restriction is the answer to the epidemic of violence in our schools, workplaces, and communities. I do not believe the answer is that simple. Violence in our society is a multilevel problem. We need to start with education at an early age to help our children deal with anger. Our children today are taught to handle their anger with violence, as evidenced in modern television, movies, and video games. The average child lacks the skills to deal with his or her frustrations. Television and movies show adults being rude and nasty to others, and this is perceived as being funny. Hitting and fighting back (getting revenge) are displayed as the right thing to do. We need to educate our children to respect others. Parents of today are often overwhelmed with material concerns and lack the energy to teach their children respect of others. Other concerns are seen as more important. Education regarding respect for others is needed at a young age, as well as how to deal with one's anger. Proper channeling of one's frustration will help prevent some of the violence in our society today. We, as health care providers, should stress the importance of stress management for our clients. We should also write our legislators to give our opinion of the violence on television and in the movies. We need to change the way our society views aggression and seek ways to help the public deal with it.

—Daria Napierkowski, MSN, RN
Stanhope, New Jersey

Source: Kaleidoscope. (1999). The American Nurse, 31(5), 4.

social factor is the increasing violence in the media. Television, movies, and video games have been declared culprits. Technology such as the Internet and satellite and cable television gives children greater access to a wide range of violent images. Studies show that the average American child watches 8,000 murders and 100,000 acts of violence before finishing elementary school (Centerwall, 1992).

The relationship between viewing violence and violent behavior is complex. The relationship is not direct, and other factors mediate the effects, with some children more susceptible than others and in different ways. Cultural norms, group norms, and family charcteristics are important in determining the effects of media violence on children's aggressive behavior. Violent portrayals most likely to influence behavior are those that show social approval, result in reward, are perceived as real, and are fast paced (Jason, Hanaway, & Brackshaw, 1999). The industry has taken steps to solve some of these issues, with rating of media and blocking options. These steps, however, only regulate content; they do not improve the material viewed by children. Parents must still play a large role and need assistance in under-

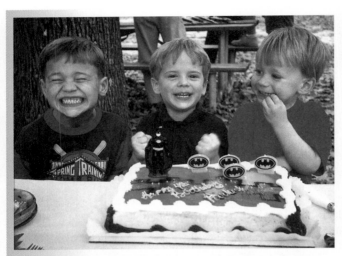

Male children raised in the United States embrace action figures who often use violence to triumph over their foes.

standing the industry classifications of films and videos and obtaining information on film and game content. They must be encouraged to monitor both the time spent and the content of viewing by children (Jason, Hanaway, & Brackshaw, 1999).

Workplace Violence

Although concerned about those who are victims of violence, nurses are increasingly aware of their own vulnerability in the workplace. Workplace violence, like domestic violence, is not new but has been hidden by much denial. It is an emerging field of study. Workplace violence exists on a continuum from verbal abuse to physical assault to homicide. It includes homicide, beatings, rape, assault, battery, theft, robbery, threats, harassment, and intimidation (McClure, 1999).

Perpetrators of violence can be frustrated or threatened coworkers, a random thief, or disgruntled clients. An average of 20 workers a week are murdered while working, and it is estimated that 1 million more are assaulted annually. Retail establishments open at night have the highest rates of homicide. In 1996, two-thirds of nonfatal assaults took place in hospitals, nursing homes, residential care facilities, and other social service locations (U.S. Department of Labor, 1996). Clients are most often responsible for these assaults, but their friends and family members can also be violent. Jobs in health care, education, and social services are the settings at highest risk of violence for women. The leading cause of occupational death for women is violence. These statistics show that nurses are a population at particular risk for workplace violence.

Some risk factors are the same for all work settings and include an increasingly violent society, availability of handguns and other weapons, and high crime neighborhoods. Also included for all work settings are organizational characteristics such as negative management practices; a culture at work that creates pressure

A CONVERSATION WITH...

Nurses care for victims of violence, perpetrators and witnesses to violent acts. The experiences of nurses who care for those affected by violence in many parts of the world point out the pervasive nature of violence. In addition, nurses themselves are at risk for violence in their personal lives, in their communities and, unfortunately, in their places of work. Violence in nursing is seldom discussed and if it is, it is in hushed tones and with a 'thank goodness it is not me' sentiment. Nurses care for and about others. It's why you are a nurse; it's why I am a nurse. We are courageous, but we don't have to suffer indignities or harm to do our jobs. All we need is respect for our professional work and to be safe. It is little enough to ask.

—**Eleanor J. Sullivan,**
RN, PhD, FAAN, President,
Sigma Theta Tau, International Nursing
Honor Society of Nursing, 1999-2000
Souce: Sullivan, E. J. (1999).
President's message, *Reflections, 25*(3), 4.

for performance; poor staffing, hiring, and retention practices; and increased diversity in the workforce, which can create conflict over differences (McClure, 1999).

Risk factors specific to nursing situations include the presence of money and drugs, working alone, poorly lit parking lots, and open exits and entrances. Also, reduced staffing levels and sicker clients with shorter lengths of stay increase the frustration levels of clients and families. The release of more acutely and chronically ill clients has increased the number of potentially dangerous clients in community health settings and emergency rooms.

Mass Violence and War

Modern nursing was born in the battlefields of the Crimean War when Nightingale revolutionized the care of the soldiers in that battle. The history since that time is marked by continuous instances in which nurses have served the wounded in battle. Nursing also has a history of peace activism among its historical leaders (Temkin, 1997). It has only been in the very recent past that public health professionals, including nurses, have begun to view the violence of war as a proper social ill to address in the public health model of prevention. Less than 10 years ago, when violence was recognized as a public health issue, very little was written in public health literature on the violence of war (Hartman, 1992a, 1992b). Groups of health professionals did have divisions of professional organizations or independent groups that had a

A CONVERSATION WITH...

Killings in Kosovo, shootings in schools, bombings in Belgrade—all extreme acts that have become the expression of our differences. Violence has invaded our homes, workplaces, communities and countries as we continue to document increases in homicide, suicide and in sexual, physical and domestic abuse. Is it not time for our society to look into its soul and ask what has gone so terribly wrong?

It seems to me there is this common theme that runs through all these acts of violence: an all-too-frequent willingness on the part of people to resort to violence when they disagree with someone or find another person's lifestyle or skin color objectionable. . . . Many nurses are not turning away from this problem. . . . While they recognize no one will provide answers or be perfect, they are taking positive, effective action. In this way they are preserving human dignity, tending to the health of populations and protecting basic societal principles while respecting differences.

—Nancy Dickenson-Hazard,
RN, MSN, CPNP, FAAN,
Executive Director, Sigma Theta Tau
International Honor Society of Nursing

BOX 22-13 MASS VIOLENCE AND WAR: SCOPE OF THE HEALTH PROBLEM

PHYSICAL HEALTH

- Increased mortality from direct violence, famine, disease
- Malnutrition from lowered food production, poverty, displacement
- Physical trauma of wounded, maimed, disfigured
- Epidemics from lowered vaccination rates and overcrowding
- Increased human immunodeficiency virus (HIV) rates from soldiers' sexual abuse and rape

PSYCHOLOGICAL HEALTH

- Persistent threat of attack
- Grief from loss of family, homes, land, possessions
- Witnessing of atrocities
- Capture and torture
- Forced to perform violence

SOLDIERS' POSTCOMBAT HEALTH

- Interpersonal and family violence
- Suicide
- Addiction
- Posttraumatic stress
- Alienation
- Psychic disintegration

IMPACT ON HEALTH DETERMINANTS

- Flight from homes creates displaced persons, abandoned and orphaned children
- Economic crisis—national resources spent on defense—no money for food, required health services, infrastructures
- Diminished health care—costs prohibitive, delivery systems destroyed, access to remaining health care system is reduced or dangerous
- Limited time and focus on parenting, caregiving as safety, basic needs, and avoidance of attack predominate
- Schools destroyed—access to education decreased and illiteracy increased, compromising both personal health education and future health manpower systems
- Health workers' morale and income decreased, thus lowering quality of health care
- Massive environmental destruction and increased hazards

---

special interest in peace, but war was not brought to the forefront until most recently.

Levy and Sidel (1997) introduced the first comprehensive examination of the relationship between war and public health. They documented the public health consequences of war, roles of health professionals, and prevention interventions. There have been cautions in social science literature about the overextension of preventive health measures to inappropriate areas, or the inappropriate role of health sciences (usually referring to medicine) as the "social guardian of morality." However, there seems to be a growing number who believe that identifying risks, developing interventions to lower risk, and implementing the interventions are possible for war. Conscious steps can be taken to measure and reduce the risk of arms, mass violence, and conflict (Foege, 1997). Mass violence of war can be claimed as a legitimate inclusion on community health prevention agendas.

Epidemiology of War

The health consequences of war are both direct and indirect. Box 22-13 details major health consequences of warfare. Nightingale is recognized as the first to do statistical analyses on the management of mass casualties during war (Garfield & Neugut, 1997; Nightingale, 1954). In recent decades, rates of mortality attributable to war have risen. World War II caused the death of 3% of the world's population of the time. The former Soviet Union lost 10% of its population in that war and the United States lost 0.3%. The number of civilian deaths in war has risen such that in 1990 civilian deaths accounted for 90% of all deaths in war. The rate of wounding during combat has decreased from 97 per 1,000 troops in the Civil War to 27 per 1,000 in World War II. Indirect effects indicate that more deaths follow from wars than occur during war itself. These deaths result from breakdown of the normal systems of sanitation, food, and other supplies and the lack of available medical care. One measure of the burden of disease, disability adjusted life years (DALYs), combines both death and suffering. In looking at the global burden of disease, violence ranked second only to respiratory disease in DALYs lost, representing its disease burden on the world (World Bank, 1993).

Roles of Nurses Related to War

Box 22-14 describes nurses' roles in relation to war and its consequences. They reflect some of the roles that have been suggested for prevention activities. Levy and Sidel (1997) list the following: surveillance and documentation of the health effects of war and factors causing war; education and awareness-raising programs on the health effects of war; advocation of preventive policies and actions; and direct action to prevent war and its consequences, such as participation in nonviolent conflict resolution and building trust. This latter role requires skills that many expert community health nurses develop. These skills include refinement of interpersonal communication skills; knowledge of conflict processes at the individual, group, and community level; understanding and using theories of conflict and conflict resolution; clarification of the history and origins of a conflict situation; and a humanitarian commitment to the pursuit of just, peaceful conflict resolution. The work suggested by Hall and Stevens (1992) for increasing appreciation and understanding of human differences is an example of direct action nurses can take to prevent war and its consequences.

The Research Brief on p. 517 illustrates the work of nurses that focuses on the experiences of war refugees. Care is provided by nurses to war refugees either by traveling to serve in relief missions or through contact with refugees who come to the United States. Refugees present unique health problems related both to previous traumatic experiences and to marginalization from the mainstream society (Allotey, 1998).

Community health nurses who work with refugee populations must manage feelings of anger, frustration, guilt, and loneliness; sleeplessness; and recurring images of suffering (Proctor, 1998). Following resettlement in countries that grant asylum, refugees often experience depression symptoms related to both premigration and postmigration experiences. Interventions for these symptoms and other health-related problems are particularly sensitive to the need for culturally congruent care (Fox, Cowell, Montgomery, & Willgerodt, 1998).

> **BOX 22-14 NURSING ACTIONS RELATED TO MASS VIOLENCE AND WAR**
>
> - Direct care of those wounded and dying from combat (Furey, 1991; Hedin, 1989; Norman, 1989; Paul & O'Neill, 1986)
> - Visible involvement in public policy related to war and its health consequences (Simpson, 1986; Stollery, 1984)
> - Networking and alliances of nursing organizations with other health organizations, peace groups, and informational networks to coordinate mass actions to humanize current policies (Hall & Stevens, 1992; Stollery, 1984)
> - Critical scholarship examining public words and images that reduce human beings to objects, incite violence, or distance citizenry from the human damage and destruction of war (Hall & Stevens, 1992, p. 114)
> - Education of the public in its perceptions and comprehension of war-related health issues (Farrell, 1992a; Stollery, 1984)
> - Consultation to countries after wars to assess effects on their peoples and health systems, identify population needs, and prepare programs for care and reconstruction (Farrell, 1992b)
> - "Advancing forms of self and group identification that do not depend on the designation and exclusion of an 'other' but embrace cultural and personal diversity" (Hall & Stevens, 1992, p. 119)

Interventions to Prevent Violence

Recognition of violence as a public health issue is a relatively recent development. Those who practice or do research in the field readily admit that knowledge of both causes and risk factors, and thus of prevention, are only beginning to be developed. Interventions related to violence can be directed to all three system levels—micro, meso, and macro—that were shown in the figure on p. 495. In addition, such interventions can be representative of the three areas of prevention: primary, secondary, and tertiary. Following the public health approach to the problem, interventions are efforts to break the causal chain between potential violence and actual violence. Although much more needs to be known about the complicated interplay of causes of violence, the factors identified in Box 22-1 and discussed throughout the chapter represent a summary of those factors that guide current intervention strategies. At the microlevel, characteristics that put individuals at risk for perpetration (e.g., use of alcohol by batterers) or victimization (e.g., children in unstable homes) can be targeted for screening and group prevention activities. Similarly, as we know more about

RESEARCH BRIEF

Berman, H. (1999). *Stories of growing up amid violence by refugee children of war and children of battered women living in Canada.* Image: The Journal of Nursing Scholarship, 31(1), 57–63.

The purpose of this study was to investigate the ways in which children ages 10 to 17 who have grown up amid violence "make sense" of their experiences. The interpretive methods used gave voice to individual experiences but placed them within the socially constructed political, economic, and cultural context in which violence is allowed. The children's exposure to violence was conceptualized, then, not as a private or individual problem, but as a public problem demanding social change.

Dialogue, reflection, and critique—methods of critical research—guided the data collection and analysis of data from 16 children of war and 16 children of battered women. All had witnessed violence but were no longer living with violence.

It was typical for the children of battered women to have no warm memories or happy moments to hold on to. Violence for them had been an everyday part of their lives in subtle and not so subtle ways. In contrast, for the children of war, the violence marked a temporary disruption in their previously happy lives.

Both groups had profound feelings of betrayal. For those who suffered war, the betrayal was from outside the home by those previously viewed as friends. The children of battered women felt betrayed from within their homes by those who were to protect them. Similar emotions of sadness, anger, and confusion were felt by both groups, but those of battered women also experienced shame and embarrassment.

Their experiences of suffering revealed the distinct ways in which war and woman abuse are socially and politically constructed. Both were in battlefields, but the battlefields of war were publicly declared and fought. They were justified, rationalized, and given legitimacy in the world. International bodies set up rules for the regulation of war. These are rules for all to abide by. In contrast, the violence directed toward women and children was conducted in secrecy, the privacy of their homes, and without rules of fair play. Rules were set by the perpetrators.

The stories of the children showed their capacity to find surprising resources. They had self-confidence, hope, and optimism for things to be better. Their "escapes" made them feel lucky, but they felt they were unlikely to forget what had happened to them.

The author concluded that although the children showed remarkable insight and strength, they faced many challenges. In spite of common conceptions that children cannot talk about deeply troubling experiences, the research demonstrated that children want to discuss their experiences and welcome the opportunity.

HEALTHY PEOPLE 2010

OBJECTIVES RELATED TO INJURY AND VIOLENCE PREVENTION

Injury Prevention

15.3   Reduce firearm-related deaths.

15.4   Reduce the proportion of persons living in homes with firearms that are loaded and unlocked.

15.5   Reduce nonfatal firearm-related injuries.

Violence and Abuse Prevention

15.32   Reduce homicides.

15.33   Reduce maltreatment and maltreatment fatalities of children.

15.34   Reduce the rate of physical assault by current or former intimate partners.

15.35   Reduce the annual rate of rape or attempted rape.

15.36   Reduce sexual assault other than rape.

15.37   Reduce physical assaults.

15.38   Reduce physical fighting among adolescents.

15.39   Reduce weapon carrying by adolescents on school property.

societal influences on development and expression of violence, macrolevel interventions directed toward laws, education, and media images are implemented. See the *Healthy People 2010* box for selected objectives related to violence.

Currently, health care practitioners' response to violence is sometimes criticized. This is related to the fairly recent recognition of violence as not just a criminal justice problem, but as a health behavior problem as well. It was just in 1999 that the membership of the American Association of Colleges of Nursing approved their position statement on domestic violence and delineated necessary competencies for nurses to provide high quality care to victims of violence (AACN, 1999). Education efforts are prevalent for all health care workers in order to raise their awareness and increase assessment and screening for abuse. Studies have indicated that physicians and nurses seldom routinely inquire about abuse. Even when treating the injuries of abused clients, psychosocial assessment or safety issues are most frequently not addressed (Family Violence Prevention Fund, 1994). Although the health care response needs to be improved, there are many ways in which community health nurses do currently initiate and collaborate in violence interventions. These are described in the following sections, according to level of intervention.

Microlevel Interventions with Individuals and Families

Community health nurses are confronted with individuals who have experienced violence in all of the many community-based settings in which they live and work. Nurses in home health, schools, clinics, religious communities, homeless shelters, and other community sites will encounter victims and potential victims of violence. Those who work in institutional settings also design protective programs for individuals who are members of populations at risk such as frail and vulnerable nursing home residents, day-care residents, and co-workers at risk for workplace violence.

Primary Prevention

Primary intervention strategies focus on strengthening the resistance of vulnerable individuals. Such efforts, including encouraging interest and involvement in school, can be successful and should begin as early as possible before young people adopt violent beliefs and behaviors (Hawkins, 1999). The general population of youth can be targeted and outreach to high-risk youth can also be extended to those who engage in physical fights, those with criminal records or history of inflicting or receiving violent injuries, drug users, gang members, and school dropouts. Relocated youth from immigrant, refugee, and mobile communities, as well as those with emotional or mental problems, are also at risk (CDC, 1992). Collaborative interventions by nurses in schools, day-care settings, after-school programs, and community youth organizations include nonviolent conflict resolution training, mediation training, coping and stress management training, life and social skills training, self-esteem and ethnic pride enhancement, mentoring programs, parenting classes, and personal safety classes that include gun safety (Jones & Selder,

1996). As part of the team that is implementing programs, nurses can ensure that gender-specific issues of power and control in male-female relationships, date rape, other dating violence, and attitudes toward women are added to the often gender-neutral and male-male focus of programs (Campbell, Harris, & Lee, 1995).

Although early intervention with youth is an optimal time for prevention, the same factors are the target for modification when working with those who are older and in situations of potential violence. Other developmental periods such as marriage, pregnancy, and retirement present opportunities for prevention by service providers. An elder's registration for Medicare could provide an opportunity for health and social service interventions to support healthy family adapting (Institute of Medicine, 1999). Further primary prevention strategies include coping, self-esteem development, early drug and mental illness treatment, realistic parenting expectations, enhanced family bonding, and development of alternatives to the use of violence for conflict resolution. The nurse should also encourage avoidance and/or protection in situations conducive to violence such as bars, high crime areas, presence of guns in homes, lone work situations, or use of alcohol in dating situations. Individual and family counseling and referral are appropriate.

Some programs have screening protocols to assess for the potential for abuse among pregnant mothers in overburdened families and to initiate home visits for those at high risk (Southern Regional Children's Advocacy Center, 1998). Hawaii's Healthy Start program of home-based services is targeted to families at risk for child abuse and neglect and uses lay home visitors trained and supervised by professional health providers (Wallach & Lister, 1995). Parental attitudes toward children and parent-child interaction patterns show measurable benefits. Programs to prevent elder abuse include efforts to reduce caregiver stress by ensuring respite care, day care, and homemaker and aid services to the family.

Secondary Prevention

Secondary prevention involves actions that are taken when violence and abuse are present. Goals include identifying the fact of abuse and intervening to aid the victim. Often, the only, or the first, practitioners to come into contact with victims are health care providers. One pressing issue is the need to increase the recognition, diagnosis, and assessment of violence by these professionals. Support for such assessment was provided when the Joint Commission on Accreditation of Healthcare Organizations set standards, in 1992 and 1994, for assessment protocols in emergency departments, alcohol abuse centers, ambulatory care centers, and all inpatient and outpatient facilities accredited by the organization. Such protocols have been developed and implemented by nurses for specific organizations (Campbell & Dienemann, 1999). General guidelines for routine screening that were released by the Family Violence Prevention Fund (FVPF) have had the support of the ANA (Family Violence Prevention Fund, 1999). The FVPF guidelines recommend routine screening of all women older than 14 years of age, whether or not symptoms or signs are present and

BOX 22-15 RECOMMENDED QUESTIONS TO SCREEN WOMEN FOR FAMILY VIOLENCE

FRAMING QUESTIONS

- Because violence is so common in many people's lives, I've begun to ask all of my patients about it.
- I'm concerned that your symptoms may have been caused by someone hurting you.

DIRECT QUESTIONS

- Are you in a direct relationship with a person who physically hurts or threatens you?
- Did someone cause these injuries? Was it your partner/husband?
- Has your partner or expartner ever hit you or physically hurt you?
- Has your partner or expartner ever threatened to hurt you or someone close to you?

Source: Family Violence Prevention Fund, 1999.

BOX 22-16 DOMESTIC VIOLENCE ASSISTANCE PROGRAMS

- Safety planning for women and children
- Help obtaining protection orders
- Support and advocacy during interviews with law enforcement, medical personnel, and legal representation
- Someone to go to court with victims
- Pretrial services
- Assistance with crime victim compensation claims
- Services for children
- Transitional housing
- Assistance and advocacy with employers regarding safety in the workplace and retention of employment
- Supportive services of clothing, food, shelter, transportation, education
- Job training or job relocation
- Counseling
- Child care
- Safety planning and other daily living needs

whether or not the provider suspects abuse has occurred. Examples of questions for screening are shown in Box 22-15.

In cases of sexual assault, increasing numbers of nurses are becoming specialized as Sexual Assault Nurse Examiners (SANEs). Their work is specialty work in forensic nursing. They work closely with law enforcement in collecting and preserving evidence of crimes. Their role is special in that they are trained to perform the necessary technical procedures during examinations, and at the same time, they can counsel and provide support in a client's time of crisis.

Reporting of abuse to authorities is an effort on behalf of victims. Health care providers in all 50 states and in the District of Columbia are required to report confirmed or suspected instances of child abuse. Most states require reporting of suspected abuse of the elderly, and state laws and procedures should be known. Mandatory reporting in the case of adults who have injuries due to domestic violence is an ongoing legal issue. At present, most states have some type of reporting of all clients who have injuries as a result of domestic violence. Some states have mandatory reporting by health care providers in instances in which the client has an injury that appears to have been caused by a gun, knife, firearm, or other deadly weapon. Some states require reporting when there is reason to believe the client's injury may have resulted from an illegal act. Other states mandate reporting when the health provider believes injuries resulted from an act of violence. Still other states require mandatory reporting when domestic violence or adult abuse is suspected (Hyman & Chez, 1994).

Laws such as those described in the previous paragraph are somewhat controversial. Some contend more harm is done than good. Ethically, there are those who argue that such mandates violate client autonomy. The stereotype of a passive/helpless victim is perpetuated. It is argued that partner abuse is not considered the same as elder abuse (cases in which there are vulnerable victims). Another potential harm is to the health care provider–client relationship by violating confidentiality and overriding informed consent of clients. There are also arguments that such reporting affects women's safety by discouraging care. Women fear risk of retaliation to themselves or their children by perpetrators, or perpetrators may restrain women from seeking care. Also, until better resources in the form of shelters, counseling, and even effective law enforcement of policy and procedures is, in fact, in place, reporting gives women false hopes of help and assistance (Hyman & Chez, 1994; Hyman, Schillinger, & Lo, 1995). Nurses need to deliberate carefully and consider the clients' best interests when making a decision to report abuse.

Victims of abuse need to be protected from further abuse, and this may require placement of children in foster care and of victims of domestic violence in shelters or safe houses. Box 22-16 outlines interventions that may be needed by victims of domestic violence and their children. For reasons discussed previously, some victims may choose not to leave the abusive situation. The nurse should support and assist the client in decision making. Contingency plans and shelter information should be provided. Interventions can also be directed to treatment for the perpetrators of abuse. Nurses can act as facilitators in group treatment sessions (Rynerson & Fishel, 1998) or make referrals to group programs or couple counseling. Often, such counseling may be court ordered. Approaches to content vary, but usually address at least anger management, skill building, and resocialization. Drop out and resistance are common in such programs.

Tertiary Prevention

Many of the same strategies that help build resistance to the use of violence are also used to rehabilitate and prevent further incidences of abuse. Education, counseling, skill building, modification of unsafe situations, stress reduction, support, and guidance are all part of the rehabilitative efforts directed toward victims and abusers.

Mesolevel Interventions: Community Structures

Prevention at this level is focused on broader factors in the larger community that contribute to violence or encourage the presence of violence. Such interventions recognize the general belief that violence prevention will not be successful unless coordinated, comprehensive, multidisciplinary, community-based approaches are initiated. These efforts must address the broader service system issues and move away from fragmented efforts. One term often used to describe such interventions is *community development*, which is action to enhance the ability of communities to meet the needs of its members. Communities are characterized as having more or less community efficacy or competence. Structures and programs must be coordinated.

One step that is needed to motivate coordinated action toward a community problem is the recognition that the problem exists. Box 22-17 outlines steps nurses can take to raise community awareness of the problem of domestic violence. Nurses working with the community often must become involved in outreach activities to promote healthier communities through partnerships with other groups, including citizens. Such work is long term, and results are not immediate. Nurses in one Washington State health department worked over a 3-year period to mobilize 17 community organizations in cooperative efforts to improve family services (Westbrook, 1999). To optimize community resources, all residents, organizations, agencies, institutions, and other components of the community must be included in the response. This makes the community response prevention and intervention oriented, not just crisis oriented.

Because each community is unique, they have different needs and resources, which means the ways to access a communitywide response to violence will be varied. What works in one community might very well not work in another. Also, consider that often there are communities within communities. For example, a neighborhood might have a Jewish ethnic group and an Italian ethnic group, each with their own traditions and sense of community. There are also self-contained communities such as Native American reservations (see the following Research Brief), prisons,

> **BOX 22-17 INTERVENTIONS TO RAISE AWARENESS ABOUT DOMESTIC VIOLENCE IN THE COMMUNITY**
>
> - Obtain *There's No Excuse for Domestic Violence* bumper stickers from the Family Violence Prevention Fund and distribute them to be placed on vehicles.
> - Ask men in the community to speak out against domestic violence and use their influence as workers and community members to let other men know that violence against women and children is wrong and will not be tolerated.
> - Place posters about domestic violence and where to go for help in business windows, gyms, laundromats, schools, and other places where women spend time. Call the Family Violence Prevention Fund to receive a free "Take Action" kit.
> - Personally speak out about domestic violence and refuse to listen to anyone make derogatory jokes or comments about women.
> - Review your community's newspaper for articles on domestic violence and determine whether there is victim-blaming language included in the articles. Speak with the newspaper editor periodically to discuss your findings and offer solutions.
> - Organize a fund-raising effort for your local family violence shelter.
> - Assess businesses' Employee Assistance Programs and determine if community businesses offer help and referrals for employees who are victims of domestic violence. If not, offer information detailing options for referrals.
> - Place stickers with the national domestic violence hotline telephone number (1-800-799-SAFE [7233]) inside stalls in women's bathrooms, on bus stop benches, on business bulletin boards, and any other places frequented by women.
> - Coordinate community educational sessions on domestic violence for both health care professionals and community citizens.

religious neighborhoods, community colleges, and senior universities. Self-contained communities may have different governing principles, needs, and resources than the community-at-large.

Collaboration and partnership of community citizens, institutions, and organizations is essential in establishing a communitywide response to domestic violence. Citizens must have ownership of the response and see themselves as playing a significant role in articulation and attainment of the response vision. Support of the members includes the support of the key leaders

RESEARCH BRIEF

Fairchild, D. G., Fairchild, M. W., & Stoner, S. (1998). Prevalence of adult domestic violence among women seeking routine care at a Native American health care facility. American Journal of Public Health, 88(10), 1514–1517.

Hamby, S. L., & Skupien, M. B. (1998). Domestic violence on the San Carlos Apache reservation. The IHS Primary Care Provider, 23(8), 102–105.

Both of these studies sought to determine the extent of domestic violence (physical only) experienced in Native American populations. Outcomes were improved documentation of the severity and high prevalence of domestic violence in the communities. In the Apache group, depression and posttraumatic stress disorder symptoms were highly associated with domestic violence. Among the Navajo, receipt of government assistance (low socioeconomic status) was associated with greater rates of domestic violence.

(both formal and informal) in the community. These are the people who are highly regarded for their knowledge and contributions to the community. Nurses can identify these leaders by doing the following:

- *Getting to know the community before any decisions are made that will impact citizens*
- *Finding out where women in the community go for help when needed*
- *Asking for advice and support from co-workers who live in the community*
- *Asking for advice and support from others who provide direct and supportive services to individuals living in the community*
- *Volunteering in a community-based organization*

After community leaders are identified, meetings and ongoing communication are necessary to develop a common definition of violence and common goals. This step will prevent the development of conflicting interventions and thus tension between participants. For instance, traditional services for battered women and their abused children have not been coordinated and are often in conflict regarding the goals of their interventions. There is a wide range of interventions, initiatives, and cooperative effort possible, limited only by the imagination and commitment of the nurse and community participants.

One outcome of awareness interventions in the community may be an increase in the demand for individual advocacy and supportive services of violence programs. Work has been suggested, for example, to improve such areas as police response, enforcement of present laws, and safer situations for reporting of cases of abuse. Community services need to be in place that increase social and psychiatric services for at-risk youth, expand alcohol and drug treatment services for pregnant and parenting women, and increase educational and employment opportunities. Child protective agencies need an increased capacity to assist clients through the provision of training, funding, and appropriate caseload assignments. Safe environments need to be created through increased surveillance, such as metal detectors at schools, and increased policing in high crime neighborhoods. Recreational facilities and programs for youth need to be available.

Macrolevel Interventions: Society and Culture

Policy issues dominate the types of interventions that nurses undertake at the macrosystem level of intervention. These interventions go far beyond reducing the virulence of the perpetrator (agent) or strengthening the victim (host) to recognize the preconditions (environment) underlying events of violence (Feldman, 1995). Action at this level is directed at large-scale efforts to address poverty, income disparity, prejudice, sexism, ageism, media violence, handgun control, and the culture of violence. These prevention efforts are attempts to change society's norms and values related to those factors that contribute to and allow violence to occur. Michael Petit, Deputy Director of the Child Welfare League, speaking at a conference on violence pointed out an indication of the nation's values. He stated that in the year 1998, the nation spent $16 billion on children's programs and $31 billion on pizza (Hattiesburg American, 1999). Such statements help us become aware of hidden social priorities.

Policy can be promoted and legislated that moves change in the right direction. Nurses, nursing organizations, and coalitions of other health care providers lobbied successfully for the comprehensive Violence Against Women Act passed in 1994 that promotes protection of women in many areas.

CONCLUSION

Community health nursing can seem daunting to some because of the broad perspective that community health nurses must address in taking on a population focus. Community health nurses by virtue of their cooperative work with many disciplines develop multiperspectival and multilingual skills. They learn to understand and communicate in many different ways (Diekemper, SmithBattle, & Drake, 1999). All public health problems challenge nursing, but the problem of violence by its very nature may be the most challenging. Alleviating all of the many forms of violence to have health, well-being, and peace for individuals in communities may be the ultimate prevention project (Temkin, 1997). The challenge has been compared with the biblical task of "taking on Goliath" because of how large it looms (Hartman, Lundy, & Janes, 1997). The following thoughts by the leader of the peaceful "Velvet" Revolution in the former Czechoslovakia, Vaclav Havel, give encouragement:

> *Hope*, in this deep and powerful sense, is not the same as joy that things are going well, or willingness to invest in enterprises that are obviously headed for success, but rather an ability to work for something because it is good, not just because it stands a chance to succeed . . . definitely not the same thing as optimism. It is not the conviction that something will turn out well, but the certainty that something makes sense, regardless of how it turns out (Havel, 1991, p. 181).

CRITICAL THINKING ACTIVITIES

1. Consider the following quotes from two famous people. How do you interpret them and how are they related?

   "The deadliest form of violence is poverty."
   Mohandas Ghandi
   "The most violent element in society is ignorance."
   Emma Goldman

2. Consider the quote below. Should war properly be considered an "ailment" of humankind, and if so, is it "curable"? How would you put military action into a prevention framework? Or could you?

   Those worthy gentlemen who look upon war, if successful, as a cause of opulence and prosperity might with equal justice . . . look upon the loss of a leg as a cause of swiftness Jeremy Bentham (1987).

3. For reference for questions 3 and 4, read Sidel, 1997. Potential ethical conflicts exist when health professionals and war intersect:

   - Conflict between caring for personnel of their own military force versus opposing forces or civilians who may need their care

   - Conflict between combatant and noncombatant roles for health personnel

   - Conflict between obligation to serve one's country in the military and broader obligation to prevent war

   Discuss these dilemmas with a military nurse and ask how they resolve their obligations.

4. Discuss the criticism of caring for victims of war as making war more tolerable.

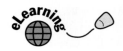

Explore Community Health Nursing on the web! To learn more about the topics in this chapter, use the passcode provided to access your exclusive web site: http://communitynursing.jbpub.com
If you do not have a passcode, you can obtain one at this site.

REFERENCES

Allotey, P. (1998). Travelling with "excess baggage": Health problems of refugee women in Western Australia. *Women and Health, 28*(1), 63-81.

American Association of Colleges of Nursing (1999). Violence as a public health issue. Washington, DC: Author.

American College of Nurse Midwives. (1997). *Position statement: Violence against women*. Washington DC: Author.

American Nurses Association (ANA). (1991). *Position statement: Physical violence against women*. Washington, DC: Author

Aron, L. Y., & Olsen, K. K. (1997). Efforts by child welfare agencies to address domestic violence. *Public Welfare,* (Summer), 4-13.

Bachman, R., & Saltzman, L. E. (1995). *Violence against women: Estimates from the redesigned survey*. Washington, DC: U.S. Department of Justice, Bureau of Justice Statistics.

Barash, D. P. (1991). *Introduction to peace studies*. Belmont, CA: Wadsworth.

Barnett, O. W., & LaViolette, A. D. (1993). *It could happen to you. Why battered women stay*. Newbury Park, CA: Sage Publications.

Bentham, J. (1987). A plan for a universal and perpetual peace. In H. P. Kainz (Ed.), *Philosophical perspectives on peace* (pp. 128-136). Athens, OH: Ohio University Press. (Originally published in 1843.)

Berliner, L., & Elliot, D. M. (1996). Sexual abuse of children. In J. Briere, L. Berliner, J. A. Bulkley, C. Jenny, & T. Reid (Eds.), *The APSAC handbook on child maltreatment*. Thousand Oaks, CA: Sage Publications.

Blackmer, J. (1994, February). Tracing teen violence and searching for solutions. *Colorado Alumnus*, 7-8. (Publication of University of Colorado, Boulder.)

Brener, N. C., Simon, T. R., Krug, E. G., & Lowery, R. (1999). Recent trends in violence-related behaviors among high school students in the United States. *Journal of the American Medical Association, 282*, 440-446.

Campbell, J. C. (1992). Violence against women. *Nursing and Health Care, 13*, 464-470.

Campbell, J. C. (1999). If I can't have you no one can. Murder linked to battery during pregnancy. *Reflections, 25*(3), 8-12, 46.

Campbell, J. C., & Dienemann, J. (1999). Symposium on violence against women. Presentation at the Sigma Theta Tau International Research Conference. London, England. June.

Campbell, J. C., Harris, M. J., & Lee, R. K. (1995). An overview of violence in America and nursing's response: Demographics, research and public policy. In H. R. Feldman (Ed.), *Nursing care in a violent society: Issues and research*. New York: Springer.

Cassidy, K. (1999). How to assess and intervene in domestic violence situations. *Home Healthcare Nurse, 17*, 665-671.

Centers for Disease Control and Prevention (CDC). (1992). The prevention of youth violence: a framework for community action. A publication of the U.S. Department of Health and Human Services. Available: http://aepo-xdv-www.epo.cdc.gov/wonder/prevguid/p0000026/entire.htm.

Centers for Disease Control and Prevention (CDC). (1998a). *Facts about suicide among black youth*. Available: www.cdc.gov/od/oc/media/fact/suicideby.htm.

Centers for Disease Control and Prevention (CDC). (1998b). Youth risk behavior surveillance —United States 1997. *Morbidity and Mortality Weekly Report Surveillance Summaries, 47*(SS-3), 1-89.

Centers for Disease Control and Prevention (CDC). (1999a). *Facts about violence among youth and violence in schools*: www.cdc.gov/ncipc/dvp/yvpt/facts.htm.

Centers for Disease Control and Prevention (CDC). (1999b). *Theories and causation of youth violence*: www.cdc.gov/ncipc/dvp/yvpt/theory.htm.

Centers for Disease Control and Prevention (CDC). (1999c). Youth violence in the United States: www.cdc.gov/ncipc/dvp/yvfacts.htm.

Centerwall, B. S. (1992). Television and violence: The scale of the problem and where to go from here. *Journal of the American Medical Society, 267*, 3059-3063.

City of Hattiesburg. (1995). *Progress report of the Hattiesburg citizen's crime task force*. Hattiesburg, MS: Author.

Davey, D. B., & Davey, P. A. (1998, November/December). Domestic violence today. What nursing students should know. *Imprint*, 41-43.

Davies, W. H., & Flannery, D. J. (1998). Post-traumatic stress disorder in children and adolescents exposed to violence. *Pediatric Clinics of North America, 45*, 341-353.

Deaths resulting from firearm- and motor-vehicle-related injuries—United States, 1968-1991. (1994). *Morbidity and Mortality Weekly Report, 43*(3), 37-42.

Department of Health and Human Services (DHHS). (2000). *Healthy People 2010: Conference edition.* Washington, DC: U.S. Government Printing Office.

Diekemper, M., SmithBattle, L., & Drake, M. A. (1999). Bringing the population into focus. A natural development in community health nursing practice. Part I. *Journal of Public Health Nursing 16*(1), p. 3–9.

DiGuiseppi, C. (1995). Counseling to prevent youth violence. In *Guide to clinical preventive services: Report of the U.S. Preventive Services Task Force* (pp. 687-698). Washington, DC: Department of Health and Human Services.

Emergency Nurses Association. (1994). *Position statement: Domestic violence.* Chicago: Author.

Family Violence Prevention Fund (FVPF) (1994). The health care response to domestic violence fact sheet. Produced by FVPF and the Trauma Foundation, San Francisco, CA. Available: http://eng.hss.cmu.edu/feminism/domestic-violence.html.

Family Violence Prevention Fund (FVPF) (1997). *What you can do: The facts.* Available: www.fvpf.org/fund.

Family Violence Prevention Fund (FVPF) (1999). *Preventing domestic violence: Clinical guidelines on routine screening.* San Francisco, CA: The authors.

Farrell, M. (1992a). The price of war. *Nursing and Health Care, 13*(8), 414-416.

Farrell, M. (1992b). After war: Long-term effects on people, their health, and the health system. *Nursing Administration Quarterly, 16*(2),4-7

Feldman, H. R. (1995). Introduction: Nursing's response to our culture of violence. In H. R. Feldman (Ed.), *Nursing care in a violent society: Issues and research.* New York: Springer.

Felitti, V. J., Anda, R. F., Nordenberg, D., Williamson, D. F., Spitz, A., Edwards, V., Koss, M. P., & Marks, J. S. (1998). Relationship of childhood abuse and household dysfunction to many of the leading causes of death in adults: The adverse childhood experiences (ACE) study. *American Journal of Preventive Medicine, 14*, 245-258.

Foege, W. (1997). Arms and public health. In B. Levy & V. Sidel (Eds.), *War and public health.* New York: Oxford University Press.

Fox, P. G., Cowell, J. M., Montgomery, A. C., & Willgerodt, M. A. (1998). Southeast Asian refugee women and depression: A nursing intervention. *International Journal of Psychiatric Nursing Research, 4*(1), 423-432.

Friedlander, B. Z. (1993). Community violence, children's development and the mass media: In pursuit of new insights, new goals, and new strategies. *Psychiatry: Interpersonal and Biological Processes, 56*(1), 66–81.

Frietag, R., Lazoritz, S., & Kini, N. (1998). Psychosocial aspects of child abuse for primary care pediatricians. *Pediatric Clinics of North America, 45*, 391-402.

Furey, J. (1991). Women Vietnam veterans: A comparison of studies. *Journal of Psychosocial Nursing and Mental Health Services, 29*(3), 11-3.

Ganley, A. L. (1996). Understanding domestic violence. In C. Warshaw & A. L. Ganley (Eds.), *Improving the health care response to domestic violence: A resource manual for health care providers.* San Francisco: The Family Violence Prevention Fund.

Garfield, R. M., & Neugut, A. I. (1997). The human consequences of war. In B. Levy & V. Sidel (Eds.), *War and public health.* New York: Oxford University Press.

Gilligan, J. (1997). *Violence. Reflections on a national epidemic.* New York: Vintage Books.

Gondolf, E. W., & Fisher, E. R. (1988). *Battered women as survivors: An alternative to treating learned helplessness.* Lexington, MA: Lexington Books.

Hall, J., & Stevens, P. (1992) A nursing view of the United States-Iraq war: Psychosocial health consequences. *Nursing Outlook, 35*(1), 113-120.

Hampton, R. L., Vandergriff-Avery, M., & Kim, J. (1999). Understanding the origins of spousal violence in North America. In T. P. Gullotta & S. J. McElhaney (Eds.), *Violence in homes and communities: Prevention, intervention and treatment* (pp. 39-70). Thousand Oaks, CA: Sage Publications.

Hartman, S. (1992a, May). *Religion, community health, and the abuse of war.* Paper presented at the International Religious Federation for World Peace, Eighth International Conference on God: The Contemporary Discussion; Peace and the Ultimate, Section on Education for Peace, Compiegne, France.

Hartman, S. (1992b, August). *Peace: The special concern of professionals.* Paper presented at Section on Spirituality, the Professions, and Peace. Assembly of the World's Religions, Seoul, Korea.

Hartman, S., Lundy, K. S., & Janes, S. (1997, June). *Taking on Goliath: Nursing's response to violence.* Paper presented at Association of Community Health Nursing Educators' Annual Spring Institute, Vancouver, British Columbia, Canada.

Hattiesburg American. (1999). Attorneys general meet to talk school violence. May 4, 9A.

Havel, V. (1991) *Disturbing the peace.* New York: Random House.

Hawkins, D. (1999). Preventing adolescent health-risk behaviors by strengthening protection during childhood. *Archives of Pediatrics and Adolescent Medicine, 153,* 226–234.

Hedin, B. (1989). Nursing education and sterile ethical fields. *Advances in Nursing Science, 11,* 43-52.

Hennes, H. (1998). A review of violence statistics among children and adolescents in the United States. *Pediatric Clinics of North America, 45,* 269-280.

Hotzworth-Monroe, A., Stuart, G. L. (1994). Typologies of male batterers: Three subtypes and the differences among them. *Psychological Bulletin, 116*(3), 476–497.

Hyman, A., & Chez, R. A. (1994). *Mandatory reporting law.* Paper for the Family Violence Prevention Fund: www.igc.org/fund/healthcare/mand_rept.html.

Hyman, A., Schillinger, D., & Lo, B. (1995). Laws mandating reporting of domestic violence: Do they promote patient well-being? *Journal of the American Medical Association, 273,* 1781-1787.

Institute of Medicine. (1999). Violence and the American family: Report of a workshop. Next steps: A guide to effective action. Available: http://uuu4.nationalacademies.org/iomhome.nsf.

Jason, L. A., Hanaway, L. K., & Brackshaw, E. (1999). Television violence and children problems and solutions. In T. P. Gullotta & S. J. McElhaney (Eds.), *Violence in homes and communities: Prevention, intervention and treatment* (pp. 133-156). Thousand Oaks, CA: Sage Publications.

Jones, F. C., & Selder, F. (1996). Psychoeducational groups to promote effective coping in school-aged children living in violent communities. *Issues in Mental Health Nursing, 17,* 559–571.

Jones, L. (1993). Can a doctor stop the violence? *USA Weekend,* November 26–28, p 9.

Kent-Wilkerson, A. (1996). Spousal abuse/homicide. A current issue in health risk management. *Journal of Psychosocial Nursing, 34*(10) 12-15.

Kotch, J. B., Muller, G. O., & Blakely, C. H. (1999). Understanding the origins and incidence of child maltreatment. In T. P. Gullotta & S. J. McElhaney (Eds.), *Violence in homes and communities: Prevention, intervention and treatment.* Thousand Oaks, CA: Sage Publications.

Levy, B. S., & Sidel, V. W. (1997). *War and public health.* New York: Oxford University Press.

Markin, D. A. (1996). Fighting the "silent epidemic." *Health Progress, 77*(2), 30-33.

McClain, P., Sacks, J., Froehlke, R., & Ewigman, D. (1993). Estimates of fatal child abuse and neglect. Unites States, 1979 through 1988. *Pediatrics, 91,* 338-343.

McClure, L. F. (1999). Origins and incidence of workplace violence in North America. In T. P. Gullotta & S. J. McElhaney (Eds.), *Violence in homes and communities: Prevention, intervention and treatment* (pp. 71-99). Thousand Oaks, CA: Sage Publications.

Mercy, J. A., Rosenberg, M. L., Powell, K. E., Broome, C. V., & Roper, W. L. (1993). Public health policy for preventing violence. *Health Affairs, 12*(4), 7-29.

Mooney, M. M., & Napierkowski, D. (1999). Are tighter gun control restrictions the answer to the epidemic of violence in schools, workplaces and communities? (Letter to the editor). *The American Nurse, 31*(5), 4.

National Black Nurses' Association. (1994). *Position statement on the reduction of violence in African American communities.* Washington, DC: Author.

National Center for Disease Control. (1999). Youth violence in the United States. Available: www.cdc.gov/ncipc/dvp/yvfacts.htm.

National Center for Health Statistics. (1998). *Fastats. Firearm mortality:* www.cdc.gov/nchswww/fastats/firearms.htm.

Nightingale, F. (1954). Notes on matters affecting the health of the British army. In F. Nightingale. *Selected writings, 1820-1910.* New York: Macmillan.

Norman, E. (1989). The wartime experiences of military nurses in Vietnam, 1965-1973. *Western Journal of Nursing Research, 11,* 219-33.

Office of Juvenile Justice and Delinquency Prevention. (1999). *Report to Congress on juvenile violence research.* Washington, DC: U.S. Department of Justice, Office of Justice Programs, Office of Juvenile Justice and Delinquency Prevention.

O'Neil, J. M., & Harway, M. (1997). A multivariate model explaining men's violence toward women: Predisposing and triggering hypotheses. *Violence against Women, 3*(2), 182-203.

Paul, E., & O'Neall, J. (1986). American nurses in Vietnam: Stressors and aftereffects. *American Journal of Nursing, 86,* 526.

Potter, L. B. (1999). Understanding the incidence and origins of community violence: Toward a comprehensive perspective on violence prevention. In T. P. Gullotta & S. J. McElhaney (Eds.), *Violence in homes and communities: Prevention, intervention and treatment.* Thousand Oaks, CA: Sage Publications.

Powell, K. B. (1997). Correlates of violent and nonviolent behavior among vulnerable inner-city youths. *Family and Community Health, 20*(2), 38-47.

Praeger, S. G., & Bernhardt, G. R. (1985). Survivors of suicide: a community in need. *Family and Community Health, 8*(3), 62-72.

Prevent Child Abuse America. (1996a). *Fact sheet: Child sexual abuse.* Chicago: Author: www.childabuse.org/fs19.html.

Prevent Child Abuse America. (1996b). *Fact sheet: Prevention of child abuse and neglect fatalities.* Chicago: Author: www.childabuse.org/fs9.html.

Proctor, N. G. (1998). Violent ethnic wars and world-wide people movement: Implications for mental health nursing practice. *Contemporary Nurse, 7*(3), 148-151.

Rynerson, B. C., & Fishel, A. H. (1998). Expressions of men who batter: Implications for nursing. *Journal of the American Psychiatric Nurses Association, 4*(2), 41–47.

Salmi, J. (1993). *Violence and a democratic society.* London: Zed Books.

Schachter, B., & Seinfeld, J. (1994). Personal violence and the culture of violence. *Social Work, 39,* 347-350.

Schafer, J., Caetano, R., & Clark, C. L. (1998). Rates of intimate partner violence in the United States. *American Journal of Public Health, 88,* 1702-1704.

Scott-Tilley, D. (1999). Nursing interventions to prevent domestic violence. *American Journal of Nursing, 99*(10), 24-27.

Sidel, V. W. (1997). *The roles and ethics of health professionals in war.* In B. S. Levy & V. W. Sidel (Eds.), *War and public health.* New York: Oxford University Press.

Simpson, R. (1986). The ultimate in preventive medicine. *The Australian Nurses Journal, 15*(10), 36.

Southern Regional Children's Advocacy Center. (1998). *Healthy families—North Alabama.* Available: www.ncac-hsv.org/hfl.html.

Stollery, R. (1984). Preventing global nuclear war! What can nurses do? *Canadian Nurse, 80*(4), 40-41.

Straus, M. A., & Gelles, R. J. (1990). *Physical violence in American families: Risk factors and adaptations to violence in 8,145 families.* New Brunswick, NJ: Transaction Publishers.

Tatara, T., Kuzemskus, L. B., Duckhorn, E., & Bivens, L. (1998). *The National Elder Abuse Incidence Study: final report.* Prepared by the National Center on Elder Abuse at the American Public Human Services Association f or the Administration on Children and Families and the Administration on Aging, United States Department of Health and Human Services: www.aoa.gov/abuse/report/default.htm.

Temkin, E. (1997). Nurses and the prevention of war: Public health nurses and the peace movement in world war I. In B. S. Levy & V. W. Sidel (Eds.), *War and public health.* New York: Oxford University Press.

The Commonwealth Fund (1999, May). *Violence and abuse. Fact sheet from the commonwealth fund 1998 survey of women's health:* www.cmwf.org/programs/women/.

United Nations Division for the Advancement of Women. (1995). Beijing declaration and platform for action: Strategic objectives and actions: Violence against women. Available: www.un.org/womenwatch/daw.

U.S. Department of Labor. (1996). *Protecting community workers against violence.* (Department of Labor Publication No. 96-53). Washington, DC: Author.

U.S. Public Health Service, Office on Women's Health. (1997). Policy recommendations of the National Nursing Summit on Violence Against Women, October 20, 1997. Washington, DC: U.S. Public Health Service, Department of Health and Human Services.

Van Soest, D. (1997). *The global crisis of violence: Common problems, universal causes, shared solutions.* Washington, DC: National Association of Social Workers.

Wakefield, M., Gardner, D. B., & Guillett, S. (1998). Contemporary issues in government. In D. J. Mason & J. K. Leavitt (Eds.), *Policy and politics in nursing and health care* (pp. 349-383). Philadelphia: W. B. Saunders.

Walker, L. E. (1984). *The battered woman syndrome.* New York: Springer.

Wallach, V. A., & Lister, L. (1995). Stages in the delivery of home-based services to parents at risk of child abuse: A Healthy Start experience. *Scholarly Inquiry for Nursing Practice: An International Journal, 9,* 159–173.

Westbrook, L. A. (1999). Effectiveness of an interdisciplinary team in public health: Implications for partnership building and collaboration in health systems. Paper presented at the 8th National Conference on Nursing Administration Research. November, San Diego, CA.

Whitlock, G. (1996). Reexamining Dr. King and Malcolm X on violence. *The Philosophical Forum, 27,* 289-319.

World Bank. (1993). *World development report, 1993.* New York: Oxford University Press.

Youth Violence and Suicide Prevention Program. (1999). *Fact sheet on dating violence:* www.cdc.gov/ncipc/dvp/yvpt/datviol.htm.

APPENDIX A

A Day in the Life of a Nurse Who Faces Violence: Sexual Assault Nurse Examiner (SANE)

Margaret M. Aiken, PhD, RN

It was 10 PM, Thursday night. As the SANE readied herself for bed, she checked to see where her pager was, her keys, and her clothes. She climbed into bed and pulled the covers up around her chin. She was exhausted. Her last thought as she drifted off to sleep was, *As tired as I am, they will probably have me out the whole damn night.* Like a knife, the pager's sound cut through the stillness of the night. She jerked herself from sleep into an upright position. She fumbled for the bedside light, toppling a glass of water to the floor as she did so. She pressed the reset button on the pager to reveal the source of the call. It was the police dispatcher calling her. By rote, she dialed the number imprinted in her brain by repetitions over 12 years.

"Communications, Smith."

"Hi! This is Donna Anthony with Rape Crisis."

"Hi Donna. They have a car in route to the center with a victim. Their ETA is approximately 2:30."

"Thanks. I will be there at about the same time."

Donna had slept in her underwear and a pair of sweats, so she had only to pull on a T-shirt, put on shoes and socks, brush teeth and hair, and leave. It was about a 20-minute drive to the center. As she drove down the street in the quiet night, she wondered just how many times she had moved through this scenario. There was always the thought, *I wonder if this will happen to me sometime when I am called out like this. What prevents it from happening?* The drive to the center was so practiced and automatic that it was not uncommon to reminisce and engage in fantasy: *I wonder what this victim will be like. A street person? A child? An addict? Or a regular person like me? One could argue the "regular" person thing. What kind of nut is cruising the streets in the middle of the night when they could be snug in a bed? I wonder which detective will be with the victim. Will it be a sympathetic one? Whoops, I almost drove right past the place. I really must pay better attention.*

As she pulled into the lot she noticed that the police car was already there. She greeted the officer, inquiring whether he had been waiting long. The officer introduced her to the victim, Anne Smithridge, who was a retired employee from one of the local banks. They went through all the rituals to gain entrance into the building and the suite of offices. Once they got inside, Donna made coffee, offered some to Ms. Smithridge and to the detective, and poured herself a large cup, thinking, *Please God, help me wake up.* Ms. Smithridge was escorted to the examining room, where she would be interviewed and examined. This woman was in her sixties, lived alone in a single family home. A man had broken into her home to rob her and then had forced her to have sex as an apparent afterthought. Donna interviewed her, examined her, collected evidence, and filled out the many forms required. She offered emotional support throughout the process. Donna was surprised at how "together" this woman was in view of what had happened. It took approximately 1 hour to complete the entire process. Donna's good work in assessment and evidence collection had contributed to the conviction of many perpetrators.

Before leaving the center, Donna called the dispatcher to see if there were any more "calls." Hearing that there were none, she informed the dispatcher that she was going home. All three left the center at the same time. As she drove home, again on "automatic pilot," she began thinking about the scores of assaulted women she had seen over the years. Each time she left the center, she made a concerted effort to forget the case. She feared that if she were to keep all the information in her active memory, she would lose her sense of balance.

The victims/survivors of rape whom she best remembered were probably those touched by either humor or horror, which likely does a disservice to all those who are abused and defiled and go unnoticed in a blur of the many. She arrived home. Wearily, she crept into the house, which was still dark. She went to the back of the house to her bedroom and again readied herself for bed, checking for the location of pager, keys, and so on. As she climbed into bed, she was reminded of the spilled water as she stepped in the puddle in her sock feet. She pulled off the socks and then padded into the bathroom to get a towel. She simply threw the towel in the pooled water, said "the hell with it," and slid between the sheets. It was now 4:30 AM

and all was well (she hoped). Donna now had to ready herself for the day at her regular full-time job at the clinic. It would be a long day, but she would make it. People often ask her why she continues in this stressful job. She invariably responds that no matter what, she feels that she does a "good thing." As she drifted off to sleep, she clicked off all the things she had to do before leaving home for her "real job." In terms of time, it would be tight, but she would make it. Indeed, it had been quite a night in the life of a SANE!

APPENDIX B

A Day in the Life of a Nurse Who Faces Violence: Prison Nursing

Miriam Cabana, RN, MSN

The nurse supervisor turned on to the blacktop road that ribboned through the 22,000-acre southern prison. As the expansive horizon of flat delta land passed on her short drive to the prison hospital, she recalled the conversation with her husband earlier in the day. He was the warden of the prison and had mused that the full moon usually means some form of violence would erupt within the prison units and that it was an "ideal" time for an escape attempt. She knew he was diligent in his efforts to protect the community as well as to maintain a safe environment for those incarcerated, which often included protecting them from violence inflicted on each other; and he shared her strong opinion about society's obligation to provide inmates with access to safe, competent health care. At the very least, there would be more physical altercations among the inmates or increased somatic complaints screened by phone from the emergency department. She instinctively knew her evening shift would be busy. Oh, for the days in her nursing career that the "full moon" myths were associated only with increased birth rates!

The transition between shifts for both nursing and security personnel was smooth. Predictably, several inmates remained in the large holding room with barred windows and door waiting their turn to see the physician. They were the last clients of the scheduled sick call. Once their assessment, diagnostic tests, or treatments were completed, the hospital correctional offi-

cers assigned to transportation would return them in handcuffs and a secured van to their respective housing units. The phone rang constantly and required the nursing supervisor and a second RN to screen the calls from officers in the housing units who reported the inmate complaints, requests for medications, refills, accidents, or any unusual behavior or symptoms observed by the officers. The nurses made the decision that required assessment in the emergency room, and two hospital officers would pick up the inmate and bring him to the hospital. The LPN and two EMTs assisted the physician. Finally, at around 8 PM, the nursing supervisor realized that the phone calls were becoming less frequent. She always felt like she was playing Russian roulette, hoping she and her staff asked the right questions or were receiving accurate replies for accurate phone assessments.

The loud ring from the "red" emergency phone jarred everyone into a state of readiness. The phone was connected to the warden's office, the central security office, and the hospital emergency department, so that all key personnel were alerted with the dialing of a single number. The ominous sound always meant an emergency of some description. As nursing and security staff gathered at the doorway to listen, the nursing supervisor quickly picked up the receiver. The excitable, stuttering voice on the other end was barely intelligible. It was obvious the officer was in trouble and had to be coaxed by the security chief to report the housing unit number. The nursing supervisor had heard the word "stabbing" and the unit number. Suddenly she heard the quivering male voice on the other end cry out, "Oh my God, he's gonna kill all of us!" before the line went dead. She immediately dispatched one of the two life-support ambulances. The second ambulance was on its way to another far-flung maximum security housing unit so the RN, a former critical care unit nurse, could assess an inmate complaining of severe chest pain. The supervisor instructed the transportation officer and RN to report to the scene of the stabbing as soon as the assessment was completed unless the inmate required further monitoring in the emergency department. She and the remaining nursing and security personnel then put into action the plan they had developed as a team shortly after her arrival. The two major trauma rooms and the staff were ready to receive victims of violence within minutes after the departure of the ambulance. The physician on call was on her way to the hospital to await their arrival.

The radio was crackling with orders and the relaying of information from security. The ambulance crew was unable to enter the housing unit until the violent rampage had been quelled and the drug-crazed inmate had been subdued by the E-squad, officers who received continuous training in confronting violence within the prison and searching for escaped felons. She could hear and feel the palpable fear and chaos; the number of victims could not be immediately determined and could not be reached because the perpetrator wielded a homemade knife, daring the officers to come near him or the victims. She had never been so close to violence. The ambulance crew described the horror of the scene to her as they arrived with the first victim removed from the unit: a young male with multiple stab wounds to the chest. A second physician was called for assistance because two other victims were reportedly arriving. She and the physician worked quickly to start IVs, insert chest tubes, and stabilize the first victim for transport to a hospital intensive care unit 30 miles away. The second victim arrived with cardiopulmonary resuscitation (CPR) in progress; he had been stabbed in the back repeatedly, then literally picked up and flipped over and

stabbed in the face, chest, and abdomen. Each time his chest was compressed, blood gushed from the multiple wounds, which totaled more than 50. After a grueling hour, the inmate, in his early twenties, was pronounced dead. She had never seen so much blood. Linens were soaked with the warm, moist liquid that continued to drip from the sides of the stretcher on which the inmate lay, and one could not avoid the pools of blood on the floor.

She silently wondered what could provoke such a hideous act of violence. She choked back the tears of anger, fear, and bewilderment. There were no family or friends to mourn or to console, since the family would be notified by phone. Her past experiences and education had not prepared her for the little value placed on life within prison and the potential for raw violence within human beings. She gently covered him with a clean sheet as she remembered her husband's frequent rebuttal to her complaints about late-night phone calls from inmates' parents: Everybody here is some mother's baby.

She entered the corridor and knew the pounding of her heart could be heard over the din of the animated conversations between officers and health care personnel. She managed to assign staff to transport the first victim to the hospital and to prepare the body of the deceased victim for the funeral home before she retreated into the quiet conference room. She could not control the violent shaking of her entire body or the feeling of revulsion that manifested as an overwhelming nausea. She knew what she had to do; but for the first time since she had become a nurse, she doubted her ability to be nonjudgmental. How could she provide care for someone who had committed such a senseless act of violence? The respect for the individuality of clients and human worth had been the foundation of her 20-year nursing career; yet, for the first time, she questioned her own ability to follow these beliefs. She also had to confront her paralyzing fear for the safety of her family as well as her own safety in her world of nursing. Finally she was able to leave the conference room and enter the noisy clinical area. Still shaking, she took a deep breath and picked up the chart of the next client to be assessed: the inmate who had stabbed the first two clients and had brought violence into her world that night.

Chronic Illness

Edith L. Hilton

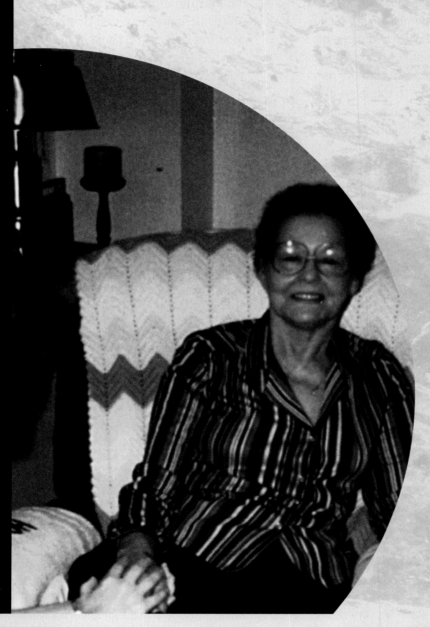

For illness runs like a thread through every life, in some it is a thin gossamer, barely discernible filament; in others it is like a heavy line which, as it grows with time, loops, bends, and strangles.

Goldfarb, 1976

QUESTIONS TO CONSIDER

After reading this chapter, answer the following questions:

1. What are the reasons for the increase in chronic illness in the United States?
2. Which population groups are most vulnerable in regard to chronic illness?
3. How do chronic illness and disability differ?
4. How do the concepts of paradox and loss relate to the experience of chronic illness?
5. What are current and future roles of the community health nurse in caring for persons with chronic illness?
6. How does the financing of chronic illness affect persons with chronic illness?
7. What are specific challenges in caring for diverse groups with chronic illness?
8. How are the health issues of caregivers of the chronically ill related to nursing management?
9. What is hospice care?
10. What role do institutions play in the management of chronically ill?

KEY TERMS

Burden
Chronic illness
Coping

Home–based caregivers
Loss
Stress

More than 50 years ago chronic illness was identified as the challenge of the era (Mayo, 1956). The expansion of community health nursing during the latter part of the 20th century results, in large part, from the development of a population of chronically ill persons who survive illnesses that were previously untreatable. Research indicates that **chronic illness** may alter individual abilities to master and participate in expected role functions (Longman, Braden, & Mishel, 1997). One of the most important responsibilities those within the community have involves participation and management of their own health (Hardy & Conway, 1978). This chapter considers aspects of chronic illness affecting individuals of different ethnic groups and of varying ages with problems arising from genetic sources to those associated with aging processes.

Chronic Illness in the United States

We have learned a great deal about infectious disease epidemics in the United States during the past two centuries; however, chronic illnesses are not well documented because large numbers of those with acute diseases perished before their diseases became chronic. During the 19th century, immigration from Europe taxed sanitary and housing resources in many East Coast cities in the United States. With repeated epidemics, health conditions for established and relocated populations dwindled. Chronic conditions such as heart disease, diabetes, neurological problems, and blood disorders are identified in literature of that time. Because drugs and therapeutic regimens were scarce, overall survival rates of these diseases were poor, especially in vulnerable populations.

Examples of chronic illness include "the dirty dozen" most common chronic illnesses: rheumatoid arthritis, ankylosing spondylitis, other related arthritic illnesses, systemic lupus erythematosus, Parkinson's disease, emphysema, multiple sclerosis, heart disease, stroke with permanent impairment, asthma and dystrophies severe enough to cause impairment, and diabetes (Wilson, 1992). See the *Healthy People 2010* box for selected objectives related to chronic illness.

Major inroads of treatment, management, and prevention occurred during the 20th century. Because of improved sanitation, use of antibiotics and technology, advances in research and communication, and better health care education, the standard of living for many Americans has improved. However, these relatively recent developments have fostered trends of developing chronic illnesses that have become more prevalent in the 20th century in the United States. An example of this trend is chronic renal failure. Until dialysis became available in the 1960s, renal failure was essentially untreatable and therefore fatal. Dialysis is now a relatively common intervention for both acute and chronic phases. Another example of the development of more recent chronicity is acquired immunodeficiency syndrome (AIDS). Initially, few survived opportunistic invaders. This is no longer true; many are surviving for years with human immunodeficiency virus (HIV), AIDS-related complex (ARC), and AIDS using newly formulated medications and combination drug regimens.

Chronically ill persons in communities include those with chemical dependency, chronic mental illness, and tuberculosis. Stable chronic conditions affecting as many as 30% of the adult population include cardiovascular disease, neurological diseases (including Alzheimer's disease), some slow developing forms of cancer, emphysema, diabetes, fetal alcohol syndrome, learning disability, adjustment disorders, and genetically linked diseases (including Down syndrome [trisomy 18 and 21], sickle cell disease, cystic fibrosis, Tay-Sachs, and schizophrenia). New medications enable individuals with these and other chronic diseases to live longer than ever before. Many chronically ill persons remain in community settings and depend on others to render all or part of their physical and/or mental care.

Vulnerable Populations

Some populations are more likely than others to develop chronic illnesses. Chronic illnesses affect various ethnic and racial groups and are gender preferential in some disease processes. The very old and the very young are susceptible to infectious processes and are at greatest risk for safety problems because of their limited defense mechanisms, such as diminished, slowed, or immature reflexes. Cancer, cardiovascular diseases (including heart attack and stroke), obesity, and diabetes are examples of disabling conditions that affect various groups.

Acute Versus Chronic Illness

Defined in 1956 by the Commission on Chronic Illness, impairments or deviations from normal having one or more of the following characteristics were recognized as *chronic illness:* (1) are permanent, (2) leave residual disability, (3) are caused by irreversible pathological alterations, (4) require special training of the client for rehabilitation, and (5) may be expected to require a long period of supervision, observation, or care. In addition to chronic illness, multiple chronic conditions per person are often noted (Strauss, 1975). A common example of this includes diabetes that affects nerve tissue, causing damage to sensory nerve pathways, diabetic-induced visual loss from retinal disease, and hypertension that coexists with diabetes.

Acute illness is defined as a disease (or process) with a sudden, dynamic onset with signs and symptoms related to the disease process itself, which either resolves shortly with complete recovery or results in death (Lubkin, 1995). Differences between acute and chronic illness are notable in treatment, duration, and perceived significance. Another important difference between acute and chronic illness relates to **coping** abilities taxed during severe and sustained illness. Acute and chronic illness also occur together. Examples of this phenomenon include asthma and diabetes in which acute manifestations emerge from chronic problems in regulating the diseases. One challenge presented by chronic illness is that of keeping clients motivated to achieve and maintain optimal levels of health. Supporting clients' efforts to learn to manage their chronic illness requires skill, creativity, and persistence to keep clients' entire life patterns in focus.

HEALTHY PEOPLE 2010

OBJECTIVES RELATED TO CHRONIC ILLNESS

Access to Quality Health Services

Primary Care

1.9   Reduce hospitalization rates for three ambulatory care–sensitive conditions— pediatric asthma, uncontrolled diabetes, and immunization-preventable pneumonia and influenza in older adults.

Long-Term Care and Rehabilitative Services

1.15   Increase the proportion of persons with long-term care needs who have access to the continuum of long-term care services.

Arthritis, Osteoporosis, and Chronic Back Conditions

Arthritis and Other Rheumatic Conditions

2.1   Increase the mean number of days without severe pain among adults who have chronic joint symptoms.

2.2   Reduce the proportion of adults with chronic joint symptoms who experience a limitation in activity due to arthritis.

2.5   Increase the employment rate among adults with arthritis in the working-age population.

2.7   Increase the proportion of adults who have seen a health care provider for their chronic joint symptoms.

Osteoporosis

2.9   Reduce the overall number of cases of osteoporosis.

2.10   Reduce the proportion of adults who are hospitalized for vertebral fractures associated with osteoporosis.

Chronic Back Conditions

2.11   Reduce activity limitation due to chronic back conditions.

Cancer

3.15   Increase the proportion of cancer survivors who are living 5 years or longer after diagnosis.

Chronic Kidney Disease

4.1   Reduce the rate of new cases of end-stage renal disease (ESRD).

4.3   Increase the proportion of treated chronic kidney failure patients who have received counseling on nutrition, treatment choices, and cardiovascular care 12 months before the start of renal replacement therapy.

4.7   Reduce kidney failure due to diabetes.

Diabetes

5.1   Increase the proportion of persons with diabetes who receive formal diabetes education.

5.2   Prevent diabetes.

5.3   Reduce the overall rate of diabetes that is clinically diagnosed.

Heart Disease and Stroke

Blood Pressure

12.9   Reduce the proportion of adults with high blood pressure.

12.10   Increase the proportion of adults with high blood pressure whose blood pressure is under control.

Cholesterol

12.13   Reduce the mean total blood cholesterol levels among adults.

12.14   Reduce the proportion of adults with high total blood cholesterol levels.

Medical Product Safety

17.3   Increase the proportion of primary care providers, pharmacists, and other health care professionals who routinely review

Continued

HEALTHY PEOPLE 2010—cont'd

with their patients all new prescribed and over-the-counter medicines.

Nutrition and Overweight

Weight Status and Growth

19.2   Reduce the proportion of adults who are obese.

19.3   Reduce the proportion of children and adolescents who are overweight or obese.

Schools, Worksites, and Nutrition Counseling

19.7   Increase the proportion of physician office visits made by patients with a diagnosis of cardiovascular disease, diabetes, or hyperlipidemia that include counseling or education related to diet and nutrition.

Respiratory Diseases

Asthma

24.2   Reduce hospitalizations for asthma.

24.3   Reduce hospital emergency department visits for asthma.

24.4   Reduce activity limitations among persons with asthma.

Chronic Obstructive Pulmonary Disease

24.9   Reduce the proportion of adults whose activity is limited due to chronic lung and breathing problems.

Source: DHHS, 2000.

Chronic Illness Versus Disability

Disabled individuals generally are unable to initiate or complete self-care activities alone because of physical impairments. To achieve independence or optimal levels of self-care, clients usually require focused rehabilitative efforts. In some cases, rehabilitation is also useful in maintaining established progress in self-care activities. Rehabilitation is also used in conditions of disability associated with chronic health problems and degenerative diseases such as epilepsy and multiple sclerosis (Hickey, 1992).

Chronic illness differs from disability in the following manner: Disability does not necessarily imply sickness or less-than-optimal health; however, chronic illness is *always* related to a permanent decrease in health status that will not, in all likelihood, result in restoration of former or normal health status. Chronic illness is contrasted with disability in the following three examples: (1) Chronic renal failure may result in chronic illness but not disability in every individual (Klang & Clyne, 1997); (2) a hip fracture may result in disability but not necessarily in chronic illness; and (3) spinal cord injury may result in both conditions, because disability immediately develops as a consequence of spinal cord damage, and chronic illness may ensue if prolonged immobility causes development of decubitus ulcers, urinary tract infections, or muscle spasms unrelieved by medications. Disability resulting from spinal cord injury may cause numerous chronic illnesses that relate to development of decubitus ulcers: Clients may require surgical interventions to enable healing. Because of inadequate sensory enervation, necessary position changes may be overlooked while individuals are in wheelchair sitting positions.

Clients with chronic disability often define themselves in terms of their illness role and diagnosis. Definitions of this type may be limiting. When persons with disabilities are viewed as striving toward higher level wellness, they may be supported by interacting with their environment in an integrated manner, thereby promoting their personhood and emphasizing their human qualities instead of their disabilities (Davidhizar & Shearer, 1997).

Experience of Chronic Illness
Paradox and Loss

In each chronic illness, disease forms a path through lives that is not always apparent at outset and that may not be clearly understood. Wellness and optimal health are subjectively described by each person experiencing those conditions, and chronic illness is best described and experienced by those living the phenomenon. An example of paradox, or a seeming contradiction associated with chronic illness, is described by a woman with chronic asthma:

> I didn't have a fever and my doctor said all my blood tests and X-rays were fine. At first my friends were sympathetic, but then they began asking whether I was really taking care of

FYI

Stable, chronic conditions affect as much as 30% of the U.S. adult population.

myself. Even my doctor seemed exasperated, and so I began to think I was crazy and had made all this up. Little did I know when this happened two years ago that I was heading for chronic asthma. My asthma finally got so bad that I had to stop teaching (Wilson, 1992, p. 42).

Many chronic disease processes involve paradox, and it contributes to feelings of loss, fear, and frustration. Johnson (1991, p. 33) explains the paradoxical nature of myocardial infarction:

The signs and symptoms of a heart attack often begin insidiously and escalate over a period of hours. Heart attacks have a paradoxical nature. Although potentially fatal, the early signs of a heart attack mimic minor and trivial complaints. Unless the heart attack is extensive, the early symptoms may be interpreted as indigestion, the flu, a pulled muscle, or food poisoning. The irony of delaying treatment is caused in part by the mixed messages given to the public. On one hand, the signs and symptoms of heart attack are well publicized because it is assumed that people will . . . seek help early. On the other hand, people are reluctant to go to the hospital emergency room or "bother" their physicians with seemingly minor complaints.

RESEARCH BRIEF

Parshall, M. B. (1999). Adult emergency visits for chronic cardiorespiratory disease: Does dyspnea matter? Nursing Research, 48(March-April), 2.

Dyspnea is among the most common reasons for those with respiratory disease to visit emergency departments (EDs). However, little is known about how characteristics of dyspnea are associated with ED visits and disposition, and how associations differ across respiratory disease diagnoses. The goal of the study was to characterize ED visits for those with chronic cardiorespiratory disease in which dyspnea was a prominent symptom. Visit urgency, medications, and disposition were all examined. Design was cross-sectional descriptive-exploratory method, with data from the 1992 National Hospital Ambulatory Care Survey used. Diagnoses examined include asthma (n = 395), chronic obstructive pulmonary disease (COPD, n = 239), and congestive heart failure (CHF, n = 329), and mixed and restrictive chronic lung diseases (n = 18 and n = 14) were analyzed. Results indicated that despite the cause, dyspnea was the most common cause for ED visits. Dyspnea associated with COPD and CHF was twice as likely to result in admissions to the hospital from ED. Dyspnea related to asthma, even when controlling for age, did not significantly affect admission rates. Further findings indicated that dyspnea resulted in two to three times greater likelihood of receiving intravenous fluids, which was significant for influencing inpatient admission. Reports of dyspnea were linked to likelihood of inpatient admission from ED.

Losses may be the first awareness of chronic disease processes taking hold. Fear of **loss** sets in quickly and is accompanied by awareness and understanding of chronic disease processes (Schaefer, 1995). Losses associated with chronic illness may include fear, social status, self-concept, self-esteem, role, family support, recognition by the health care community, and loss of independence related to financial and personal issues. Uncertainty coupled with numerous losses make chronic illness particularly devastating for clients who also face the challenges of an evolving disease process. Those with chronic heart disease describe feelings of physical incapacity that adversely affect their whole life situation. Fear, anxiety, fatigue, pain, grief, astonishment, anger, dependence, hope, and hopelessness are identified by those with chronicity.

Losses and resulting sorrow may lead to development of chronic sorrow, which evolves from grief emerging from continual loss during the trajectory of an illness or disability. For example, those with Parkinson's disease, a slowly developing, progressive neurological disorder, and their spouses often experience chronic sorrow. Losses triggering sorrow include loss of future plans, restrictions on social life, inability to travel, and decreased ability to participate in hobbies (Box 23-1) (Lindgren, 1996).

The meaning of chronic illness to individuals and to society varies widely. Individuals may undertake to control chronic physical or psychiatric illnesses using strict adherence to treatment regimens or may eschew traditional health care practices for nontraditional methods. Control of health care behaviors, however, does not always relate to successful outcomes, and some chronic diseases are difficult to manage even with current therapy. Chronic renal failure and diabetes are examples in which excellent adherence to prescribed dietary and medical regimens does not always produce either optimal control or increased life span (Miller, 1991).

Adjustment to losses becomes a recurrent theme in many chronic illnesses, but each loss may represent a singular and significant experience that must be grieved. Diagnosis of chronic illness may result in releases of powerful emotions, including

BOX 23-1 JANET RENO: A PUBLIC EXPERIENCE WITH PARKINSON'S DISEASE

Attorney General Janet Reno has served as the United States' top law enforcer, with the longest tenure in the history of the office. Since 1995, she has also lived with Parkinson's disease, with little self-acknowledgment of the affects on her demanding professional role as U.S. Attorney General. Reno makes no effort to hide her tremors and has continued to embrace her responsibility with the same vigor and tenacity. By being public with a disease that has in the past been hidden and restrictive, she has moved forward for all persons who have such a chronic illness.

denial, shock, depression, and suicidal ideation. Consider the following example of a woman with chronic illness:

> I wanted to go jump in front of a car, and I can remember one day staying home. I was just so depressed that my husband got very alarmed and took off a day of work to stay with me because he was concerned about what I might do. As I thought about jumping in front of a car, I thought it would be my luck just to be maimed (Wolf, 1994, p. 372).

By trying to protect herself from facing the reality that something is wrong, she pretends not to be ill and hopes that people will not notice her intrusive symptoms (Wolf, 1994).

• •

He who has health has hope, and he who has hope has everything.

Arabian proverb

• •

The socialization process ensures that adults will be able to assume roles recognized as necessary for members of society and for continuation of society. Socialization in children and adolescents with chronic illness can also present problems. For example, celiac disease and the dietary control it requires to maintain health have many far-reaching effects on both the ill child and the family.

Not all chronic illnesses are physical in nature; therefore, abilities and determination, which are aspects of personality, may also be compromised in cases of chronic mental illness. In addition, mental illness carries social stigma not as commonly related to physical problems, so supports that are readily available to some chronically ill persons are not universally available to those with mental illness. Geriatric depression, a commonly noted condition in elders with chronic illness, is associated with lower quality of life (Small, Birkett, Meyers, Koran, Bystritsky, & Nemeroff, 1996). Geriatric depression was found to respond well to treatment. Medication provided relief to elders with depression as frequently as younger clients in a comparison group without chronic illness.

Younger individuals also face stigma with chronic physical or mental illness. A woman with asthma shares the following:

> I was really embarrassed so I was trying to pretend that I wasn't short of breath. So I'd get up and turn around for a minute so that they wouldn't see. When I finally caught my breath, I'd start lecturing again . . . I hid the inhaler in my pocket and went to the ladies room; I always hid it from my employer and my teachers (Wolf, 1994).

Another woman with ulcerative colitis recalls her feelings:

> I never wanted to be stigmatized as someone who has a chronic problem or who is labeled as a chronic disease-type person. I've known people who just call out sick. I've never wanted to be stigmatized as one who abused sick time in that way (Wolf, 1994).

Power and Powerlessness

Power can be equated to individual possession of adequate resources enabling the chronically ill to be in control of their lives or in substantial control of important aspects of their lives (Miller, 1991). Resources include perceptions of power, which unfold with other inner attributes, and coping strategies that

emerge as a consequence of diminished health capacity and confronting of adversity (Miller, 1991).

Powerlessness is a nonadaptive coping mechanism resulting from loss of self, loss of self-esteem, loss of autonomy, and loss of hope. Chronic illness may result in additional losses without appropriate health care interventions that are sensitive to needs of individuals with ongoing challenges, uncertainty, and suffering for prolonged intervals. During illness, it is the fear of loss of the whole or a part of the body that is a focus of great psychological concern (Smith, 1974). Survival of chronically ill individuals depends, in some measure, on individual ability and determination to endure aspects of suffering for long periods. Community nurses may help alleviate powerlessness by incorporating presence, coping enhancement, and hope instillation.

Caring for Persons with Long-Term Health Problems

Knowledge of clients' perceptions of care is essential to the community health nurse who plans, coordinates, and evaluates their care. Maintaining an optimal quality of life becomes a paramount consideration when the future is uncertain, and limitations are both recognized and anticipated. Caring for a "heart attack" is very different from caring for a person with a chronic, limiting condition that imposes a major impact on lifestyle. In chronic cardiac disease, there is none of the drama associated with the emergent condition of myocardial infarction, nor is the "quick fix" available. Instead, there are implications for long-term lifestyle changes, including regaining a sense of control over one's life (Johnson, 1991). Limitations and permanent disability can be daunting prospects to those who never considered themselves to be vulnerable to long-term health issues. Facing devastating physical limitations may cause individuals to question their future and to wonder if they are able to tolerate the rigors of chronicity (Johnson, 1991). A challenging example is chronic pain resulting from development or deterioration of many conditions related to

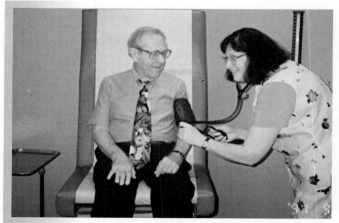

Chapter author, Dr. Edith Hilton, conducts an assessment on an elder client with heart disease.

CASE STUDY

Osteoporosis

Mrs. A., one of the 10 million women in the United States with osteoporosis, was discharged to her home 3 weeks after having her right hip replaced. She was in a long-term care facility for 2 weeks after she was released from the hospital and was happy to be home again, among familiar surroundings. Mrs. A. had just passed her 77th birthday when she fell getting out of her bathtub at home. She managed to reach the telephone and called a neighbor, who came over and helped get Mrs. A. to the hospital in an ambulance. Although always ambulatory, Mrs. A. spent the next week recovering in bed from hip replacement surgery. She had physical therapy twice daily and ambulated with assistance in her room. She was surprised to learn from her physician that she had experienced a significant overall loss of bone.

Factors contributing to loss of bone density include small bones, smoking, low calcium intake, early menopause without estrogen replacement, amenorrhea, lack of exercise, and a familial history of osteoporosis. Other factors related to osteoporosis include chronic diseases, excessive alcohol consumption, and eating disorders (Dowd & Cavalieri, 1999).

After sustaining the fracture, suspicions that Mrs. A. had weakened and fragile bones were confirmed by bone densitometry that was arranged by her community health nurse. Medicare recently added bone mass measurements to its benefits for those fitting risk criteria, so Mrs. A.'s bone density scan was covered. Her osteoporosis could have been diagnosed much earlier if she had known the risks associated with its development. Her community health nurse explained symptoms and factors contributing to development of osteoporosis. Looking back, Mrs. A. recalled one symptom in particular: losing her height. She had been 5'5" and was now just over 5'1". The community health nurse also explained how to prevent falls and directed Mrs. A. to an equipment supply store, where she ordered a metal grab-bar for her bathtub, which would reduce the possibility of future falls while bathing. Now home, Mrs. A. continued calcium supplements and estrogen replacement therapy initiated in the hospital and planned to start a walking program at the senior center near her house. Her progress will be monitored for the next few weeks by her community health nurse.

Source: Dowd & Cavalieri, 1999.

---

aging. Management of chronic pain is essential to avoid debilitating physical limitations (Dellasega & Kiser, 1997).

Nurses can be instrumental in facilitating adaptation to chronic disease processes and can promote optimal health within a framework of disease-imposed limitations. Nurses can support client-generated activities that sustain endurance and alleviate suffering (Morse & Carter, 1995). Community-based nurses are in an optimal position to identify and promote adaptation to chronic disease processes, resulting in fewer limitations.

Caring for Chronically Ill Persons in the Community

Acute phases of chronic illnesses are managed in a hospital or nursing home by health care professionals, but the majority of ongoing care takes place in the home. Because the needs of chronically ill persons often exceed resources, community health nurses must seek solutions to care for the chronically ill in the most cost-effective manner using resources of the extended family. Chronic illnesses generally are not fatal, but they are disabling by virtue of their progression and include the side effects of social isolation and fatigue. Despite the nonfatal nature of chronic diseases, they erode quality of life and diminish individual, family, and community resources.

The suffering that accompanies chronic health problems is increased by uncertainty, by remissions and exacerbations, by depleted or inadequate coping mechanisms, and by fatigue, which is a factor to consider when planning appropriate activities. The most predictable outcome to chronic illness is unpredictability (Schaefer, 1995). Client autonomy characterizes the current era of health care, which is safeguarded by nursing (Miller, 1991). Client quality of life is an appropriate consideration in chronic illness (Pearlman & Uhlmann, 1991). Assessment of quality of life is directly related to goals of nursing care, including promotion of health and restoration of maximal functioning by the client (Varricchio, 1990).

These goals become increasingly important when thinking about cancer as an acute event shifts to consideration of cancer as a chronic condition. Increasing numbers of adult cancer survivors have indicated to the health care community that related to treatment choice, quality of life is as important as overall therapeutic effect. Clients are concerned with the impact of cancer therapy on their daily lives (Varricchio, 1990). Similarly, children with spina bifida maintain quality of life through prevention of complications, minimization of additional disability, maximization of functional independence, and inclusion in society in which their developmental issues are addressed (Homan, 1997).

BOX 23-2 CURRENT ROLE FUNCTIONS: NURSING INTERVENTIONS

Active listening	Grief work facilitation	Referral
Anticipatory guidance	Health system guidance	Reminiscence therapy
Body image enhancement	Home maintenance assistance	Respite care
Body mechanics promotion	Hope installation	Risk identification
Calming technique	Humor	Role enhancement
Caregiver support	Immunization/vaccination	Security enhancement
Client education	management	Self-awareness enhancement
Client contracting	Incision site care	Self-care assistance
Client rights protection	Infant care	Self-esteem enhancement
Coping enhancement	Infection control	Sibling support
Counseling	Infection prevention	Simple guided imagery
Crisis intervention	Infection protection	Simple massage
Culture brokerage	Learning facilitation	Simple relaxation therapy
Decision-making support	Limit setting	Skin care
Discharge planning	Medication administration	Skin surveillance
Dying care	Medication management	Sleep enhancement
Emotional support	Memory training	Smoking cessation assistance
Environmental management: comfort, safety, violence prevention	Milieu therapy	Socialization enhancement
	Music therapy	Spiritual support
Exercise promotion: ambulation, balance, joint mobility, muscle control	Mutual goal setting	Support group
	Pain management	Surveillance
	Peripheral sensation management	Sustenance support
Fall prevention	Positioning	Teaching
Family integrity promotion	Preparatory sensory information	Therapy group
Family involvement	Presence	Touch
Family mobilization	Progressive muscle relaxation	Truth telling
Family process maintenance	Recreation therapy	Values clarification

Current Role Functions

Community health nurses caring for individuals with chronic illness attempt to mitigate the effects of chronic, disabling conditions for individuals and communities by functioning in many roles in established and nontraditional settings. Settings include freestanding clinics, homeless shelters, shopping malls, schools, apartments, hospitals, churches, rural settings, urban residences, and wherever health care needs occur.

Community nursing roles include caregiver, educator, counselor, advocate, case manager, researcher, and role model (Fraley, 1992). Nurses identify risk factors associated with chronic diseases and anticipate complications arising from acute illnesses superimposed on chronicity. Furthermore, nurses provide direction for modification of current health policy to reflect changing priorities and identify silent and underserved groups of chronically ill.

Community health nurses may intervene to facilitate use of adaptive coping mechanisms. Coping enhancement involves incorporation of social support, an essential coping mechanism

used by individuals with multiple sclerosis that is believed to mediate and buffer effects of stressors associated with chronic illness. Social support acts as a buffer in stroke and heart disease (Friedman, 1993; Glass, Matchar, Belyea, & Feussner, 1992). Social support and adherence/metabolic control in adolescents with insulin-dependent diabetes were found to be related, indicating that social support is essential to adherence to required diabetic regimens and produces better metabolic control than that achieved with use of metabolic regimens without social supports (Burroughs, Harris, Pontious, & Santiago, 1997).

Another nursing intervention that may mitigate feelings of hopelessness and loss is spiritual support, which is also identified as a helpful coping mechanism by chronically ill populations (Miller, 1992). Use of spiritual support may provide comfort and alleviate prolonged grieving.

One intervention that is helpful in chronic pain relief is guided imagery. The community health nurse may intervene with imagery if traditional methods fail to provide adequate pain control. *Imagery* is defined as "a mental process involving use of images or fantasy that can be used to develop cognitive control and promote stress reduction" (Miller, 1991); it has been successfully used in pain control and relaxation therapy.

Both adults and children adopt coping mechanisms in an effort to adjust or adapt to chronic illness. Childhood mechanisms include use of regressive behaviors, enhancement of self-esteem, and use of social supports (Miller, 1991).

Future Role Functions

Nurses will function as change agents, advocates, professional caregivers, managers of care, and role models in the future. The role of prevention becomes more important every year. Nursing interventions help delineate areas in which nurses have specialty knowledge and expertise. Some nursing interventions that have had limited applications in research may be explicated further in future clinical investigations, thereby providing additional support for practice (Box 23-2).

Change agent

As the number of nurse practitioners entering primary care within the community multiply, community health nurses will have increasing opportunities to identify changing needs that require immediate attention. Long waiting periods to access primary care will be shortened, and turnaround times for maintenance care activities will decrease. Nurses will be an important source of support, facilitating better and faster follow-up care and more in-depth prevention activities for all disabled and chronically ill persons.

Advocate

Advocating for chronically ill persons may result in provision and expansion of services where they are currently unavailable or are of limited availability. By increasing necessary services, additional supports and effective interventions may be identified in the future to capitalize on use of extended familial caregivers and community-based volunteers. Political activity associated with enabling increased access to health-promoting activities may be of increasing importance in the future, as the population of chronically ill persons increase in the new millennium.

Professional caregivers

An area of great need will be that of professional caregiver, who helps chronically ill persons cope. Coping with chronic illness may mean development of personal and societal resources as a means of enhancing quality of life and survival. Development of personal resources may include increasing coping abilities to endure painful or prolonged aspects of disease (Morse & Carter, 1995). Adjustment to losses associated with chronic diseases becomes essential. Adjustment entails coping with physical symptoms and uncertainty. Facilitating adjustment may include use of several nursing interventions, such as family integrity promotion, decision-making support, and mutual goal setting (Luckmann, 1997). Role modeling behaviors of

the community health nurse will include smoking cessation, weight control, and physical fitness to encourage preventive behaviors in the chronically ill. Health teaching will increase in importance, and nurses in community settings will be sought to initiate effective educational programs specifically designed to address the needs of chronically ill persons.

Interdisciplinary Roles and Responsibilities

As care providers, case managers, and advocates, community health nurses work as an integral part of interdisciplinary health care teams. Other team members include paraprofessional and professional individuals. Some of these individuals will have no direct contact with or knowledge of the chronically ill client. Others will have day-to-day contact and will depend on the community health nurse for essential information and opinions. Use of the rehabilitation interdisciplinary model frequently adds to the team concept of care that has long been in place and effectively used by health care personnel (Hickey, 1992). Rehabilitative treatments of clients depend on efforts of many health care specialists and demand that clients be actively engaged in their treatment protocols. Some treatments require a long time and are well conducted in the community (Haas & MacKenzie, 1993). Community health nurses will continue to have an active role in supporting rehabilitation efforts in chronically ill populations to optimize functional independence and self-reliance.

Financing Costs of Chronic Illness

Health care costs generally are set by formulas put forth by federal and state governments (Hickey, 1992). Medicare, Medicaid, and third-party payers are involved both in establishing fee schedules and in cost management efforts that determine "who gets what" in terms of services. Both direct and indirect health care costs are to be considered in estimating the magnitude of chronic illness. Chronic illness costs society millions of dollars annually and results in lost productivity (Clark, 1996). Many chronic illnesses are rising in cost as more people survive longer because of earlier and more accurate diagnosis. Cancer and heart disease are examples of this phenomenon, with heart disease alone affecting an estimated 68 million (Clark, 1996).

Age and chronic illness are positively related. An example of this relationship exists between age and malignant neoplasms, which are the second most common cause of death among older Americans, except in those 85 years and older, in whom cerebrovascular disease takes second place after heart disease (Valanis, 1992). Persons older than 65 represent a rapidly growing sector of the world's population. Elderly persons have the highest rates of hospitalizations and visits to physicians in the nation, even though they experience the lowest rates of acute illnesses (Valanis, 1992). The cost of caring for individuals is a substantial concern for chronically ill persons and for those who experience the long-term financial **burden** for needed care.

Funding initiatives for community-based support vary. Some private funds are available through service organizations and religious and secular groups. Public funds for community supports for home-based caregivers vary widely from region to region. In many geographic areas with well-developed support systems in place in the community, home-based caregivers do not frequently use services that may be most beneficial (Doyal, 1995). Use and availability of supports affect indirect costs of caring for chronically ill persons. Additional or indirect costs of caring for the chronically ill include time lost from work in the case of home-based caregivers, resulting in lost productivity. Cost of hospitalizations secondary to exacerbation of symptoms, as well as medications, supplies, and treatments, are also indirect costs. One example is diabetic supplies, which can cost hundreds of dollars monthly; this cost is often offset, at least in part, by federal tax dollars. Prioritizing these issues is a source of debate in political arenas, as health care costs and increasing numbers of chronically ill persons require new funding sources.

Planning for health care reform based on the current number of chronically ill persons is a complex matter. Recent discoveries in technology, pharmacology, and professional research are changing the future of chronicity. The number of chronically ill persons is expected to rise because of increasingly effective symptom control, resulting in longer lives. Health care costs appear to have decreased in the past decade with the advent of managed care; however, evidence is lacking that conclusively demonstrates that money was appropriately saved with the use of cost-cutting measures.

Many Americans continue to lack basic health insurance, and their inability to anticipate improved health care may result in additional numbers of chronically ill persons because of neglected preventive and maintenance measures. Health care is currently fragmented, and despite efforts under way to fund essential health care services for children, adults, and the elderly will continue to be uninsured and underinsured (Lubkin, 1995).

Chronically ill persons are particularly vulnerable to reforms in health care policy that may decrease or eliminate essential services, including home-based nursing care to improve and maintain health status. They are often unable to effectively advocate for themselves and rely on health care professionals to secure needed services for them. If fragmentation of health care continues, chronically ill persons will experience increased difficulties in accessing adequate health care.

Self-Determination: The Client as Partner

Chronically ill clients often experience perceptions of life quality that are not shared by physicians. Elderly, chronically ill outpatients may perceive their lives to have acceptable quality, despite their physician's perceptions to the contrary (Pearlman & Uhlmann, 1991). Research suggests that clients' perceived emotional, socioeconomic, intellectual, and physical functioning affect their perceptions of quality of life (Pearlman & Uhlmann, 1991). Quality of care may directly affect quality of life. Those who experience adequate management of symptoms and undesirable side effects may rate their quality of life as acceptable or better. However, in cases of uncontrolled relief from chronic symptoms, quality of life will decrease markedly.

Sensitivity in Community-Based Caring

Seven million American households are now involved in assisting elderly persons with either personal or household management issues (Picot, 1996). All ethnic, racial, and gender groups are involved in caring for the chronically ill. Community health nurses are in the unique position of entering private homes to render or assist in care provision. Each of these groups and individuals has issues and expectations that may present unique challenges to health care workers in provision of gender, ethnically, and racially sensitive care. Care rendered in ethnically and culturally sensitive ways will enhance nurses' efforts to individualize important interventions.

Gender-Specific Considerations

Overall, women live longer than men. In addition, more women than men function as caregivers, possibly as a result of women's more robust health and the roles that society has imposed on

A CONVERSATION WITH . . .

Rose is an 87-year-old woman who has been dependent on others for many years for her daily care. She is unable to ambulate and is in a wheelchair. She lives in a long-term care facility and experiences chronic pain from arthritis in nearly all her joints. She has been in arthritic pain for many years and has used different drugs at intervals, but she continues to experience severe pain that interrupts all other activities. She grimaces as she moves in her wheelchair, and speaks about her pain:

The pain is always there. I would like to be without it just for a day, now and then. I've really forgotten how it is to just get up and do for yourself. I never wanted to have to ask other people to help me all the time, but lately, that's how it is. I'm so tired all the time. The pain keeps me awake, and when I fall asleep, if I try to turn over, it reminds me right away by waking me up! I have the pain all the time, more or less. I take some of the arthritis medicine for it, and it helps a good bit, but it always wears off, and then it feels like the pain comes back real strong. Either sittin' or standin' it bothers me, and I can't walk any distance at all. My niece comes to take me out some, but I don't always feel like going. Course, its real nice to have her come, it's just that I can't go like I used to. We both miss getting out together, but then, at my age, I'm expecting to have pain. They all tell me you don't die from it, but it sure keeps you from doing like you want to.

—Rose

them (Doyal, 1995). Women as chronically ill individuals also tend to rely more on daughters, sisters, mothers, and friends than spouses when chronic illness occurs. Fewer women have spouses to receive care from, and women are abandoned more frequently by their spouses during chronic illness (Doyal, 1995). Accordingly, women use compensated caregivers in greater numbers than do men (Doyal, 1995). Women may have difficulty articulating preferences in aspects of care and need to be reassured, offered options, and be consulted about all facets of their care.

Issues Nurses Encounter in the Community

Professional issues encountered in providing and managing community-based care for the chronically ill include understanding long- and short-terms goals, patterns of disease progression, resource allocation, development of support systems, education, and home-based caregiver roles. In daily care, routines provide a framework and format for use of the nursing process. Continuous supervision by nurses generally is not needed by all chronically ill individuals, but activities of daily living may be supported by **home-based caregivers** (Lubkin, 1995). These individuals, who are often relatives or close friends of the individual with chronic illness, provide valuable services that enable chronically ill persons to retain autonomy in their homes. Paraprofessional caregivers who work in the community and function with a great deal of autonomy include nurse aids, therapy assistants, and transport staff, who facilitate activities of daily living, maximal independence, and travel within the community. The home setting is desirable for many chronically ill persons and supports self-identity and self-determination, whereas institutional settings may depersonalize and socially isolate some chronically ill persons from familiar surroundings, personal belongings, and cherished supports. Institutional settings may be desirable in situations in which home-based caregiving is not realistic.

Supporting Home-Based Caregivers

In addition to provision and direction of care, an additional role of importance for community health nurses is providing support to home-based caregivers. Daily provision of care to the chronically ill can be both challenging and rewarding for home-based caregivers, and support systems, both formal and informal, may be necessary for a positive experience. Anticipation of needs and understanding of disease progression make nurses invaluable assets to home-based caregivers, who may have unrealistic or unachievable goals. For example, home-based caregivers of those with chronic obstructive pulmonary disease need to understand that perceived quality of life and use of coping mechanisms may contribute more to comfort and adaptation than use of oxygen and medications (Herbert & Gregor, 1997).

Non-nursing caregivers provide care and services for chronically ill persons in numerous community and institutional settings. Familial caretakers most frequently include women in the roles of wife, mother, daughter, sibling, and grandmother. Often, these female caregivers have chronic or unmet health needs them-

selves and must subordinate their own needs to render care to their relative on a continuing basis (Doyal, 1995). Continuing care can be extremely demanding and exhausting if the familial caregiver is unrelieved. Neglect of self may develop in these circumstances, and depression, decreased overall health, and exhaustion may follow. A chronically ill woman describes her role as caretaker:

> I had angina and coronary artery disease for three years while I was taking care of my husband before he died. My problems were put on the back burner; he was a difficult man. And then after that, it did get worse. Now I think that it was just time for it to get worse (Wolf, 1994, p. 402).

It is important to anticipate caregiver burnout and suggest alternatives to prevent it from developing. Community-based programs and resources have been developed in some areas to

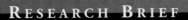

RESEARCH BRIEF

Calderon, V., & Tennstedt, S. L. (1998). Ethnic differences in the expression of caregiver burden: Results of a qualitative study. Journal of Gerontological Social Work, 30(1–2), 159–178.

A qualitative study was undertaken to detect differences in the way caregivers in three ethnic groups (African American, Puerto Rican, and Caucasian) describe their reactions to caregiving. An ethnographic method was appropriately used to focus on scientific descriptions of cultural groups. The stratified, random sample consisted of 18 caregivers who were selected from a sample of 409 caregivers. All interviews were conducted in informants' homes, with one exception. Informed consent was ensured, and data were collected through use of CES-D and guided, unstructured conversations. Data were analyzed using content analysis to discover themes and meanings expressed by caregivers.

Findings revealed differences in expression of burden, both by ethnicity and gender within ethnicity groups. Generally, caregiving was associated with negative feelings and situations. Almost all Caucasians described their situations negatively. African Americans described their situations as demanding and time-consuming. Puerto Rican caregivers reported that it was difficult to meet the demands of the care required. Several reported caregiving to be a rewarding and satisfying experience. These individuals had an extended network of support in which there were other people involved in the care and assistance of the disabled. Level of outside support was key in decreasing caregiver burden. The authors state that their findings can assist practitioners to better understand the cultural idiosyncrasies that are important in developing a culturally sensitive plan.

help familial caregivers take care of themselves. Respite and episodic care of chronically ill persons enable these caregivers to receive physical and psychological support at periodic intervals, while nurses and other members of the health care team assume responsibility for care of the chronically ill individual. Both of these options are available through some veteran's hospitals, nursing homes, public hospitals, and community health agencies. It is notable to remember, however, that these services are available only to provide temporary relief to community-based, familial caregivers. If burdens of giving full-time care exceed the abilities and resources of the familial or home-based caregiver, institutionalization becomes the primary source of care.

Parents of children with cystic fibrosis expend enormous amounts of time as familial caregivers. Caring activities can monopolize time allocated for other activities normally engaged in by caretakers. Time becomes reordered, reprioritized, and disrupted for both the ill individual and the familial caregiver (Strauss, 1975). Issues encountered by familial caregivers include other family commitments, personal physical health, recreational needs, fear of using needed equipment, stress, loss of independence, role change, loss of privacy, decreased well-being, depression, negative feelings, physical strain, anxiety, anger, guilt, loss of self, and caregiver burnout.

The effects of chronic illness on families are a major problem for some parental caregivers of children who attempt to cope with illness by adapting. Parental caregivers who lack professional help and support in the care of their children with cystic fibrosis may feel burdened and overwhelmed (Coyne, 1997). These feelings may lead to the development of abusive behaviors. Home-based caregivers of chronically ill children and adults may perpetrate abuse because of feelings of overwhelming frustration, social isolation, and powerlessness. Some family systems may have characteristics that promote abuse, including lack of family support, familial caregiver reluctance, overcrowding, isolation, family burdens, marital conflict, or differing opinions about institutionalization (Lubkin, 1995). In chronic illness, abuse may be obvious or covert. Neglect, self-neglect, exploitation, and coercion may not be readily apparent, and the community health nurse needs to be sensitive to suspected cases of abuse (Luckmann, 1997). Use of several familial caregivers may relieve frustration and feelings of isolation that underlie abuse. Another important factor in diminishing burdens of familial caregiving is engagement in social interaction, fun, and recreation, which may enhance the caregiver's sense of well-being (Thompson, Futterman, Gallagher-Thompson, Rose, & Lovett, 1993). Caregiver burnout has been linked with lack of assistance in day-to-day activities and should be examined proactively to incorporate supports necessary to benefit both familial or home-based caregiver and client.

Hospice Care

Hospice provides care and support to terminally ill persons and their families in the final stages of life and supports death with respect and dignity. For those with chronic illnesses, great comfort may be obtained by having hospice services provided within the home. This allows the familial caregiver to have a rest from caring activities and to have an opportunity to consider relevant quality-of-life issues. The role of community health nurses in hospice varies but usually includes referral through the attending physician, facilitation of transfer of care of the chronically ill client, and consultation as needed. Community-based hospice nurses may also provide education, coordination, and support services.

Institutionalization

Chronically ill persons who elect to receive institution-based care are relatively few; however, they may be frail and require care that is not available in the community. Projections of institutional provision of care, which currently includes fewer than 2 million individuals, is expected to increase rapidly over the next 40 years as Baby Boomers age and experience health problems. This number is expected to more than double to 4.6 million by 2040. Of the over-65 age group, 1% to 5% are estimated to be in long-term care facilities (Stanley & Beare, 1995).

Long-term care facilities provide essential services to some chronically ill persons, but there are several drawbacks to the current system. One of the most well-known and least desirable practices in long-term care facilities is use of physical restraints; use increases with age and degree of cognitive impairment of the client (Stanley & Beare, 1995). Both physical restraints and bed rails are used in the interest of safety and to prevent clients from wandering away to unsupervised areas. Restraints reduce falls and injuries, but they also have the effect of reducing mobility, inhibiting communication, preventing individual reorientation, and restricting patterns of socialization within and without the facility. In facilities with decreased use of physical restraints, security and safety of residents is enhanced by use of cameras, alarm systems, and staff surveillance. However, falls and client injuries continue to be a major problem in institutional settings because of staffing levels, client age, and the physical condition of clients. Many clients are frail and require frequent assistance with all activities of daily living. Other issues surrounding long-term care include loss of privacy, decreased choices in routines, diminished autonomy, and adverse relocation consequences (Stanley & Beare, 1995).

Facility selection is an important decision, and community health nurses should support consultation of the chronically ill client with family members who may assist in the process. Ideally, the chronically ill client should decide to move to a long-term care facility out of choice, rather than being forced to do so by a crisis (Stanley & Beare, 1995). The physical environment, accessibility, nurse-to-client ratio, friendliness of the staff, availability of medical and support services, cost, and location will all be of concern to the client considering placement.

Both private and publicly funded facilities for long-term care of the chronically ill exist. Long-term care facilities with religious affiliations are available in many geographic areas and may be Medicare certified for reimbursement purposes. Nonsectarian facilities are also available and may be affiliated with state or local governments. Both public and private institutions must adhere to standards of care that are put forth and monitored by local, state, and federal agencies. Areas of regulation in all long-term care facilities include resident rights; admission, transfer, and discharge rights; resident behavior and facility practice; administration; physical environment, infection control, quality of life, resident assessment; quality of care; nursing; rehabilitation; and medical services (Stanley & Beare, 1995).

Nursing home selection may cause emotional distress to chronically ill persons, who may have decreased coping skills and decreased ability to withstand a major lifestyle change. Often, the community health nurse is aware of plans to move an individual to a nursing home. Elderly persons with chronic health problems may experience severe adjustment issues related to perceived and actual losses, feelings of powerlessness, and finally, despair. Coping with these changes will require sensitive support

and time to process changes. Rapid adjustment to lifestyle changes should not be expected.

Managed care initiatives for chronically ill persons may have guidelines governing time allowed for care and services provided in nursing homes. In acute care settings, use of care maps provides tools for systematic monitoring for completeness and cost savings in care. Managed care uses a preset fee-for-service schedule in facilities that are contractually associated with the managed care company. Specific numbers of days and hours of specialty services are approved before the stay and are reviewed concurrently by managed care staff. Managed care issues are important to chronically ill persons because of its cost-restrictive features over traditional insurance and because essential services may be denied if not clearly justified.

CONCLUSION

The number of chronically ill persons is increasing and is expected to continue to rise during the next four decades as Baby Boomers age and more conditions become treatable. Women outlive men by an average of 7 years and are adversely affected by chronic illness more severely and more often than men (Stanley & Beare, 1995). Chronically ill women are more likely to lack familial caregivers than are men, and increasing numbers of chronically ill women require community-based and institutionally provided services to survive. Chronically ill persons face many issues of loss, uncertainty, isolation, and fear. Accordingly, coping abilities of chronically ill persons may be compromised, and they are less adaptable to lifestyle changes.

Because of increasing numbers of single-parent homes, working mothers, and societal mobility that contributes to

changes in extended families, fewer individuals function as caregivers for chronically ill adults and children. Home-based and familial caregivers may experience problems with resources of time, energy, conflicting responsibilities, feelings of abandonment, and social isolation.

Traditionally, community health nurses care for chronically ill persons. The current climate in health care services and distribution of health care resources makes continued provision of care to the chronically ill a challenge. As advocates and leaders in health care, community health nurses must ensure appropriate and effective provision of services to chronically ill persons expands through education, through political activity, and by involvement in health care policy and research.

CRITICAL THINKING ACTIVITIES

1. Discuss power and powerlessness. What aspects of each are essential to consider in planning care for the chronically ill? Consider how the same chronic disease may affect perceptions of power and powerlessness differently in children and adults.

2. Think of an image that would help you forget about the unpleasant sensation of nausea. Describe an image that might help you to focus on positive thoughts about disease outcomes like gaining strength or taking control.

3. Analyze health teaching strategies that enhance retention of new material. Think of two specific techniques you can use to involve chronically ill children in prevention activities. Contrast these activities with those of an elderly adult. Develop a teaching plan that incorporates use of visual aids for each population.

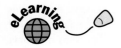

Explore Community Health Nursing on the web! To learn more about the topics in this chapter, use the passcode provided to access your exclusive web site: http://communitynursing.jbpub.com
If you do not have a passcode, you can obtain one at this site.

REFERENCES

Burroughs, T. E., Harris, M. A., Pontious, S. L., & Santiago, J. V. (1997). Research on social support in adolescents with IDDM: A critical review. *Diabetes Educator, 23*, 4.

Calderon, V., & Tennstedt, S. L. (1998). Ethnic differences in the expression of care giver burden: Results of a qualitative study. *Journal of Gerontological Social Work, 30*.

Clark, M. J. (1996). *Nursing in the community* (2nd. ed.). Stanford, CT: Appleton & Lange.

Colliton, M. A. (1981). The spiritual dimension of nursing. In I. L. Beland & J. Y. Passos, *Clinical nursing: Pathophysiological and psychosocial approaches* (4th ed.). New York: Macmillan.

Coyne, I. T. (1997). Chronic illness: The importance of support for families caring for a child with cystic fibrosis. *Journal of Clinical Nursing, 6*, 2.

Daly, J. M. (1993). *NIC Interventions Linked to NANDA Diagnoses. Iowa Intervention Project.*

Davidhizar, R., & Shearer, R. (1997). Helping the client with chronic disability achieve high-level wellness. *Rehabilitation Nursing, 22*, 3.

Dellasega, C., & Kiser, C. L. (1997). Pharmacologic approaches to chronic pain in the older adult. *Nurse Practitioner: American Journal of Primary Health Care, 22*, 5.

Department of Health and Human Services (DHHS). (2000). *Healthy People 2010: Conference edition.* Washington, DC: U.S. Government Printing Office.

Dowd, R., & Cavalieri, R. J. (1999). Help your patient live with osteoporosis. *American Journal of Nursing, 99*, 4.

Doyal, L. (1995). *What makes women sick.* New Brunswick, NJ: Rutgers University Press.

Dreher, M. C. (1996). Nursing: A cultural phenomenon. *Reflections, 22*(4), 4.

Eakes, G. G., Burke, M. L., & Hainsworth, M. A. (1998). Middle-range theory of chronic sorrow. *Image: The Journal of Nursing Scholarship, 30*(2), 179–184.

Fraley, A. M. (1992). *Nursing and the disabled across the lifespan.* Sudbury, MA: Jones & Bartlett.

Friedman, M. M. (1993). Social support sources and psychological well-being in older women with heart disease. *Research in Nursing and Health, 16*.

Gates, M. F. & Lackey, N. R. (1998). Youngsters caring for adults with cancer. *Image: The Journal of Nursing Scholarship, 30*, 1.

Glass, T. A., Matchar, D. B., Belyea, M., & Feussner, J. R. (1992). Impact of social support on outcome in first stroke. *Stroke, 24*, 1.

Haas, J. F., & MacKenzie, C. A. (1993). The role of ethics in rehabilitation medicine. *American Journal of Physical Medicine and Rehabilitation, 72*, 1.

Hardy, M. E., & Conway, M. E. (1978). *Role theory: Perspectives for health professionals.* New York: Appleton-Century-Crofts.

Harris, D. K., & Cole, W. E. (1980). *Sociology of aging.* Dallas: Houghton Mifflin.

Herbert, R., & Gregor, S. (1997). Quality of life and coping strategies of clients with COPD. *Rehabilitation Nursing, 22*, 4.

Hickey, J. (1992). *The clinical practice of neurological and neurosurgical nursing.* Philadelphia: J. B. Lippincott.

Homan, S. P. (1997). Primary care for children with spina bifida. *Nurse Practitioner: American Journal of Primary Health Care, 22*, 9.

Huff, C. (1997). Celiac disease: Helping families adapt. *Gastroenterology Nursing, 20,* 3.

Johnson, J. (1991). Adjustment following a heart attack. In J. M. Morse & J. L. Johnson (Eds.), *The illness experience* (pp. 13–88). Newbury Park, CA: Sage Publications.

Klang, B., & Clyne, N. (1997). Well-being and functional ability in uremic patients before and after having started dialysis treatment. *Scandinavian Journal of Caring Sciences, 11,* 3.

Lindgren, C. L. (1996). Chronic sorrow in persons with Parkinson's disease and their spouses. *Scholarly Inquiry for Nursing Practice, 10,* 4.

Longman, A. J., Braden, C. J., & Mishel, M. H. (1997). Pattern of association over time of side-effects burden, self-help, and self-care in women with breast cancer. *Oncology Nursing Forum, 24,* 9.

Lubkin, I. M. (1995). *Chronic Illness: Impact and Interventions* (pp. 3–568). Sudbury, MA: Jones & Bartlett.

Luckmann, J. (1997). *Saunders manual of nursing care* (pp. 10–2070). Philadelphia: W. B. Saunders.

Mayo, L. (1956). *Chronic illness.* Paper presented at the meeting of the Commission on Chronic Illness, Washington, DC.

Miller, J. F. (1992). *Coping with chronic illness: Overcoming powerlessness* (2nd ed.). Philadelphia: F. A. Davis.

Miller, M. P. (1991). Factors promoting wellness in the aged person: An ethnographic study. *Advances in Nursing Science, 13*(4), 39–51.

Morse, J. M., & Carter, B. J. (1995). Strategies of enduring and the suffering of loss: Modes of comfort used by a resilient survivor. *Holistic Nursing Practice, 9,* 3.

North American Nursing Diagnosis Association (NANDA). (1992). *NANDA nursing diagnoses: Definition and classification.* St. Louis.

Picot, S. J. (1996). Family care givers: Windows into their worlds. *Reflections, 22*(4), 13–14.

Parshall, M. B. (1999). Adult emergency visits for chronic cardiorespiratory disease: Does dyspnea matter? *Nursing Research, 48* (March-April), 2.

Pearlman, R. A., & Uhlmann, R. F. (1991). Quality of life in elderly, chronically ill outpatients. *Journal of Gerontology, 46,* 2.

President's Commission for the Study of Ethical Problems in Medicine and Biomedical and Behavioral Research (1983). *Deciding to forego life-sustaining treatment.* Washington, DC: U. S. Government Printing Office.

Schaefer, K. M. (1995). Women living in paradox: Loss and discovery in chronic illness. *Holistic Nursing Practice, 9,* 3.

Small, G. W., Birkett, M., Meyers, B. S., Koran, L. M., Bystritsky, A., & Nemeroff, C. B. (1996). Impact of physical illness on quality of life and antidepressant response in geriatric major depression. *Journal of the American Geriatric Society, 44,* 10.

Smith, S. (1974). The psychology of illness. In V. A. Christopherson, P. P Coulter, & M. O. Wolanin, *Rehabilitation Nursing,* New York: McGraw-Hill.

Stanley, M., & Beare, P. G. (1995). *Gerontological nursing.* Philadelphia: F. A. Davis.

Strauss, A. L. (1975). *Chronic illness and the quality of life.* St. Louis: Mosby.

Thompson, S. C., Futterman, A. M., Gallagher-Thompson, D., Rose, J. J., & Lovett, S. B. (1993). Social support and caregiving burden in family caregivers of frail elders. *Journals of Gerontology: Social Sciences, 48,* 5.

Valanis, B. (1992). *Epidemiology in nursing and health care.* Norwalk, CT: Appleton and Lange.

Varricchio, C. G. (1990). Relevance of quality of life to clinical nursing practice. *Seminars in Oncology Nursing, 6,* 4.

Wilson, J. S. (1992). Our nation's walking wounded: The chronically ill. *Home Healthcare Nurse, 5,* 5.

Wolf, Z. R. (1994). Seeking harmony: Chronic physical illness. In P. Munhall (Ed.), *Women's Experience* (pp. 2–410). New York: National League for Nursing.

World Health Organization. (1980). *International classification of impairment, disabilities, and handicaps.* Geneva: World Health Organization.

Chapter 24

The Role of the Community Health Nurse in Disasters

Karen Saucier Lundy and Janie B. Butts

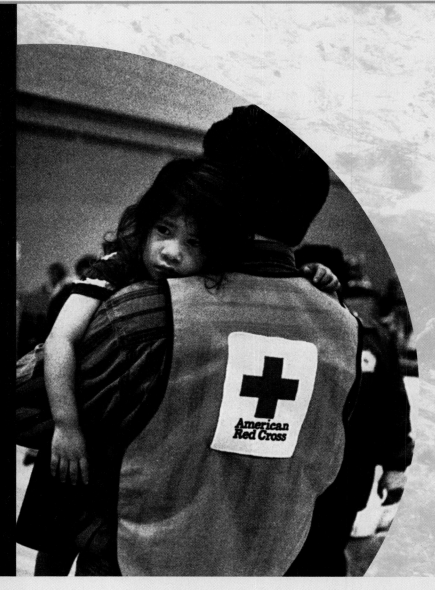

Disaster! The very word can evoke fear, panic, and a pounding heart. A major disaster occurs almost daily somewhere in the world: plane crashes, floods, hurricanes, tornadoes, fires, earthquakes, acts of terrorism, droughts, famines, and wars. The community health nurse can assist communities in preparing for disasters and limiting the damage from disasters. Communities can become stronger and healthier as a result.

QUESTIONS TO CONSIDER

After reading this chapter, answer the following questions:

1. What are the categories and types of disasters community health nurses might deal with?
2. What are the variables by which disasters can be understood?
3. What is a global disaster?
4. Who are the populations most at risk in a disaster? Why?
5. What are the stages of disaster and how does each stage impact the disaster workers and the affected population?
6. What are the steps in the disaster process?
7. What are the characteristics of a disaster plan?
8. What are the common elements of a disaster plan?
9. What is disaster response? What are the different levels of response?
10. What is disaster triage? Why and how should it be implemented?
11. What is the role of the community health nurse in the disaster relief process?
12. What specific approaches should a community health nurse use to mitigate human and material losses in a disaster?
13. What happens to the survivors in a disaster? How can a community health nurse promote recovery after a disaster?
14. What are the factors that can place individuals in a vulnerable position?
15. Why are children and elderly more at risk during a disaster? What can be done to intervene?
16. What are the sources of stress for the disaster workers and how can this be managed?

KEY TERMS

Disaster	Human-generated	Level IV response	Predisaster stage
Disaster planning	(manmade)	Major disaster	Recovery
Disaster triage	disasters	National Disaster	Reconstruction,
Emergency	Impact stage	Medical System	or rehabilitation,
Emergency stage	Interdisaster stage	(NDMS)	stage
Federal Emergency	Level I response	Natural disasters	Response
Management Agency	Level II response	Posttraumatic stress	
(FEMA)	Level III response	disorder (PTSD)	

The United States has experienced unprecedented disasters since the late 1980s, which include major earthquakes, hurricanes, tropical storms, floods, landslides, volcanic eruptions, severe winter storms, and wildfires (FEMA, 1997a). As a result of these catastrophic events, more than 500 people have lost their lives; another 4,500 people die each year in fires.

In the last two decades, natural disasters, such as earthquakes, hurricanes, floods, and volcanic eruptions, have cost approximately 32 million lives worldwide, have adversely affected the lives of at least 800 million more people, and have cost more than $50 billion in property and personal loss (Advisory Committee, 1987; Office of U.S. Foreign Disaster Assistance, 1995).

During 1998 alone, violent weather cost the world a record $89 billion, more money than was lost from weather-related disasters during the entire decade of the 1980s (Worldwatch Institute, 1998). Most of the increase in natural disaster damage was due to a combination of deforestation and climate change, including El Niño.

. . . .

Imagine that you were somehow above to watch, from a distance, a major disaster unfold. You would see suffering and devastation—but that would be only part of the story. You also would see lots of people move into action—people from government agencies, private organizations, businesses and volunteer groups. You would see them working as a team to keep essential services operating, provide first aid, food and water, clear debris, rebuild homes and businesses, and prevent the disaster from happening again.

Federal Emergency Management Agency, 1997a

. . . .

Community health nurses sometimes feel unprepared to react competently in a community disaster situation. For most practicing nurses, formal disaster education or training is not comprehensive. Therefore, the training that is received by nurses does not include the whole picture on levels of preparedness, which range from the basic emergency department response to the highest level of response from the community infrastructure. The disaster training that pertains to nurses' agency

positions is usually the only training received, which often limits their understanding of the community's perspective on preparedness and response.

Although training may not be comprehensive in many institutions, an important goal for community health nurses is for them to feel a greater sense of disaster preparedness. When community health nurses are prepared for disaster, research has indicated that communities benefit. Study after study has revealed that improved organization in nursing care, planning the disaster response, and understanding the effects of disaster on families, communities, health professionals, and ultimately society, can prevent or reduce the detrimental short- and long-term effects of disasters.

Levels of prevention are integral in planning and responding to disasters for community health nurses, as well as other key personnel in the community infrastructure. The levels of prevention are integrated at certain points in this chapter. The levels include primary, secondary, and tertiary. Primary prevention is aimed at reducing the probability of disease, death, and disability resulting from a disaster. Secondary prevention includes the immediate identification of disaster problems and the implementation of measures to treat and prevent their recurrence or complications. Tertiary prevention involves rehabilitation of disaster victims and the community to an optimal function level, with permanency of change from the disaster assumed. The goal during rehabilitation is to minimize further damage resulting from the disaster.

By increasing community health nurses' understanding, confidence, and skill in disaster planning and care, the damage to our communities during disasters can be lessened (Garcia, 1985). Not only are lives saved and human and property damage reduced, but also the overall health of the community can be strengthened.

What are the real threats of disaster? How can community health nurses be better prepared? This chapter will help you answer these questions as you develop a better understanding of the nature of disasters and learn about the various levels of disaster preparedness in which community health nurses are involved. The role of preparedness is essential to mediate the harmful effects of catastrophes, such as the Titanic disaster of 1912, described in Box 24-1.

BOX 24-1 THE MAKING OF A DISASTER: THE SINKING OF THE "UNSINKABLE" TITANIC

NONDISASTER OR INTERDISASTER PHASE

The Titanic was on its maiden voyage when it sank on April 14, 1912. This ship was the crown jewel of the White Star Line, a mammoth 46-ton British liner of incomparable luxury, three football fields long and eleven stories high, which was the world's largest and purportedly safest vessel on the water. On this maiden voyage, the Titanic had as its passengers both British and American aristocracy, along with immigrants coming to the "New World" with promises of a new life. The boat deck and bridge were 70 feet above water. According to White Star Line documentation, a "trial test" of 6 to 7

BOX 24-1 THE MAKING OF A DISASTER: THE SINKING OF THE "UNSINKABLE" TITANIC—cont'd

hours total was conducted 1 month before leaving Great Britain. This trial consisted of turning circles and compass adjustment; also, the ship sailed "a short time" at full steam, but never at full speed before passengers boarded. The crew and officers of the Titanic (numbering 899) joined the ship a few hours before the passengers and went through only one drill: They lowered two lifeboats on starboard side into water. No evidence of crew duties being delineated as to task or role in event of disaster were noted by Congress. *Congressional hearings found that the crew did not know their "proper stations" or assignment until after passengers had already boarded in Queenstown, Ireland.* There were 1,324 passengers on board the ship, and together with 899 crew members, a total of 2,223 persons were on the maiden voyage of the Titanic. Congress found no evidence of passengers having any orientation in disaster procedures. There were 1,176 lifeboats and life jackets for all persons on board. The Titanic was considered "unsinkable," having been constructed with special watertight bulkhead compartments that could be sealed off if the ship took on water. There was no evidence of a disaster plan or safety instructions posted or provided to passengers, nor were crew members prepared for their roles in the event of a disaster. *The crew staffed the Titanic round the clock and had lookouts posted in the crow's nest for any water-related hazards.*

PREDISASTER OR WARNING PHASE

The Titanic had received several ice warnings on the third day of the voyage, and the captain noted them. On the day of the disaster, a warning message cited icebergs within 5 miles of the track that the Titanic was following, very near the place where the accident occurred. Congressional hearings revealed that despite repeated warnings, no general discussion took place among the officers, no conference was called to consider these warnings, and no heed was given to them. *The speed was not reduced, the lookout was not increased, and the only extra vigilance noted was from the officer of the watch, who gave instructions to the lookouts to "keep a sharp lookout for ice." The speed of the ship had been gradually increased, and just before*

the collision, the ship was making her maximum speed of the voyage. Passengers had no advance knowledge of any possible risks of the ship related to the icebergs.

IMPACT PHASE

At 10:13 PM on Sunday, April 14, the lookout signaled the bridge and telephoned the officer of the watch with this message: "Iceberg right ahead." The officer of the watch immediately ordered the quartermaster at the wheel to put the helm "hard astarboard" and reverse the engines. The Titanic immediately struck the ice, and the impact caused the vessel to roll slightly. The impact, which ripped a hole in the steel plating of the ship, was not violent enough to disturb the crew or passengers. During this time, the damage was reported by crew members from the boiler room related to water coming in; the captain began inspecting the ship for damage. Passengers were still not aware of the accident.

EMERGENCY PHASE

The reports by the captain after various inspections of the ship revealed that the compartments were rapidly filling with water and that the bow of the ship was sinking deeper and deeper. Through the open hatches, water promptly began overflowing into the other bulkheads and decks. No emergency alarm was sounded, no whistles were blown, and no systematic warning was given the passengers. *Within approximately 15 minutes after his inspection, the captain issued a distress call to ships in the area. The call was heard by several ships in the vicinity. The Carpathia, which was 58 miles away, responded to the distress signal by turning immediately toward the sinking ship. Other ships also attempted to sail toward the sinking ship but were too far away to be of any reasonable assistance. The closest ship, the Californian, was only 19 miles north of the Titanic but did not attempt to rescue the ailing ship.* Proceedings indicate that the crew of the Titanic began firing distress rockets at frequent intervals and that the crew of the Californian saw them. The captain of the Californian failed to heed the warning signals and was chastised by Congress for "indifference or carelessness" and for not responding to the Titanic's distress calls in accordance with the dictates of international usage and law. *The*

Continued

captain immediately gave the signal to retrieve the lifeboats, with the order to put women and children in the boats first. The proceedings report that the lack of preparation at this time was most noticeable. *There was general chaos as passengers learned of the accident from each other, from some crew members who knocked on cabin doors, and from being awakened by the movement of people running on the ship.* "There was no system adopted for loading the boats; there was great indecision as to the deck from which boats were to be loaded; there was wide diversity of opinion as to the number of crew necessary to man each boat; there was no direction whatever to the number of passengers to be carried by each boat, and no uniformity in loading them" *(p. 548). In some boats, there would be only women and children; in others there would be an equal proportion of men and women. Only a few of the lifeboats were loaded to capacity; most were only partially loaded, which resulted in needless losses. If all of the lifeboats had been fully loaded at capacity for 1,176 persons, more than the 706 persons could have reasonably survived. Furthermore, the proceedings noted that if the sea had been rough (which it wasn't), it is questionable whether any of the lifeboats would have reached the water without being damaged or destroyed.* The lifeboats were suspended 70 feet above the water, and in the event of the ship's rolling (with a rough sea), the boats would have swung out from the side of the ship and then crashed back into the ship as it was being lowered. *Also, had the survivors been concentrated in fewer boats once on the water, the staff could have returned and rescued more passengers. Once the ship sank at 12:47 AM, it broke in half and people died from drowning, exposure, and trauma; 1,517 persons died, 706 survived. Survivors of the Titanic reported rowing toward the lights of a ship in the distance, which has now been established as those of the Californian.* There were questions about the way passengers were evacuated relative to whether they were in first, second, or third class accommodation. *Sixty percent of first class passengers survived, 42% of second class survived, and only 25% of the third class passengers survived. These statistics suggest that there may have been a distinction in the warning and evacuation based on class accommodation. Twenty-five percent of the crew were saved. The rescue of survivors came from the Carpathia crew and eventually from the crew of the Californian. After a thorough search, ships returned to New York and Nova Scotia with the survivors. A brief burial prayer service for the dead was held at 8:30 AM by the captain of the Carpathia. Public media notification occurred the evening of April 15, 1912.*

RECONSTRUCTION OR REHABILITATION PHASE

The wreck of the Titanic represents in myth and reality a disaster beyond human comprehension at a time when technological advances were seen as our defense against the disasters of nature. Because of lack of preparedness and lack of planning for ship disasters, technology could not have saved the passengers on the Titanic. *The recommendations that evolved from the Titanic hearings held by Congress in May of 1912 were no less than revolutionary in terms of safety preparedness. One was that* inspection certificates would be contingent on sufficient lifeboats to accommodate every passenger and every member of the crew. Inspection certificates that mandate these requirements would apply to all boats who carry passengers from ports of the United States. Lifeboats should be positioned in such a way that they would not be subject to damage from height related to water level. There would be no fewer than four members of the crew, trained in handling boats, on each lifeboat. *All crew members assigned to this duty would be drilled in lowering and rowing the lifeboats not less than twice per month and the "fact of such drill or practice should be noted in the log."* Recommendations also included assigning passengers to lifeboats before sailing and posting the shortest route to the lifeboats in each room. *Two electric searchlights were to be present on boats carrying more than 100 passengers. A radio operator must be on duty at all times, 24 hours a day. And finally, all ships from that point on would be required to meet construction standards related to watertight compartments and hulls.*

Source: Kuntz, T. (Ed.). The Titanic disaster hearings: The official transcripts of the 1912 Senate investigation. New York: Pocket Books.

The Nature of Disasters

Definitions and Types of Disasters

Some of the many definitions of disaster include the definitions of an emergency and a major disaster. An **emergency** is any hurricane, tornado, storm, flood, high water, wind-driven water, tidal wave, earthquake, volcanic eruption, landslide, mudslide, snowstorm, drought, fire, explosion, or other catastrophe in any part of the United States that requires federal emergency assistance to supplement state and local efforts to save lives and protect property, public health, and safety or to avert or lessen the threat of a disaster (U.S. Congress, Section 102, Disaster Relief Act Amendments, 1974).

A **major disaster** may be any of the events listed as an emergency in any part of the United States that, in the determination of the president, causes damage of sufficient severity above and beyond emergency services by the federal government, to supplement the efforts and available resources of states, local governments, and disaster relief organizations in alleviating the damage, loss, hardship, or suffering caused thereby (U.S. Congress, Section 102, Disaster Relief Act Amendments, 1974). Erickson (1976) gave a pictorial description of disaster:

- *A sharp and furious eruption of some kind that splinters the silence for one terrible moment and then goes away*
- *An "event" with a distinct beginning and a distinct ending that is by definition extraordinary—a freak of nature, a perversion of the natural processes of life*
- *Doing a great deal of harm*
- *Sudden, unexpected, and acute*

For the purposes of this chapter, **disaster** is an event that causes human suffering and creates unmet needs and demands exceeding the abilities of the community to cope without outside assistance. Most importantly, from a public health perspective, disasters are defined by what they do to people and are therefore relative to the context in which they occur. What results in a disaster in one community might not necessarily be considered a disaster in a different community (Noji, 1997). Disasters fall into two broad categories or types: **natural disasters** are those that arise from the forces of nature, such as hurricanes, tornadoes, earthquakes, and volcanic eruptions; **human-generated (manmade) disasters** are those in which the principal direct causes are identifiable human actions, deliberate or otherwise. These two categories can be further subdivided into different types of disasters (Box 24-2).

Floods have been the most common type of natural disaster, accounting for more than one-third of all disasters between 1980 and 1990 (Office of U.S. Foreign Disaster Assistance, 1995). One example of a horrendous flood, although not necessarily a typical disaster, was the Mississippi River Flood of 1927, which has been cited as the worst natural disaster in U.S. history. In 1927, the Mississippi River swept across a geographic area larger than Massachusetts, Connecticut, New Hampshire, and Ver-

---

BOX 24-2 CATEGORIES AND TYPES OF DISASTERS

NATURAL DISASTERS

- Meteorological: hurricanes, tornados, hailstorms, snowstorms, and droughts
- Topological: landslides, avalanches, mudslides, and floods
- Disasters that originate underground: earthquakes, volcanic eruptions, and tidal waves
- Bacteriological: communicable disease epidemics (e.g., *Ebola* virus) and insect swarms (e.g., locusts)

HUMAN-GENERATED DISASTERS

- Warfare: conventional warfare (bombardment, blockage, and siege) and nonconventional warfare (nuclear, chemical, and biological; acts of terrorism)
- Civil disasters: riots and demonstrations
- Accidents: transportation (planes, trucks, automobiles, trains, and ships); structural collapse (buildings, dams, bridges, mines, and other structures); explosion; fire; chemical (toxic waste and pollution); and biological (sanitation)

Source: Modified from Garcia, 1985; Noji, 1997.

---

mont combined and resulted in water as deep as 30 feet on the land, stretching from Illinois and Missouri south to the Gulf of Mexico and New Orleans. This flood forced almost 1 million people from their homes and resulted in thousands of deaths.

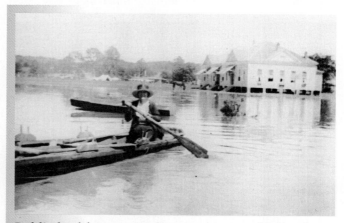

Public health nurse in disaster recovery during the worst natural disaster in the United States—the Mississippi River Flood of 1927.

Many of the dead were being pulled out of the Mississippi River at New Orleans for months after the flood. When more than 40,000 homes were destroyed close to where the dam broke in Mississippi, camps were set up in the Confederate National Park in Vicksburg. American Red Cross nurses (Box 24-3) and nurses from the Mississippi State Department of Health, as well as nurses from other states, were assigned to relief efforts for several months in the spring of 1927. A total of 383 nurses worked in the Mississippi flood disaster. Nurses worked in these refugee camps, battling typhoid and nutritional deficiencies such as pellagra. The waters from the Mississippi did not recede for 3 months (Barry, 1997; Sabin, 1998).

Although disasters can be grouped according to the stated definitions, in reality the distinction between natural and human-generated disasters is often blurred, for a natural disaster can trigger secondary disasters, such as explosions, fires, and toxins released into the air after an earthquake. Such combination-type synergistic disasters are referred to as *NA-TECH disasters*. An example of a NA-TECH disaster occurred in the former Soviet Union when windstorms spread radioactive materials across the country, increasing by up to 50% the land area contaminated in an earlier nuclear disaster at Chernobyl (see Box 24-9).

Disaster Characteristics

Disasters have different characteristics. Knowledge of these variables is necessary in disaster management and planning. Dynes, Quarentelli, and Kreps (1972) identified six variables by which disasters can be understood. The variables include predictability, controllability, speed of onset, length of forewarning, duration of impact, and scope and intensity of impact.

1. Predictability *is influenced by the type of disaster. A hurricane has a high degree of predictability in industrialized countries, and earthquakes are considerably less foreseeable than floods. Although we often assume that disasters are fairly rare occurrences, there are certain areas of the globe that are more prone to disasters, such as flood plains of the Ohio Valley or low-lying areas in the Louisiana swamp. The Gulf Coast of Mississippi, Texas, Louisiana, Florida, and Alabama are all vulnerable to the threat of hurricanes born from the warm waters of the Caribbean. Tornadoes are more common in Kansas, Texas, and Mississippi and less common in North Dakota and Idaho.*

2. Controllability *refers to the degree to which interventions can be used to control the disaster, such as using dams for flood control; earthquakes have very little controllability.*

3. Speed of onset *is great with floods and tornadoes, whereas hurricanes generally are slow to develop.*

4. Length of forewarning *is the period between warning and impact. Communities in the path of a hurricane may have the luxury of a 24-hour warning, whereas a tornado warning may provide only a few minutes of preparation.*

5. Duration of impact *also varies. A tornado may be on the ground for only a few minutes, whereas a flood's impact usually lasts for days. The worst combination of variables from the viewpoint of damage is the disaster that is rapid in onset, gives no warning, and lasts a long time. An earthquake with strong aftershocks is such a disaster.*

6. Scope and intensity of impact *refers to geographic and social space dimension. A disaster such as a tornado may be limited to a mile or two, but a flood may involve hundreds of miles. The population density of an area influences this variable and can lead to widespread consequences. An example of density is the Oklahoma City bombing, which was limited to a few city blocks but affected a large, dense population. A densely affected area can result in disruption of community functions, depending on the number of persons involved and the geographic impact.*

Global Disaster Issues

As humans continue to migrate throughout the globe and population densities continue to increase in flood plains, along vul-

---

BOX 24-3 AN EARLY FIELD TEST OF THE AMERICAN RED CROSS'S NURSE ENROLLMENT CAMPAIGN: THE PURVIS, MISSISSIPPI, TORNADO OF 1908

A devastating tornado hit the small town of Purvis, Mississippi, in April of 1908, injuring 200 persons. The American Red Cross had just undertaken its first major campaign to recruit and enroll nurses nationally for such disasters, and the Purvis tornado provided a "field test" of the newly developed communication system. In the end, a head nurse and 17 staff nurses were employed from the District of Columbia, Philadelphia, and New York. These nurses managed tent hospitals and coordinated disaster relief for 3 weeks. Although the nursing was well done, recruitment and securement of nurses with the new system had been less than successful. The ARC staff had met with considerable difficulty locating the enrolled nurses and in the end had to recruit unenrolled, volunteer nurses outside the system. The disaster served to draw attention to the need for a more collaborative effort between nursing organizations together with the American Red Cross to develop a network of disaster preparedness through local volunteer nurses.

Source: Kernodle, P. (1949). The Red Cross nurse in action 1882–1948. New York: Harper and Brothers.

nerable coastal areas, and near faults in the earth's crust, we can expect these natural disasters to worsen and affect more people. The global community continues to witness complex emergencies resulting from the breakdown of traditional state structures, armed conflict, and the upsurge of ethnicity and micronationalism (Noji, 1997). One has to look no further than today's newspaper headlines or watch CNN to find these political and cultural conflicts as they play out on a daily business, such as in Bosnia, Somalia, Rwanda, and Chechnya, to name but a few of the disaster areas. As a result of these political and cultural upheavals, refugees have become a large and vulnerable population with complex health problems.

Between 1965 and 1992, 90% of all natural disaster victims lived in Asia and Africa (IDNDR, 1994). The number of people affected (killed, injured, or displaced) by disasters worldwide rose from 100 million in 1980 to 311 million in 1991. By the mid-1990s, the number of refugees affected by a combination of natural and human-made disasters increased to an estimated 17 million throughout the world.

Earthquakes are global incidents that have been cited as causing the greatest number of deaths and the largest monetary loss of any type of natural disaster (Berz, 1984). The tragic earthquake that occurred in Istanbul, Turkey, in August 1999 is an example of high cost of human lives—thousands of deaths were reported.

Not only are these displaced vulnerable populations at risk for serious health consequences, the economic costs for their care are devastating (Noji, 1997). As United Nations Secretary General Boutros Boutros Ghali stated:

> There is no hard-and-fast division—in terms of their [disasters] effects on civilian populations—between conflicts and wars, and natural disasters. Droughts, floods, earthquakes, and cyclones are just as destructive for communities and settlements as wars and civil confrontation. Just as preventive diplomacy can foresee and prevent the outbreak of war, so the effects of natural disasters can be foreseen and contained (cited in Noji, 1997, p. xv).

Much of the destruction caused by natural disasters can be avoided. For almost every natural disaster in the world in the 1990s, "an ounce of prevention" or preparedness would have made a significant difference in terms of damage to persons and property (Noji, 1997, p. 7). Natural hazards, such as weather, earthquakes, and floods, are in fact only natural agents that "transform a vulnerable condition into a disaster" (Noji, 1997, p. 11).

People often do not know their limitations until they reach them. As technology has advanced and provided humans with opportunities to live in and explore the world without the territorial constraints of our ancestors, the probabilities that the future will be marked by periodic disasters are certainly increased. In many cases in recent disasters, building codes were ignored, communities were located in dangerous areas, warnings were not issued or followed, or plans were unknown to all community residents or were ignored (Noji, 1997).

We know much about the cause and nature of disasters, populations at risk, and the inevitable outcome when communities are not prepared for disasters. Such knowledge assists us in anticipating some of the effects a disaster may have on the health of communities. Knowing how people are injured and killed in disasters is critical prerequisite knowledge for preventing or reducing injuries and deaths during future disasters (Noji, 1997). For example, although none of the advances in science and technology have done much to arrest the force of natural disasters, we see them coming a few hours earlier and can measure their destructiveness with greater precision afterward. Yet those very advances have made us in many ways even more vulnerable to potential catastrophes, because persons often feel a "false sense of security" regarding the likelihood of serious threat from a disaster (Erickson, 1976).

International Decade for Natural Disaster Reduction

The United Nations General Assembly declared the 1990s the "International Decade for Natural Disaster Reduction" (IDNDR) and led the way in calling for a global, scientific, technical, and political effort to reduce the impact of catastrophic acts of nature (Advisory Committee, 1987). This declaration came about because both disasters and the number of their victims have increased in recent decades (Pickens, 1992). Such massive adverse impacts on the health of global populations have now been recognized as a significant public health problem. Sudden impact disasters, such as earthquakes and tornadoes, may result in large numbers of people killed, injured, or disabled for life; health facilities damaged or destroyed; and national health care development efforts in underdeveloped countries set back for years.

As human societies have become more dense with urban migration and population growth, more people are exposed and vulnerable to the hazards of disaster than ever before. Our increasingly sophisticated and technical physical infrastructure makes more developed countries, such as the United States, even more vulnerable to destruction than in past generations. For instance, a major disaster could disrupt the computer networks of the federal government or some other large organization. Damage from natural and technological disasters tends to be more and more extensive when proper planning and precautions are not taken. In the past 50 years, much has been learned about disasters and their aftereffects. Disaster preparedness involving careful and methodical planning does make a difference in mediating the destructive nature of disasters (Noji, 1997).

Disaster as a Global Public Health Problem

The Centers for Disease Control and Prevention (CDC) has led the way and has major responsibilities to prepare for and respond to public emergencies such as disasters. The CDC is also responsible for conducting investigations into the health effects and health consequences of disaster. The first major comprehensive research study of disasters was published in 1962 by Baker and Chapman in their book *Man and Society in Disaster*. Since then, many research centers have been established to study the health effects of disaster; among them are collaborative centers under the guidance and sponsorship of the World Health Organization (WHO) and the Pan American Health Organization. The major aim of these research efforts is to assess risk for death and injury and to develop strategies for preventing or mitigating the impact of future disasters.

. . . .

Will you be a hero in your daily work? . . . We may give you an institution to learn in, but it is you who must furnish the heroic feelings of doing your duty, doing your best, without which no institution is safe.

Florence Nightingale

. . . .

Disasters affect communities in myriad ways. Most effects of a disaster affect health, directly or indirectly (Noji, 1997). Communication lines, such as telephones, television, and computer links, may be disrupted, as well as transportation links, such as roads and methods of transportation. Public utilities (electricity, water, gas, water, and sewer) are often disrupted early in a mas-

---

BOX 24-5 HEALTH EFFECTS OF DISASTERS

PHYSICAL

Sleep disturbance

Poor concentration

Back pain

Tachycardia

Poor diet

PSYCHOLOGICAL

Loss of self and relationships

Emotional pain

Brooding

Aggressive thoughts

Depression

SOCIOCULTURAL

Loss of intimacy

Loss of sense of belonging to once-claimed culture

Source: Procter & Cheek, 1995.

BOX 24-4 PUBLIC HEALTH PROBLEMS THAT MAY RESULT FROM DISASTERS

- Excessive deaths and injuries can tax the local health services and therapeutic capabilities, which may require external assistance.

- Destruction or disruption of acute care health facilities, such as clinics and hospitals, may leave services and resources unable to provide care to the injured from the disaster and pre-disaster client population needs.

- Disruption of routine health services and preventive activities can lead to long-term consequences in terms of morbidity and mortality.

- Environmental hazards can lead to increased risks for communicable disease and injury from a damaged ecosystem.

- Psychological and social behavioral stressors, including panic, anxiety, neuroses, and depression, can be exacerbated.

- A shortage of safe, nutritional food sources may lead to severe nutritional deficiencies and sequelae in the very young and the very old.

- Displaced populations to overcrowded hospitals and shelter facilities may increase the dangers of communicable disease.

Sources: Adapted from Logue, Melick, & Hansen, 1981; Noji, 1997.

---

sive disaster. A substantial number of persons may be without homes. Casualties may require medical and nursing care. Damage to food, damage to food preparation and sources, and lack of sanitation resources may create serious public health threats. A long-term effect is the community's possible destruction of its industrial or economic base. A detailed summary of disasters and public health can be found in Box 24-4 and the health effects of disasters in Box 24-5.

Populations at Risk in Disasters

Not all persons in the world are equal regarding the probability of disaster occurrence or severity of consequences. The more vulnerable a population to a disaster, the more serious the outcomes of injury and damage to persons and property (Mizutani & Nakano, 1989). As far as individual health characteristics, persons with conditions that put them at risk, such as those with chronic diseases, elder persons, pregnant women, the disabled, homebound persons, or children, are among the most vulnerable in any society in regard to impact of disaster. Industrialized countries are buffered from disasters by characteristics and abilities that are summarized in Box 24-6.

The low death rate associated with recent disasters in the United States, such as hurricanes Hugo (1989), Andrew (1992), and Georges (1998), and earthquakes in San Francisco (1989)

BOX 24-6 RESOURCES FOR INDUSTRIALIZED COUNTRIES

- Sophisticated technology to forecast storms
- Development and strict enforcement of codes for earthquake-resistant and fireproof buildings
- Widespread mandatory use of communications networks to broadcast disaster warnings, alerts, and information about disaster preparedness
- Resources to provide timely and high-quality emergency health services and accommodation
- Contingency planning to prepare the population and public agencies for possible disasters
- Shelters for evacuation widely available and used by population

Source: Adapted from Garcia, 1985.

and Los Angeles (1994), are evidence of the success of the United States' resources in disaster warning and recovery (Noji, 1997). The following major factors contribute to the degree of vulnerability of populations:

- *Human vulnerability resulting from poverty and social inequality*
- *Environmental degradation resulting from poor land use*
- *Rapid population growth, especially among the poor*

Anderson (1991) estimated that 95% of the deaths that result from natural disasters occur among 66% of the world's poorest population. According to Guha-Sapir and Lechat (1986), the poor are most at risk for greatest damage for the following reasons:

- *They are likely to live in substandard housing with little structural protection.*
- *They often live in coastal locations that are at high risk for disasters.*
- *They are likely to live in flood plains and other less desirable land.*
- *They are likely to live in substandard housing built on unstable geographic slopes.*
- *They are likely to live near hazardous industrial sites.*
- *They are not usually well educated about safe and appropriate lifesaving behaviors.*
- *They are more dependent on others for transportation.*

Stages of Disaster

Disasters can be divided into five chronological stages that require specific levels of prevention and levels of response at vari-

ous points during each stage. Knowing the disaster stages will assist in the development of the disaster plan, role responsibilities, and the setting of priorities in each phase of the disaster plan. Refer to Box 24-1 as an illustration of the stages of disaster. The stages of a disaster are presented in the following list:

- *Nondisaster, or interdisaster, stage*
- *Predisaster, or warning, stage*
- *Impact stage*
- *Emergency stage*
- *Reconstruction, or rehabilitation, stage*

Disaster planning should begin before the disaster event. During the nondisaster, or **interdisaster, stage**, planning and preparation for a disaster include the two critical elements of disaster preparedness: (1) disaster training and education programs for the community and (2) the development of a disaster plan for all involved in the mitigation of a potential disaster (Noji, 1997). Mitigation is preventive in nature and defined as action taken to prevent or reduce the harmful effects of a disaster on human health and property (Malilay, 1997). Included in this critical phase of primary prevention are assessment of hazards and risks, vulnerability analysis, inventory of existing resources for coping with a disaster (human, communication, and material), and the establishment of a disaster plan. Disaster planning is discussed in more detail in a later section.

A disaster is imminent during the warning, or **predisaster, stage**. The disaster plan, when available, is implemented, which includes early warning based on predictions of impending disaster and mobilization as well as implementation of protective measures for the affected communities and populations (Garcia, 1985). Because primary prevention is the focus during this stage, disaster team members, officials, and emergency personnel prepare the population for disaster by providing information via multiple communication routes. Advisories and warnings are issued, and evacuation measures are taken where indicated. Mobilization can occur in the form of evacuation to shelters, preparation such as using sandbags around riverbanks to divert flood waters, boarding up windows and tying down boats when a hurricane is forecast, and moving to the basements or inner halls of homes and schools in the event of a tornado. Health care workers may be placed "on alert call" for health facility staffing and disaster shelter management. The effectiveness of these protective measures will depend largely on the community's preparedness and contingency plans developed in the nondisaster phase (Noji, 1997).

Problems associated with the warning include the following: first, communication systems may be inadequate in transmission and/or reception, or there may not be enough time to send warnings; second, the community must recognize the warning threat as serious and legitimate. However, some people in the targeted community may deny the need for taking action based on previous experience with the specific disaster (e.g., persons who live on a fault line or on a coastline), and the presence of false alarms in the past can desensitize persons to appropriate reaction (Garcia, 1985; Janis & Mann, 1977).

The **impact stage** involves "holding on" and enduring the impact of the disaster. This stage may last from minutes (as in earthquakes, plane crashes, tornadoes, and bomb blasts) to days or weeks (hurricanes, floods, fire, and drought). People who are directly experiencing the disaster may be unable to comprehend the scope of the disaster (Garcia, 1985). If possible, a preliminary assessment and inventory of injuries and property damage should be conducted by disaster team members during the impact phase or immediately afterward so that the implementation of secondary prevention strategies of setting priorities can be set in motion. How much the impact affects community members depends on several factors: population density, the extent of the damage, the preparedness of the community, the extent of community resiliency, and response to the consequences of the damage.

During the **emergency stage**, the community faces the consequences of the disaster's impact. This stage begins during the actual impact and continues until the immediate threat of additional hazards have passed (Garcia, 1985). Secondary prevention strategies are used to minimize damage and prevent further complications. This stage is divided into three parts—isolation, rescue, and remedy—which are presented in the following list:

1. *Isolation of the affected population can occur as a result of limited access (as a result of disaster damage, such as closed roads, downed trees, or building obstruction). The community members themselves must assume responsibility for their own needs relative to the disaster until outside help arrives.*

2. *Rescue begins when outside resources arrive and provide search-and-rescue operations. Community members are often hurried, stressed, and nonproductive in this early stage. First aid, emergency medical assistance, and a command post for disaster management are established. Restoration of means of communication begins, and regional, state, federal, and voluntary organizations and agencies converge to meet the needs of the community.*

3. *Remedy begins with the establishment of organized, professional, and voluntary relief operations and organization. The panic and confusion of the earlier phases tend to subside. Community members, disaster workers, and volunteers "get on with the task" of providing appropriate medical aid, clothing, food, and shelter to the affected population. The injured and ill are triaged, transportation becomes more organized, morgue facilities are established, reunions of family members become organized, and communication networks are established to provide early data of the disaster damage (Garcia, 1985). Later in the emergency stage, surveillance of public health effects (e.g., infectious disease, sanitation issues, safety concerns) is put in place and interventions are developed. When communities are well prepared and disaster plans are in place to help people know the "what, when, and how" of disasters for*

their population, both self-reliance and the effectiveness of early assistance saves lives and reduces injury during this critical period (Noji, 1997).

The **reconstruction**, or **rehabilitation**, **stage** begins when communities start the process of healing. Reconstruction or rehabilitation optimally restores the community to predisaster conditions (Noji, 1997). Health services are restored to normal. Damaged homes, facilities, and buildings are repaired and reconstructed. This period is also the time for evaluation and reflection by the community and disaster team members, community officials, and voluntary agencies as lessons learned from the disaster are shared and documented (Noji, 1997). This period, which may combine secondary and tertiary prevention, may take days, months, or years, depending on the nature of the disaster, the response of the community, and the extent of the damages. For persons in the impact area, the recovery can be a long course and, in some cases, can be a lifelong readjustment to life and community living after the disaster (Garcia, 1985).

It is during the rehabilitative phase that victims often suffer from posttraumatic stress disorder. **Posttraumatic stress disorder (PTSD)** is recognized by the American Psychiatric Association (APA) with the following symptoms and circumstances: The sufferer is a victim of an extremely distressing event persistently reexperiencing the event after it is over (compulsive and obsessive thoughts and details about the event), persistently avoiding stimuli that remind the victim of the event, and experiencing numbing of responsiveness and persistent symptoms of arousal not present before the trauma (APA, 1987). In conjunction with disaster, other symptoms include flashbacks, depression, inability to form close personal relationships, and sleep disturbances (Barker, 1989). Florence Nightingale is thought to have suffered from PTSD after the Crimean War. This condition, once diagnosed, requires professional mental health intervention and follow-up (Waters, Selander, & Stuart, 1992).

Disaster Planning

A planned response to disasters must occur to lessen the terror of a disaster, to cushion the impact by providing care for the greatest number of potential survivors, and to increase society's ability to survive disasters and grow more self-sufficient and self-reliant in the process (Waeckerle, 1991). Clearly, the benefits of disaster planning for society today are more significant than ever as widespread disasters become more common and more costly, in both human and property terms.

Anticipating a disaster and planning for the possibility of multiple outcomes from disasters strengthen a community's adaptability. Consequently, the disaster team develops the ability to respond more quickly and more effectively in the face of disaster (Muench, 1996). Another benefit to planning is the delineation of roles and responsibilities of the players in disaster preparedness. The result is less confusion over who does what and the roles of the multitude of organizations and volunteers once resources become available.

Once a disaster is imminent it is too late to plan a response. A clear community disaster plan for all contingencies should be coordinated by knowledgeable and experienced leaders and officials in the community. Such a plan must be as inclusive as possible, including input from health professionals; voluntary agencies; policy makers; officials from local, state, and federal levels, such as the civil defense and the Federal Emergency Management Agency (FEMA); emergency response system personnel; and all other components of the health care delivery system from acute care to home health to residential care, including medical and nursing schools (Waeckerle, 1991).

Steps in the Disaster Process

When a major disaster has occurred, such as hurricane Andrew in 1992, the president of the United States intervenes after the governor of the affected state requests the president to declare the area a major disaster. However, all major disaster declarations must follow certain steps (FEMA, 1998c).

First, local government agencies, such as the mayor and civil defense, which includes neighboring communities and volunteer agencies, must respond. Second, if the local agencies become overwhelmed, the state responds at the governor's request through state agencies and the National Guard. Third, the local, state, federal, and volunteer organizations make a damage assessment.

Fourth, when state resources have been exhausted, the governor of the state will make a request to the president for a declaration of a major disaster. The governor bases this request on the already-completed damage assessment collected by the civil defense team and commits a certain amount of state funds and resources to the long-term recovery from the disaster.

Fifth, FEMA evaluates the request and recommends action to the White House. Sixth, the president either gives the executive order for the declaration or FEMA informs the governor the request has been denied. The whole process may only take a few days. If the executive order is given, federal and financial resources are mobilized through FEMA for search and rescue and for the provision of basic human needs. Long-term federal programs are mobilized during this time.

The Disaster Plan

The purpose of **disaster planning** is to reduce a community's vulnerability to the tremendous consequences of disasters and to prevent or minimize problems resulting from system damage associated with the disaster (Drabek, 1986). Community health nurses are involved in disaster planning, as are other health care professionals in the community. Specific ways that a nurse can be more prepared for a disaster in his or her community are described in the next section.

In a disaster, the usual strategies and process for providing care may not work. Deviating from a routine plan of care may present a few problems for nurses and other health care professionals when disaster occurs. Disaster health care is very different from daily nursing practice; it is not routine (even compared with emergency department services), and the philosophy of care is based on "providing the greatest good for the greatest number." Abiding by this standard of care is often difficult for health care professionals, especially for those in routine practice settings, who practice holistic care and provide optimal care to all who need services. The disaster plan is fundamental in the preparation of health care professionals (Waeckerle, 1991). Drabek (1986) identified general

---

BOX 24-7 PRINCIPLES TO GUIDE DISASTER PREPAREDNESS FOR ALL PERSONS INVOLVED IN PLANNING

Measures used for everyday emergencies generally do not work in major disasters.
- Disasters are more uncertain, less predictable, with more unknowns, and citizens have little consensus on what needs to be done in a disaster.
- Laypersons are most likely to jump in and provide aid without direction and knowledge of prioritization and triage.

Plan for specific population needs and consider "disaster planning" as a verb, which is ongoing, rather than a noun, such as the limits of a written plan.

Provide information regularly to the community to correct misconceptions.
- Widespread looting and theft are actually quite uncommon.
- People should be given information and details about the extent of the disaster to enable them to take appropriate action, in contrast to the long-held belief of health workers that people will panic if they "know too much."

Involve the entire community in the planning process, not just officials and emergency personnel.
- Such inclusion limits confusion about who does what and where the lines of authority are.

Use routine working methods and procedures in the disaster plan, which will eliminate the need to learn new procedures and prevents confusion at the disaster site.

Disaster plans should be flexible.

Roles and responsibilities of team members should be identified by position or title, not by names of individuals, to avoid having to revise the plan when people change positions.

principles that can guide community health nurses who take part in disaster planning. These principles are listed in Box 24-7.

Waeckerle (1991) stated, "Disaster planning is an enormous undertaking" (p. 815). As in other areas of health care, enormous amounts of money are spent in the United States on disaster relief during the recovery period, with little funds available for communities to use in disaster preparedness and disaster planning. This poses very real challenges in the development of a disaster plan. Although the disaster plan is usually developed from guidelines set forth by local, state, and federal officials, communities are often on their own and must rely on local officials and volunteers to do much of the work when organizing a disaster plan and evaluating its validity through mock disaster drills (Waeckerle, 1991).

Characteristics of Disaster Plans

Through research of past disasters and presence or absence of disaster plans, disaster specialists have determined common characteristics of effective disaster plans (Drabek, 1986; Noji, 1997; Waeckerle, 1991). They are as follows:

- *The disaster plan is based on a realistic assessment of potential problems that can happen, such as destruction to property, material, and utilities; impairment of communication; and geographic isolation.*
- *Estimates of types of injuries that result from disasters most likely to occur in the area and the possible destruction of health facilities and alternative agency use are included in the plan.*
- *The plan is brief, concise, and inclusive of all who can provide disaster aid.*
- *The plan is organized by a timeline; it details the stages of a disaster, who must be involved, what must occur, and how each stage unfolds throughout the disaster process.*
- *The plan is approved by all agencies that provide authority endorsement, as well as sanctioned by those who have the*

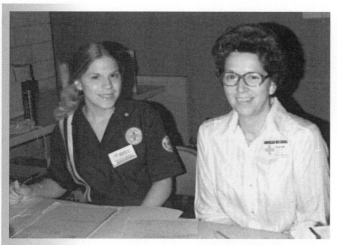

Chapter author, Dr. Karen Saucier Lundy (left), at an American Red Cross shelter after hurricane Allen in Galveston, Texas.

most power to see that the plan is updated periodically and carried out when disaster strikes.

- *The plan is regularly tested through mock drills and revised based on drill results.*
- *The plan is always considered a work in progress because needs and resources in a community relative to disaster preparedness change constantly.*

Common Elements of Disaster Plans

Although disaster plans should be targeted for the specific community, certain components should be included in all disaster plans. Each component may have more or less elaboration, detail, and specifics according to the needs of the community to which it applies. These components consist of authority; communication; supplies; equipment; human resources (health professionals, both acute and public health); emergency and disaster specialists; officials of government and voluntary agencies; engineers; weather specialists; community leaders, both lay and official; team coordination; transportation; documentation; record keeping; evacuation; rescue; acute care; supportive care; recovery; and evaluation. Details of these components are summarized in Box 24-8.

Disaster Management

The goal of disaster management is to prevent or minimize death, injury, suffering, and destruction (Taggert, 1982). Disaster management by nature is an interdisciplinary, collaborative team effort (Sullivan, 1998); however, community health nurses are integral in planning disasters and responding. Disaster management is usually coordinated by specific community officials, such as the civil defense.

Once the civil defense efforts are begun, coordination of the many networks in the community disaster infrastructure are carried out by individuals overseeing these agencies. Some examples include the mayor, chief executive officer(s) of the local hospital(s), executive officer of the local American Red Cross chapter, the emergency medical system manager, and the emergency/triage physicians and nurses.

Other agencies or resources and staff persons who make up the disaster team include local, state, and federal disaster management agencies; private relief organizations, such as churches and the Salvation Army; fire and police departments; political leaders who function under the mayor's administration; engineers, geologists, and meteorologists; sociologists, epidemiologists, and other researchers; community volunteers; and the media, including television news reporters, cable weather broadcasters, and radio communication persons (e.g., short-wave radio, HAM radio).

Disaster Response

Disaster response is a complex plan that is sometimes difficult to coordinate and carry out. All health care and other personnel should become knowledgeable about the disaster plan and their

BOX 24-8 COMMON ELEMENTS
OF A DISASTER PLAN

Authority: Issues warnings and official responses and is the central authority for disaster declarations and delegation

Communication: Warnings to public and how communicated, whether by weather sirens, television, radio, police loudspeakers; includes chain of notification, rumor control, and restriction and access to the press in the disaster area

Equipment and supplies: Sources and where located, usual and special needs, staging areas, and controlled access to supplies; dissemination of donated food, clothing, and storage

Human resources: Health professionals, both acute and public health; emergency and disaster specialists, utility officials, officials of government and voluntary agencies, engineers, weather specialists, community leaders, both lay and official

Team coordination: Central operations, staging area, chain of command

Transportation: Traffic control, access and escape routes, control of risk to victims, and rescuers related to transportation

Documentation: Details of disaster plan, how and where disseminated; procedures for managing records of injuries, deaths, supplies, and agency reporting responsibilities; development of brief forms with minimal duplication

Evacuation: Logistics and procedures, destiny of evacuees, and routes of escape

Rescue: Search and rescue operations; details the removal of victims and immediate first aid, who is responsible, and what equipment is needed

Acute care: Casualty collection points, triage, and detailed role descriptions of health care workers for immediate emergency care

Supportive care: Shelter management

Recovery: Postdisaster team meeting, debriefing, critical incident stress debriefing, press conferences, and reports to media

Evaluation: Mock disaster drills and revision of disaster plan based on results

anticipated roles. As pointed out previously, regularly evaluating the performance of all involved personnel through mock disaster drills is an important function of community health nurses and other personnel involved in coordinating disaster response (Dixon, 1986; Neff & Kidd, 1993).

Response and Recovery

The disaster team's **response** is initiated during and after the impact stage of the disaster. Local, state, regional, national, federal, and volunteer agencies assist communities in need (FEMA, 1998c). **Recovery** is a long-term process that occurs during the rehabilitation stage of the disaster. Sometimes, severe financial strain is placed on the local or state government during this time.

Levels of Disaster Response

Disasters are usually defined in terms of severity and levels of response required. Neff and Kidd (1993) identified four levels of disaster response, which are explained in the following paragraphs.

A **level I response** is limited to emergencies that require medical resources from the local hospital and community, such as minor injuries incurred in a local disaster, but also may include severe injuries incurred in multicar accidents or a plane crash. Occasionally, level I responses may include state and federal agency involvement (Neff & Kidd, 1993). In general, hospital and community resources are adequate to provide field and hospital triage, medical treatment, and stabilization for multiple casualties. All hospitals maintain a written disaster plan that corresponds with the local civil defense and community disaster plan.

Fundamental to all written level I hospital disaster plans is the assurance that a command post and chain of command will be established. Usually, the chief executive officer or a senior administrator of the hospital will be in command. Communication via telephones, cellular systems, and portable radios is limited to the commander, security, and other authorized personnel. Water conservation and backup generators are important considerations just in case they are needed. A smooth flow of clients depends on an efficient triage system in the field and within the hospital.

A **level II response** involves multiple casualties that require the use of multijurisdiction health care personnel and medical facilities across a specified region (Auf der Heide, 1989; Neff & Kidd, 1993). When more than one geographic jurisdiction is involved or required, the chain of command structure becomes unified for the sake of clarity, information flow, and minimization of duplications. Coordination and communication efforts among the agencies are emphasized at this response level.

When a mass casualty disaster occurs, a **level III response** is required (Auf der Heide, 1989; Neff & Kidd, 1993). This level of disaster, such as hurricane Andrew in South Florida in 1992, is so overwhelming that medical resources at the local and regional levels are exhausted. State and federal agencies intervene.

The **National Disaster Medical System (NDMS)** is a voluntary system that was formed through the collaborative efforts of several governmental agencies in the United States (Pretto &

Safar, 1991). The primary objective of the NDMS is to increase the mobilization of national resources in an effort to save as many lives as possible. Accomplishing this objective involves providing rapid medical responses, evacuating families and communities, and coordinating medical care. The NDMS efforts, such as recommendations and guidelines for disaster planning and response, filter down to state and local governments and officials, such as the civil defense office and the emergency medical services in the community.

Nurses are involved on every level of the NDMS. Some of the functions of community health and other nurses include serving on the NDMS's national-level task force and board; decision making regarding guidelines and policies; disaster planning on the state and local levels; collaborating with other disaster team members on plans, procedures, and tasks; coordinating the disaster team at various locations within the community; triaging victims at community and hospital locations; and managing the care of victims.

Level IV response occurs when the **Federal Emergency Management Agency (FEMA)** intervenes by providing financial and oversight assistance. FEMA is an independent agency that reports to the president of the United States. Level IV response efforts sometimes require an executive order from the president to declare the disaster a major disaster. (Discussion of the presidential response to FEMA was discussed in the section "Disaster Planning.") From 1964 to early 1998, there were 1,198 disasters, such as the earthquakes in San Francisco in 1989, declared by the president of the United States as level IV disasters (FEMA, 1998a).

Since its development in 1979, FEMA's mission essentially has remained the same, which is "to reduce loss of life and property and protect our nation's critical infrastructure from all types of hazards, through a comprehensive, risk-based emergency management program of mitigation, preparedness, response, and recovery" (FEMA, 1996, p. 2). FEMA may respond during the impact stage or the rehabilitation stage of the disaster, or both. FEMA may respond early, during impact, to increase mobilization of personnel and supplies. During recovery or rehabilitation, FEMA responds as the result of an executive order (FEMA, 1998c).

In the recovery process, FEMA assists in rebuilding communities so that communities and agencies can return to a functional status.

Project Impact was established by FEMA in an effort to build disaster-resistant communities (FEMA, 1998b). In the past 10 years, $20 billion has been spent by FEMA to assist families in repairing and rebuilding their communities after natural disasters. FEMA has responded to 43 major disasters, involving 27 states, declared by President Clinton.

Other Disaster Agencies
American and International Red Cross Disaster Services
The American Red Cross (ARC) is a humanitarian organization "led by volunteers and guided by the Congressional Charter and the Fundamental Principles of the International Red Cross Movement" (ARC, 1997, p. 1). The ARC provides relief to victims of disasters and helps people prevent, prepare for, and respond to emergencies.

On May 21, 1881, Clara Barton and a group of her friends founded the ARC as a result of her commitment to and hard work with the mass casualties of yellow fever, dysentery, and many other infections during the Spanish-American War (ARC, 1990; Frantz, 1998). Because of the efforts of the Red Cross nurses during the Spanish-American War, Cuba communicated the committed efforts of Clara Barton to important officials. Although Barton was not actually a nurse, her organizational skills were exceptional. She was a former schoolteacher and government worker from Massachusetts.

More than 100 years have passed, but the memory of Clara Barton lives. The Red Cross nurses of the Spanish-American War were responsible for the congressional decision of 1901 to establish the Army Nurse Corps.

The unique contribution that Barton made to the worldwide Red Cross movement was her organization of volunteers to help disaster victims (ARC, 1990). America became the 32nd nation to support the Red Cross international treaty at the Geneva Convention in 1882. In 1900, the U.S. Congress granted the ARC its charter.

Today the ARC is composed of more than 1.2 million adult and youth volunteers. Many nurses are considered disaster volunteers. Community health nurses should take a voluntary leader's role in the ARC's disaster preparedness, response, and shelter management. In 1995 and 1996, the ARC spent $216.5 million while assisting 125,120 families during disasters (ARC, 1998). The ARC constantly adapts to current needs (ARC, 1990). Increasingly, Red Cross volunteers are being trained for technological disasters, such as those involving toxic chemicals, explosive materials, radiation, and chemicals.

Salvation Army
The Salvation Army was founded in London in 1865 by William Booth (Salvation Army, 1997a). The Salvation Army was founded on Christian principles. The Salvation Army Act of 1980 described its mission, which is "the advancement of Christian religion . . . of education, the relief of poverty, and other charitable objects beneficial to society of the community of mankind as a whole" (Salvation Army, 1997a).

During a disaster, the Salvation Army provides food, water, shelter, and clothing and helps trace families. With the goal of carrying out God's mission, Salvationists reach out to suffering and needy people by providing the Word of God and basic human physical needs (Salvation Army, 1997b).

Evacuation
Community health nurses, among many other health care personnel, need to realize that wild panic reactions are different from fleeing from a threat (Auf der Heide, 1989). Mileti,

Drabek, and Haas (1975) stated that panic may occur but usually only when at least one of three conditions is present: (1) a perception of immediate danger, (2) encountering blocked escape routes, and/or (3) a feeling of being isolated. When panic occurs, it is usually of short duration and not contagious, depending on the response from the media (Auf der Heide, 1989).

Evacuation traditionally has been a difficult task to carry out because of people's reluctance to evacuate (Quarantelli & Dynes, 1972; Wenger, James, & Faupel, 1985). There are several reasons for this reluctance (Auf der Heide, 1989). The primary reason for hesitancy is that some people do not believe that they are in danger. Another reason is that some people want to remain at the site to protect their property. Not wanting to evacuate until the family can be removed as a unit is another reason for hesitancy. The head of the household or another member may refuse to leave until the other family members, which may also include dogs or other pets, are safe.

Besides the concern for human lives, FEMA is concerned for the lives of animals and, more specifically, the human-animal bond (Lockwood, 1997). Many owners of pets have developed a close relationship with their pets. Lockwood explored why animal owners will risk danger to themselves and not evacuate disaster areas without assurance of their animals' well-being. The most common responses are that people love their animals and treat them as part of the family.

The key to motivating people to evacuate is to improve warning effectiveness, which consists of several strategies (Auf der Heide, 1989). The credibility of the present warning and the validity of past evacuation warnings influence a person's decision of whether to evacuate. Consistency and repetition of the warning by different sources of the evacuation command always increase the chance that a person will heed the warning. Commands to evacuate by agency and community officials are taken more seriously, which promotes the belief of the message. A clear, specific message to evacuate that is understood will yield better results. Finally, an effective strategy is to ensure a course of protective actions, such as ample law enforcement officers on duty, for those people evacuating.

Role of the Media

Mass media can be a friend or foe (Auf der Heide, 1989). To enhance disaster response, the media can provide accurate information, convey instructions to the public, and stimulate donations from parts of the country not affected by the disaster.

On the other hand, the media may complicate the operations by taking a "feeding frenzy" spin on the facts. Reporters may make unreasonable demands on resources, facilities, and officials (Auf der Heide, 1989). Distortion of the facts, overreaction, and perpetuation of disaster myths are other factors that may interfere with the disaster response operations.

Good communication is vital during the evacuation operations. The Weather Bureau, radio stations, television announcements, local sirens and announcements, and computers should be used to alert the public of the impending threat. Another medium is the Emergency Broadcast System, where officials provide local, state, or national information and warnings. When the evacuation is in process, a large volume of requests place overwhelming demands on the media, as well as public officials of the city and county.

Rescue

The search-and-rescue mission is the most challenging part of the disaster operations (Silverstein, 1984; Waeckerle, 1983, 1991). Searching for and rescuing disaster victims tax the physical capabilities and emotions of rescuers. Emotional demands can be extremely traumatic to the rescuers and require psychosocial debriefing.

Teams of health care personnel, fire and security officials, and volunteers comb the designated area many times in search of casualties. Once the casualties are located, quick triage actions are necessary. After the victims are categorized by way of triage, rescue workers need to continue to search the area for undiscovered injured people or dead bodies.

Triage

The triage system normally practiced in emergency departments across the country is not the same triage system used during a disaster (Kitt, Selfridge-Thomas, Proehl, & Kaiser, 1995). Field (disaster) triage is used when mass casualties result from disaster. The initial triage that takes place in the field is called the *primary triage*. *Secondary triage* occurs at the point of entry into the medical facility, and *tertiary triage* occurs in the specified area where the client is located, such as the emergency department, pediatrics, and so on.

Disaster triage allows health care personnel to identify the most salvageable clients so that treatment can be initiated immediately. Colored tags with symbols are attached to disaster victims so that level of triage can be readily seen by health care personnel (Kitt, Selfridge-Thomas, Proehl, & Kaiser, 1995).

Several factors may affect the triage system (Dixon, 1986). The client's general state of health is one factor. For example, an elderly person may have a poor cardiovascular status, which may decrease the person's survival expectation. Another factor that may affect the outcome of triage is the health care worker's inexperience in triage and assessment. Lack of supplies or equipment is another factor. Not having proper supplies and equipment in sufficient quantities can adversely influence the disaster victim's triage status (Neff & Kidd, 1993)

Disaster Shelters

Shelters are managed by trained volunteers and/or Red Cross nurses. When help is needed, the executive director of the affected local chapter of the Red Cross calls upon nurses and other volunteers. Shelters are opened by volunteers in the community

Hurricane Camille

Hurricane Camille was a category 5 hurricane that hit the coasts of Mississippi, Alabama, and Louisiana with winds in excess of 200 mph. Hurricane Camille resulted in the deaths of 141 persons, 9,472 injuries, property loss and damage for 74,000 families, and more than $1 billion total damage. At the 30-year anniversary of the storm, the scars and influence of Camille still exist on the Mississippi Gulf Coast, where the most severe damage occurred. The storm produced 24-foot tidal waves in August of 1969 and remains one of the deadliest storms of the 20th century.

Comments from Survivors

"Afterwards, it looked like we had been bombed. My house was 'caddywhompas' on its foundation. All you could hear were helicopters and people crying. It was the most horrible experience I have ever had."

"The thing that I remember were the dead cows on the beach."

"The beach looked like a holocaust. A woman slipping and sliding through mud and muck clutching a lifeless child to her chest."

Source: Hattiesburg American, August 14, 1994, p. 7A.

---

through coordination efforts of the ARC, the mayor, civil defense, and other officials of the community. Churches, schools, civic centers, and community centers are used as shelters.

It is sometimes difficult to determine or anticipate shelter needs during disasters. The local Red Cross depends on other ARC chapters, the mayor, and civil defense teams to report anticipated numbers of persons that are evacuating their premises and reporting to a shelter. In widespread disasters, shelters are opened in a number of areas that house the local residents as well as victims who have traveled a long distance to escape more immediate danger. An example of a widespread disaster was hurricane Camille in 1969, which traveled from the Mississippi Gulf Coast to North Mississippi and beyond (see box above). Persons in the most danger were on the Mississippi Gulf Coast, so they evacuated to cities and towns north of the coast, while the local residents of those areas also were evacuating their premises and relocating to the same shelters. In instances such as this, anticipating the correct number of shelter residents is difficult. However, good communication between city officials and remote areas regarding evacuation numbers should be a priority.

For each shelter, there is one team manager, at least one nurse volunteer, multiple people to keep records, and numerous volunteers trained to assist victims. Activities include keeping thorough records; coordinating meals; providing snacks, cots, blankets, and other essentials; providing health care, such as first aid treatment and over-the-counter medications that have been authorized by a physician; acting as a liaison between victims and resource agencies and their families; and protecting the victims from harm by keeping alert to possible fire outbreaks, accidents, and other mishaps.

The ARC's motto is "Help Can't Wait" (ARC, 1995). When help is needed, mass recruitment of supplies, equipment, food, and shelter is coordinated by the ARC. For example, in 1993 after the summer Midwest floods, Wal-Mart Stores, Inc., loaned the ARC a large warehouse, forklifts, and staff to expedite distribution of urgently needed supplies to the shelters (ARC, 1995). Other retail stores and pharmaceutical companies offered many supplies and a large amount of monetary assistance.

Role of the Community Health Nurse in Disasters

Why should community health nurses be involved in disaster? Aren't trauma and hospital nurses better qualified to work in disasters than nurses in the community?

Good questions—ones that many student nurses and practicing nurses alike may ask. Our ideas about disasters, what happens, and who is involved—both victims and rescuers—are often shaped by the media. The disaster movie formula developed as a major box office draw in the 1970s with such movies as *The Poseidon Adventure* (1972), about a sinking cruise ship; the *Airport* movie series about jet liner crashes; *The Towering Inferno* (1974), about a burning skyscraper; *The Hindenburg* (1975), about the real-life zeppelin airship disaster of 1937; and *The China Syndrome* (1979), about a fictitious nuclear power plant accident, which became an eerie prelude to the actual Three Mile Island nuclear accident that same year. During the past 30 years, U.S. and international moviegoers have been fascinated by disasters and continue to line up for top movies, such as *Armageddon* (1998), *Deep Impact* (1998), and *Titanic* (1997), the biggest movie money-maker of all time.

These movies, as well as television programs such as *ER*, portray disasters as a backdrop for story lines and romances, heroes and villains, and greatly influence the way we visualize disasters. As a result, disaster planning and disaster preparedness are given very little attention.

Community health nurses are much better prepared than most other health care professionals to manage disasters in the community, because emergency treatment and triage are but two of many activities that help people cope with disaster.

Successful strategies often pair a community health nurse with a trauma nurse in the disaster setting. One of the major determinants of how well a disaster is managed is not only how well we carry out our individual roles in a disaster but also how well we allow others to carry out their roles (Suserud & Haljamae, 1997).

General Functions of the Community Health Nurse

Community health nurses, as well as other nurses, are involved in emergency treatment and triage during the impact stage of the disaster. Good physical assessment skills are vital for success. Only health care personnel highly skilled in assessment should triage. Most health care personnel are not trained in advanced assessment skills and cannot make acuity judgments proficiently. However, baccalaureate-prepared personnel and emergency paramedics are trained to triage and then give emergency treatment.

Because nursing is specialized, as are most health professions, community health nurses often are more knowledgeable about teamwork and interdisciplinary effort than nurses in other specialties because they rely on group efforts daily in community health nursing practice. Community health nurses are experts in program planning, community assessment, and group dynamics, skills that are critical to the effective management of a disaster crisis. Because community health nurses are population focused, assessing and intervening with vulnerable populations are second nature.

Other functions that enable community health nurses to work effectively in disasters include working with the media to inform and educate, the use of public health interventions to minimize risks from communicable diseases, and the securing of community resources for victims. These functions are accomplished while coordinating multiagency efforts in the mediation of health risks at the disaster site (Garcia, 1985). The background work of disaster management, for which community health nurses are perfectly suited, may not make it to the big screen, but such activities are what ultimately influence how well a community survives and heals from disaster.

Specific Nursing Approaches

A major goal of community health nurses is to be an asset to the community, not a burden. Specific approaches that community health nurses should accomplish to mitigate human and material losses in a community disaster include the following strategies:

1. *Personal preparedness:*
   * *Be disaster-prepared and disaster-aware.*
   * *Maintain your own emergency equipment, supplies, and skills.*
   * *Be certain that your family knows what to do during a disaster, when to do it, who to call, and where to go.*
   * *Use caution and prudence when selecting the location of your home.*

2. *Community involvement:*
   * *Become familiar with local disaster plans and emergency evacuation procedures.*
   * *Get involved in the political issues in your community that relate to disaster preparedness and recovery.*
   * *Support leaders who choose long-term, focused solutions in loss reduction and emergency preparedness rather than those who choose short-sighted, politically expedient solutions.*
   * *Help modify land use and develop ordinances that reflect the best knowledge of geography and water hazards.*
   * *Support local emergency assistance organizations by serving on advisory boards.*
   * *Assist in the education of the public in personal disaster preparedness.*
   * *Visit schools to help prepare children for assuming the lifetime responsibility of being prepared for disasters in the community.*

3. *Professional preparedness:*
   * *Become trained and certified in professional disaster nursing by the local ARC chapter.*
   * *Get involved in the development of agency and community disaster plans.*
   * *Attend continuing education classes and disaster skills updates to keep current in disaster management skills.*
   * *Be supportive of administrative efforts to increase disaster preparedness.*
   * *Write new stories, volunteer to speak at community meetings, write letters to the editor of local newspapers, and publish articles in nursing journals about the nursing role in disaster preparedness (Garcia, 1985).*

Shelter Management and Care

Pickens (1992) emphasized the importance in roles of health care workers in disasters. Community health nurses play a vital role in disaster preparedness and response. In fact, the leadership administered by community health nurses may greatly impact the public's reception and comprehension of disaster education and warnings. See the Case Study on p. 567 for examples of successful shelter management.

The general public, as well as many nurses, do not realize the impact that nurses have before, during, and after a disaster (Demi & Miles, 1984). The leadership role that community health nurses can take may prevent deaths and property damage.

Red Cross disaster nurses and other volunteers are often trained to coordinate and manage shelters, conduct tertiary triage within the shelter, and administer first aid to sick or wounded people. Currently, the Red Cross has a pool of more than 15,000 trained disaster volunteers, many of whom are nurses (ARC, 1995). Volunteers are ready for immediate assignment for damage assessment, case management, and shelter management at a moment's notice.

The ARC shelter manager, often a community health nurse, organizes and manages the shelter operations by fulfilling the roles

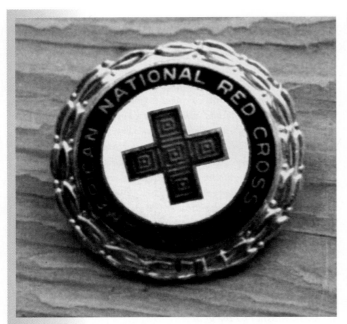

American Red Cross nursing pin.

of administrator, leader, and supervisor (Garcia, 1985). The way the manager conducts operations impacts the flow of operations and activities within the shelter. Functions of the manager include allocating space, obtaining supplies and equipment, scheduling staff, completing reports and records, and attending to problems.

If the community health nurse volunteer happens to be the manager and the nurse on duty, the dual roles and functions can become overwhelming. Care should be coordinated by application of the nursing process (Garcia, 1985). Good assessment and planning skills are among the most important functions of the community health nurse volunteer. Interventions in this setting include preventing disease and illness, providing emotional support, protecting health, and providing intermittent, temporary care to this vulnerable population.

Anticipation of certain problems will facilitate the operations and care of the community health nurse volunteer. For instance, in the shelter population, the nurse should expect some everyday, normal occurrences, which will include chronically ill people who are dependent on medications and equipment, normal episodes of illness and infection, communicable disease, and emotional stress reactions. Evaluation of the shelter population should be ongoing, including one-on-one conferences with shelter families and staff members.

Disaster Recovery

Toffler, in his classic study *Future Shock* (1970), described future shock as "the response to overstimulation" (p. 344). He described numerous examples of stress in situations requiring constant change; among them are persons in disasters. Toffler described persons who experienced a disaster as being trapped in environments

A CONVERSATION WITH...

Because of the tremendous response from caring volunteers at the Oklahoma City bombing disaster, the first critical step was to establish a centralized system to manage the number of individuals calling to report to the emergency site. Once established, we were able to schedule, validate licenses, and orient volunteers from the Oklahoma State Medical Association, Oklahoma Nurses Association, American Red Cross, hospitals, and other entities to the expectations and limitations of the bomb site.

There was tremendous generosity from everyone. Medical supplies, equipment, and medication were immediately available and continued to be delivered at the site for many days. Public health was responsible for centralizing and assuring that these supplies were used appropriately and responsibly by licensed providers. It was important to assure that the appropriate practice guidelines were in place.

Providing disaster services as a public health function doesn't end with just providing emergency services. Public health is also responsible for ensuring that volunteers that provide ongoing emergency health services are competent and properly licensed. It is important to be familiar with your state's nurse practice act and knowledgeable regarding any actions that might be needed to invoke licensure reciprocity in the event that the disaster is such magnitude that volunteers arrive from other states or countries to assist.

Planning and ongoing networking with all players in the emergency response team is very important. While personnel may change, the fundamental needs in an emergency generally do not. Having a public health work force that is prepared in disaster response is very beneficial.

Any coordination and networking that can be in place with state and local American Red Cross chapters prior to a disaster benefits both the public health agency and the American Red Cross.

—**Toni D. Frioux,**
MS, CNS, ARNP, Chief, Nursing Service,
Oklahoma State Department of Health

that are rapidly changing, unfamiliar, and unpredictable. Results of such situations can be devastating, even for the most stable and well-prepared person. Victims of disasters may be hurled into antiadaptive states and be incapable of the most elementary decision making (Toffler, 1970). Evidence of this reaction can be seen in pictures of a woman, after a destructive earthquake, strolling down a dangerous, debris-filled road with a dead or wounded baby in her arms, her face blank and numb, appearing impervious to the danger around her. Persons can be overwhelmed and become paralyzed as familiar objects and relationships are transformed. Where a person's house once stood, a tornado can within minutes change the environment into an unrecognizable pile of rubble and gushing water pipes. The Oklahoma City bombing destroyed life and property within minutes, replacing familiar landmarks with images of unimaginable horror and destruction.

Simple acts taken for granted hours before, such as making a telephone call or pouring a cup of coffee, are no longer appropriate or possible. Signs, sounds, and other psychological and cultural cues surround disaster victims without meaning, without recognition during and immediately after the impact. Every word, every action, every movement is characterized by uncertainty. Even in a crowd, victims often experience a sense of isolation and loneliness, abandonment, and an overwhelming sense of loss—loss of the world as they know it. Confusion, disorientation, and distortion of reality occur spontaneously; fatigue, anxiety, tenseness, and extreme irritability follow. Apathy, emotional withdrawal, and pessimism result when victims develop a sense of little hope for the future or when they see themselves as never being safe or stable again (Toffler, 1970).

In the classic study *Everything in its Path*, sociologist Kai Erickson described the 1972 Buffalo Creek flood and its aftermath in terms of disaster impact and the destruction of community (Erickson, 1976). This study provided a detailed and analyzed view of a disaster and the resulting conflict between individualism and dependency, self-assertion and resignation, and self-centeredness and community orientation. The results of this devastating disaster included loss of community connection, declining morality, rise in crime, and the rise in out-migration from the sudden loss of neighborhood and community. Organized disaster activity was largely provided by outsiders.

Collective deaths, like those in a disaster, do not permit persons to set up the usual barriers between the living and the dead, as is customary in the deaths of the hospital, where "death is screened from view, sanitized, muffled, tidied up" (Erickson, 1976, p. 169). In disaster, "death lies out there at its inescapable worst. There are no wreckers to rush the crushed vehicle away, no physicians to shroud death in a crisp white sheet or to give it a clean medical name, no undertakers to wash away the evidence of death and to knead out the creases of pain or fear . . . and the sight does not go away easily" (Erickson, 1976, p. 169).

Effects on Survivors

When death is experienced on a wide scale, such as in a disaster, survivors often experience guilt as a result of their own survival

(Erickson, 1976). They may even come to regret their own survival, when others around them were killed in what seems like a meaningless and capricious way, in part because "they cannot understand by what logic they came to be spared" (p. 170). Survivor guilt has often been described in disaster research literature. Lifton (1967), in his classic study of the psychological effects of the atomic bomb in Hiroshima, found that survivors described the open eyes of corpses as evoking guilt: It was as if the eyes were saying, "Why me, why not you?"

Lifton and Olson (1976) identified five major elements that may be found in some type of combination in all disasters. Psychological difficulty or maladaptive response is more likely to occur if all five elements are found in a single disaster, as in the Buffalo Creek flood. The five elements are suddenness of the event, human callousness in causation (human-made rather than natural causation), continuing relationship of survivors to the disaster, isolation of the community, and totality of destruction.

The experience of the disaster can have both short- and long-term effects on mental health and functioning, such as dissociation, depression, and PTSD (Gerrity & Flynn, 1997). Refer to Box 24-5 for other health effects associated with disasters. Meichenbaum (1994) has compiled from disaster research a list of factors that can place individuals in a vulnerable position for developing psychological problems when all five of Lifton and Olson's (1976) elements are present in a disaster. They include the following:

- *Objective and subjective characteristics of the disaster, such as proximity of the victim to the disaster site, the duration, the degree of physical injury, and the witnessing of grotesque, graphic scenes*
- *The characteristics in the community of postdisaster response and recovery environment, such as cohesiveness of community and disruption of social support systems*
- *The characteristics of the individual or group; for example, elders, unemployed persons, single parents, children, those with previous history of mental disorders, and those with marital conflict before the disaster*

Most studies on the aftermath of disasters have reported that the first reaction of survivors is a state of dazed shock and numbness. The "disaster syndrome" consists of classic symptoms of mourning and bereavement on a communitywide scale: grief for lost community members and homes and grief for lost culture and familiar surroundings (which will never be the same again, no matter what form the recovery takes). To make this reaction worse, government and rescue workers often control access to the disaster area, keeping residents from their own homes and cleaning up wreckage without consulting the community members. Often, such work by disaster workers, although necessary, further distances the survivors from their need to be a part of the recovery process and exacerbates feelings of loss of control caused by the disaster itself.

Among the symptoms of extreme trauma that can affect an entire society, such as the Oklahoma City bombing, is a sense of vulnerability, a feeling that one has lost a certain natural immunity to misfortune, a growing conviction that the world is no longer a

BOX 24-9 THE CHERNOBYL NUCLEAR DISASTER: WILL IT EVER BE OVER?

On April 26, 1986, a reactor blew up in Chernobyl in the former Soviet Union, resulting in an explosion that threw out 100 million curies of dangerous radionuclides to surrounding areas of the Ukraine, Belarus, and Russia. The World Health Organization estimates that 4.9 million persons were affected, making it the largest nuclear disaster in history. The results: Livestock, vegetables, grains, the soil, and the environment continue to be hazardous for human existence, although a large population still inhabit these areas. Cancer, rare pediatric cancers, leukemia, chromosomal damage, and stress-related disorders plague the region and result in premature death and disability among all age groups. Scientists even now do not know how long the nuclear danger will remain or if it ever again the region will be safe to live in.

Source: Edwards, 1994.

safe place to be (see Box 24-10 and Case Study on p. 567). A lingering thought grows into a prediction of sorts: If this can happen, something even more terrible is bound to happen—the line has been crossed (Erickson, 1976). Box 24-9 describes an example of the far-reaching effects of the Chernobyl disaster, which continues to threaten the well-being of affected communities.

Special Survivor Populations: Elders and Children

Children are at special risk during a disaster because of their immaturity—they have not yet developed adult coping strategies and do not yet have the life experiences to help them understand what has happened to them. Also, we know that children rely on routine and consistency in their environment, relationships, and home life for a sense of security and identity. These areas are often disrupted in a disaster. Problems can emerge at school and last for much longer periods when compared with adults (Gerrity & Flynn, 1997). Children may suffer from fears, phobias, sleep disorders, nightmares, excessive dependence, fear of being alone, hypersensitivity to noise and weather conditions, and regression, such as thumbsucking, bedwetting, and "baby talk" or stuttering (Laube & Murphy, 1985).

Elders often experience significant depression and despair from losing homes and being uprooted from familiar surroundings. Many of the elderly had already lost primary family members and friends before the disaster. Among their valuables are family photos and mementos, Bibles, and keepsakes. Loss of this sort has a considerably greater effect on elders than others. There are also the compounded problems of more chronic diseases and health problems, making them more vulnerable to disaster stress (Gerrity

& Flynn, 1997). Disorientation and memory disturbances have also been noted in this population (Laube & Murphy, 1985). Again, refer to Box 24-5 to review health effects in disasters.

Simple intervention methods, such as group work for children and elders and short-term counseling immediately after the disaster, have proven quite effective in helping the recovery process. Community health nurses are in an excellent position to intervene with these vulnerable populations. Community health nurses must be able to locate children and elders so that immediate action can be taken. The most likely place to find these populations are in community shelters.

Traditional healers and informal community resource persons have also been used effectively by recovery teams to assist the community in looking within for healing energy. Women's associations, community development schemes, family welfare workers, and church volunteers have all had significant success in mobilizing community resources to promote community healing and recovery. Such strategies reduce the need for outside resources, as well as helping the community regain its stability using its own assets of solidarity (Richman, 1993).

Collective Trauma: The Loss of Community

Erickson (1976) detailed the loss of not only the sense of community, which occurs in a mass disaster, but also the loss of communality, which consists of a network of relationships that make up their general human surround. Erickson (1976) described communality as a "state of mind shared among a particular gathering of people" (p. 189). In a sense, this community is one that cushions the pain, provides a context for intimacy, represents morality, and serves as the repository of old traditions and culture.

When a disaster demolishes a community, people find that they no longer have the collective reservoir of pooled resources, both physical and emotional, from which to draw. Communities act as a "cluster of people acting in concert and moving to the same collective rhythms who allocate their personal resources in such a way that the whole comes to have more humanity than its constituent parts. In effect, people put their own individual resources at the disposal of the group—placing them in the communal store and then drawing on that reserve supply for the demands of everyday life" (p. 194).

When a community is destroyed, people find themselves without the reservoir on which they have relied in the past. They find that they are almost empty of feeling, empty of affection, and empty of confidence and assurance. Residents feel abandoned, often expressing feelings of fear, apathy, and demoralization. Comments from survivors often reflect despair: "I thought this was the end of the world" or "It looked like Dooms Day" (Erickson, 1976, p. 199).

. . . .

Whoever fights monsters should see to it that in the process he does not become the monster. And when you look into the abyss, the abyss looks into you.

Nietzsche

. . . .

Nurses' Reactions to Disasters

Nurses also should attend to the needs of the disaster workers themselves during and after a disaster to reduce the possibility of producing secondary victims. Rescue personnel are often reluctant to take breaks to replenish food, water, and rest when time is of essence in the search and recovery phase when they are needed. Nevertheless, nurses should be firm in reminding workers that in order to remain useful, they must not exhaust themselves in the process. Seeing that workers are rotated and providing rest, nourishment, and relaxation for the rescuers should be considered essential responsibilities of the community health nurse.

Nurses often experience the same disturbing, and sometimes dramatic, emotional problems as those found in their clients who were victims. Nurses may experience difficulty concentrating, fatigue, irritability, insomnia, and other unique symptoms of stress. The unique symptoms include depersonalization of the victim, a macabre sense of dark humor, hypervigilance, and excessive unwillingness to disengage or leave the disaster scene or the helping role (e.g., refusal to leave after the arrival of a relief shift) (Gerrity & Flynn, 1997). Reactions of nurses are magnified when the nurse is a member of the affected community and when the nurse may have endured property and community damage, as well as

CASE STUDY

The Oklahoma City Bombing, April 19, 1995

On the morning of April 19, 1995, the Alfred P. Murrah Federal Building in Oklahoma City was the site of a devastating terrorist bomb. In addition to federal employees and other government workers, the building was the site of a day-care center. Because of the effectiveness of the city's disaster plan, rescue and recovery began within minutes after the explosion. Oklahoma experiences frequent, deadly tornadoes throughout the state and consequently maintains a highly organized disaster planning response.

Initial priorities the morning of the bombing included getting people out of the building, triaging injuries, and transporting the injured to six nearby hospitals. Nurses in hospitals, home health agencies, and public health and other facilities in the community quickly responded to the needs of the victims. By midafternoon of that day, the four trauma departments had seen 40 to 80 persons each. Victims were transported by ambulances, private vehicles, cabs, and vans. A family communication center was quickly set up at a local church, 5 miles from the bomb site, by the American Red Cross and FEMA. This center, which "wrapped its arms around the families of the victims of the blast," provided mental health professionals, hospice nurses, psychiatric nurses, and counselors 24 hours a day for 2 weeks after the bombing. The medical examiner's office communicated with the families of the victims there, and rescue workers from the bomb site frequently reported back to the families concerning the progress of the search teams.

A play area for children was set up, and the Salvation Army provided comfort services, including food and clothing. Pets were brought by local groups to provide solace for the victims. A Native American healer was present for tribal members. Toll-free numbers were provided by the state mental health department for direct and indirect victims' use to prevent and treat posttraumatic stress disorder. Support groups were set up, television talk shows featured survivors and disaster workers, and articles were printed in the local newspapers, all directed toward giving the people of Oklahoma a chance to talk through the horror of their collective experiences. The city's convention center became a huge hostel that fed, clothed, and housed thousands of rescue workers during this period. Roses and chocolates appeared on the pillows of disaster workers, stress management was available, massages were provided for sore muscles, and there was "always a listening ear for sore souls."

Nurses were involved at all levels of the disaster, including triage at the command center, accompanying surgeons as they removed the legs of a child in the bombed building, providing grief counseling for the families of victims and for the disaster workers themselves, providing direct care at hospitals to the injured, and visiting the families of victims in their homes for forensic identification and later on as follow-up.

According to Wilson (1996), an "important reason why the people here worked so well was because of disaster planning. When people live in an area that is nicknamed 'tornado alley,' they plan for disaster" (p. 24). "Though we will never rectify the loss of life incurred in a disaster by planning ahead, we can be ready to mobilize the resources to make all of us a little less vulnerable" (p. 25).

Source: Wilson, 1996.

stress related to family well-being. According to Laube-Morgan (1992), nurses should be considered "normal persons reacting in a very normal manner to an abnormal condition" (p. 19).

Sources of stress for the disaster nurse can be generally classified into three categories: (1) event stressors, the trauma and fatigue associated with the extreme intensity of the disaster event, of the highest intensity if the nurse lives in the affected community and has family who are potential victims; (2) occupational stress—stress related to role conflict, role overload, and role confusion; and (3) organizational stressors—factors that emerge from the organizational response itself, multiagency demands, and the complex tangle of bureaucracy that emerges in a major disaster (Hartsough & Myers, 1985). With every disaster victim treated, nurses often experience an unconscious fear that the victim could just as easily have been one of their loved ones.

Nurses are educated to maintain professional composure in any type of stressful situation, even in the face of grief, suffering, and death. This composure has been termed *detached concern* by Coombs and Goldman (1973). Detached concern is the adaptive

ability to care for critically ill and injured clients while maintaining an acceptable emotional detachment. Research has revealed that nurses function effectively in disasters, and very few have long-term emotional difficulties after the disaster.

In Laube's (1973) study of the hurricane Celia disaster, the majority of nurses functioned in their role without impairment from anxiety. Major stressors that nurses may experience during disasters have been identified by researchers as excessive physical demands, concerns for personal safety, inadequate supplies, seeing people suffer and not being able to meet basic needs of all, hurt children, disorganization, and concern for their own family's welfare (Waters, Selander, & Stuart, 1992).

Family roles seem to play a critical part in the nurse's response to disaster. Health care workers who are from the disaster area have exceptional stress, because not only must they work through their own reactions to and losses of the community from the disaster, but they also must resolve the family/community role conflict (Waters, Selander, & Stuart, 1992). In other words, when the nurse's family well-being is jeopardized, professional effectiveness decreases and

A CONVERSATION WITH...

How did you become interested in disaster research?

In 1970 I was fresh out of my master's program at the University of Colorado and was asked by the local American Red Cross Chapter in Dallas to give a talk to their nurses on the psychological effects of disaster. I thought they wanted me to talk about the psychological effects of disaster on nurses (later learned that they just wanted the effects in general). I had no experience so I went to the library to research the subject and found only one reference specific to the effect on nurses—Jeannette Rayner's article written in 1958. By generalizing from publications about army nursing, plus Rayner's article, I managed to meet my assignment but felt a great need for an in depth study of the psychological effects of disaster on nurses. I later wrote a small grant to the American Red Cross for funding to survey nurses' reactions in a recent tornado close to home. While waiting on that response, Hurricane Celia hit the coast of Texas. I immediately called and requested that I be sent to that area. This was granted and I was on site within 24 hours of the disaster. That study was published in Nursing Research. I later broadened my area of study to cover all health care providers in disaster. Not long after my first study I was invited to be a part of a task force to revise the Disaster Act to include assistance for psychological aspects of disaster. That was completed and has been carried forth ever since.

Should BSN nurses be prepared in disaster response and recovery?

Students in baccalaureate programs should have classes and simulated experience in reducing the impact of disaster. If available, collaboration with the local Red Cross chapter is ideal. Nursing students that take their courses can earn hours toward Red Cross certification, thus shortening the time after graduation to become a Red Cross nurse.

Why do you believe BSN nurses should be prepared in disaster nursing?

Nurses are uniquely qualified by the nature or their education and experience. Nurses are prepared to work with the whole patient—physically and psychologically. They work both in crisis and chronic conditions which is necessary because a disaster victim, definitely in crisis, may also have a chronic illness. Thus, they have the basic qualifications. Updating their knowledge and skills should continue through workshops and disaster drills sponsored by/through their place of work.

—Jerri Laube, RN, PhD, FAAN

Dr. Jerri Laube is co-author, with Dr. Shirley A. Murphy, of *Perspectives on Disaster Recovery* (1985, Appleton-Century-Crofts).

stress more likely will impact the nurse's role. This finding means that outside disaster workers are indicated early in the course of disasters and should continue until the local health care providers can be assured of their own family's safety (Laube, 1985).

• •

It's when Mother Nature gets so angry at man and his arrogance that she whips up a little humble pie.
Jimmy Buffett, 1998, on a tornado in Brookings, South Dakota

• •

Stuhlmiller (1996) contended that because nurses are typically involved with suffering and disruption of lives of their clients, they in fact may be in a better position than other disaster workers to mediate the effects of the disaster. By participating in debriefings, nurses are healing themselves as they help others begin their own process of healing. Stuhlmiller contended that we often assume that workers are at risk for post-traumatic stress and proceed with negative assumptions about how they should react. By doing so, we unwittingly hamper their "natural restorative capacities" (p. 19). In other words, looking for the negative effects may overshadow the positive outcomes on which nurses tend to focus—the positive outcomes that come from helping people in extreme need.

"Disasters challenge self-understanding and meanings just as illness does . . . what the rescuers need most then is what nurses are particularly good at providing. Nurses can foster emotional recovery and growth by attending to what approaches work best and by acknowledging the validity of the person's expressed pain, fear and grief" (p. 19). Such a view is consistent with Laube's (1973) conclusion that with all of the possible stressors nurses face with disasters, studies consistently reveal the nurses' responses to disaster do not interfere with their effectiveness as professionals (Laube, 1973).

As a result of these findings, it can be concluded that nurses are extremely vulnerable to PTSD in the aftermath of a disaster. The following Research Brief describes the nurses' reactions and feelings during and after hurricane Hugo. Box 24-10 consists of actual quotes from nurses who expressed their feelings about their work in a disaster.

Prevention Strategies for Nurses

By being prepared for a disaster through specialized training and anticipatory stress counseling, nurses can reduce the damage of a disaster to self. Simple measures such as appreciating the intensity of emotions and dealing with them; taking breaks; eating nutritious foods with smaller, more frequent meals; avoiding drinking large amounts of caffeine and alcohol; exercising; and sleeping as much as possible have given nurses the added strength to not only

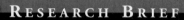

RESEARCH BRIEF

Chubon, S. J. (1992). Home care during the aftermath of hurricane Hugo. Public Health Nursing, 9(2), 97–102.

Chubon was in the midst of an ethnographic study of home care nurses' job stress when hurricane Hugo struck the South Carolina coast in 1989. The home health agency was heavily damaged by wind and water and was uninhabitable for more than a week. Because the nurse researcher had observed the nurses for 10 weeks before the hurricane, she was able to collect data about their response to the disaster in the context of their usual role of home health nurse. The nurses in the agency were simultaneously victims and caregivers for their home health clients. They experienced grief, anger, and frustration about their losses, as well as conflict between family responsibilities and work responsibilities. Chubon's work supported the findings of previous studies in which nurses continued to function effectively in their work roles despite their emotional responses. Because baseline data were available before the hurricane struck, this study indicated that the nurses' functioning was generally consistent with their predisaster work patterns. Sources of stress consistently related to the safety of their own loved ones and family. Suggested interventions were (1) to bring outside nurses from other home health agencies to care for assigned clients until the local nurses stabilize their own family situations and (2) to make mental health resources available in the immediate postrecovery period for the nurses in the agency.

BOX 24-10 WORDS OF WISDOM FROM NURSES WORKING THE OKLAHOMA CITY BOMBING

"I realized that in the midst of the organized chaos, I had found the focus which nurses have had since Florence Nightingale, when she attended wounded soldiers of the Crimean War. I found that my degree of specialization no longer mattered. I had become a trauma nurse for one patient when he needed me."

—Melissa Craft, RN

"These memories are hard to forget. But I will remember the strength and goodness that could not be extinguished even by such devastation. For its part, nursing as a caring profession was made manifest during this time."

—Karen Bradford, RN

Source: The Many Graces, 1996.

survive but flourish in a disaster. Seldom can as much attention be given to the victims as the nurse believes is necessary.

Although nurses seem to be fairly effective in mediating stressors in the disaster setting, they are certainly not immune to possible ill effects. Laube-Morgan (1992) suggested from her research of the 1989 Loma Prieta earthquake in California that prevention programs for disaster workers should be included in disaster preparedness. For primary level prevention, a crisis team should work with the disaster staff before a disaster strikes. The crisis team should include a social worker, minister, psychiatric nurse, and other mental health professionals as available. This team should have input into the disaster plan and be included in disaster drill critiques and debriefing. At a secondary level of prevention, the same team should be highly visible during the impact of the disaster. They could provide emotional support and monitor the emotional stability of the workers, intervening as necessary. At the tertiary level of prevention, after the disaster, the team should take an active role in organizing and conducting mandatory disaster debriefing sessions. Counseling referrals should be made at this time and should, again, have input into the critique of the disaster plan's effectiveness related to worker response and recovery (Laube-Morgan, 1992). Such strategic interventions can prevent burnout and emotional casualties of the health care provider.

CONCLUSION

As disasters are increasing in number and, many times, severity each year, community health nurses need to be adequately prepared more now than ever before. Lillian Wald, a famous nursing theorist and community activist, responded to her societal needs by developing the Henry Street Settlement House in 1893. Wald stated, "Nurses not only serve the individual but promote the interest of a collective society" (as cited in Kippenbrock, 1991, p. 209). This statement also applies today, especially in the face of disasters.

Being prepared for future disasters means that community health nurses must plan disaster care for multicultural populations. The hallmark of American society is multiculturalism (Sobier, 1995). The major disaster goal for nurses now and in the future is to retain maximum wellness of individuals and populations in communities (Procter & Cheek, 1995). Learning to work with appropriate resources and placing emphasis on specific approaches to enhance individuals, families, and communities are integral to protection and healing from a disaster.

Melanie Dreher, past President of Sigma Theta Tau International (1996), pointed out that nurses are very resilient and can be called *everyday heroes*. There have been numerous nurses who were outstanding in heroic acts, such as Nightingale, Alcott, and Cavell. Dreher contended that nurses with "heroine" status are recognizable by traits and actions. She stated: "They define their life's work not in terms of paychecks, working conditions and employment benefits, but in terms of the number of lives saved, families in crisis who were counseled, and patients comforted" (p. 5).

CRITICAL THINKING ACTIVITIES

1. Based on the Case Study on p. 567, answer the following questions:
   - What are the primary, secondary, and tertiary prevention disaster interventions carried out by nurses during the Oklahoma City bombing?
   - Identify activities in each of the stages of disaster recovery.
   - Give examples of the three categories of stressors that disaster nurses faced in Oklahoma.
   - Identify the components of the Oklahoma City disaster plan. What would be your recommendations for the disaster team, based on the information above?

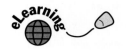

Explore Community Health Nursing on the web! To learn more about the topics in this chapter, use the passcode provided to access your exclusive web site:
http://communitynursing.jbpub.com
If you do not have a passcode, you can obtain one at this site.

REFERENCES

Advisory Committee on the International Decade for Natural Hazard Reduction. (1987). *Confronting natural disasters: An international decade for natural hazard reduction*. Washington, DC: National Academy Press.

American Psychiatric Association (APA). (1987). *Diagnostic and statistical manual of mental disorders* (3rd ed. rev.). Washington, DC: Author.

American Red Cross (ARC). (1990). *A history of helping others* (ARC Publication No. 4627). Washington, DC: ARC National Headquarters.

American Red Cross (ARC). (1991). *Coping with disaster: Emotional health issues for disaster workers on assignment* (ARC Publication No. 4472). Washington, DC: ARC National Headquarters.

American Red Cross (ARC). (1995). *Disaster is everybody's business* (ARC Publication No. 5061). Washington, DC: ARC National Headquarters.

American Red Cross (ARC). (1996). *Disaster services: We're there when you need us* (ARC Publication No. 4450). Washington, DC: ARC National Headquarters.

American Red Cross (ARC). (1997). *Our mission statement*: www.redcross.org/mission.html.

American Red Cross (ARC). (1998). *Disaster facts*: www.fema.gov/library/df_5.htm.

Anderson, M. B. (1991). Which costs more: prevention or recovery? In A. Kreimer & M. Munasinghe (Eds.), *Managing natural disasters and the environment*. Washington, DC: World Bank.

Auf der Heide, E. (1989). *Disaster response: Principles of preparation and coordination*. St. Louis: Mosby.

Baker, G, & Chapman, R. (1962). *Man and society in disaster*. New York: Basic Books.

Barker, E. (1989). Care givers as casualties. *Western Journal of Nursing Research, 11*, 5.

Barry J. M. (1997). *Rising tide: The great Mississippi flood of 1927 and how it changed America*. Simon & Schuster: New York.

Berz, G. (1984). Research and statistics on natural disasters in insurance and reinsurance companies. *The Geneva Papers on Risk and Insurance, 9*, 135–157.

Buffett, J. (1998). *A pirate looks at fifty*. New York: Random House.

Chubon, S. J. (1992). Home care during the aftermath of Hurricane Hugo. *Public Health Nursing 9*(2), 97–102.

Coombs, R. H., & Goldman, L. J. (1973). Maintenance and discontinuity of coping mechanisms in an intensive care unit. *Social Problems, 20*, 342–355.

Demi, A. S., & Miles, M. S. (1984). An examination of nursing leadership following a disaster. *Topics in clinical nursing*. Rockville, MD: Aspen Publishing.

Dixon, M. (1986). Disaster planning—Medical response: Organization and preparation. *American Association of Occupational Health Nurses, 34*(12), 580–584.

Drabek, T. E. (1986). *Human system response to disaster: An inventory of sociological findings*. New York: Springer-Verlag.

Dreher, M. C. (1996, First Quarter). Heroism. *Reflections*, 4–5.

Dynes, R. R., Quarantelli, E. L., & Kreps, G. A. (1972, December). *A perspective on disaster planning, TR-77* (pp. 6–8). Washington, DC: Defense Civil Preparedness Agency.

Edwards, M. (1994, August). Living with the monster—Chernobyl. *National Geographic, 186*, 2.

Epstein, P. R. (1998). Watching El Nino, *Public Health Reports, 113*, 330–333.

Erickson, K. (1976). *Everything in its path: Destruction of community in the Buffalo Creek flood*. Simon & Schuster: New York.

Federal Emergency Management Agency (FEMA). (1996). *This is FEMA*. Washington, DC: FEMA Headquarters.

Federal Emergency Management Agency (FEMA). (1997a). *FEMA highlights and statistics for 1997*: www.fema.gov/library/fact97.htm.

Federal Emergency Management Agency (FEMA). (1997b). *The strategic plan: Partnership for a safer future*. Washington, DC: FEMA Headquarters.

Federal Emergency Management Agency (FEMA). (1998a). *Historical presidential disaster declarations*: www.fema.gov/library/dd-1964.gif.

Federal Emergency Management Agency (FEMA). (1998b). *Project impact*: www.fema.gov/impact/.

Federal Emergency Management Agency (FEMA). (1998c). *The federal disaster declaration process and disaster aid programs: Response and recovery*: www.fema.gov/declara/.

Frantz, A. K. (1998). Nursing pride: Clara Barton in the Spanish-American War. *American Journal of Nursing, 98*(10), 39–41.

Garcia, L. M. (1985). *Disaster nursing: Planning, assessment, and intervention.* Rockville, MD: Aspen Publishing.

Gerrity, E. T., & Flynn, B. W. (1997). Mental health consequences of disasters. In E. K. Noji (Ed.), *The public health consequences of disasters* (pp. 101–121). New York: Oxford University Press.

Guha-Sapir, D., & Lechat, M. F. (1986). Reducing the impact of natural disasters: Why aren't we better prepared? *Health Policy and Planning, 1,* 118–126.

Hartsough, D. M., & Myers, D. G. (1985). *Disaster work and mental health: Prevention and control of stress among workers.* Rockville, MD: National Institute of Mental Health.

International Decade for Natural Disaster Reduction Promotion Office (IDNDR) (1994). *Natural disasters in the world: Statistical trends on natural disasters.* Tokyo: National Land Agency.

Janis, I. L., & Mann, L. (1977, June). Emergency decision making: A theoretical analysis of responses to disaster warnings. *Journal of Human Stress,* 35–48.

Kippenbrock, T. A. (1991). Wishing I'd been there. *Nursing and Health Care, 12*(4), 209.

Kitt, S., Selfridge-Thomas, J., Proehl, J. A., & Kaiser, J. (1995). *Emergency nursing: A physiologic and clinical perspective* (2nd ed.). Philadelphia: W. B. Saunders.

Laube, J. (1973). Psychological reactions to nurses in disaster. *Nursing Research, 22,* 343–347.

Laube-Morgan, J. (1992). The professional's psychological response in disaster: Implications for practice. *Journal of Psychosocial Nursing, 30*(2), 17–22.

Laube, J., & Murphy, S. A. (1985). *Perspectives on disaster recovery.* Norwalk, CT: Appleton-Century-Crofts.

Lifton, R. J. (1967). *Death in life: Survivors in Hiroshima.* New York: Random House.

Lifton, R. J., & Olson, E. (1976). The human meaning of disaster. *Psychiatry, 39,* 1–7.

Lockwood, R. (1997). *FEMA: Through hell and high water: Disasters and the human-animal bond.* Washington, DC: FEMA and the Humane Society of the United States.

Logue, J. N., Melick, M. E., & Hansen, H. (1981). Research issues and directions in the epidemiology of health effects of disasters. *Epidemiological Review, 3,* 140–162.

Malilay, J. (1997). Floods. In E. K. Noji (Ed.), *The public health consequences of disasters* (pp. 287–301). New York: Oxford University Press.

Meichenbaum, D. (1994, June 14–18). *Disasters, stress, and cognition.* Paper presented for the NATO Workshop on Stress and Communities, Chateau da Bonas, France.

Mileti, D. S., Drabek, T. E., & Haas, J. E. (1975). *Human systems in extreme environments: A sociological perspective* (Monograph No. 21). Boulder, CO: Program on Technology, Environment, and Man, Institute of Behavioral Science, University of Colorado.

Mizutani, T., & Nakano, T. (1989). The impact of natural disasters on the population of Japan. In J. I. Clarke, P. Curson, S. L. Kayastha, & P. Nag (Eds.), *Population and disaster.* Cambridge, MA: Basil Blackwell.

Muench, J. (1996). Disaster training pays off for Juneau nurses. *Alaska Nurse, 46*(5), 1.

Neff, J. A., & Kidd, P. S. (1993). *Trauma nursing: The art and science.* St. Louis: Mosby.

Noji, E. K. (1997). *The public health consequences of disasters.* New York: Oxford University Press.

Office of U.S. Foreign Disaster Assistance. (1995). *Disaster history: Significant data on major disasters worldwide, 1900-present.* Washington, DC: Agency for International Development.

Pickens, S. (1992). The decade for natural disaster reduction. *Nursing & Health Care, 13,* 192–195.

Pretto, E. A., & Safar, P. (1991). National medical response to mass disaster in the United States: Are we prepared? *Journal of the American Medical Association, 266,* 1259–1262.

Procter, N. G., & Cheek, J. (1995). Nurses' role in world catastrophic events: War dislocation effects on Serbian Australians. In B. Neuman (Ed.), *The Neuman systems model* (3rd ed.). Norwalk, CT: Appleton & Lange.

Quarantelli, E. L., & Dynes, R. R. (1972, February). When disaster strikes (it isn't much like what you've heard about or read about). *Psychology Today,* p. 72.

Richman, N. (1993). After the flood. *American Journal of Public Health, 83*(11), 1522–1524.

Sabin, L. (1998) *Struggles and triumphs: The story of Mississippi nurses.* Jackson, MS: Mississippi Hospital Association Foundation.

Salvation Army. (1997a). *The Salvation Army international headquarters: About us:* http://salvationarmy.org/aboutus.htm.

Salvation Army. (1997b). *The Salvation Army international headquarters: International spiritual life commission:* www.salvationarmy.org/slc.htm.

Silverstein, M. E. (1984). *Triage decision trees and triage protocols.* Washington, DC: FEMA Headquarters.

Sklar, D. P. (1987). Casualty patterns and disasters. *Journal of the World Association of Emergency Disaster Medicine, 3,* 49–51.

Sobier, R. (1995). Nursing care for the people of a small planet: Culture and the Neuman systems model. In B. Neuman (Ed.), *The Neuman systems model* (3rd ed.). Norwalk, CT: Appleton & Lange.

Stuhlmiller, C. M. (1996, First Quarter). Studying the rescuers. *Reflections,* 18–19.

Sullivan, T. J. (1998). *Collaboration: A health care imperative.* New York: McGraw-Hill.

Suserud, B., & Haljamae, H. (1997). Acting at a disaster site: Experiences expressed by Swedish nurses. *Journal of Advanced Nursing, 25*(1), 155–162.

Taggert, S. D. (1982). *Emergency preparedness manual.* Salt Lake City: University of Utah.

The anniversary of hurricane Camille. (1994, August 14). *Hattiesburg American,* p. 7a.

The many graces of Oklahoma City nurses. (1996). *Reflections, 22*(1), 10–12.

Toffler, A. (1970). *Future shock.* New York: Random House.

Waeckerle, J. F. (1983). The skywalk collapse: A personal response. *Annals of Emergency Medicine, 12,* 651.

Waeckerle, J. F. (1991). Disaster planning and response. *New England Journal of Medicine, 324,* 815–821.

Waters, K. A., Selander, J., & Stuart, G. W. (1992). Psychological adaptation of nurses post-disaster. *Issues in Mental Health Nursing, 13,* 177–190.

Wenger, D. E., James, T. F., & Faupel, C. E. (1985). *Disaster beliefs and emergency planning.* New York: Irving Publishers.

Wilson, J. S. (1996). Healing Oklahoma's wounds. *Home Healthcare Nurse, 14*(1), 23–25.

Unit V
Vulnerable Populations

Chapter 25

Vulnerability: An Overview

Angeline Bushy

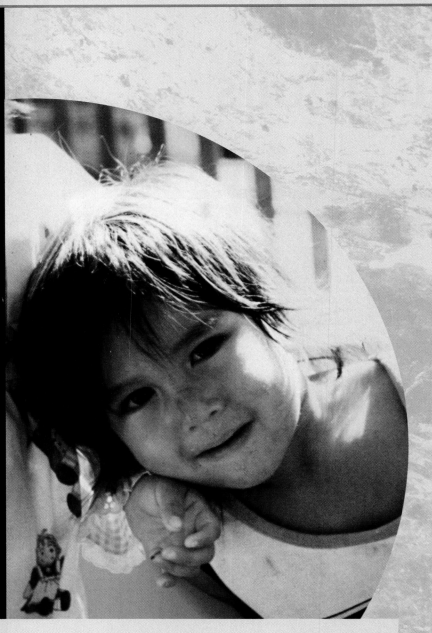

Community health nurses traditionally have been recognized as cru-saders and advocates for populations described as vulnerable and at risk. Compared with the general population, persons in these groups experience disparities in access and uneven quality of care, which contributes to poorer health outcomes.

QUESTIONS TO CONSIDER

After reading this chapter, answer the following questions:
1. What is vulnerability?
2. What are the risk factors that contribute to vulnerability and poor health?
3. What is the relationship between poverty and vulnerability?
4. What are some examples of vulnerable populations?
5. What are the some characteristics of specific vulnerable populations?
6. How can nurses intervene to bring about positive health outcomes for vulnerable populations?

KEY TERMS

Access to care	Hardiness	Risk	Vulnerable families
At risk	Medically indigent	Underinsured	Vulnerable populations
Disadvantaged	Near poor	Uninsured	Working poor
Disenfranchised	Poverty index	Vulnerability	

Healthy People 2010 (DHHS, 2000) lists specific objectives for illness prevention and health promotion that target populations described by some as at risk and vulnerable. Specifically cited are the poor, homeless, very young, elderly, adolescents who are pregnant, severely mentally ill persons, substance abusers, victims of abuse, and the disabled. Also targeted in this policy-guiding document are persons at risk for, or who already have, communicable diseases, specifically human immunodeficiency virus (HIV), hepatitis B virus (HBV), and other sexually transmitted diseases. The interaction effect of multiple risk factors results in co-morbidity among people who are vulnerable. Therefore, the epidemiological web of causation model is useful for nurses to understand the interrelationship of risks and vulnerability. Poverty is a recurring theme and an important intervening factor in health status but surely not the only one. Furthermore, nurses must examine clients' hardiness and level of resilience, their strengths, access to community resources, and social support systems because these can counterbalance other risk factors that promote vulnerability.

Basic Concepts Related to Risk and Vulnerability

The concepts of **risk** and **vulnerability** are sometimes difficult for nurses to fully understand because of the multiple factors that contribute to them. Moreover, not all people experience these factors in the same way. While one person may thrive after experiencing certain risks, for example, another individual may have less favorable outcomes. Essentially, understanding the interrelationship of the two concepts is influenced by personal beliefs, cultural values, and societal attitudes about dependency. The terms *risk* and *vulnerability* often are interchanged in health policy discussions and in the nursing literature. Even though the two concepts are closely related, there are some differences in their meanings and what the words refer to (ANA, 1991, 1997; NRHA, 1997, 1998, 1999; Sebastian & Bushy, 1999).

Risk

The term *risk* emerges from writings on the natural history of diseases. In epidemiological models, *risk* refers to health conditions that result from the interaction of many factors, including a person's genetic makeup, lifestyle, and the physical and social environments in which he or she lives and works. The effect of the integration of multiple factors subsequently makes it more or less likely that a person will develop a particular health problem (Provan & Sebastian, 1998).

Vulnerability

The term *vulnerability* has it origins in the Latin word *vulnerare,* which means "to wound." Broad definitions of the term include the notions of susceptibility to injury and lack of protection from danger, that is, a potential for physical attack and being insufficiently defended; being liable to censure and criticism; or being more liable to succumb to persuasion and temptation. More specially, in reference to health policy and community health nursing, *vulnerability* refers to a person or group that is more likely to develop a health-related problem and have more serious outcomes stemming from their exposure to multiple risks (Sebastian & Bushy, 1999).

Persons with Special Needs

The notion of special needs is used in reference to individuals, groups, families, and communities who manifest social service and health care needs that are distinct, exceptional, and different from what is considered "ordinary" or "usual" (National Center for Health Statistics, 1999). These individuals often are forgotten, discounted, or misunderstood and may or may not be at risk, vulnerable, or disenfranchised. In most cases, the community and families of persons with special needs have additional challenges in meeting their health care needs, which may be emotional, economic, physical, or social (Aday, 1993, 1994; Conger & Elder, 1994; Dever, 1997; Garrison, 1998; Kotch, 1997).

Vulnerable Populations

It is important to stress that the vulnerable are not a homogenous group, but rather represent all segments of society. **Vulnerable populations** are a (sub)group that shares common risks or combinations of risk factors; one that is pervasive is poverty or low socioeconomic status (DHHS, 1991, 2000). Vulnerability implies that, compared with the general population, some people are more sensitive to risk factors; this can impact their health, usually for the worse. Those who are vulnerable are particularly sensitive to risks that originate from economic, physical, social, biological, and genetic factors, along with their lifestyle behaviors.

Rarely does one risk factor act in isolation, as shown in the web of causation model (see the figure on p. 579). For example, a person with a chronic mental illness or a physical disability, such as a seizure disorder or respiratory condition that is difficult to manage, may not be able to maintain a full-time job. Therefore, the person probably will not have a regular or adequate salary. In turn, this has an impact on his or her ability to secure adequate and/or safe housing, essential health care, and pharmacological services, and perhaps prevents the person from pursuing further education to seek a job that will pay a higher wage. Associated with chronic symptoms and the inability to be financially self-sufficient, the person may experience chronic depression and lowered self-esteem. To deal with the seemingly overwhelming emotional issues, and in an effort to self-manage the physical symptoms, the person may resort to using over-the-counter medications or alcohol or increasing the dosage of prescribed medications. The interaction of these multiple risks results in the person's becoming even more susceptible (vulnerable) to additional factors that can negatively impact the person's health status (Sebastian & Bushy, 2000).

Vulnerable families is another phrase often found in the health policy literature. These families are at particular risk be-

THE WEB OF CAUSATION MODEL.
....

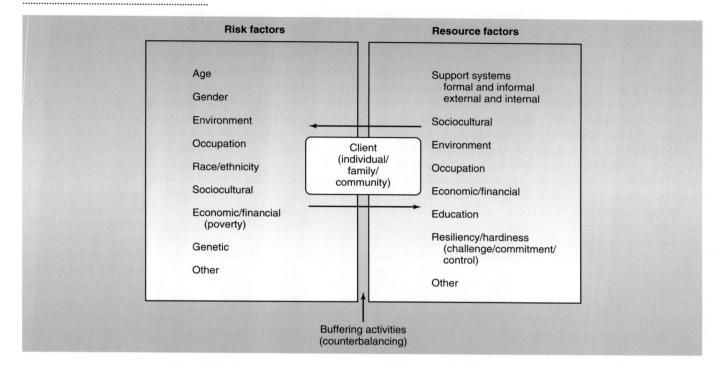

cause of the intensity or clustering of multiple stressors associated with unanticipated life events and normal maturational changes. Examples of families at high risk and who are particularly vulnerable to future health problems include those who have a member who is chronically ill or disabled, has a chronic mental illness, or abuses alcohol or other mind-altering substances. Families with a pregnant teenager are also considered vulnerable. Special or unexpected events can promote vulnerability, too, such as a family member receiving a diagnosis of a fatal disease, the sudden death of a child, unemployment, and natural or manmade disasters such as a devastating fire, flood, hurricane, tornado, or earthquake. Trauma-related events such as auto accidents, domestic violence, sexual abuse, and violent crimes also predispose a family, as well as a community, to subsequent physical, emotional, and social problems. An increasing combination of intense and multiple stressors (risks) coupled with the depletion of resources can push the family or a community beyond its ability to cope, hence intensifying vulnerability. Therefore, nurses in community health practice must closely listen to clients to learn about their personal stories. What words are used to describe a health problem in relation to their lifestyle and activities of daily living? Understanding the client's perspective is essential for instructing, counseling, advocating, developing, and evaluating nursing interventions that are deemed appropriate and acceptable by a targeted population (Kudzma, 1999; Leininger, 1997).

Web of Causation: The Interrelationship of Risk and Vulnerability

From the preceding discussion it becomes obvious that numerous antecedents (risks) contribute to vulnerability. It also fits the web of causation model that is used in epidemiology to understand and approach health and illness (Dever, 1997; Friis & Sellers, 1999; Stanhope & Knollmueller, 1997). This schematic model can assist nurses in the community to understand the interrelationship among multiple factors that contribute to the choices made by individuals, families, and communities that ultimately affect their health status. Factors commonly associated with vulnerability that could be included in a web of causation model include disadvantaged socioeconomic status, lifestyle behaviors, low self-esteem, feelings of powerlessness, and disenfranchisement. Consistent with the web of causation model, the interaction between individual assets, social assets, and demographic factors contributes to a higher likelihood of poorer versus better health. Moreover, age, race, ethnicity, and gender are demographic variables associated with variations in health outcomes. Even more noteworthy is the role that social, economic, and cultural factors play in developing vulnerability or resilience. The web of causation also is useful in determining areas where nursing interventions can most effectively be focused to prevent or manage particular risks that predispose a person, family, or even a community to a particular health risk.

For example, a variation that results from genetic predisposition is breast cancer. Or, for instance, race and ethnicity are associated with an intricate set of socioeconomic variables that correlate to chronic illnesses such as hypertension, diabetes, and cardiovascular diseases (Hamburg, 1998; Kochanek, Maurer, & Rosenberg, 1994; Sebastian & Bushy, 1999). Health disparities are examined in greater detail later in this chapter. Individual assets include skills and resources that contribute to one's ability to be economically self-sufficient, such as education and employment. Social assets are characteristics of one's social network that provide emotional and instrumental support, such as family structure, friendship ties, neighborhood connections, and religious organizations. These are but a few of the many risk factors and intervening variables that contribute to vulnerability and resilience.

In applying the web of causation model to teenage pregnancy, for example, nurses in community health settings are able to reflect on the multiple factors that contribute to this costly public health problem (Sebastian & Bushy, 1999). It is important to emphasize that this problem cannot be viewed from an isolated perspective such as not using birth control or the lack of morals of teenage girls. The risk factor of **disadvantaged** status partly is attributable to adolescents' lack of physical and emotional maturity, which predisposes them to impulsive lifestyle choices and poorer pregnancy outcomes than women who are several years older. Low self-esteem is another characteristic shared by many adolescents, resulting in some emulating peers to feel accepted. Unprotected sex is a risky lifestyle behavior that often is fostered by the use of mind-altering substances such as alcohol and street drugs. These behaviors increase the risk of exposure to communicable infections such as HIV, hepatitis, and other sexually transmitted disease, all of which contribute to less than optimal pregnancy outcomes.

Risky lifestyle behaviors are reinforced or discouraged by community as well as family attitudes regarding sex education and family planning in school curricula. Low socioeconomic status is closely related to level of education and employment opportunities, characteristics that are common themes among adolescent parents. Poverty persists because a young, single mother cannot get a job that provides an adequate salary to support herself, much less a family. As for political and social factors, these are reflected in policies related to public assistance programs (welfare) and child care programs. Ultimately, these can enable, or deter, an adolescent from obtaining the necessary skills to secure a job that can provide an adequate wage to support a family (NRHA, 1997, 1998, 1999).

In brief, adolescent pregnancy is a complex problem involving many risk factors that makes a highly susceptible group even more vulnerable. Moreover, it has a direct impact on the children of adolescent parents, who are the future. The interaction of these factors, as well as many others, are determinants in the rate of adolescent pregnancies in a particular community. Other vulnerable groups similarly are caught up in a web of causation composed of many risk factors.

Poverty: Impact on Risk and Vulnerability

Poverty is closely associated with risk, even though it is not the only contributing factor to vulnerability. Being poor affects the health and well-being of individuals of all ages as well as families and communities. Although it often is hidden in a community, poverty exists even within areas that seem affluent. Poverty significantly contributes to other health risk factors, thereby increasing the vulnerability of all community residents, especially other poor residents (DHHS, 1991, 2000; USDA, 1997).

Most health professionals and policy makers contend that poverty is associated with poorer health. Yet one of the greatest obstacles in addressing the problem is the multitude of definitions and individual perspectives about poverty and who truly is "poor." Almost everyone has an idea about poverty; however, it tends to be a relative concept based on personal experiences and cultural values (Sebastian & Bushy, 1999). To understand the meaning of poverty and its impact on the daily lives of families, community health nurses should first examine their own perspectives about the issues as well as personal beliefs in relation to others' views. The self-appraisal process can be an effective approach to glean insights on what being poor can mean to others, especially vulnerable clients and their families. In addition, the self-appraisal should include reflecting on social, cultural, and environmental factors and how these contribute to poverty for a particular at-risk group, such as the homeless, single parents, elderly, children, or persons infected with a communicable disease. Insights about another's life situation can go a long way to helping nurses become more accepting and nonjudgmental when working with clients whose personal choices and life situations are different from their own.

Historical Perspectives

It also can be useful for nurses to understand the historical evolution of society's attitudes about poverty and people who are poor and dependent (Sebastian, 1996). Historically, people in the United States have been rather ambivalent in their views on the topic. Over the centuries, two common themes consistently emerge: a strong work ethic and religious/moral beliefs. When our nation was first established, the view of poverty held by some groups was that it was a temporary condition that could and would be overcome with commitment and hard work. Then, citizens believed that poor people were worthy of assistance and displayed a sense of responsibility to help the needy. The notion that poverty could be a permanent state did not fit with the ideals of our founding fathers, however, who embraced self-sufficiency and individual achievement. Therefore, people were willing to help others who were afflicted with poverty, but it was assumed that persons in need would be on their own, sooner rather than later.

With the Industrial Revolution at the end of the 19th century, the public's frame of reference changed about poverty and assisting those in financial need. At that time, the prevailing attitude was that poor and dependent persons were deserving of their plight in life. Affluence was seen as a moral issue. In other words, it was a just reward for hardworking individuals and a punishment for those who did not work hard. This perspective corresponded with the lack of public assistance programs for the poor and disadvantaged in our nation. In fact, it was not until the mid-1930s, after the Great Depression, that the Social Security program went into effect in our nation. The Medicare program, which focused on the health care of the elderly, went into effect about 30 years after that.

Ambivalence toward the poor and dependent continues even today (Sebastian & Bushy, 1999). Persons who are seen as "temporarily" poor are considered to be worthy of public assistance. This view became a central theme in the 1995 debates leading to the enactment of welfare reform legislation in 1996. Since then, eligibility criteria have become quite stringent as to who does and who does not qualify for public assistance, and for how long. Greater financial responsibility in caring for the poor has shifted from the federal government to the state governments and the private sector. The long-term effect of the welfare-to-work legislation has been mixed. Short term, on the one hand, the actual number of recipients of welfare has dropped in most states. On the other hand, there has been an increase in the number of families that are classified as "near-poor" and children living in poverty, many of whom are single mothers with children.

In addition, educational and job opportunities in small towns and rural areas often are limited. In turn, this means that persons receiving public assistance may need to move out of their community to develop the necessary work skills and to obtain employment, often part-time and at the minimum wage. For some, it means leaving behind family and other support systems. The situation can become even more complicated because child care in many instances is nonexistent or inadequate for women who must work outside of the home. Another approach to help reduce the cost of public assistance to single mothers with children has been a concerted effort to ensure that child support is paid by fathers who are not present in the home. In brief, long-range consequences for vulnerable families of the welfare-to-work program remain to be seen. Current public sentiment for the most part is to reduce financial entitlements to people who are perceived as not wanting to help themselves.

Cultural Perspectives

The meaning of poverty and how to deal with it is culturally based and varies widely among societies and individuals. Often, the cultural beliefs of a particular subgroup or community may conflict or even contradict public sentiment (NRHA, 1998, 1999). For example, some people give poverty spiritual relevance by believing that poor people on earth will earn riches in heaven. Still others view most aspects of poverty quite negatively and believe that if poor people would get motivated and work for a living they would be better off and others wouldn't have to support them and their children for the rest of their lives.

Professional groups describe poverty in terms related to the culture of their various disciplines. For instance, social scientists often use the term *impoverished* to describe a variety of conditions related to the lack of a home, relationships, or material possessions. This term also can refer to limited educational, occupational, and financial resources. Health care providers tend to define poverty in terms of not having sufficient financial resources to meet basic living expenses such as food, clothing, shelter, transportation, and health care. Therefore, adequate or inadequate financial resources can either counterbalance or intensify other risk factors that contribute to vulnerability.

Economists and policy developers use the phrase *persistent poverty* to categorize individuals, families, communities, and counties that are very poor for an extended time (National Center for Health Statistics, 1999; USDA, 1997). For instance, a number of rural counties across the nation have been classified as having persistent poverty for nearly half a century. In persistent poverty families, poverty is transmitted from one generation to another. Community planners talk about *neighborhood poverty*, which refers to geographically defined urban areas that characteristically are poor, with substandard housing and high levels of unemployment. *Underclass poverty* refers to the display of negative attitudes and behaviors that are associated with poverty and indicate a deviance from social norms. Essentially, each person, family, community, and professional discipline has a perspective on the definition, cause, and cure of poverty. A community health nurse may find these frames of reference useful in examining personal attitudes and biases about poverty, people who are poor, and the risks that promote and sustain vulnerability.

Policy Perspectives

The federal and state governments use an absolute economic standard to delineate poverty based on the criteria of an "adequate living wage" for a family with a certain number of members (DHHS, 1991, 2000; Federal Register, 2000; USDA, 1997). People who fall below this standard are considered poor; hence, they qualify for public assistance programs. This standard is referred to as the **poverty index**, which is determined by calculating the cost of specific goods and services within a given time frame. The federal poverty index takes into consideration the cost of food for a minimum/adequate diet for an individual. This rate is then adjusted for the number (size) and ages of members in a household and place of residence. In 2000, for example, the poverty threshold for a family of four was $17,050. In other words, a family of four whose income falls below this economic index is considered poor; those above the threshold are not. Families who have a slightly higher income sometimes are referred to as the **near poor**. Poverty guidelines are issued by the U.S. Department of Health and Human Services and revised annually based on the consumer price index. Subsequently, the guidelines are used to determine whether a person or family qualifies for assistance or services under a particular federal or state entitlement program, such as Medicaid, WIC, Head Start, Welfare-to-Work

Program, Children's Health Insurance Program (CHIP), and Pell educational grants. The U.S. Bureau of the Census uses this index for statistical purposes to compare national, state, and county socioeconomic and other quality-of-life factors (National Center for Health Statistics, 1999).

There is some question as to the adequacy of the federal poverty index as a tool used in determining services for poor families. Standards that are used to derive the index are disputed, in particular by health professionals (Sebastian & Bushy, 1999). Criticism centers on conceptual and measurement approaches that are used to calculate the index, specifically the diet plan and substance indicators. These are proposed to be an adequate measure of poverty. A broader measure is recommended by advocates for the poor, because the standard of living that is offered by the financial resources of the poverty index is far from adequate. Others suggest that reluctance to revise the poverty index has political implications. In other words, if new measures are adopted or higher inflation adjustments are used, substantially more people would be added to the national poverty rolls. No one in federal and state governments, particularly elected officials, wants to be held responsible for an increase in the number of people receiving public assistance. Regardless, community health nurses will often encounter the poverty index and poverty thresholds, because these have implications for planning, coordinating, and evaluating services for at-risk clients who are vulnerable and also poor.

Health-Related Perspectives

Compared with those with a higher socioeconomic status, health care generally is less available and accessible to the poor, as evidenced by wide health disparities, especially among underrepresented ethnic groups (DHHS, 1991, 2000; NRHA, 1997, 1998, 1999). For example, the poor have higher rates of infant mortality, complex health problems, and physical limitations resulting from chronic illness. Furthermore, they are hospitalized three times more often than people in higher income brackets. Common hospital admission diagnoses for the poor are asthma, diabetes, hypertension, and other chronic illnesses that in many instances could be better managed with education and routine health care.

Low socioeconomic status can have an impact on the health of people in other ways too. For example, some types of cancer have significantly higher morbidity and mortality rates among people who are poor, especially if they are members of an underrepresented ethnic group. Likewise, poor people are more vulnerable to trauma-induced injuries and death by violence. Injuries to children in poor families most often are associated with fires, drowning, and suffocation. In impoverished communities, infant mortality rates create additional acute and chronic health concern. Also, there is a higher incidence of adolescents who become parents. Patterns of risk exposure that contribute to vulnerability continue throughout adulthood, as evidenced by a higher incidence of chronic diseases that are not managed, trauma-related injuries, and early death. Even though low socioeconomic status is not a direct cause of vulnerability, it certainly is a stressor that can intensify the impact of other risk factors.

Community Perspectives

Rural and urban communities of all sizes and cultures have poor people in their midst. Poor communities and neighborhoods share several commonalties, including a higher proportion of underrepresented ethnic groups and single mothers, higher rates of unemployment, and lower wages for those who are employed. In poor communities, children in single-parent households are poorer in income and other resources compared with counterparts in communities with higher average family incomes (NRHA, 1998, 1999; USDA, 1997). People of color who also are poor are more likely to experience violence, discrimination, and police brutality than more affluent counterparts. Other correlates of poverty include increased rates of communicable disease (especially tuberculosis and HIV), premature death, occupational hazards, unsafe housing, and homelessness. Especially unfortunate correlates for impoverished children include delayed development, depression, anxiety with increased incidences of separation from families, and placement in foster care. Using the web of causation model, nurses can visualize how poverty intensifies other risk factors that contribute to and sustain vulnerability in an individual, family, and community.

Poor neighborhoods have higher rates of crime and substance abuse with lower-quality levels of education. Housing often is less than adequate—sometimes even deplorable. Community health nurses should not be surprised to find poor individuals and families living in condemned buildings, on the street, in cardboard boxes, under highway viaducts, in stalled vehicles, or in storage sheds. It is not unusual for poor families to be intermittently homeless (DHHS, 1991, 1998). Substandard living conditions result in residents being exposed to a range of environmental hazards (risks), including inadequate heating, sanitation, and bathing facilities; vermin and other pests; and unsafe drinking water. Poor neighborhoods are more likely to be situated near highly industrialized areas, landfills, and toxic waste sites and have gang-related activity. Thus, living in a poor neighborhood poses an additional risk that contributes to increased morbidity and mortality independent of an individual's lifestyle, behaviors, and occupation.

Living in a resource-depleted environment impacts vulnerability in other ways too. Poor people continually are faced with multiple risks associated with chronic stressors such as frustration over employment options, inadequate and unsafe housing conditions, repeated exposure to violence and crime, inadequate child care assistance, and the insensitive attitudes of health and social service agencies (ANA, 1997). Bombardment of stressful situations on an already vulnerable client, family, or community perpetuates feelings of powerlessness, hopelessness, and helplessness; poor self-esteem; anxiety; chronic depression; and physical illness. It is not unusual for an individual, family, neighborhood, or community to become immobilized. In other words, they do not have the ability to effectively respond to even the routine activities of daily living. They go from crises to crises and try to cope as best they can. As coping abilities are strained by unpredictable and unrelenting events, vulnerable individuals, families, and communities lose their ability to master multiple stress-producing situations, which can be a detriment to their health.

Vulnerable Populations with Special Needs

There are many at-risk vulnerable populations with special needs in this nation. The needs of the vulnerable populations that are receiving the most public attention are discussed here—specifically children, elders, underrepresented ethnic groups, women, the **disenfranchised,** and the **uninsured** and **underinsured** (Sebastian & Bushy, 1999). As mentioned earlier, at-risk individuals usually experience co-morbidity and fall into more than one of these groups, thereby intensifying their degree of vulnerability. Other chapters in this text offer greater detail for some of these groups.

Children and Adolescents

Compared with adults, nearly twice as many children live in poverty. In recent years, the number of adults and elderly living in poverty has decreased while the number of children living in poverty has dramatically increased. Of all persons in the United States who are poor, nearly 40% are younger than 18 years of age, and about 11% are older than 65. One in five American children younger than 6 years of age and one in four children younger than 18 is poor. Children in single-parent households are twice as likely to be poor as those who live in two-parent

homes. Of all children who are poor, about one-third are African American. In recent years, poverty among Latinos has increased more than any other group. Native American children, however, probably are the poorest and the most likely to be in substandard living conditions, especially those who live on Indian Reservations (DHHS, 1991, 2000; National Center for Health Statistics, 1999; U.S. Bureau of the Census, 1997). Despite these statistics, many Americans do not see poverty as a major problem for children (see Research Brief on p. 584).

Dr. Jocelyn Elders, a former U.S. Surgeon General, stated that many of these children are members of the 5-H Club; that is, they are hungry, homeless, hugless, hopeless, and without health care. Furthermore, low income, low educational level, and low-wage occupations correlate with infant mortality, low birth weight, birth defects, and infant deaths (DHHS, 1998). Poverty also increases the risk in young children for developing chronic diseases, trauma-induced injuries and death, developmental delays, poor nutrition, inadequate immunizations, iron deficiency anemia, and elevated serum lead levels. Compared with nonpoor children, their poor counterparts are more likely to go hungry and suffer from fatigue, dizziness, irritability, headache, and ear infections. Poor children have a higher incidence of upper respiratory infections, weight loss, inability to concentrate, and absenteeism from school. The youngest are at the greatest risk and are more vulnerable to developmental delays associated with inadequate nutrition and lack of routine preventive health care.

As for disadvantaged adolescents, usually they do not have the opportunity to acquire the skills and knowledge that are associated with success in adulthood. Correspondingly, they lack a sense of personal mastery and self-esteem. Compared with more affluent teens, those who are poor are more likely to have below

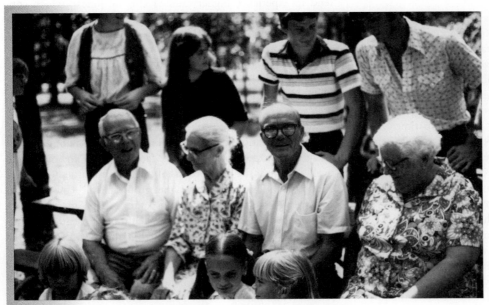

Elders and children have greater risks for many diseases.

RESEARCH BRIEF

Blendon, R. (1998). Survey: Americans don't see poverty, health care as children's most pressing problems. APHA—the Nation's Health, 1, 6.

A survey conducted by Harvard University, The Robert Woods Johnson Foundation, and the University of Maryland asked Americans to list the "two or three most serious problems facing children in America today." Respondents overwhelmingly cited drug abuse (56%), crime (24%), home life and related problems (22%), and poor quality education (17%). Poverty was rarely cited (2%), and health care even less often (1%). Of the parents who were surveyed, only 29% had read or seen anything about a new government program to provide health insurance for uninsured children; this figure was even smaller (26%) for parents whose children were uninsured. When asked how their states should extend aid to children, of the respondents 43% said expand government-funded clinics; 31% said to give vouchers for private insurance; only 16% said expand Medicaid. These findings demonstrate that overall our nation is unaware of and does not support legislation to allocate billions of dollars in federal matching funds to help states extend health care to uninsured children. Initiatives to help vulnerable children could fail because of the lack of public knowledge and support.

average academic skills and subsequently to drop out of school (National Center for Health Statistics, 1998; NRHA, 1994, 1997, 1998, 1999).

Regardless of race, poor adolescents are about six times more likely to have children than their nonpoor counterparts. A number of reasons are cited for this demographic variance, including the lack of knowledge about sexual development and practicing safe sex, limited access to family planning services, and the lack of responsible adult role models. With welfare reform (e.g., welfare-to-work programs), there are restrictions on the length of time that one can receive public assistance. During this time frame, the welfare recipient is expected to make significant life changes that will lead to financial independence. Most often, this entails the person's completing the necessary education to obtain a job. Usually, these are entry-level positions in the service industry offering the minimum hourly wage. Many times, it is only a part-time job that does not provide health insurance benefits. Although single-parent women may eventually be removed from state's welfare rolls, they often do not make an adequate living wage to support themselves and their children. Community health nurses should be aware that poor money management skills, along with the costs of child care, contribute to the problem of sustained poverty among single-parent families. A variety of innovative programs are being implemented across the nation

to help address the special needs of vulnerable children and adolescents, such as after-school recreational programs and employer-sponsored child care services. Community health nurses have an important role in health promotion, anticipatory guidance, and illness prevention strategies in these initiatives.

Elders

Elderly persons constitute another vulnerable group who are at risk (DHHS, 1991, 2000; NRHA, 1997, 1998, 1999; Sebastian & Bushy, 1999). Many of them live on fixed incomes, have chronic health problems, live alone, and are unable to manage their own affairs. For example, elders in many instances do not have transportation because they do not own a vehicle, cannot drive, and have no access to public transportation or anyone to transport them. The elderly who are in long-term care or extended care facilities are particularly vulnerable because of the additional stress (risk) of being displaced from their home and family. Even though the poverty rate among elders has decreased in the last two decades, many experience numerous risks that predispose them to health problems, including environmental, nutritional, and sociocultural factors. The decline in poverty is partly attributable to changes in Social Security benefits, coupled with the increased availability of other federal and state entitlement programs that focus on the elderly population. A few elders, even though they are eligible for entitlement benefits, are not aware that these programs exist, and others may not know how to access these services. This phenomenon occurs most often in rural areas, where a person may be socially or geographically isolated, and among individuals who cannot speak or read English or for whom English is their second language. Elderly people who are members of underrepresented ethnic groups, particularly African Americans, Latinos, and Native Americans, tend to experience higher rates of chronic illness, which contributes to the health disparities that have been identified within these groups.

Underrepresented Ethnic Groups

Race and ethnicity are related to risk and vulnerability (DHHS, 2000; National Center for Health Statistics, 1999; NRHA, 1994, 1997, 1998, 1999; Sebastian & Bushy, 1999; USDA, 1997). Similar to poverty, the factors of race and ethnicity do not operate in isolation. People of color who are also poor are more likely to be exposed to other risk factors, which interact negatively to impact the health status of their communities. (The predominant underrepresented ethnic groups in the United States are African Americans, Latinos/Hispanics, Asian Americans, Native Americans, and Alaska Natives.) Although health status in the United States improved throughout the 20th century, disparities still exist across various segments of the population. Health disparities among underrepresented ethnic groups are rooted in economic, environmental, and socioeconomic circumstances (National Center for Health Statistics, 1999).

Essentially, those having a low socioeconomic status and fewer years of education do not fare as well in terms of morbidity, mortality, injuries, exposure to environmental hazards, and access to health care as do people with more financial resources and higher educational backgrounds. For example, the infant mortality rate for whites declined from 7.3 per 1,000 live births to 6.3 per 1,000 live births between 1990 and 1995, representing a 14% decline in infant mortality. This all-time low for infant mortality rate represents substantial progress in a leading national health indicator. The infant mortality rate for African Americans also declined by 14% during this time; however, comparing 1990 rates of 16.9 per 1,000 live births with 1995 rates of 14.6 per 1,000 live births, African Americans continue to have a very high infant mortality rate. In fact, it is more than 100% higher for African Americans than European Americans. Infant mortality among Hispanics actually increased from 1990 (7.5 per 1,000 live births) to 1995 (7.6 per 1,000 per live births).

Studies have shown that it is not race or ethnicity that is the primary contributor to these poor outcomes, but lower socioeconomic status. Kochanek, Maurer, and Rosenberg (1994) evaluated the gap in life expectancies between African Americans and Caucasians in the United States. They found that the gaps (disparities) were related to socioeconomic status rather than to race. Thus, members of certain subsets of the population are at higher risk or are more vulnerable to poor health than the population as a whole, and these vulnerabilities have much to do with economic and social circumstances. The view that health is an outcome of both personal assets, such as heredity and lifestyle, and social and environmental context (e.g., access to health care, healthy living and working environments, access to nutritious foods) is not a new one but is receiving increasing attention in policy and research arenas (Krieger, 1996; Sebastian & Bushy, 1999).

The goal for the United States is elimination of "the disparities in six areas of health status experienced by racial and ethnic minority populations while continuing the progress we have made in improving the overall health of the American people" (Hamburg, 1998). These six areas are infant mortality, cancer screening and management, cardiovascular disease, diabetes, HIV and acquired immunodeficiency syndrome (AIDS) infection, and immunizations. *Healthy People 2010* (DHHS, 2000) called for a reduction in health disparities between the majority population and special populations in the United States, particularly for people of color (Hamburg, 1998). Communities that are particularly vulnerable are those in persistent poverty counties, especially Native Americans living on reservations, African Americans living in the rural South, and migrating farm workers of Latino origin. Many in these communities experience living standards and health outcomes that compare with those in Third World countries (Christoffel & Gallagher, 1999; NRHA, 1997, 1998, 1999).

Women

Another highly vulnerable group is women who are poor. The term *triple jeopardy* is used in reference to poor women of color. Another risk factor that could be added to those three is age (DHHS, 1991, 2000; National Center for Health Statistics, 1999; Sebastian & Bushy, 1999). Women tend to outlive their spouses, often by more than a decade. This further contributes to the increase in poverty and isolation, especially among women of color.

Poverty has particularly serious negative consequences for women of childbearing age (NRHA, 1997, 1998, 1999). Poor women are more likely than nonpoor women to receive late or no prenatal care, resulting in poorer pregnancy outcomes. More precisely, a significant indicator of the health of a nation is infant mortality and morbidity rates. The health status of women has a direct effect on perinatal outcomes and an indirect effect on the health and well-being of their families. Women who are mothers tend to be the primary caregivers and decision makers regarding health care choices. In addition, women play a very important role in transmitting health information from professional sources to their families. Community health nurses may find that interventions that focus on women provide the greatest potential for success in changing health behaviors of a vulnerable population.

Disenfranchised Populations

Some people who are disenfranchised may be vulnerable, but that is not necessarily true in all cases. Disenfranchisement refers to feelings of separation from mainstream society (DHHS, 1991, 2000; O'Connor, 1994; Sebastian & Bushy, 1999). When this phenomenon occurs, an individual or group does not experience an emotional connection with the rest of society. The disenfranchised include the chronic mentally ill, the homeless, prisoners, persons with HIV/AIDS, refugees, and immigrants.

Some veterans of the Vietnam War, for example, are disenfranchised as a result of serving in the military for a war that was not supported by the American public. A few of the veterans experienced public criticism for participating in the war, even though they were required to do so. The conflicting political environment of the time, exacerbated by posttraumatic stress disorders that often develop as a result of intense combat experiences, contributed to their feelings of isolation from society. Some believe that no one else understands their plight. Interestingly, Vietnam veterans make up a significant proportion of the homeless population in this nation.

Disenfranchisement also suggests that a person or group may not have the necessary support systems to effectively cope with stress or to manage a healthful lifestyle. In part this can be attributed to the reality that some vulnerable people do not have well-established links with formal organizations in their community such as social service agencies, churches, or schools. Sometimes, they have fewer informal sources of support, too, such as family, friends, or neighbors. For example, homeless people often have few people whom they can call on for assistance. However, all vulnerable people are not without social support or other kinds of resources. In fact, many families report that they have reliable and even consistent support from churches, extended families, neighbors, and the community even though they may feel disenfranchised from society as a whole. Coupled with the perceived disenfranchisement, certain vulnerable groups, such as poor children, older women, the homeless, and migrant farm workers, are hidden and essentially remain invisible to society.

Hence, these groups may be disregarded and often are forgotten by health professionals and in social planning initiatives. Nurses in community health settings often are the principal contact for many of these individuals.

Uninsured and Underinsured Populations

Even though vulnerable populations are more likely to need health care services, many are not able to access them (DHHS, 1991, 2000; NRHA, 1997, 1998, 1999; Sebastian & Bushy, 1999). A number of reasons are cited for this phenomenon (Box 25-1), but one of the most problematic is the lack of health care insurance. More precisely, in 1998 there were more than 43 million people who did not have health insurance benefits. Three groups are particularly affected by escalating health care costs and reductions in service within a community—the elderly, poor children, and growing numbers of individuals who do not have health insurance or do not receive public assistance, specifically Medicaid. Of these, some may qualify for public assistance, but the family does not have the ability to apply or lacks the motivation to do so. Some of the **medically indigent** fall in the category of **working poor** or near poor. That is, there are working adults in the family, but they do not have enough money to purchase health care insurance, yet their income is too high (above the federal poverty index), so they are disqualified from obtaining public assistance. A number of families have health insurance but do not have adequate coverage (underinsured) with low reimbursement rates, high co-payments, or prohibitive clauses in their contracts for preexisting medical conditions.

Although the elderly, poor children, and the near poor have been in the public spotlight, other populations are also affected.

BOX 25-1 SELECT DIMENSIONS OF LIMITED ACCESS TO CARE

- Lack of adequate health care insurance
- Inability to pay for services
- Language and cultural barriers
- Inequitable distribution of health care providers (more often in inner cities and remote rural counties)
- Geographic and social isolation
- Challenges associated with transportation and communication infrastructures (great distances to providers, poor travel conditions, lack of telephone services)
- No public transportation
- Inconvenient hours to see clients at clinic or health center
- Insensitive attitudes by health care providers toward clients who are poor or of another racial/ethnic/cultural background

As cost containment strategies are implemented by employers, many employees find that their insurance benefits have been reduced or eliminated. Families often assume they have adequate coverage until a family member experiences a catastrophic illness or chronic disability, and subsequently, they are confronted with excessive medical expenses. Community health nurses should also be sensitive to the fact that the working poor/near poor are likely to underuse preventive services. For many of them, illnesses often go untreated until there is an acute manifestation of symptoms or an emergency. This behavior has implications for designing, implementing, and evaluating nursing services that target **at-risk** vulnerable groups and populations with special needs.

Nursing Considerations

Limited Access to Care

At-risk and vulnerable individuals, families, and populations tend to have numerous nursing care needs. For example, poor health conditions often are exacerbated because the vulnerable, especially those who also are poor, have limited access to health care professionals and primary health care services (DHHS, 1991, 2000; NRHA, 1997, 1998, 1999). **Access to care** means more than having health services available in a neighborhood or a community. Existing health care or social services must fit with the needs and preferences of the population for these to be deemed as acceptable and appropriate. Achieving "fit of service" implies that community health nurses must partner and work with the community. The following strategies have been found useful in designing appropriate and acceptable services for vulnerable clients in diverse settings.

- *Getting to know the community and working with residents to identify what services are needed and the best way to provide those services*
- *Scheduling clinic visits for clients at times that are convenient for vulnerable populations, such as after finishing field work or at times when public transportation is operational*
- *Having bilingual nurses available in the health care facility for the convenience of clients who do not speak English*
- *Having staff members who reflect the cultural, racial, and ethnic background of the clients who use the health care facility*
- *Ensuring that all employees are sensitive to the plight of others, especially the poor and those having other belief systems. This may involve offering sensitivity programs for employees*
- *Demonstrating a nonjudgmental attitude when working with people who are poor and of another culture*

Ethical and Legal Considerations

There are innumerable ethical and legal issues accompanying poverty and providing care to vulnerable and at-risk population (ANA, 1991, 1997; Sebastian & Bushy, 1999). Community health nurses often find themselves in key positions to advocate for vulnerable populations and help them effectively solve their problems and become contributing members of society. Associated with this responsibility are ethical and legal considerations that must be understood. One of the most common ethical issues encountered is the allocation of scarce resources. At the core of this value-laden issue are a number of questions. For example, who is most needy, worthy, or deserving to receive scarce resources? Who decides? Where does enabling dependent behavior end? Where does helping the needy to become more self-sufficient start? As resources become scarcer, grappling with ethical issues will become paramount in our society, especially when designing nursing services for vulnerable populations in medically underserved regions.

There also are an array of corresponding legal issues associated with poverty. For instance, poor neighborhoods often experience more violence and crime. Consequently, legal situations may arise related to maintaining confidentiality versus reporting criminal activity that nurses may encounter, such as domestic abuse, child neglect, and gang- and drug-related activities. Community health nurses are encouraged to become familiar with ethical and legal issues related to their nursing practice and to reflect on approaches to prevent and deal with such situations in an appropriate manner.

Clients' Strengths and Resources

Successful nursing interventions build on resources that are available to and acknowledged by the client. Moreover, health promotion research focuses on factors that contribute to health and maintain long-term well-being. Specifically, negative risk factors must be balanced against health-enhancing factors such as hardiness and support systems. The concepts of hardiness and support systems are best understood as interfacing catalysts, one enhancing the effects of the other.

Hardiness

Hardiness is a term used to describe aspects of human resilience (Baer & Bowers, 1998; Lancaster, 1998; Lee, 1993, 1998; Low, 1996). Theoretically, hardiness alludes to a combination of factors that keep some people from developing a problem, even with exposure to a health risk. It is identified as a potential intervening factor in individuals and families (perhaps communities too) who seem to overcome the most adverse conditions and still lead meaningful lives. For example, hardiness may be a factor in why some persons with HIV infections survive for decades, whereas others become very ill or even die within a short time after becoming infected. Dimensions of the concept of hardiness include control, commitment, and challenge. The interrelationship among the three dimensions is the essence of hardiness. Essentially, faced with stressful life events, the hardy person will attempt to change or modify the event (control) into something that is consistent with his or her life purpose (commitment), which will result in learning and personal growth (challenge). There may be additional aspects related to all three dimensions that are relevant to community health nursing, in particular that of "control," or the lack of it, among at-risk and vulnerable groups.

Support Networks

Support networks also can be counterbalancing and mediating forces to risk factors that contribute to vulnerability. Support can be formal or informal in nature. Furthermore, there is no prescription as to who should be included in the individual's network or the family's or community's circle of support (Lee, 1998; Magilvy, Congdon, & Martinez, 1994; Sebastian & Bushy, 1999). Preference and use of support varies by individuals, families, and communities and is culturally defined. For instance, some cultures have extensive social support networks, as is the case for many Native American, African American, and Latino families. The extent of these networks often becomes evident when a client visits the clinic or is hospitalized, accompanied by a contingent of relatives representing several generations. Such an extensive network is not the case for everyone, however. Community health nurses will find that some clients are unable to identify even one person in their support network. For these people, the health care system becomes even more significant.

For example, a middle-aged homeless man, recently released from prison after being incarcerated for several decades, lost all contact with his family. In another case, a 25-year-old homosexual man was diagnosed with HIV/AIDS in a large city located in another state. Upon visiting his parents in a very small town, he told them about his diagnosis and how the infection probably was acquired. They responded by asking him never to come back to their home or their town. Their religious belief system does not condone homosexuality. More than likely they would be extremely ashamed if the community found out about their son's diagnosis or sexual orientation. Increasingly, many faith communities are identifying and supporting vulnerable congregation members. Parish nurses, along with other community health nurses, assume a variety of roles in developing and sustaining support networks for the most vulnerable individuals, families, and populations.

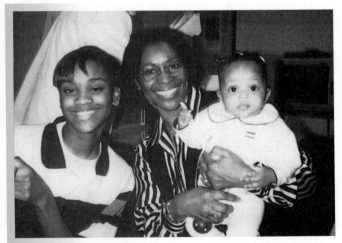

Vulnerable populations include women and children.

Nursing Roles

Nurses in community health settings assume a variety of roles in coordinating services and developing interventions for at-risk and vulnerable individuals, families, and communities. When developing a plan of care, it is important for nurses not only to assess the multiple risk factors but also to identify mediating resources, such as the individual's, family's, or community's resiliency and the quantity and quality of their support networks. Assessment goes beyond helping to identify formal and informal resources, however. It implies the use of specific nursing roles, including advocate, activist, case manager, educator, counselor, partner, collaborator, and researcher. The roles change when developing, implementing, and evaluating interventions to fit vulnerable clients' particular needs and preferences (ANA, 1997; Lancaster, 1998; Sebastian & Bushy, 1999).

Advocate and Activist

In the role of advocate, the nurse must first be sensitive to the health care needs of the vulnerable individual, family, or community, in addition to having a broad knowledge of community resources and how to access them. The nurse also must possess the ability to communicate in a professional manner with and for a client to coordinate a continuum of services. Persistence is needed on the part of the nurse when acting on behalf of a vulnerable client. Time and patience often are necessary to maintain contact with these clients and direct them to the appropriate resources. Political activism at the local, state, and national levels is another aspect of the advocacy role. Nurses can make a difference in the lives of those who are vulnerable and poor by getting involved in the policy arena and by working with elected officials. Community health nurses are in positions to work with public and private entities to provide the necessary resources for new or more comprehensive services (Blendon, 1998; Brownson, Baker, & Novick, 1998; Flynn, 1996, 1997). An example of this is using formal and informal opportunities to discuss issues relevant to public health with legislators and policy makers. Remember, during these interactions the nurse is seen first and foremost as a professional role model having expert power. Nurses in community health practice are in a unique position to advocate for improving the economic and health status of vulnerable populations and for those having special needs.

Advocacy involves representing special consumer groups to regulatory organizations and even local health commissions. The nurse advocate publicly supports and sometimes opposes federal and state initiatives. Advocacy may entail grassroots lobbying for legislation that provides a financial safety net for people with catastrophic costs that are not covered by Medicare or health insurance. Sometimes, it involves a nurse testifying against the views of an elected official who does not support a safe house for abused women, or a residential home for the mentally challenged, or a halfway house for youth offenders. The overall goal of a nurse advocate is to represent vulnerable populations and help these clients solve problems and develop appropriate solutions for their concerns. Advocacy and activism does not mean taking care of, enabling, or promoting long-term dependency. It means teaching people how to help themselves by developing greater resilience and more effective coping skills to deal with their concerns (Sebastian & Bushy, 1999).

Case Manager

A case manager is another role for nurses who work with clients having special needs. This role usually involves the nurse in partnership with an individual client. Case management is a process in which services are organized and coordinated to meet a client's particular needs and to use scarce resources more effectively. In community health nursing centers, case managing a client can extend over a very long period, sometimes months or even years. Moreover, case managers will find that the need for formal and informal services often increase in intensity and complexity as clients are exposed to other health risks and stressful situations. Nurses in the role of case manager, especially those working with vulnerable clients who experience multiple risks, must ensure that needed services are used and care plans are modified to reflect changes. Effective case management requires a broad knowledge base of nursing roles, formal resources, and informal community support networks and an innate ability to integrate all three. Case managers are crucial in preventing and resolving confusion that can arise when clients have multiple members on their health care teams. Confusion is especially problematic among clients in very large agencies. Inherent in case management are the activist and advocacy roles described earlier, along with the nurse educator and counselor roles (Sebastian & Bushy, 1999).

Educator and Counselor

Two other important, often overlapping roles for nurses are teacher and counselor. People might change risky lifestyle behaviors if they learn about the detrimental impact on their health (Dever, 1997; Lancaster, 1998). Education can be one of the most cost-effective and noninvasive interventions to inform consumers, regardless of their socioeconomic status, about pharmacotherapy protocols, health promotion, stress management, developmental changes, and symptom management of chronic health problems. Education, accompanied by counseling interventions, can be used by nurses in supporting clients through the grief process; in adjusting to anticipated, and unanticipated, life events; and for improving communication skills between family members and with health professionals. Education and counseling, in some instances, can be used to teach high-risk clients to ask appropriate questions of investigating agencies they encounter. The educator and counselor roles are important to enable clients to locate and access community resources. However, nurses cannot do it all alone. Community-focused interventions must be developed to expand a nurse's span of effectiveness using resources that are available and acceptable to the client.

Partnership Exemplar: Fighting Violence with Knowledge

The following exemplar highlights two vulnerable groups: adolescents and Vietnam veterans, that formed a partnership in one community to address the problem of violence.

Shortly after finding two pipe bombs in a locker at a junior high school in Massachusetts, school officials looked for assistance from a local nonprofit group, the Veterans Education Project (VEP). This group was organized in 1982 by several veterans of the Vietnam War who were concerned about the glamorous and inaccurate portrayal of war in the media, especially in movies. The overall mission of VEP was to give young people an accurate portrayal of war and its impact on people. Subsequently, members of VEP were invited by the school to address the students, and now they speak regularly to the student body on a subject with which they were are all too familiar, violence and its consequences. One of the VEP speakers, a former U.S.

Marine, said, "War is an extreme example of violence. By talking about it we try to draw some parallels between the violence of war and violence in the street." In 1990, VEP started addressing the growing epidemic of teenage brutality and violence in the United States. According to the Children's Defense Fund, more than 60,000 children have died from gunshot wounds since 1979. This is more than the number of American soldiers who died in the conflicts in Vietnam, the Persian Gulf, Haiti, Somalia, and Bosnia combined. Members of VEP know they cannot completely stop violence by talking about it; however, by describing how violence adversely affected them and the people they love, members of VEP believe they can give vulnerable kids hope.

1. As a school nurse, what could be your role in this partnership?

2. What kind of community activities could this group organize to promote their message of nonviolence?

Source: Wexler, 1998.

Collaborator and Partner

Nurses can collaborate with providers from community-based agencies and citizen groups to address the particular concerns of vulnerable and at-risk populations with special needs to create a seamless continuum of care (Flynn, 1997; Lasker, 1997). Nurses in community health settings must learn to partner with administrators and others from institutions outside the health care system, specifically education, housing, and employment bureaus. Collaboration can be useful to extend and enhance scarce resources, especially in medically underserved and persistent poverty communities. Nurses should also learn to collaborate with private and not-for-profit entities on community projects that focus on the needs of groups who are at risk for poor health outcomes. Even if community health nurses are not involved directly in partnerships, they can serve as liaisons or facilitators to promote collaboration between community groups (see the Case Study above). The challenge for community health nurses is to become as proficient in partnering/collaborating roles as in direct caregiving skills.

Researcher

The role of the nurse as a researcher has become very important in recent years. The needs of vulnerable and at-risk populations can be significant, and there are no easy answers to meet them, especially in communities with seemingly few resources (Flaskerud & Winslow, 1998; Leininger, 1997; NRHA, 1997, 1999; Sebastian & Bushy, 1999; Siegal & Doner, 1998). There is an urgent need for nursing research on implementing and evaluating interventions that can be used with vulnerable and medically underserved segments of society. In many instances, vulnerable populations with special needs must first be identified, because they may be hidden or forgotten. In addition, outcome studies are needed to measure the health-related effects of existing community-based nursing interventions within a targeted population. Nurse scholars report that the sky is the limit for studying health concerns of particular populations that experience multiple risk factors that promote vulnerability. Likewise, there is a need for evidence-based and cost-effective nursing practice models that target selected at-risk groups and lead to favorable health outcomes.

CONCLUSION

This chapter examined the issues surrounding risk and vulnerability and its impact on health. Definitions were examined as well as risk factors that contribute to vulnerability and poor health status. *Healthy People 2010* objectives (DHHS, 2000) specifically address the factors that contribute to health disparities among vulnerable groups, including the homeless, children, elders, pregnant adolescents, the chronic mentally ill, substance abusers, victims of abuse, and those with disabilities. Community health nurses should be aware that vulnerability is precipitated by a multitude of interrelated risk factors. Perhaps the one risk that most exacerbates the effect of others is poverty. In other words, not having enough money to procure safe housing, adequate nutrition, preventive health care, and the education to de-velop the skills to work in a job that provides a living wage all can contribute to level of vulnerability. Community health nurses must learn to accept, respect, and understand how these risk factors contribute to vulnerability and influence a client's lifestyle and health care behaviors. Sensitivity entails recognizing health risks as well as the person's, family's, or community's strengths and resources when designing a holistic nursing care plan.

. . . .

It is increasingly evident that violations of dignity are pervasive events with potential severe and sustained negative effects on physical, mental, and social well-being.

Jonathon Mann, 1999

. . . .

CRITICAL THINKING ACTIVITIES

1. How do you define poverty? What words are used in your family when talking about poor or dependent families and individuals?

2. What characteristics or attributes do you associate with a family or individual who is poor? On what experiences or situations do you base your ideas? Family? Friends? Classmates? Personal experience?

3. What resources are available in your community to address the needs of the poor or vulnerable? Make a list of formal and informal resources to refer to when referring clients. If possible, contact one or two agencies or providers to discuss the criteria that are used to determine who can receive entitlements.

4. Interview an elderly person or a single mother who is on a fixed income that is provided by an entitlement program, such as Social Security or a welfare-to-work program. Ask the person to share personal insights on what it means to be dependent, with very limited financial resources. What at-risk or vulnerable group do they fall into? Is this group cited in *Healthy People 2010*? How does the person/family feel about public services that they are enrolled in, and how do they describe health care providers attitudes toward them or their family?

5. Ask someone you know to share his or her life story with you. Identify risk factors that contribute to vulnerability. What strengths and resources are used to cope with those risk factors? Describe the person's health care–seeking behaviors when he or she needs professional care for a health problem. What suggestions does the person have to make health care services more accessible? Reflect on potential ethical and legal implications that contribute to vulnerability in this person's lifestyle. How can these best be addressed?

6. The Case Study on p. 589 is an example of collaboration among two vulnerable groups. Learn about partnership models in your community. Ask local school officials, the ministerial association, law enforcement, and public safety officials if similar initiatives exist. Describe these and share your findings with peers. Develop strategies to give credit to the partners, and encourage other groups to assume a proactive role in dealing with the special populations who are at risk in your area; for instance, interview participants for the school newspaper or invite them to speak to peers.

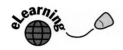 Explore Community Health Nursing on the web! To learn more about the topics in this chapter, use the passcode provided to access your exclusive web site:
http://communitynursing.jbpub.com
If you do not have a passcode, you can obtain one at this site.

REFERENCES

Aday, L. A. (1993). *At risk in America: The health and health care needs of vulnerable populations in the United States.* San Francisco: Jossey-Bass.

Aday, L. A. (1994). Health status of vulnerable populations in the United States. *Annual Review of Public Health, 15,* 457–509.

American Nurses Association. (ANA). (1991). *Community-based nursing services. Innovative models.* Washington, DC: Author.

American Nurses Association. (ANA). (1997). President embraces quality commission's consumer "Bill of Rights." *The American Nurse, 29*(6),18–19.

Baer, M., & Bowers, C. (1998). Using a nursing framework to measure client satisfaction at a nurse-managed clinic. *Public Health Nursing, 15*(1), 50–59.

Blendon, R. (1998). Survey: Americans don't see poverty, health care as children's most pressing problems. *APHA—the Nation's Health,* 1, 6

Brownson, R., Baker, E., & Novick, L. (1998). *Community-based prevention: Programs that work.* Gaithersberg, MD: Aspen Publishers.

Christoffel, T., & Gallagher, S. (1999). *Injury prevention and public health: Practical knowledge, skills and strategies.* Gaithersberg, MD: Aspen Publishers.

Conger, R., & Elder, G. (1994). *Families in troubled times: Adapting to changes in rural America.* New York: Aldine.

Department of Health and Human Services (DHHS). (1991). *Healthy people 2000: National health promotion and disease prevention objectives.* Washington, DC: Government Printing Office.

Department of Health and Human Services (DHHS). (1998). *Health United States: 1997.* Washington, DC: U.S. Government Printing Office.

Department of Health and Human Services (DHHS). (2000). *Healthy people 2010: Conference edition.* Washington, DC: U.S. Government Printing Office.

Dever, A. (1997). *Improving outcomes in public health practice.* Gaithersberg, MD: Aspen Publishers.

Federal Register. (2000, February 15). *The 2000 HHS poverty guidelines, 65*(31), 7555–7557.

Flaskerud, J., & Winslow, B. (1998). Conceptualizing vulnerable populations health-related research. *Nursing Research, 47*(2), 69–78.

Flynn, B. (1996). Healthy cities: Toward worldwide health promotion. *Annual Review of Public Health, 17,* 299–309.

Flynn, B. (1997). Partnerships in healthy cities and communities: A social commitment for advanced practice nurses. *Advanced Practice Nursing Quarterly, 2*(4), 1–6.

Friis, R., & Sellers, T. (1999). *Epidemiology for public health practice.* Gaithersberg, MD: Aspen Publishers.

Garrison, M (1998). Determinants of the quality of life for rural families. *The Journal of Rural Health, 14*(2), 146–153.

Hamburg, M. (1998). Eliminating racial and ethnic disparities in health: Response to the Presidential Initiative on Race. *Public Health Reports, 113,* 372–375.

Kochanek, K., Maurer, J., & Rosenberg, H. (1994). Why did black life expectancy decline from 1984 through 1989 in the United States? *American Journal of Public Health, 84*(6), 938–944.

Kotch, J. (1997). *Maternal and child health: Programs, problems and policy in public health.* Gaithersberg, MD: Aspen Publishers.

Krieger, N. (1996). Inequality, diversity and health: Thoughts on "race/ethnicity," and "gender." *Journal of the American Medical Women's Association, 51*(4), 133–136.

Kudzma, E. (1999). Culturally competent drug administration. *American Journal of Nursing, 99*(8), 46–52.

Lancaster, J. (1998). *Nursing issues in leading and managing change.* St. Louis: Mosby.

Lasker, R. (1997). *Medicine & public health: The power of collaboration.* New York: The New York Academy of Medicine.

Lee H. (1993). Comparison of selected health behavior variables in elderly women with osteoarthritis in different environments. *Arthritis Care Research, 6*(1), 31–7.

Lee, H. (Ed.).(1998). *Conceptual basis for rural nursing.* New York: Springer.

Leininger, M. (1997). Transcultural nursing research to transform nursing education and practice: 40 years. *Image: The Journal of Nursing Scholarship, 29*(4), 341–347.

Low J. (1996). The concept of hardiness: a brief but critical commentary. *Journal of Advances in Nursing, 24*(3), 588–590.

Magilvy, J., Congdon, J., & Martinez, R. (1994). Circles of care: Home care and community support for rural older Adults. *Advances in Nursing Science, 16*(3), 22–33.

Mann, J. (1999). Dignity and health: The UDHR's revolutionary first article. *Health and Human Rights International Journal, 8,* 31–38.

National Center for Health Statistics. (1999). *Health, United States, 1998.* Hyattsville, MD: U.S. Public Health Service.

National Rural Health Association (NRHA). (1994). *A shared vision: Building bridges for rural health access: Conference Proceedings.* Kansas City, MO: Author.

National Rural Health Association (NRHA). (1997). A national agenda for rural minority health: A strategic planning document. Kansas City, MO: Author.

National Rural Health Association (NRHA). (1998). *Bringing resources to bear on the changing care system: Conference proceedings for 2nd annual rural minority health conference.* Kansas City, MO: Author.

National Rural Health Association (NRHA). (1999). *A national agenda for rural minority health.* Kansas City, MO: Author.

O'Connor, F. (1994). A vulnerability-stress framework for evaluating interventions in schizophrenia. *Image: The Journal of Nursing Scholarship*, *26*, 231–237.

Provan, K., & Sebastian, J. (1998). Networks within networks: Service link overlap, organizational cliques, and client outcomes in community mental health. *Academy of Management Journal*, *41*(4), 453–463.

Sebastian, J. (1996). Vulnerability and vulnerable populations: An introduction. In M. Stanhope & J. Lancaster (Eds.), *Community health nursing: Promoting the health of aggregates, families, and individuals* (4th ed., pp. 623–646). St. Louis: Mosby.

Sebastian, J. G., & Bushy, A. (1999). *Special populations in the community.* Gaithersberg, MD: Aspen Publishers.

Siegal, M., & Doner, L. (1998). *Marketing public health: Strategies to promote social change.* Gaithersberg, MD: Aspen Publishers.

Stanhope, M., & Knollmueller, R. (1997). *Public health and community health nurse's consultant: A health promotion guide* (pp. 623–646). St. Louis: Mosby.

U.S. Bureau of the Census. (1997). Population profile of the United States: Annual report. Washington, DC: Government Printing Office.

U.S. Department of Agriculture (USDA). (1997). *Agriculture fact book.* Washington, DC: USDA, Office of Communications.

Wexler, M. (1998). Front Line-F.Y.I.: Fighting violence with knowledge. *Modern Maturity*, *41R*(1), 68.

Chapter 26

Urban and Homeless Populations

Janie B. Butts

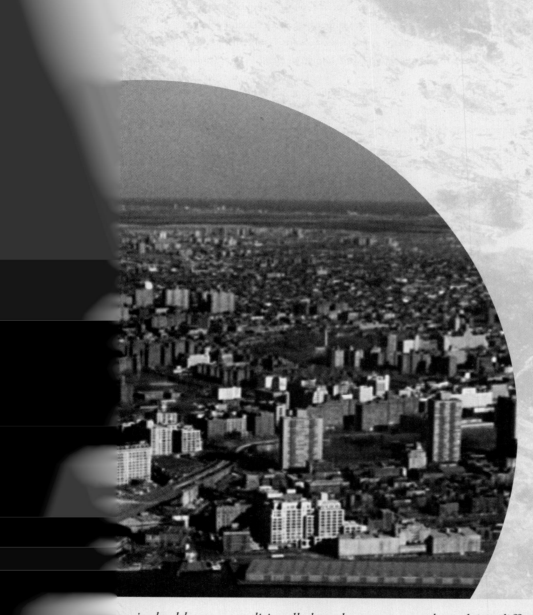

Community health nurses traditionally have been accustomed to solving difficult health and social problems in various populations. Today, problems associated with urban and homeless people pose challenges requiring every skill that can be mustered by community health nurses. Strong community leadership for dealing with these problems is essential. Community health nurses can be the leaders on the forefront in preventing and managing these problems.

CHAPTER FOCUS

Urban Populations
Health and Social Problems of Urban People
Programs for Healthier Urban People

The Homeless Population
Scope of the Problem
Definitions of Homeless People
Historical Perspective
The Health Problems of Homeless People

Nursing Care of Urban and Homeless People
Be Committed
Use Leadership Skills
Use Available Resources
Be an Advocate
Foster Communication and Trust
Assess the Problem
Plan and Give Care

QUESTIONS TO CONSIDER

After reading this chapter, answer the following questions:
1. What are the major factors contributing to homelessness today?
2. How is poverty related to homelessness?
3. What is the Healthy Cities movement?
4. What is the Federal Emergency Relief Organization?
5. What was the first federal legislation specifically passed to aid the homeless?
6. What are barriers to health care for the homeless?
7. What are some of the most common health problems of the homeless?
8. What is the role of the community health nurse in addressing the needs of urban homeless persons?

KEY TERMS

Federal Emergency Relief
  Administration (FERA)
Ghetto counterculture
Healthy Cities
Homeless

Stewart B. McKinney
  Homeless Assistance
  Act of 1987
Urban population

Urban Populations

America's urban people are under siege in neighborhoods across the country (Pantera, 1996). Communities are exposed to diseases, health disorders, violence, crime, hunger, poverty, drug abuse, and homelessness at alarming rates. Although homelessness is a problem in both rural and urban areas, most homeless people exist in urban areas.

An **urban population** is at least 50,000 people in an incorporated or unincorporated area (U.S. Department of Commerce, 1992). Cities have continued to increase in population as people, especially young adults, have migrated to cities from rural areas in hopes of fulfilling their dreams of success. With the promise of wealth and a new way of life, young people are charmed, sometimes only to find disappointment in their careers, poverty, and stress (Goldstein & Kickbusch, 1996). Some have been unable to find jobs. Not only do many people migrate to the city, but many people are born and remain in the city for the duration of their lives.

Poor income and jobless situations perpetuate urban poverty and its problems. With a rapidly growing population, urban officials cannot keep pace with the needs of the people. In fact, a majority of urban problems are associated with rapid growth, such as diminishing supplies of clean water, air pollution, crime and violence, poverty, diseases, overcrowding, racial discrimination, and inadequate housing (Goldstein & Kickbusch, 1996).

Health and Social Problems of Urban People

People in urban areas face many stressors that are different from those in rural areas. Although many of the same problems exist in rural areas, the health and social problems associated with living in urban areas usually are more pronounced.

Poverty in urban populations has been the source of many problems that have developed in cities, especially hunger, health problems, communicable diseases because of overcrowded con-

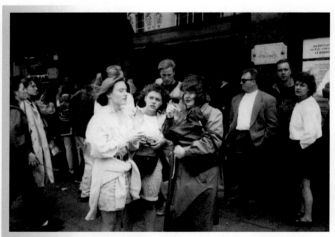

Urban life usually involves existing in crowds and waiting in line for service.

ditions, violence and crime, homelessness, and inadequate housing (Polednak, 1997).

Lack of steady jobs remains a problem. However, many Americans continue to view welfare and other support programs for the poor as the main cause of the social problems in America (Polednak, 1997). As a result, the public, as well as many governmental policy makers, increasingly rejects such programs. The consequence of these attitudes has been a deterioration of health and welfare programs for poor people.

Racial discrimination remains an unsettling issue. A "color line," described by Lewis (1993, p. 251), has caused whites and nonwhites to remain segregated. Major income and health care differences exist between whites and nonwhites overall. Poverty and overcrowding in nonwhite populations have been linked to the exacerbation of communicable diseases (Polednak, 1997).

Poverty in inner cities is also linked to a poor quality of life and increased health problems among adults of all ages (Polednak, 1997). A substantially higher infant mortality rate among nonwhites was found in 38 metropolitan areas (Polednak, 1997). Among African Americans, 10 to 25 deaths per 1,000 live births were noted, compared with 5 to 10 deaths per 1,000 live births among whites. Lack of access to health care, poor prenatal care, adolescent pregnancy, substance abuse, and an overall poor quality of life are consequences of poverty. Causes of mortality among African Americans and other nonwhites in urban areas included cardiovascular diseases, renal diseases, and homicides at higher rates than whites.

Ghetto counterculture is a term that has been used to label a phenomenon in urban America (Massey & Denton, 1993, p. 48). Ghetto counterculture is used to describe the racial segregation that has taken place in residential areas. This residential segregation has created nonwhite urban underclass communities, producing "concentration" effects in these areas (p. 48). The concentration of nonwhites in high-poverty areas, such as inner cities, has resulted in a spiraling decline in the human condition. Concentration effects lead to increased social problems such as crime and drugs, physical deterioration of buildings, and poor access to health care facilities and other services. Respiratory infections, tuberculosis (TB), skin infections, and many other illnesses occur in concentrated areas. The Research Brief on p. 597 highlights the public health threat of adult pertussis in urban people.

Another health problem associated with urban living in the United States is the reemergence of measles. The Centers for Disease Control and Prevention (CDC) (1995) documented a 20-fold increase in measles from 1989 to 1991, which was largely attributed to failure to vaccinate children in accordance with established public health guidelines. In fact, the CDC recently found that only 50% of all children living in the inner cities were vaccinated by their second birthday.

Other health problems have emerged in the last decade. Contamination of community water supplies has contributed to many outbreaks of infectious diseases in urban areas, such as the

RESEARCH BRIEF

Nennig, M. E., Shinefield, H. R., Edwards, K. M., Black, S. B., & Fireman, B. H. (1998). Prevalence and incidence of adult pertussis in an urban population. Journal of the American Medical Association, 275, 1672–1674.

Bordetella pertussis has been found to be a significant public health threat in urban populations. A study was conducted to determine the prevalence of adult pertussis infection in urban people with a prolonged cold for 2 weeks or longer. Of 153 adult subjects in San Francisco, the researchers found that 12.4% of them had *Bordetella* (or adult) *pertussis*, which translates to 176 cases in every 100,000 people in the United States. The researchers recommended that booster shots be initiated for all persons older than 7 years of age.

Cryptosporidium infection in Milwaukee (MacKenzie et al., 1994). There has been the reappearance of plague, cholera, and dengue fever in many parts of the world, especially in the "megacities" of 10 million or more people (Global Report on Human Settlements, 1996).

Programs for Healthier Urban People

Healthy People 2010 specified two major goals to improve the health of Americans (DHHS, 2000). Although the goals do not specifically mention urban populations, they can be applied to urban populations. One goal is to eliminate health disparities. A large percentage of the population in inner cities is nonwhite. Mortality, morbidity, and lack of health care access and utilization continue to soar among nonwhites, especially in inner cities (DHHS, 2000). As a result, several national health programs have been targeted for African Americans and other nonwhites. Many of the national programs have stemmed from the Public Health Service. Community health nurses are in an excellent position to help manage these health programs or coordinate the health care.

The **Healthy Cities** movement was initiated by the World Health Organization (WHO) in Europe in 1984. It was brought about by a speech given at an international meeting in Canada with a theme that "health is much more than medical care" (IHCF, 1995, p. 1). Soon after the initiation of Europe's Healthy Cities project, others followed, including Canada, the United States, Latin America, Africa, and Asia.

The International Healthy Cities Foundation (IHCF) was established in August 1994 (IHCF, 1995). From the beginning, this organization was envisioned by global advisory boards as a dynamic interconnection of people, organizations, and networks involving many disciplines and interest groups. The goal of IHCF and the WHO is to increase the level of health for all citizens of the world.

IHCF's mission is to facilitate linkages among people, issues, and resources to support the development of the Healthy Cities movement (IHCF, 1995). With this mission in mind, IHCF developed an infrastructure of three programs: communications, resource tools, and training and advisory services. Many people at various levels are involved in IHCF, including partners from public health and safety; educators; religious groups; alcohol and drug programs; and community groups focusing on civil and human rights, volunteerism, housing, labor, business, environment, occupation, and many others. Virtually every discipline on the global front has a voice in IHCF.

WHO recognized that urban cities held almost half the world's population. Through the Healthy Cities program, local individuals and local resources are recruited to work together to identify and help resolve health problems in their community. There are numerous participating cities throughout the United States and the world. In the Healthy Cities program, attention is given to modifying the physical, social, and economic environment of the community to improve the health of individuals.

One of the first major United States cities to launch a Healthy Cities project was Boston. Since its inception in 1992, Boston has served as a leader of the Healthy Cities movement in the United States (Office of Community Partnerships, 1996). After an extensive evaluation of the Healthy Boston project, the Office of Community Partnerships realized that the project had been very successful in reaching its goals, which were to create a collective community voice, serve as a catalyst to optimize services, create new partnerships, embrace multicultural and collaborative values, embrace health issues, and create healthy communities. Only four recommendations for improvement came from the evaluation. One of those recommendations was for the improvement of leadership development and more support for coalitions. Community health nurses could fill this role by becoming leaders and providing support and coordination of health and political coalitions. Community health nurses need to realize the potential healthy outcomes for urban populations when a Healthy Cities project has been successfully undertaken.

At the International Healthy Cities Conference in Athens, Greece, in June 1998, the third phase of the Healthy Cities movement was launched. Jo Asvall, WHO's Regional Director for Europe, stated at this conference, "WHO is emphasizing the diversity and seriousness of urban health issues and the need for action at the local level" (WHO, 1998, p. 1). At this conference, the members evaluated outcomes and the impact of the movement for the previous 10 years.

Several other programs have been specially targeted at the African American population in inner cities, such as the Harlem Health Connection and the Safe Kids/Healthy Neighborhoods Injury Prevention Program in Harlem (Polednak, 1997). African American inner-city churches and community groups have also been committed to improving living conditions in urban areas.

Urban development projects across U.S. cities have provided health opportunities for urban populations (Bates, 1997; Polednak, 1997). Improving the health outcomes of these people through better access to health care with an emphasis on health promotion and prevention of disease is a result of urban development efforts. Many problems still exist, but the urban development efforts of communities are becoming beneficial to the urban residents. Many of these projects start at the grassroots level and are coordinated and managed by city officials and community leaders.

One urban development project that began at the local level and has spread rapidly throughout the United States is the Atlanta Project, which has now become the America Project (TAP, 1995). This project was developed by former President Jimmy Carter in an effort to promote hope and healing and to unite the Atlanta people to improve the quality of life in neighborhoods. The success of the project spread quickly throughout the United States and has been adopted by many major city officials. The project's mission required several elements for success, which included having a vision, planning well, empowering the community, collaborating, volunteering, and communicating effectively.

West (1994) emphasized that young African American urban people are faced with despair and are fighting the forces of death, destruction, and disease. With consistent efforts, programs such as the Healthy Cities movement and other urban development programs can provide the resources for health promotion and healing. Community health nurses have a responsibility to become involved in urban policy making, urban development projects, and urban health care.

The Homeless Population

Today the United States is faced with overwhelming social problems (Family and Youth Services Bureau, 1996). However, none of the problems has threatened the human condition as much as homelessness. Interwoven throughout the homeless population are the social problems of substance abuse, racism, violence, limited education, crime, and poverty.

A new culture of homeless people has emerged. The number and composition of homeless people during the last two decades of the 20th century have grasped the attention of the American people. The individuals comprising the homeless populations are no longer the "skid row bums," "hobos," and "tramps" found years ago. Now women, adolescents, families with children, and elderly people represent a large portion of the homeless population (Institute of Medicine, 1988). It has been projected that single women with children will soon make up the majority of homeless people (Vladeck, 1990).

The homeless lifestyle is a barrier to good health practices and thus leads to more prevalent health problems (Flynn, 1997; Hatton, 1997). Community health nurses play a vital role in breaking down the barriers that prevent positive health practices in this new culture of homeless women, men, and children. As

we will see later, outreach to nontraditional service locations and case management are key strategies on which community health nurses can focus (Cousineau, Wittenberg, & Pollatsek, 1995). Although the *Healthy People 2010* objectives do not specifically address the issue of homelessness, they address all of the conditions, problems, and population groups affected.

••••••••••••••••••••••••••••••

RESCUE MISSION

THEY'LL SIT LIKE THAT FOR HOURS
for a ticket away from
their hunger rack ribs
with their shirts off
in summer lined up
as if waiting on
Buck Rogers' next
scuffle
those racks look
like evil fingers
closing around
empty innards
when the bell chimes
Jesus saves
and the door flings open
they file in like boys
returning from an
exhausting recess
it's bread that saves now
as they sit quietly
almost broken of old habits
although a few
(perhaps toothless?)
still neatly trim
the crust away

James A. Lopresti, Denver, Colorado, 1977

••••••••••••••••••••••••••••••

Scope of the Problem

In 1997, cities all across America had unmet needs for shelter and food. Approximately 27% of the requests for shelters by homeless persons and thirty-five percent of shelter requests by homeless families were unmet in 1997 (U.S. Conference of Mayors, 1997). The problem is growing every year. In 1998, officials of the nation's major cities expected a 92% increase in requests for food and shelter (U.S. Conference of Mayors, 1997). No city officials expected a decline in requests for the following year. In fact, in 1998, a survey revealed that there was a startling increase in emergency food and shelter across America (Rosenblum & Imgrund, 1999).

Homelessness is a growing problem that is more than local (Appel & Boden, 1999). Homelessness is a global problem. The homeless population is located in both urban and rural areas. Women, adolescents, substance abusers, families with children, and people with mental illness or who are deinstitutionalized make up the homeless population (Interagency Council on the Homeless, 1994; Lezak & Edgar, 1996; DHHS, 1995). The es-

A CONVERSATION WITH...

Donald, a Homeless Man in Gulfport, Mississippi

"You never know, it could be your brother...out there needing your help."

Nurse: Donald, you told me you were from New York and that you came here. Do you have any family down here?

Donald: No, no family at all, like a bird I fly south for the warm weather, this time in New York right now it's freezing and it's really crowded in the line of business I'm in.

Nurse: What line of business is that?

Donald: I do a little everything, I am over here now a couple of days cause people give me a lot of yard work over here, and they feed me, give me a little change of clothes, I sprinkle a little water on myself.

Nurse: You don't find this weather cold down here right now? It's like forty something degrees out here.

Donald: Yeah, it's like forty something degrees here and maybe twenty something degrees in New York City. I'm pretty well prepared, I got about four layers of clothing on, most of the time down here I have to strip some of this off.

Nurse: Well, let me ask you something, Donald. Like I explained to you, I'm a nurse and I'm studying health care. Where do you go when you get sick, how do you go about getting some help, about seeing a doctor?

Donald: Well, most of the hospitals here, they've been all right, they direct me to the emergency room... they'll fix you up, say if I just have a cold.

Nurse: Well you look fairly young anyway...

Donald: Yeah, I am in pretty good health.

Nurse: Well, I see that you got some stuff with you.

Donald: This is just basic essentials, you know sneakers, a little change of clothes; I have my blanket, I have been running into some cold nights, I have some utensils, and things, nothing much, just everyday homeless persons' things. People give me this, I go to shelters. I have been lucky to catch a few shelters down here, but you know last night it was a little crowded and I had to stay outside, but I am pretty much prepared for it.

Nurse: How long do you plan to stay down here?

Donald: As long as business is good, I say that as long as I can make a meal, work somewhere and make a meal; I'll stay.

Nurse: You say you don't have any family down here, but do you have any family up in New York?

Donald: I have a sister, last address unknown. I don't bother anybody, I am self-sufficient, I try to take care of myself, I don't ask for much, I lead a simple life.

Nurse: Like I said before, if I ask you anything personal and you don't want to answer, you don't have to. Do you drink any alcohol?

Donald: Very little, very little...like my sign reads here "Will work for food," it doesn't say, "for alcohol"....Now occasionally I have been known to take a good sip, it warms the innards.

Nurse: How about the people who you meet at the shelters, do you notice that they drink much alcohol?

Donald: The majority of them are heavy wine drinkers, well they drink whatever they can get a hold of, anything that's over one percent alcohol they drink it.

I am basically a loner, I travel alone, I've been all over this country, I've been by myself, I've been making it.

Nurse: You're not scared out on the roads...the violence?

Donald: Yeah, there's times I'm scared, but, you know, luckily people know I don't have anything. They don't bother me. I have run into a lot of good people. They just don't bother me ever.

Nurse: Was there anything you think would be helpful for me to know about people who live on the roads?

Donald: Yes, if you could get to talk to some more people or if more people would talk openly I think that you would find that the homeless situation is really bad and people who could lend a hand in any kind of way, just donating some old clothes to Salvation Army or Goodwill, they should really look into it. I think the states should look more into the homeless situation 'cause it's really out there and it's really bad, it could be your brother, one of your relatives—out there needing your help.

—Interviewer: James Ryan, RN, BSN

Mr. Ryan found Donald under a freeway underpass in Mississippi holding a sign that said "Will work for food." Interview used with permission.

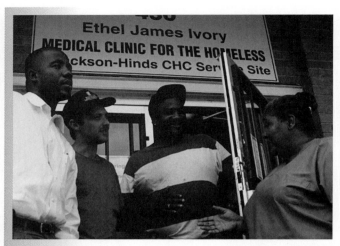

Homeless clinics in inner-city locations can provide essential care for the homeless population.

timate of homeless children is 100,000 at any given day or night (Institute of Medicine, 1988). Still more astounding are the facts that each year 30% to 50% of all homeless people are families with children and 22% of all homeless people are children (Milhaly, 1991; Reyes & Waxman, 1989).

A problem exists in counting accurate numbers of homeless people because of the "one point in time" reference. The group of homeless persons may be different people and different numbers from one night to another. During a 7-day period in March 1987, statistics revealed that more than 600,000 homeless peo-

ple sought shelter from the outside environment (Burt & Cohen, 1989). During the 1990 Census, the U.S. Department of Commerce (1992) attempted to gather statistics on numbers of homeless people. The department was unable to obtain specific numbers across the country but gathered data in certain cities over a specific number of days and nights. Currently, the U.S. Conference of Mayors studies specific U.S. cities every year to draw conclusions about the scope of the problem and characteristics of the population of homeless people. In 1997, 29 cities were evaluated by the U.S. Conference of Mayors for their status regarding hunger and homelessness. The statistics for 1997 are very similar to estimates of previous years. Table 26-1 characterizes the 1997 homeless population in more detail.

Researchers have estimated the number of homeless people across America, suggesting that the number of individuals experiencing homelessness is even greater than previously expected. In the latter part of the 1980s, as many as 9.32 million persons were believed to have been homeless at least once (Culhane, Dejowski, Ibanex, Needham, & Macchia, 1993; Interagency Council on the Homeless, 1994; Link, Phelan, Breshan, Stueve, Moore, & Susser, 1995). Even more disturbing is that families are the fastest growing segment of the homeless population (U.S. Conference of Mayors, 1989). Box 26-1 delineates the composition of homeless people.

The estimated number of homeless people does not include the growing segment of people who are on the verge of homelessness (Interagency Council on the Homeless, 1994). More than 1 million families are on waiting lists for public housing at any given time. Many more people have moved in with friends or

---

TABLE 26-1   **CHARACTERISTICS OF HOMELESS PEOPLE IN 1997**

CHARACTERISTICS	FINDINGS IN THE HOMELESS POPULATION
Family status	47% are single men
	36% are families with children; of these families, 76% are headed by a single parent, and 59% are children
	14% are single women
	25% are children; of these children, 4% are unaccompanied youth
Race and ethnicity	58% are African American
	29% are Caucasian
	10% are Hispanic
	2% are Native American
	1% are Asian American
Institutional history	27% are considered mentally ill
Health/social status	43% are substance abusers
	9% have AIDS or HIV-related illness
Employment	17% are employed in full- or part-time jobs
Homeless veterans	22% are veterans

Source: U.S. Conference of Mayors, 1997.

BOX 26-1 WHO ARE THE NEW HOMELESS PEOPLE?

- Single adults unaccompanied by children
- Single mothers with children
- Families with children
- Individuals who have been deinstitutionalized
- Persons who are diagnosed with mental illness
- Runaway and throwaway youths
- Abandoned children
- Unemployed, impoverished adults
- Immigrants
- Veterans
- Elderly people

BOX 26-2 USE OF THE TERM HOMELESS

In the latter part of the 1970s, the term homeless became a trendy way to refer to individuals living on the streets or in shelters (Interagency Council on the Homeless, 1994). At that time, homeless individuals were predominantly males who had been deinstitutionalized. The term was popularized by proponents as a way to describe homeless people in a nonstigmatizing, nonjudgmental way. However, the term became synonymous with bums. A new kind of homelessness has placed a strain on the use of the term. In the last two decades, poverty has brought families, women, and children in record numbers to face homelessness.

relatives. Increasing numbers of people are paying more than half their income for rent, making them at risk for homelessness at any time.

Definitions of Homeless People

An official definition of **homeless** was offered by the federal government in the Stewart B. McKinney Homeless Assistance Act of 1987 (U.S. Congress, House, 1987). Any individual lacking a fixed, regular, and adequate nighttime residence is defined as a homeless person. The definition includes any individual with a primary nighttime residence at shelters, missions, welfare hotels, and public or private places not designated for sleeping quarters. Any person needing institutionalization but instead residing in an institution providing only temporary residence for homeless people is also considered homeless. Box 26-2 provides an insight into the way the term *homeless* has been used in the past.

Other definitions of homeless include individuals with no mailing address or place to sleep; people who sleep outdoors on streets or in parks, at train stations, at subways, underground, or in cars; and people on the verge of homelessness (Bean, Stefl, & Howe, 1987; Benda & Dattalo, 1988; Phillips, Pauley, & Rudolph, 1997; Interagency Council on the Homeless, 1994; Rivlin, 1986; Stark, 1987).

Homelessness has also been described in terms of three stages (Belcher, Scholler-Jaquish, & Drummond, 1991). *Episodic homelessness* characterizes people who live below the poverty line and who are on the verge of homelessness or may actually experience one or more episodes of homelessness for short periods. *Temporary homelessness* describes people who have recently become homeless but still view themselves as part of their community. *Chronic homelessness* describes people who have adopted their state of being as a way of life and have declined in social status, financial status, and interpersonal and family connections.

Historical Perspective
The Beginning of Homelessness in America

As long as can be remembered, homeless people have been inhabitants of America (Institute of Medicine, 1988). English people who settled on North American soil segregated themselves by classes. The workers and the more affluent people gave assistance to poor people (Trattner, 1984). During the 1600s, colonists adopted England's ideology and many principles of England's law, which was written to protect the welfare of families and communities. Therefore, adult white men, "free" African Americans, and Indians were left to wander aimlessly and beg for food, clothing, and other assistance. The only individuals who warranted assistance at that time were white women, children, and disabled people.

As the mid-1800s approached, a new generation of poor people surfaced in the United States during the industrialization and farming era. Sporadic and transient labor became essential (Hoch & Slayton, 1989). Most of the homeless populations consisted of men because they were the providers and often had to leave home to find work. Some who traveled the land by railways to look for transient work were labeled as "hobos." Other men who sought transient work on foot were labeled as "tramps." Then there were "bums," who usually traveled by railways, stole from others, and begged for money and food. The Civil War and migration to the West created another mass of homeless people, who were labeled "cowboys," "Indian scouts," and "gold seekers" (Hoffman, 1953).

Not long after the turn of the 20th century, "skid rows" surfaced in major cities, where homeless and indigent people gathered for food, assistance, and word-of-mouth information at diners, bars, mission homes, and old hotels. Most of these people were older white men. The skid row population fluctuated with the status of the American economy (Momeni & Wiegand, 1989). Shantytowns, where homeless people colonized, sprang up across the United States after the crash of the stock market in

1929. The skid row population continued to increase until World War II brought new jobs.

Societal and Governmental Influences Through the 1970s

Because manifestations of mental illness place persons at high risk for homelessness, a large proportion of the homeless population was believed to be mentally ill in the 1800s. In 1890, New York was the first state to enact a law allowing the state government to assume full responsibility for individuals classified as the "insane poor" (Anderson, 1934).

A federal plan was not initiated until 1933, when the **Federal Emergency Relief Administration (FERA)** supplied food, shelter, clothing, money, jobs, and health care to homeless individuals (Anderson, 1940). In 1935, FERA was replaced by the Works Progress Administration (WPA) federal program, which was aimed at creating jobs only for people who could meet strict residency standards. Because a residence was required to receive assistance, homeless people were not included in this plan.

The 1940s and World War II created new jobs and decreased poverty and homelessness for a few years, but the 1960s brought a substantial increase in the homeless population. In 1963, the Community Health Centers Act was enacted, which deinstitutionalized approximately 430,000 people with mental illness (Rossi, 1989). These people were released from the institutions in which they lived, and many of them had nowhere to live and no job. Deinstitutionalizing thousands of people was cited as a humane act but detrimentally expanded the homeless population.

The combination of deinstitutionalization and the declining economy in the 1970s forced courts to rule on homelessness for the first time. In 1972, the U.S. Supreme Court ruled that vagrancy was no longer a crime (Cook, 1979). The Court also declared that governmental assistance provided only to people who claimed a permanent residence was unconstitutional. In the same decade, the New York Supreme Court ruled that homeless people should be provided a clean place to sleep, nutritious food, supervision, and security. Efforts were made to comply with the court ruling. Many, but not all, homeless people in New York were given assistance.

Societal and Governmental Influences in the 1980s

The state of New York's move toward improving homeless conditions contributed to the federal government's actions toward homeless programs. Several other major events occurred in the United States during the 1980s that drove the federal government into action to provide federal assistance (Interagency Council on the Homeless, 1994). A dramatic increase in poverty and the shrinking of affordable housing were major forces that led to the homeless epidemic.

Racial discrimination in the job market presented another concern. By 1985, less than 45% of African American men ages 16 to 24 were able to find employment, compared with 70% of white men of the same age range (Interagency Council on the Homeless, 1994). Other situations that contributed to homelessness and poverty were substance abuse, disabilities, chronic health problems, and changes in the family structure that led to a shift toward female-headed households.

Also in the 1980s, a shift in the labor market from a focus on goods production to a focus on services caused plants to relocate or close and farms to shrink or cease to operate. Laborers were no longer in high demand. Rather, the demand was for

---

TABLE 26-2   **GOVERNMENTAL ACTIVITIES FOR HOMELESS PEOPLE IN THE 1980S**

DATE	ACTIVITIES OF THE 1980S
1982	The Community for Creative Non-Violence in Washington, DC, estimated that 2.2 million Americans lacked shelter.
1982	The U.S. Conference of Mayors reported that the demand for emergency services for the homeless far outweighed the capabilities to provide services. In fact, only 43% of the demand was met.
1983	The Emergency Food and Shelter (EFS) Program of the Federal Emergency Management Agency (FEMA) allocated $100 million to the U.S. Department of Agriculture's Temporary Emergency Food Assistance Program (TEFAP) to reduce the impact of the homeless crisis.
1984 to 1987	FEMA allocated $325 million for continued relief. Other agencies that allocated money for relief efforts included the Health and Human Services Emergency Assistance Program and the HUD Community Development Block Grant Program.
1987	The Stewart B. McKinney Homeless Assistance Act was enacted to provide emergency shelters, job training, and other assistance to homeless people providing $490 million.
1988	The National Resource Center on Homelessness and Mental Illness was established by the Policy Research Associates (PSA) in order to provide on-site technical assistance, targeted workshops, publications, databases, and instant access to homeless people with mental illness.

TABLE 26-3	GOVERNMENTAL ACTIVITIES FOR HOMELESS PEOPLE IN THE 1990S

DATE	ACTIVITIES OF THE 1990S
1992	Funding was set aside to provide rental assistance to 4,750 disabled homeless households annually for 3 years.
1993	President Clinton committed to make homelessness a top priority in the White House.
1994	The Interagency Council on the Homeless (1994) published a proposal to reduce the homeless population. The main objective was to find "a decent home and a suitable living environment" for every American, which would become known as the "Continuum of Care." The reality was that the council hoped to reduce homelessness by one-third.
1995	President Clinton proposed a reorganization of the HUD McKinney programs under a single account. Homeless projects continued as a high priority in the Oval Office.
1995	President Clinton vetoed the balanced budget bill, which would have cut federal welfare by $81.5 billion and virtually eliminated homeless assistance programs provided by the McKinney Act. The President's budget proposed consolidating three runaway and homeless programs. The budget also focused on disadvantaged groups, including veterans and other homeless people.
1995	The National Law Center on Homelessness and Poverty published a report that evaluated NIMBY (Not In My Backyard!) opposition to services for homeless people in 36 jurisdictions across the United States
1995	Funding was set aside to provide rental assistance to 15,000 homeless households annually for 5 years.

highly skilled and educated people. A way of life had disappeared; jobs were gone; a new culture of homeless people existed.

The combined tensions created by all of these problems placed at-risk people at serious disadvantages and thus strained many households to the point of homelessness.

Table 26-2 provides a list of governmental activities during the 1980s. Historically, the assistance offered by government programs and local groups has provided only immediate relief and has failed to address the long-term problems of homelessness (Fuchs & McAllister, 1996). The **Stewart B. McKinney Homeless Assistance Act of 1987** and the grassroots efforts of local relief groups were instrumental in prompting the federal government to make a commitment to reduce homelessness (Interagency Council on the Homeless, 1994).

Societal and Governmental Influences in the 1990s
Many programs were born during the 1990s. Once the initial Stewart B. McKinney Homeless Assistance Act of 1987 was developed, the program branched into numerous programs throughout the federal government (Interagency Council on the Homeless, 1994). Table 26-3 outlines a few of those programs in the 1990s. By 1994, the McKinney programs had expanded to $1.2 billion. Numerous non-McKinney programs also were created. Today almost a dozen of these non-McKinney programs target homeless people. Many federal programs, although not targeted to the homeless, provide indirect assistance to homeless people. The McKinney Act has been the major federal vehicle to assist homeless people (Interagency Council on the Homeless, 1994).

The 1990s brought about unprecedented growth and complexity in the homeless population. As a result, nurses, social workers, agencies, and others have gained rich, abundant experiences in trying to manage homelessness. The same social problems leading to homelessness persist: declining wages, poor education, persistent illiteracy, racial discrimination, chronic health problems, violence, crime, and poverty.

Americans must face that even as new programs have sprung up, the problem of homelessness has grown because economical, health, and social forces are ever-present. Organizations have historically looked for easy solutions to seemingly unresolvable problems. Homelessness remains a problem without a solution, just as it has always been. America is now faced with even more complex human problems: newer, stronger, and more addictive drugs, such as heroin and cocaine; socially stigmatizing infections such as tuberculosis, sexually transmitted diseases, and human immunodeficiency virus (HIV); and decline of family support, which means that relatives often do not take in family members needing assistance anymore. Box 26-3 delineates several factors that may contribute to an individual's homelessness.

The Health Problems of Homeless People
Common Health Problems
Homelessness in the United States translates into major health problems. People who are homeless are faced with myriad health problems, which fall into three basic categories: health problems that contribute to a state of homelessness, health problems that are the consequence of homelessness, and treatment of health problems that is complicated by homelessness (Institute of Medicine, 1988).

The first category involves health problems that contribute to a state of homelessness. Most people with chronic health problems

> ### BOX 26-3 WHY ARE PEOPLE HOMELESS?
>
> - Poverty
> - Changes in the labor market from focus on goods production to services
> - Lack of affordable housing
> - Devaluation of the dollar and devaluation of federal income assistance
> - Unemployment
> - Street violence, domestic violence, and crime
> - Crisis in families; abuse, neglect, and incestuous relationships
> - Lack of kin support
> - Mental illness
> - Deinstitutionalization
> - Substance abuse
> - Socially stigmatizing infectious diseases (e.g., HIV, tuberculosis)
>
> *Sources: Interagency Council on the Homeless, 1994; Jahiel, 1992; Sumerlin & Bundrick, 1997; Susser, Struening, & Conover, 1997.*

that lead to a state of homelessness suffer from lack of employment because of their disabling state of health (Berne, Dato, Mason, & Rafferty, 1993; Institute of Medicine, 1988). These homeless persons usually do not have a support network of family members and friends. Chronic schizophrenia, dementia, and personality disorders are examples of mental illnesses that may actually contribute to a state of homelessness and financial insecurity. Relationships with family and friends may become excessively strained when an individual's ability to cope with everyday life situations diminishes. Family members may become so stressed trying to deal with everyday problems that they abandon or throw out the mentally ill family member into the streets.

Individuals with acquired immunodeficiency syndrome (AIDS) may become homeless when they are no longer able to work because of illness and opportunistic infections (Institute of Medicine, 1988). They often lose their houses or apartments and face overwhelming medical expenses. Living on the street or in a shelter becomes a way of life for them. Alcoholism, drug dependency, and other disabling health problems (e.g., accidental injuries or degenerative diseases) may lead to similar life situations. In 15 studies on alcoholism in the homeless population (as cited in Rossi, 1989), 33% of homeless people abused alcohol and were homeless as a result of alcoholism. These people suffered from health problems as a result of the alcoholism.

The second category includes many disorders and illnesses that result from living on the streets or in shelters. Examples of physical problems include skin and blood vessel diseases, respira-

tory disorders and infections, malnutrition, parasitic infestations, foot and lower extremity problems, physical assault, rape, trauma, periodontal disease, tooth decay, degenerative joint disease, sexually transmitted diseases, cirrhosis, and hepatitis (Institute of Medicine, 1988). Psychological and social problems that may be triggered include personality disorders, alcohol and drug dependence, prostitution, poor oral and body hygiene, hunger, adolescent pregnancy, developmental and learning delays in children, violence, criminal convictions, depression, low self-esteem, and other mental illnesses (Institute of Medicine, 1988; Interagency Council on the Homeless, 1994; Rossi, 1989). Table 26-4 reflects specific health problems associated with homelessness.

Skin, blood vessel, and traumatic problems that homeless people experience are often related to strenuous walking and wandering, inadequate clothing, improper fitting of shoes, and exposure to infections and parasites. Some of these problems include venous stasis, varicose veins, peripheral vascular disease, cellulitis, skin ulcerations, skin infestations, bruises, contusions, lacerations, abrasions, abscesses, and burns of all severities (Rossi, 1989).

Communicable diseases affect scores of homeless people and are cause for a major public health concern (Rossi, 1989). Living on the streets or in shelters subjects homeless people to poor sanitary conditions, poor hygiene, and inadequate, if any, sleeping quarters. Communicable diseases (e.g., tuberculosis) are easily transmitted in these living conditions.

The third category results from complications associated with the treatment of acute or chronic health problems in homeless people (Institute of Medicine, 1989). One major chronic disease that is complicated by inadequate treatment is diabetes mellitus. Daily injections and a diabetic exchange diet are difficult, if not impossible, to maintain. Protecting syringes from theft or contamination, for example, is challenging. Hypertension, renal disease, liver disease, peripheral vascular disease, and schizophrenia are other chronic problems that are complicated by homelessness. Inability to follow medical regimen, lack of money to cover medical and health expenses, or inability to follow the prescribed dietary regimen complicate these health problems.

Homeless families have similar acute and chronic physical and mental problems. Homeless children also are at risk for developing chronic physical disorders. In a study conducted by Wright and Weber (1987), 16% of the homeless children were reported to have a variety of chronic physical disorders. Some of the most common disorders included asthma, anemia, and malnutrition. Some other disorders reported at high rates were various types of respiratory infections, skin infections, ear and eye infections, dental problems, and gastrointestinal problems.

In another study of homelessness in New York City in 1985 (Chavkin, Kristal, Seabron, & Guigli, 1987), the infant mortality rate of the homeless population (24.9 per 1,000 live births) was more than twice the overall infant mortality rate in New York City (12 per 1,000 live births). In the same study, the researchers found that homeless pregnant women were more likely to give birth to infants of low weight than nonhomeless pregnant women.

TABLE 26-4   **COMMON HEALTH PROBLEMS OF HOMELESS PEOPLE**

CLASSIFICATION	SPECIFIC HEALTH PROBLEMS
Skin and traumatic disorders	Skin ulcerations
	Skin infestations (e.g., lice, scabies, worms)
	Peripheral vascular disease, varicose veins
	Cellulitis
	Carbuncles
	Bunions, corns
	Abrasions, lacerations
	Wounds
	Bruises, contusions
	Sprains, strains
	Burns
Acute disorders/diseases	Tuberculosis, pneumonia, influenza, asthma
	Bladder and renal infections
	Female-specific genitourinary infections
	Male-specific genitourinary infections
	Diabetes mellitus complications
Chronic disorders/diseases	Psychosocial disorders/problems
	Cancer of all types
	Endocrine disorders (e.g., diabetes mellitus)
	Anemia and other nutritional deficiencies
	Eye, ear, mouth, and dental disorders
	Cardiovascular disorders (hypertension, heart, and circulatory disorders)
	Arthritis and other musculoskeletal disorders
	Pregnancy
	HIV/AIDS and other sexually transmitted diseases
	Seizures and other neurological disorders
	Obstructive pulmonary disease
	Gastrointestinal disorders
Mental illnesses	Personality disorders
	Criminal convictions
	Jail, prison, or detention sentencing
	Drug and alcohol abuse
	Lack of family or friends support system
	Poverty

Source: Rossi, 1989.

HIV transmission is a primary concern for all homeless people, especially homeless adult and adolescent women. In a survey of homeless adults who were entering a storefront medical clinic, 69% were found to be at risk for acquiring HIV infection because of several at-risk behaviors: unprotected sex with multiple partners, injection drug use, sex with a partner who injects drugs, or exchanging sex for money or drugs, primarily crack (St. Lawrence & Brasfield, 1995). Safe, intimate relationships may be difficult, if not impossible, for homeless people to maintain because of drug use, mental illness, violence, survival sex (sex in exchange for food, money, or drugs), and transient living conditions. In their survey, Fisher, Hovell, and Hofstetter (1995) found that 91% of homeless women experienced battery and 56% experienced sexual assault.

Homeless mothers have been a forgotten population in terms of research or published literature. Berne, Dato, Mason, and Rafferty (1993) noted that homeless mothers traditionally have waited to seek health care until their conditions developed into emergency situations. Chronic stressors, physical and sexual abuse, lack of family ties, poverty, lack of coping abilities, domestic violence, street violence, overcrowded conditions, poor hygiene, and poor nutrition predispose homeless mothers to chronic physical, social, and mental problems. Tuberculosis, depression, sexually transmitted diseases, HIV/AIDS, drug abuse, prostitution for money or drugs, and poor parenting skills often result.

• •

RESCUE MISSION 2

THEY GATHER THEMSELVES IN GROUPS OF TWELVE

around shakey cardtables
some unvarnished wood
and others metal and formica

they're here for another supper
for some the last one
before they lean slowly
toward another side of town

here they all gather at the Riverside mission
apostles of the alleys
sheltered in boxes and
doorways opened onto the
promised streets and rails

lord, are these bones hungry
these tweeds and wools shine
but not with grace from the father
a dull halo of wear

in the seat where a man
can rub thin with contact
from concrete and unpainted benches
and still turn the other cheek

some bring their own wine
refusing the coffee or tea
and milk can no longer faithfully
support these crumbling bones

no one will be betrayed here
though some have thought of a sellout
at times for thirty cents to luck
onto more wine or cigarettes

the bread is passed around again
wholly for the sake of one's almighty health
a man's got to eat to save himself
though the word wasn't made flesh
enough to bless them with a small
taste of steak

after supper they file out on
the thin soles of unpolished shoes

the moon rests like a large stone
rolled to close a room where a brother
waits with a good steak, new tweed
a cigarette and a rousing story of
how when he was hungry there was always
someone to share their bread

James A. Lopresti, Denver, Colorado, 1977

• •

Adolescents are also vulnerable to a variety of social and health problems, including violence, prostitution, drug abuse, and physical and mental disorders. The following Research Brief summarizes research findings about homeless youth and their exposure to and involvement in violence while living on the streets.

The accumulation of problems that homeless people experience is overwhelming to say the least. Reducing or alleviating homelessness is critical to the general health and human condition in our society. Public policies are needed to meet two goals: to reduce or combat the short-term problems of pain and suffering in homeless individuals and to address the long-term problems by reducing the risk of becoming homeless. By becoming a political advocate for the basic rights and health of the homeless population, community health nurses can help create or change public policies involving homelessness.

Barriers to Health Care

Researchers have indicated that lack of access is a major barrier to health care for homeless people (e.g., Hunter, Getty, Kemsley, & Skelly, 1991; Wood & Valdez, 1991). Homeless people cannot afford health insurance, and not surprisingly, homeless people experience even more problems in accessing health care than nonhomeless people with or without insurance. Homeless people typically do not have a regular family practitioner. They seek care from emergency departments more often than poor people who are not homeless. Homeless people may also be discouraged from obtaining health care services or even turned away by health care personnel from private clinics (Freeman, Blendon, Aiken, Sudman, Mullinix, & Corey, 1987). Other barriers to health care include the following (Flynn, 1997; Hatton, 1997; Institute of Medicine, 1988; Nyamathi, Flaskerud, & Leake, 1997; Percy, 1995):

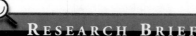

RESEARCH BRIEF

Kipke, M. D., Simon, T. R., Montgomery, S. B., Unger, J. B., & Iversen, E. F. (1997). *Homeless youth and their exposure to and involvement in violence while living on the streets.* Journal of Adolescent Health, 20, 360–367.

A survey of 432 youth between the ages of 13 and 23 years old, who were homeless or at imminent risk for homelessness, revealed that males and females were exposed to equally high levels of violence on the streets. Females were more likely to have been sexually assaulted but less likely to report it or report any other violent acts. Ethnic identity was not a significant predictor of exposure to violence. The overall findings revealed that these youth were exposed to violence at a significantly higher level than other youth in national surveys.

- *Lack of systematic communication with health care professionals*
- *Lack of transportation to a health care facility*
- *Lack of social and family support*
- *Psychological depression; hard-to-reach homeless people*
- *Lack of motivation by the homeless person to seek health care*

Nursing Care of Urban and Homeless People

Community health nurses function on all three levels of prevention—primary, secondary, and tertiary—regarding the care of urban and homeless aggregate populations. Homeless people have generated a culture all their own, enriched with diverse customs and backgrounds that should be taken into consideration when managing care for them (Family and Youth Services Bureau, 1994). Managing health and social problems for urban and homeless individuals and populations is among the most challenging functions of the community health nurse.

Homeless people suffer from myriad emotional and physical ups and downs. The Research Brief below reflects a summary of research findings on the experiences of homeless female-headed families.

Both young and old homeless people need what everyone needs—opportunities, advantages, and services that help them live healthier lives. Ed DeBerri, Assistant Director at the National Resource Center on Homelessness and Mental Illness (1997), stated that the most effective programs and policies have human dignity as their guiding principle. Through hands-on experience with homeless individuals, DeBerri (1997) learned five important principles about homeless people and their needs.

RESEARCH BRIEF

Menke, E. M., & Wagner, J. D. (1997). The experience of homeless female-headed families. Issues in Mental Health Nursing, 18, 315–330.

Homeless families are at high risk for severe physical, emotional, and social health problems. Eighty-five percent of all homeless families are headed by single women. Sixteen of these women were asked to describe their experiences of being the head of the homeless family. The themes that emerged were: loss of freedom, a sense of being different, feeling down, maternal survival (motherhood), and living under pressure. They described being homeless as a nightmare, not knowing what will happen to them or where they will be from day to day.

· ·

"IF I'M LUCKY"

Buddy, can you spare me a quarter?
I've got an important call to make.
And maybe if I bum enough quarters
A little drink will help me heal my heartache.
You see, I'm drowning
In a river of liquor.
I'm going down for the last time.
I'm a loser . . .
I'm a boozer . . .
On lower Broadway.
If I'm lucky
I won't see the sun rise.
Years ago, I hopped a Greyhound to Nashville.
A big country star would I be.
And if I must confess
I met with some success
But success got the better of me.
So tonight I'll wrap my arms around my bottle
In an old cardboard box
We will lie.
I'm a loser . . .
I'm a boozer . . .
On lower Broadway.
If I'm lucky
I won't see the sun rise.
So don't preach to me
About Jesus.
Cause Jesus don't live on the streets.
He lives in a white ivory tower
in the heart of someplace
called Belle Meade.
You see, there's one thing in life
I've got faith in,
Is this warm toasty feeling inside.
I'm a loser . . .
I'm a boozer . . .
On lower Broadway.
If I'm lucky
I won't see the sun rise.
If I'm lucky
I won't see the sun rise.

Music and Lyrics by Felton Keyes, BSN, RN, 1985
Used with permission

· ·

First and foremost, DeBerri found that homeless people have talents, needs, and desires. They want to be shown respect for who they are and what they know. Second, shelters and case management traditionally have not been sufficient to prevent the problems of homelessness or to end homelessness. Housing, financial support, and social and family support are needed to improve the conditions. Third, providing comprehensive health care, social services, and housing can reduce homelessness. Fourth, helping to find work for homeless individuals is essential. Homeless people need to feel productive and useful, just like all people. Fifth, new resources need to be developed and used creatively; then the successes of these programs need to be publicized.

These five principles also can be applied to the care of urban populations. Drawing on the strengths of urban or homeless individuals and the resources available in the community will enable community health nurses to implement appropriate interventions that can actually work. An example of drawing on the strength of a homeless person would be to find a homeless person who can sew and asking him or her to teach a group of people in the shelter how to mend their clothes. Another example is to recruit a person from the shelter to teach good hygiene and hand washing techniques to the children in the shelter. The community health nurse's interventions will help create social and economic viability, build diversity in skills and resources, strengthen the community, and contribute to healthier people in the community.

However, improving the conditions of urban people and reducing the rate of homelessness are outcomes that need a collaborative effort among multidisciplinary agencies in the community. Without communitywide participation, poor conditions among the urban and homeless populations and increased incidence of homelessness will persist. Furthermore, without communitywide efforts to eliminate poverty, prejudice, violence, and discrimination, the nurse's attempts to improve the health and human conditions among urban and homeless populations will be fruitless.

Specific interventions that the community health nurse should implement are described in the following sections. The interventions are aimed at managing health and social problems of urban and homeless populations.

Be Committed

Be committed to make a difference in the community. To properly intervene, community health nurses first need to be committed enough to help make a difference in the community. A high level of commitment will facilitate the nurses' care of urban and homeless clients in the community. In fact, all three levels of prevention interventions will follow more easily if commitment to make a difference in the community has already been established. Commitment from community health nurses translates to hope and healing among the urban and homeless populations.

A paramount example of one person's commitment to make a difference is former President Jimmy Carter. The Atlanta Project (TAP) was initiated by Carter in 1991 (TAP, 1995). The central mission of this project was to bring the "two Atlantas" (the affluent and poverty groups) together to improve the quality of life in Atlanta's neighborhoods, especially urban areas. TAP has been somewhat successful since its induction in decreasing the gap between the rich and the poor. In fact, Carter became committed to spreading TAP to all of America, thus be-

coming The America Project. By 1995, more than 100 official delegations from numerous cities across America had begun modeling their urban enhancement and development programs after TAP.

Use Leadership Skills

Become an enthusiastic leader and an encourager. Being committed to enthusiastically leading the way in solving problems for urban and homeless people will help others catch on, pitch in, and follow. Once others start contributing their time and efforts into this mission, specialized expertise areas will start to develop among the workers. Acting as a leader and encourager can be used at all three levels of prevention. One example of using excellent leadership skills is when, upon recognizing the need for a community health center, the community health nurse promotes and sells the idea to key people in the community and political officials, leads the way in planning and organizing, and then coordinates the activities. Before long, the nurse's dream will be realized through hard work and commitment.

Good, effective leadership provides the glue to pull everything together (TAP, 1995). Community health nurses are in a position to become leaders of the community. However, they need a vision, effective communication, effective delegation, and commitment to follow through to the end of the project.

Another effective leadership characteristic involves recognizing the talents of those populations being served. Urban and homeless people are people with numerous talents. Caring, concern, and good communication skills may be talents that urban and homeless people can contribute. Other talents include artistic and musical talents. The community health nurse needs to recognize and use those talents to expand available resources. Also, by recognizing value in others' contributions, self-esteem among the people will be increased and an atmosphere of team effort will be established. One example of using a person's strengths is to ask a homeless person, who has been recognized as having a team attitude and leadership abilities, to help plan and coordinate an activity or event at a homeless shelter.

Use Available Resources

Draw on every federal and community resource available to you. Community health nurses should realize that to make a difference, they need to network with other agencies and draw on existing community and federal resources. The management of care involved in this level of intervention is secondary prevention. Drawing on federal and community resources to provide outreach programs mandates that the community health nurse maximize the use of collaborative partnerships with disciplines and agencies within the community.

One of the fundamental elements that contributed to the success of TAP was its personnel's realizing that everything and every resource needed to make a difference in Atlanta was within reach. Mark O'Connell, president of the United Way of Metro Atlanta, speaking about one solution for improving urban life, stated, "The answer is in how we use the resources we already have and in how we value people" (TAP, 1995). In this regard, community health nurses can equate O'Connell's statement about valuing people to caring about urban and homeless people, which takes a high level of commitment to help with improving the community.

Local resources can help supply meals, hygiene products, clothing, and even health care. Food missions, local free clinics, churches, Salvation Army, and American Red Cross are valuable resources that the community health nurse can use. State and federal resources can be drawn upon for financial, health, education, and shelter programs, as well as other types of programs. Medicare, welfare, Medicaid, Head Start, and food stamps include a variety of state and federal programs that can be used.

Be an Advocate

Become a political advocate for preventing homelessness and the problems associated with the urban population. Intervention at this level is primary prevention, which involves taking political action. Talking to politicians and speaking out in favor of prevention of homelessness and the problems associated with urban populations are essential to effecting change in the community. Even more important is for community health nurses to speak out in numbers through their professional organizations, such as the American Nurses Association and the American Public Health Association, in order for new public policies to be adopted. Being a united voice through large numbers of community health nurses is powerful and grabs the attention of politicians across the country.

In becoming politically involved, community health nurses need to remember not to become overwhelmed or take on too many issues at one time. It is more effective to concentrate on one or two problems at a time. Promoting ideas and attitudes and selling a political viewpoint or solution can go a long way toward reducing the problems associated with homelessness or the urban poverty population. Writing letters to local, state, and federal officials and congressmen is an effective way to capture attention. Other ways include presenting concerns at public meetings, getting elected as a lobbyist through organizations, interacting with congresspersons on a one-on-one basis, and publicizing the needs and concerns of these populations through brochures, newspapers, radio, and television.

To better persuade policy makers and city officials of specific needed interventions, community health nurses should learn exactly what needs and concerns exist in their community. The National Law Center on Homelessness and Poverty (1999a) stated that permanent solutions to homelessness must address the fundamental cause—that homeless people cannot pay for housing. The Law Center stated that permanent solutions to prevent homelessness include ensuring affordable housing, adequate income, and social services, as well as prohibiting discrimination.

These solutions are issues that community health nurses can address when speaking out politically.

••••••••••••••••••••••••••••••

VAGRANT

he floated like a guppy once
didn't need to care
didn't care to need

it's all there in the sac
the warmth and cushion
the belly always filled first

but he still had to let go
though stubborn; a caesarian
and make his way in the world

there was a breast for a spell
and he grew into a plump little
pear on buttermilk bisquits and gravy

he stole apples and squash
sneaking in and hiding the plunder
in the crowded cupboards

it doesn't take long for years
to rot and ripe and rot again
and jobs came and went

why, once not long back he even
sold carnations-fullblown white ones-
on street corners for change

he's shrunk and wrinkled like a
sunbaked codfish now
wandering from mission to mission

turning up on doorsteps like some
crazy orphaned bouquet of lillies-
of-the-valley

not caring to need
not needing to care

James A. Lopresti, 1977

••••••••••••••••••••••••••••••

The National Law Center on Homelessness and Poverty (1999b) also listed selected rights of homeless people. Community health nurses should become familiar with the rights of homeless people to detect violations of these rights by certain groups, organizations, or individuals. Preserving the rights of homeless people through political advocacy is an important intervention for community health nurses. The rights include but are not limited to the following (National Law Center on Homelessness and Poverty, 1999b, pp. 1–2):

- *Homeless children have a right to attend school.*
- *Homeless children have the right to participate in mainstream federal, state, and local programs.*

CASE STUDY

Descent of a Woman: From Rags to Riches to Rags

"You're about to enter a secret world, hidden from thousands carrying on the business of the day just steps away. It's a dark world of broken lives and shattered dreams. And if you don't think you could wind up there, wait until you meet the woman about to guide you through this twilight zone. . . . What could possibly make a woman who had it all leave her home, her life, her children, for a terrifying existence underground?" (Phillips, Pauley, & Rudolph, 1997, p. 8).

By age 26, Nadine had a husband, three healthy sons, a prosperous clothing boutique in New York's trendy Soho district, and a lifestyle she had always wanted. Her life as a child was saddened by the abandonment of her mother, who turned to drugs and prostitution. Nadine, by age 8, was herself experiencing the effects of alcohol. Later, she turned to marijuana and cocaine, often smoking marijuana with her father.

She temporarily cleaned up her life. But taking care of a family and attending to a business with all its financial demands resulted in too much pressure for Nadine. Nadine and her husband sometimes experimented with cocaine as they celebrated their newfound success. The drugs, the money, and the success pushed Nadine and her husband to vicious fights. Soon the money was gone. Nadine left her family. Nadine's drug use became excessive—from pot and cocaine to, finally, a powerful addiction to heroin. The drug had so much power over her that she turned to prostitution to support a $100-a-day habit.

When she had exhausted all of her resources, her boyfriend (a drug pusher) introduced her to "the condo," an underground subway escape in New York where thousands of homeless people live to stay high on drugs and to escape life, family, and the law. People refer to the underground people as the "mole people." After unsuccessfully trying drug rehabilitation 20 times, Nadine felt she had hit rock bottom. She had even been pronounced clinically dead once in an emergency department in New York.

"She joined a band of drug addicts descending under an iron plate literally into the bowels of New York city, down 13 metal steps, then around and around a grimy concrete staircase . . . just a few blocks and a world away from her old life. Instead of a bathroom . . . the subway tracks were her toilet. The kitchen? Whatever they could beg, borrow, or steal. And this soot-filled platform right next to the roaring train, her bedroom. [Under New York] there's another city. . . . This one has about 45,000 people in it . . . the homeless who are sleeping underground" (Phillips, Pauley, & Rudolph, 1997, p. 16).

After a long time living homeless and like a mole underground, Nadine's break came. She crossed paths with Renny Chun, a journalist. Chun pushed Nadine, through numerous contacts, to rehabilitation. Nadine wanted help but was afraid of being sober and of failure. She desperately wanted to see her sons, which provided her the strength she needed to kick the habit cold turkey. Now Nadine lives one day at a time and hopes to never be in the condo again. She reunited for a short while with her sons. Dateline NBC reported that she was seeking legal visiting rights for the future. Nadine's courage has helped her to be clean and sober today and hopefully tomorrow.

Underground living is a reality for homeless people in major cities where subway escapes exist. Rudolph (Phillips, Pauley, & Rudolph, 1997) discussed the nightmare that Nadine experienced and related the magnitude of the problem of the underground. Nadine took Rudolph and the television viewers to "the condo" to see the drug addicts lying with the rats, the human waste, the garbage, and the sewer. She noticed that the same people she had previously known were still underground.

1. What are some factors, psychological and external, that led Nadine to homelessness? As you answer this question, think about her life as a child and as an adult.

2. What health problems/infections would you anticipate Nadine to have while exposed to underground living? As a prostitute? As a homeless person? If Nadine had been homeless in your city, list resources that would have been available to her.

3. How would you, as a community health nurse, help Nadine? Include how you could intervene using a holistic approach. Include as many physical, psychosocial, cultural, developmental, and spiritual factors that you should take into consideration when planning Nadine's care.

Source: Phillips, Pauley, & Rudolph, 1997.

- *Homeless people have the right to apply for the Earned Income Tax Credit.*
- *Homeless people have the right to vote.*
- *Homeless people have the right to sleep in public if there is nowhere else to sleep.*
- *Homeless people have the right to apply for food stamps, Medicaid, and Supplemental Security Income.*

Purposefully exposing themselves to urban and homeless people by placing themselves in strategic locations within the community is an excellent way for community health nurses to learn about the needs of urban and homeless people. Meeting these individuals face to face and interacting with them will help community health nurses to see individualized problems. The broad picture of health and social problems among these people also will become more focused. Ultimately, the community health nurse can communicate these health and social problems and prevention strategies to policy makers at all levels of government.

Foster Communication and Trust

Develop open communication and trust among the urban and homeless populations. A climate of open communication and trust is pivotal to developing an environment of security and support. Violation of trust and conveying a false sense of security have serious consequences and should be avoided when interacting with urban and homeless people. Nurses need to remember not to make promises of hope that will never be met. Trust is built on truth, reliability, and open communication. For a leader to be effective, trustworthiness is critical. Following through on a project or goal and being dependable are ways that the community health nurse can establish trust and open communication.

Assess the Problem

Develop and practice good assessment skills. For primary prevention, assessment is aimed at identifying factors that play a role in the problems of urban living and problems that contribute to

FYI

Homeless as a term was first used in 1981 by Mitch Snyder and Robert Hayes to describe the growing number of persons living in boxes and eating out of garbage cans in urban areas as a result of the worst recession in half a century.

Source: Jencks, 1994.

homelessness. At this level of prevention, community health nurses need to assess the political structure of the city and state and resources available in the community at all levels of government.

Secondary prevention assessment involves evaluating the health and social problems associated with urban poverty and homelessness. A good understanding of these problems will help the community health nurse to develop a strong and purposeful plan for outreach. Also involved at this level is an assessment of access to health care, screening programs, food missions, and other resources.

Tertiary prevention assessment is aimed at evaluating available resources to help people cope with the chronic problems associated with urban poverty and homelessness. Health care, mental health, and social services that take referrals for indigent people are important resources to assess. Identifying the needs of urban and homeless people is also considered assessment at the tertiary prevention level. Free clinic access, alcohol and drug detoxification programs, protection from communicable diseases, and care of chronic mental and physical problems are some specific needs that will be identified. Social needs that will be identified include protection from violence and sexual assault, literacy programs, job training programs, and housing/shelter programs.

Plan and Give Care

Develop and implement an effective plan of care. Planning care for urban and homeless populations means that community health nurses will need to focus on basic life care needs as well as aggregate needs. First, short-term and long-term goals need to be identified at the primary, secondary, and tertiary levels. Needs should also be prioritized from most urgent human needs to least urgent.

However, an effective plan of care is futile if the plan does not lead to action on the part of the community health nurse and other community resource providers. Actually following through with an effective plan goes back to maintaining a high level of commitment. Resource agencies and people are available and ready to help. The community health nurse must be committed to finding these resources and then using them. Although referral agencies are critical to good outcomes for homeless people, community health nurses need to realize the importance of the nursing role. The community health nurse provides a continuity of care that no other discipline offers. While providing continuity, the nurse's quality of care has an excellent chance to improve health and holistic outcomes for the person.

....

Most Americans want the homeless off the streets but no one wants them next door.

Jencks, 1994, p. 117

....

Conclusion

Inner cities cannot keep pace with the needs of the rapidly growing population. Many problems existing in inner cities are the result of the rapid increase in population, not necessarily the result of poverty. Poverty remains the culprit for many problems in urbanized areas, including hunger, homelessness, health problems, communicable diseases, overcrowded living conditions, violence and crime, and inadequate housing. Poverty in inner cities is directly related to higher infant mortality rates among African Americans, a poor quality of life, and increased health problems among all adults in inner cities. Several massive efforts have been under way to help improve the quality of life in urbanized areas. Many of the programs have been the result of *Healthy People 2000* and *2010*. Some specific programs include the Healthy Cities movement, urban development projects, and the America Project. Several other programs have been targeted for African American urban populations.

Today, America is faced with an overwhelming problem of homelessness. A new culture of homeless people has emerged—whole families, single mothers with children, and teens. Families are the fastest growing segment of homeless people in the United States.

Barriers to health care of homeless individuals include poverty, lack of access to health care, lack of communication with health care professionals, lack of transportation to a health care facility, lack of family and social support, psychological depression, lack of motivation to seek health care, and difficulty in locating homeless people for follow-up care. The homeless population experiences many health and social problems, some of which include communicable diseases, foot and leg ulcerations, arthritis, poor hygiene, malnutrition, respiratory and cardiovascular problems, substance abuse, chronic health problems that are poorly managed, HIV/AIDS, mental illness, prostitution because of sex-for-drug swaps, violence, crime, and assault.

Community health nurses need to function at all three level of prevention—primary, secondary, and tertiary—to be effective in managing care of urban and homeless people.

All urban and homeless people need what everyone else needs—opportunities, advantages, and services that help them live more healthful lives.

CRITICAL THINKING ACTIVITIES

1. Think about Nadine's state of homelessness as described in the Case Study on p. 610. Consider her desire for drugs and the life she was living during her period of homelessness. What views/attitudes should you, a community health nurse, take as a logical and ethical approach toward Nadine?

2. Discuss the way each of the following six ethical principles might apply to Nadine, her situation, and her health care. See chapter 11 for ethical issues in community health nursing.

Autonomy	Privacy
Freedom	Beneficence
Veracity	Fidelity

3. John, 36 years old, is a homeless man with a history of intravenous drug use and AIDS. He is wasting away and has multidrug-resistant tuberculosis. He went to the free neighborhood health clinic where you work, presenting with fever, cough, and purulent blood-tinged sputum. As a community health nurse, discuss four health outcomes that John and you would plan for his care. Give the rationale for each.

4. Discuss some therapeutic communication strategies the community health nurse might use with a single mother with two children, all of whom are homeless. The mother has a crack addiction, and you have reason to believe that she swaps sex for drugs while the children, ages 2 and 8, are alone on the street.

5. Select nursing interventions at the primary, secondary, and tertiary levels for an elderly homeless female with a history of congestive heart failure and insulin-dependent diabetes mellitus. Include interventions that address the holistic nature of the individual.

6. Yolanda, a homeless African American adolescent, 16 years old, has presented to a shelter for food, clothing, and sleep. You are the community health nurse assisting her. You learned through your assessment that she has had morning sickness and has been very sick, to the point that she slept on the streets for 7 nights because she did not have the strength to walk 2 miles to the shelter. She had become dehydrated and weak. She admitted to using crack cocaine on a regular basis and stated that she could not control her desire to use the drug. She has not seen a family practitioner for her morning sickness and dehydration or to receive a pregnancy test. She thinks that she is at least 3 months pregnant by a young man she met on the streets. He has since been imprisoned for selling drugs. She ran away from home several months ago to escape a poor family relationship with her mother.

   - Based on what you have learned about Yolanda, list the risk factors that may have contributed to Yolanda's homelessness and her situation.

   - Knowing that shelter care would not be enough for Yolanda, what would be your plan of care for her? Include resources, social support, family, and other agencies you may use.

   - Yolanda receives medical attention and is stabilized for now. What can you do in the first few days at the shelter to instill in Yolanda a sense of competence, a sense of usefulness, a sense of belonging, and a sense of power and control? Include cultural considerations and values.

   - What barriers will Yolanda face when she makes any decisions concerning her well-being? Obtaining a primary practitioner? Returning to her environment? Returning to school?

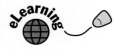

Explore Community Health Nursing on the web! To learn more about the topics in this chapter, use the passcode provided to access your exclusive web site: http://communitynursing.jbpub.com
If you do not have a passcode, you can obtain one at this site.

REFERENCES

Anderson, N. (1934). *Homeless in New York City.* New York: Board of Charity.

Anderson, N. (1940). Highlights of the migrant problem today. *Proceedings of the National Conference of Social Work.* New York: National Conference of Social Work.

Appel, J., & Boden, P. (1999, March 11). More than a local problem: Homelessness needs attention of whole nation. *San Francisco Chronicle,* PSA 2301, Editorial Section: http://library.northernlight.com/AC19990312010051852.html.

Bates, T. (1997). Response: Michael Porter's conservative urban agenda will not revitalize America's inner cities: What will? *Economic Development Quarterly, 11*(1), 39–49.

Bean, G., Stefl, M., & Howe, S. (1987). Mental health and homelessness: Issues and findings. *Social Work, 32,* 411–416.

Belcher, J. R., Scholler-Jaquish A., & Drummond, M. (1991). Three stages of homelessness: A conceptual model for social workers in health care. *Health and Social Work, 16*(2), 87–93.

Benda, B. B., & Dattalo, P. (1988). Homelessness: Consequence of a crisis or long-term process? *Hospital and Community Psychiatry, 39,* 884–886.

Berne, A. S., Dato, C., Mason, D. J., & Rafferty, M. (1993). A nursing model for addressing the health needs of homeless families. In G. D. Wegner & R. J. Alexander (Eds.), *Readings in family nursing.* Philadelphia: J. B. Lippincott.

Burt, M., & Cohen, B. (1989). *America's homeless: Numbers, characteristics, and the numbers that serve them.* Washington, DC: Urban Institute.

Centers for Disease Control and Prevention (CDC). (1995). Measles—United States, 1994. *Morbidity and Mortality Weekly Report, 44*(26), 486–494.

Chavkin, W., Kristal, A., Seabron, C., & Guigli, P. (1987). The reproductive experience of women living in hotels for the homeless in New York City. *New York State Journal of Medicine, 371,* 10–13.

Cook, T. (Ed.). (1979). *Vagrancy: Some new perspectives.* New York: Academic Press.

Cousineau, M. R., Wittenberg, E., & Pollatsek, J. (1995). *Study of the health care for the homeless program.* (HV 4505). Bethesda, MD: Department of Health and Human Services, Bureau of Primary Health Care.

Culhane, D. P., Dejowski, E. F., Ibanex, J., Needham, E., & Macchia, I. (1993). *Public shelter admission rates in Philadelphia and New York City: The implications of turnover for sheltered population counts.* Washington, DC: Fannie Mae Office of Housing Research.

DeBerri, E. (1997). Listening to the voice of homelessness. *Access, 9*(1), 2.

Department of Health and Human Services. (1991). *Healthy People 2000: National health promotion and disease prevention objectives.* Washington, DC: U.S. Government Printing Office.

Department of Health and Human Services. (1995). *Strengthening homeless families: An annotated resource guide for homeless shelters.* (DHHS Contract No. 105-94-2016). Washington, DC: U.S. Government Printing Office.

Department of Health and Human Services. (2000). *Healthy People 2010: Conference edition.* Washington, DC: U.S. Government Printing Office.

Family and Youth Services Bureau. (1994). *A guide to enhancing the cultural competence of runaway and homeless youth programs.* (DHHS Contract No. 105-92-1709). Silver Spring, MD: U.S. Government Printing Office.

Family and Youth Services Bureau. (1996). *Reconnecting youth & community: A youth development approach.* (DHSS Contract No. 105-92-1709). Silver Spring, MD: U.S. Government Printing Office.

Fisher, B., Hovell, M., & Hofstetter, C. R. (1995). Risks associated with long-term homelessness among women: Battery, rape, and HIV infection. *International Journal of Health Services, 25,* 351–369.

Flynn, L. (1997). The health practices of homeless women: A causal model. *Nursing Research, 46*(2), 72–77.

Freeman, H. E., Blendon, R. J., Aiken, L. H., Sudman, S., Mullinix, C. F., & Corey, C. R. (1987). Americans report on their access to care. *Health Affairs, 6*(1), 6–18.

Fuchs, E., & McAllister, W. (1996). *A continuum of care: A report on the new federal policy to address homelessness* (HUD Contract No. DU100C000018360). Washington, DC: Department of Housing and Urban Development, Center for Urban Policy.

26 Urban and Homeless Populations   615

Global report on human settlements. (1996). United Nations Centre for Human Settlements. Nairobi, Kenya: United Nations Centre for Human Settlements.

Goldstein, G., & Kickbusch, I. (1996). A healthy city is a better city. *World Health Organization.* Geneva, Switzerland: World Health Organization.

Hatton, D. C. (1997). Managing health problems among homeless women with children in a transitional shelter. *Image: Journal of Nursing Scholarship, 29*(1), 33–37.

Hoch, C., & Slayton, R. A. (1989). *New homeless and old: Community and the skid row.* Philadelphia: Temple University Press.

Hoffman, V. F. (1953). *The American tramp, 1870–1900.* Unpublished master's thesis, University of Chicago, Chicago, IL.

Hunter, J. K., Getty, C., Kemsley, M., & Skelly, A. H. (1991). Barriers to providing health care to homeless persons: A survey of providers' perceptions. *Health Values, 15*(5), 3–11.

Institute of Medicine. (1988). *Homelessness, health and human needs.* Washington, DC: National Academy Press.

Interagency Council on the Homeless. (1994). *Priority home: The federal plan to break the cycle of homelessness.* (HUD Publication No. 1454-CPD[1]). Washington, DC: Department of Housing and Urban Development.

International Healthy Cities Foundation (IHCF). (1995a). *International healthy cities foundation information page:* www.oneworld.org/cities/cities_info.html.

International Healthy Cities Foundation. (1995b). *What is the healthy cities movement?:* www.oneworld.org/cities/cities_healthy. html.

Jahiel, R. I. (Ed.). (1992). *Homelessness: A prevention-oriented approach.* Baltimore, MD: Johns Hopkins University Press.

Jencks, C. (1994). *The homeless.* Cambridge, MA: Harvard University Press.

Kipke, M. D., Simon, T. R., Montgomery, S. B., Unger, J. B., & Iversen, E. F. (1997). Homeless youth and their exposure to and involvement in violence while living on the streets. *Journal of Adolescent Health, 20,* 360–367.

Lezak, A. D., & Edgar, E. (1996). *Preventing homelessness among people with serious mental illnesses: A guide for states.* (DHHS Publication No. 3106). Rockville, MD: Department of Health and Human Services, Center for Mental Health Services.

Lewis, D. L. (1993). *W. E. B. DuBois: Biography of a race, 1868–1919.* New York: Henry Holt.

Link, B., Phelan, J., Breshan, M., Stueve, A., Moore, R., & Susser, E. (1995). Lifetime and five-year prevalence of homelessness in the United States: New evidence on an old debate. *American Journal of Orthopsychiatry, 65,* 347–354.

MacKenzie, W. R. et al. (1994). A massive outbreak in Milwaukee of cryptosporidium infection transmitted through the public water supply. *New England Journal of Medicine, 331*(3), 161–167.

Massey, D. S., & Denton, N. A. (1993). *American apartheid: Segregation and the making of the underclass.* Cambridge, MA: Harvard University Press.

Menke, E. M., & Wagner, J. D. (1997). The experience of homeless female-headed families. *Issues in Mental Health Nursing, 18,* 315–330.

Milhaly, L. K. (1991). *Homeless families: Failed policies and young victims.* Washington, DC: Children's Defense Fund.

Momeni, J. A., & Wiegand, G. (1989). *Homelessness in the United States.* New York: Greenwood Press.

National Law Center on Homelessness and Poverty. (1999a). Solutions to homelessness in America: www.nlchp.org.solution.htm.

National Law Center on Homelessness and Poverty. (1999b). Selected rights of homeless persons: http://www.nlchp.org/rights2/htm.

Nennig, M. E., Shinefield, H. R., Edwards, K. M., Black, S. B., & Fireman, B. H. (1998). Prevalence and incidence of adult pertussis in an urban population. *Journal of the American Medical Association, 275,* 1672–1674.

Nyamathi, A., Flaskerud, J., & Leake, B. (1997). HIV-risk behaviors and mental health characteristics among homeless or drug-recovering women and their closest sources of social support. *Nursing Research, 46,* 133–137.

Office of Community Partnerships. (1996). *Healthy Boston evaluation: Final report:* http://www.cpn.org/sections/topics/community/stories-studies/healthy_boston_eval1.html.

Pantera, M. J. (1996). Collaborative partnerships—forgotten amidst urban chaos. *Parks & Recreations, 31*(3), 48–53.

Percy, M. S. (1995). Children from homeless families describe what is special in their lives. *Holistic Nursing Practice Journal, 9*(4), 24–33.

Phillips, S. (Announcer), Pauley, J. (Announcer), & Rudolph, L. (Reporter). (1997, August 19). *Dateline NBC.* New York: National Broadcasting System. Transcript from Burrelle Publishing, Livingston, NJ.

Polednak, A. P. (1997). *Segregation, poverty, and mortality in urban African Americans.* New York: Oxford University Press.

Policy Research Associates. (1988). *The national resource center on homelessness and mental illness.* Delmar, NY: Author.

Reyes, L. M., & Waxman, L. D. (1989). *A status report on hunger and homelessness in America's cities, 1989.* Washington, DC: U.S. Conference of Mayors.

Rivilin, L. G. (1986). A new look at the homeless. *Social Policy, 16*(4), 3–10.

Rosenblum, S. B., & Imgrund, J. (1999, January 4). Survey shown hunger, homelessness on rise. *Nation's Cities Weekly, 10*(1): http://www.library.northernlight.com/PN1999011800005106.html.

Rossi, P. H. (1989). *Down and out in America: The origin of homelessness.* Chicago: University of Chicago Press.

St. Lawrence, J. S., & Brasfield, T. L. (1995). HIV risk behavior among homeless adults. *AIDS Education and Prevention, 7,* 22–31.

Stark, L. (1987). A century of alcohol and homelessness: Demographics and stereotypes. *Alcohol, Health and Research, 11,* 8–13.

Sumerlin, J. R., & Bundrick, C. M. (1997). Research on homeless men and women: Existential-humanistic and clinical thinking. *Psychological Reports, 80,* 1303–1314.

Susser, E., Struening, E., & Conover, S. (1987). Childhood experiences of homeless men. *American Journal of Psychiatry, 144,* 1599–1601.

The America Project (TAP). (1995). *Because there is hope: Gearing up to renew urban America.* Atlanta: Carter Collaboration Center.

Trattner, W. I. (1984). *From poor law to welfare state: A history of social welfare in America* (3rd ed.). New York: Free Press.

U.S. Conference of Mayors. (1989). *Status report on the Stewart B. McKinney Homeless Assistance Act of 1987.* Washington, DC: Author.

U.S. Conference of Mayors. (1997). *A status report on hunger and homelessness in America's cities: 1997.* Washington, DC: Author.

U.S. Congress, House. (1987). *Stewart B. McKinney Homeless Assistance Act, conference report to accompany H.R. 558.* Washington, DC: 100th Congress, First Session.

U.S. Department of Commerce. (1992). *1990 Census of population: General population characteristics, United States* (CP-1-1). Washington, DC: Department of Health and Human Services, U.S. Government Printing Office.

Vladeck, B. C. (1990). Health care and the homeless: A political parable for our time. *Journal of Health Politics, Policy, and Law, 15,* 305–317.

West, C. (1994). *Race matters.* New York: Vintage.

Wood, D., & Valdez, R. B. (1991). Barriers to medical care for homeless families compared with housed poor families. *American Journal of Diseases of Children, 145,* 1109–1115.

World Health Organization (WHO). (1994). *Briefings on multi-city action plans: WHO healthy cities project, phase II 1993–1997.* Copenhagen, Denmark: WHO Regional Office for Europe.

World Health Organization Regional Office for Europe (WHO). (1998). *International healthy cities conference: Athens, 20–23 June 1998*: http://www.who.dk/cpa/pr98/pr9806e.htm.

Wright, J. D., & Weber, E. (1987). *Homelessness and health.* New York: McGraw-Hill.

Chapter 27
Rural Populations
Gale A. Spencer and Lindsay Lake Morgan

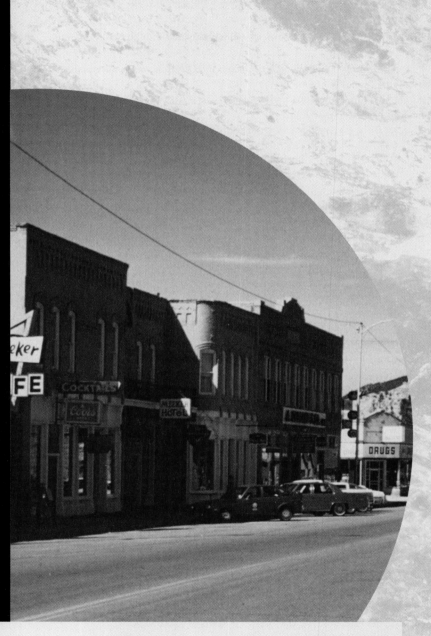

Eighty-four percent of the land area in the United States is considered rural, but only 25% of the total U.S. population lives in those rural areas. Although this is a small percentage of the population, people living in these areas have many special health needs. Community health nurses are a significant source of health care for rural people.

QUESTIONS TO CONSIDER

After reading this chapter, answer the following questions:
1. What are the various definitions of rural health?
2. How do rural populations differ from urban populations?
3. What lifestyles and behaviors of rural adolescent populations put them at risk for illness or injury?
4. What specific characteristics of rural life increase isolation for rural elders?
5. What specific cultural characteristics of migrant workers provide a challenge for community health nurses?
6. What are the differences between rural and urban homeless populations?

KEY TERMS

Access to health care	Housing	Metropolitan statistical areas	Sexual activity
Agricultural hazards	Intentional injury		Substance use and abuse
Confidentiality	Isolation	Migrant farm workers	Unintentional injury
Culture	Lifestyle	Rural-urban continuum	

Definitions of Rural

Definitions of *rural* are based on geographic, demographic, sociological, and economic perspectives. A simple definition of rural is "country." If you don't see many houses or buildings but you do see nature—mountains, plains, forests, or other scenery—you are in a rural area. This definition is based on geography and the environment. It is the most subjective definition.

In the United States, initial formal attempts at defining rural are based on sparse population. The U.S. Bureau of the Census (1993) defines urban as "all territory, population, and housing units in urbanized areas and in places of 2,500 or more persons outside urban areas." Although towns the size of 2,500 people may have characteristics more like rural places than urban places, they are considered urban by this definition.

When the characteristics of a place are taken into consideration, sociological ideas are applied to the definition. The availability of services such as libraries, colleges, newspapers, transportation, and health care affect people's perceptions regarding how urban or rural life seems. One commonly used definition of rural combines demographics and proximity to services. Proximity to services is assumed when a place is near an urbanized center. The **rural-urban continuum** (USDA, 1995) describes counties by both population and proximity to services. The continuum identifies **metropolitan statistical areas** (MSAs) as one or more counties that are considered metropolitan. Counties that are not in MSAs are all rural, but they range on a continuum based on their urbanization, population, and adjacency to an MSA. Counties are described as fol-

SCHEMATIC OF RURAL COUNTIES.

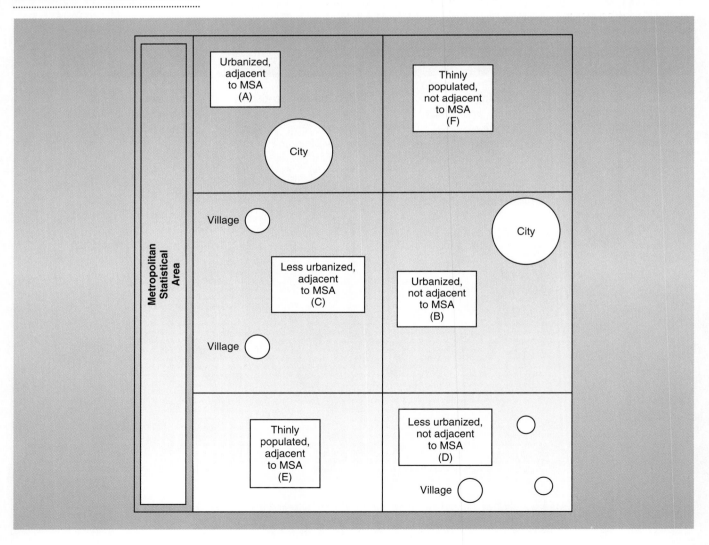

lows (North Carolina Rural Health Research and Policy Analysis Center, 1998):

- *Urbanized, adjacent to MSA (A)*
- *Urbanized, not adjacent to MSA (B)*
- *Less urbanized, adjacent to MSA (C)*
- *Less urbanized, not adjacent to MSA (D)*
- *Thinly populated, adjacent to MSA (E)*
- *Thinly populated, not adjacent to MSA (F)*

Examples of rural counties are seen in the schematic drawing on p. 620 and are given letters according to their urbanization and adjacency to an MSA.

Economists have defined rural counties in terms of their economic base. This way of defining a rural area helps in predicting the impact of events. For example, if an area is dependent on farming and the weather interferes with crop growth, economists can project earnings and losses for the region. When the major income of an area declines, it can be expected that services (e.g., car sales, new construction) in that area will also suffer. Some types of counties defined by their economic base include the following:

- *Farming-dependent counties: remotely located, sparsely populated, geographically concentrated in the Midwest*
- *Mining-dependent counties: most are in the South or West*
- *Manufacturing-dependent counties: account for 31% of the nonmetropolitan population; three-fifths are in the Southeast, with a more urban orientation*
- *Government-dependent counties: approximately 75% are state and local government jobs, whereas 25% are federal; evenly distributed across the country*
- *Services-dependent counties: serve as centers for trade, services, or recreation; evenly distributed across the country*
- *Nonspecialized counties: may have economic activities such as construction, agricultural services, forestry, or fisheries; found across the country, but most are in the South (Cook & Mizer, 1994)*

Using all of the definitions together will help community health nurses get the most complete picture of the area. Combining the concepts of population density, resources, access and distance to services, and predominant economic base guides the nurse in identifying the barriers to health and health care.

In general, rural areas are sparsely populated, isolated from services, and have limited services from which to choose. Rural people sometimes have multiple roles such as farmer, judge, rotary president, and church elder. This is because there are fewer people to fulfill all the necessary functions of a community.

There are many other ways to define rural, depending on the professional discipline and the purpose of the definition. Twenty-six different definitions of *rural* were used by authors who published articles in *The Journal of Rural Health* between 1993 and 1995 (Ricketts & Johnson-Webb, 1997). It is important to know what definition is being used when evaluating literature or programs. An area that an author defines as rural may have more services available than the community for which you are planning interventions.

Rural Population Characteristics

In 1997, 25% of the U.S. population resided in rural areas (What is rural?, 1999). This represents an increase of 6.6% since 1990. Although the reported growth of the rural population was still below the 7.8% growth identified in urban areas, it represents renewed growth in rural populations (Table 27-1). This growth was not seen during the 1980s, when urban growth was more than four times that of rural growth (3% rural compared with 12.7% urban) (USDA, 1999, pp. 20–21). The growth in rural populations from 1990 to 1997 is attributed to the rebound of population growth, the movement of newcomers from metropolitan areas and foreign immigrants. From 1995 to 1997, approximately 400,000 people moved from urban to rural areas, and another 100,000 came directly from foreign immigration (USDA, 1999, p. 20). The reason for the rebound in the rural population itself was that the birth rate was greater than the death rate during this period.

Rural populations differ demographically from urban populations in the following ways. Elders make up a larger proportion of rural populations. In 1997, 18% of the rural population was

TABLE 27-1 **REGIONAL POPULATION CHANGE 1990–1997**

	POPULATION PER THOUSAND		
REGION	1990	1997	% CHANGE
United States	248,765	267,636	7.6%
Rural (nonmetro)	50,904	54,276	6.6%
Urban (metro)	197,861	213,360	7.8%

Source: Adapted from USDA, 1999, p. 21.

composed of people 60 years and older compared with 15% of the urban population (USDA, 1999, p. 35).

Although rural counties have had a slower growth in elderly populations from 1990 to 1997, elders continue to make up a larger proportion of the population. Rural elders have characteristics and needs that differ from their urban counterparts. Health and social services are deficient for 25% of all older persons living in rural areas. Nearly 6% of rural elders are age 75 or older compared with 5% of urban elders. The older population found in rural areas is predominately white (Table 27-2). The older population is concentrated in the rural South (44%), with a substantial older population also found in the rural Midwest (33%). Rural elders are more likely to be married than their urban counterparts (61% rural to 57% urban). However, widowhood increases with age, and by age 75, 49% of rural women are likely to be widowed. Rural elders are also more likely to assess their health as fair or poor, and 43% of rural elders older than 75 years reported health problems compared with 30% of urban elders at the same age (USDA, 1999, pp. 35–37).

There are also key ethnic differences in elder populations living in rural and urban areas. The following are just a few of these differences (USDA, 1999, p. 35):

- *Elders who are members of underrepresented ethnic groups make up a smaller proportion of the elderly population living in rural than in urban areas.*

- *Rural African American elders are more likely to be widowed and live alone than their urban counterparts.*

- *Elders who are members of underrepresented ethnic groups in rural areas are less educated and less healthy than white elders living in both rural and urban areas.*

- *Elders who are members of underrepresented ethnic groups living in rural areas tend to be poorer than their urban counterparts.*

The rural population of the United States is predominately non-Hispanic white, which represents 83% of the rural population and 73% of the urban population. Hispanics represent 12% of the urban population and only 5% of the rural population

(U.S. Bureau of the Census, 1996). Although African Americans make up approximately 14% of the urban population, they account for only 9% of the rural population (U.S. Bureau of the Census, 1997).

Poverty is more extensive in rural areas. In 1996, the poverty rate was 16% in rural areas and 13% in urban areas (USDA, 1999, p. 81). The poverty gap of 2 to 3 percentage points between rural and urban areas remained quite stable during the 1990s, which suggests that the downward spiral into poverty in rural areas has either stopped or reversed (USDA, 1999, p. 81). However, in rural areas, 26% of the residents live in households with income just above the poverty guideline (Box 27-1), compared with 18% of urban households (USDA, 1997, pp. 31–33). This fact makes rural residents vulnerable to downturns in the national or regional economies, as well as to personal or family economic setbacks.

Poverty rates for underrepresented ethnic groups in rural areas are approximately three times higher than those of rural whites and are significantly higher than those of underrepresented ethnic groups in urban areas (USDA, 1999, p. 81). The poverty rate was highest for rural African Americans (35%), followed by rural Native Americans (34%) and rural Hispanics (33%), and lowest for non-Hispanic rural whites (12%) (USDA, 1999, p. 82) (see the figure on p. 623). Although a higher rate of poverty was found in underrepresented ethnic groups in rural areas, almost two-thirds of the rural poor are non-Hispanic whites. This finding results from the fact that non-Hispanic whites make up the majority of the rural population.

Rural children also live in poverty at higher rates than do urban children. In 1996, 3.2 million rural children younger than 18 lived in homes with incomes below the poverty threshold. In 1996, the poverty rate for all rural children regardless of race was 24%. The poverty rate for African American children in rural areas was 50%, and for both rural Hispanic children and Native American children, it was just above 40%, compared with 17%

TABLE 27-2	RACIAL COMPARISONS OF RURAL AND URBAN ELDERS IN 1997	

	RURAL/ NONMETRO	URBAN/ METRO
White/Non-Hispanic	92%	84%
Hispanic	2%	6%
African American	6%	10%

Source: Adapted from USDA, 1999, p. 35.

BOX 27-1 WHAT DOES THE POVERTY GUIDELINE MEAN?

Poverty guidelines are the minimum income level needed by a family or individual to meet basic needs of food, shelter, clothing, and other essential goods and services. The official poverty guidelines are adjusted for family size and are set by the Department of Health and Human Services for use by all federal agencies. They are adjusted every year for inflation. In 2000, the poverty guideline was $17,050 for a family of four, $11,250 for a family of two, and $8,350 for a single individual.

Source: Federal Register, 2000.

COMPARISON OF RURAL-URBAN POVERTY RATES BY RACE/ETHNICITY.

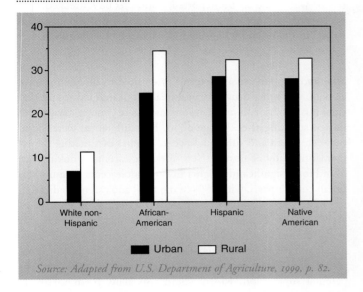

Source: Adapted from U.S. Department of Agriculture, 1999, p. 82.

for rural white children (USDA, 1999, p. 89). The majority (62%) of rural poor children lived in single-parent families, and females headed 55% of these families (USDA, 1999, p. 83).

Rural elders also have a substantially higher poverty rate than urban elders (13% rural to 10% urban). This rate essentially was the same as that of working adults. Underrepresented ethnic groups also make up a larger share of poor elders than would be expected based on their smaller percentage of the population. Poverty rates for older women are also higher than those for men. Sixteen percent of older women are poor; 14% of them are white, 40% are African American, and 34% are Hispanic (USDA, 1999, p. 40). In 1997, of the elderly population living in rural areas, more than 66% were women, nearly 50% were widows, and approximately 66% lived alone (USDA, 1999, p. 40). This population is more likely to be less healthy and to have less access to good housing, adequate nutrition, transportation, and support services than their healthier and wealthier urban counterparts (USDA, 1999, p. 40).

Perspectives and Stereotypes

The word *rural* means many different things to people. It may bring to mind a place where a person can be close to nature and a place where people rely on honesty and hard work. To others, *rural* may be a place where tiny trailers surrounded by rusting automobiles express the poverty of country life.

Learning about our personal biases and preexisting ideas is a lifelong process. We learn as professional nurses to put aside our impressions to give the best care possible to our clients. Even when we try to overcome our biases about people, however, these thoughts may still underlie our behaviors. Constantly con-

fronting what we think and asking where these beliefs come from will always enlighten our behaviors. Recognizing the power of the media and the biases expressed in them helps us stay alert to subtle influences in our lives.

Issues, Concepts, and Populations

Rural life is associated with certain issues and concepts that nurses need to be aware of when caring for rural populations. Because rural populations are diverse, it is difficult to find similarities for discussion. For example, elderly Amish people present very different health needs than elderly coal miners. For this reason, special at-risk populations are discussed in relation to more broad issues and concepts found in rural life. See p. 632 for selected *Healthy People 2010* objectives related to rural life. Some of the more important issues and concepts identified in rural health care are **lifestyle, isolation, culture, housing, confidentiality,** and **access to health care.** These concepts serve as the framework for the following discussion of at-risk populations in rural areas. Each concept is identified and related to a selected at-risk population. These are examples upon which to add your own experience and study of issues, concepts, and populations in rural areas.

Lifestyle: Adolescents

Health behaviors and lifestyle profoundly affect the health of all people. Rural people especially lack opportunities for health promotion and health education because of limited access to health care providers. Although rural adolescents face many of the same health problems as adolescents in urban areas, they also face unique barriers to health promotion, which include limited access to appropriate health services (DHHS, 1991, 2000). There is a limited amount of research specifically on the health status of rural adolescents; however, the risks that have been identified for all adolescents will be discussed as they relate to rural adolescents and rural lifestyle. These risks include **unintentional injury** from bicycles and automobiles, particularly in combination with alcohol consumption; **intentional injury,** including homicide, suicide, and dating violence; **substance use and abuse** and its related consequences of delinquency and human immunodeficiency virus (HIV) disease; and **sexual activity,** with the risks of sexually transmitted diseases and unintended pregnancy. One additional risk for rural adolescents that is not identified for urban adolescents is that of **agricultural hazards.**

Unintentional Injuries

Unintentional injuries are found to occur most often when driving or riding in a moving vehicle, whether it be a bicycle, all-terrain vehicle, snowmobile, or automobile. Bicycle helmets have been proven to be effective in preventing head injuries, but many adolescents still are not using helmets. In rural areas, bicycles may be the only source of transportation because of poverty, isolation, or multiple roles of family members who must share one car. Thus, bicycle safety issues are of great importance. There may also be more hazards in the rural areas because there are no designated bicycle paths, which results in riding on country roads. The roads are often rough and have no shoulders to allow the rider to get out of the way of automobile and truck traffic.

Automobile driving behaviors of adolescents have always been of concern in rural areas. A study by Kidd and Holton (1993) found that risky driving practices in rural areas were correlated with alcohol use, risk-taking motivations, a low grade point average in school, and male gender. Rural adolescents often drive all types of vehicles at a much younger age than in urban areas because they can drive without a license on private property. In addition, poor roads and using the car to cruise for entertainment put rural adolescents at greater risk.

All-terrain vehicles and snowmobiles are also more common in rural areas. These vehicles represent special safety risks because of exposure of the rider, likelihood of turnover, limited safety requirements, and rough terrain. Muellman, Walker, and Edney (1993) investigated the magnitude of difference in death rates between rural and urban areas. Age-adjusted unintentional injury death rates were higher in rural areas, with motor vehicle accidents being the main contributor.

Intentional Injury

Violence resulting in intentional injury most often results from the use of firearms. Intentional injuries can be against oneself or against others. In a study by Brent, Perper, Moritz, Baugher, Schweers, and Roth (1993), access to a gun by an adolescent was associated with suicide, thus increasing the risk of intentional injury to oneself. In another study by Kingerly, Mirzaee, Pruitt, Hurley, and Heuberger (1991), violence against others was found to be widespread among eighth- and ninth-grade boys in rural Texas. Fifty-three percent of the boys in the study had been in at least one fight in the previous year.

Alcohol and other risk behaviors such as carrying weapons have been correlated with violence against others. In a study by Spencer and Bryant (1997), high school students in rural school districts were found to carry a weapon to school and in the community more often than students in urban or suburban school districts. It might be expected that the rural students would carry guns in the community more often because hunting is an acceptable sport in rural areas. The significant differences found between rural, urban, and suburban students carrying weapons to school is of concern, particularly in light of the 1998 and 1999 school shootings in small rural communities.

Dating violence is most frequently studied in college populations; however, a study by Symons, Groer, Kepler-Youngblood, and Slater (1993) examined self-reported incidence of dating violence in rural adolescents. This study found that most of the students had been involved in at least one incident of dating violence, and a quarter of the students had been involved in dating violence two or more times. Dating violence, including date rape, occurs more often than expected in high school students. However, most adolescents are not able to accurately label date rape even when they can clearly report the incident (Fahs, Smith, Atav, Britten, Collins, Morgan, & Spencer,1999). Violent behavior was found in the reported studies to be correlated with adolescents who took more drug risks, carried weapons, were involved in fights, and who were more likely to be victimized.

Substance Use

Substance use and *abuse* are terms often used to discuss tobacco, alcohol, and other drugs. Most available research has found that smoking cessation is much more successful among those who started smoking after the age of 13. Few differences were found between urban and rural adolescents in rates of smoking. However, in a study of upstate New York adolescents, smoking was found to be significantly higher in rural adolescents than in their urban counterparts, with 58% of the rural adolescents indicating use of tobacco, compared with 43% of the urban adolescents (Spencer, Atav, & Collins, 1997). From the data collected in this study, the parents of the rural adolescents were not as well educated, and many smoked themselves, making the behavior more acceptable. These adolescents also spent more time without parental supervision, which would also allow them to smoke without parental censure.

Rural adolescents appear to have alcohol use rates higher than the national average. Alcohol use among adolescents increases significantly as adolescents get older. Adolescents in rural areas often participate in large outdoor drinking parties in secluded areas that are not monitored by adults. Older adolescents often initiate younger adolescents to these parties by getting them drunk. Many older adolescents reportedly purchase alcohol

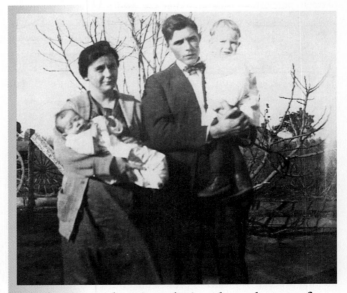

Families in rural settings during the early part of the 20th century experienced a high infant and maternal mortality rate.

for younger adolescents (Wagenaar, Finnegan, Wolfson, Anstine, Williams, & Perry, 1993).

Although cocaine has not been found to be in common use by rural adolescents, use of other drugs, especially marijuana, by adolescents continues to be a problem (Fahs et al., 1999). Anabolic steroids appear to be used equally in both rural and urban areas (Whitehead, Chillag, & Elliot, 1992).

Sexual Activity

The birth rate has been declining over the past several years. However, even with this decline, every year more than 1 million adolescents give birth. Of these births, approximately 200,000 occur to teens in rural areas (Yawn & Yawn, 1993) (Table 27-3). Although less than one-third of unmarried mothers were younger than 20 in 1994, unmarried motherhood is thought of as a teenage problem. In the rural areas, however, more unmarried mothers are likely to be adolescents (USDA, 1997, p. 67). In 1994, 1 of every 10 infants in urban areas was born to an unmarried teen mother, as compared with the rural areas, where 1 in every 9 infants was born to an unmarried adolescent.

Births to unmarried adolescent mothers have become a community problem because they require additional support from community agencies (USDA, 1997). This support takes the form of additional economic resources from welfare agencies or from families who do not have monies to finance a new family unit, and from schools who must teach not only academic subjects to the young mother but parenting skills. Many rural schools have found that the best way to keep adolescent mothers in school is to provide home tutoring for them during the later stages of the pregnancy and child care later at the school. Although both require additional funds from the community, they are cost-effective because these services often make the difference between young mothers' finishing or not finishing high school. Many rural schools have found that having the school nurse participate in teaching child care as part of the curriculum for adolescents returning to school with their babies enhances parenting and assists in preventing additional teen pregnancies.

Community health nurses are often the health care professional most consistently seen by the rural adolescents during their pregnancies. This requires community health nurses to serve in the following roles:

* *An educator to prepare the adolescent and her family about the changes that will occur through out the pregnancy*
* *A counselor regarding family concerns and disagreement regarding the pregnancy*
* *An advocate for services for the adolescent and her newborn*

Research conducted on sexually transmitted diseases in both rural and urban adolescent populations found no differences. A study of rural and urban high school students by Svenson, Varnhagen, Godin, and Salmon (1992) found no differences in knowledge, attitudes, and behaviors regarding sexually transmitted diseases. Engaging in risky behaviors such as unprotected intercourse was also not found to be different between the two groups. However, the 1997 study by Spencer, Atav, and Collins found that sexual activity was significantly different between urban and rural adolescents. Rural adolescents reported sexual activity beginning at a younger age (9.6% of rural adolescents reporting 11 years or younger as age at first intercourse compared with 7.4% of urban adolescents). Participation in sexual activity was also significantly different between rural and urban adolescents, with 49% of rural adolescents stating they participated in sexual activity, compared with 35% of urban adolescents. Many rural school districts do not address the issue of sexually transmitted diseases or teen pregnancy because of the more conservative nature of the school boards, whose members are representatives of these districts. Community health nurses and school nurses must be advocates in rural communities for health education on these topics to be introduced in the school and at community-sponsored activities such as church groups, scouts, or 4-H Clubs (Spencer, Atav, & Collins, 1997).

Agricultural Hazards

Adolescent workers on farms are at particular risk of injury as a result of the hazardous nature of agriculture and the lack of safety regulations (see Research Brief on p. 626). Estimates indicate that, in the United States, at least 23,000 injuries and 300 fatalities on farms involve children and that approximately 20% of all fatalities each year occur on U.S. farms (National Committee for Childhood Agricultural Injury Prevention, 1996). Because the Occupational Safety and Health Administration (OSHA) regulates only businesses employing 11 or more people and the majority of family farms have a small labor force, children/adolescents working on farms are not subject to regulatory protections. Older adolescents and males have higher injury and death rates than do younger adolescents and females (Wilk, 1992). The traditional division of labor by gender on the farm also is an important social influence on work hazards and injury rates. With increasing age, adolescents are channeled into gender-specific tasks, such as males using machines and females doing household tasks (Bartlett, 1993).

Community health nurses need to find ways to target rural adolescents for health promotion. One way is to work with

TABLE 27-3	NONMARITAL BIRTHS BY MOTHER'S AGE, 1994

AGE OF UNMARRIED MOTHER	URBAN	RURAL
<20 years	29.2%	36.2%
20–23 years	34.4%	36.6%
24–49 years	36.4%	27.2%

Source: Adapted from USDA, 1997, p. 68.

RESEARCH BRIEF

Schulman, M. D., Evensen, C. T., Runyan, C. W., Cohen, L. R., & Dunn, K. A. (1997). Farm work is dangerous for teens: Agricultural hazards and injuries among North Carolina teens. The Journal of Rural Health, 13(4), 295–305.

Survey data were collected from a random sample of teens working on farms in North Carolina. The teens ranged in age from 14 to 17. The researchers analyzed the data for farm-based hazard exposure and injury. The sample consisted of 141 teens (72% male) whose mean age was 16.6 years. The data indicated that these North Carolina teens were exposed to significant safety hazards throughout their farming experience. The teens in the sample were exposed to tractors, large animals, all-terrain vehicles, farm trucks, and rotary mowers. More than one-third of the sample was exposed to pesticides and tobacco harvesting equipment. Commonly reported injuries ranged from insect stings to cuts, burns, and falls.

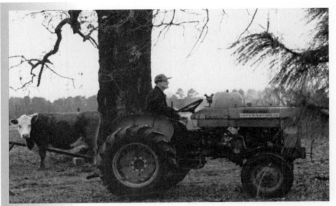

Tractor accidents are a leading cause of injuries in rural areas.

and death limit opportunities for human connections. Disease processes further isolate elders. For example, diabetes that requires a special diet and frequent blood glucose testing and insulin injections may prohibit participation in some social events.

Other problems that rural people experience can be more complex if they are older. On average, rural elders have approximately 20% lower incomes than metropolitan elderly because of lower social security payments, smaller savings, fewer opportunities for part-time work, and infrequent enrollment in Supplemental Security Income (SSI) (Krout, 1994). Most (80%) rural elders own their homes, but these homes are likely to have been built before 1940. These homes may lack modern heating,

school nurses in junior and senior high schools to advocate for current information to be included in school health curricula. Many rural schools are linked with the Internet, which can be a way to engage many adolescents in innovative health programming. Clubs, church youth groups, scouts, and 4-H are other arenas where young adolescents in rural areas gather, and many of these groups are often in need of programs for these teens. Community health nurses often are members of the rural community and are asked to present programs on health; they should take full advantage of these opportunities.

Isolation: Rural Elders

Isolation is fundamental to rural life. Isolation encompasses the ideas of sparse population, limited contact with others, greater distances between people, and limited transportation. Sometimes, people choose the isolation of rural life because they feel it gives them independence and opportunity for self-sufficiency. Isolation is neither a positive nor negative feature, but a reality that community health nurses need to take into account when planning and implementing health care.

Elderly people in rural areas present challenges to community health nurses that arise from both the isolation of rural life and the isolation of elderly life. Multiple losses, both physical and psychosocial, add to the isolation elderly people can experience. Physical changes of normal aging can contribute to isolation. Sensory losses such as diminished hearing and vision result in distancing from the normal experience of life. Decreased mobility resulting from skeletal changes and disease may cause elderly people to stay at home. Fear of falling and other safety issues limit social interaction. Loss of friends because of relocation

RESEARCH BRIEF

Johnson, J. E. (1996). Social support and physical health in the rural elderly. Applied Nursing Research, 9(2), 61–66.

Johnson (1996) studied the social support of 82 elderly people who lived in an isolated community with a population of less than 2,500 or on a farm or ranch. Thirty-five percent reported that they had no one available to assist them. Johnson found that 47.51% had a low level of social support and only 21.22% had a high level of support. Although the sample size was small, this study suggests that elderly people living in isolated rural areas have few people in their social support networks. Of the elders who had help available, one-fourth had only one person in the "network." The supportive persons were most often spouses, adult children, friends, and spiritual advisors. Johnson noted that health professionals, ministers, and social workers were not named as part of the support network.

plumbing, and insulation and may be in need of other repairs. Rural elders often need to relocate, but there are limited alternative housing opportunities in rural areas (Krout, 1994). Their houses may resell at a low price, creating another financial loss for the rural elder.

Elderly people residing anywhere may find themselves unable to drive their own cars. Lack of alternative transportation in rural areas is a problem that has wide-reaching effects on rural people. Elders have difficulty obtaining supplies, accessing health care, and meeting psychosocial needs.

Many research studies have been conducted that examine the unique characteristics and needs of this at-risk population. Community health nurses are challenged to design interventions that recognize the independence of older rural people but maintain their safety and health. Community-based services for rural elders must meet the criteria of availability, accessibility, awareness, acceptability, affordability, appropriateness, and adequacy. Parish nurse programs have had great success in rural areas because they meet these criteria. Nurses serve church members by "organizing health fairs, writing health articles for church newsletters, making presentations, providing blood pressure screening, referring to community health and social service resources, making home visits, and coordinating support groups" (Mockenhaupt & Muchow, 1994, p. 195). Health care providers must find a way to reduce the isolation experienced by rural elders by providing transportation, enhancing communication systems, and creating additional opportunities to bring elders together (see Research Brief on p. 626).

Culture: Migrant Farm Workers

Migrant farm workers represent a unique culture arising from ethnic background and a distinctive lifestyle. The migrant farm worker population is estimated to be approximately 5 million (DHHS, 1990; Lambert, 1995; Sandhaus, 1998). There are three primary streams in which they travel. The West Coast and midcontinent (or central) streams consist mostly of people of Mexican heritage. The East Coast stream is the most ethnically diverse, consisting of African Americans, Haitians, Puerto Ricans, whites, and some Mexican Americans (Lambert, 1995; Smith & Gentry, 1987).

Migrant farm workers "follow the crops." That is, they move north with the spring, living in temporary housing for days or weeks. The housing is often substandard and crowded, from shacks to mobile homes, rarely with furnishings. Sanitation and drinking water provision are also variable and often not available in the fields where the migrants work. Entire families make the season-long trip, with those who are unfit for fieldwork (elders and preteens) caring for the young children. Some areas make an effort to provide schooling for the young children, even though it is summer. Farm work provides the income that the family lives on for the entire year. Pay is hourly, at or below minimum wage, and for only the duration of the farming season.

Often, local communities react with hostility to migrant farm workers who are commonly seen as markedly different and potential carriers of disease. Thus, living apart from the local communities, this population becomes more vulnerable to isolation and neglect. Fear of deportation, poverty, and limited education only serve to intensify feelings of distrust. As a result, migrant workers form cohesive communities of their own based on language, food, music, religion, social interactions, and beneficial folk practices. It is critical that community health nurses acknowledge their cultural differences and include family and social support networks when planning care for this population (Sandhaus, 1998).

In addition to understanding the culture of migrant farm workers, health care providers are confronted with their difficult health care needs. The major health care problems include women's health issues, high infant mortality, delayed immunization, poor dental health, mental health problems, substance abuse, family violence, malnutrition, diabetes, hypertension, respiratory illness (especially tuberculosis), anemia, and parasites. The infant mortality rate for migrant workers is 25 times higher than the national average. Parasitic infections occur 11 to 59 times more often in migrant workers than in the general population. Deaths from tuberculosis, influenza, and pneumonia are 25% higher. The life expectancy for migrant workers is 49 years, compared with a national average of 75 years (Sandhaus, 1998).

Occupation-specific health problems are also worse for migrant workers than for other farm workers. These problems include risk of motor vehicle accident caused by high annual mileage, pesticide exposure, poor sanitation, farm accidents, skin

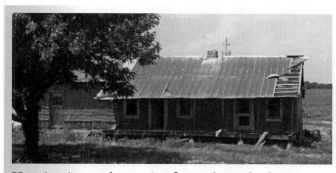
Housing in rural areas is often substandard.

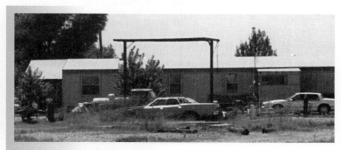
Common rural housing.

diseases, and frequent and severe heat and cold exposures (Rust; 1990; Sandhaus, 1998). The fact that the population does not stay in one place for very long interferes with diagnosis, follow-up, and referral for any health problem.

Community health nurses have led the way in designing health care delivery models that respond to cultural differences, mobility, and the fundamental health care needs of migrant farm workers. Recognizing that migrant farm workers cannot rely on the consistency of one health care provider to oversee care, nursing models that emphasize education, self-care, empowerment, and responsibility for one's own health have found success with this population (Poss & Meeks, 1994; Stein, 1993; Watkins, Larson, Harlan, & Young, 1990). Successful programs often include mobile clinics with hours appropriate to migrant work schedules, sensitivity to cultural preferences, bilingual workers, and use of lay workers and peers.

The health care of migrant farm workers must be supported at the local, state, and national levels. With the identified health concerns of migrants ranging from infant mortality to communicable disease, funds must be found to support the following:

- *The provision of adequate and accessible health care*
- *Adequate living wages*
- *Migrant education programs*

Housing: Homeless People

Poverty in rural areas is most reflected in available housing. Rural homes are in worse condition than those in urban areas. Some have incomplete plumbing facilities, and others have structural problems such as inadequate heating, faulty electric, leaking roofs, and holes in the walls. Home ownership, however, is higher in rural areas than in urban areas (USDA, 1999). These two facts combined lead to rural homelessness. People have difficulty finding adequate housing to rent.

Homelessness in urban populations has been extensively examined (see chapter 26); however, little attention has been given to the problem of homelessness in rural populations. Research studies at both the state and national levels have noted that rural homelessness appears to be growing (First, Rife, & Tooney, 1990; Fitchen, 1991; Lindsey, 1995). The Housing Assistance Council, a Washington advocacy group, estimates up to 12.5% of homeless persons in the United States live in rural areas (NRHA, 1994, p. 1.) The National Rural Health Association (NRHA) (1996) defines a family as homeless if they have no fixed place of residence. This includes living temporarily in shelters, with friends or relatives, in informal church-sponsored arrangements, in automobiles, in abandoned buildings, on the street, in campgrounds, and in the case of farm families, those facing eminent eviction (NRHA, 1996, p. 1).

Homeless families are the largest growing subgroup of the homeless (Bassak, 1991; Helvie, 1999 Lindsey, 1995). Homeless families are often single-parent families with the woman as head of household. Approximately 3.5% of poor workers in rural ar-

eas have at least three barriers to earning a livable wage: low educational level, female head of household, and a child younger than 6 at home (USDA, 1997). These workers are at grave risk of becoming homeless. Wagner, Menke, and Ciccone conducted a study in 1995 to examine the health of rural homeless families. Their study found the following similarities to previous urban studies:

- *Most families were female headed.*
- *The ethnic distribution of homeless families mirrored the percentage of poor people in the area under study.*
- *Poverty was more extensive in rural than in urban areas as a greater percentage of the population was below the poverty line, and thus poverty was more difficult to escape.*

Wagner, Menke, and Ciccone (1995) also found the following differences between rural and urban homeless families:

- *The average number of rural homeless children was lower than reported in urban studies.*
- *Rural families were more likely to have been homeless for 4 to 12 months, which is longer than found for urban homeless families.*
- *Rural families were more likely to have doubled up with another family, which has been found to mask the degree of homelessness present in rural areas.*
- *Fewer rural families were found to stay in shelters, which may be attributed to the fact that fewer shelters were available.*

Community health nurses who practice in rural areas are likely to encounter homeless families daily. These nurses must have an understanding of the needs of rural homeless families and be prepared to provide accessible, adequate, and appropriate care. This is not a simple task as homeless rural families are not easily identifiable, and each family will have different needs based on the length of time that they have been homeless. Case management has been found to be a particularly helpful tool in assisting homeless families or those who are near homeless find solutions. Rural community health nurse, acting as case managers, are challenged to identify what services (health care or social services) are available in the community, to creatively piece together other types of services available to fill in the gaps that exist, and to make these services acceptable to the families.

Multidisciplinary teams are often created to meet the needs of homeless families identified in the rural area. These teams may be composed of health care professionals, clergy, local politicians, community organizations, and other social support groups available in the rural community. The community health nurse is in a perfect position to develop and lead these teams as a member of the community who is knowledgeable about community support systems and able to broker a coalition of various community members.

The need for housing for homeless families in rural areas is at crisis proportion. With the number of poor single-parent families that are now found to be homeless, affordable housing must be a prime concern for rural policy.

CASE STUDY

As a community health nurse, you are running the once-a-week well-child clinic in a rural town. As you call in the first young mother, Mrs. Boone, you recognize the strong odor of dirty clothing, soiled diapers, and unwashed children. Mrs. Boone sits down and places her youngest child, a small, pale girl, on her lap. The other two children, boys who appear to be preschool age, sit quietly on the floor at the end of the room. Mrs. Boone and the three children all are wearing grimy clothes. Mrs. Boone looks at the floor and says, "We come over from the emergency room—they sent us over here because we don't have health insurance and the baby is sick. The nurse in the emergency room said you would see us even if we don't have no money."

You ask, "Tell me what's been going on?" as you take a seat opposite Mrs. Boone.

"We just come here last week from Little County with my boyfriend. We're staying with his brother but we've got to find another place to live because there isn't enough room. A couple of days ago Melanie, that's the baby's name, started being real fussy and she feels hot. She didn't sleep at all last night and kept us all awake. My boyfriend got real mad and told me to do something about her. Kids drive him crazy. Anyway, it seemed like she was pulling on her ear. She had the same thing about a month ago, and we got some medicine from the nurse where we lived before and it got better. Can you give me some medicine?"

You ask, "What was wrong with Melanie when the nurse saw her, and what kind of medicine did she get?"

"The nurse said her ear was infected and gave her some kind of medicine for the infection and for the fever. I gave her the medicine until she felt better. I lost the rest of the bottle when we were getting ready to move or I could have given her the rest of it now. I've really got to do something to make her be quiet—she is driving my boyfriend crazy." The older of the two boys on the floor begin to whine "I'm hungry." Mrs. Boone quickly turns to him and yells, "I told you to be quiet. Shut up before I smack you."

You take a deep breath and begin to get a health history on Mrs. Boone and the children. Mrs. Boone tells you that Melanie, the youngest, is 18 months old. The other two children, Travis and Jack, are 3 and 5, respectively. Mrs. Boone is 19. She did not finish high school but got married at 14, when she found that she was pregnant with Jack. She has been at home with the children, and her husband had been supporting the family with his earnings from two part-time jobs. About 2 months ago, her husband abandoned her and the children; she did not know where he was. Mr. Boone did not believe in welfare and had not let Mrs. Boone apply for any government assistance. After Mr. Boone left, Mrs. Boone managed to get some emergency food from a church food pantry and was thinking about applying for emergency assistance from welfare. Instead, she met her current boyfriend, Ashford, about 4 weeks ago, and they decided to come to Big County to see if they could find work. Mrs. Boone states that both the boys are quite healthy but that Melanie has been sick on and off since birth.

After you examine Melanie, you find that she has an ear infection and anemia. There is no money for medication for Melanie's ear infection.

1. What should you do?
2. Would you consider this family homeless?
3. What community supports should be sought to help them?

Confidentiality: Persons with HIV/AIDS

Although most HIV/AIDS cases are still found in major metropolitan areas of the United States, the incidence of HIV/AIDS in rural areas is increasing at a greater rate than in metropolitan centers. Data from the Centers for Disease Control and Prevention (CDC) reveal that among the more than 500,000 new AIDS cases reported through 1995, 16% were from rural areas and small towns. Between 1992 and 1995, the greatest rate of increase in AIDS cases occurred in rural areas, 30% in comparison with 25.8 % in the largest metropolitan regions. Three reasons for this increase have been discussed in the literature:

1. The escalation of intravenous drug use (Steel, Fleming, & Needle, 1993)
2. An increase in homosexual activity (Berry, 1993)
3. The migration of already infected people who return to their families of origin in rural areas for care and support as their disease progresses (Buehler, Frey, & Chu, 1995; Davis & Stapleton, 1991)

The migration of AIDS-infected people increases the rural numbers as a result of the shift in the numbers of cases from urban to rural. Unfortunately, funding to support HIV and AIDS programs is usually provided to the county of diagnosis rather than to the county of current residence; thus, rural counties often do not benefit from state programs (Buehler, Frey, & Chu, 1995). In addition, transient migrant workers who harvest crops for rural farmers have also been identified as a population who spreads HIV infection in rural areas.

The spread of HIV and AIDS to rural communities has been described as the "second wave" of the epidemic (Berry, 1993). The demographic characteristics of the rural HIV and AIDS population also differ from those of the urban population. They are more likely to be young, nonwhite, and female and to have acquired their infection through heterosexual behaviors (Rumbly, Shappley, Waivers, & Esinhart, 1991).

A qualitative study (Atav, 1995) was conducted in upstate New York to assess the needs of rural AIDS support organizations and to articulate policy priorities. Six priorities were identified:

1. Number of cases versus the rate of cases: *The supportive agencies stated that rural communities do not want to deal with AIDS-related issues because the actual number of cases is small. These small numbers make the disease invisible. Another reason for not wanting to take responsibility for HIV/AIDS is that the payment and funding formulas do not take into consideration the special service needs of rural communities. Although small rural communities continue to deny the problem, the rate of HIV/AIDS cases continues to skyrocket.*

FYI

Facts About Rural AIDS

Rural populations (fewer than 50,000) have the highest rates of increase in AIDS cases, representing 6.7% of all cases in the United States in 1996, with heterosexual contact accounting for most of the cases in many areas.

In rural areas, homosexual men often are not openly gay and tend to engage in unprotected sex with strangers.

Homophobia, racism, and AIDS stigmas make HIV prevention efforts nearly impossible in some rural areas.

Source: NRHA, 1998.

2. Continuation of funding: *HIV/AIDS programs were well funded, but because the state was the largest supporter of these programs, they were extremely vulnerable to political and fiscal changes in the state capital.*

3. Funding for education: *There is little funding for education and prevention activities. Education and prevention funds are raised from donations and grants. Accessing school-age*

CASE STUDY

Nina is a 30-year-old HIV-infected woman. When she was 17 years old, she lived with a man in New York City. Once into the relationship, she found that he was using intravenous drugs and selling drugs to supply his habit. After trying without success to get him to go for treatment, she left the relationship of 3 years. At age 22, she met and married James. They now have three children. James Jr. is 7 years old, Sheldon is 5, and Latisha is 3.

Once they started their family, they decided to move to rural Vermont, where James' mother, sister, and brother-in-law lived. When Sheldon was 3 months old, he began to have one infection after another. After almost 2 years of continuing antibiotics, the family practitioner suggested that they take Sheldon to a pediatrician. The pediatrician was located in an urban center about 45 miles from their home. The pediatrician, after reviewing the records and taking an in-depth history, requested that Sheldon be tested for HIV infection. When Sheldon tested positive for HIV, the

pediatrician asked that all members of the family be tested. James, James Jr., and Latisha tested negative for HIV, and Nina tested positive. The pediatrician sat down with both James and Nina to discuss treatment and follow-up care for the family. Nina was adamant that all care should come from health care providers in the urban area because she did not want anyone in her community to know of the HIV diagnoses. The pediatrician suggested a referral to an infectious disease specialist from the urban center. After meeting with the infectious disease specialist, a referral was made to her local public health department, where you will be the case manager for the family.

1. Did the infectious disease specialist ignore Nina's request for services from the urban area by referring her to the local public health department?

2. What plans will you make for Nina and for Sheldon?

3. What will you advise regarding notification of the elementary school that James and Sheldon attend?

4. How will you support the family?

populations is also difficult because parents in rural school districts tend to be more conservative regarding sensitive topics.

4. Level of expertise of health care workers: *In remote rural towns, the level of expertise is lacking. Clients with AIDS are almost always transported to urban centers for care. Rural physicians want case managers to assume the role of the AIDS expert in the community. One of the most significant problems is the lack of alternative treatments.*

5. Transportation: *Distance to health care facilities for clients and to client homes for health care providers makes service delivery and access both expensive and difficult. Public transportation is either absent or inadequate in rural areas.*

6. Confidentiality: *Confidentiality is difficult to maintain. In small communities, everyone knows one another. Being known to have HIV/AIDS creates many problems for rural clients. The stigma is often so strong that some rural clients will not even allow case managers to visit their homes (Atav, 1995).*

Rural community nurses are critical to the management of persons living with AIDS (PLWAs) because they are the largest group of health care professionals in nonmetropolitan parts of the country. Furthermore, they are the health care professionals who provide the most regular, prolonged, and intimate care for rural HIV/AIDS clients. Because of geographic distances, lack of public transportation systems, a shortage of social and support services, fewer health care providers, and limited technological resources, care of the AIDS client in rural America has become increasingly difficult. In addition, the poverty found in rural areas and the lack of health insurance are also barriers to care (Graham, Forrester, Wysong, Rosenthal, & James, 1995).

Confidentiality is a concern for anyone; however, it is especially important to the rural population infected with HIV/AIDS. Rural community health nurses caring for HIV-infected clients will probably be known to both the clients and their families as neighbors, friends, or friends of friends. This informality contributes to a fear regarding lack of privacy. This fear often results in HIV-infected per-

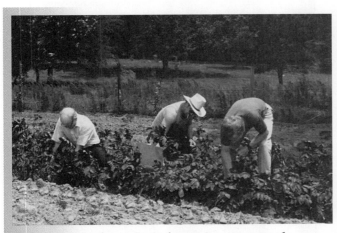

Agriculture is the main industry in many rural areas.

sons driving long distances for treatment rather than risk disclosure of their HIV status (Levi, 2000). It also results in lack of education for both the HIV-infected person and the family members about the disease. "Fear of personal safety, loss of employment, and stigmatizing family members are strong motivators for persons who delay treatment" (Sowell & Christiansen, 1996, p. 112). The concern over confidentiality is almost as great as the fear of HIV itself (The National Commission on AIDS, 1990).

Access to Health Care: Agricultural Workers

Agricultural workers are exposed to distinct health risks. The annual occupation-related death rate for all workers is 9 per 100,000 workers, and the death rate for farmers is 42 per 100,000 (Gerberich, 1995). Compared with blue-collar and white-collar workers, farmers have a higher rate of amputations, arthritis, cardiovascular diseases, ischemic heart disease, hypertension, skin cancer, chronic respiratory diseases, asthma, and back pain (Schenker, 1996). Farmers are exposed to excessive noise from machinery. They sometimes resist wearing the protective equipment required because it is bulky and hot and prevents them from hearing mechanical problems and warning cries (Marvel, Pratt, Marvel, Regan, & May, 1991). Entanglements in machinery, falls, and electrocution are common injuries (Ehlers, Connon, Themann, Myers, & Ballard, 1993). Chemical hazards for the farmer include pesticides, fertilizers, fumes, solvents, and sanitizing solutions. They can also experience allergic reactions to substances. Respiratory diseases arising from dusts, gases, and chemicals are prevalent in farm workers. Exposure to these hazards can occur during almost all the phases of farm work. Work with animals creates risk for communicable diseases as well as injury.

Mental health is a serious problem for farmers. They report high stress levels caused by the responsibilities placed on one person, the risks in farm work, the necessity to maintain a great store of current knowledge, and the unpredictability of factors such as the weather, market prices, and land value. Suicide rates for farmers are nearly twice that of the general population (Ehlers, Connon, Themann, Myers, & Ballard, 1993).

Farm families also experience special risks. Farm wives often help on the farm as well as having jobs out of the home. Children are at very high risk of injury on the farm. Approximately 300 children die every year on American farms, and thousands more are injured (National Committee for Childhood Agricultural Injury and Prevention, 1996). Farm family members demonstrate higher than expected rates of some cancers, respiratory illnesses, and adverse reproduction outcomes (Ehlers et al., 1993). Finally, migrant farm workers are exposed to all of the same risks, but potentially without the knowledge, skills, and safety equipment that is recommended.

Many farmers face an issue of access to health care. Distance from metropolitan areas and services is definitive of rurality. Travel may be over poor roads and involve geographic barriers. When one bridge is out, the travel necessary to get to the next bridge may be prohibitive.

Farmers define *health* as "the ability to work" (Lee cited in Weinert & Long, 1994). Because farmers may be indispensable

HEALTHY PEOPLE 2010

OBJECTIVES RELATED TO RURAL LIFE

Cancer

3.9 Increase the proportion of persons who use at least one of the following protective measures that may reduce the risk of skin cancer: avoid the sun between 10 AM and 4 PM, wear sun-protective clothing when exposed to sunlight, use sunscreen with a sun protective factor (SPF) of 15 or higher, and avoid artificial sources of ultraviolet light.

Environmental Health

Toxics and Waste

8.13 Reduce pesticide exposures that result in visits to a health care facility.

Infrastructure and Surveillance

8.25 Reduce exposure of the population to pesticides, heavy metals, and other toxic chemicals, as measured by blood and urine concentrations of the substances or their metabolites.

Injury and Violence Protection

Unintentional Injury Prevention

15.23 Increase use of helmets by bicyclists.

15.24 Increase the number of states and the District of Columbia with laws requiring bicycle helmets for bicycle riders.

Source: DHHS, 2000.

---

to their work, they push themselves to work when they are ill or injured. They will seek health care only when they are unable to ignore the health problem. Under these circumstances, farmers often seek health care in almost an emergency state. Sometimes, they need a higher level of care because they wait until the health problem demands action. Because they are self-employed, farmers may forego buying health insurance for themselves and their families. Furthermore, there is no law that requires farmers as employers to insure their workers. Lack of insurance also may inhibit farm workers from seeking health care.

. . . .

I've seen it all in a small town. . . .
I can be myself here in this small town.
People let me be just what I what to be.
John Mellencamp, "Small Town," 1985

. . . .

Emergency rescue of farmers presents several barriers. Farmers work independently and their absence may not be noticed for several hours. Notification systems to call for emergency help are sporadic through rural America. The terrain and distance may delay rescue vehicles. Rescue equipment such as "the jaws of life" may be unsuited for farm machinery (Staff, 1995).

Health care delivery to farmers and other rural residents requires innovation that recognizes their special needs. Mobile clinics, flexible hours, prevention and screening programs, and networks

for peer education and assistance are possibilities. Throughout the country, there are agricultural health and safety centers that provide grant funding, report research findings, and support community health workers' efforts to protect farm workers (see following Research Brief).

RESEARCH BRIEF

Dewar, D. M. (1996). Farm health and safety issues: Do men and women differ in their perceptions? American Association of Occupational Health Nursing Journal, 44(8), 391–401.

A farm family survey was conducted to learn the differences between men's and women's health concerns. The women's predominant farm health and safety concerns were (in order of importance) general physical problems, occupational hazard screening, service provider integrity, and the economic benefits of using farm health and safety services. Men's predominant concerns were (in order of importance) counseling needs, skin problems, convenience of farm health and safety services, and economic benefits of using farm health and safety services. Dewar stated that "programs lack imaginative ways to provide services reflecting cultural characteristics of the community" (p. 400).

CONCLUSION

In conclusion, rural life is often idealized as one of peacefulness and health. Although there are rewards associated with rural living, research is just beginning to reveal the realities of health care needs in this population. Health care planners and providers must develop innovative acceptable programs and educate health care providers to give accessible, acceptable, appropriate, and better than adequate care.

Community health nurses lead the way in understanding diverse rural populations and communities by recognizing the effects of lifestyle, isolation, culture, poverty/housing, confidentiality, specific health needs, and access to health care. The community nurse is capable of reaching these unique populations because often he or she is part of the rural culture and is accepted as an insider by the people for whom they care.

FYI

The National Farmworker Program provides information for centers, providers, and patients in support of migrant health:

  National Farmworker Program, Inc.
  1515 Capitol of Texas Highway, South
  Suite 221
  Austin, TX 78746
  512-328-7682

A CONVERSATION WITH . . .

There is a somewhat bipolar aspect of being a small town clinic in winter and a very busy primary care/emergency room/triage center in summer. That particular aspect requires an elasticity and ability to reprioritize and change gears that takes one to the edge. My friend and I have also found that the severity of climatic change here also puts a lot of challenge into life; however, it seems that the most energy is found in the edges of greatest challenge. I find a relationship with this land to be essential to my practice and to my humanity in sharing healing with others. In short, I love my life!

—Lynne Cameron, ANP
Skagway Medical Center,
Skagway, Alaska, June 21, 1999

CRITICAL THINKING ACTIVITIES

1. Richford, New York, is a rural community with a population of approximately 1,150. Most of the residents work elsewhere, and those who do not are mostly self-employed in farming. There is no local industry, grocery store, restaurant, hotel, bank, library, school, or police department. There is one outreach clinic operated by a hospital system about 30 miles away, and a volunteer fire/EMS department. There is a closer community hospital (22 miles), but the residents prefer traveling the 30 miles to the metropolitan area for health services. There is very limited public transportation (twice daily stops) and no taxi services. According to the rural-urban continuum, in what type of county is Richford located? How does this understanding affect your health planning?

2. A rural community health nurse has been asked to participate on a community task force to develop a plan to stop underage drinking in the community. They receive $10,000 from their state senator to be used in the development and implementation of the plan. If you were the community health nurse, what would your role be as community health educator and consultant for this group?

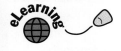

Explore Community Health Nursing on the web! To learn more about the topics in this chapter, use the passcode provided to access your exclusive web site:
http://communitynursing.jbpub.com
If you do not have a passcode, you can obtain one at this site.

REFERENCES

Atav, A. S. (1995) *AIDS in rural upstate New York: An assessment of needs and priorities.* Unpublished manuscript. Binghamton University, Binghamton, NY.

Bartlett, P. F. (1993). *American dreams, rural realities: Family farms in crisis.* Chapel Hill, NC: University of North Carolina Press.

Bassak, E. L. (1991). Homeless families. *Science America, 265*(6), 66–74.

Berry, D. E. (1993). The emerging epidemiology of rural AIDS. *Journal of Rural Health, 9*, 293.

Brent, D. A., Perper, J. A., Moritz, G., Baugher, M., Schweers, J., & Roth, C. (1993). Firearms and adolescent suicide. A community case control. *American Journal of Diseases in Children, 147*(10), 1066–1071.

Buehler, J. W., Frey, R. L., & Chu, S. Y. (1995). The migration of persons with AIDS: Data from 12 states, 1985 to 1992. *American Journal of Public Health, 85*(11), 1552–1555.

Cook, P. J. & Mizer, K. L. (1994, December). *The revised ERS county typology: An overview.* Rural Development Research Report Number 89. Economic Research Service, U. S. Department of Agriculture.

Davis, K., & Stapleton, J. (1991). Migration to rural areas by HIV patients: Impact on HIV-related healthcare use. *Infection Control and Hospital Epidemiology, 12*(9), 540–543.

Department of Health and Human Services (DHHS). (1990). *Atlas of state profiles.* Washington, DC: Author.

Department of Health and Human Services (DHHS). (1991). *Healthy people 2000.* Washington, DC: Author.

Department of Health and Human Services (DHHS). (2000). *Healthy people 2010: Conference edition.* Washington, DC: U.S. Government Printing Office.

Dewar, D. M. (1996). Farm health and safety issues. Do men and women differ in their perceptions? *American Association of Occupational Health Nursing Journal, 44*(8), 391–401.

Ehlers, J. K., Connon, C., Themann, C. L., Myers, J. R., & Ballard, T. (1993). Health and safety hazards associated with farming. *American Association of Occupational Health Nursing Journal, 41*(9), 414–421.

Fahs, P. S. S., Smith, B. E., Atav, A. S., Britten, M. X., Collins, M. S., Morgan, L. L., & Spencer, G. A. (1999). Integrative research review of risk behaviors among adolescents in rural, suburban, and urban areas. *Journal of Adolescent Health, 24*(4), 230–243.

Federal Register. (2000, February 15). *The 2000 HHS poverty guidelines, 65*(31), 7555–7557.

First, R. J., Rife, J. C., & Tooney, B. G. (1994). Homelessness in rural areas: Causes, patterns, and trends. *Social Work, 39*(1), 97–108.

Fitchen, J. M. (1991). Homelessness in rural places: Perspectives from upstate New York. *Urban Anthropology and Studies of Cultural Systems, 20*(2), 177.

Gerberich, S. G. (1995). Prevention of death and disability in farming. In H. H. McDuffie, J. A. Dosman, K. M. Semchuk, S. A. Olenchock, & A. Senthilselvan (Eds.), *Agricultural health and safety.* Boca Raton, FL: Lewis.

Graham, R. P., Forrester, M. L., Wysong, J. A., Rosenthal, T. C., & James, P. A. (1995). HIV/AIDS in the rural United States: Epidemiology and health services delivery. *Medical Care Research and Review, 52*(4), 435–52.

Helvie, C. O. (1999, Spring). Nursing the homeless—A vulnerable population. *American Public Health Association Public Health Nursing Newsletter*, pp. 8–9.

1999 HHS poverty guidelines. (1999, March 18). *Federal Register*, pp. 13428–13430.

Johnson, J. E. (1996). Social support and physical health in the rural elderly. *Applied Nursing Research, 9*(2), 61–66.

Kidd, P. S., & Holton, C. (1993). Driving practices, risk-taking motivations, an alcohol use among adolescent drivers: A pilot study. *Journal of Emergency Nursing, 19*(4), 292–296.

Kingerly, P. M., Mirzaee, E., Pruitt, .B. E., Hurley, R. S., & Heuberger, G. (1991). Rural communities near large metropolitan areas: Safe havens from adolescent violence and drug use? *Health Values, 15*(4), 39–48.

Krout, J. A. (1994). An overview of older rural populations and community-based services. In J. A. Krout (Ed.), *Providing community-based services to the rural elderly* (pp. 3–18). Thousand Oaks, CA: Sage Publications.

Lambert, M. I. (1995). Migrant and seasonal farm worker women. *Journal of Obstetric, Gynecologic, and Neonatal Nursing, 24*(3), 265–268.

Levi, J. (2000). The public health challenges of the HIV epidemic. *American Journal of Public Health, 90*(7), 1023–1024.

Lindsey, A. M. (1995). Physical health of homeless adults. *Annual Review of Nursing Research, 13*, 31–61.

Marvel, M. E., Pratt, D. S., Marvel, L. H., Regan, M., & May, J. J. (1991). Occupational hearing loss in New York dairy farmers. *American Journal of Industrial Medicine, 20*, 517–531.

Mockenhaupt, R. E., & Muchow, J. A. (1994). Disease and disability prevention and health promotion for rural elders. In J. A. Krout (Ed.), *Providing community-based services to the rural elderly* (pp. 183–201). Thousand Oaks, CA: Sage Publications.

Muellman, R. L., Walker, R. A., & Edney, J. A. (1993). Motor vehicle deaths: A rural epidemic. *Journal of Trauma, 35*(5), 717–719.

National Committee for Childhood Agriculture Injury and Prevention. (1996). *Children and agriculture: Opportunities for safety and health.* Marshfield, WI: Marshfield Clinic.

National Rural Health Association (NRHA). (1994, Fall). *Rural Clinician Quarterly.*

National Rural Health Association (NRHA) (1996). *The Rural Homeless: America's Lost Population.* Kansas City, MO.

National Rural Health Association (NRHA). (1998, Winter). *Rural Clinician Quarterly, 8*(1), 5.

North Carolina Rural Health Research and Policy Analysis Center. (1998). *Mapping rural health: The geography of health care and health resources in rural America*. Chapel Hill, NC: Author.

Poss, J. E., & Meeks, B. H. (1994). Meeting the health care needs of migrant farmworkers: The experience of the Niagara County Migrant Clinic. *Journal of Community Health Nursing, 11*(4), 219–228.

Ricketts, T. C., & Johnson-Webb, K. D. (1997). *What is "rural" and how to measure "rurality": A focus on health care delivery and health policy*. Chapel Hill, NC: Federal Office of Rural Health Policy, North Carolina Rural Health Research and Policy Analysis Center, Cecil G. Sheps Center for Health Services Research.

Rumbly, R. L., Shappley, N. C., Waivers, L. E., & Esinhart, J. D. (1991). AIDS in rural eastern North Carolina—patient migration: A rural AIDS burden. *AIDS, 5*(11), 1373–1378.

Rust, G. S. (1990). Health status of migrant farmworkers: A literature review and commentary. *American Journal of Public Health, 80*(10), 1213–1217.

Sandhaus, S. (1998). Migrant health: A harvest of poverty. *American Journal of Nursing, 98* (9), 52–54.

Schenker, M. B. (1996). Preventive medicine and health promotion are overdue in the agricultural workplace. *Journal of Public Health Policy, 17*(3), 275–305.

Schulman, M. D., Evensen, C. T., Runyan, C. W., Cohen, L. R., & Dunn, K. A. (1997). Farm work is dangerous for teens: Agricultural hazards and injuries among North Carolina teens. *The Journal of Rural Health, 13*(4), 295–305.

Smith, L. S., & Gentry, D. (1987). Migrant farm workers' perceptions of support persons in a descriptive community survey. *Public Health Nursing, 4*(1), 21–28.

Sowell, R. L., & Christensen, P. (1996). HIV infection in rural communities. *Nursing Clinics of North America, 31*(1), 107–123.

Spencer, G. A., Atav, A. S., & Collins, M. S. (1997). *A comparison of health risk behaviors of rural, suburban and urban adolescents*. Unpublished manuscript. Binghamton, NY.

Spencer, G. A., & Bryant, S. A.(1997). A comparison of dating and other violent behaviors of rural, suburban and urban adolescents. Unpublished manuscript. Binghamton, NY.

Staff. (1995). *Topics in Emergency Medicine, 17*(3).

Steel, E., Fleming, P. L., & Needle, R. (1993). The HIV rates of injection drug users in less-populated areas. *American Journal of Public Health, 83*(2), 286–287.

Stein, L. M. L. (1993). Health care delivery to farmworkers in the southwest: An innovative nursing clinic. *Journal of the American Academy of Nurse Practitioners, 5*(3), 119–124.

Svenson, L. W., Varnhagen, C. K., Godin, A. M., & Salmon, T. L. (1992). Rural high school students' knowledge, attitudes, and behaviors related to sexually transmitted diseases. *Canadian Journal of Public Health, 83*(4), 260–263.

Symons, P. Y., Groer, M. W., Kepler-Youngblood, P., & Slater, V. (1993). Prevalence and predictors of adolescent dating violence. *Journal of Child and Psychiatric Nursing, 7*, 14–23.

The National Commission on AIDS Report Number Three in Rural America. (1990). http://hivinsite.ucsf.edu/social/natl_comm_aids/2098.25ff.html.

U.S. Bureau of the Census. (1993). *Census of population and housing, 1990: Public use microdata samples, technical documentation*. Washington, DC: U. S. Government Printing Office.

U.S. Bureau of the Census. (1996, March). Table 4. Residence and Region by Household Relationship, Race and Hispanic Origin—Poverty Status of Persons in 1995. In *CPS Annual Demographic Survey, March Supplement*: http://ferret.bls.census.gov/macro/ 0301996/pov/4_001.htm.

U.S. Bureau of the Census. (1997, June 26). *Table 3. Distribution of the Population, by Region, Residence, Sex, and Race: March 1996*: www.census.gov/population/ socdemo/race/black/tabs96/tab03-96.txt.

U.S. Department of Agriculture (USDA). (1995). *Understanding rural America*. Washington, DC: Author.

U.S. Department of Agriculture, Economic Research Service (USDA). (1997). *Rural Conditions and Trends, 8*(2).

U.S. Department of Agriculture, Economic Research Service (USDA). (1999). *Rural Conditions and Trends, 9*(2).

Ventura, S. J., Martin, J. A., Mathews, M. S., & Clarke, S. C. (1996). Advance report of final natality statistics, 1994. *Monthly Vital Statistics Report, 44*(11): www.cdc.gov/nchswww.data.mv44_11s.pdf

Wagner, J. D., Menke, E. M., & Ciccone, J. K. (1995). What is known about the health of rural homeless families? *Public Health Nursing, 12*(6), 400–408.

Wagenaar, A. C., Finnegan, J. R., Wolfson, M., Anstine, P. S., Williams, C. L., & Perry, C. L. (1993). Where and how adolescents obtain alcohol beverages. *Public Health Reports, 108*(4), 459–464.

Waller, J. A. (1993). Injuries to farmers and farm families in a dairy state. *Journal of Occupational Medicine, 34*(3), 414–421.

Watkins, E. L., Larson, K., Harlan, C., & Young, S. (1990). A model program for providing health services for migrant farmworker mothers and children. *Public Health Reports, 105*(6), 567–575.

Weinert, C., & Long, K. (1994). Rural health and health seeking behaviors. *Annual Review of Nursing Research, 12*, 65–92.

What is rural? (1999, March 2): www.Nal.usda.gov/ric/faqs/ruralfaq/html).

Whitehead, R., Chillag, S., & Elliot, D. (1992). Anabolic steroid use among adolescents in a rural state. *Journal of Family Practice, 35*(4), 401–405.

Wilk, V. A. (1992). Injuries to farmers and farm families in a dairy state. *Journal of Occupational Medicine, 34*(3), 283–290.

Yawn, B. P., & Yawn, R. A. (1993). Adolescent pregnancies in rural America: A review of the literature and strategies for primary prevention. *Community Health, 16*(1), 36–45.

Chapter 28
Adolescent Pregnancy

Loretta Sweet Jemmott, Michelle Cousins Mott, and Susan Oliver Dodds

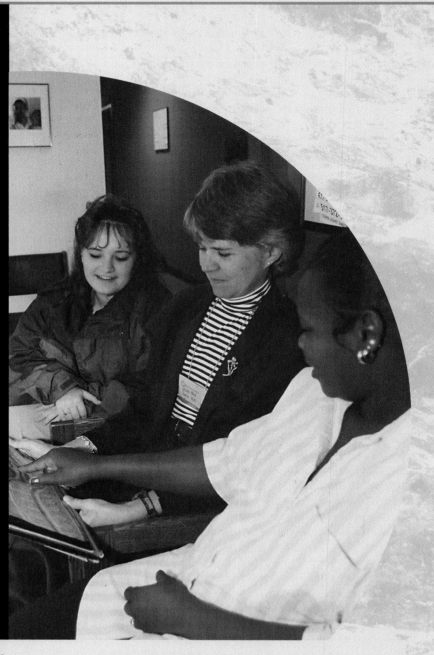

Adolescent pregnancy is a major public health problem, affecting not only the pregnant adolescent and her infant, but also families and communities nationwide.

CHAPTER FOCUS

Sexual Behavior and Pregnancy Rates

Factors Contributing to Adolescent Pregnancy
Developmental Stage
Social and Environmental Factors

Impact of Adolescent Pregnancy
Psychosocial and Health Outcomes
of the Mother
Impact on the Family
Impact on the Adolescent Father
Psychosocial and Health Outcomes
of the Newborn

Role of the Nurse
Primary Prevention
Adolescent Pregnancy Prevention Community-Based
Programs
Program Evaluation
Secondary and Tertiary Prevention

*Healthy People 2010: Objectives Related to
Family Planning*

QUESTIONS TO CONSIDER

After reading this chapter, answer the following questions:
1. What are the factors contributing to adolescent pregnancy?
2. What are the health outcomes for adolescent mothers?
3. What is the effect of adolescent pregnancy on the family?
4. How are adolescent fathers affected by their partner's pregnancy?
5. What are the health outcomes for babies born to adolescent mothers?
6. What kinds of community-based prevention programs are available?
7. What is the role of the community health nurse in primary, secondary, and tertiary prevention efforts for
adolescent pregnancy?

KEY TERMS

Abortion
Abstinence
Acculturation
Adolescent fathers
Adoption

Childhood victimization
Condoms
Contraception
Family dynamics
Health outcomes

Gynecological age
Peer educators
Low birth weight (LBW)
Prenatal care

Repeat pregnancy
Primary prevention
Secondary prevention
Tertiary prevention

Adolescent pregnancy has often been depicted as affecting only poor, urban, minority teens, but the problem extends across all ethnic groups, socioeconomic classes, and geographic boundaries. Adolescents living in rural areas are affected at rates comparable to their urban peers (Loda, Speizer, Martin, Skatrud, & Bennett, 1997). Despite our investment of a significant amount of attention, time, research, and money on prevention efforts, the results remain discouraging, as adolescent pregnancy rates in the United States remain higher than those in most other industrialized countries (Foster, 1997).

Community health nurses can play a significant role in reducing the incidence of adolescent pregnancy and improving the quality of **health outcomes** of adolescent mothers, their children, and communities overburdened by this problem. By implementing creative interventions that address adolescents, families, and the community, community health nurses can be important weapons in the battle against pregnancy prevention. However, it is important for the community health nurse to understand the contributing factors to adolescent pregnancy, the impact of adolescent pregnancy on adolescents and families, and the role of the community health nurse before these interventions are implemented.

Sexual Behavior and Pregnancy Rates

More than three-fourths of American adolescents have had sexual intercourse by the time they are 19 years of age, and adolescents are initiating sex at earlier ages (AGI, 1994, 1998; CDC, 1991; Hatcher, Trussell, Stewart, Stewart, Kowal, Guest, Cates, & Policar, 1994; Sonenstein, Pleck, & Leighton, 1989). Much of this sexual activity occurs without the use of safer sex measures, and consequently, adolescents are at risk for becoming pregnant and acquiring sexually transmitted diseases (STDs), including human immunodeficiency virus (HIV). Lack of protection is more likely among younger teens and adolescents, who have less sexual experience, making pregnancy particularly likely during the initial sexual intercourse encounters (AGI, 1998; Polaneczky,

FYI

One in eight adolescents in the United States ages 15 to 19 becomes pregnant each year.

Half of all initial adolescent premarital pregnancies occur within the first 6 months after initiation of coitus; 20% occur in the first month alone.

Media images of adolescent pregnancy often show minority adolescent teens, but adolescent pregnancy is not only a minority issue. Caucasian teenagers consistently account for the largest percentage of adolescent pregnancies and births.

Source: AGI, 1994, 1998; Pittman & Adams, 1988.

1998; Pratt, Mosher, Bachrach, & Horn, 1984; Spitz, Velebil, Koonin, Strauss, Goodman, Wingo, Wilson, Morris, & Marks, 1996; Taylor, Kagay, & Leichenko, 1986; Zabin, Kantner, & Zelnik, 1979; Zelnik, Kantner, & Ford, 1981).

More than 1 million adolescents become pregnant each year, with the majority of those pregnancies being unintended. Recent statistics report that, overall, adolescents account for 30% of all nonmarital births in the United States and 25% of unplanned pregnancies (AGI, 1998). Eighty-three percent of low-income adolescents become pregnant (Kirby, 1997), and many of these pregnancies are linked to negative future educational and employment outcomes (Coyle, Kirby, Parcel, Basen-Engquist, Banspach, Rugg, & Weil, 1996). The phenomenon of closely spaced (repeat) births among teens is also significant. More than 25% of adolescents who become pregnant will become pregnant again within 2 years (AGI, 1998; Campaign for Our Children, 1996). Multiple pregnancies intensify the negative consequences associated with adolescent pregnancy.

Factors Contributing to Adolescent Pregnancy

Many factors have been associated with adolescent pregnancy. Factors including earlier age of onset of puberty, earlier age of initiation of intercourse, increased sexual activity, nonuse or inconsistent use of contraceptives, lack of knowledge about sex and conception, developmental age, and social/environmental status have contributed to an increased risk for teenage pregnancy. For the community health nurse to develop appropriate interventions to prevent adolescent pregnancy, it is essential to understand the contributing factors.

Developmental Stage

Adolescence is a time of uncertainty and experimentation, as young people strive to develop their identity in preparation for adulthood. For many young people, it is a time of sexual experimentation. This experimentation is in response to the adolescents' physical, hormonal, cognitive, and psychosocial development. Unfortunately, the consequences of such experimentation far too often include increased risk of pregnancy.

Psychosocial Development

Adolescent psychosocial development progresses through three stages: early, middle, and late adolescence. Early adolescence (ages 11 to 13) is characterized by turmoil stemming from physical changes and emotional fluctuation influenced by changing hormone levels (Drake, 1996). In this stage, adolescents are often seeking control, may show defiance to authority figures, and may use sex as an outlet for the expression of their perceived control (Drake, 1996; Flavell, Miller, & Miller, 1993). Middle adolescence (ages 14 to 16) is characterized by development of self-identity and sexual identity. In search of their identity, adolescents may imitate the behaviors they see around them from media, older peers, parents, and other adults (Foster, 1997; Males, 1993). Late adolescence (ages 17 to 20) is characterized by the adaptation of self-identity and development of coping strategies that will be used in adulthood (Drake, 1996). Adolescents who do not have a strong self-identity and sexual identity may not be able to assert themselves and apply coping strategies such as the sexual negotiation skills that are used with a sexual partner (Flavell, Miller, & Miller, 1993). As a result, adolescents may give in to sexual pressure from their peers and sexual partners.

Intrapersonal Issues and Development

The development of self-concept is a major task of adolescence. For adolescents who have a poor sense of self and have a history of unsuccessful life experience, the need for love and attention may lead to sexual intercourse and pregnancy. As a mother, the adolescent may sense that she will be the center of attention in the family and have a feeling of importance and belonging (Fisher, 1984).

Adolescents may view sexual intercourse and pregnancy as a link to a sexual partner. They may believe that having sex or becoming pregnant is a way that they can ensure a continued, exclusive, caring relationship with that partner. As a result, some adolescents may feel pressured into sexual relations because they fear losing their partner if they do not comply (Davis, 1980; Toledo-Dreves, Zabin, & Emerson, 1995). This is a particularly important factor for adolescents who do not feel needed or cared for within the family unit.

In general, pregnancy as a strategy to compensate for unmet needs, to have self-esteem, or to assert independence is not particularly beneficial or successful. Parenting provides ample opportunity for failures, which are not helpful to adolescents already faced with repeated failures in their lives. An infant cannot meet all the nurturing expectations of the adolescent and has significant nurturing and attention needs of its own.

Social and Environmental Factors

Environment significantly influences adolescent ideas about sex and pregnancy and their resulting behavior. Each society has implied messages about sexuality, social behavior, and pregnancy. The clarity of the messages the community provides influences the sexual behaviors and expectations of its members (Foster, 1997). Several social and environmental factors have been identified as contributing to the high rates of adolescent pregnancy in the United States. Influences from family, culture, socioeconomic status, peers, sexual partners, drugs/alcohol use, previous sexual abuse, and STDs have all been identified (Kenney, Reinholtz, & Angelini, 1997; Plouffe & White, 1996; Robinson & Frank, 1994; Toledo-Dreves, Zabin, & Emerson, 1995; Widom & Kuhns, 1996; Zoccolillo, Meyers, & Assiter, 1997).

The Family of the Adolescent

An understanding of **family dynamics** is essential for the community nurse to work effectively with the pregnant adolescent and her family. Every family is governed by its own rules and ex-

pectations, which determine expected behavior for its members (Bowen, 1971). Problems occur when there is poor communication and conflicting messages about sex and pregnancy (DiIorio, Hockenbeery-Eaton, Maibach, Rivero, & Miller, 1996). Adolescents may hear mixed messages from the family, which often come from the family's own discomfort and embarrassment about sex and pregnancy. As a result, adolescents may perceive affirming attitudes about adolescent sexuality.

The Ethnicity/Culture of the Adolescent

Differences in culture may affect the family and peer reactions to adolescent pregnancy, which in turn influences an adolescent's perception of pregnancy. Many factors contribute to cultural identity, and it is not suggested that all members of a particular cultural group will behave in an identical fashion; however, the community nurse must be aware of and sensitive to cultural influences on adolescent pregnancy.

Mainstream American culture has a negative view toward adolescent pregnancy, yet the rates of adolescent pregnancy remain higher in the United States than in other industrialized nations (Desmond, 1994; Trad, 1999). The existence of many subcultures and various culturally based beliefs may contribute to the higher rates of adolescent pregnancy. For example, in traditional, patriarchal Latino culture, females are expected to respond to male demands, and marriage and motherhood/fatherhood are viewed as catalysts to adulthood (Orshan, 1996). As a result, Latino adolescents may have a positive attitude toward pregnancy. However, the extent to which these common culturally based beliefs impact attitudes toward pregnancy may depend on the adolescent's level of acculturation. **Acculturation** is a dynamic, multidimensional phenomenon in which the ideals and beliefs of one culture are incorporated into that of another (Orshan, 1996; Reynoso, Felice, & Shragg, 1993). Acculturated American Latino adolescents from traditional Latino families may receive contradictory sexual messages from mainstream American society and the more traditional messages of their Latino culture. To the adolescent who is developing an identity, these conflicting views may lead to inconsistent feelings about sexual activity and contraceptive use.

Similarly, African American adolescents who grow up in single-parent families may receive mixed messages about adolescent pregnancy. These adolescents may see a pattern of intergenerational out-of-wedlock teen pregnancies but hear disapproving messages about adolescent pregnancy (Desmond, 1994). Compounding the issue, there may be poor communication between the adolescent and parent about sexual issues.

Cultural influences are not limited to adolescents in minority cultures. Caucasian adolescents may also be influenced by cultural issues. In some European American cultures, discussion about sex and pregnancy is taboo. Adolescents who live in these environments may look to their peers and the media for rules of acceptable sexual conduct. Uneducated peers may provide misinformation, and the media may provide a false image of sex and pregnancy risks.

Socioeconomic Factors

There exists a vicious cycle between lower economic status and adolescent pregnancy (Males, 1993). Lower socioeconomic status has been correlated with higher rates of sexual activity and adolescent pregnancy, and adolescent pregnancy is associated with higher rates of school dropout. Adolescents who drop out of school have a decreased likelihood of attaining gainful employment. Data have shown that few adolescent parents are adequately prepared to assume the economic, social, and psychological responsibility of child care and child rearing (Stevens-Simon, Kelly, Singer, & Cox, 1996). This phenomenon has been seen across the various cultures and ethnic groups in the United States (Desmond, 1994; Farber, 1994).

Lower socioeconomic status may be linked to decreased access to care, which translates to decreased access to family planning and prevention information. Decreased access to care and contraceptive information may contribute to a higher rate of **repeat pregnancy** in the adolescent and may impact the health of the child (AGI, 1994).

The Adolescent's Peers

One of the single most influential factors in adolescent sexual activity and pregnancy is the influence of peers (Coyle et al., 1996). Formation of peer groups and an increased need for peer acceptance are normal developmental milestones of adolescence. However, this increased need for acceptance may cause adolescents to give in to the requests of their peers or imitate the actions of their peers, which may include sexual experimentation and risky sexual behavior. Moreover, sexual information is often exchanged by adolescent peers and may lead to misconceptions and result in unintended pregnancy.

The Adolescent's Sexual Partner

It is important to understand the male partner of female adolescents because female adolescent sexual activity often is submissive to male sexual desire (Jemmott & Jemmott, 1990). In addition, the typical contraceptive methods on which adolescents rely before seeking prescription contraceptives are male methods, such as condoms and withdrawal before ejaculation (Morrison, 1985).

Male attitudes toward contraceptive use, especially **condoms**, have been described as negative (Jemmott & Jemmott, 1990, 1992; Jemmott, Jemmott, & Fong, 1998; Morrison, 1985; Sorensen, 1973). For instance, many males view condom use unfavorably because they believe it reduces the pleasure or spontaneity of sexual activities. Adolescent males commonly believe that **contraception** is a female's responsibility (Jemmott & Jemmott, 1990).

Little attention has been paid to the age of sexual partners of adolescents. It has been reported that the majority of male sexual partners of adolescent females are approximately 5 years older (average age 20 to 24) (AGI, 1998), with only 30% of adolescent pregnancies resulting from **adolescent fathers**. Adolescent females may view their relationships with older partners as providing an escape from poverty, a show of defiance, a display of sexuality, and a boost to self-esteem. However, adolescent females with an in-complete perception of self may not feel able to negotiate and assert sexual boundaries, such as condom use with their older partners, and may submit to the older partner's sexual demands. Consequently, many adult-adolescent relationships result in an adolescent pregnancy (Toledo-Dreves, Zabin, & Emerson, 1995).

Adolescent males have similar risk factors for pregnancy as their female peers. Often, adolescent males struggle with development and may attempt to demonstrate independence, belong to peer groups, and demonstrate physical and sexual maturity by engaging in sexual activity. As adolescents, males may also lack future-oriented thinking and concrete thinking abilities. Together, these factors contribute to increased potential for participating in risky sexual behaviors that may lead to pregnancy (Jemmott, 1993). Adolescent males may also view pregnancy as a catalyst toward manhood and may purposely have unprotected intercourse. In the African American community, the risk for an adolescent-fathered, teenage pregnancy may be higher. The mean age for sexual initiation among African American males has been estimated to be as low as 11.1 years (Jemmott, 1993; Jemmott & Jemmott, 1990). See the Research Brief below.

Substance Use Among Adolescents

Several studies have found that the use of alcohol or drugs during sexual activity is associated with risky sexual behavior, such as intercourse with multiple partners and failure to use condoms (Jemmott & Jemmott, 1992). Alcohol and drug use may change the nature of the sexual behavior in which people engage because

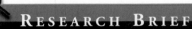

RESEARCH BRIEF

Robinson, R. B., & Frank, D. L. (1994). The relation between self-esteem, sexual activity, and pregnancy. Adolescence, 29(113), 26–35.

A study by nurse researchers examined self-esteem in relation to sexual behaviors for adolescents. A sample of 141 male and 172 female adolescents of diverse ethnic backgrounds was surveyed to determine levels of self-esteem, sexual activity, pregnancy, and fatherhood status. The Coopersmith Self-Esteem Inventory was also used to obtain qualitative data related to self-esteem, demographics, and sexual activity. Analysis revealed no differences in the self-esteem of males versus females. Sexual activity or virginity had no relationship to self-esteem in males or females. Self-esteem levels were no different for pregnant teens in comparison with nonpregnant teens. However, males who had fathered a child had lower self-esteem than nonfathers. The findings support a multifocused approach to sex education for pregnancy prevention and also emphasize a need to include males in both pregnancy intervention efforts and further research on adolescent pregnancy.

logic and good judgment are clouded and inhibitions are loosened when people are "high" or because intoxication provides an excuse to engage in risky behavior (Crowe & George, 1989; Fortenberry, Orr, Katz, Brizendine, & Blythe, 1997; Jemmott & Jemmott, 1992; Kokotailo, Langhough, Cox, Davidson, & Fleming, 1994). However, there is a second, simpler explanation of the relationship between alcohol and drug use and risky sexual behavior. Adolescents who use alcohol and drugs more frequently than their peers may also engage in more sexual activity than their peers; consequently, they may engage in more risky sexual activity compared with their peers. The argument is not that alcohol and drug use causes adolescents to engage in different, more risky sexual behavior, but rather that adolescents who use alcohol and drugs engage in sexual activity more frequently (Jemmott & Jemmott, 1992).

Sexual and Physical Abuse of Adolescent Females

Childhood victimization may be linked to promiscuity and adolescent pregnancy. Adolescent females who were physically and/or sexually abused may be more likely to initiate sexual intercourse at a younger age, use drugs and alcohol, and engage in more promiscuous relationships than nonabused adolescents (Kenney, Reinholtz, & Angelini, 1997). Childhood abuse has been associated with low socioeconomic status, unemployment, family dysfunction, substance use, and psychological dysfunction. Because many of the risk factors for childhood abuse are interrelated and linked to adolescent pregnancy, it is difficult to separate the effect of each factor in a child's environment that may influence behavior (Fiscella, Kitzman, Cole, Sidora, & Olds, 1998).

Adolescents who have experienced physical or sexual abuse may use sex in an effort to attain loving nonabusive relationships or may view pregnancy as a way out of the abusive environment at home (Widom & Kuhns, 1996). However, the adolescent who has not fully developed emotionally may not be in the position to be assertive and use sexual negotiation skills, leaving them at greater risk for experiencing further sexual exploitation by present and future partners.

Knowledge Deficit Regarding Sex, Conception, and Contraception

The increased sexual activity among adolescents has not been accompanied by increased knowledge about sexual function, procreation, or birth control. Studies indicate that many adolescents remain woefully ignorant about conception and the menstrual cycle (Darabi, Jones, Varga, & Hourse, 1982; Davis & Harris, 1982; Jemmott & Jemmott, 1990; Landry, Bertrand, Cherry, & Rich, 1986). In addition to lack of information on sex and conception, adolescents lack correct information on birth control methods and the correct use of contraceptives (Morrison, 1985; Pollack, 1992).

Even though contraceptive information has become more available, many adolescents do not use birth control on a regular basis (Box 28-1). Adolescents generally engage in sexual intercourse for some time before obtaining reliable contraception. Reluctance to obtain and use contraception is associated with certain attitudes and psychological and social factors. Stevens-Simon,

FYI

One of five pregnant adolescents is physically and/or sexually abused (hitting, unwanted touching, sexual advances, or intercourse) by a family member or partner during their pregnancies.

BOX 28-1 WHY ADOLESCENTS DO NOT USE CONTRACEPTION IN THEIR OWN WORDS

- I didn't mind getting pregnant.
- I didn't want to appear to my partner to be prepared to have sex.
- I wanted to get pregnant.
- I wasn't planning to have sex.
- I didn't know how to get birth control.
- I thought my boyfriend was sterile.
- I didn't think that I could get pregnant.
- I didn't know how to use birth control.
- I wanted to have a baby so my boyfriend would love me.
- I thought my partner would be angry with me if I used birth control.
- I was afraid my family would find out.
- I wanted a baby to love.
- I was afraid of the side effects.
- I thought other people would find out that I was using birth control.
- It's hard to talk to my partner about birth control.
- I was embarrassed about using birth control.
- My boyfriend wanted me to get pregnant.
- I just did not get around to it.
- My partner didn't want to use birth control.
- Birth control can be expensive.
- Using a condom interferes with sexual pleasure.
- Getting birth control is inconvenient.

Source: Adapted from AGI, 1981; Howard & McCabe, 1992; Jemmott & Jemmott, 1990, 1992; Jemmott, Jemmott, & Fong, 1998; Loda et al., 1997; Zelnik & Kantner, 1979.

Kelly, Singer, and Cox (1996) reported that adolescents' attitudes include "I don't mind getting pregnant" or "I want to get pregnant." Adolescents who feel this way may neglect to use contraception or be inconsistent users of contraception.

Impact of Adolescent Pregnancy

Adolescent pregnancy has significant, far-reaching consequences. Pregnancy can affect the adolescent's health, development, education, and socioeconomic status. The family and community may also feel the effects because the majority of adolescents are unwed, live with their families, and depend on public assistance (Coley & Chase-Lansdale, 1998). In addition to psychosocial and economical outcomes, the adolescent mother experiences physical consequences that may affect her health.

Psychosocial and Health Outcomes of the Mother

Pregnancy is a time of increased demands on a woman's body. These demands can be harmful to a developing adolescent, especially if there is no focus on the increased needs of pregnancy such as nutrition and rest. In general, adolescents experience greater health problems with pregnancy than do women older than 20 years of age. The consequences are especially severe to the youngest adolescents, those 12 to 15 years of age (Levy, Perhats, Nash-Johnson, & Welter, 1992; Trad, 1999).

Adolescents are at greater risk for developing pregnancy-induced hypertension and toxemia (AGI, 1981), anemia, nutritional deficiencies, and urinary tract infections (Bulcholz & Gol, 1986). Adolescent girls are more likely to deliver prematurely, experience rapid or prolonged labor, develop abruptio placenta, or have fetal or maternal infections (Mott, 1990).

Lack of Prenatal Care

One of the major reasons for negative health outcomes for mothers and infants is lack of **prenatal care.** More pregnant adolescents delay seeking prenatal care, access less prenatal care, or do not receive regular care as often as adult women (Cockey, 1997; Geronimus, 1986). The same teenagers at greatest risk for pregnancy—those from poor families—are also at greatest risk for poor prenatal care. This lack of care contributes to poorer health outcomes for both mother and infant. Most adolescents do not receive prenatal care in the first trimester, with nearly 20% accessing care in the last trimester only. In general, this group tends to be more illness-oriented than prevention-oriented in their health practices. The reasons for this delayed initiation of prenatal care are varied and include denial of the pregnancy, lack of knowledge, lack of access to health care, concern about concealing the pregnancy, developmental immaturity (Cockney, 1997; Zuckerman, Walker, Frank, Chase, & Hamburg, 1984), and an orientation toward concrete, present-centered reasoning (Geronimus, 1986).

Repeated Pregnancy

Several studies have shown that many young mothers have more than one child during their teen years. Obtaining exact numbers is difficult because U.S. Census data does not report repeat pregnancy rates, but estimates range from 15% to 60%, depending on the study (Brown, Saunders, & Dick, 1999; Cockey, 1997).

Adolescent mothers who have repeat pregnancies continue to be at higher risk for poor outcomes. Although it might be reasonably assumed that adolescent mothers would be more savvy in a second pregnancy, seeking and receiving more timely prenatal care, this is often not the case. One study examined the outcomes of first and second adolescent pregnancies among Caucasian and African American teenagers. The results revealed that a poor outcome in the first pregnancy was associated with a three times greater risk of repeating that outcome in the second pregnancy. The recurrence rate of preterm delivery was especially severe for African American adolescents (Blankson, Cliver, Goldenberg, Hickey, Jin, & Dubard, 1993). These results are critical because they provide a specific target for the **secondary prevention** efforts of nurses working in the community.

Psychosocial Outcomes

Although pregnancy can become a stimulus for positive growth in an adolescent, generally the results are more negative than positive. Motherhood or fatherhood in the adolescent years can cause severe disruption in the normal psychosocial development of adolescents. Pregnancy places an additional psychosocial burden on teenagers, who are already attempting to cope with the normal maturational crisis of adolescence (Bulcholz & Gol, 1986; Trad, 1999).

Adolescents typically cope with the confusion and conflict in their lives by finding safety and acceptance in their peer groups. However, adolescent parents, especially mothers, may find them-

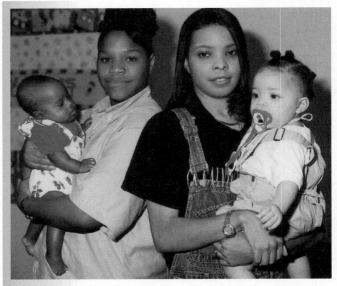

Parenting classes help teen mothers bond with their babies.

selves isolated from their peer groups at a critical time in their development. The degree of isolation may vary depending on the norms accepted by different cultural peer groups.

A primary goal of adolescence is attainment of independence. Although pregnancy may enhance independence in some ways by forcing the adolescent to take charge of a difficult situation, this forced rapid ascension into adulthood certainly is not without negative consequences. After delivery, as adolescent parents cope with the demands of a new infant, their own needs and desires are no longer first priority. The increased stress of being an adolescent parent can lead to more self-doubt, uncertainty, loneliness, and helplessness (Lieberman, 1980). The adolescent's inability to effectively cope with these feelings is reflected in the increased incidence of child abuse and neglect within this cohort (Marshall, Buckner, & Powell, 1991).

Education and Economic Disruption

Adolescents who become pregnant are less likely than their nonpregnant peers to complete their education. For example, whereas 90% of women who delay childbearing beyond adolescence complete a high school education, only 70% of adolescent mothers ultimately reach this goal (AGI, 1994). Without a complete education, many adolescent mothers find employment opportunities out of their reach and rely on low-paying jobs or public assistance programs (Grogger & Bronars, 1993).

Impact on the Family

An unplanned adolescent pregnancy can seriously jeopardize quality of life not only for the young mother and infant but also for the extended families. Families are often called on to shoulder considerable economic and emotional burdens. The strain on the family is often intensified because adolescent mothers are more likely to live in single-parent households (AGI, 1994). The long-term impact on the family is unknown, but as families compensate to deal with adolescent pregnancy, they may normalize the experience and set the stage for future adolescent pregnancy. From generation to generation, this trend may develop into a cycle. The children of adolescent parents are at increased risk of perpetuating the cycle by becoming adolescent parents themselves and dropping out of school (Campaign for Our Children, 1996).

Impact on the Adolescent Father

For every adolescent conception that occurs outside marriage, there is a father as well as a pregnant mother, yet there is limited research focusing on adolescent males who become fathers. The impact of adolescent pregnancy has been largely focused on adolescent females despite the obvious involvement of males. Even though adolescent males are the fathers in only 30% of adolescent pregnancies, it is important for the community health nurse to address the problem of teenage pregnancy with this group. Adolescent fathers may be more at risk for continued educational and social problems. Fagot, Pears, Capaldi, Crosby, and Leve (1998)

found that adolescent fathers had more arrests and substance use problems than did nonfathers of the same age. The adolescent father's reaction to the pregnancy, his own psychosocial developmental issues and needs, and his behavior as a young father are critical to developing positive health outcomes for the child and impacting the behaviors of these young men before adulthood.

The adolescent father's reaction to the pregnancy is a crucial factor in determining what role he will play in the pregnancy and delivery and in the child's life. Some adolescent males react positively, but others do not. Reactions to pregnancy are influenced by many factors, including family reaction, peer group reaction, and relationship with the mother of the child. Another factor that may influence the reaction is the developmental stage of the father, because many may not be able to cope effectively with a pregnancy. Problems that impact the adolescent male revolve around the acknowledgment of the child, his financial responsibility, his school commitment, and his work situation (Males, 1993). Adolescent fathers report feeling frightened and disturbed by the responsibilities and neglected in the decision-making process, although few abandon the mother during pregnancy. Unfortunately, the young father may abandon the adolescent mother after pregnancy.

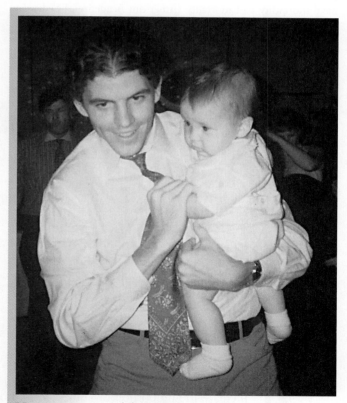

Nurses can use celebrity role models like Will Turpin, bass guitarist for Collective Soul (shown here with his son, Tristan), to demonstrate the rewards of waiting for marriage and fatherhood.

Regardless of the good intentions of most men, the fate of most adolescent fathers is similar to that of teenage mothers. Most are ill prepared to assume the role of fatherhood, and few relish the opportunity. Generally, having come from poor, relatively uneducated backgrounds, they experience serious social and economic disadvantages compared with young men who postpone fatherhood until a later age (Sonenstein, Stewart, Lindberg, Pernas, & Williams, 1997). Most of the fathers lack the necessary skills to provide a stable home environment for their families even if they want to. In short, poverty is the tie that binds most adolescent fathers and mothers. Although some manage to cope with their situation, continue educational and vocational pursuits, and mature into self-sufficient, productive members of society, the odds are stacked against them.

Psychosocial and Health Outcomes of the Newborn

Infants born to adolescents are at risk for various health problems as a result of complications with the adolescent mother's pregnancy and with the birth. These health problems include the increased incidence of preterm deliveries (before 38 weeks' gestation), increased incidence of **low-birth-weight (LBW)** infants (birth weight of less than 2,500 g), and increased incidence of perinatal morbidity and mortality (American Academy of Pediatrics, 1989; Blankson et al.,1993; Leppert, Namerow, & Barker, 1986).

There has been considerable debate over whether young maternal age alone is an independent risk factor for complications, and the results are still unclear (DuPlessis, Bell, & Richards, 1997). More recent research suggests that other mediating factors (e.g., low socioeconomic status, poor prenatal care, race/ethnicity, unfavorable sociocultural circumstances) play a critical role (Plouffe & White, 1996; Yoder & Young, 1997).

Role of the Nurse

It is apparent that pregnancy during the adolescent years presents some unique risks and special needs for the adolescent, her pregnancy, and her infant. Obviously, **primary prevention** of pregnancy is a crucial component of any adolescent intervention program. However, if young girls become pregnant, it is imperative that they receive secondary and tertiary preventive care, including adequate prenatal care coupled with long-term postpartum follow-up to ensure a healthy outcome for both mother and child. Community health nurses, because of their expertise in assessment, health teaching, and program development, are well suited to this task. Their accessibility to adolescent populations places them in a pivotal position to play a significant role in the delivery of care before sexual activity, during pregnancy, and during long-term follow-up with the parents and child.

Healthy People 2010 addresses specific goals for adolescent pregnancy prevention (see the *Healthy People 2010* box below for selected objectives). The community health nurse may use these national objectives to guide the development of individual, local, and regional nursing interventions.

HEALTHY PEOPLE 2010

OBJECTIVES RELATED TO FAMILY PLANNING

9.2   Reduce the proportion of births occurring within 24 months of a previous birth.

9.6   Increase male involvement in pregnancy prevention and family planning efforts.

9.7   Reduce pregnancies among adolescent females.

9.8   Increase the proportion of adolescents who have never engaged in sexual intercourse before age 15 years.

9.9   Increase the proportion of adolescents who have never engaged in sexual intercourse.

9.10   Increase the proportion of sexually active, unmarried adolescents aged 15 to 17 years who use contraception that both effectively prevents pregnancy and provides barrier protection against disease.

9.11   Increase the proportion of young adults who receive formal instruction before turning age 18 years on reproductive health issues, including all of the following topics: birth control methods, safer sex to prevent HIV, prevention of sexually transmitted diseases, and abstinence.

Source: DHHS, 2000.

••••••••••••••••••••••••••••••••

The majority of adolescents behave as if their states were that of moratorium. That is, adolescence is a time for experimenting with how one might want to be as an adult.

Rew (1998) quoted in Frisch and Frisch (1998)

••••••••••••••••••••••••••••••••

Primary Prevention

Because primary prevention is a critical component of effective community health nursing, there are tremendous opportunities for nurses to address the multifaceted problem of teen pregnancy and make important contributions to developing and implementing interventions to reduce the incidence of adolescent pregnancy. Table 28-1 provides a list of issues to be considered when planning nursing interventions. An example of primary prevention is education and counseling for adolescents about sexual health issues, including, but not limited to, pregnancy prevention, family life education, family planning, and the postponement of pregnancy into adulthood. A comprehensive program in primary prevention targeting adolescent pregnancy includes three goals:

1. *Delaying or halting participation in sexual activity*
2. *Providing access to contraception and sufficient knowledge and skills to use contraception appropriately*
3. *Strengthening life goals and encouraging long-term planning*

Some prevention programs focus selectively on one goal, whereas others address all three.

One task in primary prevention is contraceptive education targeted at both males and females, encouraging adolescents to practice responsible sexual behavior. For adolescents to use contraceptives (including condoms) consistently, they need not only the correct knowledge on how to use the method, but also technical skills on how to use them correctly and on how to negotiate contraceptive use, especially condoms, with their partners. Adolescents need confidence and self-efficacy in their ability to use contraceptive methods, and the desired method must be available and accessible. Finally, adolescents need positive attitudes toward contraceptive use, especially condoms (Jemmott & Jemmott, 1992, 1998). Community health nurses should carefully explore an adolescent's knowledge base and correct any misconceptions about birth control methods. This is the important first step in providing adolescents with clear, accurate directions regarding the use of birth control. Some recent trends in contraceptive use among adolescents are encouraging. For example, two-thirds of adolescents reportedly use some form of contraception at first intercourse, with a significant increase in prevalence of use at first intercourse among 15- to 19-year-old females (AGI, 1994, 1998). Kahn, Brindis, and Glei (1999) claim that more than 1 million adolescent pregnancies were averted in 1995 because of consistent contraceptive use. These pregnancies

would have led to approximately 480,000 live births, 390,000 abortions, 120,000 miscarriages, 10,000 ectopic pregnancies, and 37 maternal deaths.

The two most popular methods of contraception used by adolescents have traditionally been the birth control pill and the condom (USPHS, 1997). Although it is beyond the scope of this chapter to fully discuss contraceptive options, it is particularly important for nurses working with adolescents to recognize the type of methods, side effects, and potential barriers that influence contraceptive choice.

Considering the variety of factors that contribute to an adolescent's increased risk for pregnancy, it is clear that there is not one reason why teens become pregnant. However, there are clear solutions and programs. These solutions and programs differ according to their target and the problem identified.

Adolescent Pregnancy Prevention Community-Based Programs

A comprehensive review of adolescent pregnancy prevention research reveals many successes and failures. Kirby (1997) concludes that programs with positive outcomes share important characteristics (Box 28-2). There is no clear agreement on what exact combination of these elements makes up the ideal prevention program. Clearly, programs must be tailored to match the needs of the particular target population. Ideally, members of the target population should be involved in the program development and implementation. There is a pressing need for prevention programs that are culturally sensitive and relevant, addressing the norms, attitudes, and beliefs of the target population. There are various types of programs with different approaches to pregnancy prevention, such as peer education, life options, working with parents, and working in schools and other settings.

Lessons Learned

Important lessons have been learned in the area of adolescent pregnancy prevention. For example, although some prevention efforts focus solely on the importance of **abstinence** from sexual intercourse, the bulk of current evidence indicates that this approach is not successful in delaying the onset of intercourse (Kirby, 1997). Furthermore, education alone is generally not sufficient to change risky behavior such as inconsistent contraceptive use (Howard & Mitchell, 1993). Multidisciplinary programs are needed that combine elements such as sexuality education, enhanced negotiation and communication skills, and access to services and contraceptives (AGI, 1994; Howard & Mitchell, 1993; Plouffe & White, 1996). Finally, although some have expressed concern that sexuality education and/or contraceptive distribution might encourage sexual activity among teens, recent research reviews have concluded that the opposite is actually true (Kirby, 1997; Kirby, Resnick, Downes, Kocher, Gunderson, Potthoff, Zelterman, & Blum, 1993).

TABLE 28-1	CONSIDERATIONS FOR NURSING INTERVENTIONS

ISSUE	CONSIDERATIONS
Adolescent father	Acknowledge the risk factors for adolescent fatherhood and encourage involvement in the prenatal and postnatal periods. In speaking with adolescent males, it is important for the nurse to identify and assess beliefs and diagnose problems that may be specific to the adolescent male. Personalize interventions to adolescent males, both in terms of preventing adolescent pregnancy through responsible sex and in terms of coping with the consequences of being a young father. Interventions that positively affect adolescent fathers may indirectly benefit their partners by enhancing partner support (Roye & Balk, 1996). Talking in a nonthreatening, engaging manner with the male adolescent will facilitate effective communication that will address risk factors and beliefs and promote healthy outcomes for the father, mother, their families, and their child (Roye & Balk, 1996; Sonenstein et al., 1997). Stress male responsibility in birth control. Increase his role in pregnancy and child care. Improve his parenting skills and support his lifestyle changes (completing school, job training, and working).
Developmental stage	Nurses who are knowledgeable about factors in adolescent development can better design developmentally appropriate primary interventions to prevent pregnancy, STD, and HIV in their community. Recognize the developmental tasks and stages of adolescence in order to recognize the influence that those developmental factors have on adolescent sexual behavior. Consider the biophysical, cognitive, and psychosocial theories of development. Answer questions and educate the adolescent about physical development and sexual issues.
Culture/ethnicity	Assess and diagnose each adolescent client and family in order to develop culturally sensitive interventions that are tailored to address cultural factors that impact sexual behavior, contraception, and potential pregnancy.
Peer	Take advantage of the powerfully influential peer group to reach adolescents; trained **peer educators** may be used to deliver safer sex and abstinence messages.
Intrapersonal	Be aware that the adolescent is in a stage where she is developing self-identity and self-esteem and that the adolescent may use sexual activity and pregnancy to bolster her identity.
Attitudes	Explore nonjudgmentally the adolescent's attitudes about pregnancy.
Socioeconomic status	Assess the adolescent's economic situation and intervene to connect the adolescent and family with needed community resources.
Sexual abuse	Identify adolescents in potentially abusive situations and assess both the adolescent and the adolescent's family for abuse.
Positive health outcomes	Conduct home visits to adolescents during pregnancy and after birth to improve pregnancy outcomes and infant health status and to delay repeat pregnancies (Olds, 1992; Olds, Henderson, & Kitzman, 1994; Olds, Henderson, Tatelbaum, & Chamberlin, 1988).

BOX 28-2 CHARACTERISTICS OF EFFECTIVE ADOLESCENT PREGNANCY PREVENTION PROGRAMS

Effective programs should do the following:

- Focus clearly on reducing one or more sexual behaviors that lead to unintended pregnancy or HIV/STD infection

- Incorporate behavioral goals, teaching methods, and materials that are appropriate to the age, sexual experience, and culture of the students

- Be based on theoretical approaches that have been demonstrated to be effective in influencing other health-related risky behaviors

- Last long enough to allow participants to complete important activities

- Provide basic, accurate information about the risks of unprotected intercourse and methods of avoiding unprotected intercourse

- Use a variety of teaching methods designed to involve the participants and have them personalize the information

- Include activities that address social pressures related to sex

- Provide models of and practice in communication, negotiation, and refusal skills

- Select teachers or peers who believe in the program and then provide them with training, which often includes practice sessions

Source: Kirby, 1997.

Peer Education Approach

The peer education model shows great promise for use in adolescent pregnancy prevention (Minter, 1990) because the peer group is a common source for information about sex. In this model, peers are trained to lead prevention programs within their peer group. Community health nurses may serve as trainers and facilitators in these programs. Some of the advantages of peer education are that it provides positive role models, reinforces norms, empowers youth, and encourages personal responsibility (Coyle et al., 1996).

Life Option Approach

A promising approach that is worthy of additional study is programs that shift the focus to enriching an adolescent's life options across the board by addressing concerns such as academic performance, self-esteem, substance abuse, and long-term goal realization. These programs may include one-on-one mentoring and role modeling with successful adults, community service participation, remedial education, tutoring services, counseling by both professional and peer groups, self-worth enhancement techniques, and exposure to new experiences to expand life options (e.g., concerts, museums, travel). This approach attempts to expand an adolescent's future goals and expectations by improving educational and employment prospects. Because future-oriented, goal-directed adolescents are less likely to become pregnant, the expected result is a reduction in the rate of adolescent pregnancies. Although this approach does not directly address adolescent pregnancy, it targets many of the factors that contribute to an adolescent's risk for unintended pregnancy (Kirby, 1997; Loda, Speizer, Martin, Skatrud, & Bennett, 1997). Because the community health nurse is familiar with the community and its members, he or she may serve as a trusted mentor, educator, community liaison, and coordinator of such programs. In addition, for these programs to be effective, community health nurses must be aware of programs and resources that target adolescents in a broader sense, not only in terms of pregnancy prevention and contraception.

Working with Parents and Adults

Community health nurses may work with parents and other adults significant to the adolescent, such as adult relatives, teachers, coaches, and neighbors. This approach may be a promising avenue for prevention because parents and significant adults influence the behavior of adolescents, including sexual behavior, in their everyday interactions. Although there is no single way for parents to effectively communicate with their children, the nurse may suggest that parents follow the guidelines provided by the National Campaign to Prevent Teen Pregnancy outlined in Box 28-3.

School-Based Programs

A large number pregnancy prevention programs target teens through school programs. Some of the programs in school may include sex education, family life education, and contraception education. Sex education is provided by some private schools and by public schools in approximately 70% of the states (Norr, 1991); however, most family life programs are offered at the junior or senior high school level as an elective course, which means they do not reach many adolescents and cannot target those at greatest risk. Also, most sex education teachers have little training in sex education, and it is not their primary focus. In school systems with school nurses, the nurse is involved in both sex and family life education. Nurses can also provide factual sex education to teenagers as they provide other health services. Nurses are effective sex educators because they are equipped to provide sexual content in a factual, nonjudgmental approach. They are also proficient at encouraging and guiding client discussion, characteristics helpful in addressing sex education with adolescents. These and other school-based programs receive limited funding, and access is limited for most students. However,

A Conversation With...

This teenage mom was 17 when she had her first child. She married the father of the child, finished high school, and is pursuing a college education.

On learning I was pregnant, I was really sad. My world was coming to an end. Many changes took place. My boyfriend and I both wanted to finish high school. So we were married and moved in with my in-laws.

After the baby was born, we graduated and soon moved into a trailer. I was overwhelmed with the responsibility. I lost so much sleep I thought I would never feel rested again!

We made the choice to stay married and I chose to go on to college against all odds. Now that college graduation is only a little over a year away, and I've grown up a lot, my future has hope! It has taken us more than three years, but I can truthfully say the last four months have been happy for us as a family.

Two major factors that have helped me keep from giving up on education and my marriage were the support of my mother and the teen-mom support group leader who became a real friend to me. They gave me something to hang on to and hope for when the winds of strife seemed capable of blowing me over.

After almost four years, we are beginning to see ourselves as a family mostly because of two concepts learned in the support group. The first was that I realized decisions in life were mine to make. I was responsible for my life. The second concept was learning how to effectively communicate love to my husband and son. He and I are the two people in the world that will love our son more than anyone else. We are partners in our responsibility for his nurturance, guidance, and support. How different my life might have been if I had not involved myself with this community service.

—A Teen Mother
Source: A. McFarland. (1998, May 5). "Family Matters." Fort Payne, AL: *The Times Journal*, p. 4.

BOX 28-3 Ten Tips for Parents to Help Their Children Avoid Teen Pregnancy

1. Be clear about your own sexual values and attitudes.
2. Talk with your children early and often about sex, and be specific.
3. Supervise and monitor your children's behaviors, setting rules, curfews, standards, and so on.
4. Know your children's friends and their families.
5. Discourage early, frequent, and steady dating.
6. Take a strong stand against your daughter dating a significantly older boy; do not allow your son to develop an intense relationship with a much younger girl.
7. Help your teenager to have options for the future that are more attractive than early parenthood.
8. Let your kids know that you value education highly.
9. Know that your kids are influenced by the media; pay attention to what they are watching, listening, and reading.
10. Develop strong, close relationships with your children at an early age.

Source: National Campaign to Prevent Teen Pregnancy, 1998.

school-based programs operate within a highly politicized environment. Decisions to include or exclude certain program elements within school-based programs may be made in an effort to minimize controversy rather than to maximize positive outcomes. As a result, community health nurses may need to broaden the focus of their prevention efforts beyond the domain of the school.

Working in Various Settings

Rather than limit the discussion of sexuality and pregnancy prevention to any one setting or a particular type of visit, community health nurses are uniquely positioned to seize opportunities to provide education and implement prevention in numerous settings. These settings, such as family planning clinics, primary health care clinics, school health clinics, and community-based health clinics, are all ideal settings for adolescent pregnancy prevention, even when the adolescent does not present for contraceptive services. Interventions targeting adolescents who use the services of family planning clinics appear to be particularly promising in that they can effectively reach a high-risk group, adolescent females (and potentially their partners) who come to the clinic for a pregnancy test (Zabin, Emerson, Ringers, & Sedivy, 1996). These clinics are logical sites because of the population that they serve: More than 60% of adolescents younger than 17 use family planning clinics (Zabin & Clark, 1981), and more than 82% of young African American adolescents use them (Mosher, 1990). In addition, they provide the opportunity to reach a population of vulnerable, high-risk adolescents at a timely moment.

Program Evaluation

Evaluation is an important part of the nursing process. Programs must be continually evaluated and modified by the community health nurse to ensure their effectiveness and appropriateness for preventing adolescent pregnancy. New prevention programs are constantly in the process of being designed; however, few programs are carefully and consistently developed and evaluated. Thus, efforts may be wasted on interventions that are not effective. One measure of a sound design is the incorporation of theory in the design. Community nurses should have a knowledge base that includes an understanding of various behavioral theories such as the health belief model (Becker, 1974), social cognitive theory (Bandura, 1986), and the theory of reasoned action (Azjen & Fishbein, 1980). These theories can be used to understand the factors that encourage or discourage health promotion behaviors and can guide both program design and evaluation. The lack of meaningful program evaluation is a major defect in the primary prevention of adolescent pregnancy. Evaluation by the community health nurse is critical not only to identify ineffective programs or program elements but also to identify effective interventions and provide the impetus for replication and reevaluation in a different population. An effective prevention intervention is one that makes positive behavioral changes in

measurable outcomes such as decreased incidence of unprotected sex or decreased number of sexual partners.

Secondary and Tertiary Prevention

Prevention efforts may not reach all adolescents because the risk of pregnancy may not be associated with extremely negative outcomes (Stevens-Simon, Kelly, Singer, & Cox, 1996). Therefore, the community health nurse must implement secondary and **tertiary prevention** techniques. In secondary and tertiary prevention, the community health nurse focuses attention on the health care, prevention needs, and long-term development of pregnant adolescents and adolescents who are already young mothers or fathers (Table 28-2). Secondary prevention efforts are designed to promote healthier outcomes from adolescent pregnancy. Its efforts are aimed at improving participation in prenatal care, childbirth preparation, and parenting activities. Interventions may include early detection of pregnancy, options counseling, prenatal care, childbirth education, parenting education, and safer sex education. Community health nurses may also be involved on a more global scale in secondary prevention efforts by working to increase access of pregnant adolescents to care. These efforts may include developing policies relevant to adolescent pregnancy in various organizations, working through coalitions and in other professional organizations.

Early Detection

A goal for the community health nurse is to identify pregnant adolescents early in their pregnancies, because many teens wait until they are visibly pregnant before they initiate prenatal care (Baker, 1996). Factors such as shame, denial, self-esteem issues, low value and knowledge of health, limited access to care, lack of future-oriented thinking, and lack of symptoms have all been linked to failure to receive early diagnosis and care (Baker, 1996; Lee & Grubbs, 1995; Thompson, Powell, Patterson, & Ellerbee,

TABLE 28-2   **SECONDARY AND TERTIARY PREVENTION: NURSING INTERVENTION**

ISSUE	CONSIDERATIONS FOR NURSING INTERVENTIONS
Early detection	Identify pregnant adolescents early in their pregnancies.
	Recognize factors linked to failure to receive early diagnosis and care.
Pregnancy options	Assess knowledge about pregnancy options.
	Be sensitive to the factors that impact her decision.
	Assess the support the adolescent receives throughout the pregnancy.
	Facilitate therapeutic relationships with the adolescent mother and father and their social support networks.
	Include the father of the baby. A comprehensive assessment should include identification of his attitudes, emotional reactions, plans for education, and plans for involvement with the pregnancy, his partner, and the child.
	Provide options counseling.

Continued

TABLE 28-2   SECONDARY AND TERTIARY PREVENTION: NURSING INTERVENTION—CONT'D

ISSUE	CONSIDERATIONS FOR NURSING INTERVENTIONS
Prenatal care	Encourage early and consistent prenatal care to reduce neonatal and maternal complications.
	Teach the adolescent and her partner about the special needs of pregnancy.
	Assess barriers to adolescent prenatal care.
	Provide health screening assessments, counseling, and education for pregnant clients.
The adolescent father	Encourage the father's participation in prenatal visits.
	Invite the father to prenatal classes, encourage questions and participation in prenatal visits, and acknowledge the father's role as a partner in the pregnancy.
	Encourage fathers to participate in the delivery.
Parenting education	Assess knowledge about parenting.
	Provide education about positioning and handling of infants, nutrition, hygiene, elimination, growth and development, immunization, and recognition of illnesses.
	When doing health teaching it is important to be sensitive to the ethnicity and culture of the client and integrate it into the care of the infant.
Postpartum care	Focus on the standard postpartum areas as well as on specific concerns of the adolescent, such as body image, weight loss, and fatigue.
	Assess the adolescent's adjustment to her new role and the emotional support systems available to her.
	Provide a health assessment of both the mother and infant, newborn care education and supervision, prenatal education on growth and development and parenting skills, review of role adjustment and available supports, and sex education and birth control information.
	Encourage the adolescent to continue developing as an individual (e.g., to continue her education, participate in some social activities, to explore relationships with peers) and at the same time increase her proficiency and confidence in parenting.
Support	Assess available physical and emotional support.
	Refer adolescents to other possible resources, such as parenting programs, cooperative day care, or programs that pair the new mother with an older adolescent mother with a successful experience.
Status of the newborn	Provide a newborn assessment/well-baby check.
	Assess for signs of adequate maternal-infant bonding.
	Provide information about child care.
Sexual activity and contraceptive use	Assess adolescents' plans for sexual activity and need for contraceptive methods.
	Initiate discussion about birth control while the adolescent is pregnant so that both partners have an opportunity to identify contraceptive and safer sex methods that they will use after the pregnancy.
	Provide instruction on condom use during pregnancy in your discussion of disease prevention in pregnancy.
	Help the adolescent explore the risks involved if they have sex without adequate protection.
	Help the adolescent select the most appropriate form of contraception from several alternatives
	If the adolescent has already used birth control, it is helpful to identify the method, how it was used, and the reason for discontinuance.
	Make sure that the adolescent is aware of community resources (family planning clinics) where she may be supplied with contraceptives.
	Encourage clinic attendance, promote access to contraception, and provide referrals to appropriate contraceptive services when counseling individuals or teaching sex education classes; emphasize the importance of contraceptive use by all sexually active adolescents.
	Monitor compliance and encourage cooperation with adolescents.

BOX 28-4 ADOLESCENTS AND ABORTION

Nearly 4 in 10 teen pregnancies (excluding miscarriages) end in abortion. There were about 289,000 abortions among teens in 1994.

Since 1980, abortion rates among sexually experienced teens have declined steadily because fewer teens are becoming pregnant, and in recent years fewer pregnant teens have chosen to have an abortion.

The reasons most often given by teens for choosing to have an abortion are concern about how having a baby would change their lives, feeling that they are not mature enough to have a child, and having financial problems.

Twenty-nine states currently have mandatory parental involvement laws in effect for a minor seeking an abortion: AL, AR, DE, GA, ID, IN, IO, KS, KY, LA, MD, MA, MI, MN, MS, MO, NE, NC, ND, OH, PA, RI, SC, SD, UT, VA, WV, WI, and WY.

Sixty-one percent of minors who have abortions do so with at least one parent's knowledge; 45% of parents know about their daughter's abortion. The great majority of parents support their daughter's decision to have an abortion.

Source: Alan Guttmacher Institute, 1998.

1995). Community health nurses can work to identify teens early in their pregnancies by using community outreach techniques such as advertisement for prenatal services in malls, schools, public transportation, and churches.

Options Counseling

In counseling the pregnant adolescent, the nurse must be aware that the adolescent's decisions about her pregnancy and subsequent pregnancy prevention will affect both the adolescent mother and her entire family. Once pregnancy is confirmed, the adolescent faces an important decision about her options, which include **abortion, adoption,** or keeping the baby (Box 28-4). The nurse has the responsibility to provide (or refer to someone who will provide) the adolescent with information about pregnancy options. Among adolescents, the most common outcome (55%) is a live birth. Only 1 in 20 pregnant adolescents chooses to place her infant for adoption, whereas 35% of adolescent pregnancies end in abortion (National Center for Health Statistics, 1990).

The community health nurse must recognize that many factors play a role in the decision the adolescent makes about the pregnancy. These factors may include cultural and religious upbringing, family attitude toward the pregnancy (perceived or real), partner attitude, and state law. Partner age plays an important role, as the data has shown that adolescent females with younger partners tend to terminate their pregnancies at a higher rate than adolescent females with adult partners (AGI, 1994).

Prenatal Care

Once an adolescent decides to continue the pregnancy, effort is directed toward ensuring a healthy outcome for the mother and infant. Early initiation and regular continuance of prenatal care significantly reduce the risk for both adolescents and their infants (ANA, 1987). The nurse should educate the adolescent and her partner about the special needs of pregnancy as they relate to adolescence, such as the following:

- *Special nutritional needs (Box 28-5)*
- *Physical changes and demands of pregnancy*
- *How pregnancy affects the female adolescent's growth and development*
- *Emotional changes during pregnancy for both parents*
- *What to expect during delivery*

BOX 28-5 ADOLESCENT PREGNANCY AND NUTRITION REQUIREMENTS

The nutritional needs of the pregnant adolescent are often different from those of adult women. Many adolescents are experiencing rapid physical growth and maturation during their teenage years. Pregnancy increases the nutritional requirements of the adolescent.

*The recommended nutritional goals of the adolescent depend on the **gynecological age** of the adolescent. (Gynecological age is the number of years between the chronological age and the age of menarche.) Adolescents with a gynecological age less than or equal to 2 years have increased nutritional needs because of their own physical growth requirements. When the gynecological age is less than 2 years, the pregnant teen may compete with the nutritional requirements of the fetus to meet those of the adolescent.*

Because adolescent diets are often high in salt, sugar, and fatty foods and low in protein, vitamins, and minerals, the nurse must be diligent about assessing and diagnosing deficits in the pregnant adolescent's diet.

- *Preterm labor*
- *Signs and symptoms of pregnancy complications*

Programs that address barriers to adolescent prenatal care have demonstrated positive outcomes, including reduced neonatal and maternal complications (Rogers, Peoples-Sheps, & Suchindran, 1996; Yoder & Young, 1997).

Prenatal care services that prove successful in getting teenagers to use and comply with the overall program of care are those that provide an accepting, caring atmosphere and work to reduce obstacles to beginning or continuing care. These results have been in comprehensive community-based programs with a heavy outreach and educational emphasis, using multidisciplinary health care teams, especially community health nurse involvement, and home visits. The community health nurse acts as the case manager of prenatal care and sees that clients are provided with needed services. The nurse is the team member who spends the most time with the adolescent, providing most of the health screening assessments, counseling, and education for pregnant clients.

Prenatal programs should also aim to improve the quality and duration of the father-child relationship. Community health nurses can assist in these efforts by encouraging the father's participation in prenatal visits. Most fathers are curious and interested in the process of gestation and delivery but are uncomfortable asking questions and hesitant in interacting with health care providers. The community health nurse can invite the father to prenatal classes, encourage questions and participation in prenatal visits, and acknowledge the father's role as a partner in the pregnancy. Fathers can be encouraged, but not forced, into participation in the baby's delivery.

Three types of programs offer prenatal care to adolescents: private medical services, clinic programs, and school-based prenatal programs. The choice of program depends on the accessibility and the financial circumstances of the adolescent and her family. Private medical services are provided by physicians in single or group practices or associated with health maintenance organizations. These services are available to people who have a medical insurance plan or can afford to pay. Clinic programs are for families without insurance or the financial resources to pay for prenatal care. School-based programs provide services in connection with other school-run clinic services or in separate schools designed for the exclusive use of pregnant adolescents (Olds, 1992). School-based prenatal services provide a comprehensive approach to care and are usually found in large school districts with high rates of adolescent pregnancy.

Parenting Education and Contraceptive Education

Adolescent parents typically need more structured education focusing on newborn care, parenting skills, and fostering developmentally appropriate interactions. Discussion about birth control should also be initiated while the adolescent is pregnant so that both partners have an opportunity to identify contraceptive methods that they will use after the pregnancy. The community

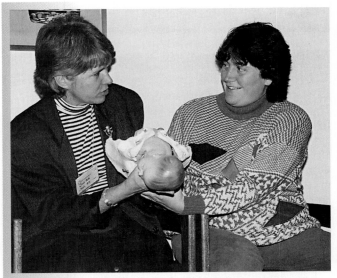

Nurse role modeling appropriate infant care with teen mother.

health nurse is in a unique position to provide these services at a group or individual level and promote continuity of care that focuses on the new family.

Transition from Prenatal to Postpartum Care

After delivery of the baby, the focus is on postpartum care, which varies widely in scope and duration of services. All prenatal programs provide a postpartum check for the mother. A well-baby check is included in most services, although a private obstetrical practice may rely on the mother to make her own arrangements for all infant care. The most extensive postpartum care is delivered in community programs that rely heavily on nurses. These programs usually include the following:

- *Health assessment of both the mother and infant*
- *Newborn care education and supervision*
- *Prenatal education on growth and development and parenting skills*
- *Review of role adjustment and available supports*
- *Sex education and birth control information*

One valuable component of these programs is the emphasis on regular contact with the new mothers, starting the first week after delivery. Studies show that regular nurse visits reduce anxiety and increase infant health as measured by fewer accidents and emergency department visits (Olds, 1992; Olds, Henderson, & Kitzman, 1994; Olds, Henderson, Tatelbaum, & Chamberlin, 1988). Mothers experience many concerns or problems before the first scheduled clinic or physician visit. Earlier contacts allow the adolescent and nurse to address these issues and reduce anxiety. Contact need not always be in person; some care can be provided by telephone monitoring of the new mother.

Health and Psychosocial Status of the Mother

At a minimum, the mother should have a 6-week postpartum examination. Some community health programs start home visits at about 2 weeks postpartum. The physical assessment should focus on the standard postpartum areas as well as on specific concerns of the adolescent, such as body image, weight loss, and fatigue. In addition, the nurses should assess the adolescent's adjustment to her new role and the emotional support systems available to her. Adjusting to the role of parent during adolescence is difficult. Conflict is not unusual. Family members may expect the adolescent to instantly become an adult and mother, or the opposite, to remain a child and allow her parents to assume all the responsibilities for the infant. Ideally, the adolescent should be encouraged to continue developing as an individual (e.g., to continue her education, participate in some social activities, to explore relationships with peers). The adolescent mother needs support in increasing her proficiency and confidence in parenting and integrating her new responsibilities into her daily routine. She may be juggling school, social activities, and infant care. Fatigue and stress are common.

The community health nurse can help the new mother look at the immediate family, other relatives, significant others, and the father of the infant and his family for support. The adolescent mother could also be referred to other possible resources, such as parenting programs, cooperative day-care programs, or programs that pair the new mother with an older adolescent mother with a successful experience. Even if support systems are adequate, the family may need some help in understanding and supporting the adolescent as a maturing individual. Adequate physical and emotional support, along with health teaching and realistic expectations for their children, successfully reduces the incidence of abuse and neglect from at-risk mothers (Marshall, Buckner, & Powell, 1991; Olds, 1992; Olds, Henderson, & Kitzman, 1994; Olds, Henderson, Tatelbaum, & Chamberlin, 1988).

Sexual Activity and Contraceptive Use

Ideally, the idea of future contraception should be introduced as part of the prenatal program. The adolescent must decide whether she will continue sexual activity after delivery and must be encouraged to be honest with the nurse about her decision. Sometimes, the mother is no longer involved with the father of the infant and announces that she does not intend to be sexually active or to have another child. In this case, the adolescent mother should be helped to explore the risks involved if she changes her mind without adequate protection. Once an adolescent has been pregnant, she risks repeating the situation (AGI, 1981; Brown, Saunders, & Dick, 1999).

Access to and regular use of birth control is the goal of contraceptive services for adolescents. Family planning clinics and private physicians are one source; school-based clinics are a more recent effort. Community health nurses can encourage clinic attendance, promote access to contraception, and provide referrals to appropriate contraceptive services when counseling individuals or teaching sex education classes. The nurse must emphasize the importance of contraceptive use by all sexually active adolescents (Kahn, Brindis, & Glei, 1999).

Health Status and Care of the Newborn

In addition to the usual newborn assessment, the community heath nurse should look for signs of adequate maternal-infant

CASE STUDY

You are a school nurse at Hilton High School. You have carefully followed several of your students who have become pregnant and helped them find resources for support both during and after their pregnancies. You have noticed, however, that several of your students have decided to discontinue breast-feeding. In speaking with Arlene Johnston, a 15-year-old sophomore with a 3-month-old son, Antonio, you find out that she too is reconsidering breast-feeding. She understands the benefits of breast-feeding and is able to discuss them with you. Both Arlene and her mom think that breast-feeding is good for Antonio. However, upon further questioning, you discover that her new partner, Sam, and her friends at school think that breast-feeding is "nasty." Arlene feels embarrassed that her friends know she breast-feeds, and she is afraid that she will lose her friends and boyfriend.

1. What factors in Arlene's (and the other adolescents') cognitive development support her decision to discontinue breast-feeding?

2. How can you address this to continue to promote Arlene's breast-feeding Antonio?

You decide that one means to addressing attitudes toward breast-feeding is to address the attitudes of all students at Hilton High.

1. Consider different ways that you, as the school (community) health nurse, can address the students at Hilton High.

2. Think about what special considerations there are for such an intervention.

bonding. Evidence of attachment includes calling a child by its name, cuddling, talking to the infant, and demonstrating an interest in infant care and development. Adolescents sometimes demonstrate difficulty in bonding simply because they have had no previous experience with infants and are afraid to do anything. Sometimes, another person has assumed the role of caregiver and the adolescent becomes an observer rather than caregiver. Bonding can be assessed in clinic settings, but home visits by the community health nurse allow for a more accurate picture of the nature and scope of the mother-infant relationship. Considering the current trend of short postpartum length of stay, the community health nurse has the opportunity to observe the interaction among the infant, teenager, and other caregivers for a longer time than nurses in the clinical setting.

Tertiary Prevention

Tertiary prevention efforts may include prevention of additional adolescent pregnancies, support of positive parent-infant interaction, support groups for adolescent parents, and programs that support the adolescents while they pursue educational goals. The techniques discussed previously that are used in primary prevention may be used to prevent repeat pregnancies in adolescents. The nurse may work collaboratively with organizations that provide support such as child care and allowing adolescent parents to complete and pursue further education (Smith & Hanks, 1994). Other nursing interventions may include long-term child development education and parenting classes. Programs that foster maternal education, father involvement, and increased self-esteem show significant promise for better maternal and infant development (Diehl, 1997; Roye & Balk, 1996).

CONCLUSION

Despite the proliferation of prevention efforts, adolescent pregnancy is a significant and enduring community health problem. It has been linked to various problems such as increased poverty, decreased educational attainment, increased psychological stress, potential isolation from peers, and increased reliance on public funds. Multiple pregnancies among adolescents are not uncommon and are particularly disturbing because the negative effect of pregnancy increases dramatically.

Many factors contribute to adolescent pregnancy, and community health nurses must be aware of potential risk factors and understand the complex interaction of these factors. Without this awareness and understanding, the nurse will not be able to adequately perform the nursing process to develop and evaluate age-appropriate, culturally sensitive, convenient, comprehensive, and affordable interventions that will meet the special needs of adolescents. It is clear that unless community health nurses and other health professionals make an effort to provide information, few adolescents will actively seek out nurses or other professionals as resources. Nurses are well suited to address the issues of adolescent pregnancy. The professional roles in schools, clinics, screening programs, health departments, and community outreach centers provide access to at-risk populations. Community health nurses have the opportunity, sensitivity, and commitment to work to achieve positive outcomes for adolescents and their children.

Beyond the scope of care to individuals, community health nurses are sensitive to the community in which they practice. Community health nurses are uniquely equipped to assess communities, identify needs and special risk groups, and formulate solutions. Nurses have an obligation to meet the special needs of pregnant adolescents by designing programs, organizing community support, and advocating for funding and policy changes to enhance positive health outcomes for adolescents and their infants.

CRITICAL THINKING ACTIVITIES

1. What are the social norms and cultural beliefs about adolescent pregnancy and sexuality in your community? How do you think that these beliefs affect adolescent behavior?

2. What strategies can the community health nurse implement to help the pregnant adolescent and her family cope with the changes in the family structure?

3. You are planning a pregnancy prevention intervention for adolescents in your community. Identify program characteristics that you might include in your intervention that have been shown to be effective in adolescent pregnancy prevention programs.

4. It is important for the community health nurse to be aware of community resources to appropriately refer clients. What resources are available in your community for pregnant adolescents? adolescents with children? adolescent fathers?

5. Does your school district provide child care for adolescents with children? Do you believe they should? Why?

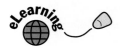

Explore Community Health Nursing on the web! To learn more about the topics in this chapter, use the passcode provided to access your exclusive web site: http://communitynursing.jbpub.com
If you do not have a passcode, you can obtain one at this site.

REFERENCES

Alan Guttmacher Institute (AGI). (1981). *Teenage pregnancy: The problem that hasn't gone away.* New York: Author.

Alan Guttmacher Institute (AGI). (1994). Sex and America's teenagers. New York: Author.

Alan Guttmacher Institute (AGI). (1998). *Facts in brief: Teens and pregnancy:* http://www.agi-usa.org/pubs/fb_teen_sex.html.

American Academy of Pediatrics, Committee on Adolescence. (1989). Adolescent pregnancy. *Pediatrics, 83,* 132–135.

American Nurses Association (ANA). (1987). *Access to prenatal care: Key to prevention of low-birth weight.* Kansas City, MO: Author.

Azjen, I., & Fishbein, M. (1980). *Understanding attitudes and predicting social behavior.* Englewood Cliffs, NJ: Prentice Hall.

Baker, T. J. (1996). Factors related to the initiation of prenatal care in the adolescent nullipara. *The Nurse Practitioner, 21*(2), 29–42.

Bandura, A. (1986). *Social learning theory.* Englewood Cliffs, NJ: Prentice Hall.

Becker, M. H. (1974). The health belief model and personal health behaviors. *Health Education Monographs, 2,* 324–508.

Blankson, M. L., Cliver, S. P., Goldenberg, R. L., Hickey, C. A., Jin, J., & Dubard, M. B. (1993). Health behavior and outcomes in sequential pregnancies of black and white adolescents. *Journal of the American Medical Association, 269*(11), 1401–1403.

Bowen, M. (1971). The use of family theory in clinical practice. In J. Haley (Ed.), *Changing families.* New York: Grune & Stratton.

Brown, H. N., Saunders, R. B., & Dick, M. J. (1999). Preventing secondary pregnancy in adolescents: A model program. *Health Care for Women International, 20*(1), 5–15.

Bulcholz, E. S., & Gol, B. (1986). More than playing house: A developmental perspective on the strengths in teenage motherhood. *Theory and Review,* 347–357.

Campaign for Our Children. (1996). *Fact sheet on adolescents who have babies:* http://www.cfoc.org/statsfactsheet.html.

Centers for Disease Control and Prevention (CDC). (1991). Premarital sexual experience among adolescent women—United States, 1970–1988. *Morbidity and Mortality Weekly Report, 39,* 929–932.

Cockey, C. D. (1997, June). Preventing teen pregnancy. It's time to stop kidding around. *Lifelines,* 32–40.

Coley, R. L., & Chase-Lansdale, P. L. (1998). Adolescent pregnancy and parenthood. Recent evidence and future directions. *American Psychologist, 53*(2), 152–166.

Coyle, K., Kirby, D., Parcel, G., Basen-Engquist, K., Banspach, S., Rugg, D., & Weil, M. (1996). Safer choices: A multicomponent school-based HIV/STD and pregnancy prevention program for adolescents. *Journal of School Health, 66*(3), 89–94.

Crowe, L. C., & George, W. H. (1989). Alcohol and human sexuality: Review and integration. *Psychological Bulletin, 102*, 374–386.

Darabi, K. F., Jones, J., Varga, P. L., & Hourse, M. (1982). Evaluation of sex education outreach. *Adolescence, 17*(65), 57–64.

Davis, K. A. (1980). *A theory of teenage pregnancy in the U.S. adolescent. Pregnancy and childbearing*. Washington, DC: Department of Health and Human Services.

Davis, S. M., & Harris, M. B. (1982). Sexual knowledge, sexual interests, and sources of sexual information of rural and urban adolescents from three cultures. *Adolescence, 18*(66), 471–492.

Department of Health and Human Services (DHHS). (1990). *Healthy People 2000: National health objectives* (Publication No. 91-50213). Washington, DC: U.S. Government Printing Office.

Desmond, A. M. (1994). Adolescent pregnancy in the United States: Not a minority issue. *Health Care for Women International, 15*(4), 325–331.

Diehl, K. (1997). Adolescent mothers: What produces positive mother-infant interaction? *Maternal Child Nursing, 22*, 89–95.

DiIorio, C., Hockenbeery-Eaton, M., Maibach, E., Rivero, S., & Miller, K. (1996). The content of African American mothers' discussions with their adolescents about sex. *Journal of Family Nursing, 2*(4), 365–382.

Drake, P. (1996). Addressing the needs of pregnant adolescents. *Journal of Gynecological and Neonatal Nursing, 25*(6), 518–524.

DuPlessis, H. M., Bell, R., & Richards, T. (1997). Adolescent pregnancy: Understanding the impact of age and race on outcomes. *Journal of Adolescent Health, 20*, 187–197.

Fagot, B., Pears, K., Capaldi, D., Crosby, L., & Leve, C. (1998). Becoming an adolescent father: precursors and parenting. *Developmental Psychology, 34*(6), 1209–1219.

Farber, N. (1994). Perception of pregnancy risk: A comparison by class and race. *American Journal of Orthopsychiatry, 64*(3), 479–484.

Fiscella, K., Kitzman, H. J., Cole, R. E., Sidora, K. J., & Olds, D. (1998). Does child abuse predict adolescent pregnancy? *Pediatrics, 101* (4 Pt. 1), 620–624.

Fisher, S. M. (1984). The psychodynamics of teenage pregnancy and motherhood. In M. Sugar (Ed.), *Adolescent parenthood*. Jamaica, NY: Spectrum Publications.

Flavell, J. H., Miller, P. H., & Miller, S. A. (1993). *Cognitive development* (3rd ed.). Englewood Cliffs, NJ: Prentice Hall.

Fortenberry, J. D., Orr, D. P., Katz, B. P., Brizendine, E. J., & Blythe, M. J. (1997). Sex under the influence. *Sexually Transmitted Diseases, 24*(6), 313–319.

Foster, H. W. (1997). The campaign to prevent teen pregnancy. *Journal of Pediatric Nursing, 12*(2), 120–121.

Geronimus, A. (1986). The effects of race, residence and prenatal care on the relationship of maternal age to neonatal mortality. *American Journal of Public Health, 76*(12), 1412–1421.

Grogger, J., & Bronars, S. (1993). The socioeconomic consequences of teenage childbearing: Finding from a natural experiment. *Family Planning Perspectives, 25*(4), 156–161, 174.

Hatcher, R. A., Trussell, J., Stewart, F., Stewart, G. K., Kowal, D., Guest, F., Cates, W., Jr., & Policar, M. S. (1994). *Contraceptive technology* (16th ed., rev.). New York: Irvington.

Howard, M., & McCabe, J. A. (1992). An information and skills approach for younger teens: Postponing sexual involvement program. In B. C. Miller, J. T. Card, R. L. Paifoff, & J. I. Peterson (Eds.), *Preventing adolescent pregnancy*. Newbury Park, CA: Sage Publications.

Howard, M., & Mitchell, M. E. (1993). Prevention teenage pregnancy: Some questions to be answered and some answers to be questioned. *Pediatric Annals, 22*(2), 109–118.

Jemmott, L. S. (1993) AIDS risk among black male adolescents: Implications for nursing intervention. *Journal of Pediatric Health Care, 7*, 3–11.

Jemmott, L. S., & Jemmott, J. B., III. (1990). Sexual knowledge, attitudes, and risky sexual behavior among inner-city black male adolescents. *Journal of Adolescent Research, 5*, 346–369.

Jemmott, L. S. & Jemmott, J. B., III. (1992). Increasing condom-use intentions among sexually active inner city black adolescent women: Effects of an AIDS prevention program. *Nursing Research, 41*, 273–279.

Jemmott, J., Jemmott, L., & Fong, G. (1998). Abstinence and safer sex HIV risk-reduction interventions for African American adolescents: A randomized controlled trial. *Journal of the American Medical Association, 279*(19), 1529–1536.

Kahn, J. G., Brindis, C. D., & Glei, D. A. (1999). Pregnancies averted among U.S. teenagers by the use of contraceptives. *Family Planning Perspectives, 31*(1), 29–34.

Kenney, J. W., Reinholtz, C., & Angelini, P. J. (1997). Ethnic differences in childhood sexual abuse and teenage pregnancy. *Journal of Adolescent Health, 21*(1), 3–10.

Kirby, D. (1997). *No easy answers: Research findings on programs to reduce teen pregnancy* (Summary). Washington, DC: The National Campaign to Prevent Teen Pregnancy.

Kirby, D., Resnick, M. D., Downes, B., Kocher, T., Gunderson, P., Potthoff, S., Zelterman, D., & Blum, R. W. (1993). The effects of school-based health clinics in St. Paul on school-wide birthrates. *Family Planning Perspectives, 25*(1), 12–16.

Kokotailo, P. K., Langhough, R. E., Cox, N. S., Davidson, S. R., & Fleming, M. F. (1994). Cigarette, alcohol and other drug use among small city pregnant adolescents. *Journal of Adolescent Health, 15*, 366–373.

Landry, E., Bertrand, J., Cherry, F., & Rich, J. (1986). Teenage pregnancy in New Orleans: Factors that differentiate teens who deliver, abort, and successfully contracept. *Journal of Youth and Adolescence, 15*, 259–274.

Lee, S. H., & Grubbs, L. M. (1995). Pregnant teenagers' reasons for seeking or delaying prenatal care. *Clinical Nursing Research, 4*(1), 38–49.

Leppert, P. C., Namerow, P. B., & Barker, D. (1986). Pregnancy outcomes among adolescents and older women receiving comprehensive prenatal care. *Journal of Adolescent Health Care, 7*, 112–117.

Levy, S. R., Perhats, C., Nash-Johnson, M., & Welter, J. F. (1992). Reducing the risks in pregnant teens who are very young and those with mild mental retardation. *Mental Retardation, 30*(4), 195–203.

Lieberman, E. J. (1980). *The psychological consequences of adolescent pregnancy and abortion: Adolescent pregnancy and childbearing.* Washington, DC: Department of Health and Human Services.

Loda, F. A., Speizer, I. S., Martin, K. L., Skatrud, J. D., & Bennett, T. A. (1997). Programs and services to prevent pregnancy, childbearing, and poor birth outcomes among adolescents in rural areas of the Southeastern United States. *Journal of Adolescent Health, 21*, 157–166.

Males, M. (1993). School-age pregnancy: why hasn't prevention worked? *Journal of School Health, 63*(10), 429–432.

Marshall, E., Buckner, E., & Powell, K. (1991). Evaluation of a teen parent program designed to reduce child abuse and neglect and to strengthen families. *Journal of Child Adolescent Psychiatric and Mental Health Nursing, 4*(3), 96–100.

McFarland, A. (1998, May 5). "Family Matters." Fort Payne, AL: *The Times Journal,* p. 4.

Minter, P. (1990). Teen talk: Peer groups addressing teen pregnancy. *American Journal of Public Health, 80,* 349–350.

Morrison, D. (1985). Adolescent contraceptive behavior: A review. *Psychological Bulletin, 98,* 538–568.

Mosher, W. D. (1990). *Use of family planning services in the United States: 1982 and 1988.* Hyattsville, MD: National Center for Health Statistics.

Mott, S. (1990). Adolescence. In S. Mott, S. James, & A. Sperhac (Eds.), *Care of children and families.* Redwood City, CA: Addison-Wesley.

National Campaign to Prevent Teen Pregnancy (1998). *Ten tips for parents to help their children avoid teen pregnancy.* Washington, DC: Author.

National Center for Health Statistics (NCHS). (1990). Advance report of final natality statistics, 1990. *Monthly Vital Statistics Report, 41*(9), Supplement.

Norr, K. (1991). Community-based primary prevention of adolescent pregnancy. *Birth Defects: Original Article Series, 27*(1), 175–199.

Olds D. (1992). Home visitation for pregnant women and parents of young children. *American Journal of Diseases of Children, 146*(6), 704–708.

Olds, D., Henderson, C., & Kitzman, H. (1994). Does prenatal and infancy nurse home visitation have enduring effects on qualities of parental caregiving and child health at 25 to 50 months of life? *Pediatrics, 93*(1), 89–98.

Olds, D., Henderson, C., Tatelbaum, R., & Chamberlin, R. (1988). Improving the life-course development of socially disadvantaged mothers: A randomized trial of nurse home visitation. *American Journal of Public Health, 78*(11), 1436–1445.

Orshan, S. A. (1996). Acculturation, perceived social support, and self-esteem in primigravida Puerto Rican teenagers. *Western Journal of Nursing Research, 18*(4), 460–473.

Pittman, K., & Adams, G. (1988). *Teenage pregnancy: An advocate's guide to the numbers.* Washington, DC: Children's Defense Fund.

Plouffe, L., & White, E. W. (1996). Adolescent obstetrics and gynecology: Children having children—Can it be controlled? *Current Opinion in Obstetrics and Gynecology, 8*(5), 335–338.

Polaneczky, M. (1998). Adolescent contraception. *Current Opinion in Obstetrics & Gynecology, 10*(3), 213–219.

Pollack, A. E. (1992). Teen contraception in the 1990s. *Journal of School Health, 62*(7), 288–293.

Pratt, W., Mosher, W., Bachrach, C., & Horn, M. (1984). Understanding U.S. fertility: Findings from the National Survey of Family Growth, Cycle III. *Population Bulletin, 39,* 1–42.

Rew, L. (1998). The adolescent. In N. C. Frisch & L. E. Frisch (Eds.), *Psychiatric mental health nursing.* Albany, NY: Delmar Publishers.

Reynoso, T.C., Felice, M. E., & Shragg, G. P. (1993). Does American acculturation affect outcome of Mexican-American teenage pregnancy? *Journal of Adolescent Health, 14,* 257–261.

Robinson, R. B., & Frank, D. L. (1994). The relation between self-esteem, sexual activity, and pregnancy. *Adolescence, 29*(113), 26–35.

Rogers, M. M., Peoples-Sheps, M. D., & Suchindran, C. (1996). Impact of a social support program on teenage prenatal care use and pregnancy outcomes. *Journal of Adolescent Health, 19*, 132–140.

Roye, C. F., & Balk, S. J. (1996). The relationship of partner support to outcomes for teenage mothers and their children: A review. *Journal of Adolescent Health, 19*, 86–93.

Smith, J. B., & Hanks, C. A. (1994). Reaching out to mothers at risk. *RN*, 42–46.

Sonenstein, F. L., Pleck, J. H., & Leighton, C. K. (1989). Sexual activity, condom use, and AIDS awareness among adolescent males. *Family Planning Perspectives, 21*, 152–158.

Sonenstein, F., Stewart, K., Lindberg, L., Pernas, M., & Williams, S. (1997). Practical advice and program philosophy. *Involving males in preventing teen pregnancy*

Sorenson, D. (1973). *Adolescent sexuality in contemporary America.* New York: World Press.

Spitz, A. M., Velebil, P., Koonin, L. M., Strauss, L. T., Goodman, K. A., Wingo, P. Wilson, J. B., Morris, L., & Marks, J. S. (1996). Pregnancy, abortion, and birth rates among US adolescents—1980, 1985, and 1990. *Journal of the American Medical Association, 275*(13), 989–994.

Stevens-Simon, C., Kelly, L., Singer, D., & Cox, A. (1996). Why pregnant adolescents say they did not use contraceptives prior to contraception. *Journal of Adolescent Health, 19*, 48–53.

Taylor, H., Kagay, M., & Leichenko, S. (1986). *American teens speak: Sex myths, TV, and birth control.* New York: Planned Parenthood Federation of America.

Thompson, P. J., Powell, M. J., Patterson, R. J., & Ellerbee, S. M. (1995). Adolescent parenting: outcomes and maternal perceptions. *Journal of Obstetrical, Gynecological and Neonatal Nursing, 24*(8), 713–717.

Toledo-Dreves, V., Zabin, L. S., & Emerson, M. (1995). Duration of adolescent sexual relationships before and after conception. *Journal of Adolescent Health, 17*, 163–172.

Trad, P. V. (1999). Assessing the patterns that prevent teenage pregnancy. *Adolescence, 34*(133), 221–240.

U.S. Public Health Service (USPHS). (1997). Put prevention into practice: Unintended pregnancy. *Journal of the American Academy of Nurse Practitioners, 9*(4), 193–198.

Widom, C. S., & Kuhns, J. B. (1996). Childhood victimization and subsequent risk for promiscuity, prostitution, and teenage pregnancy: a prospective study. *American Journal of Public Health, 86*(11), 1607–1612.

Yoder, B. A., & Young, M. K. (1997). Neonatal outcomes of teenage pregnancy in a military population. *Obstetrics & Gynecology, 90*(4), 500–506.

Zabin, L. S., Kantner, J., & Zelnik, M. (1979). The risk of adolescent pregnancy in the first months of intercourse. *Family Planning Perspectives, 11*, 215–226.

Zabin, L. S., & Clark, S. D. (1981). Why they delay: A study of teenage family planning clinic patients. *Family Planning Perspective, 13*, 205–217.

Zabin, L. S., Emerson, M. R., & Ringers, P. A., & Sedivy, V. (1996). Adolescents with negative pregnancy test results: An accessible at-risk group. *Journal of the American Medical Association, 275*(2), 113–117.

Zelnik, M., & Kantner, J. F. (1979). Reasons for nonuse of contraception by sexually active women age 15–19. *Family Planning Perspectives, 11*(5), 289–296.

Zelnik, M, Kantner, J. F., & Ford, K. (1981). *Sex and pregnancy in adolescence.* Beverly Hills, CA: Sage Publications.

Zoccolillo, M., Meyers, J., & Assiter, S. (1997). Conduct disorder, substance dependence, and adolescent motherhood. *American Journal of Orthopsychiatry, 67*(1), 152–157.

Zuckerman, B. S., Walker, D. K., Frank, D. A., Chase, C., & Hamburg, B. (1984). Adolescent pregnancy: Biobehavioral determinants of outcome. *Journal of Pediatrics, 105*(6), 857–863.

Chapter 29
Disabilities and Health
Valerie M. DeCoux and Linda G. McDowell

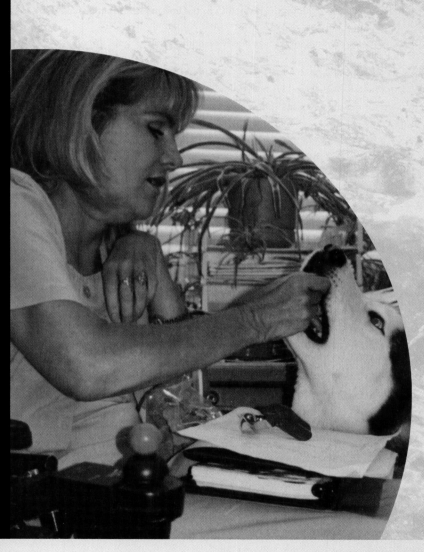

The move toward community services for individuals with disabilities has greatly expanded the role of the community health nurse. Although in the past this population was served primarily by nurses and physicians in institutional settings (hospitals, rehabilitation centers, nursing homes, or state residential facilities), there has been a strong movement to include people with disabilities in community life and offer a comprehensive array of individualized, community-based services.

QUESTIONS TO CONSIDER

After reading this chapter, answer the following questions:
1. What is a disability?
2. What are the legal protections for a person with disabilities?
3. How should we communicate with a person with disabilities?
4. What are community living needs related to caring for a population with disabilities?
5. What services are available for persons with disabilities?
6. Are there ethical issues that still influence the care of persons with disabilities?
7. What are specific roles for the community health nurse in caring for a population with disabilities?

KEY TERMS

Assistive technology
  device
Case management
Disability
Early intervention

Individualized education
  plans
Individualized family
  service plan
Informed consent

Medical assistive devices
Mental impairment
People-first language
Personal care attendant
Person-centered planning

Physical impairment
Rehabilitation
Respite care

Approximately 20% of individuals in the United States have some kind of a disability, and 10% have a severe disability. We can expect an increase in the number of people with disabilities (incidence of disability increases with age) as the baby boom generation ages and the life expectancy of the general population increases. Primarily through development of advanced surgical techniques and medications, medicine has made great strides in increasing the survival of infants, children, and adults with disabilities. Now, the more difficult task of improving the overall quality of life for these individuals is at hand. Society, including members with disabilities, has come to expect not only a long life, but a rich, fulfilling life as well.

Community health nursing is poised as the key profession to integrate knowledge of the health care needs of people with disabilities with the often more challenging needs related to full inclusion in community life. In addition to possessing the knowledge required to serve in the traditional role of caregiver, the community health nurse must be well versed in disability legislation; issues of accessibility, work, housing, transportation, and recreation; use of technology; and case management strategies required to navigate the complex and inconsistent service system presently in place.

....

The only disability in life is a bad attitude.

Scott Hamilton

....

Definitions

Terms can be useful when people who share something in common are grouped together for easier communication about them. Terms can be harmful, however, when the focus is on the label and anticipated problems rather than on the unique capabilities of each individual. Labels usually generate predictions of what a person can or cannot do, and a person tends to act based on the expectations of others. Each person within a particular disability category has different abilities and will require varying levels of assistance and support. To offer appropriate help, the community health nurse should get to know the capabilities and needs of each person before making assumptions about their needs based on a disability label (DiLeo, 1993).

The term **disability** "is now being used to indicate that an individual has some functional limitation due to an alteration in anatomy (internal or external physical configuration, such as short stature or missing limbs) or physiology (organic processes, such as paralysis, decreased cardiac function, or ineffectiveness of the immune system)" (Hablutzel & McMahon, 1992). For the purposes of protection by the Americans with Disabilities Act (ADA, 1990), *disability* is defined as "(a) a physical or mental impairment that substantially limits one or more of the major life activities of such individual; (b) a record of such an impairment; or (c) being regarded as having such an impairment" (U.S. Department of Justice, 1992, p. 8). If an individual meets any one of these three criteria, he or she is considered an individual with a disability for the purposes covered by the ADA. When enacting the ADA in 1990, Congress adopted the same basic definition of disability first used in the Rehabilitation Act of 1973 and the Fair Housing Amendments of 1988. Congress used the term *disability* rather than *handicap* in an effort to use up-to-date, currently accepted terminology. The term *handicap* is not a synonym for disability and is now rarely used other than to describe parking places and facility accessibility.

Physical impairment according to the ADA is "any physiological disorder or condition, cosmetic disfigurement, or anatomical loss affecting one or more of the . . . body systems," including, for example, orthopedic, visual, and hearing impairments; cerebral palsy; epilepsy; muscular dystrophy; multiple sclerosis; and human immunodeficiency virus (HIV) disease (symptomatic or asymptomatic) (U.S. Department of Justice, 1992, p. 8).

Mental impairment "is any mental or psychological disorder, such as mental retardation, organic brain syndrome, emotional or mental illness, and specific learning disabilities" (U.S. Department of Justice, 1992, p. 8).

Incidence of Disabilities

Approximately 1 in 5 Americans have some type of disability causing difficulty in performing certain functions (e.g., seeing, hearing, walking, talking, climbing stairs, lifting, carrying), have difficulty with activities of daily living (e.g., bathing, dressing, toileting, feeding), or have difficulty with certain social roles (e.g., doing schoolwork, performing household chores, working). About 1 in 10 Americans have a disability so severe that he or she is unable to perform certain basic activities, such as walking, dressing, or speaking; must use assistive devices such as a wheelchair or scooter for mobility; or need personal assistance to perform basic activities. Among children ages 6 to 14, about 1 in 8 has some type of disability. The number or percentage of adults with a disability is more difficult to determine and will not represent the same percentages as in the school-age population. Some disabilities, recognized during the school years, become difficult to detect in adult settings, even though the impact may be significant. For instance, individuals with learning disabilities or mental illness may go unidentified for long periods and are often not counted in studies reporting the incidence of disabilities in adulthood. The incidence of disability increases significantly with age; about half of adults age 65 and older have a disability. As the population continues to age, we can expect the proportion of the population having disabilities to increase accordingly (U.S. Department of Commerce, 1997). Table 29-1 provides examples of disabling conditions, and their etiologies, incidence,

TABLE 29-1   **EXAMPLES OF DISABILITY, ETIOLOGY, INCIDENCE, AND EFFECTS**

DISABILITY	ETIOLOGY	FREQUENCY	EFFECTS (SELECTED)
Amputation	Trauma, bone cancer, diabetes	Not available	Impaired mobility
Autism	Brain damage, abnormality in brain development, genetic predisposition	10/10,000 live births[1]	Impaired reciprocal social interaction, impaired communication and imaginative activity, markedly restricted repertoire of interests and activities
Cerebral palsy	Perinatal anoxia, trauma, intraventricular hemorrhage, or stroke; trauma, meningitis in early childhood	1.4–2.4/ 1,000 births[1]	Difficulty with balance, coordination and movement, hypertonicity. Associated with sensory impairments, seizures, mental retardation
Down syndrome	Genetic; extra chromosome 21	1/700–1/1,000 live births[1]	Mental retardation, hypotonia, physical characteristics, sensory impairments, decreased immunity, frequent respiratory infections and otitis media, increased incidence of leukemia, thyroid problems, early onset Alzheimer-type dementia
Duchenne's muscular dystrophy (MD)	Genetic, inherited as a sex-linked trait, affects males	1/3,500 males[1]	Increasing muscle weakness beginning with waddling gait and resulting in need for crutches or wheelchair; eventually heart and diaphragm are affected; usually causes death before adulthood
Fetal alcohol syndrome (FAS)	Maternal alcohol ingestion resulting in prenatal exposure (leading known cause of mental retardation)	1–2/1,000 births[1]	Mental retardation, decreased height and weight, facial characteristics, behavior problems including hyperactivity and noncompliance
Fragile X syndrome	Genetic; inherited as a sex-linked trait	1/1,500 males 1/500 females[1]	Mental retardation, hypotonia, physical characteristics, behavior problems such as self-stimulatory behavior, self-injurious behavior, and aggression
Hearing impairment	Otitis media (middle ear infections), congenital malformation, genetic, prenatal exposure to maternal virus or drug, meningitis, head trauma	1/1,000 infants born with severe to profound hearing loss[1]	Ranges from mild hearing impairment to deafness; developmental delay, language impairment, need for hearing aid, FM trainer, speech-language therapy, sign language.
Polio	Polio virus causes paralysis below part of spinal column damaged by virus	Eliminated since 1991 but 16,316 cases of paralytic polio occurred from 1951–1954[3]	Paralysis, complications related to immobility (decubiti, fractures), postpolio syndrome in mid to late adulthood causing increased severity of symptoms
Spina bifida (myelomeningocele)	Multifactorial etiology; environmental causes including folic acid deficiency and genetic influences	60/100,000 births[1]	Paralysis below level of defect, impaired ambulation requiring crutches, walker or wheelchair, lack of bowel & bladder control, hydrocephalus requiring shunt, seizures, vision problems, mental retardation, complications related to immobility

Continued

TABLE 29-1   EXAMPLES OF DISABILITY, ETIOLOGY, INCIDENCE, AND EFFECTS—CONT'D

DISABILITY	ETIOLOGY	FREQUENCY	EFFECTS (SELECTED)
Spinal cord injury (SCI)	Trauma from diving accidents and motor vehicle accidents	250,000 individuals with SCI in the United States[2]	Paralysis, hypotonia and muscle wasting, incontinence, complications related to immobility and repeated catheterization; high-level injuries can also cause inability to breathe without assistance
Traumatic brain injury (TBI)	Trauma from motor vehicle accidents, gunshots, child abuse	71–125 per 100,000 (22% of those died)[2]	Motor, communication, cognitive, sensory, and behavioral deficits
Vision impairment	Prenatal exposure to viruses or bacteria, prematurity and oxygen treatment, eye trauma, chemical burns, diabetes, glaucoma, cataracts	1/3,000 children are blind[1]; vision impairment increases significantly in older adults	Ranges from poor sight to total blindness

[1]Batshaw, 1997.
[2]Marino, 1999.
[3]CDC, 1999.

and effects on the individual. Table 29-2 lists recommended popular films that portray main characters with disabilities.

The effects of disability on the individual, family, and community vary and are related to a number of variables, including age and rapidity of onset, cause, and severity of the disability. Personal characteristics such as determination and resiliency along with available family and community support also play a role in determining the impact of a disability.

TABLE 29-2   POPULAR FILMS PORTRAYING CHARACTERS WITH DISABILITIES

FILM	DISABILITY	FILM	DISABILITY
As Good As It Gets	Obsessive-compulsive disorder	Man Without a Face, The Mask	Craniofacial defect
Benny & Joon	Schizophrenia	The Miracle Worker	Deaf/blind
Best Boy	Mental retardation	My Left Foot	Cerebral palsy
Born on the Fourth of July	Spinal cord injury	One Flew over the Cuckoo's Nest	Mental illness/institutional care
Charley	Mental retardation	Philadelphia	AIDS
Children of a Lesser God	Hearing impairment	Rain Man	Autism
The Elephant Man	Physical disability	Rear Window	Spinal cord injury
First Do No Harm	Epilepsy	Regarding Henry	Traumatic brain injury
The Fisher King	Schizophrenia	Scent of a Woman	Visual impairment
Forrest Gump	Mental retardation	Sling Blade	Mental retardation
The Heart Is a Lonely Hunter	Hearing impairment	There's Something About Mary	Mental retardation
La Strada	Mental retardation	What About Bob?	Anxiety disorder
The Last Picture Show	Mental retardation	What's Eating Gilbert Grape	Mental retardation
Lorenzo's Oil	Adrenoleukodystrophy (ALD)		

Historical Context of Disability Services and Disability Legislation

Beirne-Smith, Patton, and Ittenbach (1994) paint a clear picture of how society's values and historical events have influenced the lives of people with disabilities. Before the 1700s, services for persons with disabilities were virtually nonexistent. In the United States, the family unit was of prime importance, so most of the responsibility for caring for a member with a disability rested on the family. The colonies also enacted laws that provided some support in the forms of poorhouses and workhouses. During the first part of the 1800s, there was an attitude of optimism, and it was believed that children with mental retardation or other disabilities could be trained, "cured," and returned to the community as productive citizens. By the late 1800s, however, society recognized that these individuals could not be "cured." People with disabilities were then pitied, resulting in decreased opportunities for systematic training and increased formation of institutions. By the end of the 1800s, the general attitude of pity shifted to fear. Citizens became concerned that "mentally defective" people were dangerous, and society responded with restricted marriages, mandatory sterilization, and institutionalization (Cegelka & Prehm, 1982). This alarmist attitude was based on a fear of the inheritability of mental defectiveness and its perceived relationship to poverty, crime, incorrigibility, and disease.

One ironically positive occurrence in the early 1900s was the return of World War I veterans with war-caused disabilities. As a result, in 1920, the Vocational Rehabilitation Act brought medical and rehabilitation services not only to veterans, but also to others who displayed a need. President Franklin D. Roosevelt's administration improved the situation somewhat with passage of the Social Security Act of 1935 and a supportive attitude toward public welfare programs. As more veterans with disabilities returned home during World War II, a concern for the rights of citizens with disabilities grew. Although government services had finally become available for individuals with disabilities in the 1920s, these services continued to be provided in ways that segregated people with disabilities from others until the 1970s (Berkowitz, 1987). During most of the 20th century, "literally, through institutionalization, and subtly, through negative attitudes and behaviors, people with disabilities have been isolated from the social mainstream and denied the benefits and opportunities available to people without disabilities" (Ward, 1996, p. 4).

Fortunately, advances in medical care such as the development of antibiotics in the 1940s and 1950s and increasingly successful surgical procedures for spina bifida, hydrocephalus, and congenital heart defects since the 1970s, coupled with developmental and rehabilitation services, have enabled people with disabilities to live longer. Public outrage and court involvement in response to abusive conditions in institutions, along with research on the negative impact of institutionalization, led to the development of services in local communities in the 1960s and 1970s.

With the expectation that most individuals with disabilities will live to adulthood, society and policy makers have been forced to consider strategies to protect the rights of these individuals.

Current Situation for People with Disabilities

In 1998, the Harris survey of Americans with disabilities reported a number of facts related to the quality of life for people with disabilities in the United States. Although a majority of Americans with disabilities believe that life has improved for people with disabilities over the past 10 years, adults with disabilities still lag behind other adults in most aspects of life. Examining the areas of employment, housing/income, education, and health care highlights how the existence of a disability continues to place an individual at risk in many aspects of life. In the area of employment, 3 of 10 adults with disabilities are working (29%), compared with 8 out of 10 adults without disabilities (79%); this statistic has remained the same for the past 10 years. For housing/income, 1 in 3 (34%) adults with disabilities are in very–low-income housing with annual incomes of less than $15,000, compared with 1 in 8 (12%) of those without disabilities. When examining the area of education, data show that 1 in 5 adults with disabilities (25%) have not completed high school, compared with 1 in 10 adults without disabilities (9%). Finally, in the area of health care, 1 in 5 adults with disabilities (21%) did not get the medical care that they needed on at least one occasion during the past year, compared with 1 in 10 adults without disabilities (11%) (National Organization on Disability, 1998).

Despite these areas of difficulty, many people with disabilities reported improvement over the past 10 years in access to public facilities and transportation, quality of life, public attitudes toward people with disabilities, and how the media portray people with disabilities (National Organization on Disability, 1998). These improvements may in part be due to increased awareness of the Americans with Disabilities Act of 1990 or additional laws passed in recent years to protect people with disabilities.

....

We who live with disabilities have been silenced by those who did not want to hear what have to say. We have also been silenced by our own fear.

Kenny Fries

....

Legislation Protecting the Rights of People with Disabilities

Strongly influenced by the civil rights movements of the 1960s, the disability community began to fight for the right to integration and meaningful equality of opportunity. Although the U.S.

Constitution protects the rights of all citizens, individuals with disabilities have needed additional protection under the law from exploitation, abuse, and neglect. Specific rights (affirmative rights and protection from mistreatment) of citizens with disabilities have been defined in federal and state laws and are represented in state agency policies and procedures. Affirmative rights, which are designed to meet individual needs and promote independence, include the right to effective and appropriate services as close as possible to home. Eligible individuals with disabilities and their family members have the right to participate in service planning meetings, to be notified if and why services are terminated, and to be informed of the process for challenging the decision. Adults with disabilities have the right to manage their own affairs, including the decision of how to spend money, how to use their free time, how to manage their own possessions, where and with whom to live and work, how to worship, and whether to vote.

Some individuals with disabilities will need assistance in making effective decisions about their lives. Information about options and consequences of choices should be presented in ways the person will understand. Once educated decisions have been made, they should be respected and supported (DiLeo, 1993).

Laws are also in place to protect individuals with disabilities from mistreatment, including acts of negligence or intentional acts such as corporal punishment or abuse (physical, sexual, verbal, or mental) leading to physical or emotional harm. Courts may appoint a guardian to intervene in the choices (i.e., certain medical treatment decisions) an individual with disabilities might otherwise make in accordance with their affirmative rights. The Social Security Administration may establish a payee of funds if it is determined that an individual with disabilities receiving Social Security benefits is unable to manage his or her own income.

Congress passed several critical pieces of disability legislation that began to protect the rights of people with disabilities. See Table 29-3 for a summary of legislative milestones for people with disabilities in the United States. The most significant piece of legislation has been Public Law (P.L.) No. 101-336, the ADA, which reaffirmed the rights of individuals with disabilities to equal access to facilities and opportunities and expanded these rights to all services offered to the public, not just those receiving federal funds.

The ADA is the most significant disability-related legislation to date, including provisions affecting employment, state and

---

TABLE 29-3   **LEGISLATIVE MILESTONES FOR PEOPLE WITH DISABILITIES**

TITLE	PURPOSE
P.L. 93-112 Sec. 504 of the Rehabilitation Act (1973)	Initiated legislation to prohibit discrimination against and to provide access to persons with disabilities in programs receiving federal funds. Amendments ensured no discrimination in education and employment. Also known as the "Bill of Rights for People with Disabilities."
P.L. 94-103 (1974)	The Developmental Disabilities Assistance and Bill of Rights Act defined the term *developmental disabilities* and provided funding to states and university-affiliated programs.
P.L. 94-142 (1975)	The Education for All Handicapped Children Act required states to provide a free appropriate education for all children with disabilities between the ages of 3 and 18.
P.L. 99-457, Part H (1986)	Amended P.L. 94-142 to include children from birth through age 2 and their families.
P.L. 101-476 (1990)	The Individuals with Disabilities Education Act (IDEA) was the reauthorization of P.L. 94-142 and entitles all students ages 3–21 with disabilities a free, appropriate public education in the least restricted environment. Included incentives for providing services for children from birth to 2 years old. School districts are required to identify and evaluate children with disabilities at no cost to families. The law added a further requirement for schools to provide transition services to students with disabilities.
P.L. 101-336 (1991)	The Americans with Disabilities Act (ADA) reaffirmed the rights of individuals with disabilities to equal access to facilities and opportunities and expanded this right to all services offered to the public, not just those receiving federal funds.
P.L. 102-569 (1992)	The 1992 Amendments to the Rehabilitation Act emphasized competitive employment outcomes, integrated settings, helping students make transitions from school to work, using profit-making organizations for on-the-job training, and the assumption that persons with disabilities can benefit from vocational rehabilitation services.
P.L. 103-218 (1994)	The Technology-Related Assistance Act for Individuals with Disabilities provided grant funding for programs providing technology assistance that is responsive to consumer needs.

local government services, public transportation, public accommodations, and telecommunications. Provisions stipulate that employers may not discriminate against individuals with disabilities in hiring or promotion and must provide reasonable accommodations. All government facilities, services, and communications must be accessible, as must new buses and rail cars. Places of public accommodation, including restaurants, hotels, and stores, may not discriminate against individuals with disabilities, and in fact must proactively make efforts to include people with disabilities in services offered. All new construction or alteration of facilities must be accessible, and telephone companies must offer telephone relay services to persons who use telecommunication devices (Jenkins, Patterson, & Szymanski, 1992).

Unfortunately, the presence of policy and legislation offering protections to individuals with disabilities does not ensure compliance or positive outcomes (Sands & Wehmeyer, 1996). In fact, their very existence is worthless unless people with disabilities and their advocates demand enforcement. In addition, attitudes toward people with disabilities cannot be legislated, and negative attitudes remain a barrier to full inclusion in all aspects of community life.

Appropriate Language for Communicating About Persons with Disabilities

The community health nurse should use language that is current and endorsed by the disability community when speaking or writing about people with disabilities. The words we choose and the way we structure sentences can create a clear, positive view of persons with disabilities or a negative, discriminatory portrayal that reinforces common stereotypes. One of the best known guidelines is that of **people-first language**, with which the speaker puts the person first, not the disability. For example, the community health nurse should refer to "the child with mental retardation" or "a man with Down syndrome." One exception to the people-first language guideline is when speaking about deaf people. Many deaf people do not consider themselves disabled and prefer to be called a "deaf person" rather than a "person who is deaf" or a "person with a hearing impairment." Deaf people often see themselves as members of a subculture with their own language, customs, and ways of perceiving their roles in the hearing world (Craft, 1995). When in doubt, the community health nurse should ask clients how they wish to be described.

The community health nurse must avoid using language that characterizes the person with a disability as pitiable. Do not say "afflicted with," "crippled with," or "suffers from." Rather, say "the person *has* a spinal cord injury" or speak about "the person *with* spina bifida." Words such as *crippled* or *deformed* are never acceptable. The word *handicapped,* which was once used to refer to a person with a disability, has been redefined. *Handicap* now refers to a functional limitation that varies based on the conditions in the environment of the individual. For example, although a person with a spinal cord injury has a disability, whether or not that individual has a handicap in a certain situation would depend on conditions such as lack of a ramp to a building entrance. Finally, emphasize abilities, not limitations. Health care providers should never say "confined to a wheelchair" or "wheelchair-bound." These negative phrases connote pity and can encourage dependency. Instead, the professional should say "uses a wheelchair" or "uses crutches." (Research and Training Center on Independent Living, 1996).

Community Living Needs of People Who Have Disabilities

Legislation has been passed to ensure that environments in which people with disabilities live and work follow the patterns of life and conditions that most people experience. Children and adults with disabilities have the right to live in homes and attend school or work within integrated settings with nondisabled peers. For example, most adults live in settings of their choosing, with people of their choice, getting up and going to bed at "normal" times, eating three meals a day about five hours apart, going to work, and choosing their own recreational activities and friends. Social movements (e.g., "normalization" and now "inclusion") have urged the provision of opportunities and supports for individuals with disabilities to enable them to live and work in their communities (DiLeo, 1993; Wehman, 1996).

Similar to individualized family services plans and individualized education plans, which are discussed later in this chapter as plans of service for children, individual service plans of assistance and skill enhancement can be written for adolescents and adults to identify the supports needed to transition to work, further education, or other living arrangements. These plans are written with the individual with a disability and/or family members as the most important members of the team. An approach called **person-centered planning** brings a team of people together who care about the individual with disabilities to listen, learn, and help him or her plan for the future. Family members, who generally know the person best, are viewed as not only a source of critical information about that individual but also as a valued decision maker. The team's job is to discover resources, within the person and in the community; help access these resources; and determine support roles necessary for promoting positive community living. Those support roles may be an advocate, a bridge builder, and/or a network creator. These roles are especially critical in systems where empowerment of individuals and their family members in decision making for community living and work is not a priority of service provision (DiLeo, 1993; Wehman, 1996).

Unfortunately, service plans are still being written that segregate individuals with disabilities. Segregated situations are often established under the premise that people need to "get ready" for living and working in the community. Work and living skills, however, are best learned in real jobs, homes, and communities. Program activities with self-contained groups of people with disabilities in perpetual preparation for the real world by traveling, recreating, working, and living together do not promote the uniqueness and value of each individual with a disability, nor do they prepare individuals for life in the community (DiLeo, 1993; Wehman, 1996).

Our society, with cultural values of productivity, skill, attractiveness, and affluence, still views people with disabilities as different in a negative way, perceived as incompetent or as children who never grew up, "funny looking," or even dangerous. The most powerful way to change negative societal attitudes is for individuals with disabilities to participate successfully in their communities, as skilled and productive workers and managers of their own homes (with the right supports). As neighbors, co-workers, and friends, people with disabilities demonstrate their adult needs for expression of personal accomplishment, responsibility, interdependence, privacy, and sexuality. The more opportunities for choice and the more competencies an individual possesses, the more self-esteem and status he or she will have in the community. Community health nurses who provide assistance should show care in interactions, choosing moments to teach and methods of support provision that are professionally appropriate and demonstrate personal respect. For example, the community health nurse should use minimal cues, gestures, and words (the less assistance the better, to counteract dependency), watching tone and volume, to promote the dignity of the individual and not convey an attitude of pity or assume a parental role.

Homes of Their Own

Historically, people with significant disabilities, particularly those with mental impairments, had two living options. Either the family could care for the individual at home indefinitely, with little, if any, public assistance, or the family could place the individual in a state residential facility. Current beliefs about the rights of people with disabilities support that (1) all children, including those with severe disabilities, have the right to live at home with their family; and (2) adults with disabilities have the right to the supports necessary to live in a home in the community, either alone or with another adult of their choosing.

Living options for people with disabilities are often presented on a continuum from large segregated facilities at one end to group homes or homes of their own at the other. Such a continuum reinforces the past belief that large residential institutions or large group homes can be legitimate options as places to live. Most professionals believe that "the people who were most often viewed as needing to live in larger, specialized facilities, such as institutions and group homes, were often the very people who most benefited from the opportunities a smaller place offered" (Racino & Taylor, 1993, p. 36). When these smaller group homes are managed based on the same model of services as the large facilities, however, people with disabilities are still shortchanged. The pseudo-home can be highly routinized, "run" by service providers, and "homelike" in atmosphere, but it is not truly a home.

Living arrangements can vary from a home of one's own, a semi-independent or supported apartment (with staff available to assist), a home with one's family, a foster home, or a group home (Kirk, Gallagher, & Anastasiow, 1993; Wehman, 1996). Regardless of the type of living arrangement a person wants, needs, and can reasonably afford, there should be opportunity for choice, ownership of personal property, and privacy. For example, the individual should choose the type of neighborhood, style of home, landscaping, furnishings, and decorations, all choices demonstrating the individual is a competent adult. Also, a person should own his or her possessions, make choices in how to spend his or her own money, and choose activities he or she wishes to participate in. If there is a roommate (by choice of the individual), arrangements should be made for privacy, such as providing personal space and securing private items.

Housing must be accessible for the individual with a disability. Contractors and builders may be unaware of modifications or regulations involving accessibility, and few accessible houses or apartments are available, particularly in rural areas. The community health nurse can educate community members and leaders regarding housing needs of adults with disabilities, which in many ways overlap the needs of older adults in the community: the need for safe, affordable, and accessible housing choices. Information related to accessibility is available through each state's Department of Rehabilitation Services or Office of Vocational Rehabilitation Services, along with ample information available on the Internet.

A person with a disability may require assistance in the home to carry out activities of daily living such as bathing, dressing, cooking, eating, and toileting. It is estimated that about 9 million individuals in the United States (approximately 3% of the population) need personal assistance to carry out typical daily activities. Although most of these helpers are relatives (80%), in many cases, the individual with a disability must hire a helper to come into the home (U.S. Department of Commerce, 1997). A **personal care attendant** can be employed to assist with activities of daily living, transportation, pet care, and household chores and maintenance. Personal assistant services also include interpreting, mobility assistance, social support, medical assistance, reading, and recreation. Unfortunately, availability of attendants, coordinating agencies, and public funding options vary greatly from state to state.

Families who may be caring for a child or adult with a significant disability 24 hours a day need the option of **respite care** to prevent caregiver burnout. Respite care provides another caregiver to assume the round-the-clock care of the family member with a disability, allowing the caretaker a vacation, a mental health break, time to recover from illness, or merely time to oneself. Because of the significant medical problems that individuals with severe disabilities may have, the respite provider (e.g., church, civic group, the Association for the Rights of Citizens) often will recruit nurses in the community to serve as respite caregivers. Respite may be provided in the client's home, at a group home, in a private home, or at an organization's facility.

An Accessible Community

Accessibility to all that a community offers is critical if persons with disabilities are to participate to the fullest extent possible in community life. Many individuals with disabilities cannot afford to own customized vehicles to drive or may be physically or mentally unable to drive. Accessible public transportation is needed by many persons who are disabled so that they may work, recreate, worship, seek medical attention, socialize, and so on, as we all do on a daily basis. Inadequate transportation was cited as a problem by 30% of adults with disabilities in a 1998 Harris poll. Many areas are lacking adequate public transportation, particularly in rural areas of the country. By the year 2002, all public busses must be accessible. Facility accessibility is also necessary and required by the ADA. It is accomplished by accommodations such as curb cuts, ramps, large doorways with easily opened doors, elevators, and wide hallways. The community health nurse can educate community leaders about these needs for access and may become involved in advocating for individual clients or working with legislators for policy reform. Individuals who use wheelchairs for mobility are often frustrated with the inadequate involvement of people with disabilities in the development of facilities that comply with ADA accessibility requirements (Pierce, 1998). Ideally, a person who uses a wheelchair should serve on committees involved in designing buildings to ensure that they not only meet ADA requirements, but also are functional for those who use wheelchairs or who have other types of disabilities.

Meaningful Work

In addition to the obvious benefit of work as a way to earn money, meaningful work allows individuals to be contributing members of society and to enjoy social contact. Many people with disabilities have limited opportunity for friendships. Adults with mental retardation often do not have the opportunity to develop meaningful, reciprocated friendships and instead must rely entirely on paid caretakers, family members, or other obligated people as their friends (Green & Schleien, 1991). Work offers the opportunity to develop working relationships with other workers while interacting to solve problems, complete assignments, and express oneself.

Vocational options for individuals with mild to severe disabilities range from day treatment programs and sheltered workshops to supportive employment and competitive employment in community businesses. Each of the options represents less and less supervision and assistance for the individual with disabilities in a work setting. Box 29-1 presents an array of employment opportunities for persons with disabilities.

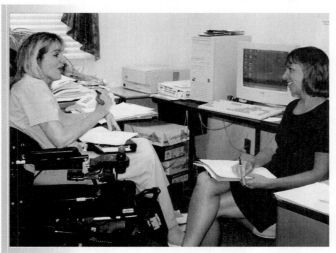

Dr. Valerie DeCoux, chapter author, consults with faculty member with disability.

BOX 29-1 VOCATIONAL SERVICES FOR PERSONS WITH DISABILITIES

Nonvocational day treatment programs focus on daily living skills and therapy. Partly vocational day activity services combine training in daily living skills with some vocational experiences, typically in a simulated environment. Vocational experiences are usually based on manual skills such as sorting, cleaning, or assembling. Sheltered workshops offer the individual with a disability pay for piece work in a facility that usually does subcontract work for a company. All employees in such a work environment have disabilities. Semi-sheltered group enclaves or work crews are small groups of individuals with disabilities who perform paid work for real businesses. Rather than being employed by the business, however, the employees work under the auspices of a human services agency, which bills the business. Individual supported or transitional jobs offer, with ongoing support of a human service agency, a paid job in which the person with a disability is hired and supervised by a business, much as a typical employee would be. Competitive (unsupported) employment is paid employment in which an individual with a disability is hired and directly supervised by an employer. Support from a human service agency is gradually phased out, and the employee works without support or intrusion from human service professionals.

Adapted from Hagner & DiLeo, 1993.

Competitive community employment not only provides wages to support a lifestyle of choice, means of purchasing desired items, and funds for recreational pursuits, but it also brings self-esteem, respect from others, a sense of accomplishment, and personal growth. For example, a downtown office job can promote self-esteem and respect for an individual with disabilities. A job may bring about more attention to personal appearance, new friends, and pride in a new role contributing to an organization. In time, the individual may receive better paying, long-term, higher status positions. A job and relationships built on a job can also help co-workers and employers view the individual as an individual, rather than as a representative of a particular disability category (DiLeo, 1993; Wehman, 1996).

A recent 1998 Harris survey cited a number of factors that facilitated beginning or continuing employment for people with disabilities. Three major factors identified as helpful were assistance from vocational rehabilitation (23%); getting equipment or a device that they needed to do their work, talk with other workers, or get around at work (21%); and getting an interpreter or personal care attendant (7%). For those individuals with disabilities who did not work full-time, reasons given included the following: employers do not recognize they are capable of doing the job (42%); they lack skills, education, or training needed to get the job (33%); they need a personal assistant to help get to work or to do the job (32%); they risk losing benefits or insurance (31%); no work is available in the line of work respondent could do (29%); and special equipment or devices are needed to do the work, talk to or hear other workers, or get around at work (28%) (National Organization on Disability, 1998).

Years of research verify that individuals with disabilities who need long-term employment assistance fare better in supported employment than in sheltered workshops (Noble & Conley, 1987). To assist individuals with severe disabilities to succeed in employment, professionals must identify suitable opportunities within community businesses and develop the supports that those individuals need. Inclusive employment within the community is the right of all people, including those with significant disabilities.

Relationships

All people experience sexual feelings, and individuals with disabilities are no exception. Sexual activity is one of the most controversial issues pertaining to the lives of individuals with disabilities, particularly mental retardation. Sexual development for individuals with mental retardation is for the most part similar to persons without mental retardation. Many professionals argue that individuals have the right to socially appropriate sexual expression. Others disagree and are concerned about outcomes, including unwanted advances (e.g., rape, incest) and sexually transmitted diseases. Appropriate sexual expression is more difficult for individuals with mental retardation who have higher levels of supervision and support. They may not have information about sexual development and functioning and typically have fewer socialization opportunities in which to practice appropriate behav-

iors, roles, and expectations (Beirne-Smith, Patton, & Ittenbach, 1994).

Individuals with physical disabilities such as spinal cord injuries or cerebral palsy also may need education regarding sexuality. The community health nurse and other professionals assisting individuals with disabilities may have to set aside their own sexual values in order not to deny, limit, or inhibit an individual's interest in romance and sex. People with disabilities should receive sex education, sexual health care information, and opportunities for socializing, sexual expression, and intimacy.

Recreation

Participating in recreational activities is an important aspect of life for individuals with disabilities, just as it is for others in our society. Recreation may take the form of individual or team games, athletic programs in schools, college-sponsored recreational sports, employer-sponsored activities, church-sponsored activities, and family recreation. Specific activities include outdoor recreation (e.g., birding, hiking, bike riding, canoeing, softball) and indoor activities (e.g., ceramics, painting, aerobics, weight lifting, racquetball). Ideally, recreational activities in the community serve to promote physical health and conditioning, improve social skills, facilitate friendships, and develop specific skills. Although achieving a balance between work and leisure is important for everyone, it is especially critical for people with disabilities. Many individuals with disabilities who work do not have recreational outlets for evenings and weekends. Community recreation programs have been slow to accept responsibility for offering programming that includes people with disabilities. "It is not enough merely to open programs to people with disabilities; the professionals in charge of the programs must go further and actively recruit and encourage the participation of people with disabilities and provide them with successful and ongoing mechanisms of support" (Schleien, Ray, & Green, 1997, p. 19). Community recreational opportunities ranging from individual skill building to competitive international competition are becoming increasingly available to people with disabilities and are supported by recreational specialists and special equipment (e.g., modified bowling balls, walkers for ice skating, sit-skis for snow skiing). In addition to group participation in community-based opportunities for recreation, home-centered hobbies such as card games, board games, collections, and other leisure interests should be encouraged.

Adults with disabilities may attend fewer social and cultural activities than adults without disabilities. Although they attend a place of worship almost as often as individuals without disabilities (54% as compared with 57%), their participation in other social events is typically less. For example, only 33% of adults with disabilities go to a restaurant at least once a week, compared with 60% of those without disabilities; 70% of people with disabilities did not go to a sporting event in the past year; only 48% went to the movies or the theater during the past year; and only 27% attended a live music performance at least once during the year (National Organization on Disability, 1998).

Services for Individuals with Disabilities

Case Management

The vast array of services required by many individuals with disabilities requires some system of central coordination. This system is called *case management*. **Case management** has been defined as "the collaborative provision of coordinated care by professionals from multiple disciplines, in one or more settings, over a period of time, to achieve specific outcomes" (Trachtenberg & Lewis, 1996, p. 203). After its inception in the mental health field, case management was later adopted in the rehabilitation field in the 1960s and 1970s. The intent of current disability legislation, along with the special interests of third-party payers, has driven the development of case management as a way not only to coordinate services but also to allocate resources. Persons with disabilities often have complex problems requiring services from a multitude of agencies. An interdisciplinary case management team identifies problems, formulates goals, and coordinates the services needed. In the process, gaps and redundancies in the community service system may be identified and dealt with. Case management teams therefore not only serve the targeted client, but also have the potential to improve the overall service system for persons with disabilities in the community.

The case manager may be the individual with the disability, a family member, or an agency service provider, such as the community health nurse. Although the case manager may represent a particular agency, he or she must look beyond the agency's prescribed services to address the broad range of client needs across all possible support agencies. To complicate matters further, an individual receiving services through several different agencies may have multiple case managers, assigned by health service agencies, social service agencies, or insurance companies. Communication among these case managers is essential to avoid the risk of duplication or omission of services. At this time, there are no requirements for certification of case managers. A case manager for one agency may be master's degree–prepared social worker, and another agency may use nonprofessionals with varying educational backgrounds. Some clients, to ensure that their needs and not the needs of the agencies are being met, may contract with a private case manager on a fee-for-service basis. Whether initiated to better meet the client's needs, to better allocate scarce resources, or to ensure adherence to a treatment plan, case management has the potential to encourage communication between the parties involved in order to meet clearly defined client-generated goals.

Educational Programming

For young children with disabilities, promoting optimal development in the gross motor, fine motor, language, cognition, adaptive/self-help, and social areas is the focus of intervention. **Early intervention** is the term used to refer to specialized services for infants and toddlers who are at risk for or are experiencing a developmental delay. Early intervention services are provided at no cost to families through each state's early intervention system, usually through the state's local education agencies (public school system) or health department. An interdisciplinary team along with the parents develop an **individualized family service plan** (IFSP), which is a documented plan of care to meet the child's and family's needs. For instance, an infant born with Down syndrome could benefit from physical therapy in the first months of life to begin working on emerging gross motor skills such as head control, upper body strength, and rolling over. (Infants with Down syndrome have hypotonia and delayed gross motor skill development.) Speech language therapy would also be needed to work on sucking, spoon feeding, and making sounds in the early months. (Infants with Down syndrome have a small osseous orbit of the mouth, large protruding tongue, and poor muscle tone, causing feeding problems and delayed language development.)

Public schools are the primary agency for serving children with disabilities from 3 years of age (or younger) until 21 years of age. Schools are required by law to provide every child with a disability a free appropriate public education in the least restrictive environment. For most children with disabilities, this means integration, or education within regular education classrooms of same-age peers without disabilities. Public school districts have made varying degrees of movement toward this goal. In addition to education, public schools must provide related services needed by the child for the child to benefit from education and may include physical therapy, occupational therapy, speech language therapy, nursing, and therapeutic recreation. Documented plans called **individualized education plans** (IEPs), developed by the parents and an interdisciplinary team provided by the school, provide direction for the child's care and a means of enforcing accountability.

The community health nurse, when serving as a school health nurse, can play a critical role in preventing disabilities and ensuring a safe and supportive school experience for children with disabilities. The school health nurse may collaborate with teachers to develop and present an injury prevention curriculum aimed at specific age groups (e.g., poisoning and preschoolers or head injuries and elementary/middle school children). Teachers will rely on the school health nurse for guidance and assistance in working with children who have physical disabilities such as spina bifida or cerebral palsy, children taking medications for behavior problems, children with compromised immune systems, and children with seizure disorders. The school nurse may also serve on an interdisciplinary team to assess children with disabilities for eligibility for special education services or conduct annual vision and hearing screening for at-risk children.

Transition from Education to Work and Living in the Community

Students with disabilities are now placed in regular education programs as much as possible because the best preparation for living and working in an integrated environment is to be taught in an inclusive school setting. Educational programming available to students with disabilities includes four major areas: (1) general education academic content, (2) basic academic skills and social skills, (3) learning strategies, and (4) vocational and life skills. A balance of these instructional areas should also address relevant adolescent issues such as biological changes and sexuality; social values and behavioral competence; identification of personal interests, talents, and areas of need; and a desire for emotional independence (Patton, Blackbourn, & Fad, 1996; Wehman, 1996).

Educational systems are expanding their roles in preparing students for transition to work and living in the community. Employers and employees of industries and businesses should be invited to address school systems about their workforce needs. Business connections and alliances offering students opportunities for work experiences and employment before graduation are having success. Many students with disabilities are staying employed upon graduation and are not remaining dependent on their families or the social service system.

To facilitate successful transition from the school environment to more independent living and work environments, key connections should be built with community businesses, community colleges, recreation centers, and adult supports for living. Appropriate planning focusing on student/family choice is also critical. Major options for students with disabilities include (1) employment (full-time or part-time, supported or nonsupported), (2) further education (2- and 4-year colleges, technical schools, trade schools, adult education), (3) military service, (4) volunteer work, (5) "domestic engineering" (house husband/wife), or (6) absence of gainful employment or purposeful activity (Patton, Blackbourn, & Fad, 1996).

Transition planning is shifting the decision making to individuals with disabilities and their families. Students are now learning to make choices, be more self-determined, and be self-advocates assuming control and management responsibilities for their own lives. Professionals are shifting away from "curing" individuals with disabilities to supporting them for improved quality of life. Before students leave the school environment, they and their family members must learn how to access the supports (informal and unpaid or formal and paid) they need and want in the communities. Person-centered planning focuses on the desires of the individuals and their families and identifies the formal and informal supports the individuals will need to achieve their future dreams. A planning meeting focuses on the individual's abilities and preferences and identifies possible resources in order to provide desired assistance and support for adult living and work.

Rehabilitation

Rehabilitation is a term used for interventions aimed at restoring or optimizing functioning after an injury or significant medical problem. Rehabilitation nurses work to reduce the stigma associated with disabilities, restore maximum levels of independent

functioning, advocate for optimal quality of life, help the individual and family adapt to an altered lifestyle, and improve the overall outcome for the client. Individuals having experienced spinal cord injuries or cerebrovascular accidents are examples of types of clients who would be involved in rehabilitation. Initially, after a significant injury, the client is involved in inpatient rehabilitation, which may use nursing, physical therapy (PT), occupational therapy (OT), speech language therapy, recreation therapy, music therapy, and counseling. Later, after discharge from the facility, the client may receive home visits from a home health nurse and PT or OT sessions at an outpatient rehabilitation facility. Both the length of the initial hospital stay and the number of outpatient rehabilitation visits permitted after discharge have been severely curtailed in recent years by insurance providers.

Medical Technology

Many individuals with disabilities require technology assistance, nonmedical or medical, immediately after an injury, during rehabilitation, and/or throughout their lives. **Medical assistive devices** assist or replace necessary body functions and are necessary to keep the individual alive or prevent further disability. Clients using medical technologies also typically require daily skilled nursing care. Medical technology is used to assist with respiration, nutrition, excretion, and surveillance of vital functions and oxygen levels.

Individuals with chronic respiratory failure may require oxygen supplementation by nasal cannula, face mask, oxygen tent or hood, or a tracheostomy. These individuals often may require chest physiotherapy and suctioning several times a day to clear pulmonary secretions. When assistance is needed to replace or

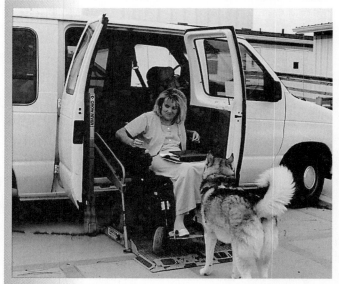

Faculty member with disability uses service dog to function more independently.

augment the individual's own breathing, mechanical ventilation and tracheostomy are used. Training nurses in rehabilitation facilities about ventilators can expedite the discharge of ventilator-dependent clients from the hospital acute care unit to rehabilitation facilities.

Clients with chronic serious respiratory problems may be discharged to home from an acute care setting while still using a ventilator. Home ventilator care is one of the most expensive, time-consuming, and risky types of home therapies. Equipment failure or poor judgment of the caregiver can result in immediate death of the client (Capen & Dedlow, 1998). Young children receiving long-term mechanical ventilation are at high risk for language deficits, feeding problems, and behavior problems. A speech-language pathologist should be consulted to devise a developmentally appropriate alternative mode of communication for the individual with a tracheostomy receiving long-term oxygen supplementation or ventilation. Alternative methods of communication such as sign language, language boards, or computers can promote expressive language development and help prevent potential behavior problems stemming from frustration.

Neurological impairments such as cerebral palsy can cause numerous problems with feeding such as a weak suck, poor lip closure, poor tongue control, uncoordinated suck-swallow reflex, and gastroesophageal reflux. In addition, some individuals may lack the stamina to chew, swallow, and breathe without becoming totally exhausted or risking aspiration. Nasogastric tubes may be used as a short-term method to deliver food directly to the stomach but are not used for long-term feeding because of the irritation to the nose and throat and the unappealing appearance. Individuals who cannot take in enough food by mouth to be adequately nourished can benefit from a gastrostomy. A gastrostomy is an opening through the abdominal wall directly to the stomach. A gastrostomy tube or button is inserted into this opening to allow for feeding. Occasionally, the gastrointestinal tract is not able to digest or absorb nutrients, and the individual is nourished with total parenteral nutrition (TPN). TPN is infused in a central venous catheter placed in the vena cava or right atrial area to provide adequate dilution of the hypertonic solution (Krzywda, 1998).

Medical technology or equipment may be necessary to promote excretion of wastes. Indwelling urinary catheters may be used to empty the bladder and keep the individual dry. Two main problems with long-term indwelling catheters are frequent urinary tract infections, which can cause permanent kidney damage, and the bulkiness and unsightliness of the urine collection bag. Many persons with spina bifida (accompanied by paralysis below the level of the defect) or spinal cord injuries prefer to perform clean intermittent self-catheterization throughout the day, eliminating the need for the urine collection bag and indwelling catheter. An ostomy or opening in the abdominal wall may also be used, either to empty the bladder or to allow evacuation of the bowel contents through the abdominal wall. In the past, adults with kidney failure could re-

ceive hemodialysis at home, and now children with kidney failure can receive peritoneal dialysis at home and avoid hospitalization. Peritoneal dialysis, in which fluid is passed into the abdominal cavity via an abdominal catheter and allowed to drain back out, takes several hours to complete and may be needed up to 3 to 5 days per week (Batshaw, 1997).

A final common category of medical technology used at home or in rehabilitation settings includes monitoring devices such as cardiorespiratory monitors and pulse oximeters. Monitors are important for alerting caregivers to problems requiring prompt intervention, such as a kink in the oxygen tubing or an occluded airway, but the beeping and alarms of the monitors can unfortunately compete with the client as the focus of the caregiver.

Nonmedical Assistive Technology

Nonmedical assistive technology is often a critical part of the continuum of services needed by a person with a disability. An **assistive technology device** is "any item, piece of equipment, or product system, whether acquired commercially off the shelf, modified, or customized that is used to increase, maintain, or improve functional capabilities of individuals with disabilities" (P.L. 100-407, the Technology Related Assistance for Individuals with Disabilities Act, 1988). Areas in which assistive technology is helpful include activities of daily living, environmental control, communication, mobility, transportation, and recreation. Within each of these areas, technology can be either low tech (easy to make and inexpensive) or high tech (more difficult to make, often computerized or electronic, and expensive).

Technology for everyday living, or those adaptations and devices that will enable the individual to perform activities of daily living, are the first needs of consumers. These needs must be met before other needs like transportation can be attended to. Examples of technology to help with activities of daily living include "grabbers," adapted eating utensils, shower chairs, and Braille or large-print labels on appliances. Environmental control can be achieved through the use of switch extenders to place light switches within reach of a person in a wheelchair, adapters to convert lamps into "touch" lamps, or voice-controlled lights and heating/cooling. According to a Harris poll (1998), personal computers are owned by 30% of people with disabilities, up from only 20% in 1994. Voice recognition software is available that enables a person with vision, motor, or coordination problems to use a computer strictly by voice commands and dictation, without ever having to touch the keyboard. The ability to communicate is a basic need of all individuals, regardless of disability or age. Communication systems (which may be based on sign language, gesturing, or Braille) may require low-tech devices such as simple communication boards at which to point or gaze, or high-tech computers that "talk" for the person such as the Liberator. TDDs (telecommunication devices for the deaf) allow individuals with severe hearing impairments to transmit and receive typed messages over the telephone. Mobility devices include the traditional walkers, canes, and crutches along with scooters and wheelchairs. Scooters and wheelchairs have become costly and highly technical pieces of equipment that are custom-made to fit the size, posture, and lifestyle of the person with a disability. In addition to manual wheelchairs, power wheelchairs with joystick control and tilt and recline options are available. For persons without upper extremity control, sip and puff or breath-controlled power chairs are available. Specialized wheelchairs have also been developed for rough outdoor terrain and for specific sports such as wheelchair basketball, track, or rugby. Technological adaptations for vehicles include wheelchair lifts for vans, mechanical or electronic hand controls, and steering devices.

Ideally, evaluations for assistive technology devices should be conducted by appropriate interdisciplinary teams that include the client as a key member. Individuals on the team may include physical therapists, occupational therapists, nurses, speech-language pathologists, rehabilitation engineers, vocational rehabilitation counselors, teachers, and technology suppliers. Although many of the low-tech devices can be made or purchased for a moderate price, other pieces of technology such as computerized communication devices, specialized wheelchairs, and customized vans require significant financial resources (Box 29-2).

Advances in technology are enhancing the possibilities for individuals with disabilities to communicate and move more effectively. With the knowledge of technology, service providers can provide solutions to everyday problems in school and workplace settings. However, adequate funding to make the best tech-

nology available to citizens with disabilities has still not been allocated. For example, grocery stores have laser scanners and voice synthesizers on their computers, yet people with disabilities have difficulty accessing voice synthesizers of this quality for themselves (Patton, Blackbourn, & Fad, 1996).

Adaptive/assistive devices have moved some individuals from dependence to independence but include sometimes costly equipment such as customized electric wheelchairs and electronic communication systems. Because of the considerable expense, school systems, insurance companies, and public assistance programs often disagree on who should pay for the devices (Kirk, Gallagher, & Anastasiow, 1993).

It has been estimated that more than 2.5 million Americans need assistive technology devices that they are unable to acquire, primarily because of the high cost of the products (Laplante, Hendershot, & Moss, 1992). Technology, both low and high tech, has made the difference for many people with disabilities between a life of dependency and limited options and an independent, productive life in which the person is included in all aspects of community life.

Assistance Animals

In addition to technological assistance, individuals with disabilities may also benefit from animal assistance. Using pets to enhance health status dates back to the 18th and 19th centuries, when pets were used in Britain to give institutionalized people with mental retardation a sense of purpose and meaning. Caring for pets has been shown to help individuals improve mood, lower blood pressure, overcome physical limitations, and increase social skills (DeLaune & Ladner, 1998). A variety of animals can be used to provide companionship and give purpose to daily living (e.g., cats, dogs, rabbits, guinea pigs, birds) or to assist clients in daily activities (e.g., dogs, monkeys).

The most commonly used animal to assist clients with disabilities is the dog. Assistance dogs, although commonly thought to include only guide dogs for people who are blind, actually include several types of dogs serving a variety of purposes. Guide dogs are specially trained dogs who, when working, stay at their owner's side and provide behavioral cues about the environment. Examples would be warnings of steps, streets, or other obstacles in the path of movement. Hearing dogs, also specially trained, may be used by individuals with significant hearing impairments to cue the individual about meaningful sounds in the environment such as a doorbell, telephone, smoke detector, or an approaching person. Service dogs for persons with physical disabilities are especially useful to persons using wheelchairs. These dogs are trained to be helpful by picking up dropped objects (e.g., a pen, car keys, a wallet), carrying items in a dog backpack, and retrieving objects (e.g., a telephone) for the owner. For an individual who can walk short distances between a chair and a nearby bathroom, for instance, a large dog can help the person balance and provide stability for the short walk. A lesser-known type of assistance dog is the seizure detection dog. Certain dogs

---

BOX 29-2 MEANS OF FINANCING ASSISTIVE TECHNOLOGY

PUBLIC SOURCES

Medicaid
Medicare
CHAMPUS
Private insurance
Social Security Administration work incentive
Veterans Administration
State vocational rehabilitation agencies
State education agencies

PRIVATE SOURCES

Lions Club
Easter Seals
United Way
Sororities and fraternities
Muscular Dystrophy Association
Credit financing

seem to have an innate ability to sense an impending seizure. Dogs with this ability can be trained to warn the owner that a seizure is about to begin, enabling the owner to position himself or herself in a safe position away from sharp and hard objects and to summon help. Once the seizure begins, if no one else is present, the dog is trained to bark to get help. All of the aforementioned types of assistance dogs require specialized training for both the dog and the prospective owner, funds to purchase the dog (often available through a civic organization), and owner commitment.

The ADA (1990) protects the rights of a person with a disability who uses an assistance dog to have full access to any public facility, including hospitals and outpatient rehabilitation facilities. The community health nurse may be involved in developing or revising a health care agency's policies regarding service animals to ensure that the facility is in compliance with ADA guidelines (Eames & Eames, 1997). Questions about access to places of public accommodation can be directed to the U.S. Department of Justice's ADA hot line (800-514-0301).

Ethical Issues Related to Disabilities

A number of ethical issues exist in the disability field. Newborn screening for diseases such as phenylketonuria (PKU) is one area of question. Presently, in many states, newborn screening is conducted without parental consent. This screening detects several diseases, including PKU, which respond profoundly to early treatment. It is more economical for states to detect and treat a disease such as PKU early rather than provide lifelong support for an untreated child who will develop severe mental retardation. Does this law violate parents' rights to give informed consent? Would it be ethical to expand mandatory screening of newborns for other genetic diseases such as cystic fibrosis when the disease course will not be significantly improved by newborn diagnosis?

Prenatal diagnosis is now readily available to most women in the United States and raises a number of concerns for those in the disability field. It is feared that women could be pressured to undergo abortions of fetuses with disabilities because of society's devaluing of people with disabilities and its unwillingness to pay for their care. Although the goal of prenatal diagnosis is to give information to expectant parents so that they can make an informed choice, the high rates of abortion following diagnosis of a disability suggests that service providers are biased in the information that they share. It is critical that prenatal diagnostic information be shared through a genetic counselor and that parents receive accurate information about a disabling condition before making any decisions.

Historically, another ethical debate centered around the relatively common occurrence of withholding lifesaving surgical treatment of newborns with obvious disabilities such as Down syndrome, hydrocephalus, or spina bifida. Although withholding treatment from infants with disabilities had been common, the

1982 birth of "Baby Doe" in Indiana brought this practice under public scrutiny. An infant was born with Down syndrome and tracheoesophageal fistula, a connection between the trachea and esophagus. Without corrective surgery, oral feedings would be routed into the baby's lungs via the fistula. Following the advice of their obstetrician, the parents refused to consent to the corrective surgery and the infant was not given food or water. A consulting pediatrician tried to stop the starvation of the infant, but the courts upheld the parents' decision and the infant died a number of days later. In response to the public outrage resulting from the death of this infant, the federal government enacted the "Baby Doe" ruling and notified all hospitals that such activity would be penalized. Since 1982, it has been unlawful to withhold treatment from a baby born with a disability; however, violation of this "Baby Doe" ruling carries minor penalties such as loss of federal dollars, rather than criminal or civil actions.

Professionals need to be aware of their own biases and consciously strive to prevent them from coloring the information shared with parents about the risks and benefits of procedures. Research has shown that nurses and physicians are often not supportive of treating infants with severe disabilities because of quality-of-life issues, cost of care, and impact on the family. Nurses and physicians have been shown to be less optimistic about achieving a positive outcome than parents, teachers, social workers, physical therapists, and occupational therapists. Because of these biases, nurses may unknowingly accentuate certain risks or underestimate the potential quality of life of an infant with a disability, thereby influencing the parents' treatment decision (Batshaw & Cho, 1997). Other ethical issues, including do not resuscitate orders or withdrawing life support, are based on similar issues as the withholding treatment issue discussed earlier. Personal beliefs about the value of an individual with a disability and what an acceptable quality of life is influence the recommendations made by medical professionals when parents face decisions about resuscitation and life support.

Another ethical issue involves the use of organs from infants born with anencephaly, a congenital absence of the brain except for a brainstem. These infants typically live only a few days, and the condition is uniformly fatal. Because of an extreme shortage of organs available for transplant in infants, newborns with anencephaly were used as organ donors (with parental consent). This practice came under scrutiny because the donor infants were not technically brain dead before the organs were harvested; allowing the infant to die first would have resulted in damage to the organs to be harvested. Since 1988, this practice has not been permitted, and there are virtually no organs available for infants in need of transplants. Ethical concerns included the fear that this practice encouraged the use of a human solely as an organ donor, that it used euthanasia by taking the organs before the donor had died, and that it could be the beginning of the harvesting of organs from the terminally ill, prisoners, institutionalized individuals, the poor, and other devalued populations.

Sexual and reproductive rights of individuals with disabilities have been another area of ethical debate. Not only have people with disabilities reported feeling violated by the personnel caring for them (see the following Research Brief), but in individuals with mental retardation, the person may not learn appropriate physical boundaries. In the past, programs for individuals with mental retardation separated males and females and punished sexual acting out behavior such as masturbation. These methods are now considered questionable because they forbid individuals to express their autonomy through activities that are pleasurable and potentially harmless to others. Of course, individuals with mental retardation need to be taught appropriate times and places to engage in sexual behaviors such as masturbation. In addition, these individuals should receive instruction in using judgment in choosing when and with whom to engage in sexual activity, in the use of birth control, and in the prevention of sexually transmitted diseases. Sterilization is considered in some cases in which the individual is unable to learn to use birth control, would be unable to competently raise a child, or would ex-

perience a serious health risk if pregnant. Sterilization should not be done, however, strictly for the convenience of parents, schools, or institutions. If it is determined that sterilization is necessary, the individual should participate to the fullest extent possible to obtain informed consent.

Informed consent means that the individual understands the risks and benefits of the procedure, is presented with alternatives, and is given the opportunity to express a choice. Acquiring informed consent from an individual with mental retardation can be time-consuming, requiring simplification of information and multiple meetings. Informed consent is a sensitive issue in the United States because of the eugenics policies of the 1920s and 1930s. These policies were in some cases a model for the eugenics programs in Nazi Germany and required compulsory, involuntary sterilization of individuals who were "feeble-minded" or "mental defectives" in an effort to improve public health and the gene pool. A 1927 U.S. Supreme Court ruling defending sterilization resulted in more than 60,000 persons with mental retardation being sterilized without consent. Before sterilization is performed, the motives of those in favor of the procedure along with documented efforts to use a less restrictive alternative must be examined (Batshaw & Cho, 1997).

Healthy People 2010 Objectives Related to Disabilities

Although people with disabilities are targeted by *Healthy People 2010* as a special population, objectives related to people with disabilities are found throughout the document. The health promotion and disease prevention needs of people with disabilities are critical. People with disabilities are at high risk for developing additional health problems, which will only further decrease their level of functioning. Secondary conditions such as decubitus ulcers or urinary tract disorders are associated with the decreased mobility experienced by many individuals with physical disabilities and are often preventable. People with disabilities are also more likely to develop musculoskeletal disorders caused by lack of physical activity or respiratory problems caused by lack of physical activity or tobacco use. In addition, people with disabilities encounter many of the same risks as the rest of the population, such as drug and alcohol abuse, poor nutrition, and stress. The box on p. 677 lists selected objectives related to people with disabilities found in *Healthy People 2010*.

Roles of the Community Health Nurse

The roles of the community health nurse in working with individuals with disabilities are varied. These roles include client partner, change agent, researcher, case finder, case manager, referral agent, advocate, educator, and caregiver.

In working with individuals with disabilities, the community health nurse may assume the role of *client partner*. The

RESEARCH BRIEF

Lillest, B. (1997). Violation in caring for the physically disabled. Western Journal of Nursing Research, 19, 282–296.

This study used in-depth interviews to explore how people with disabilities perceive and experience the care they receive from public health personnel. The methodology was based on a phenomenological hermeneutic framework that focuses on the subjects themselves to convey the essential meaning of human experience. The participants in the study were 6 men and 10 women ages 21 to 85, living in Norway, who had physical disabilities (multiple sclerosis, tumors, cerebral hemorrhage, and spinal cord injuries) and used wheelchairs for mobility. All participants required some type of help from health care personnel in their home.

"A major and disturbing finding is that the informants describe feelings of being violated, transgressed, and infringed upon by the personnel in charge of their care" (p. 282). Through interviews, it was revealed that some of the participants constructed specific body boundaries in an effort to cope with the violation of their bodies and body zones. Many informants reported the feeling of being only a body or an object to the health care personnel.

This study concludes that serving individuals with chronic conditions within the framework of care designed for acute illnesses is inappropriate. Lillest sees the authority of the community health nurse serving to undermine clients' autonomy and strip them of their status—a distinctive feature of institutions but not expected in primary health service.

HEALTHY PEOPLE 2010

OBJECTIVES RELATED TO DISABILITY

Disability and Secondary Conditions

6.1   Include in the core of all relevant *Healthy People 2010* surveillance instruments a standardized set of questions that identify "people with disabilities."

6.2   Reduce the proportion of children and adolescents with disabilities who are reported to be sad, unhappy, or depressed.

6.3   Reduce the proportion of adults with disabilities who report feelings such as sadness, unhappiness, or depression that prevent them from being active.

6.4   Increase the proportion of adults with disabilities who participate in social activities.

6.5   Increase the proportion of adults with disabilities reporting sufficient emotional support.

6.6   Increase the proportion of adults with disabilities reporting satisfaction with life.

6.7   Reduce the number of people with disabilities in congregate care facilities, consistent with permanency planning principles.

6.8   Eliminate disparities in employment rates between working-aged adults with and without disabilities.

6.9   Increase the proportion of children and youth with disabilities who spend at least 80% of their time in regular education programs.

6.10   Increase the proportion of health and wellness and treatment and facilities that provide full access for people with disabilities.

6.11   Reduce the proportion of people with disabilities who report not having the assistive devices and technology needed.

6.12   Reduce the proportion of people with disabilities reporting environmental barriers to participation in home, school, work, or community activities.

6.13   Increase the number of tribes, states, and the District of Columbia that have public health surveillance and health promotion programs for people with disabilities and caregivers.

Source: DHHS, 2000.

community health nurse can enhance client competence by developing equal partnerships with clients that do not place the community health nurse in the dominant role. The nurse can share professional knowledge with clients but also assist clients in recognizing and building on their own experiential knowledge (Paavilainen & Astedt-Kurki, 1997).

Often experiencing the flaws in the service system alongside families, the nurse may be moved to serve as a *change agent* for the service system. One nurse joined a certified therapeutic recreation specialist (CTRS) to change a community recreation program's policy of excluding children with disabilities from its youth basketball program. By educating the director and staff about the ADA requirements and strategies for inclusion, a child with spina bifida who used a wheelchair was placed on one of the teams and enjoyed several years of competitive basketball play with his same-age nondisabled peers. In the roles of *researchers,* the nurse and CTRS went on to examine the extent of the child's participation on the team, the extent of his contribution to team

FYI

President George Bush signed the Americans with Disabilities Act on July 26, 1990, the landmark law that advanced the rights of persons with disabilities.

success, and the extent of his social acceptance by his teammates (Green & DeCoux, 1994).

The role of *casefinder* is a more traditional role of the public health nurse. In the disability field, locating young children with or at risk for disabilities is especially important. *Childfind*, or locating, assessing, and offering services to such children, is required by federal law in all states. Both the states' early intervention system and public school system are responsible for Childfind. The community health nurse may work with a developmental screening team through the public school system or the state's early intervention system to identify children ages birth to 5 years with or at risk for disabilities. Typically, the nurse's role in developmental screening includes eliciting a family medical history and the child's medical and developmental history, conducting a physical examination, and assessing hearing and vision. The developmental component may be conducted by a specially trained nurse, early childhood special educator, developmental pediatrician, or psychologist.

Case management, or coordinating the client's care, is another role that may be assumed by the community health nurse. Knowledge of both community services and eligibility requirements is essential for effective case management. This knowledge is also used in the role of *referral agent.* The nurse can direct clients to agencies that can meet their needs by providing a contact person's name and the phone number of the agency. Some clients, however, may need assistance with contacting agencies. The parents of a child who has recently experienced a traumatic brain injury may be emotionally and physically exhausted and in a state of denial regarding the likelihood of long-term disability, necessitating that the nurse be active in contacting potentially helpful agencies, groups, and individuals.

Serving as an *advocate,* or speaking on behalf of people with disabilities who are unable to speak for themselves, is an important role of the community health nurse. This advocacy may be on the community level, with the community health nurse advocating for a medically fragile child to be included in a regular classroom rather than served "homebound" by a local public school system. At the policy level, the community health nurse could speak before a legislative hearing about the need for small group homes for adults with mental retardation in local communities or the need for public assistance with the cost of personal care attendants needed to allow people with disabilities to remain in their own homes. In some cases, the nurse may need to refer clients to the state's protection and advocacy program.

FYI

Theresa Uchytil, Miss Iowa, was born without a left hand and adopted as her slogan for the 2000 Miss America contest: "Americans with disabilities, think ability."

The role of the community health nurse as *educator* continues to be a cornerstone of community health nursing when working with clients with disabilities. The nurse may educate an entire community on prevention of fetal alcohol syndrome or an individual client with a spinal cord injury about preventing decubiti formation. The community health nurse can motivate adults with disabilities who have completed rehabilitation programs and returned home to resume an active productive life. Education by the nurse was credited as the key to self-care and responsibility by all clients with spinal cord injuries participating in a study looking at motivation of adults with disabilities (Box 29-3) (Brillhart & Johnson, 1997).

The role of *caregiver* is another historic role of the community health nurse. In this role, the nurse applies the nursing process by assessing, implementing, and evaluating care of a client with a disability. For clients with significant disabilities, this care may require familiarity with medical and assistive technological devices such as ventilators and computerized communication systems.

BOX 29-3 AUTONOMIC DYSREFLEXIA: WOULD YOU RECOGNIZE THE SIGNS?

What is it?
A life-threatening condition that can occur in a person with a spinal cord injury at or above the T6 level.

Is it very common?
Approximately 48% to 90% of people with high-level spinal cord injuries will experience autonomic dysreflexia.

What causes it?
It is triggered by painful stimuli below the level of the injury, such as bladder distension, bowel overdistension (impaction, constipation), pressure ulcers.

What should the caregiver do?
Raise the person's head, remove the noxious stimuli (check bowel, bladder, skin), and give antihypertensive medication as ordered.

Source: Travers, 1999.

FYI

Runner Marla Runyan became the first blind athlete to qualify for the 2000 U.S. Olympic team.

CONCLUSION

Persons with disabilities are living longer and more productive lives than ever. Community health nurses are in settings where the opportunity to promote the health of persons, families, and populations with disabilities are ample. Using knowledge gained from this chapter, community health nurses can assist these populations with preventing health problems and enhancing their ability to make informed health decisions.

A CONVERSATION WITH...

Put a disabled person in the middle of a group of workers and they complain less and are more productive. Hire the disabled. They'll motivate the rest of your workforce.

(Actor Christopher Reeve was critically injured in a horse riding accident in May of 1995 and sustained a spinal cord injury. He is paralyzed from the neck down. Mr. Reeve continues to speak, direct, and act and has written his autobiography Still Me *about his experiences with disability.)*

Source: Zaslow, J. (2000, May).
The uncommon strength of
Christopher Reeve. *USM Weekend*, 4–5.

CRITICAL THINKING ACTIVITIES

1. How does having a disability affect a person's self-concept?
2. Can a person with a disability ever be autonomous? Why or why not?
3. When community health nurses assist clients with disabilities in areas of health promotion, what are the most difficult challenges in regard to self-care and independence?
4. How can community health nurses promote positive self-regard for persons with disabilities in the media? Give some examples of projects that could enhance the perception of "abilities" rather than disabilities for this vulnerable population group.

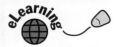

Explore Community Health Nursing on the web! To learn more about the topics in this chapter, use the passcode provided to access your exclusive web site: http://communitynursing.jbpub.com
If you do not have a passcode, you can obtain one at this site.

REFERENCES

Batshaw, M. L. (1997). *Children with disabilities* (4th ed.). Baltimore: Paul H. Brookes.

Batshaw, M. L., & Cho, M. K. (1997). Ethical choices: Questions of care. In M. L. Batshaw (Ed.), *Children with disabilities* (4th ed., pp. 727–742). Baltimore: Paul H. Brookes.

Beirne-Smith, M., Patton, J., & Ittenbach, R. (1994). Historical perspective. In *Mental retardation* (4th ed., pp. 25–55). Upper Saddle River, NJ: Prentice-Hall

Berkowitz, E. D. (1987). *Disabled policy: America's policy for the handicapped.* Cambridge, MA: Cambridge University Press.

Brillhart, B., & Johnson, K. (1997). Motivation and the coping process of adults with disabilities: A qualitative study. *Rehabilitation Nursing, 22,* 249–256.

Capen, C. L., & Dedlow, E. R. (1998). Discharging ventilator-dependent children: A continuing challenge. *Journal of Pediatric Nursing, 13,* 175–184.

Centers for Disease Control and Prevention (CDC). (1999, April 2). Achievements in public health, 1900–1999; Impact of vaccines universally recommended for children, United States, 1900–1998. *Morbidity and Mortality Weekly Report, 48*(12), 243–248: www.cdc.gov/epo/mmwr/preview/mmwrhtml/00056803.htm.

Craft, D. H. (1995). Visual impairments and hearing losses. In J. P. Winnick (Ed.), *Adapted physical education and sport* (2nd ed., pp. 143–166). Champaign, IL: Human Kinetics.

DeLaune, S. C., & Ladner, P. K. (1998). *Fundamentals of nursing: Standards and practice.* Albany, NY: Delmar.

Department of Health and Human Services, Public Health Service (DHHS). (1991). *Healthy people 2000: National health promotion and disease prevention objectives, full report with commentary.* (Publication No. PHS 91-50212). Washington, DC: U.S. Government Printing Office.

DiLeo, D. (1993). *Enhancing the lives of adults with disabilities: An orientation manual* (2nd ed.). St. Augustine, FL: Training Resource Network.

Eames, E., & Eames, T. (1997). Interpreting legal mandates: Assistance dogs in medical facilities. *Nursing Management, 28*(6), 49–51.

Green, F. P., & DeCoux, V. (1994). A procedure for evaluating the effectiveness of a community recreation integration program. *Therapeutic Recreation Journal, 28*(1), 41–47.

Green, F. P., & Schleien, S. J. (1991). Understanding friendship and recreation: A theoretical sampling. *Therapeutic Recreation Journal, 25*(4), 29–40.

Hablutzel, N., & McMahon, B. T. (1992). *The Americans with Disabilities Act: Access and accommodations.* Orlando: Paul M. Deutsch Press.

Hagner, D., & Dileo, D. (1993). *Working together: Workplace culture, supported employment, and persons with disabilities.* Cambridge, MA: Brookline.

Jenkins, W. M., Patterson, J. B., & Szymanski, E. M. (1992). Philosophical, historical, and legislative aspects of the rehabilitation counseling profession In R. M. Parker & E. M. Szymanski (Eds.), *Rehabilitation counseling: Basics and beyond* (2nd ed., pp. 1–41). Austin, TX: PRO-ED.

Kirk, S. A., Gallagher, J. J., & Anastasiow, N. J. (1993). *Educating exceptional children* (7th ed.). Boston: Houghton Mifflin.

Krzywda, E. A. (1998). Central venous access: Catheters, technology, and physiology. *Medical-Surgical Nursing, 7,* 132–141.

Laplante, M., Hendershot, G., & Moss, A. (1992). *Assistive technology devices and home accessibility features: Prevalence, payment, need, and trends.* Washington, DC: National Center for Health Statistics.

Marino, M. J. (1999, June/July). CDC report shows prevalence of brain injury. *TBI Challenge, 3*(3).

National Organization on Disability. (1998). *The 1998 N. O. D./Harris survey of Americans with disabilities.* New York: Louis Harris & Associates.

Noble, J., & Conley, R (1987). Accumulating evidence on the benefits and costs of supported and transitional employment for people with severe disabilities. *Journal of the Association for Persons with Severe Handicaps, 12,* 163–174.

Paavilainen, E., & Astedt-Kurki, P. (1997). The client-nurse relationship as experienced by public health nurses: Toward better collaboration. *Public Health Nursing, 14,* 137–150.

Patton, J. R., Blackbourn, J. M., & Fad, K. (1996). *Exceptional individuals in focus.* Englewood Cliffs, NJ: Prentice-Hall:

Pierce, L. L. (1998). Barriers to access: Frustrations of people who use a wheelchair for full-time mobility. *Rehabilitation Nursing, 23,* 120–125.

Racino, J. A., & Taylor, S. J. (1993). People first: Approaches to housing and support. In J. A. Racino, P. Walker, S. O'Connor, & S. J. Taylor (Eds.), *Housing, support, and community: Choices and strategies for adults with disabilities* (vol. 2, pp. 33–56). Baltimore: Paul H. Brookes.

Research and Training Center on Independent Living. (1996). *Guidelines for reporting and writing about people with disabilities* (5th ed.). Lawrence, KS: Research and Training Center on Independent Living, Bureau of Child Research, University of Kansas.

Roman, M., Miller, L., Maculuso, S., Dempsey, R., & Golden-Baker, S. (1998). Breaking the boundaries: Collaborating to develop a model ventilator training program. *Medical-Surgical Nursing, 7,* 9–18.

Sands, D. J., & Wehmeyer, M. L. (Eds.). (1996). *Self-determination across the life span: Independence and choice for people with disabilities.* Baltimore: Paul H. Brookes.

Sands, D. J., & Wehmeyer, M. L. (1996). Future directions in self-determination: Articulating values and policies, reorganizing organizational structures, and implementing professional practices. In D. J. Sands & M. L. Wehmeyer (Eds.), *Self-determination across the life span: Independence and choice for people with disabilities* (pp. 331–344). Baltimore: Paul H. Brookes.

Schleien, S. J., Ray, M. T., & Green, F. P. (1997). *Community recreation and people with disabilities: Strategies for inclusion* (2nd ed.). Baltimore: Paul H. Brookes.

Trachtenberg, S. W., & Lewis, D. F. (1996). Case management. In L. A. Kurtz, P. W. Dowrick, S. E. Levy, & M. L. Batshaw (Eds.), *Handbook of developmental disabilities: Resources for interdisciplinary care* (pp. 203–208). Gaithersburg, MD: Aspen.

Travers, P. L. (1999). Autonomic dysreflexia: A clinical rehabilitation problem. *Rehabilitation Nursing, 24,* 19–23.

U.S. Department of Commerce, Economics and Statistics Administration. (1997). *Census brief: Disabilities affect one-fifth of all Americans*: www.census.gov/prod/3/97pubs/cenbr975.pdf.U.S. Department of Justice (1992). *Nondiscrimination on the basis of disability in state and local government services*: www.usdoj.gov/crt/ada/reg2.

Ward, M. J. (1996). Coming of age in the age of self-determination: A historical and personal perspective. In D. J. Sands & M. L. Wehmeyer (Eds.), *Self-determination across the lifespan: Independence and choice for people with disabilities* (pp. 3–16). Baltimore, MD: Paul H. Brookes.

Wehman, P. (1996). *Life beyond the classroom: Transition strategies for young people with disabilities* (2nd ed.). Baltimore: Paul. H. Brookes.

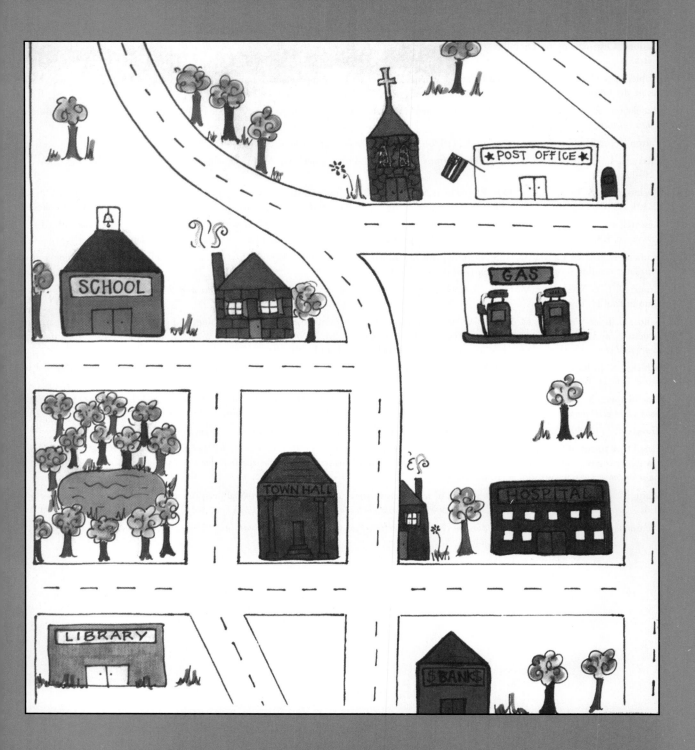

PART TWO

Community-Based Nursing Care

Recent changes in society have had a profound impact on the health care delivery system in the United States. There has been an explosion of technology accompanied by an increase in health care costs to the consumer, with resulting changes in the *setting* and *focus* of health care delivery. Managed care and controlling health care costs are primary foci of the health care industry. The family, as the oldest and most basic of all social institutions, has undergone dramatic change in structure and function. Through the family, health care needs are identified and addressed, from birth to death. The portion of the U.S. population that is older than 65 is the fastest growing segment, as well as the group that requires the most health care dollars. Individuals with higher acuity levels, that in the past were treated in acute care institutions, are now being discharged to the community and treated in the home. The nurse of the 21st century will require a firm foundation in both acute and community-based/community-focused nursing health care to assist individuals in making the transition not only from acute care to home care but to and from other community settings, such as school and work.

Through the family, children are socialized to norms, values, and behavior. As such, the family is a powerful influence on the health beliefs and behavior of its members. The assessment of family functioning and its ability to meet the health needs of its members is a critical aspect of the community health nurse role.

Research indicates that gender influences the seeking, acquisition, and use of health services and health behavior. Women are less likely to be diagnosed with heart disease because it has long been associated as a male health problem. Men, in turn, often seek health care later than their female counterparts, which often results in less successful outcomes.

When children receive appropriate health-promotion and disease-prevention services, they are less likely to develop health problems. Nursing has a role in providing anticipatory guidance to parents and children regarding health-promotion and disease-prevention activities.

Community-based settings for mental health care have dominated for several decades. With the mental health clients, this is more cost-effective than institutionalization, and outcomes for the family are positive. Local community mental health centers provide care for all levels of mental health care needs. Lack of reimbursement and appropriate identification mechanisms for locating the mentally ill require creativity on the part of the community health nurse to meet community mental health needs.

Because Americans are living longer, myriad age-appropriate additional health care services for the aging population will be necessary. The health and care of the elder client is but one of the challenges associated with this age group. Ample research has documented that the caregiver is also at high risk from impaired health. Poor health of the caregiver is often a deciding factor in making the decision to place an elderly family member into institutionalized care. Community health nurses must develop and implement strategies that promote physical and mental health for both the elder and the caregiver.

Unit VI
Care of Families

Chapter 30

Foundations of Family Care

Ruth A. O'Brien

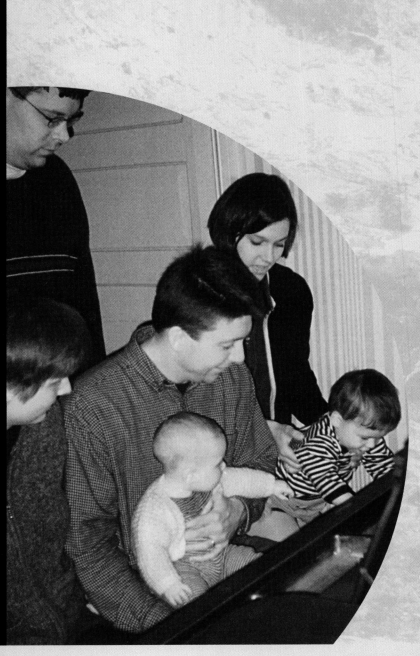

The family is two or more individuals who manifest some degree of interdependence in their interactions with each other and their environment in meeting basic human needs for affection and meaning. Moreover, our family is who we think it is.

QUESTIONS TO CONSIDER

After reading this chapter, answer the following questions:
1. How is *family* defined?
2. What are the health responsibilities of the family?
3. What is the difference between family-oriented and family-focused nursing care?
4. What is an example of a conceptual framework for family assessment?
5. How is the self-efficacy model of family interventions used in promoting the health of families?

KEY TERMS

Affect	Family	Interdependence	Positive feedback
Beliefs	Family developmental	Meaning	Power
Communication	tasks	Negative feedback	Self-regulation
Contracting	Function	Nonsummativity	Structure
Environment			

Joyce Williams, a school nurse at Sagebrush Elementary, reflected on her recent meeting with Mrs. Carson, the first grade teacher for Kevin Johnson. Mrs. Carson had contacted her to discuss Kevin's increasing episodes of toileting accidents and inattention in class over the past 2 months. Mrs. Carson questioned whether Kevin's behavior was indicative of problems coping with his parents' divorce; she told Joyce that the third grade teacher who had Kevin's sister in class related that the children's father recently remarried and moved to another city about 50 miles away. According to Kevin's school file, Mrs. Johnson was a legal secretary for a large law firm downtown. Recognizing the strains that a single, working parent raising two children, 6 and 8 years old, might be experiencing, Joyce decided that she would call Mrs. Johnson to schedule a home visit to talk with her about the problems Kevin's teacher had reported. A home visit, rather than a conference at the school, would provide an opportunity for her to observe parent-child interaction and also to gain a better appreciation of how Mrs. Johnson is handling being a single parent and what other supports are available.

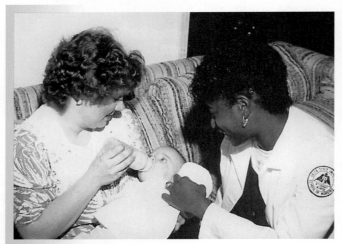

The single-mother family has increased in number during the past decade. These families are at special risks for poverty and a lack of health insurance.

FYI

Two-thirds of women work for pay during the same years that they are bearing and raising children.

Source: International Law Office. (1999). Maternity Protection at Work. *Geneva, Switzerland: International Labor Office.*

Definition of Family

Dramatic changes in family structure over the past few decades are highlighted in contrasting media images portrayed in popular television sitcoms, such as *Ozzie and Harriet* and *Father Knows Best* in the 1950s and 1960s and *Murphy Brown* in the 1990s. The popular image of the family as a nuclear two-parent unit raising their own children, with father as the breadwinner and mother as the homemaker, as portrayed in *Ozzie and Harriet* and *Father Knows Best,* is no longer the dominant pattern in American society. In fact, only 1 in 5 families of the 1990s fits this popular stereotype (Ahlburg & De Vita, 1992).

Single-parent, stepfamilies or blended families, dual-career families in which both parents work, married couples without children, cohabitating couples, and gay and lesbian families were typical of the diverse family patterns of the 1990s (Bianchi & Spain, 1996). *Murphy Brown,* the popular sitcom featuring a successful career woman who chooses to have a baby without a husband, illustrates one of the changes in the demography of the family over the past 40 years. And the Johnson family described in the case vignette at the beginning of the chapter represents yet another form of family diversity resulting from divorce and remarriage.

Social, demographic, and economic factors have all contributed to the changing composition of the family. U.S. Census Bureau statistics indicate that 1 in 3 births in 1995 were to unmarried women. Contrary to common perceptions that teens are responsible for most of the out-of-wedlock births, rates of out-of-wedlock births are highest among single women in their 20s (Snyder & Moore, 1996). Based on the trend toward a higher proportion of births to single women, coupled with the higher incidence of divorce, about half of all children today are expected to spend some part of their time in a single-parent home (Bianchi & Spain, 1996). And given that more than 75% of people who divorce remarry, demographers estimate that stepfamilies or blended families (approximately 19% in 1990) will become the norm in the 2000s (Ahlburg & De Vita, 1992). The number of dual-career families also has markedly increased, with almost three-fourths of married mothers with children in 1996 reporting some paid employment. Furthermore, the continued growth of the older population will increase both the number of elderly couples and the number of frail elderly persons living alone who will require supportive services in an era when adult daughters hold jobs and are not as readily available as earlier generations to be family caregivers (Bianchi & Spain, 1996).

Heightened attention to demographic changes in the composition of the family over the past 40 years has generated considerable debate among social scientists on whether the family is declining in importance in our society. In reflecting on the passion that often surrounds the debate, Cowan, Field, Hansen, Skolnick, and Swanson (1992) asserted, "Families mattered in the past; they continue to matter in the present; and they will matter still, in the uncertain years of our future" (p. 481). Valuing the family, however, should not be confused with valuing a particular family form. They urged that rather than viewing demographic changes in the composition of the family unit as indicative of family decline, we need to reconsider traditional definitions of family that emphasize legal and biological ties between members and conceptualize how diverse types of families fulfill different functions to address the complexity of their health needs.

How should we define the family for community health nursing assessment and intervention? Although community health nursing's primary target of service is the community (Williams, 1996), work with the family as a population is one strategy that nurses may use to improve the health of communities. Thus, community health nurses need a broad conceptual perspective of the family that recognizes diverse compositions. **Family** in this chapter refers to two or more individuals who identify themselves as family and manifest some degree of interdependence in interactions with each other and their **environment** in meeting basic human needs for affection and meaning. Themes central to this definition are members' **interdependence** in meeting basic needs and members' **beliefs** that they are a family. This purposefully broad view of family encompasses the traditional two-parent nuclear family, single-parent families, stepfamilies or blended families, and childless couples, as well as relationships that are not built on legal or biological ties, such as gay or lesbian families.

Health Responsibilities of the Family

How well the family functions has a great impact on individual family members' well-being and health behaviors. Health professionals' encounters with the family are episodic, with the family assuming responsibility for a least 75% of the health care of its members (Duffy, 1988). An assessment of family functioning in promoting and protecting its members' health requires a clear understanding of its responsibilities in this arena. Five major responsibilities of the family for members' health are presented.

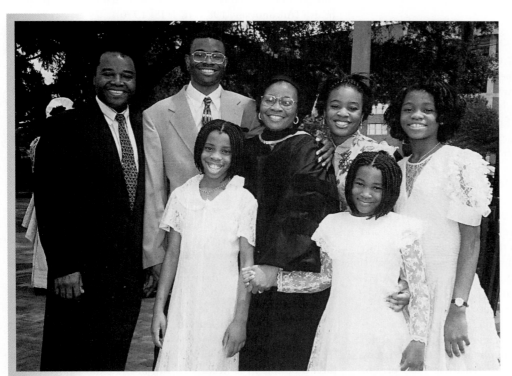

The family provides security where children can get a sense of who they are and what they can accomplish.

Development of Members' Sense of Personal Identity and Self-Worth

The family plays a significant role in the development of one's mental health (Hanson & Boyd, 1996; Loveland-Cherry, 1996). Family interactions may facilitate or impede members' access to (1) **affect,** the sense of loving and being loved; (2) **power,** the freedom to decide what one wants and the ability to obtain it; and (3) **meaning,** a sense of who and what one is. The functionally healthy family is one that maintains a balance between all members' access to affect, power, and meaning so that no member consistently and systematically is denied actualization of these basic human needs. Community health nurses often receive referrals to conduct a family assessment in situations in which parents have experienced difficulties in meeting the socioemotional needs of infants and young children, resulting in impaired attachment and inadequate weight gain associated with the syndrome referred to as *failure to thrive.* Early parent-infant attachment is critical to the development of trust and ability to form intimate relationships with others later in life. Parents who have difficulty forming appropriate attachments with their infants may have lacked appropriate role models as young children themselves. Such individuals often are suspicious of professionals, and much interpersonal skill and patience is needed to establish working relationships with them. By conveying warmth and caring, coupled with a nonjudgmental attitude, nurses can assist parents in learning how to meet the socioemotional needs of their children.

Emotional Support and Guidance During Life Cycle Transitions

As individuals grow and mature, they are expected to meet new performance expectations consistent with their current life stage. For example, a child is expected to learn to read when he or she goes to school. Should the child find reading difficult, school progress is slowed and the child's sense of personal worth is threatened. Support and guidance from the family is essential in helping individuals achieve their developmental tasks across the life cycle (Duvall & Miller, 1985). In fact, the family as a whole is described as having responsibilities, goals, and developmental tasks that parallel the developmental tasks of individual family members. Thus, while children are expected to learn to read and develop other cognitive skills when they go to school, the family has the corresponding developmental task of encouraging children's educational achievement and learning to relate to the educational system in an effective manner.

Community health nurses have many opportunities to provide guidance to families undergoing life cycle transitions. Prenatal and postpartum visits for new parents can offer health teaching to ease the transition to parenthood. Changes in family structure as a result of divorce and/or remarriage also present new developmental tasks for family members, such as single par-

enthood and the addition of stepparent into children's lives. As noted in the introductory paragraph, Kevin's teacher in making a referral to the school nurse questioned whether his toileting accidents in school might be symptomatic of difficulty in coping with his parents' divorce and the subsequent move and remarriage of his father.

• •

For good or ill, our families and the environment in which we live are the backdrop against which we play out our entire lives. Families shape our futures; our early family experiences heavily influence and to a degree determine how we forever after think and behave.
Hillary Rodham Clinton, *It takes a village and other lessons children teach us,* 1996

• •

Socialization of Family Members to Value and Maintain Health

Family members acquire values about health and learn personal health practices relative to nutrition, exercise, smoking, alcohol consumption, and hygiene through their family of origin and later transmit these values and beliefs to children as they become parents. Recognition that lifestyle factors are the single most important determinant of most of our chronic diseases has focused attention on the importance of the family's responsibility to teach its members how to maintain and preserve health (Antonovsky, 1987; DHHS, 1990).

Healthy People 2010 (DHHS, 2000) offers a vision for preventing unnecessary death and disability, enhancing the quality of life for all Americans through the establishment of specific health promotion and disease prevention objectives. Many of the objectives focus on lifestyle risks that have their origin in health practices learned within the family context. In their interactions with families, nurses may assist members to assess health risks and to incorporate health promotion into their lifestyle (Duffy, 1988). Schools and the workplace also offer natural loci for helping children and adults to improve their health knowledge and develop attitudes that facilitate healthier behaviors.

Education About When and How to Use the Health Care System

The family also serves as the basic referent for defining illness and what should be done about it (Doherty & Campbell, 1988). The process by which the ill person seeks information and advice from family, friends, neighbors, and other nonprofessionals has been labeled the "lay referral network." Whether a family member's symptoms should be treated with home remedies and over-the-counter medications or professional help should be sought is negotiated within the family based on interpretations of the seriousness of the symptoms, the possible cause, and the impact that illness may have on the member's fulfillment of role responsibilities (Doherty, 1992). While *Healthy People 2010* has shifted national attention toward primary prevention by emphasizing health promotion and health protection activities, secondary prevention, which involves early detection and treatment of illness, also is recognized as another important approach for fostering healthy communities. In some families, one is defined as ill only when symptoms are severe enough to impact role performance. Teaching women the importance of breast self-examinations and having yearly Pap smears and a mammogram after age 50 or teaching males the importance of regular testicular and digital rectal examinations are examples of ways nurses can encourage family members to value the early detection of disease and to use the health care system in a more proactive way.

Care Provision and Management for Chronically Ill, Disabled, and Aging Family Members

Families assume a major share of the responsibility for intergenerational support and assistance. Among older disabled persons who live in the community, more than 90% relied in part on family for care (Ahlburg & De Vita, 1992). Two distinct caregiving roles that may be assumed by the family are direct care provider and indirect care manager. The direct care provider actively assists family members with those activities and tasks that they are no longer able to perform independently. Stevenson (1990) reported that 80% of family caregivers provided care for the impaired relative 7 days a week for an average of 4 hours per day. In contrast, the indirect care manager identifies the needed services an impaired relative requires and manages their provision by others. Problems in meeting societal expectations of families for caring for disabled and aging members are emerging because the caregiving role previously filled by women has dramatically changed as a result of the increase in dual-career families. Recognition of the latter has led to the rapid expansion of home health services and hospice programs to facilitate care of family members within their home environment.

Theoretical Approaches to the Family

Theory provides the practitioner with a systematic way of viewing a particular phenomenon. There are varied theoretical frameworks that have been used to describe family interaction and behavior. No single theory is sufficiently broad to deal with the complex dynamics that undergird the family's competence to fulfill its health responsibilities. Thus, an integrated approach that blends family systems theory with family development and human ecology theory will be used. This ecological systems perspective is particularly relevant to the discipline of nursing because it considers interrelationships between individuals within the family as well as between the family unit and the community over time.

Human Ecology Theory

Human ecology theory emphasizes the importance of social contexts as influences on human development. Bronfenbrenner (1986) notes that the parent-child relationship is enhanced as a context for development to the extent that the family's interrelationships with social networks, neighborhoods, communities, institutions, and cultures are supportive of its efforts to care for children. A similar perspective is presented by Hillary Rodham Clinton in her book, *It Takes A Village: And Other Lessons Children Teach Us.* Thus, the extent to which work settings provide quality day care or flexible working hours can strongly influence the success of dual-career couples in fulfilling their child-rearing functions. Similarly, adolescent parents are more likely to be able to continue to meet their own developmental needs for education when school policies support pregnant teens' remaining in school throughout the pregnancy and/or provide child care for teens returning to school after the baby's birth.

· ·

Nothing is more important to our shared future than the well-being of children. For children are at our core—not only as vulnerable beings in need of love and care but as a moral touchstone amidst the complexity and contentiousness of modern life. Just as it takes a village to raise a child, it takes children to raise up a village to become all it should be. The village we build with them in mind will be a better place for us all.
Hillary Rodham Clinton, 1996
It takes a village and other lessons children teach us

· ·

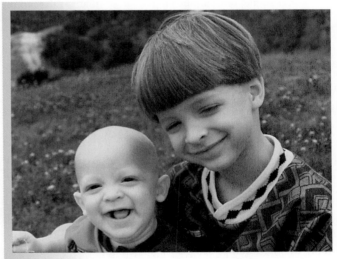

The socialization of children is one of the most important functions of the family.

Another distinctive feature of human ecology theory is its recognition that the family is both influenced by and actively influences the larger social systems with which it interacts. This perspective of human ecology theory encourages us to look at interactions between the family and its multilevel environment as reciprocal rather than unidirectional processes. For example, although governmental policies often strongly impact the health care services available to a family, families can impact and shape policy. Parents concerned about pressures from health maintenance organizations (HMOs) and insurance companies, which often forced mothers and their newborns to be discharged within 24 hours of birth, joined professional and citizen lobby groups to help pass a 1996 law titled "The Newborns' and Mothers' Health Protection Act." This bill requires insurers to cover a minimum stay of 48 hours for mothers and their newborns.

Family Systems Theory

Although human ecology theory provides us with a conception of how interrelationships between the family and its social context influence the family's capacity to foster health, it does not address how internal processes within the family may facilitate or impede health. Family systems theory, however, does provides us with several key concepts to understand the role of internal family processes on health. First is the concept of **nonsummativity,** which states that the family as a whole is greater than the sum of its parts; a change in one family member affects all family members (Wright & Leahey, 1994). Because the whole is more than and different from the sum of its parts, the family's ability to fulfill its health responsibilities cannot be predicted from knowledge about an individual's behavior and health practices. Rather the nurse must assess how family relationships and their social environments either impede or foster health (see the Research Brief above).

For example, one cannot judge that an infant is developing adequate attachment without assessing the relationships between the parent and infant. Are bids of the infant to mother for attention when distressed responded to with soothing behaviors on the part of the mother? Healthfulness is reflected in the dyad's capacity to achieve patterns of interaction that are mutually rewarding (Robinson, Emde, & Korfmacher, 1997). Another example of the principle of nonsummativity is illustrated in the brief vignette presented at the beginning of this chapter. Rather than simply viewing Jimmy's toileting accidents and inattention as indicators only of a potential underlying physical health problem, the school nurse and teacher recognize the importance of considering that Jimmy's symptoms may reflect problems he is having in coping with changes in family relationships. Moreover, the school nurse chooses to follow up on the problem by scheduling a home visit to gather more data on how the mother is handling the transition to being a single parent.

Two other concepts important in understanding how the family operates as a system are structure and function. **Structure** refers to the organization of relationships among family mem-

RESEARCH BRIEF

Deatrick, J. A., Brennan, D., & Cameron, M. E. (1998). Mothers with multiple sclerosis and their children: Effects of fatigue and exacerbations on maternal support. Nursing Research, 47(4), 205–210.

A study of 35 mothers with multiple sclerosis and their children found that both mothers and children perceived that mothers were less physically affectionate when mothers' symptoms of illness were exacerbated. Mothers, however, significantly underestimated the changes in their physical affection compared with children's perceptions. Qualitative data further revealed that affective issues were linked with tremendous fears of the children, particularly the younger children, as reflected in the following comments: "I cry when she's sick. Sometimes I think that she is going to die."

bers (i.e., roles), whereas **function** defines the purposes or goals of the family, such as activities necessary to ensure health and growth of its members (Walsh, 1982). Structure and function are interrelated in that the structure of a family influences how well it is able to fulfill its purposes or goals. Roles within a family must be integrated much as the meshing of gears in a finely tuned engine to facilitate attainment of common goals. Nurses working in the community often encounter families who are struggling with children's behavioral problems because the parents cannot agree on what are reasonable bedtimes for young children or how to consistently set limits, and consequently each defines different expectations for the child. Although adults may learn to balance multiple role expectations (e.g., spouse, parent, worker, volunteer), young children need clarity in role expectations to begin to develop a sense of identity and self-worth (one of the family's five health responsibilities).

Finally, understanding the role that **self-regulation** processes play in how the family functions in meeting its health responsibilities is important for nurses working in the community. A balance between stability and change is needed for a family to effectively address the differing needs of its members over time (Klein & White, 1996). Self-regulation involves processing the internal as well as external feedback that a family receives regarding its behavior. Feedback can be positive or negative. **Positive feedback** moves the family toward change, whereas **negative feedback** tends to promote stability. In assessing a family, the nurse seeks to identify those behaviors that are detrimental to health and provides feedback in the form of health teaching. In the previous example in which parents are having difficulty in agreeing on limits for their children, teaching by the nurse about realistic expectations for the child's developmental age and the importance of consistency in parental discipline would be directed toward behavioral change. On the other hand, in working with a mother who the nurse observes reads to her toddler, teaching about how parents can facilitate language development of toddlers would reinforce and expand on the mother's existing behaviors.

Family Development Theory

Family development theory highlights that change is an inherent aspect of family life. The family life cycle is described in terms of developmental stages characterized by major family events—in particular, the addition and exiting of members (Carter & McGoldrick, 1989). The concept of **family developmental tasks** refers to growth responsibilities that must be achieved by a family during each stage of its life cycle to successively meet the health and developmental needs of its members. For example, the birth of a child necessitates that other family members learn new role behaviors for protecting and fostering the health and development of the infant. Variations in the family life cycle and its developmental tasks are changing with the increasing diversity of family types. Although the single-parent family experiences the same life cycle changes as the traditional two-parent nuclear family, the absence of the second parent to carry a share of the family tasks with respect to support, child rearing, companionship, and gender role modeling for children may result in increased stressors for single parents. Divorce and possibly remarriage, with their losses and shifts in family membership, create new developmental tasks. For example, after divorce, spouses need to work through resolution of the attachment to one another while promoting ongoing parental contact between the ex-spouse and children (Carter & McGoldrick, 1989). With stepparent or blended families, crucial developmental tasks involve the restructuring of family boundaries and roles to allow for inclusion of new family members (stepparent and possibly stepchildren). Bain (1978) has advanced a theory to predict the capacity of families to cope with life cycle transitions that helps integrate human ecology and family systems with family development theory. According to his theory, families who are likely to have the least capacity to cope with life cycle transitions, or who are at most risk, are (1) those who are experiencing a greater number of concurrent life cycle changes involving (2) role transitions of great magnitude (e.g., blended families) and who (3) have a social support network that is small and nonsupportive, and (4) live in a community that has few available services to assist them with the transitions confronting them.

Family-Oriented Versus Family-Focused Nursing Role

Nurses working in the community generally advocate a family approach in the delivery of services. In reality, a family approach has varied meanings in practice. Many times, nursing interventions are directed toward the health concerns of referred individuals, with other family members being considered only as a support system for helping the individual cope with his or her health concerns. This family-oriented approach is most typical of nurses working in ambulatory care centers and home health agencies. For example, in working with a newly diagnosed diabetic, the nurse may assess the extent to which other family members understand and support the diabetic individual's need to modify dietary patterns to manage the disease effectively and prevent further complications. The complexity of health issues confronting families may, at times, necessitate a more sophisticated holistic approach. With a family-focused approach, as contrasted with a family-oriented approach, the family as a whole is viewed as having specific health responsibilities, and the extent to which family processes support these functions is the nursing focus. Assessments of the family as a group are made and interventions are directed toward helping the family grow in its abilities to meet its health responsibilities. A typical example often encountered by nurses working in public health departments is the family with a 13-year-old pregnant adolescent. From an ecological systems perspective, the adolescent's pregnancy necessitates role changes for all family members as the new baby is incorporated into the family. Hence a family-focused approach is needed to help family members deal effectively with the life cycle transitions triggered by the adolescent's pregnancy.

As nurses move into community settings, they need to be aware of the differences between a family-oriented and family-focused approach and select the one that is best suited to the needs of the health care situations they encounter. The mission of the health care delivery system in which the nurse works also may influence the choice of approach. For example, where the mission of the organization is disease control or rehabilitation, the family-oriented approach may be a better fit. Nurses working in organizations such as health departments, which have a population-focused perspective and emphasize health promotion and disease reduction, are likely to find more support for a family-focused approach.

A Conceptual Framework for Family Assessment

A conceptual framework provides direction to the collection, organization, and interpretation of data about the family's health situation. The conceptual framework for family assessment presented in this chapter builds on the perspective of the family as an ecological system and is designed to assist nurses in evaluating the extent to which a family is able to fulfill its health responsibilities (Box 30-1). The conclusion reached by conducting the assessment is an evaluation that the family is functioning more or less optimally in meeting its health responsibilities, as opposed to an evaluation regarding the health status of a particular family member.

To meet its health responsibilities, a family needs to be conscious of the health needs of its members at varying stages in the

Promote mental health of family members by providing opportunities for each to achieve a satisfactory sense of personal identity and self-worth.

Provide support and cognitive guidance for family members to achieve developmental tasks associated with life cycle transitions.

Socialize family members to adopt health practices that foster health and reduce risks for disease.

Educate family members about when and how to use health care services when disruptions in health occur.

Assist ill, disabled, and aging family members to meet their basic needs either through direct care provision or through helping them access community services.

EXPANDING FAMILY HEALTH POTENTIAL.

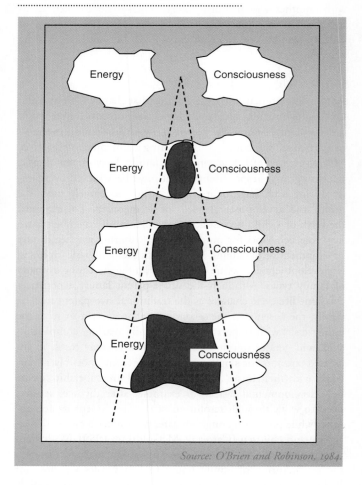

Source: O'Brien and Robinson, 1984.

life cycle and have sufficient energy to undertake the desired healthful behaviors (O'Brien, 1979; O'Brien & Robinson, 1984). At times, a family may have sufficient energy but lack the necessary awareness of members' needs to use its energy constructively to attain desired goals. The reverse also may be true. Thus, it is only when energy and consciousness interface and overlap that the family has the potential to effectively fulfill its health responsibilities (see the figure on the right).

A more detailed discussion of these two core concepts as well as those family attributes and processes that may influence the level of energy and consciousness within a family system is presented below.

Energy

To teach family members good health practices, to use the professional care system to foster health maintenance, to provide members with supportive and effective relationships necessary for positive mental health, and to actively cope with life cycle transitions all require the investment of energy (Newman, 1994; Rogers, 1983). A critical issue in family functioning is the regulation of energy flow to attain balance as opposed to imbalance—too much or too little energy (O'Brien & Robinson, 1984). When the energy flow within families is too much, behavior is likely to be chaotic and ineffectual, resulting in crisis-oriented problem solving when members' needs or concerns become too great to ignore. The latter is often the case in families that lack clear boundaries and where extended kin, neighbors, and friends move in and out of the household at will. In contrast, when energy is low or depleted, family members' needs are likely to be unmet, as illustrated in the following experience related by a mother suffering from postpartum depression.

My husband and son got back from the store. I think my 3-year-old son wanted to tell me about something that happened. It was physically so hard to listen that I really remember just trying to pull up some kind of wall so that I wouldn't be battered to death. At this point I was really sitting on the couch trying to figure out whether I could ever move again, and I started to cry. My son started hitting me with his fists, and he said, "Where are you, Mom?" It was really painful because I didn't have a clue as to where I was either. He was really trying to wake something up, but it was just too far gone. There was no way that I could retrieve the mom that he remembered and hoped he would find, let alone the mother I wanted to be for my new baby.

Beck, 1996

In addition to assessing the energy that the family has available to invest in meeting members' health needs, it is important to identify how it replenishes its energy. The potential sources of energy vary from family to family, from individual to individual. For some, the source may be religious beliefs, cultural traditions, shared time together, school or work activities, or social relationships with friends. The nature of the sources is unimportant, provided that the family acquires sufficient energy to meet the demands placed on it. With a family that manifests a low energy level, nursing intervention may take the form of helping the family identify new ways of acquiring energy.

Pertinent questions to consider in assessing a family's energy level include the following:

- *How does the family acquire energy?*
- *What are its sources?*
- *Is there sufficient energy to meet the varying needs of its members? If not, where is the family's energy directed?*
- *Does the expenditure of energy in meeting family demands occur repeatedly at the expense of one particular family member?*

Consciousness

Consciousness is being aware of one's own feelings, needs, and actions as well as what is happening with others; in essence, it is the information that a system has available to effectively fulfill its functions (Newman, 1994). Growth and change within a family are directly linked to the family's level of consciousness, because it enables knowledge to be translated into goal-directed behavior. That is, the greater the consciousness, the more aware the family will be of its health responsibilities at any given stage of the life cycle, and the repertoire of choices generated for meeting those responsibilities will be more refined (Newman, 1994; O'Brien & Robinson, 1984). A thoughtful assessment of the family's level of consciousness provides the foundation for planning health promotion activities.

Another important aspect of the family's consciousness is the myths it creates about how it operates as a family (O'Brien & Robinson, 1984). For example, a family may describe relationships among members as close and intimate because all members spend a lot of time watching television together. Yet an observer might note that family members hardly ever communicate with one another during the time spent in the same room. Quite obviously, family myths may at times impede addressing family members' needs because the family is unable to recognize the need for behavioral change as a result of the belief that it is already behaving in the desired way. A useful assessment technique to begin to help family members become more aware of their own behavior is to engage them in reflective exercises. For example, in responding to a mother who complains that her son is "always misbehaving and won't listen" to her, the nurse might ask the mother to describe in detail a typical incident, including what her son was doing at the time and how she responded to his behavior. A common error that parents make in setting limits is to tell the child what not to do but offer no explanation for why the behavior is unacceptable.

Pertinent questions to consider in assessing a family's level of consciousness include the following:

- *How aware and knowledgeable is the family of specific health and developmental needs of its members?*
- *Does it hold incorrect beliefs that are likely to lead to unsound health practices?*
- *Is its perception of how it functions congruent with reality?*
- *What are the sources that the family utilizes in acquiring knowledge?*
- *How do past family experiences influence its consciousness of health issues?*
- *Does it actively seek to expand its level of consciousness or does it respond only to crisis demands?*

Role Structure

Roles define the goals and actions that are expected to characterize the occupant of a specific position such as mother or father (Hardy & Conway, 1988). Identification of the varying roles of family members provides the nurse with important information about the organization of relationships among family members, such as who is expected to do what and for whom. Flexibility of role definitions enables the family to deal more effectively with developmental transitions and situational crises resulting from illness or disability of one of its members (Boss, 1988).

Difficulty in the performance of one's role is defined as role insufficiency. A basic concept in role theory is that roles are reciprocal in that they are patterned to complement that of a role partner. Thus, the mothering role cannot be understood without looking at the corresponding role of the child at a particular developmental stage. Role behaviors expected of mothers of infants will differ from those expected of mothers whose children are in their adolescent years. When role insufficiency occurs, one or more family members' health and developmental needs are likely to be unmet.

In assessing family members' role performance, nurses need to be aware that role behaviors are learned according to the cultural values of the family. Collecting information about the family's customs and traditions is important for interpreting whether family members' roles are appropriate within their social context. For example, the maternal grandmother often assumes the mothering role for young children in African American single-parent families (Burton & deVries, 1995). Furthermore, it often is helpful to gather information about their early role models and how these experiences have affected present role behaviors (Friedman, 1998). It is not uncommon for parents' expectations and behaviors toward children to be similar to those they experienced in their families of origin (see the Research Brief on p. 696).

Role overload leading to increased stress and reduced levels of wellness has been cited as an issue for single-parent families (Burden, 1986; Popenoe, 1995). The single parent must fulfill

RESEARCH BRIEF

Hall, L. A., Sachs, B., & Rayens, M. K. (1998). Mothers' potential for child abuse: The roles of childhood abuse and social resources. Nursing Research, 47, 87–95.

A study of 206 low-income single mothers of young children found that the mothers' child abuse potential was positively associated with the levels of physical and sexual abuse experienced in their own childhood; sexual abuse displayed the strongest association. Compared with mothers who were not sexually abused in childhood, those reporting violent sexual abuse as children were almost six times more likely to have high potential for physically abusing their children.

both mother and father roles, often in addition to the work role, whereas role ambiguity and conflict are often major sources of stress in stepparent and blended families as members attempt to define whether the stepparent should assume the role of parent or nonparent and how children of the respective parents should relate as siblings. A typical example of resulting role conflict is the stepfather who disciplines his wife's child for misbehavior and is confronted by his wife for "overstepping" the boundaries of his role as a stepfather. In addition, ongoing relationships with the biological parent and the addition of relationships with the kin of the stepparent further compound the clear definition of family roles (Carter & McGoldrick, 1989). It is important for the nurse to carefully assess role strain and conflict occurring within the family because tension and conflict may negatively impact members' emotional well-being. Clarity of role expectations is crucial to helping family members develop a sense of personal identity and self-worth. Moreover, role strain and conflict, if left unresolved, may deplete the usable energy available for meeting the family's other health responsibilities, such as teaching members basic health practices to maintain health and how to use health care services appropriately (Pratt, 1976, 1982).

Pertinent questions to consider in assessing a family's role structure include the following:

- *What roles do each of the family members fulfill? How competently do members perform their roles?*

- *How do past family experiences influence members' role performance?*

- *If role strain or conflict exists, what are the contributing factors?*

- *Is there flexibility in roles when needed?*

Decision-Making Processes

Decision making is central to the fulfillment of family responsibilities in meeting members' health and developmental needs. It is a process that involves (1) recognizing the need for a decision,

(2) identifying and weighing alternatives, and (3) selecting an alternative and facilitating its implementation. Central to effective decision making is the processing of information; the decision maker must be able to discriminate between what is important and what is not, between what is relevant and what is irrelevant, between actions that will achieve goals and those that will not. The family's use of health care services often provides insight into their decision-making processes. As noted, families often seek the advice of extended kin and friends about how to interpret untoward symptoms and whether they are sufficiently serious to warrant professional care. In some families, illness may be equated with inability to perform one's expected roles, resulting in a delay in seeking health care until symptoms are advanced. Studies have shown that poor health-related decision-making skills often reflect difficulty in decision making in other areas of family life. On the other hand, parents who make general lifestyle decisions that are growth-oriented and motivated toward change are more likely to practice and encourage health promotion behaviors for themselves and their children (Duffy, 1988). Nursing assessment of the family's decision-making processes focuses on identifying strengths or limitations in the information-processing function as well as the generation of alternative solutions. Immediate closure through the selection of a single option without explicit ranking or elimination of alternatives is characteristic of dysfunctional families, whereas healthy, functioning families explore numerous options, and if one alternative does not work, the family backs off and tries another, instead of trying to just make one option work (O'Brien & Robinson, 1984; Walsh, 1982). Of equal importance to note are those situations in which families arrive at no decision. Discussions finish inconclusively and are then decided by events, as with a couple who argues about what form of birth control to use until the wife discovers she is pregnant. Such an event is called *de facto decision making* in that things are allowed to happen without planning. De facto decision making is characteristic of multiproblem fam-

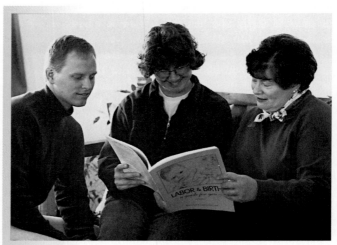

Chapter author, Dr. Ruth O'Brien (right), counsels prenatal family about birth options.

ilies, many of whose members feel powerless and/or lack the energy to actively manage their lives. It also may occur in healthy families dealing with highly stressful situations when members' abilities to process information is reduced (Friedman, 1998).

Observations about family decision-making processes also help clarify its power structure. Families tend to reach decisions either by consensus or accommodation (Friedman, 1998). With consensus, a particular course of action is mutually agreed on by all concerned. With accommodation, some members assent to allow a decision to be reached. Accommodation occurs by use of compromising, bargaining, and coercion. Thus, by recognizing situations involving accommodation and who was identified with the decision reached, the nurse can identify the "power" brokers in the family. Identification of who has the power in family decision making is crucial for nurses working with families because interventions must be designed to include these family members (see the following Research Brief).

Pertinent questions to consider in assessing family decision making include the following:

- *Who makes what decisions?*
- *Are there particular health needs/issues that are not recognized or addressed?*
- *Is the family able to discriminate between information that is relevant and that which is irrelevant to the decision?*
- *Are alternative solutions generated and weighed? Is the selected alternative implemented?*
- *Who holds the power in family decision making? To what extent do family decisions involve consensus or coercion?*

RESEARCH BRIEF

Cole, R., Kitzman, H., Olds, D., & Sidora, K. (1998). Family context as a moderator of program effects in prenatal and early childhood home visitation. Journal of Community Psychology, 26(1), 37–48.

The ability of a nurse home visitation program for first-time mothers and their infants to affect changes in the quality of the caregiving environment was found to vary with household structure. Mothers who lived alone and those who lived with their husbands or boyfriends were able to create safer and more stimulating child-rearing environments than mothers who lived with grandmothers or with other adults. The investigators interpreted these findings as suggesting that where the mother is able to plan and take a course of action on her own, or in concert with someone over whom she is likely to exert some decision-making influence such as a husband or boyfriend, she is more able to implement changes in the home suggested by nurse home visitors.

Communication Patterns

Observation of a family's communication patterns yields valuable information about the meaning accorded to various family members as well as the clarity of interpersonal boundaries (Sieburg, 1985). **Communication** is a transactional process between two or more individuals in which feelings, needs, information, and opinions are shared. One of the most basic assessments regarding the family's communication patterns is the identification of who communicates what with whom. Individuals within the family may selectively disclose feelings, needs, and information to other members. Thus, communication patterns are linked to the family's level of consciousness. When individuals share their ideas and feelings freely and completely, they have a broad base of cues and provisional solutions on which to base their final actions. Problem solving is more effective in such families because members contribute to the solution of concern and are more likely to be committed to the decisions reached.

Still another important assessment is the identification of covert rules governing communication among family members. Satir (1983) defines rules as the "shoulds" and "should nots" of family life. For example, a family rule may be that only positive feelings should be expressed or that sex is not an appropriate topic of discussion. An illustration of the importance that family rules play in understanding communication exchanges among family members may be found in a spousal argument over the wife's allowing the couple's 10-year-old son to attend a movie with a group of friends. After much heated discussion, the husband acknowledges that he did not object to his son's having gone to the movies with his friends, but he felt his wife should have consulted him before giving the son permission. In reality, the argument between husband and wife stems from the husband's perception that his wife violated a family rule, namely that decisions about the son's peer activities are joint parental decisions. One fundamental principle of communication theory is that every exchange not only conveys information or content, but a definitional meaning of how one views self and others (Sieburg, 1985). In fact, the recognition accorded to the other is more crucial than the content. By attending to the recognition accorded to others, the nurse can gain an understanding of how communication shapes member's feelings of self-worth and self-efficacy. Confirming messages validate the intrinsic worth of the person and endorses the other's self-experience as unique and valuable. Confirmation is conveyed by direct verbal acknowledgment of the other's message, expanding or elaborating on its content, requesting clarification of what another has said—all behaviors reflective of active listening.

Child: "Mom, look I tied my own sneakers."

Mother: "Let me see. Yes, you did do a fine job of tying your laces. You have worked very hard at learning to do that. I'm proud of you."

In contrast, disconfirming messages question the other's perception or validity of self-experience through such behaviors as looking away from the other when speaking, interrupting the other, turning to speak to a third person while the other is still talking, interjecting comments that are irrelevant, engaging in other activities while talking, exiting while another is talking, or remaining silent when a response is required or expected (Sieburg, 1985). Obviously, such behaviors leave the recipient with a feeling of powerlessness and, over time, result in lowered self-esteem.

Child: "Mom, look I tied my own sneakers."

Mother: "Don't bother me now. Can't you see that I'm reading the newspaper?"

Another important principle of communication relates to the congruence between the verbal and nonverbal aspects of the exchange. Verbal language conveys the substance of the message, whereas nonverbal language transmits the more subtle nature of the intent of the message. The degree of congruence and balance between the verbal and nonverbal portions of an exchange define the degree of clarity of the message for the recipient. Given that much verbal conflict among family members often stems from faulty interpretation of nonverbal aspects of communication, it is particularly important to assess the extent to which family members are able to elicit feedback and validate messages to minimize misinterpretation of cues and faulty mind reading (Sieburg, 1985).

Communication patterns also are the most observable indicators of the clarity of interpersonal boundaries among family members. The use of "I" statements as opposed to "we" statements and the extent of mind reading and censorship (e.g., "You shouldn't say that," "You have no reason to feel angry") present in members' communications with one another provide important clues to the clarity of interpersonal boundaries and members' sense of separateness and personal autonomy (Sieburg, 1985). Clear and functional communication among family members is considered a cornerstone of the healthy family (Goldenberg & Goldenberg, 1996; Janosik & Green, 1992; Satir, 1983). It is foundational in enabling the family to fulfill its health responsibility in assisting members to develop a sense of personal identity and self-worth. Moreover, clarity and openness of communication among family members facilitates effective decision making when disruptions to health arise. Families whose members lack good communications skills also often have difficulty accessing community services to help with their needs.

Pertinent questions to consider in assessing a family's communication patterns include the following:

* *Who talks to whom?*
* *What feelings or issues are closed to discussion?*
* *Are members able to clearly state their needs and feelings?*
* *Is there congruence between verbal and nonverbal aspects of communication?*
* *How well do members listen when others are communicating?*
* *Do members elicit feedback and validation in communicating with one another?*
* *What are the predominant patterns of acknowledgment accorded various members?*
* *Is communication among members age appropriate?*

Values

Knowledge of the value orientations of the family provides direction to understanding the why of family dynamics. A family's configuration of values ascribes meaning to certain health events and suggests ways to respond to them (Friedman, 1998). The identification of family values, however, is often compounded by the family's own lack of awareness of how it ascribes worth to people, events, and things. It is important to distinguish both the overt and covert values operative in family behavior.

A particularly important value orientation to assess is how the family views itself in relation to the environment. The family that feels it has little control over what happens does not take the initiative to seek out new ideas, information, or resources and apply them to the solution of family problems or to minimize health risks (Boss, 1988). Similarly, the time orientation of the family impacts the extent to which it actively addresses life cycle transitions and change. Families that emphasize past traditions may experience life cycle transitions as more stressful (Carter & McGoldrick, 1989). Likewise, a predominant focus on the present is likely to minimize anticipatory planning and emphasize de facto decision making (Duffy, 1988). As noted in the discussion of family decision making, families that rely on de facto decision making are less likely to engage in health promotion activities or use preventive health services.

Furthermore, there is a hierarchical nature to family values that influences the family's perceptions of risks and benefits of taking certain actions. The relative ranking of health in the family's hierarchy of values is important in determining the extent to which forces within the family tend to sustain or undermine health care behaviors. For example, the family who places a high value on home ownership may choose to forego preventive health care if economic resources are limited. An accurate assessment of a family's value system should help tailor interventions to goals that are important to the family.

A family's values are a reflection of its subculture, as well as of the community in which it resides. Obviously, the greater the degree of congruence between a family's subcultural values and the community's values, the more the community supports the family's identity. Incompatibility in values between the family and community generates conflict that increases stress within the family as a whole or between varying members of the family who have assimilated the community's values in differing degrees. Such stress may deplete the energy available to meet health responsibilities as well as negatively affect members' self-esteem (Friedman, 1998; Pratt, 1982).

It is equally important to recognize that nurses often have their own personal as well as professional values that define how the "ideal family" should behave. Unless nurses are aware of their own values, interactions with families may become conflictual as they pursue interventions directed toward expectations they hold for the family that are incongruent with its own values and beliefs. Generally, nursing's code of ethics encourages respect for the family's autonomy to make its own choices involving health matters unless such choices are likely to result in serious harm for others, such as spread of communicable disease and physical or sexual abuse of children.

Given that values cannot be seen directly, Friedman (1998) advocates the use of a "compare and contrast" method to assist the nurse in identifying specific family values. The compare and contrast method involves using a list of central values of the dominant culture or the family's subcultural reference group to engage the family in a discussion of their own values. Through discussion with the family, the nurse seeks not only to identify values held by the family and their overall relative importance to one another, but also to identify value differences and clashes between family members.

Pertinent questions to consider in assessing a family's values include the following:

- *What are the important values held by the family?*
- *To what extent do family values foster active coping and mastery of concerns?*
- *What is the family's orientation to the past, present, and future?*
- *What is the relative ranking of health in the family's hierarchy of values?*
- *Are there value conflicts evident within the family, between the family and subculture/community, or between the family and nurse?*

Family Boundaries

Family boundaries serve to distinguish the family from the social contexts or environments with which it interacts. In essence, family boundaries serve as a conceptual filter controlling the degree of exchange that family members have with their environ-

ment (Klein & White, 1996). Having selectively permeable boundaries allows for family growth and change, because the use of resources outside the family is enhanced (see the Research Brief below). The latter can contribute to family functioning by developing awareness of alternative courses of action (e.g., greater consciousness) and by increasing understanding of personal health practices and the value of self-directed action for promoting health (Pratt, 1982). Conversely, the amount of information a family can handle adequately is limited, and loose boundaries that result in an excess of information or conflicting information from the environment may amplify and create family disorganization (Walsh, 1982).

Markedly restricted interchange with the environment creates a greater reliance on inner family resources. Relatively closed families may exhibit more energy, in the form of tension, than they can discharge in constructive ways. Studies repeatedly have noted that child abuse clusters in families that are isolated from other families, neighbors, and society. In healthier isolated families, the members tend to believe that all or most of the needs of the members can be met within the family or the family's reference group (Sedgwick, 1981). Yet such exclusive reliance on internal resources may occur to the detriment of one or more family members in situations involving long-term chronic illness or disability, as evidenced by caregiver burden (Kramer & Kipnis, 1995; Smith, Tobin, & Fullmer, 1995).

Pertinent questions to consider in assessing family boundaries include the following:

- *Are family boundaries overly rigid or overly loose?*
- *What ongoing relationships does the family maintain with extended kin, friends, or other social groups?*
- *Do interactions with its support network foster or impede the family's ability to cope with its health responsibilities?*
- *Is the family satisfied with its support network?*
- *Is the family willing and able to access community services?*

Although the framework for family assessment presented in this chapter emphasizes critical areas of family functioning that have been found to contribute to the family's effectiveness in meeting its health responsibilities, one usually begins by obtaining basic identifying data about the family and its immediate environment: names and ages of family members, health history of each family member, racial/ethnic background, education, employment, income, health insurance, housing, characteristics of the immediate neighborhood, and availability of health and other basic services in the neighborhood (e.g., grocery stores, schools, churches, transportation). The purpose or reason for the nurse's contact with the family guides the initial information collected about pertinent areas of family functioning. For example, in making a home visit to the Johnson family to follow up on Kevin's toileting accidents and inattention in school, the nurse might begin by asking Mrs. Johnson what she thinks may be contributing to the changes in Kevin's behavior. Initial

RESEARCH BRIEF

Jepson, C., McCorkle, R., Adler, D., Nuamah, I., & Lusk, E. (1999). Effects of home care on caregivers' psychosocial status. Image: The Journal of Nursing Scholarship, 31(2), 115–120.

A sample of 161 caregivers of cancer patients were randomly assigned to a home care nursing intervention or to a control group that received no home care. At 3 and 6 months, caregivers in the home care intervention group showed improved psychosocial functioning (fewer depressive symptoms) compared with caregivers in the control group.

Family Life Cycle Transition: Teenage Pregnancy

Nancy, a 16-year-old unmarried Caucasian teen, lives in a housing project with her mother, her mother's current boyfriend, and two brothers—Jerome, 17 years old, and Derrick, 3 years old. She is 25 weeks pregnant. The pregnancy was unplanned; she was not using any form of contraception. Ronald, her 26-year-old boyfriend, is the father of the expectant child. Ronald has two previous children (ages 2 and 4 years) by another woman whom he rarely sees.

Nancy did not seek prenatal care until the beginning of her second trimester of pregnancy. To date, she has gained 13 pounds. Her health practices include the use of home remedies and self-comfort measures that she learned from her grandmother. She began smoking at age 13 and now smokes 1 to 2 packs of cigarettes a day. A frequent problem is urinary tract infections. Nancy told the clinic nurse who made the referral, "I can hardly get up in the morning to face the day now that I am pregnant. Sometimes life just doesn't seem worth it."

The two-bedroom apartment is too small for the five-person family; Nancy sleeps on a pull-out couch in the living room. She complains that she never has any privacy. The home is cluttered and in need of cleaning. Much cigarette smoke permeates the environment. Nancy says she feels unsafe in her neighborhood, where groups of males congregate outside the project complex; thus, she stays indoors most of the day.

Nancy dropped out of school in the ninth grade to stay home and care for Derrick while her mother works. She states that she knows that she will not be able to get a very good job in the future without finishing high school and wishes she could find a way to continue her education. Her mother works long hours as a certified care assistant in a nursing home trying to support herself and her children. The mother's current boyfriend is looking for employment because he had to quit his job in construction as a result of a back injury from an automobile accident.

Nancy is ambivalent about her pregnancy. She reports that Ronald has become more distant as her pregnancy has progressed; she is concerned that he may not assume financial responsibility for the baby and that this will be a further strain on her mother. She expresses confidence about being able to take care of a baby because she has had significant responsibility for her younger brother. The nurse observes that Nancy displays much warmth and patience in interactions with Derrick during the visit.

Nancy receives Medicaid and help from the Women, Infants and Children (WIC) Program. Although she could not be specific as to how Ronald makes a living, she states, "He always seems to have plenty of money." He has given her some money to buy baby equipment and clothes.

1. What initial family diagnosis would you make?
2. What other information would you need to know to assist Nancy in promoting a healthy pregnancy?
3. What community resources could you use to promote family health in this family?

---

information shared by the family will help guide the nurse in determining what other data to collect. The data are synthesized to identify family strengths in meeting its health responsibilities and areas where the family could use help to cope more effectively. The latter serves as a guide for negotiating the nurse's continuing role and activities with the family.

A Self-Efficacy Model for Nurse-Family Intervention

Because the family's ability to effectively fulfill its health responsibilities requires self-direction and self-governance, the nurse-family intervention should facilitate the family's active

participation in dealing with the health concerns or issues that it is experiencing. Indeed, the family's active participation in nurse-family interactions may be a significant variable in determining the effectiveness of nursing intervention (O'Brien & Robinson, 1984). The **contracting** process provides a means for enhancing family participation in its own health maintenance. Contracting is based on the belief that families have the potential for self-growth and the right to self-determination. It calls for an active participative as well as a collaborative role for both family and nurse because the goal is to build family self-efficacy in addressing its needs. The contracting process may be subdivided into five interlinking, sequenced phases (Sloan & Schommer, 1982). As with any relationship, the phases denote an ebb and flow of movement rather than discrete points at which something begins or ends. In the description that follows, each phase is discussed separately, although in reality they may overlap.

Identification of Family Health Concerns and Needs

This phase begins with the initial contact between the family and the nurse. Data, both subjective and objective, are gained about each other through observation and exchange of information. The use of a conceptual framework for assessing family functioning facilitates a clear identification of how the family is meeting its health responsibilities and any accompanying concerns (see appendix A). The preferable outcome of this first phase is an agreement between the nurse and family on the definition of the problems, needs, and concerns to be addressed in subsequent interactions. Two other outcomes are also possible: (1) referral to a more appropriate service or (2) termination because congruence between nurse and family does not exist and effective problem solving is not feasible (Williamson, 1981).

Mutual Setting of Goals

What does the family hope to accomplish? This is a crucial question, and one that is not asked often enough by nurses. By asking what the family hopes to gain from the intervention, the nurse assists the family to focus on its own goals and priorities. The nurse also can gain a sense of congruency between individual member and family goals, often a source of potential conflict (Lynch & Tiedje, 1991). In essence, this phase involves collaborative negotiations and democratic compromise rather than the nurse deciding goals. The nurse, however, expands the family's consciousness by sharing observations and knowledge that can facilitate the family's identification of goals.

The communication style used by the nurse can foster or hinder the family's acceptance of a suggested goal. For instance, "Perhaps we need to work on ways to reduce the distress your son's behavior is causing" is likely to be met with a more favorable response than, "You need to work on improving your relationships with one another." The second approach will invariably raise the family's defenses, whereas the first fosters its willingness to allow the nurse to help them work toward a solution to their concern. Helping the family to set realistic, attainable goals is one of the nurse's key functions. Goals should be stated in a precise manner capable of being monitored and a time frame for accomplishment specified. For example, "Mother will spend half an hour each evening in some planned activity with children" is a more measurable goal than, "Mother will improve attention given to children." Even when specific goals are set, there may be lack of progress. The family's prioritizing of goals may conflict with the nurse's. The nurse may need to support the family's priorities to free its energy for other goal attainment. If the nurse cannot offer such support because of possible injury to a particular family member, the family needs to be informed of what action will be taken.

Delineation of Alternatives

Once the goals are established, the nurse and family need to discuss how they can be attained. This process involves (1) the exploration and determination of the family's strengths and available resources, (2) the steps or actions needed to attain the goals, (3) the negotiation and division of responsibilities of the family and nurse for goal attainment, and (4) the establishment of a reasonable time limit for implementing the plan.

Emphasizing the already existing family strengths reinforces the family's belief in its own ability to solve problems and meet goals. In working with a mother having difficulty with limit setting and discipline with a toddler, the nurse might begin by acknowledging the attempts the mother has made to solve the problem and emphasize how well she is managing other areas of child care. Such an approach fosters esteem and confidence in the mother and facilitates her acceptance of the nurse as a helping person. A temptation to be avoided is the offering of numerous suggestions about how to do something better or differently before recognizing and drawing out the family's estimation of its own resources and potential solutions. The nurse can then supplement the family's developing knowledge base by introducing family and/or community resources not identified for its consideration.

Equally important in the planning process are decisions on the sequence of activities and the time frame needed to achieve the goal. The nurse generally plays a supportive role in this process, encouraging the family to make specific and detailed plans that are likely to maximize goal attainment. Agreement on the nurse's role and ways to monitor progress are crucial outcomes of this phase.

Implementation of the Plan

The plan and division of responsibilities mutually agreed on are tried. The nurse plays particularly vital roles during this phase. First is the anticipation of problems or setbacks that may arise, followed by helping the family recognize and deal with them in as positive a way as possible. A series of minor setbacks can discourage and demoralize family members to the extent that the carefully negotiated plan may be prematurely abandoned. Frequent contacts for guidance and support during the implementation phase can help individual family members accomplish their tasks. Second, the nurse has an important role-modeling function in that nursing responsibilities are carried out as agreed, within the given time limit. If problems are encountered in fulfilling the agreed-on nursing activities, the nurse should communicate them openly to the family and seek help in making alternative plans.

Evaluation

Evaluation is an ongoing process throughout all phases of the nurse-family transaction as well as an end phase. Results may range from successful goal attainment to discovering that the selected solution is not acceptable to the family. The latter may happen when the family and nurse fail to identify the "real" problem,

Application of Nurse–Family Intervention Model: Johnson Family

Mrs. Williams, the school nurse at Sagebrush Elementary, called Mrs. Johnson and scheduled a home visit for 5:30 PM. She began the visit by clarifying for Mrs. Johnson the changes in Kevin's behavior that his teacher had noted in recent months and asked her if she had observed similar problems at home. Mrs. Johnson reported that Kevin had begun to have episodes of nighttime bedwetting and she felt he was more moody and at times, quite argumentative with her when she would not let him "have his way." She stated that she had spoken with Kevin's pediatrician about the bedwetting, and he felt that Kevin was probably having trouble with the changes with his father. Kevin had no history of bedwetting or toileting accidents since about 3 years of age. The pediatrician encouraged her not to scold Kevin for his accidents and to try to give him a little more attention to help him deal with his separation from his father.

When asked what she thought of the pediatrician's advice, Mrs. Johnson acknowledged that she knew the divorce had been hard for the children. Their father's former job had made it possible for him to be home with them after school, and he had spent a lot of time with Kevin, helping him with schoolwork, games, and other activities. Since her ex-husband's remarriage, he has spent less time visiting with the children. She knew that Kevin missed his father's attention, but planning time to do all the things his dad had done was difficult for her along with working and managing the home. Moreover, she knew Kevin resented going to the "after-school program" because of her work hours. In fact, she sometimes had to ask her mother-in-law to pick up the children from the child-care center because she had to work late. Mrs. Johnson indicated that she didn't want to refuse her boss's request to work late because she was hoping to qualify for a promotion. One of the women she worked with was retiring in another 6 months, and her position as office manager would need to be filled. Although her mother-in-law was always willing to be helpful with caring for the children, she didn't like to ask too often. She felt that her in-laws might have

some feelings that she contributed to the divorce because of her interest in "getting ahead in her career." Her own parents did not live close.

During the visit, Mrs. Williams observed that Mrs. Johnson often seemed impatient with Kevin, responding rather sharply to him when he came into the room where they were meeting to ask questions. She often redirected him to go to his sister for help. At one point, Mrs. Johnson even remarked to the nurse that she had difficulty coping with Kevin's many requests of her and that it hurt her when he made comments to her about how things were different "when Daddy lived here." When she set limits with him, he often remarked, "I want to go live with my Daddy."

Using Mrs. Johnson's descriptions of the problems she was facing in dealing with Kevin at the time of the divorce (Kevin's bedwetting and increased demands for her attention, his remark that "things were different when Daddy lived here") and her own observations about parent-child interactions, and Mrs. Johnson's hesitation to turn down requests for overtime work and to ask for too much help from in-laws, the nurse felt it appeared that the family was experiencing difficulty with new family developmental tasks resulting from the divorce and remarriage of the father, such as learning to be a single parent and promoting ongoing parental contact between the ex-spouse and children. In discussing with Mrs. Johnson ways that she thought the nurse might be helpful, they identified the goal as helping Mrs. Johnson to assist her children with the divorce and developed the following immediate plan:

- The nurse would set up a conference with the school psychologist for Mrs. Johnson to have some counseling about how to deal with Kevin's reaction to the divorce and his behavior.

- Mrs. Johnson would take children to neighborhood library on the weekend and borrow some children's books that deal with parental divorce. Together she and children would read the books.

- Mrs. Johnson would try to spend half an hour each evening with children in some planned activity that the children helped choose.

- The nurse would revisit in 2 weeks to follow up on Mrs. Johnson's meeting with the school psychologist and to assess how children had responded to books on parental divorce and the mother's efforts to plan some activity with them each evening.

they select unrealistic solutions, or unforeseen outcomes occur. As in other phases, the family should be encouraged to participate equally by sharing feelings and concerns about its course as well as about the nurse's role in accomplishing outlined responsibilities. Emphasis on positive strides, although they may be small, can bolster the family's sense of self-efficacy.

Crucial questions to consider in end-phase evaluation include the following:

- *Was the goal(s) achieved?*
- *Was the selected solution(s) appropriate?*
- *What factors facilitated or impeded goal attainment?*

- *Should the nurse-family relationship be terminated or should other goals and plans be developed?*

The manner in which the nurse-family relationship is concluded is as vital as the way in which it is begun. The establishment of a plan for continuity of care, if needed, is crucial. Often, after a period of intensive nursing supervision, a plan for periodic reassessment of the situation is warranted. This is particularly applicable to families dealing with long-term chronic illness or disability. The family should know how to contact the nurse should unanticipated changes occur before the scheduled interval for reappraisal.

CONCLUSION

Understanding the family as a focal unit for nursing care will become more important in the future as health care delivery increasingly takes place in community settings. A family is two or more individuals who manifest some degree of interdependence in their interaction with each other and their environment in meeting basic needs for affection and meaning. The family life cycle is described in terms of developmental stages corresponding to major family events–in particular, the addition and exiting of members.

Families who are likely to have the most difficulty coping with life cycle transitions are those who experience a large number of concurrent life cycle changes involving transitions of great magnitude; who have a small, nonsupportive social network; and who live in a community with few resources to assist them.

Health responsibilities of the family include the (1) provision of opportunities for members to achieve a sense of personal identity and work, (2) emotional support and cognitive guidance for members experiencing life cycle transitions, (3) education of members about how to maintain health and when and how to use professional services, (4) the socialization of members to value health and to accept personal responsibility for its maintenance, and (5) care provision for chronically ill, disabled, or aging family members. To fulfill its health responsibilities, the family needs sufficient energy and knowledge to invest in goal-directed behavior.

Nurses' work with families is facilitated through the use of a conceptual framework for collecting, organizing, and interpreting data about how the family is fulfilling its health responsibilities and issues and concerns they are experiencing. The self-efficacy model for nurse-family intervention involves a contracting process in which the nurse and family pursue mutually established goals.

CRITICAL THINKING ACTIVITIES

1. Reflect on your own experience in growing up in a family. Identify how your family met each of the five health responsibilities. How are your beliefs about health and ways to maintain your health similar to or different from those practiced in your family?

2. Using the case study on *Family Lifecycle Transitions: Teenage Pregnancy*, address the following questions.

   • What are some factors that may have led Nancy to become pregnant? As you answer this question, think about her life history.

   • What are the potential health threats to Nancy and her unborn baby, given her current health habits and living situation?

   • Using the framework for assessment presented in this chapter, how would you assess the family's current capacity to deal with this life cycle transition given the information provided?

   • What additional information would you want to gather?

   • What ethical principles should guide your interactions with Nancy and her family?

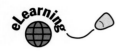

Explore Community Health Nursing on the web! To learn more about the topics in this chapter, use the passcode provided to access your exclusive web site:
http://communitynursing.jbpub.com
If you do not have a passcode, you can obtain one at this site.

REFERENCES

Ahlburg, D. A., and De Vita, C. J. (1992). New realities of the American family. *Population Bulletin, 47*(2), 1–44.

Antonovsky, A. (1987). *Unraveling the mystery of health: How people manage stress and stay well.* San Francisco: Jossey-Bass.

Bain, A. (1978). The capacity of families to cope with transition: A theoretical essay. *Human Relations, 8,* 675.

Beck, C. T. (1996). Postpartum depressed mothers' experiences interacting with their children. *Nursing Research, 45*(2), 98.

Bianchi, S. M., & Spain, D. (1996). Women, work, and family in America. *Population Bulletin, 51*(3), 1–48.

Boss, P. (1988). *Family stress management.* Newbury Park, CA: Sage Publications.

Bronfenbrenner, U. (1986). Ecology of the family as a context for human development. Research Perspectives. *Developmental Psychology, 22*(6), 723–742.

Burden, D. S. (1986). Single parents and the work setting: The impact of multiple job and homelife responsibilities. *Family Relations, 35*(1), 37–43.

Burton, L., & deVries, C. (1995). Challenges and rewards: African-American grandparents as surrogate parents. In L. M. Burton (Ed.), *Families and aging.* Amityville, NY: Baywood.

Carter, E. A., & McGoldrick, M. (Eds.). (1989). *The changing family life cycle: A framework for family therapists* (2nd ed.) New York: Gardner Press.

Clinton, H. R. (1996). *It takes a village: And other lessons children teach us.* New York: Simon & Schuster.

Cole, R., Kitzman, H., Olds, D., & Korfmacher, J. (1998). Family context as a moderator of program effects in prenatal and early childhood home visitation. *Journal of Community Psychology, 26*(1), 37–48.

Cowan, P. A., Field, D., Hansen, D. A., Skolnick, A., & Swanson, G. E. (Eds.). (1992). *Family, self, and society: Toward a new agenda for family research.* Hillsdale, N.J.: Lawrence Erlbaum.

Deatrick, J. A., Brennan, D., & Cameron, M. E. (1998). Mothers with multiple sclerosis and their children: Effects of fatigue and exacerbations on maternal support. *Nursing Research, 47*(4), 205–210.

Department of Health and Human Services (DHHS). (2000). *Healthy People 2010: Conference edition.* Washington, DC: U.S. Government Printing Office.

Doherty, W. J. (1992). Linkages between family theories and primary health care. In R. Sawa (Ed.), *Family health care* (pp. 30–39). Newbury Park, CA: Sage Publications.

Doherty, W. J., & Campbell, T. L. (1988). Families and health. Newbury Park, CA: Sage Publications.

Duffy, M. E. (1988). Health promotion in the family: Current findings and directives for nursing research. *Journal of Advanced Nursing, 13.*

Duvall, E. M., & Miller, B. L. (1985). *Marriage and family development* (6th ed.). New York: Harper & Row.

Friedman, M. M. (1998). *Family nursing: Research, theory and practice* (4th ed.). Stamford, CT: Appleton & Lange.

Goldenberg, I., & Goldenberg, H. (1996). *Family therapy: An overview* (4th ed.). Monterey, CA: Brooks/Cole.

Hall, L. A., Sachs, B., & Rayens, M. K. (1998). Mothers' potential for child abuse: The roles of childhood abuse and social resources. *Nursing Research, 47,* 87–95.

Hanson, S. M. H., & Boyd, S. T. (Eds.). (1996). *Family health nursing: Theory, practice and research.* Philadelphia: Davis.

Hardy, M. E., & Conway, M. (1988). *Role theory: Perspectives for health professionals.* New York: Appleton-Century-Crofts.

Janosik, E. H., & Green, E. (1992). *Family life.* Boston: Jones & Bartlett.

Jepson, C., McCorkle, R., Adler, D., Nuamah, I., & Lusk, E. (1999). Effects of home care on caregivers' psychosocial status. *Image: The Journal of Nursing Scholarship, 31*(2), 115–120.

Klein, D. M., & White, J. M. (1996). *Family theories: An introduction.* Thousand Oaks, CA: Sage Publications.

Kramer, B. J., & Kipnis, S. (1995). Eldercare and work-role conflict: Toward an understanding of gender differences in caregiving burden. *The Gerontologist, 35*(3), 273–278.

Loveland-Cherry, C. (1996). Family health promotion and health protection. In P. J. Bomar (Ed.), *Nurses and family health promotion* (2nd ed., pp. 22–35). Philadelphia: W. B. Saunders.

Lynch, I., & Tiedje, L. B. (1991). Working with multiproblem families: An intervention model for community health nurses. *Public Health Nursing, 8*(3), 147–153.

Newman, M. A. (1994). *Health as expanding consciousness* (2nd ed.). New York: National League for Nursing Press.

O'Brien, R. A. (1979). *A conceptualization of family health. Clinical and scientific sessions.* Kansas City: ANA.

O'Brien, R. A., & Robinson, A. G. (1984). Family as client. In J. A. Sullivan (Ed.), *Directions in community health nursing.* Boston: Blackwell Scientific.

Popenoe, D. (1995). The American family crisis. *National Forum, 75*(3), 15–19.

Pratt, L. (1976). *Family structure and effective health behavior: The energized family.* Boston: Houghton Mifflin.

Pratt, L. (1982). Family structure and health work: Coping in the context of social change. In H. I. McCubbin, A. E. Cauble, & J. M. Patterson (Eds.), *Family stress, coping, and social support* (pp. 73–89). Springfield, IL: Charles C. Thomas.

Robinson, J. L., Emde, R. N., & Korfmacher, J. (1997). Integrating an emotional regulation perspective in a program of prenatal and early childhood home visitation. *Journal of Community Psychology, 25*(1), 59–75.

Rogers, M. E. (1983). Analysis and application of Rogers' theory of nursing. In J. W. Clements & F. B. Roberts (Eds.), *Family health: A theoretical approach to nursing care* (pp. 219–228). New York: Wiley.

Satir, V. (1983). Conjoint family therapy (3rd ed.). Palo Alto, CA: Science and Behavior Books.

Sedgwick, R. (1981). *Family mental health: Theory and practice.* St. Louis: Mosby.

Sieburg, E. (1985). *Family communication: An integrated systems approach.* New York: Gardner Press.

Sloan, M. R., & Schommer, B. T. (1982). The process of contracting in community health nursing. In B. W. Spradley (Ed.), *Readings in community health nursing* (2nd ed., pp. 197–204). New York: Little, Brown.

Smith, G. C., Tobin, S. S., & Fullmer, E. M. (1995). Elderly mothers caring at home for offspring with mental retardation: A model of permanency planning. *American Journal on Mental Retardation, 99*(5), 487–499.

Snyder, N. O., & Moore, K. A. (1996). *Facts at a glance.* Washington, DC: Child Trends.

Stevenson, J. P. (1990). Family stress related to home care of Alzheimer's disease patients and implications for support. *Journal of Neuroscience Nursing, 22*(3), 179–188.

Walsh, F. (Ed.). (1982). *Normal family processes.* New York: The Guilford Press.

Williams, C. A. (1996). Community-based, population focused practice: The foundation of specialization in public health nursing. In M. Stanhope & J. Lancaster (Eds.), *Community health nursing: Promoting health of aggregates, families and individuals* (4th ed., pp.21–34). St. Louis: Mosby.

Williamson, J. A. (1981). Mutual interaction: A model of nursing practice. *Nursing Outlook, 29*, 104.

Wright, L. M., & Leahey, M. (1994). *Nurses and families: A guide to family assessment and intervention* (2nd ed.). Philadelphia: Davis.

APPENDIX A

FAMILY ASSESSMENT GUIDE

1. Family Composition and Identifying Data
   - *Names, ages of family members*
   - *Address*
   - *Racial/ethnic background*
   - *Education/school attendance*
   - *Employment*
   - *Income*
   - *Health insurance*

2. Environmental Data
   - *Is housing adequate to meet family's needs?*
   - *What are the characteristics of the immediate neighborhood and community?*
   - *What health and other basic services are available in the neighborhood? in the community?*
   - *What is the availability of public transportation?*

3. Energy
   - *What are the sources of energy for the family?*
   - *Is there sufficient energy to meet the varying health needs of its members? If not, where is the family's energy directed?*
   - *Does the expenditure of energy in meeting family demands occur repeatedly at the expense of one particular family member?*

4. Consciousness
   - *How aware and knowledgeable is the family of specific health and developmental needs of its members?*
   - *Does it hold incorrect beliefs that are likely to lead to unsound health care practices?*
   - *Is its perception of how it functions congruent with reality?*
   - *What are the sources that the family utilizes in acquiring knowledge?*
   - *Does it actively seek to expand its level of consciousness or does it respond only to crisis demands?*
   - *How do past family experiences influence its consciousness about health issues?*

5. Role Structure
   - *What roles do each of the family members fulfill?*
   - *How competently do members perform their roles?*
   - *How do past family experiences influence members' role performance?*
   - *If role strain or conflict exists, what are the contributing factors?*
   - *How are role conflicts resolved?*
   - *Is there flexibility in roles when needed?*

6. Decision-Making Processes
   - *Who makes what decisions?*
   - *Are there particular needs/issues that are not recognized or addressed?*
   - *Is the family able to discriminate between information that is relevant and that which is irrelevant to the decision?*
   - *Are alternative solutions generated and weighed?*
   - *Is the selected alternative implemented?*
   - *To what extent does family decision making involve consensus or coercion?*

- *Does the mode of decision making affect its implementation?*
- *Is the family satisfied with the results of their choices?*

7. Communication Patterns
   - *Who talks to whom?*
   - *What feelings or issues are closed to discussion?*
   - *Are members able to clearly state their needs and feelings?*
   - *Is there congruence between verbal and nonverbal aspects of communication?*
   - *How well do members listen when others are communicating?*
   - *Do members elicit feedback and validation in communicating with one another?*
   - *What are the predominant patterns of acknowledgment accorded varying members?*
   - *Is communication among members age appropriate?*

8. Values
   - *What are the important values held by the family?*
   - *To what extent do family values foster active coping and mastery of concerns?*
   - *What is the family's orientation to the past, present, and future?*
   - *What is the relative ranking of health in the family's hierarchy of values?*
   - *Are there value conflicts evident within the family, between the family and subculture/community, or between the family and nurse?*

9. System Boundaries
   - *Are family boundaries overly rigid or overly loose?*
   - *What ongoing relationships does the family maintain with extended kin, friends, or other social groups?*
   - *To what degree do interactions with its support network foster or impede the family's abilities to cope with its health responsibilities?*
   - *Is the family satisfied with its support network?*
   - *To what extent is the family willing and able to access community services?*

Chapter 31

Caring for the Family in Health and Illness

Linda Beth Tiedje

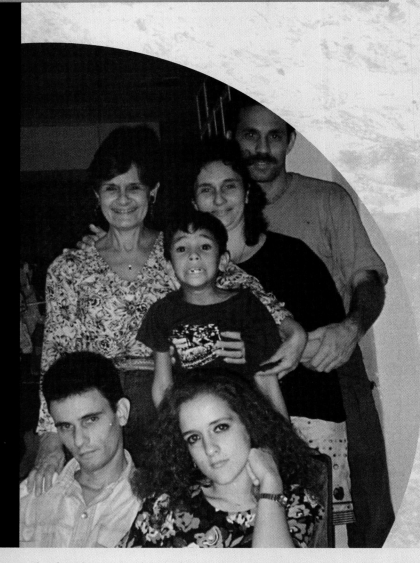

Caring for families in health and illness is not new to nurses. Lillian Wald, Margaret Sanger, and Mary Breckinridge are a few of the nurses who helped establish a tradition of family care. Indeed, some count public health nurses as one of the unique contributions America has made to the cause of public health. Much has changed in the social and economic system since the days of Wald, Sanger, and Breckinridge. Each generation of nurses must reclaim this tradition of family care: keeping relevant wisdom from the past and learning new ways to help families in the ever-changing world in which we live.

CHAPTER FOCUS

Thinking Differently About Family Health
- Thinking Upstream
- Thinking of a Bottom-Down Health System
- The Human Ecology Model: Thinking in Layers

Community-Based Services for Promoting Family Health
- Preventive Support Services for All Families
- Targeted Programs for More Vulnerable Families
- Families in Crisis

Characteristics of Successful Interventions: Creating Healthy Families and Communities
- Relationship-Focused Care
- Intensity and Timing of Interventions
- Nursing Skills and Strategies

Issues in Family Nursing Today

Values: A Challenge for the Future

Healthy People 2010: Objectives Related to Families

QUESTIONS TO CONSIDER

After reading this chapter, answer the following questions:

1. What is thinking upstream and relevance to caring for families?
2. What are community-based services in the promotion of health for families?
3. What are characteristics of successful family interventions?
4. What is the nurse role in relationship-focused care?
5. What are necessary nursing skills and strategies in promoting positive family interventions?
6. What are current issues in family nursing?
7. What are current nursing values?

KEY TERMS

Ad Hoc Committee to Defend Health Care
Bottom-down health system
Caring
Comprehensive community initiatives (CCIs)

Courage
Human ecology model
Inclusion
Intensity
Intensive services
Least possible contribution theory

Nursing skills and strategies
Preventive support services
Social responsibility
Strength-based approach

Reflective thinking
Relationship-focused care
Targeted programs
Think upstream
Timing

What is family health, and what does it mean to care for the family in health and illness? Family health is a whole series of activities that are designed to promote health, to prevent disease and injury, to prevent premature death, and to create conditions in which we can all be safe and healthy (Levy, 1998). There are many examples of activities nurses do every day to promote family health:

- *Supporting a family with a chronically ill child to find community resources and respite care*
- *Working with a family with a schizophrenic young adult to establish consistent drug therapy and vocational training*
- *Discussing eating patterns learned in families of origin when providing support and information for weight reduction*
- *Reflecting on family learned values as we attempt to understand others for whom health is not a priority*
- *Assessing whether other women in the family have breast-fed in the process of helping a new mother initiate breast-feeding*
- *Working for the enforcement of laws that prohibit sales of tobacco to minors and eliminating cigarette vending machines*
- *Being part of school curriculum committees to ensure a focus on social skills so that students learn skills such as sharing, listening to others, and working cooperatively in groups*
- *Teaching parenting competency skills in parent education classes*
- *Participating in community-based sex education committees*

A more specific example of family nursing to prevent disease, injury, and premature death occurred in Hawaii. A group of emergency department (ED) nurses there noted the numbers of individual children who were coming to the ED as a result of drownings and near drownings. Some of the children were resuscitated; others died. Over time the nurses collected data from families and found that none of the pools in which the children drowned had fences. Working with families, the fire department, and other community groups, they raised funds to help families fence their private pools, and the accidental drownings among children decreased. This is an example of a family-focused, community-targeted intervention that served to prevent disease and injury and premature death. Nurses in EDs each day save children in tertiary care settings; they can also move beyond this "downstream" approach, to thinking about how to work with families in *preventing* such accidents from occurring in the first place.

Thinking Differently About Family Health

As novice health care providers, we may view provision of health care to families as an "extra," a nonessential part of individually focused, technically oriented care. As we become more confident of our physical assessment, communication, and psychomotor skills, we learn that health care is more than the provision of individual-level physical care. Indeed, we begin to appreciate that

factors at the level of the family, group, and society affect the health of individuals within them. Overall family health challenges us to think in new ways about influences on the family. Specifically, this new way of thinking challenges us to (1) **think upstream**, always asking, "What would have prevented this in the first place?" (Butterfield, 1991; McKinlay, 1979); (2) think of working with families in a **bottom-down health system** (Hancock, 1993) where homes and neighborhood meeting places are the basis of health care delivery, not hospitals; and (3) to use the **human ecology model** (Bronfenbrenner, 1986) in thinking beyond what happens within individual families to factors outside families that influence family health.

Thinking Upstream

If we think of illness as people drowning in swiftly flowing water, thinking upstream means we have to think beyond rescuing people from the water and look upstream to see what is "pushing" the people into the dangerous water in the first place (McKinlay, 1979). Rescuing people is a "downstream endeavor." In health care, downstream endeavors are short-term, individually focused interventions such as lung transplants for two-pack-a-day smokers or treating myocardial infarctions instead of the sedentary, stressful lifestyles that lead to them. Upstream interventions focus on the social and physical environments in which families live. Upstream interventions focus on changing the behavioral, social, political, and environmental factors that lead to poor health, not waiting "downstream" for poor health to occur (Butterfield, 1991).

In the late 1990s, school violence erupted throughout the United States: Springfield, Oregon; Littleton, Colorado; Pearl, Mississippi; Paducah, Kentucky; Fayetteville, Tennessee; Jonesboro, Arkansas; and Edinboro, Pennsylvania. School violence was a rare and unpredictable phenomenon that fueled a search for "answers." The answers and the causes, of course, were multifaceted. A steady diet of violent media, the availability of guns, increasing feelings of alienation and unchecked rage, racism, and a lack of communication within families all were implicated as causes. School violence is a complicated phenomenon with no easy answers. In the real world, downstream thinking (dealing with consequences of school violence) and upstream thinking (dealing with its prevention) are both required. To focus only on downstream thinking is a mistake. The other mistake often made is to focus blame on singular causes. President Bill Clinton, in a radio address to the nation (May 1, 1999), urged all citizens to focus on responsibility instead of blame. What responsibility could be taken by each citizen to help prevent such violence in the future? Thinking responsibly means thinking upstream about what would prevent such school violence in the first place. Consider these comments taken from a *USA Today* story the week of the Littleton, Colorado, shootings. Recall that in Littleton the student gunmen targeted people of color and athletes:

> "I think one of our jobs as students is to include everybody; I would want to do that." Mario Francisco Penaiver, 18-year-old student from Puyallup, Washington.

HEALTHY PEOPLE 2010

OBJECTIVES RELATED TO FAMILIES

Educational and Community-Based Programs

Health Care Setting

7.7 Increase the proportion of health care organizations that provide patient and family education.

Maternal, Infant, and Child Health

Breast-Feeding, Newborn Screening, and Service Systems

16.19 Increase the proportion of mothers who breast-feed their babies.

Nutrition and Overweight

Food Security

19.18 Increase food security among U.S. households and in doing so reduce hunger.

Source: DHHS, 2000.

"These kids were not genetically programmed to be racist. They have been taught by the people around them." Stanley Wilson, 39, Montgomery, Alabama.

"We, as a society, have to ask, 'What is the impact of a steady diet of violent media content on a growing child?'" Kathryn Montgomery, the Center for Media Education.

Urging parents to take any guns in their homes to the police, Rosie O'Donnell, talk show host, said, "If you have a gun in the house, you are 43 times more likely to be a victim of gun violence."

The National Association of Attorneys General and the National School Boards Association have also published a manual with tips on preventing violence in schools, focusing on parents as a key in prevention. Some of the upstream thinking includes encouraging parents to participate and volunteer at school and encouraging students and teachers to talk about problems. The National School Safety Center also encourages parents to talk with their children about fears and feelings and to be part of their children's lives. Community health nurses, in the spirit of such upstream thinking, could start school-based parent groups. If parental involvement is one of the keys to prevention, parents need to know *how* to communicate, offer support, and open the dialog. Community health nurse–led parent groups would be a preventive start. See above for selected *Healthy People 2010* objectives focusing on families.

Thinking of a Bottom-Down Health System

Hancock (1993) suggests that instead of thinking of a health care delivery system based in tertiary or hospital-/specialty-based care, we should focus on how to keep people healthy (see the figure to the right). Such a system would be a health system, as opposed to the current illness-focused system. Most resources would then be prevention-focused at the neighborhood and community level. In a bottom-down health system, the services

link people and families with others in support groups, neighborhood activities, parent training groups, early childhood education, and after-school recreation programs. Such services can be provided by primary care teams in the home and primary health centers based in schools and neighborhoods.

A bottom-down health system is based on the concept of social capital (Kawachi, Kennedy, Lochner, & Prothrow-Stith, 1997; Lomas, 1998) and the importance of increasing social cohesion in communities. Features of social capital in communities

BOTTOM-DOWN HEALTH SYSTEM.

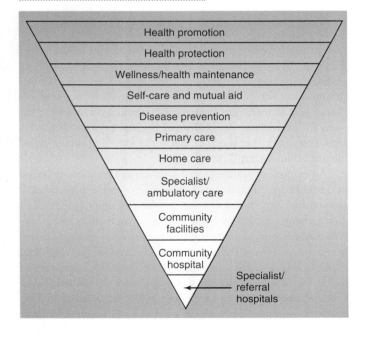

RESEARCH BRIEF

Lantz, P. M., House, J. S., Lepkowski, J. M., Williams, D. R., Mero, R. P., & Chen, J. (1998). Socioeconomic factors, health behaviors, and mortality: Results from a nationally representative prospective study of US adults. Journal of the American Medical Association, 279(21), 1703–1708.

A recent study investigated the difference in mortality rates (death) between those with higher and lower levels of education and income. Four behaviors were examined in the low- and high-income group. The four behaviors were cigarette smoking, alcohol drinking, sedentary lifestyle, and weight. It was thought that the differences in mortality between the groups would be due to a higher rate of these behaviors in those with low education and income. Results indicated that the risk of dying was higher in the lower-income group. However, the four health behaviors together only explained 12% to 13% of the effect of income on mortality, a modest amount. This means that differences in death rates between the rich and poor would persist even with improved health behaviors.

If health risk behaviors do not explain higher mortality in people of lower education and income, what does? Several factors have been suggested: more exposure to occupational and environmental health hazards in poor neighborhoods; differential access to health care; social variables such as lack of social support; a lost sense of mastery, optimism, control, and self-esteem; heightened levels of anger and hostility; and chronic stress at home and work, including racism and classism.

The Human Ecology Model: Thinking in Layers

In chapter 30, the family was presented as an ecological system using general systems and human ecology theories. These theories focus on the external influences that affect families and their ability to function. These forces outside the family have a powerful influence on what goes on inside the family. Some of these systems outside the family are neighborhoods, institutions, the media, and government. The human ecology model (see the following figure) shows how individual and family health are nested within and influenced by these macro-level forces, like Russian dolls stacked neatly one inside the other (Bronfenbrenner, 1986).

In this human ecology model, many factors inside and outside the family influence family health. Are community factors more important than family factors? Are individual factors more important than family factors? Are community factors more important than individual factors? Each of the three broad categories of factors—community, family, and individual—contributes about the same amount to making people within families, especially children, resilient and resistant to stress.

Most traditional interventions focus mainly on individuals, occasionally on families, and less often on institutions and communities. For example, when a community health nurse makes a home visit to an adolescent mother, her baby, and her extended family, traditionally, the primary focus has been on individuals within that family, such as how much the baby weighs and health follow-up for mother and baby. Bronenfenbrenner (1986) would encourage us also to look at the family and community: Does the workplace or school have a designated place to pump breast milk? Do friends support the adolescent mother by providing child care from time to time? What encouragement is the mother

include "social organization such as networks, norms and trust that facilitate coordination and cooperation for mutual benefit" (Putnam, 1995, p. 66). This can be done by creating meeting places, sports leagues, clubs, and associations. Creating spaces in communities for people to come together allows for idea exchange and fosters trust. Building a community structure is the focus for health, not the individual (Minkler, 1998). Some experts now think that social capital is the most important determinant of our health (Lomas, 1998).

An example of building social cohesion in a community occurs in Grand Ledge, Michigan, each spring. On a spring weekend, several activities are planned to bring people of all ages together. Children gather to make May baskets to deliver to friends, and a May Pole dance is held at a city park. Other activities include a teddy bear tea, a quilt show, and a pie contest. Such community building is "for health" because it increases social contact. A vast group of studies has already linked social support networks to health outcomes (House, Landis, & Umberson, 1988). But more than that, a new body of research is emerging that supports the additional health benefits of cohesive, caring communities (Lomas, 1998).

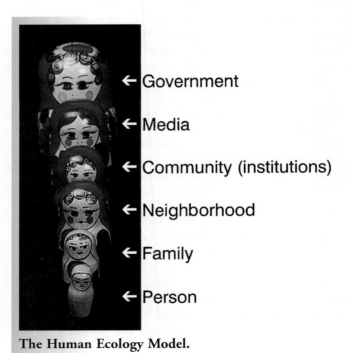

The Human Ecology Model.

← Government
← Media
← Community (institutions)
← Neighborhood
← Family
← Person

FACTORS THAT CONTRIBUTE TO INVULNERABILITY OR RESISTANCE OF STRESS IN CHILDREN.

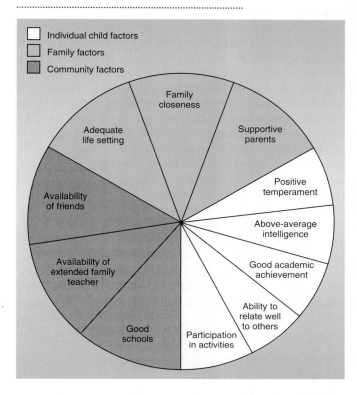

receiving to return to school? Does the mother have a list of friends she can keep by the phone to call when she needs to talk? What messages do the media (e.g., television, magazines) provide to adolescent women? Do local churches provide quality drop-in child care? What are school policies regarding child care for adolescent parents? What are government programs for employment or educational support for teen parents? Does this adolescent mother have access to contraceptive services?

The human ecology model emphasizes that "the way we organize our society, the extent to which we encourage interaction among the citizenry, and the degree to which we trust and associate with each other in caring communities is probably the most important determinant of our health" (Lomas, 1998, p. 1181).

Community-Based Services for Promoting Family Health

Recall that in the introduction to this chapter one aspect of family health was to create conditions in which we can all be safe and healthy. "Every community must have a range of family-based programs, starting with **preventive support services** for all families, continuing through **targeted programs** for more vulnerable families, and ending with highly **intensive services** for families in crisis" (Children's Defense Fund, 1994, p. 4, emphasis added).

KEY CONCEPT: THE HUMAN ECOLOGY MODEL

Think of an individual client you have taken care of in the past. List family, neighborhood, community, media, and government factors that influence his or her health or illness. Then identify one prevention-targeted intervention that would help prevent disease and injury or promote health. For example, research has established connections between asthma and the exposure to environmental chemicals and passive smoke. In addition to treating asthma (tertiary care), a more prevention-oriented approach would examine family, neighborhood, community, media, and government factors that influence asthma and then develop interventions targeted at prevention of these factors. For instance:

- *Government:* E-mail legislators about air quality standards.
- *Media:* Use principles of marketing, public relations, and advertising to design a public service campaign working with the state health department, such as public service announcements to increase awareness of asthma and who is affected. Use experts such as William DeJong and Jay Winsten, who have written *The Media and the Message: Lessons Learned from Past Public Service Campaigns.* (This book provides guidelines and is available from the National Campaign to Prevent Teen Pregnancy, 2100 M Street NW, Suite 300, Washington DC, 20037).
- *Community:* Petition local restaurants to provide no smoking sections.
- *Neighborhood:* Plan test cigarette buys using teens to see which businesses are not enforcing bans on cigarette sales to minors.
- *Family:* Role-play with clients ways to persuade those they live with not to expose them to passive smoke.
- *Individual:* Encourage those with asthma to write about their stressful experiences. A recent study documented the positive effects of such a writing intervention for people with asthma (Smyth, Stone, Hurewitz, & Kaell, 1999).

Preventive Support Services for All Families

In contrast to the United States, where programs are most commonly developed for "at-risk" groups with problems, in other parts of the world, community-based social support for all families is part of a comprehensive program of health care. *All* families

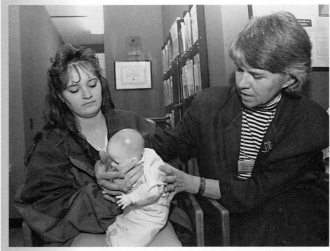

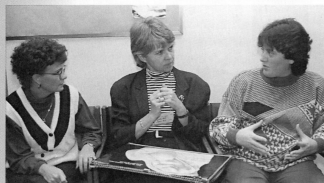

Chapter author, Dr. Linda Beth Tiedje, works to promote health with teen mothers through hands-on education and by including family members in interventions.

receive postpartum home visits after they leave the hospital, and health visitors continue to see *all* families of preschool children on a regular basis (Crockenberg, 1985).

Another example of preventive support services for all families is a preterm birth prevention program begun in France, based on a communitywide public health approach. In contrast to approaches in the United States, which have unsuccessfully attempted to identify women at risk for preterm birth, in France all families, regardless of income, were targeted by a national media campaign. The purpose of the campaign was to make everyone more aware of symptoms of preterm labor. In addition, the effects of employment, such as long-term standing, were also widely publicized as affecting preterm labor. This universal preterm birth prevention approach has become a successful national policy in France and has markedly reduced infant mortality there (Papiernik, Bouyer, Yaffe, Winisdorffer, Collin, & Dreyfus, 1986).

Another example of preventive support services for all families is a widely disseminated program created by the Search Institute in Minneapolis. The program uses a **strength-based approach** and focuses on building assets broadly in all individuals, families, and communities (Roehlkepartain, 1995). The assumptions include that all people and environments possess strengths that can be used toward improving their quality of life and that all environments, even the most bleak, contain resources.

Targeted Programs for More Vulnerable Families

What does an "at-risk" family look like? Who is vulnerable? Some define vulnerable populations as groups who experience limited resources and have a consequent high risk for morbidity and premature mortality (Flaskerud & Winslow, 1998), such as families with a chronically ill child who do not have respite care. Families who are least likely to cope with life cycle transitions are

CASE STUDY

Strength-Based Approaches

At a prenatal clinic, a nurse approached a teenage mother and her boyfriend with their new baby who seemed thin for her age of 6 weeks. The father was holding the baby and burping her, vigorously pounding on her back. Overcoming her urge to negatively comment on the father's burping technique, the nurse asked how things were going. The family related that the baby had already had surgery for pyloric stenosis and had several repeat visits at child health clinic to check on her small head circumference. Later in a discussion with other families in the clinic waiting room, the father strongly voiced his opinion that babies needed lots of holding and "couldn't be spoiled." Reflecting back on this encounter, if the nurse had acted on her initial impulse to judge this teen couple and their child-care techniques, she would have missed the opportunity to see their real strengths: attentiveness at keeping health care appointments, shared care of the child, and knowing that the child needed holding and touch. This strength-based approach is in keeping with Search Institute programs.

1. How could the nurse be most effective in working with this young family?

2. What might be a priority intervention for these parents?

those defined to be most at risk, such as families with a history of abuse who are moving to a new city with a new baby. Vulnerable families might also have a small and nonsupportive social network or live in communities with few available services. All of these factors may make families at risk from time to time.

Economic factors also help define risk in families, poverty being an especially potent factor. One-third of all children in the United States will live in poverty at some time before reaching adulthood. Surprisingly, fewer than 20% of poor families live in inner-city urban areas (Federman, Garner, Short, Cutter, Kiely, Levine, McGough, & McMillen, 1996). Individuals in these poor families are indeed vulnerable, facing multiple problems such as joblessness, substance use, crime, violence, and poor schools. These multiproblem families vary in size, composition, location, and the nature of problems they present (Lynch & Tiedje, 1991).

Although not all poor families are multiproblem families, certain family qualities help define families as multiproblem. Women in multiproblem families often feel exploited and powerless in relationships with males. Men in these families, if present, often do not see themselves as responsible for taking care of children either physically or emotionally. Children in multiproblem families depend on proximal control and lack home orientation to school norms (Lynch & Tiedje, 1991). These defining qualities are not intended as value judgments or descriptors for *each* family in this category. Multiproblem families have problems both within the family and between the family

FYI

Refugee Families

In 1999 in Kosovo, thousands of families were displaced causing crisis and chaos. Once refugee camps were established to provide for basic needs, schools were set up to provide education and a unifying social support for the families. Finally, the United Nations trained preventive mental health workers to work with groups of children. Health care workers assisted the children in playing games, telling stories, and expressing their grief, because many of them were separated from parents. The components of these interventions are common to interventions for all families in crisis.

and the wider community. They often feel insecure and fearful in the wider community. Multiproblem families span both vulnerable and crisis family categories and are known for both the chronic problems that make them vulnerable and the crises they frequently experience. Comprehensive, community-based services targeting family economics, social support, and education are more successful with multiproblem families than services that focus narrowly on one type of problem at a time.

Families in Crisis

A family may be in crisis for several reasons. Families may run out of food. Home fires may leave a family without shelter. Families in which physical and emotional abuse occur are certainly families in crisis. Families displaced by war are also families in crisis. Regardless of the cause, interventions to help families in crisis share common components. First, their basic needs of food, clothing, and shelter must be provided for and their safety ensured. Next, both social and community support networks must be initiated or maintained. Finally, longer term mental health prevention programs must be referred to or established.

Characteristics of Successful Interventions: Creating Healthy Families and Communities

Launching and sustaining work with families is difficult. Successful nursing interventions with families contain several similar components: (1) **relationship-focused care**, (2) attention to **intensity** and **timing** of the interventions, and (3) particular **nursing skills and strategies**.

Relationship-Focused Care

The ability of sensitive nurses to develop ongoing, meaningful relationships with families makes a difference in the ultimate

RESEARCH BRIEF

Byrd, M. E. (1999). Questioning the quality of maternal caregiving during home visiting. Image: The Journal of Nursing Scholarship, 31(1), 27–32.

Field research examined 53 maternal-child home visits made by one nurse over a period of 8 months during 1995 and 1996. The nurse provided information about infant feeding, sleeping, elimination, and development. Although the visits were not exclusively with multiproblem families, two issues emerged that have implications for services to these families. With the most vulnerable of the families, the nurse's visits were primarily "child-focused," and the mother-nurse interactions centered on assessing, then doubting, the ability of the mother's caregiving. Both factors may limit positive outcomes, particularly when maternal caregiving behaviors are doubted. A more successful strategy is to form a supportive interpersonal relationship with the mother. The approach advocated is one of caring and supporting the mother so that she can care for the child.

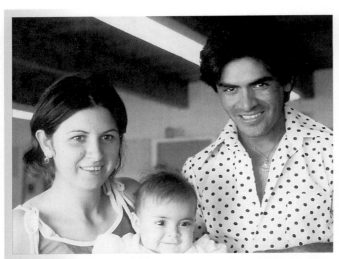

The family provides the framework for learning about health risks and health behavior.

RESEARCH BRIEF

Heinicke, C. M. (1993). Factors affecting the efficacy of early family intervention. In N. J. Anastasiow & S. Harel (Eds.), At-risk infants: Interventions, families and research (pp. 91–100), Baltimore: Paul H. Brookes.

Using intervention studies available addressing the family formation period, Heinicke and his colleagues concluded that the most effective programs provided 11 or more contacts with parents over at least a 3-month period. The intensity of the intervention allowed for an ongoing, nurturing, and supportive relationship with staff delivering the intervention.

effectiveness of an intervention. Nursing is more than a series of tasks to be performed "on" families or information delivered to educate them. Through interactions with families nurses weave a "tapestry of care" (Gordon, 1997). Interpersonal connections become the foundation for effectively influencing health behaviors and helping people take charge of their health and healing (Remen, 1996; Tanner, 1995; Zerwekh, 1997).

Intensity and Timing of Interventions

Programs with successful results offer opportunities for multiple contacts with families over a short time. Programs during the childbearing years are particularly useful because they furnish potential continuity over time and multiple contacts. Multiple contacts in and of themselves do not ensure success, however. Other factors, such as provider credibility, are also important for successful results.

School-based clubs and groups offer opportunities for multiple contacts over time. One such group, begun by a school nurse, targeted preadolescent girls, who during the second decade of life appear to be substantially more vulnerable than boys to environmental and psychological stressors (Pipher, 1994). A school nurse started a girls club with girls from the fourth grade. The girls met weekly over the noon hour at school, at first to talk. A softball team, field trips to sporting and cultural events, and a presentation on grooming and hygiene were soon club activities. Such a club, building assets such as self-esteem

CASE STUDY

Establishing Trust for Relationship-Focused Care

At the request of a children's clinic, a nurse made a home visit because clinic personnel were concerned that a 6-month-old child had not been brought in for cast changes. The cast was the result of treatment for congenital foot deformities. At the first home visit, the mother was guarded and uncommunicative and admitted the nurse to her home with obvious reluctance. The dominant feature in the dark, cluttered room was a slate pool table. The nurse, sensing that so costly an item in all probability was highly prized, shared that observation with the mother. The nurse then admired the pool table,

noting its many features. The mother responded immediately. She explained at length about how much it meant to the family to have it, how friends and neighbors gathered to use it, and its contribution to her life. She then angrily described the previous nurse who had scolded her for spending money foolishly instead of using her resources to better meet the needs of her children. She was grateful to the current nurse for being a more understanding person and immediately switched the conversation to questions she had about her children. She then proceeded to plan with the nurse how she could arrange for necessary clinic follow-up for the 6-month-old, thanked the nurse for all her help, and asked when she would return.

Source: Lynch & Tiedje, 1991.

and communication skills, is health promoting and helps prevent adolescent pregnancy. Positive, asset-building activities with preadolescent girls are prime examples of intensive interventions.

In addition to intensity, most family interventions require time and living through difficulties. Unlike quiz shows, family interventions do not provide immediate answers. It takes time for families to experiment with new ideas and strategies. It takes time for families to come to their own solutions.

For example, there is a growing number of community-based programs for couples who present for domestic violence counseling and want to be treated jointly (Johannson & Tutty, 1998). Although controversial, in cases of domestic abuse, the conjoint treatment of couples is increasing because unless both men and women are treated, the cycle of abuse repeats even when a relationship with a particular abusive partner ends. Conjoint treatment requires patience and time. Most conjoint groups last 12 weeks and are preceded by gender-specific (all-men or all-women groups) 24-week treatment groups. The conjoint groups are often held in community centers, schools, or YWCAs and emphasize alternatives to domestic violence. Cessation of physical violence between the partners is a condition for group membership.

• •

Most people learn how to avoid emotional hijackings from the time they are infants. If they have supportive and caring adults around them, they pick up the social cues that enable them to develop self-discipline and empathy.

Hillary Rodham Clinton, 1996

• •

Nursing Skills and Strategies

Nurses delivering interventions to families must have skills specific to the intervention delivered. Five skills are particularly important: communicating, problem solving, listening, connecting, and evaluating.

Communicating

In addition to the skills nurses need to communicate, communication is also a core issue in families and communities. Community health nurses can facilitate communication and also teach particular communication skills to people in families and groups. The following program example is one way nurses may provide parents with practical advice about ways of communicating with their children. The content area is human sexuality.

In New York, Jo Leonard and Marcia Siegel (1998) implemented a workshop for mothers and daughters called "Mother-Daughter Workshop: Getting Your Period." Offering the class to girls ages 9 to 13, no class is bigger than eight mother-daughter pairs. The class is based on the premise that parents are the first and most important sexuality educators and that family support and guidance have a significant effect on sexual activity. The class provides opportunities for parents and children to practice communicating about sexuality. It also provides opportunities to ask questions about sexuality in a neutral atmosphere. The class is a prime example of a strategy nurses may use to enhance family communication.

• •

At work, you think of the children you've left at home. At home, you think of the work you've left unfinished. Such a struggle is unleashed within yourself; your heart is rent.

Golda Meir, Former Prime Minister of Israel

• •

Problem Solving

Problem solving is a skill that must be done with and not for families and communities. Nurses may have "rescue fantasies" as helpers, wanting to take on the problem and tell others what to do. Coming to terms with who owns the problem leads to mutual goal setting and gives clients the power of solving their own problems.

For example, a nurse in a prenatal clinic was discussing the importance of finishing high school with a pregnant mother who had dropped out of school. The pregnant woman was accompanied by her mother, who also was a high school dropout. As the nurse talked with both women, it was obvious that the grandmother was proud of her longstanding job as a hotel maid. She also believes high school had been unnecessary for her achievement. For the nurse to assume an authoritarian, directive role in this situation and insist on high school completion would have been unproductive. Instead, talking with the mother and daughter about education, jobs, and life success over the course of the pregnancy helped the nurse better understand the mother-daughter perspective. The mutual problem solving that evolved enabled the daughter to "own the problem" of high school completion and take the necessary steps for it to happen.

Listening

Nurses have vast amounts of health information to share with families and communities in an effort to improve health outcomes. Often, our first impulse is to give advice and information. Sometimes, especially in response to particular client questions, advice is appropriate. However, we have entered an era in which health information is no longer a commodity exclusively owned by health systems. Many individuals, families, and communities can access health information from many sources. Self-care and wellness reflect a growing awareness that maintaining and enhancing health is a shared enterprise between providers and consumers. In such a shared enterprise, listening becomes a more vital skill. What does the client already know? What experiences has the client already had? Listening through storytelling has recently been reclaimed as a powerful educational and therapeutic tool (Banks-Wallace, 1998). When a nurse truly listens to clients' or families' stories, he or she can more fully understand where they are coming from. Storytelling can reveal the way clients and families think about health issues, as well as gaps in their understanding. The use of storytelling as an educational tool also has been expanded to include groups of clients within prenatal and other clinic settings (Banks-Wallace, 1999).

Connecting

Caring for families in health and illness requires the ability to connect with other agencies and programs, to coordinate and reinforce interventions. Being assertive, phoning other providers, planning family meetings—all this requires skill and a definite lack of shyness! Nurses often know the many other agencies involved with a family and initiate care conferences to coordinate services. Long before case managers were popular, community health nurses were coordinating services for individuals and families. It is nurses who often are the best client advocates, articulating family needs for and with families.

During the late 1980s and the early 1990s, an approach emerged to facilitate connecting: **comprehensive community initiatives (CCIs)**. Instead of focusing on one type of problem at a time, CCIs focus on creating systems of comprehensive services (e.g., health care, social services, education, housing) through a variety of programs and community building to better the lives of urban poor families (Stagner & Duran, 1997). The overall purpose is to provide neighborhood conditions in which families can succeed. CCIs share certain attributes such as emphasizing participation and providing a variety of services with their predecessors: settlement houses (early 1900s), neighborhood programs (1930s), war on poverty programs (1960s), and community action agencies (1970s).

Evaluating

Outcomes of what community health nurses do are important. To measure those outcomes, evaluation knowledge and skills are especially critical. In addition to evaluating interventions with individuals and families, nurses are often asked to serve on evaluation teams to review the impact of community planning or intervention efforts. Traditional evaluation methods include pretesting and post-testing, interviews, surveys, record review, and focus groups (Minkler, 1998). A new approach that expands on some of these traditional methods is called *empowerment evaluation*. It is used as a tool for both evaluation and community building (Fetterman, Kaftarian, & Wandersman, 1996).

Empowerment evaluation was used in the evaluation of a human immunodeficiency virus (HIV) prevention community planning effort funded by the Centers for Disease Control and Prevention in 1994 and consists of four steps. The first step in the empowerment evaluation process is taking stock. This involves a review of documents (e.g., budgets, reports, organizational charts) and interviews and focus groups with community participants to uncover background experiences. The purpose of this step is to reveal a common history and broad shared experience. In the second step, setting goals, the evaluator helps community group members identify where they want to go and the

kind of evaluation they want to create. Note that the evaluation process is not a preconceived idea of the evaluator.

The third step, that of developing strategies, is often difficult. Uneasy group dynamics and underfunding often create hassles and obstacles as communities struggle to decide on particular strategies to meet high expectations. In the example of the HIV prevention planning, one team encountered many difficulties when generating strategies. In an effort to overcome these difficulties, participants were asked to name the biggest hassle of community planning and to identify what they particularly appreciated in each of the other participants. The written responses were then organized into hassles, uplifts, and ways of changing course. These responses were circulated and then discussed at a community meeting. This helped the participants move beyond the difficulties to the work they needed to do: developing strategies.

The fourth and final step of empowering evaluation is documenting the process, that is, keeping a written record of what occurred and why, in a way accessible to all participants. The usefulness of this step was apparent in the HIV prevention planning process when the planning group, after nearly a year, faced some difficult decisions. Planning group members were on a 3-day retreat and faced a vote about how to proceed. Behind-the-scenes maneuvering, miscommunication, and longstanding alliances left the planners angry and divided. The empowering evaluation team found some data collected after an ice breaker exercise early in the planning process when participants had been asked to share their personal mottoes and messages for the world. One of the messages was from a group member who had died of acquired immunodeficiency syndrome (AIDS) just a few months before. Stunned, the group was reminded of their collective vision, and they were then able to vote in a more unified spirit. This use of data is a prime example of how documenting the process can be used to empower communities in evaluation efforts (Roe, Berenstein, Goette, & Roe, 1996).

The five nursing skills and strategies of communicating, problem solving, listening, connecting, and evaluating are a necessary foundation for community health nurses as they seek to provide services to individuals, families, and communities. These skills are necessary but not sufficient in a health care system where changes are massive, swift, and without precedent. Therefore, in the next section, issues in family nursing resulting from large-scale integrated health care enterprises, managed care plans, intense market competition, and a pervasive concern for operational efficiency and cost reduction are discussed.

Issues in Family Nursing Today

The health care climate in which we practice may constrain what we want to do with families and communities. For example, many states have community programs in which nursing visits are reimbursed in a fragmented way for childbearing families: maternal support services for mothers, infant support services for children, Women, Infants and Children (WIC) for nutrition, and family planning services for contraception. The "family" sees many health care providers, with little concern for coordination of services. As nurses in that situation, we may find ourselves in situations we have not created and without much power. It is difficult to provide family-centered care in an environment that reimburses for individual services and that is not designed for time with families. Difficult, but not impossible. The nation's estimated 2.5 million nurses make up the clinical backbone of the care delivery system. Nurses are uniquely suited in this emerging health care system. We have the exact skills the health care delivery system needs: communicating, problem solving, listening, connecting, and evaluating.

Nursing reinvented itself in the past when social changes demanded it. Before the Depression, most nurses worked in private duty. As the Depression grew worse, nurses moved into hospitals and were employed at a salary. We can reinvent ourselves again, as we have done before (Sharts-Hopko, 1998). How do we accomplish this reinvention?

One strategy is based on the **least possible contribution theory** (Weisman, 1981). A little can go a long way, and the least

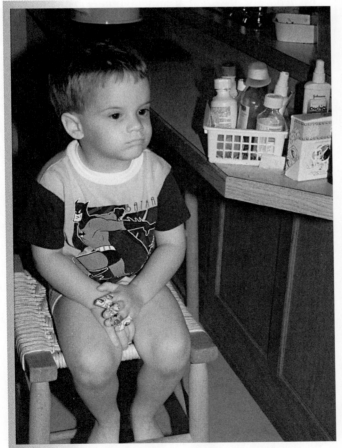

Children learn how to care for themselves in the family.

possible contribution is the one with the best chance of making a difference, however small. Making one small, insignificant contribution furnishes a foundation on which one can continue to add other contributions until something surprising but substantial results. Of course, least possible contribution does not mean doing as little as possible. Least possible contribution means doing something that the nurse is really good at and something that is only a little bit beyond the ordinary (Weisman, 1981).

An example of the least possible contribution theory in action occurred in 1997 when a group of Massachusetts health care providers created the **Ad Hoc Committee to Defend Health Care.** Together these physicians and nurses worked to reestablish caregiving from those who were trying to make health care a business driven by the bottom line. This committee has become a national movement against "a corporate-driven health care system" (Shindul-Rothschild, 1998). The committee's agenda is based on the following legislative initiatives: (1) Give the public information so that they can make informed choices; (2) assure patients that they will be cared for by registered nurses; and (3) extend whistle-blower protection to all health care workers so that they are not put in the position of choosing between a job and advocacy for clients. Only through such group efforts can the health care delivery scale be tilted back toward care instead of profits. Human and capital resources can then be put back into direct client care instead of where the true inefficiencies lie in the delivery system—in the huge administrative overhead.

Values: A Challenge for the Future

The value of inclusion rather than exclusion and the embracing of diversity as a means of enriching the social fabric remain two of our greatest challenges in community health. To deliver relationship-focused care to families, nurses must get emotionally free to focus on the family without judgment or bias. As nurses we may perceive people's situations differently because of our own value systems, which are created by our own experiences. We live in a heterogeneous society, a society with many different kinds of people and families. There are recent immigrant families from all over the world, as well as families whose ancestors came from Northern Europe, England, Eastern and Southern Europe, and Scandinavia. We must not only assess minorities for cultural norms, customs, and rituals; the majority culture also has cultural norms, customs, and rituals that must be owned. To ignore cultural assessment of everyone is to imply that the majority culture is the "norm" and is beyond assessing.

The structure of families is also increasingly diverse: single parent, two parent, gay or lesbian parent, and so on. Therefore, health care providers often find themselves relating to families that are different from the ones they grew up in either in culture or structure. It is common when confronting such differences to feel strange or uncomfortable. Sometimes, health care providers react by thinking of ways all people and families are alike, such as that we all have similar needs (e.g., food, clothing, shelter) and we all need love and affection. As health care providers, we also need to preserve the differences in people and families. That is more difficult. At times, we may just want everyone to be like us.

To better meet the values challenges of a diverse culture, three activities are outlined in this section. The first is a self-assessment quiz in Box 31-2 to increase value and community awareness. The second is a critical thinking exercise in Box 31-3 about providing support for families when there are scarce resources. Decisions about such family support ultimately involve values. The third activity is to recall how core nursing values may help us meet the challenges of a diverse society.

In the area of values, looking where we have come from may help us in where we are going. Nursing may provide guidance to

meeting the values challenges in providing care to families and communities in a diverse culture. Salmon (1999) reminds us that there are five core values in nursing: **caring, courage, inclusion, reflective thinking,** and **social responsibility.** The value of caring is what has allowed us to move from the "doing for" approach to the current focus on enabling and empowering. The second value of courage needs to be shared and taught with exemplars and living models. We need to share and call attention to the daily courageous acts of nurses, particularly as they care for diverse groups. The third nursing value of inclusion seems most appropriate for the values challenge of working with diverse

---

BOX 31-2 SELF-ASSESSMENT QUIZ FOR PROVIDERS WORKING WITH FAMILIES AND COMMUNITIES

In the spirit of thinking of similarities and differences in people, this self-assessment is intended as a means for you as a provider to become more aware of your values. In addition, questions 4 to 9 are intended to assess your awareness of your community, because community cohesion and the degree to which you associate with others in creating caring communities will be important to your success as a community health nurse.

1. Do you respect others' beliefs?
2. Do you believe that life is good and positive?
3. What is your ethnic/cultural heritage? List some norms/customs/rituals.
4. When was the last time you took public transportation?
5. Have you given blood recently?
6. Have you ever served on a jury?
7. How many of your neighbors do you know by name?
8. When was the last time you went to a free public event or amusement like a museum or the zoo?
9. When was the last time you checked a book out of the local library?
10. Do you do volunteer work in your community?

Source: Questions 1 to 3 are based on Benson, 1996; questions 4 to 10 are based on a community quotient quiz adapted by the Utne Reader (Cordes & Walljasper, 1997).

BOX 31-3 VALUE CHECKPOINT: CRITICAL THINKING

The issue of who is responsible for children affects not only how we as health care providers care for families, but also how resources get allocated in our society. People from widely different points of view can agree that valuing families is important in our society. What is harder is agreeing on how much the family needs to be supported by social institutions, including churches, schools, community agencies, and government (Schorr, 1989).

The conservative view is that families should be self-reliant and self-sufficient, not relying on community and government support. The liberal view is that "parents are and should be the most important people in their children's lives. But that doesn't mean they can or should raise their children without any help" (Children's Defense Fund, 1994). Liberals maintain that many forms of assistance are needed to maintain strong families, including sufficient family income and access to health care, child care, and adequate housing.

Think for a moment about your attitudes and beliefs regarding family support. How much family support is needed? What kind of support is needed? Should government ensure basic health care for all families, including children and parents? How does increasing the supply of affordable housing promote health in families? What is the best environment for families if we want to create families who are self-reliant, self-sufficient, and responsible? At what point does the conservative model threaten the overall health of the community? At what point does the liberal model threaten self-reliance in families?

CONTINUUM OF SERVICES.

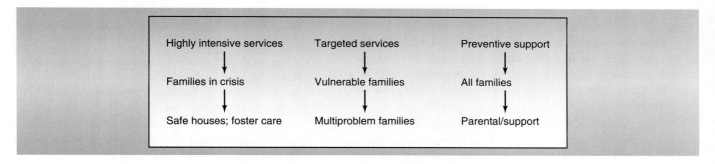

groups. But have we as nurses, so long marginalized and excluded, learned our lessons so well that we in turn oppress others? Listen to Salmon on this point: "I wonder what we teach our students about inclusion. Do they understand that our health care system serves only some people, and that more than 40 million others have no real access to care? . . . Does our science teach students to care only for those who are part of the system? . . . Or do we convey the value that nursing's job is not complete until all receive the care they need?" (p. 23).

The fourth nursing core value is that of reflective thinking, not easy to come by in our fast-paced lives. However, as community health nurses, we must become more than just technicians. "We must also educate people who are equipped intellectually to deal with the meaning of what they do and who they are in the context of humanity" (Salmon, 1999, p. 24). It is reflection that is needed as we deal with the issues of value conflicts in a complex and diverse society.

Finally, the last core value, the linchpin for all the others, is social responsibility. Nightingale's vision of nursing's responsibility to the common good was based on social responsibility. She saw a society like ours in which certain groups were marginalized and in poor health because of unjust systems. "Her response was to engage nursing in addressing these injustices" (Salmon, 1999, p. 25). Nursing is only as good as what it does for all the people. Do we, like Lillian Wald, have a firm grasp of the way in which society functions to impact the health of individuals? Our sense of social responsibility will help us meet the challenges of values conflicts in a diverse culture.

CONCLUSION

Community health nurses must not only care for individuals and families, but also create caring and cohesive communities. Key concepts highlighted in this chapter, which serve as a foundation for a community-based family nursing, include the following:

- *Family health is a series of activities designed to promote health, to prevent disease and injury, to prevent premature death, and to create conditions in which we all can be safe and healthy.*

- *Family health challenges us to think in new, broader ways. Thinking differently about family health means (1) thinking upstream about prevention, (2) thinking of a bottom-down health system focused on increasing cohesion in communities and providing services at the neighborhood level, and (3) thinking in layers in terms of the human ecology model about the many external influences on family health.*

- *There are three general strategies for promoting family health: preventive services for all families, targeted pro-grams for more vulnerable families, and intensive services for families in crisis.*

- *There are three characteristics of all successful interventions with families embedded in neighborhoods and larger social systems. Successful interventions involve (1) relationship-focused care, (2) attention to intensity and timing of interventions, and (3) the use of the nursing skills and strategies of communicating, problem solving, listening, connecting, and evaluating.*

- *The issues in family nursing today are varied and complex. Most important are the constraints of the health care delivery system.*

- *There are many challenges facing community health nurses as they build and organize communities for health. A special challenge is the value conflicts that result when we work with diverse families and communities.*

- *Salmon's five core values of nursing are proposed as ways to meet the value conflicts of diversity. The five core values are caring, courage, inclusion, reflective thinking, and social responsibility.*

CRITICAL THINKING ACTIVITIES

1. As a community health nurse, you have been assigned to a community action committee to design a parent support group for parents of teens in your local high school. The purpose of the group is to teach communication, conflict resolution, and problem-solving skills and to provide a forum for social support for parents. A major emphasis will be on practicing skills. Explore the following questions and give rationales for your decisions:

   - Would you have a group for parents only, for parents and teens, or separate groups for parents and teens?

   - What resources would you use to teach communication, conflict resolution, and problem-solving skills? Remember that a major emphasis of the groups is to practice these skills.

   - The teaching of social skills to children is important, especially children who feel alienated and left out. In a recent book, *Why Doesn't Anybody Like Me?*,

Hara Estroff Marano gives several suggestions to parents. How would you incorporate some of these suggestions into your parent group? What activities would you use to make the suggestions come alive?

- How many weeks will the groups meet, when (e.g., evening, weekend), and how long (e.g., 1 hour, 2 hours)?

- Who would you have lead the groups? What experts in your community would you utilize to help you if you were chosen to lead the groups?

2. Using the research of Lantz, House, Lepkowski, Williams, Mero, and Chen (see the Research Brief on p. 712), explore the factors contributing to the gap in mortality between the rich and the poor. Especially look at factors other than health behaviors. Explain how some of the other factors suggested by the research might contribute to increased mortality in the poor. How might these factors affect physical health? What are interventions that would address these other factors?

Other factors: *Intervention:*

- Lack of social relationships and social supports

- Personality factors such as a lost sense of mastery, optimism, sense of control, and self-esteem

- Factors such as a heightened level of anger and hostility

- Chronic and acute stress in jobs and at home as a result of lack of resources

- The stress of racism and classism and other stresses related to the unequal distribution of power and resources

- Differences in exposure to occupational and environmental health hazards (poor people tend to have more exposure to these hazards, e.g., lead)

- Differences in access to health care

3. Think of a family you are currently working with. Name one skill that each family member possesses that is a strength. Does the documentation system used in your nursing agency, hospital, or community clinic have a place for listing strengths of individuals and families?

4. Most conjoint domestic abuse after-treatment groups are co-led by a man and a woman. Leaders should have experience in counseling, group work, and family violence. Assume you are co-leading a conjoint after-treatment group.

- What safety considerations would you have for the formerly abused women in the group?

- What skills would be particularly important for couples to practice in the groups?

- What built-in strategies would you use to monitor current physical abuse in these relationships?

- What system would you have in place for crisis intervention if abuse developed between sessions?

Continued

CRITICAL THINKING ACTIVITIES—CONT'D

5. Explain why someone in a family or community would respond differently to a problem than you do. Discuss the following questions with the family/community to enhance their problem solving (adapted from Schorr, 1997).

- What do you think is the problem?
- What do you think you should do?
- What would help?
- What have you done in the past when this happened? Did it work?
- What are your options?
- Who might help you?

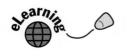

Explore Community Health Nursing on the web! To learn more about the topics in this chapter, use the passcode provided to access your exclusive web site: http://communitynursing.jbpub.com
If you do not have a passcode, you can obtain one at this site.

REFERENCES

Banks-Wallace, J. (1998). Emancipatory potential of storytelling in a group. *Image: The Journal of Nursing Scholarship, 30*(1), 17–21.

Banks-Wallace, J. (1999). Storytelling as a tool for providing holistic care to women. *American Journal of Maternal Child Nursing, 24*(1), 20–24.

Benson, H. (1996). *Timeless healing. The power and biology of belief.* New York: Simon & Schuster.

Bronfenbrenner, U. (1986). Ecology of the family as a context for human development. Research Perspectives. *Developmental Psychology, 22*(6), 723–742.

Butterfield, P. G. (1991). Thinking upstream: Nurturing a conceptual understanding of the societal context of health behavior. In K. A. Saucier (Ed.), *Perspectives in family and community health* (pp. 66–71). St. Louis: Mosby.

Byrd, M. E. (1999). Questioning the quality of maternal caregiving during home visiting. *Image: The Journal of Nursing Scholarship, 31*(1), 27–32.

Children's Defense Fund. (1994). *Helping children by strengthening families: A look at family support programs.* Washington, DC: Author.

Clinton, H. R. (1996). *It takes a village: And other lessons children teach us* (p. 65). Touchstone Books.

Cordes, H., & Walljasper, J. (Eds.). (1997). *Goodlife: Mastering the art of everyday living.* Minneapolis: Utne Reader.

Crockenberg, S. B. (1985). Professional support and care of infants by adolescent mothers in England and the United States. *Journal of Pediatric Psychology, 10,* 413–428.

Federman, M., Garner, T. I., Short, K., Cutter, W. M. IV, Kiely, J., Levine, D., McGough, D., & McMillen, M. (1996). What does it mean to be poor in America? *Monthly Labor Review, 119*(5), 3–17.

Fetterman, D. M., Kaftarian, S. J., & Wandersman, A. (Eds.). (1996). *Empowerment evaluation: Knowledge and tools for self-assessment and accountability.* Thousand Oaks, CA: Sage Publications.

Flaskerud, J. H., & Winslow, B. J. (1998). Conceptualizing vulnerable populations: Health-related research. *Nursing Research, 47*(2), 69–78.

Gordon, S. (1997). *Life support: Three nurses on the front lines.* Boston: Little, Brown.

Hancock, T. (1993). Re-designing healthcare from the bottom down. In *Healthier communities action kit* (vol. 2). San Francisco: The Healthcare Forum.

Heinicke, C. M. (1993). Factors affecting the efficacy of early family intervention. In N. J. Anastasiow & S. Harel (Eds.), *At-risk infants: Interventions, families and research* (pp. 91–100), Baltimore, MD: Paul H. Brookes.

House, J. S., Landis, K. R., & Umberson, D. (1988). Social relationships and health. *Science, 241*(4865), 540–545.

Johannson, M. A., & Tutty, L. M. (1998). An evaluation of after-treatment couples' groups for wife abuse. *Family Relations, 47*(1), 27–35.

Kawachi, I, Kennedy, B. P., Lochner, K., & Prothrow-Stith, D. (1997). Social capital, income inequality, and mortality. *American Journal of Public Health, 87*(9), 1491–1498.

Lantz, P. M., House, J. S., Lepkowski, J. M., Williams, D. R., Mero, R. P., & Chen, J. (1998). Socioeconomic factors, health behaviors, and mortality: Results from a nationally representative prospective study of US adults. *Journal of the American Medical Association, 279*(21), 1703–1708.

Leonard, J., & Siegel, M. (1998). Mother and daughter workshops. *Childbirth Instructor Magazine, March/April,* 34–35.

Levy, B. S. (1998). Creating the future of public health: Values, vision, and leadership. *American Journal of Public Health, 88*(2), 188–192.

Lomas, J. (1998). Social capital and health: Implications for public health and epidemiology. *Social Science and Medicine, 47*(9), 1181–1188.

Lynch, I., & Tiedje, L. B. (1991). Working with multiproblem families: An intervention model for community health nurses. *Public Health Nursing, 8*(3), 147–153.

McKinlay, J. B. (1979). A case for refocusing upstream: The political economy of illness. In E. G. Jaco (Ed.), *Patients, physicians, and illness* (3rd ed., pp. 9–25). New York: The Free Press.

Minkler, M. (Ed.). (1998). *Community organizing & community building for health.* New Brunswick, NJ: Rutgers University Press.

Papiernik, E., Bouyer, J., & Yaffe, K., Winisdorffer, G., Collin, D., & Dreyfus, J. (1986). Women's acceptance of a preterm birth prevention program. *American Journal of Obstetrics and Gynecology, 155,* 939–946.

Pipher, M. (1994). *Reviving Ophelia: Saving the selves of adolescent girls.* New York: Ballantine.

Putnam, R. D. (1995). Bowling alone. American's declining social capital. *Journal of Democracy, 6,* 65–78.

Remen, R. N. (1996). *Kitchen table wisdom.* New York: Riverhead Books.

Roe, K. M., Berenstein, C., Goette, C., & Roe, K. (1996). Community building through empowering evaluation. In Meredith Winkler (Ed.), *Community organizing & community building for health* (pp. 308–322). New Brunswick, NJ: Rutgers University Press.

Roehlkepartain, J. L. (1995). *Building assets together.* Minneapolis: The Search Institute.

Salmon, M. E. (1999). Thoughts on nursing: Where it has been and where it is going. *Nursing and Health Care Perspectives, 20*(1), 20–25.

Schorr, L. B. (1997). *Common purpose: Strengthening families and neighborhoods to rebuild America.* New York: Anchor Books.

Schorr, L. B. (1989). *Within our reach: Breaking the cycle of disadvantage.* New York: Anchor Books.

Sharts-Hopko, N. C. (1998). On chaos, wholeness, and long-standing values: Direction for nursing's future. *American Journal of Maternal Child Nursing, 23,* 11–14.

Shindul-Rothschild, J. (1998). Nurses week tribute: A nursing call to action. *American Journal of Nursing, 98*(5), 36.

Smyth, J., Stone, A. A., Hurewitz, A., & Kaell, A. (1999). Effects of writing about stressful experiences on symptom reduction in patients with asthma or rheumatoid arthritis. *Journal of the American Medical Association, 281*(14), 1304–1309.

Stagner, M. W., & Duran, M. A. (1997). Comprehensive community initiatives: Principles, practice, and lessons learned. In R. E. Behrman (Ed.), *The future of children: Children and poverty* (vol. 7[2]). Los Altos, CA: The Center for the Future of Children.

Tanner, C. A. (1995). Living in the midst of a paradigm shift. *Journal of Nursing Education, 34*(2), 51–52.

University of Massachusetts, Cooperative Extension. (1990). *Building communities of support for families in poverty.* Amherst, MA: Author.

U.S. Public Health Service (USPHS). (1991). *Healthy People 2000: National health promotion and disease prevention objectives.* (Publication No. PHS 91-50213). Washington, DC: Dept. of Health and Human Services.

Weisman, A. D. (1981). Understanding the cancer patient: The syndrome of caregiver's plight. *Psychiatry, 44,* 161–168.

Zerwekh, J. V. (1997). Making the connection during home visits: Narratives of expert nurses. *International Journal for Human Caring, 1*(1), 25–29.

Unit VII
Care of Individuals

Chapter 32
Women's Health

Norma G. Cuellar, Karen Saucier Lundy, and Venus Callahan

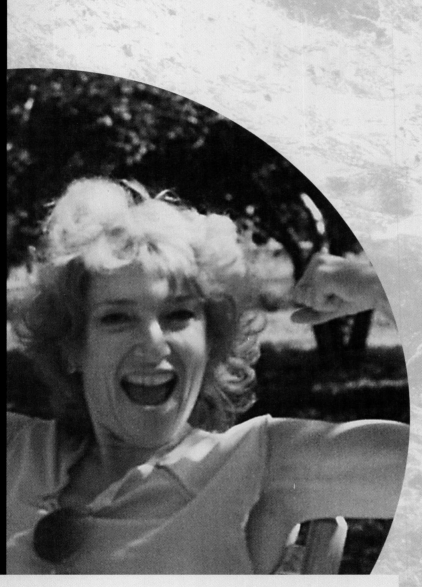

Women now live an average of 30 years longer than they did 100 years ago. A woman born in 1900 was expected to live 49 years; today's baby girl can expect a life span of 79 years. Significant changes and increased opportunities in the lives of American women have broadened the focus of women's health to include physiological, emotional, social, cultural, and economic well-being.

QUESTIONS TO CONSIDER

After reading this chapter, answer the following questions:
1. How are demographic variables related to women's health status?
2. As women age, what specific health concerns and issues are most prevalent?
3. What are special health concerns of lesbians, women of color, and elder women?
4. What are the special ethical issues related to health that concern women?
5. What populations of women are more vulnerable to health risks?
6. How can nurses provide preventive-based care to the diverse population of women in the promotion of health?
7. What are sources of empowerment for women related to improved health?
8. What future issues will likely influence the health of women?

KEY TERMS

Caregivers
Commission on the Status
  of Women
Constructed knowledge
Empowerment

Feminism
Feminization of
  poverty
Heterosexism
Homophobia

Hormone replacement
  therapy
Mammography
Perimenopausal period
Procedural knowledge

United Nations Platforms
  for Action for Women
Urinary incontinence
World Conference
  on Women

For much of the 20th century, women's health focused almost exclusively on reproductive functions such as menstruation, childbearing, and menopause. In 1990, a landmark report by the General Accounting Office (GAO) revealed shocking gaps in research on women's health issues. During the 20th century, women had been left out of most research on cancer, heart disease, and interventions, such as the development of new technology and medications. Such inequities resulted in women's health being considerably behind in advances known to benefit men (Allen & Phillip, 1997).

In the 1990s, the federal government mobilized the greatest effort ever to improve women's health through research and services. We now have better and safer **mammography** and breast cancer treatment, more effective ways to prevent and treat osteoporosis, and we know more about alternatives for women during the **perimenopausal period.** As the lives of women have been extended, chronic diseases and disabilities have taken the place of acute illness and childbirth as leading causes of death. Women are living longer lives, challenging community health nurses to help women improve the quality of these added years.

Women, as the primary **caregivers** of families, are key to achieving the goal of healthy communities. However, women face significant barriers in gaining access to health care. Often, inadequate education and low socioeconomic status prevent women from assuming the responsibilities of their own health and well-being. As consumers of health services, women must be involved in the development of health policy to achieve parity in availability and access to health care resources for women. Community health nurses play key roles in collaborating with women to achieve the national goal of health care for all. This chapter provides information about the context of women's health and how community health nurses can assist women of all ages to meet health needs.

Demographic Profile of Women's Health

Population Characteristics

Currently, 84% of women in the United States are Caucasian (Phillips, Sexton, & Blackman, 1996). In subsequent generations, however, the racial and ethnic diversity of women is expected to increase markedly. The mean age for women in the

United States is currently 34 years. As baby boomers begin to age, the care of the elderly population, who will be predominantly women, will have a significant impact on health care.

Proportion of Women

The U.S. Census Bureau (1999) reports a ratio at birth of 105 males to 100 females. However, in most countries, women typically have longer life spans than men and consequently make up 52% of the world's population. In the United States, the average life span for a woman is 78.6, compared with 72.3 for men. Because males are more likely to die at any given age, the proportion of females to males increases over the life span (U.S. Census Bureau, 1997). This fact should alert the community health nurse that special needs for the elderly may predominantly center around women's gerontological issues.

· ·

We grow neither better nor worse as we get old, but more like ourselves.

Mary Lamberton Becker

· ·

Education

Education is positively correlated with health status (National Center for Health Statistics, 1993). According to the U. S. Census Bureau (1999), more women are completing educational degrees, although a higher percentage of women than men are only graduating from high school and community colleges. Above this educational level, the numbers reverse, with more men than women completing baccalaureate programs (16.8% and 15.4%, respectively), master's programs (5.9% and 4.9%, respectively), and doctoral programs (1.5% and 0.6%, respectively). In the

FYI

In the United States, women live on average 7 years longer than men.

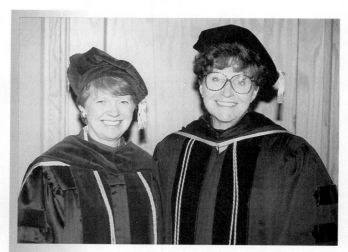

As women become better educated, health indicators improve also.

past, the predominant roles women chose were in education, nursing, library science, and social work. However, in the last two decades, more women have entered professions traditionally held by men such as engineering, theology, medicine, law, and dentistry, making up 50% of student enrollment. A continuing concern is that ethnic minority women have been slow to enter these major areas of study (Pollard & Tordella, 1993). An emerging trend, according to the U.S. Census Bureau, reflects an overall increase in college enrollment among African Americans and Hispanics since 1970 (Allen & Phillips, 1997). Such a trend holds promise for increasing the number of women pursing advanced specialty degrees as these cohorts move through the educational ranks.

Employment

More women are in the workforce than ever before and are entering the workforce at an earlier age. However, increased opportunities in the workforce are creating more challenges and risks for their families, such as child and elder caregiving issues. The job market remains male dominated, with average annual salaries differing by gender. Recent data indicate that women earn $0.71 to every $1.00 earned by men (U.S. Census Bureau, 1997).

....

Since every woman's problem occurs in part because of the nature of being female in this culture, which programs us to put the needs of others ahead of our own, we need to make radical changes in our minds and in our lives to get and stay healthy.

Christine Northrup

....

Traditional female occupations generally pay less than comparable men's jobs and have fewer benefits. Sixty-five percent of women are in the workforce as librarians, teachers, social workers, and nurses with low salaries. Working women continue to assume responsibility for child care, housework, and elder care (Wuest, 1993). More than 50% of women with an infant are in the workforce, up 35.3% since 1978. The percentage of new mothers who work tends to increase both with age and education (Taeuber, 1991). Men are more likely to be employed in higher-level management positions, with jobs that offer health benefits, medical leave, and insurance. Women with limited health benefits may not seek out health care when needed and are less likely to practice preventive health care.

Poverty

Women earn less than men and, as a result, make up two-thirds of all poor adults. In 1996, 24% of women lived in poverty, a number increasing every year (U.S. Census Bureau, 1997). This statistic is greatly influenced by culture and race, with the largest increases among African American and Hispanic women.

Women in poverty are usually 18 to 24 years old, live in the south (50% of the U.S. women in poverty live in this region), and reside outside central cities. Many factors contribute to poverty, including the gender wage gap, single mothers as heads of households, teenage birth rates, lack of adequate child care, and lack of enforcement of child support payments. Of all the countries in the industrialized world, the United States is the only country without a system that provides subsidized child care for working parents.

Dual-earner families are least likely to live in poverty, with a median salary reported at $36,389, compared with families headed by a man at $26,827 and by a woman at $15,346 (U.S. Census Bureau, 1999). These factors have been called the **feminization of poverty**. In the community setting, women should be aware of social services, child-care programs, nutritional resources, and other resources for family needs.

Marital Status/Family Configuration

Women's roles in marriage and the family are in a state of transition and have been since the 1960s. The traditional role of the unemployed mother working in the home has become a small minority. Only 6% of households have a male working full-time supporting a full-time homemaker with children in the home. The necessary goal of any family, however defined, is to maintain the integrity of self and members, including safety, well-being, and health of the family. In today's society, 28% of married couples do not have children; 32% of families are headed by single women, with an increase seen in female heads of households in all racial groups; and 25% of families live in single-dwelling homes (U.S. Census Bureau, 1999).

Racial differences in lifestyles can affect attitudes and beliefs about health. African Americans, as compared with Caucasians, are more often single or married with no spouse present or living with extended families. More Caucasians are divorced or widowed and tend to have fewer children than African Americans and Hispanics. Families maintained by women with no husband present are more likely to be poor. Among those men who are present in their families, African American and Hispanic men tend to spend more time with their family tasks than Caucasian men (Lawton, Rajagopal, Brody, & Kleban, 1992).

Childbearing

Trends in U.S. birth rates have major implications for the growth of the population and future trends in health care. Fertility rates dropped in 1997, with an overall decline in birth rates (U.S. Census Bureau, 1999). The numbers of births are expected to decline further as the baby boomers age and pass their childbearing years. More women are delaying childbearing or choosing to remain childless. Birth rates vary by age and ethnicity, with the number of births for unmarried women declining in all age groups. Table 32-1 illustrates the birth rate by age and race in 1996.

TABLE 32-1   1996 PERCENTAGE OF BIRTH RATES OF WOMEN BY AGE AND RACE

AGE GROUP	TOTAL BIRTHS	CAUCASIAN	AFRICAN AMERICAN	AMERICAN INDIAN	ASIAN OR PACIFIC ISLANDER
10–14	11,242	50%	46%	2%	2%
15–19	494,272	70%	26%	2%	2%
20–24	951,247	77%	19%	>1%	3%
25–34	1,982,740	83%	11%	>1%	5%
35–44	472,473	82%	11%	>1%	6%
45–49	2,980	80%	9%	>1%	10%

Source: CDC, 1997.

There are 6 million pregnancies in the United States each year. Three million of these pregnancies are unplanned, with 1.5 million ending in abortion (Pasquale, 1994). The leading method of contraception remains female sterilization, followed by the oral contraceptive pill (U.S. Census Bureau, 1997).

In 1995, 81.3% of mothers began prenatal care within the first trimester, the highest ever recorded. Twice as many African American women deliver low-birth-weight babies compared with Caucasian women. Of women of childbearing age, 25% are not covered by insurance and 25% are insured but without maternity insurance coverage. Medicaid is used to help pay for 34% of all deliveries, and approximately 15% of childbearing mothers receive food stamps (U.S. Census Bureau, 1997). Parenting classes, health care for children, quality day-care facilities, and flexible employment opportunities for working mothers are not consistently available to women in the United States; the health and well-being of working families has not been a national funding priority. Many countries throughout the world have established policies that ensure protection and support of mothers, infants, and families and can serve as role models for such positive family investments.

Health Status

Life expectancy steadily increased for both men and women in the 20th century. The life expectancy of women has increased to nearly 80 years, with women older than 50 making up the fastest growing segment of the U.S. population (U.S. Census Bureau, 1999). With a decline in mortality in certain diseases for men (e.g., cardiovascular disease) and an increase in the numbers of women who assume many lifestyle behaviors and health habits previously characteristic of men (e.g., cigarette smoking, alcohol use, full-time work in the labor force, head of household responsibilities), the differences in life spans for women and men (currently 78.6 and 72.3 years, respectively) may not be so great in the future.

Morbidity

Women experience higher morbidity than men and use acute care health services at a higher rate than men. Women are hospitalized more than men and experience more chronic conditions, including arthritis, depression, orthopedic problems, diabetes, chronic obstructive pulmonary disease (COPD), hemorrhoids, hypertension, chronic bronchitis, asthma, and chronic sinusitis. Although research has shed some light, these gender differences are still not fully understood. Twice as many women as men are

Most women have contact with the health care system during their reproductive years. Venus Callahan, chapter author, examines an expectant mother.

FYI

For all persons who live to be 100 years of age, there will be five women for every two men.

limited in physical activity, reporting more missed days from work or school, and in research studies they report their health conditions as worse than those of men.

The three major chronic conditions women experience are heart conditions, arthritis, and hypertension, which all increase with age (U.S. Census Bureau, 1999). Differences in morbidity exist by age. The leading chronic condition in younger women is chronic sinusitis and hay fever, followed by orthopedic problems. For middle-aged women, arthritis, hypertension, and COPD are the most common. For women older than 65, arthritis and hypertension remain the leading chronic illnesses. However, older women also have all the consequences of aging, including sensory impairments, heart disease, and mobility impairments.

Mortality

The leading causes of death in women are heart disease, cancer, and stroke, with differences by age and across racial groups. The leading causes of death for young women younger than 24 are accidents, homicide, suicide, human immunodeficiency virus/acquired immunodeficiency syndrome (HIV/AIDS), and complications of pregnancy. For women ages 25 to 64, the leading causes of death are cancer, HIV/AIDS, heart disease, and COPD. The leading causes of death in women older than 65 are heart disease, cancer, cerebrovascular accident (CVA), pneumonia, and influenza. These diseases can be caused by lifestyle and environmental and social factors and are often preventable. Alcohol and drug use and abuse, unprotected sex, cigarette smoking, lack of exercise, obesity, and environmental threats are all implications in the mortality rate (Allen & Phillips, 1997).

Some investigators claim that the mortality of women may be influenced by their own perceptions of health. Some women may delay seeking care when sick because of family and work obligations, may not take symptoms of pain seriously, and may not pursue health care. Also, physicians have been accused of minimizing women's complaints and not treating women as aggressively as their male cohorts (Mark, Shaw, & DeLong, 1994). All of this may contribute to women entering the health care system at a high acuity level.

• •

Aging is very much a woman's issue. That's because women are most valued for their childbearing capacities. Once we've used up those capacities and our supposed sexual attractiveness, our social worth is gone.

Gloria Steinem, 1999

• •

Reproductive Risks

Women are uniquely at risk during pregnancy and childbirth, including the risks of induced and spontaneous abortions. Even now in the 21st century, women die during childbirth, with pulmonary embolism the leading cause of death in pregnant women. However, through partnerships between community health nurses and the health care system, maternal mortality has been dramatically reduced through prenatal care, education related to maternal risk factors, blood transfusions, anesthesia, and antibiotics. Racial discrepancies persist in number of deaths, with women of color having a threefold greater incidence of death during pregnancy than Caucasian women (Williams & Thomas, 1997). This is attributed to lack of prenatal care, poor nutrition, and substandard living conditions. Concurrent infant death rates are also disproportionate among races, with twice the number of infants of color dying than Caucasian infants.

Health Promotion and Prevention Across the Life Span

Community health nurses, because of their unique relationship to clients and their awareness of community problems and resources, occupy a pivotal role in influencing women's beliefs and practices for health promotion and illness prevention. Community health nurses, as educators of women about health issues, incorporate the health promotion and disease prevention of *Healthy People 2010* (see the *Healthy People 2010* box on p. 736 for selected objectives) to accomplish the primary goal of identifying and implementing behavioral and social interventions that are effective in motivating women to use preventive health services across the life span.

Adolescence (12 to 18 Years Old)

Community health nurses can play an important role in promoting the health of adolescent females through teaching, counseling, and role modeling. Community health nurses need to establish trusting relationships with adolescents, thereby gaining their confidence. Nurses need to be able to ask questions that might reveal alcohol and other drug abuse, high-risk sexual activity, or emotional distress. Community health nurses working with adolescents face challenges in communication, peer influences, and the stigma of being seen in local health clinics or settings. Effective programs that have a positive impact on the health of adolescents are often specifically targeted to teens in schools, night clinics, and malls, as well as through celebrity and teen role model spokespersons.

Young women in adolescence have many issues to deal with, including puberty; menarche; body image; eating disorders; and sexual issues, including sexual identity, contraception decisions, and sexually transmitted diseases (STDs). Attitudes about these issues are influenced by peers, society, and family relationships. *Healthy People 2010* objectives should guide direction for efforts in this age group. School-based health programs for health promotion, exercise and fitness, sex education, and prevention of drug use should address social concerns for this age group. Because the greatest number of new smokers are adolescent females, primary lung cancer prevention must start at the elementary school level with aggressive counseling programs to decrease the number of new smokers among young girls. Successful programs with teen

HEALTHY PEOPLE 2010

OBJECTIVES RELATED TO WOMEN'S HEALTH

Arthritis, Osteoporosis, and Chronic Back Conditions

Osteoporosis

2.9 Reduce the overall number of cases of osteoporosis.

2.10 Reduce the proportion of adults who are hospitalized for vertebral fractures associated with osteoporosis.

Cancer

3.3 Reduce the breast cancer death rate.

3.4 Reduce the death rate from cancer of the uterine cervix.

3.11 Increase the proportion of women who receive a Pap test.

3.13 Increase the proportion of women aged 40 years and older who have received a mammogram within the preceding 2 years.

Family Planning

9.4 Reduce the proportion of females experiencing pregnancy despite use of a reversible contraceptive method.

9.11 Increase the proportion of young adults who have received formal instruction before turning age 18 years on reproductive issues, including all of the following topics: birth control methods, safer sex to prevent HIV, prevention of sexually transmitted diseases, and abstinence.

9.12 Reduce the proportion of married couples whose ability to conceive or maintain a pregnancy is impaired.

9.13 Increase the proportion of health insurance policies that cover contraceptive supplies and services.

HIV

13.3 Reduce the number of AIDS cases among females and males who inject drugs.

Injury and Violence Prevention

Violence and Abuse Prevention

15.34 Reduce the rate of physical assault by current or former intimate partners.

15.35 Reduce the annual rate of rape or attempted rape.

Maternal, Infant, and Child Health

Maternal Death and Illness

16.4 Reduce maternal deaths.

16.5 Reduce maternal illness and complications due to pregnancy.

Prenatal Care

16.6 Increase the proportion of pregnant women who receive early and adequate prenatal care.

Nutrition and Overweight

Iron Deficiency Anemia

19.12 Reduce iron deficiency among young children and females of childbearing age.

19.14 Reduce iron deficiency among pregnant females.

Sexually Transmitted Diseases

STD Complications Affecting Females

25.6 Reduce the proportion of females who have never required treatment for pelvic inflammatory disease (PID).

25.7 Reduce the proportion of childless females with fertility problems who have had a sexually transmitted disease or who have required treatment for pelvic inflammatory disease.

25.8 Reduce HIV infections in adolescent and young adult females aged 13 to 24 years that are associated with heterosexual contact.

Source: DHHS, 2000.

girls and the prevention of smoking initiation have focused on assertiveness training and decision-making models of accountability.

The Youth Risk Behavior Surveillance System under the auspices of the Centers for Disease Control and Prevention (CDC, 1993) monitors health-risk behaviors among youth and young adults. These health-risk behaviors contribute to unintentional and intentional injuries, tobacco use, alcohol and other drug use, sexual behaviors, dietary behaviors, and physical activity and should guide the community health nurse in planning interventions directed toward the female adolescent. Schools, churches, and recreational groups all provide the community health nurse with opportunities to influence health decisions through education (U.S. Adolescent Health Summary, 1997).

Young Adulthood (19 to 35 Years Old)

Two main concerns of women in this age group include making career choices and establishing relationships that may lead to marriage and pregnancy (Allen & Phillips, 1997). Community health nurses can address health promotion interventions in the context of these two life tasks. Nurses need to be knowledgeable regarding the various resources that are available in the community to assist women in this age range with such decisions. The nurse can be an effective model/mentor for young women in this developmental stage and should be able to address such concerns as fertility counseling, parenting skills, contraception options, domestic violence, and occupational health issues. Women in young adulthood face concerns such as STDs, contraceptive choices, safety, intentional and unintentional injury, stress management, alcohol and drug abuse, unhealthy dietary behaviors, physical activity, and role stress and strain. As women marry and establish families, they face issues such as learning to balance work and children, sexual harassment in the workplace, and establishing habits of self-care. The community health nurse must be cognizant of the problems of this age group and skillful in locating and accessing the resources available to therapeutically intervene.

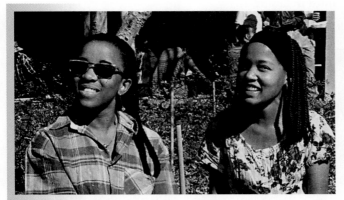

African American women have higher risks for cancer and hypertension and are less likely to use preventive health service.

Perimenopausal/Menopausal (36 to 55 Years Old)

The community health nurse must address health priorities with this age group of women, which include the following:

- *Benefits and risks of **hormone replacement therapy** (HRT)*
- *Early signs and symptoms of a cardiovascular disease*
- *Benefits of monitoring and controlling cholesterol and blood pressure levels*
- *Maintaining bone strength and density*
- *Maintaining healthy weight*
- *Exercising regularly*
- *Benefits of a regular mammogram*

It is during this time that breast cancer becomes a greater threat to a woman's longevity (Allen & Phillips, 1997). As women delay childbearing and with advanced reproductive technology, more and more women may be having their first child during this late reproductive stage. Women may also be caring for their own parents during this time while building careers, creating even greater time and energy demands. Table 32-2 is the recommended preventive health care calendar for adult women according to the American Medical Association (AMA, 1997).

The perimenopausal years are ages 36 to 50. During this period of a woman's life, the ovaries begin to slow down and eventually cease production of estrogen. Because of this decrease in estrogen, women may experience symptoms such as hot flashes, vaginal dryness, or night sweats. All perimenopausal women should be counseled about the benefits of taking hormone replacement therapy. Without estrogen, bones will begin to lose density and become thinner, weaker, brittle, and more prone to fracture. The lack of estrogen also decreases the high-density lipoprotein (HDL) cholesterol and raises the low-density lipoproteins (LDL) cholesterol, which increases the risk of cardiovascular problems such as myocardial infarction and CVA.

Women may react differently to these premenopausal physiological changes in the body. During this time, a woman may reexamine her life, which may result in a new self-identity. Women must explore what aging means to them and go through an acceptance of what their life has been and what it may still become. Sexuality of women changes during this time. Despite the fact that the public does not consider older women to be sexually active, most report positive experiences with sex during this time (Fogel & Woods, 1995). Many women view this time as the best years of their lives—children are grown, job is secure, and acceptance of self-identity has been established. For women who have devoted early years to childrearing, they may be returning to school or reentering the career market.

Mature (55 and Older)

As more women are reaching the mature stage of the life cycle, the community health nurse must realize that a shift of health emphasis from infectious and acute diseases to chronic diseases

TABLE 32-2   **RECOMMENDED HEALTH CARE CALENDAR**

TEST OR PROCEDURE	WHO NEEDS IT?	HOW OFTEN?
General physical exam (including blood pressure and lifestyle counseling)	Everyone	Every year
Pelvic examination	Everyone	Every year
Dental examination	Everyone	Every year
Eye examination	Everyone	Every year
Breast examination	Everyone	Every year
Breast self-examination (BSE)	Everyone	Every month
Skin cancer check	Everyone	Every 3 years
Rectal examination	Everyone	Every year
Pap smear	Everyone	Every year
Blood cholesterol	Everyone	Every 3 years (if first test was normal); as recommended by doctor if level is elevated
Mammogram	Everyone	Every 1 to 2 years between ages 40 and 49; once a year after age 50
Tests for sexually transmitted diseases	Anyone who is sexually active	Every 6–12 months if multiple partners otherwise as recommended by doctor
Electrocardiogram	Anyone with two or more of the following risk factors for heart disease: family history, smoking, high cholesterol, diabetes, high blood pressure	Every 3 to 5 years
Sigmoidoscopy	Anyone over 50	Every 3 years
Fecal occult-blood test	Everyone	Every year
Tuberculin skin test	Anyone who is at increased risk	Every year or as recommended by doctor
Tetanus booster	Everyone	Every 10 years
Diphtheria booster	Everyone	Every 10 years

Source: AMA, 1998.

occurs in this age group of women. Because of the chronic nature of diseases in this age group, the historical definition of health (absence of disease) is less applicable. Rather, an emphasis should be placed on functional health, independence, and autonomy. Health promotion should be aimed at preserving the mature woman's ability to function at the highest spectrum of wellness. Health-promoting activities to enhance wellness are listed in Box 32-1.

BOX 32-1 HEALTH PROMOTION ACTIVITIES FOR THE MATURE WOMAN

HEALTH SCREENINGS

Blood pressure, early cancer detection, hearing and vision screenings

HEALTH EDUCATION

Stress reduction, nutrition, general health, smoking cessation, classes about seasonal health issues such as hypothermia, heart related illness, colds/flu

IMMUNIZATIONS

Influenza shots

SAFETY

Safe driving courses, self-protection measures

EXERCISE

Walking, aerobics, water aerobics, weight lifting, weight-bearing exercise

Health Concerns Across the Life Span

Adolescence (12 to 18 Years Old)

Violent deaths, homicide, suicide, and accidents, particularly motor vehicle accidents, are responsible for the majority of deaths in this age group. Adolescents' misconception that they are "immortal" leads to risk-taking behaviors that make them more susceptible to injury and death. Female adolescents face potential threats to health such as substance abuse, pregnancy, acne, menstrual disorders, eating disorders, and STDs. Every year, nearly one-fourth of all new HIV infections, one-fourth of all new STD infections, and 1 million pregnancies occur among our nation's teenagers (U.S. Adolescent Health Summary, 1997).

The community health nurse can be a pivotal force in promoting the health of adolescents through health assessment, risk analysis, screening, anticipatory guidance, health teaching, and counseling with the adolescent as well as the parents. The most common health care request of adolescent females is related to pregnancy. Included in this visit, the community health nurse must conduct a health screening assessment, including last missed menstrual period, contraception being used, living arrangements, and financial status. If an adolescent is pregnant, anticipatory guidance is needed. This includes referral to a local prenatal health clinic or health department, encouragement of open communication regarding pregnancy with family or significant other, and referral to local department of human services for Medicaid enrollment if necessary. Health teaching must include the effects of alcohol and drugs on the fetus, the potential side effects of x-rays on the fetus, nutrition, and Women, Infant and Children (WIC) nutrition program enrollment. The counseling services of the nurse must include conducting a meeting with the adolescent and parent to inform them of the pregnancy. For sexually active adolescents who are not pregnant, the nurse should encourage enrollment in family planning clinic for contraceptives and STD education.

....

I'm not the usual celebrity size. And I think that people who like to see images of themselves reflected back feel strongly connected to me.

Rosie O'Donnell, 1997

....

Young Adulthood (19 to 35 Years Old)

For young adults and college students, as for adolescents, violent death or injury, alcohol and substance abuse, unwanted pregnancies, and STDs are major health threats. Most health problems in this stage are related to lifestyle behaviors. Weight concerns and eating problems are often reported as concerns for young women. Media images and social influences pressure young women desiring to be thin into abusive habits, such as purging, vomiting, laxative and diuretic abuse, and poor nutrition (Fogel & Woods, 1995). Young women should be aware of

interventions to delay onset of osteoporosis, including increasing calcium intake and weight-bearing exercises to promote bone density and decreasing cola intake, which decreases reabsorption of calcium.

The community health nurse can play a vital role in educating this group regarding behaviors that will positively affect their lifestyles. The proper use of condoms to help prevent STDs and the availability and variety of different contraceptive choices to prevent an unwanted pregnancy must be discussed with the young adult. Addressing these concerns and seeking a solution together will accomplish the ultimate goal of improved health.

Perimenopausal/Menopausal (36 to 55 Years Old)

A comprehensive assessment of women in this age group should include the changes of life that this woman goes through, including physiological, psychological, and emotional changes. The community health nurse must assess the woman's knowledge regarding the changes in her body, including her beliefs about menopause and the implications for her health. The nurse must be aware of complementary therapies women may chose for their health care and should be open-minded about what is acceptable for their client. Cardiovascular disease, cancer, and osteoporosis are the three major diseases that occur during the perimenopausal/menopausal period of a woman's life.

Cardiovascular Disease

Cardiovascular disease is the leading cause of death in American women, accounting for more than 359,000 deaths from coronary heart disease and 87,000 deaths from strokes in 1990 (Smith, 1995). Most effective for disease reduction is primary prevention through risk factor modification. The modifiable risk factors are cigarette smoking, hypertension, hypercholesterolemia, and physical inactivity, with less direct but still important risk factors of obesity, diabetes, stress, and menopause.

Community health nurses need to first be aware of the modifiable risk factors and then develop a cardiovascular health plan with an emphasis on prevention. When a woman seeks health care, either for herself or a family member, the community health nurse should seize the opportunity to emphasize heart health. The relationship between estrogen and cardiovascular disease, along with cardiac risk factors, must be discussed and assessed. The use of medications in the home should be reinforced by client teaching, including when to take prescribed nitroglycerin and when to seek medical attention for chest pains. By empowering the woman with knowledge, she will be able to seek medical care early and hopefully extend not only her longevity but her quality of life as well.

Cancer

Cancer is the second leading cause of death for women (Allen & Phillips, 1997). The most common types of cancer in women are lung, breast, colorectal, ovarian, and pancreatic. Lung cancer has surpassed breast cancer as the leading cause of cancer deaths. Tobacco is the single most toxic carcinogenic substance responsible for the occurrence of lung cancer and has been linked to cancers of the mouth, pharynx, larynx, esophagus, pancreas, uterine cervix, kidney, and bladder (McGinn & Haylock, 1993). Smoking cessation programs for women who smoke need to be readily accessible (see the following Research Brief).

. . . .

Cancer got me over unimportant fears, like growing old.
Olivia Newton John, 1998
Actress, singer, and breast cancer survivor
who had a modified radical mastectomy
to remove a cancerous tumor in July 1992

. . . .

Breast cancer is the second leading cause of cancer death in women overall and is the leading cause of cancer deaths in women aged 50 to 54. It is imperative that community health nurses educate women regarding signs and symptoms of breast cancer such as a lump, thickening or swelling, dimpling, skin irritation, distortion, retraction, scaliness, pain, and nipple tenderness, discharge, or inversion (American Cancer Society, 1995). A trained health care provider must investigate these

symptoms as soon as possible. If cancer is detected in the early stages (localized), the 5-year survival rate is 94%.

When a woman is receiving chemotherapy for cancer, the nurse should be aware of the side effects of chemotherapy and what can be done in the home to decrease or alleviate symptoms of discomfort (e.g., nausea, vomiting, pain). They must also be aware of local resources to ensure that women have prompt access to care as soon as a definite cancer diagnosis has been obtained, along with support groups and referral agencies for cancer victims. See Box 32-2 for Cancer Support Groups.

Osteoporosis

Bone mass peaks at the end of the growth period, usually around age 17. There are some small gains in bone mass up to age 30; this is then followed by a progressive loss of bone mass. Twenty-eight million Americans, 80% of whom are women, have osteo-

---

RESEARCH BRIEF

Marcus, B., & Albrecht, A. (1999). The efficacy of exercise as an aid for smoking cessation in women. Archives of Internal Medicine, *159(11), 1229–1235.*

This descriptive research study examined the effectiveness of exercise as an aid for smoking cessation in women. The sample was composed of 281 healthy but sedentary female smokers between the ages of 18 and 65 who had smoked routinely for at least 1 year. The subjects were followed in a 12-week smoking cessation program. Of the 134 women who exercised three times a week, 19.4% gave up smoking for at least 2 months after their program ended, compared with 10.2% of the 147 nonexercisers. Three months later, 16.4% of the exercisers were still not smoking, compared with 8.2% of the nonexercisers. One year after the study, the different was 11.9% and 5.4%, respectively. The study provides evidence that vigorous exercise leads to improved rates of continuous abstinence from smoking in women.

BOX 32-2 CANCER SUPPORT GROUPS

American Cancer Society
1599 Clifton Rd. NE
Atlanta, GA 30329
800-ACS-2345

Candlelighters Childhood Cancer Foundation
1312 18th St. NW, 2nd Floor
Washington, DC 20036-1808
800-366-2223

National Alliance of Breast Cancer Organizations
1180 Avenue of the Americas, 2nd Floor
New York, NY 10036
212-719-0154

National Coalition for Cancer Survivorship
323 8th St. SW
Albuquerque, NM 87102
505-764-9956

SHARE: Self-Help for Women With Breast Cancer
19 W. 44th St.
New York, NY 10036
212-719-0364
Hot line 212-382-2111

Y-ME National Organization for
    Breast Cancer Information and Support
18220 Harwood Ave.
Homewood, IL 60430
800-221-2141
24-hour hot line 708-799-8228

TABLE 32-3	OSTEOPOROSIS RISK FACTOR PROFILE FOR WOMEN	

RISKS	MODIFIABLE FACTORS
65 years and older	Slender build
Family history of osteo-porosis	Estrogen deficiency
	Sedentary lifestyle
Caucasian or Asian	Low calcium intake
Postmenopausal, espe-cially premature	Failure to achieve peak bone mass
History of atraumatic fracture	Cigarette smoking
	High alcohol consumption
Loss of 1 inch or more in height	Weight below normal
	Steroid use

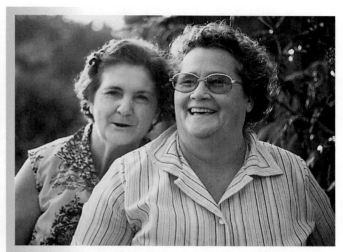

As women age, friendships become more important in promoting a sense of well-being.

porosis, representing a major public health problem in the United States. Vertebral fractures generally occur in women 55 years and older, and result in back pain, height loss and kyphosis, anterior rib pain, negatively changed body image, difficulty in fitting clothes, a protuberant abdomen, and abdominal discomfort (as a result of reduced lumbar vertebral height). Hip fractures occur twice as often in women older than 75 than in men and are associated with excess mortality of 5% to 20% as a result of preoperative and postoperative complications, such as deep vein thrombosis, pulmonary embolism, and pneumonia.

The community nurse must be aware of the lifestyle changes to prevent osteoporosis, including calcium intake, weight control, and weight-bearing exercise, as well as hormone replacement therapy used to treat osteoporosis. The osteoporosis profile (Table 32-3) can be used by nurses to identify risk factors for women.

Mature (55 and Older)

Mature women deal with many health care issues as they age. Many of the illnesses discussed in the section on menopausal women apply here also. However, as women live longer, their chronic conditions may increase in severity. Depression, dementia, and **urinary incontinence** are some of the illnesses that occur later in life. Arthritis, osteoporosis, hypertension, and cardiovascular disease continue to be health concerns for women in this age group (Fogel & Woods, 1995).

Community health nurses often must deal with depression in mature women. Many may have outlived their spouses and are dealing with the loss daily. This depression often goes untreated. Many medications may also contribute to the depression. If dementia is present, safety considerations in the surrounding environment should be made. Urinary incontinence is seen twice as often in women than in men; it is found in 30% of elderly women (Fogel & Woods, 1995). Nurses must also be aware of

medications that may cause urinary retention or urinary incontinence, possibly leading to urinary tract infections.

Diversity and Women's Health
Cultural Influences

The impact of culture on women is imperative for the community health nurse to understand. Gender roles are influenced by culture. An awareness of family dominance patterns is essential when teaching clients and communicating with family members. In some cultures, women may not speak unless they are given permission by a spouse or father. It is also important to understand how men and women interact in each culture (Lipson, Dibble, & Minarik, 1996; Purnell & Paulanka, 1998). Although most cultures are still largely patriarchal, matriarchal influences are also important. Acceptable ways of communicating and touching should be assessed by community health nurses and included in any interventions for the client. Guidelines for a cultural communication assessment appear in Box 32-3.

Sexual Orientation

As lesbianism has become more accepted, its impact on families and health care should be acknowledged by the community health nurse. Family structures are no longer made up only of the typical married couple with children. Gay and lesbian couples have openly taken residence together and may live with other persons, including communal communities where responsibilities are shared based on common beliefs. Many lesbian women choose to adopt children or conceive a child through artificial insemination or heterosexual intercourse (Zeidenstein, 1990). However, most cultures continue to stigmatize homosexuality, forcing homosexuals to remain "in the closet" (Giger & Davidhizar, 1995). Health care continues to be prejudiced toward heterosex-

BOX 32-3 QUESTIONS FOR ASSESSING CULTURAL COMMUNICATION PATTERNS

1. Is the individual willing to share thoughts, feelings, and ideas?

2. What does touching mean in the culture? Is touching certain body parts appropriate?

3. What does silence mean in the culture? a loud voice?

4. What spatial and distancing characteristics when communicating are observed for family members versus strangers?

5. What eye contact is used (avoidance, changes among family, friends, strangers, or socioeconomic groups)? Is it a sign of respect or insult?

6. What facial expressions are used? Do they smile a lot, show emotions?

7. How are people greeted?

Source: Adapted from Purnell & Paulanka, 1998.

ual relationships by ignoring specific health care considerations of this population.

Lesbian women are more likely to neglect their own health care needs and avoid examinations by health care providers because of the stigma and humiliation that often goes along with the disclosure of being a lesbian. They are more likely to reveal their identity to practitioners who are open and nonjudgmental (Stevens, Tatum, & White, 1996). Lesbians are at low risk for vaginal infections, STDs, and HIV. In contrast, they are at higher risk for breast and uterine cancer than their heterosexual cohorts (Rosser, 1994). They also are more likely to experience stress and depression because of social isolation. Substance abuse is reported in 30% of lesbian women, compared with 7% in the general population (Deevey & Wall, 1992). **Heterosexism** and **homophobia** contribute to prejudice, fear, and continued discrimination against lesbians.

The community health nurse should learn to communicate without bias with women of all sexual orientations. Lesbians are often insulted when health care workers assume they are heterosexual and ask questions gender specific, such as "What form of birth control do you use?" Alternative questions should be phrased in the form of open-ended, nongender statements like "Tell me about your sexual activity." The nurse should encourage lesbian women to have regular pelvic examinations and to avoid unprotected oral sex by using latex barriers (Zeidenstin, 1990). Mental health counseling and support networks are also options for dealing with the psychosocial issues, sexual practices associated with relationships.

Women and Aging

The elderly population will more than double by the year 2050, with the oldest old—those older than 85—the most rapidly growing segment. Twenty percent of elders will be from underrepresented populations (U.S. Census Bureau, 1997). These women are much more likely to be widowed, live alone, and live in poverty. Women belonging to underrepresented racial and ethnic groups have been termed "quadruple jeopardy" because they are elderly, minority, female, and poor. Elderly women are also reported to have high levels of depression related to loneliness (Bennett, 1987).

Differences have been identified regarding why women are living longer, including differences by gender, exposure to environmental hazards, health habits, personality styles, and reactions to illness. Men have traditionally held jobs that expose them to more hazardous environmental factors, such as asbestos and carcinogens. Women have traditionally smoked less and managed stress better (Golub & Freedman, 1985). These differences are expected to narrow in the future as a result of changes in our society, equal rights for women, and greater participation of women in the workforce.

· ·

Freedom is what you do with what's been done to you.

Jean-Paul Sartre

· ·

Because women generally outlive men, more women live alone or live in long-term care facilities. Women currently outnumber elderly men by 6 to 5 from age 65 to 69, and by 5 to 2 over age 85 (U.S. Census Bureau, 1997). More families are opting to care for their elderly parents at home; however, women (especially Caucasian women) continue to make up a larger percentage in nursing homes, with 50% childless or having outlived their own children (Golub & Freedman, 1985). The financial consequences for elderly women are of major concern. Elderly women often have saved little, because many grew up in a male-dominated time in which women did not have to consider financial affairs. The few resources that these women have must be used for a longer period. With rising health care costs, many elderly women rely on Medicare and Medicaid resources (Benderly, 1997).

Elderly women often report they are disappointed with health care and their treatment by health care personnel. As the women age, they report that physicians often dismiss their complaints as compared with their male cohorts. An example of this is often seen in women with cardiac conditions. Until recently, women have been ignored in cardiovascular research and have not been offered the same interventions that men traditionally have—

such as cardiac rehabilitation. Many elderly women report feeling disrespected and mistreated. Discrimination by race and sexual orientation is also a concern. Elderly lesbian women are often discounted in health care practices, with their significant other being eliminated from major health care decisions. Elderly women may not have been socialized to deal with finances, and this may place them at significant risk. Rural elderly women may also be disadvantaged because a large number of them have a low educational and socioeconomic status (Golub & Freedman, 1985).

Community health nurses must acknowledge the diverse needs of elderly women. Health promotion should be encouraged, including sleeping, exercising, weight control, and diet. Nurses in the community should work with elderly women, listening to their needs and problems, making life less stressful for these women. The cultural prejudices against the elderly in the United States influence the way women perceive themselves as they age, how they care for themselves, and how they relate to health care providers.

Global Issues and Women's Health

The **Commission on the Status of Women** is one of the first bodies established by the United Nations Economic and Social Council to monitor the situation of women and promote their rights in all societies around the world. The United Nations Fourth **World Conference on Women** was held in Beijing, China, in 1995. Ethical issues related to women were determined, setting universal standards regarding equality between women and men. Women's concerns should be brought to the forefront with issues related to human rights. Mutilation of female body parts, prostitution for survival, and female child slavery are all considered culturally acceptable in some countries. Women must participate in the political arena and in decision making related to legislation to fully address these ethical concerns. Women should also have a role in the contribution of development of their countries, including policy, employment, education, the economy, and the environment. Above all, women must have a voice in the fight against poverty and violence against women.

Issues Affecting Women's Health

Violence

Violence can take many forms, including physical assault, sexual assault, and homicide. Age has been identified as the most significant trait that puts women at risk for a violent attack, because younger women are more likely to be victims of sexual and domestic abuse (Allen & Phillips, 1997). The health consequences of violence against women include physical, psychological, and social effects. Violence touches 1 in 4 families and is responsible for more than 1 in 3 female murder victims. It involves 6 out of every 10 couples and kills as many women every 5 years as the total number of Americans killed in the Vietnam War. Violence is the single largest cause of injury to women in the United States—more common than automobile accidents and muggings combined, creating 100,000 days of hospitalization, 30,000 emergency department visits, and 40,000 trips to the doctor's office each year. Thirty-five percent of hospital visits by women are attributed to violence, with the women seeking treatment for symptoms related to ongoing abuse. However, only 5% of these domestic violence victims are so identified (AMA, 1998).

The cost to business is perhaps as much as $5 billion annually in lost productivity as a result of absenteeism. Community health nurses should be aware of "red flag" identifiers associated with domestic violence, such as women who (1) always seem to have bruises on the limbs, torso, and face; (2) come to the clinic with vague symptoms of illness such as pain in lower abdomen, chronic diarrhea, or pain of undetermined origin; (3) have trouble making eye contact; (4) have controlling partners; and (5) consistently wear sunglasses, even indoors.

Community health nurses should be aware of local resources that can be accessed to assist women who find themselves in an abusive situation. National crisis lines such as the Domestic Violence Crisis Line and the Sexual Assault Crisis Line are accessible nationwide.

Homelessness

Homelessness is a growing problem in all urban and rural regions. Single women head approximately 40% of the homeless families (Allens & Phillips, 1997). For women, many factors can lead to homelessness, such as divorce, poverty, eroding work opportunities, decline in public assistance, domestic violence, substance abuse, and mental illness. Substance abuse often accompanies homelessness and increases the risk of homeless women for prostitution and other health-related conditions such as HIV, STDs, tuberculosis, and malnutrition.

The community health nurse can assist homeless women and families through primary, secondary, and tertiary prevention interventions at the individual, community, and national levels. The community health nurse may be the referral for financial assistance and act as an advocate to assist the client through the

FYI

An excellent resource, the National Resource Center on Homelessness and Mental Illness provides technical assistance and information about services and housing for the homeless and mentally ill population. It is sponsored by the Center for Mental Health Services, Substance Abuse and Mental Health Services Administration at 800-444-7415.

"red tape" of the bureaucratic process. Nurses must work in the community by challenging government officials to examine the homeless problem and soliciting concerned citizens to develop shelters and programs for homeless individuals and families.

Incarceration

In the last few years, as a result of the decline in economic conditions and the crackdown on drugs and crime, the number of women in prison has increased. In the last 10 years, due to the decline in economic conditions and the crack down on drugs and crime, the number of women in prison has increased to 138,000 (Wheeler, 2000). Women account for 5.8:% of the prison population and 9.3% of the jail population (Gilliard & Beck, 1994). The typical conviction is for property crimes, for example, check forgery and illegal credit card use. About 80% of women in prison report an income of $2,000 per year before being incarcerated. Ninety-two percent report incomes under $10,000. Single mothers account for 90% of the women incarcerated, with 54% being women of color. (www.igc.apc.org/justice/prisons/women/women-in-prison.html).

The majority of incarcerated women have a dependency on drugs and/or alcohol and are usually from a low socioeconomic group. With these lifestyle patterns, health care has usually been neglected before they are incarcerated. Many of the women have a host of chronic medical problems such as tuberculosis, HIV, and other STDs. Historically, the prison systems have not had the resources to provide sufficient health care for these women. Community health nurses need to be politically active and petition legislative bodies to allocate monies for health care for this vulnerable population. The community health nurse needs to assume the role of client advocate in regard to child care and visitation while incarcerated. Parenting and child-care classes should be made available to the inmates. Programs that provide occupational training and promote self-esteem and assertiveness have been linked with better outcomes for women who are released from prison.

Poverty

Poverty dramatically affects women's health. Poor women have limited access to health care and preventive health care services, which results in delay of diagnosis of disease and injury, and consequently, shorter life spans. Factors unique to women in regard to poverty include the following:

- *Women are usually responsible for children, and many are single parents with no extended support.*
- *Women are not traditionally trained to assume the bread winner role and usually accept lower-paying jobs, often leading to a choice between public assistance and inadequate child care while they work.*

- *Health care is an expendable luxury when placed alongside child care, food, and lodging.*
- *Jobs women take may not have health care benefits comparable to men's jobs.*

Community health nurses need to be knowledgeable about local resources to assist women who are poor to gain access to health care. Ways to reach women in poverty for preventive health care, such as church-based programs, should be identified. Some local resources that are available in most areas include county and state health departments, federal health clinics, The United Way, Medicaid, and Social Security Administration.

Workplace Health

Women represent almost half of the current workforce. Many factors have contributed to this increasing number of women in the workforce, including economic necessity, fewer women having children, changes in women's attitudes of work, and changes in society. Women face a variety of concerns in the workplace, including reproductive risks, job stress, role conflict, sexual harassment, discrimination, and salary inequality. Women make up the largest percentage of health care workers in this country, including nurses, technologists, physicians, therapists, dietitians, and clerical workers. Major occupational hazards for health care workers include biological, chemical, environmental, physical, and psychosocial hazards (Fogel & Woods, 1995).

RESEARCH BRIEF

Trossman, S. (1999, May/June). RN Explores Agent Orange's Lasting Effects on Women Vets. American Nurse, *p. 24.*

Eighty-nine percent of female veterans who served in the Vietnam War were nurses. Agent Orange, a toxin used in Vietnam to clear out dense vegetation and crops, is well known for its serious adverse health affects and role in cancer and Hodgkin's disease in men. Virtually no research had been conducted on the women who were exposed to Agent Orange. Dr. Linda Schwartz has studied this "forgotten population" and found that they are at great risk for increased cancer rates and miscarriages. Agent Orange was used to keep down weeds around the camps, and the empty containers often used to store supplies and as barbecue grills. Nurses handled the containers and were exposed to the toxin as well. The outcome of this study has been to influence policy in the Veteran's Association to compensate women for these damages.

All of these factors may influence a woman's health, both physically and mentally, in the workplace. The community health nurse in the occupational setting must address sensitive issues for women, including effects of cancer, reproductive problems (e.g., menstrual disorders, reduced fertility, genetic damage, spontaneous abortion, stillbirths), back problems, and carpal tunnel syndrome (Fogel & Woods). At-risk occupations for women must be identified. Even though many factors affect women's health in the workplace, very little research has been conducted with regard to women. Most research has been based on males as workers, resulting in biased research findings. This has led to designs and practices that compromise the working woman's health and safety. Community health nurses must be advocates for women in the workplace by conducting research based on female workers and educating women about specific gender risks associated with work.

Toward the Future
Women's Ways of Knowing

Women must play a major role in their acquisition of knowledge to make informed health decisions. Historically, most women have not been as well educated as men in basic or health sciences. The way in which women have been educated directly influences their health knowledge. Poorly educated women may participate in the health care system in silence—afraid to ask questions, feeling inadequate, with minimal knowledge of their own health care. They may accept answers without question. They may not be able to understand the complex health care system or understand why they are expected to change from old patterns. Some distrust anyone of authority and reject science and medicine, relying on tradition or family influence.

As women become better educated through college, life and work experiences they learn **procedural knowledge,** including critical thinking and logical reasoning skills. Some women will acquire **constructed knowledge** and are able to synthesize knowledge from many areas. The logic of women's ways of knowing stems from the fact that fewer women than men graduate from baccalaureate or higher degree programs (Rosser, 1994). Education can play a key role in eliminating the subservient way women react to the health care industry. Community health nurses play a critical role in the education of women throughout the life span.

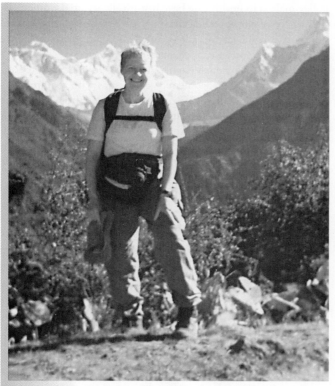

Research indicates that women can enjoy good health and an active lifestyle over a lifetime with attention to regular exercise and strength training.

When you don't like a thing, change it. If you can't change it, change the way you think about it and stop complaining and whining. Whining is not only graceless, it is hazardous—it can alert a brute that a victim is in the neighborhood.

Maya Angelou

Feminism

The politics of women's health care issues have long been in the forefront of the feminist movement. Until recently, few women have been invited to attend or participate in legislative forums related to women's health. Women have often been absent in the establishment of research priorities related to their health. Feminism and the promotion of women's rights in society today are closely associated with the promotion of a national women's health agenda.

I myself have never been able to find out precisely what feminism is: I only know that people call me a feminist whenever I express sentiments that differentiate me from a door mat.

Rebecca West, 1913

....

Feminism's agenda is basic . . . .It asks that women be free to define themselves—instead of having their identity defined for them, time and again, by their culture and their men.

Susan Faludi

....

Feminist theory deals with gender by race and class, along with individuals, groups, and communities. There are many feminist theories, including liberal feminism, Marxist feminism, socialist feminism, African American feminism, lesbian separatist feminism, conservative feminism, existential feminism, psychoanalytic feminism, and radical feminism.

Women's issues focus on economics, health care, and violence toward women. The correlation between the feminist movement and the political arena and the impact on women's health are clearly obvious. Women must continue in their quest for a voice in health care policy and the implementation of policies that affect women (Rosser, 1995). Community health nurses can promote the feminist agenda through public policy activism and serving on boards where women's health issues are concerned.

....

For us who nurse, our nursing is a thing, which unless we are making progress every year, every month, every week, take my word for it, we are going back.

Florence Nightingale,
1872, graduation address, St. Thomas School of Nursing

....

FYI

The Pill That Launched a Social Revolution

Some medical historians say that the development of a foolproof contraceptive for women in 1960 influenced the role of women more than any single factor in the history of humankind. In 1950, the Planned Parenthood Federation provided funds to conduct research on the development of a safe, reliable oral contraceptive to a biologist, Gregory Pincus. Ten years later, the oral contraceptive, marketed under the name Enovid-10, was approved by the U.S. Food and Drug Administration, in 1960. Within 2 years, 1.2 million women were taking it to control the size of their families. In 1999, 10 million women used an oral contraceptive. The "pill" was indeed revolutionary in changing lives, attitudes, values, and society of women and men.

Empowerment

Empowerment is based on the assumption that all people are created equal. Each person has the opportunity to recognize his or her own assets and develop from them on a professional, physical, spiritual, and emotional level. Recognizing and respecting the fact that all people have assets supports humility and dismisses the threat that others are better, eliminating any jealousy or threats of insecurity. People feel powerful in themselves when they feel secure. Community health nurses can be the "mirror" that reflects the woman's steps toward recognizing her own special assets. By affirming and reinforcing the woman's ability to recognize these assets, the woman gains confidence to move forward in the search for security and improved self-esteem.

One of the most empowering events for women has been the formation of the **United Nations Platforms for Action for Women** with the purpose to challenge governments to raise the status of women. The most recent conference was the 1995 Fourth World Conference on Women in Beijing, China, and identified commonly held beliefs about women's rights to health care. The four strategic objectives for women's health are listed in Box 32-4. A specific action plan has been specified by the U.S. Congress to achieve each of the four objectives.

Health Care Policy

Policy makers in health care have historically ignored women's issues when developing health care policy. However, many policies were made in the last decade of the 20th century that influence the health promotion and well-being of women.

The Women's Health Equity Act of 1990 identified the inequality of research in women's health issues with requirements that women and underrepresented racial and ethnic groups be included in research. At the same time, the National Institutes of Health established the Office of Research in Women's Health based on the concept that women's research must expand from the traditional focus of women's reproductive systems to include

BOX 32-4 STRATEGIC OBJECTIVES OF THE WORLD CONFERENCE ON WOMEN

1. Increase women's access throughout the life span to appropriate, affordable, and quality health care, information, and related services.
2. Strengthen preventive programs that promote women's health.
3. Undertake gender-sensitive initiatives that address sexually transmitted diseases, HIV/AIDS, and sexual and reproductive health issues.
4. Increase resources and monitor follow-up for women's health.

While the education of girls and women is obviously desirable for its own sake, it is especially crucial to lowering birthrates because of the different possible futures it opens up. . . . By opening the doors of education and social participation for the world's women and children, we can not only help our human family to a better life, but reduce our pressure on the planet as well.

—Carl Pope,
Executive Director of the Sierra Club.
Source: Pope, C. (1999). Solving the population problem: The key is to improve the lives of women. *Sierra Magazine, 84*(5), 14–15.

BOX 32-5 RESEARCH AREAS FOR WOMEN ACROSS THE LIFE SPAN

Adolescence	*Prevention of accidents, suicide prevention, HIV, sexuality, alcohol, tobacco, diet and exercise*
Young adult/ college	*Low-birth-weight babies, pregnancies dangerously complicated by hypertension, ectopic pregnancies resulting in death, infertility, sexuality transmitted diseases, cancer prevention (breast), safety (alcohol/drugs), health education, contraception, eating disorders, discomforts of pregnancy, obesity, HIV, family planning*
Midlife	*Disease prevention (cancer, hypertension, stroke, heart disease), health promotion, health education, strengths of single family head of households, multiple role adaptation, obesity, influence of diet on osteoporosis, domestic violence, early detection of cancer, arthritis, pain*
Perimeno- pausal	*Heart disease, health promotion, health education, impact of diet on osteoporosis, domestic violence, urinary incontinence, hormone replacement therapy, dietary influence on breast cancer, calcium and vitamin D supplements*
Mature	*Coping with chronic illnesses and disability, urinary incontinence, depression, institutionalization, respite care, social and economic contributions to health status, older women and health policy, racial/cultural influences on health care, caregivers, cost-effectiveness of health care to elder women*

all body systems and behavioral factors that influence women's health care. Recommendations for priority research for the next two decades for women include health promotion and wellness, eliminating barriers to health care services, prevention of illness, health education, and recognizing differences among women. In 1993, the Women's Health Initiative, a 14-year descriptive and intervention study of women and diseases, was launched to examine postmenopausal women of all races and socioeconomic levels, with specific considerations of the effects of interventions on heart disease, stroke, cancer, and osteoporosis. Box 32-5 identifies areas of research needed for women across the life span.

The Family Medical Leave Act was passed in 1993, allowing for 12 weeks of unpaid leave time from work for family or medical reasons. Employees are guaranteed the same job, pay, and benefits when they return to work after a leave. Because women are the primary family caregivers in the United States, this legislation is considered of major benefit for women.

Women are the dominant caregivers in our society, making up 75% of caregivers in the home (Biegel, Sales, & Schulz, 1991). Caring for family members has long been an expectation of women. In addition to working outside the home, women are required to care for children, spouses, and aging parents. Women often must give up their employment to care for family members, with loss of wages, employee benefits—health and retirement—and social support. Many women who lack health insurance may not have adequate resources for health care. With the extra stresses of caregiving, women may end up divorced, with the added loss of security from the employee benefits of their spouses (e.g., health insurance) (Hogan, 1990). To address these issues, in 1991, the Family Caregiver Support Act was proposed entitling a caregiver to $2,400 a year for support services;

however, this bill was not passed (Riggs, 1991). Health care policy for female caregivers must not be ignored, but rather mandated, including monetary reimbursement and respite services. Changes in health care policy that relate to the problems of female caregivers could help these women improve their quality of life.

Health behaviors of women are affected by the availability of health care resources and influenced by education and income. Women get health insurance either through employment or marriage. Well-educated women are more likely to practice positive health promotion such as healthy eating, exercising, not smoking, and drinking less alcohol (Fogel & Woods, 1995). Poverty and lack of education have a negative influence on health, with an increase in stress, depression, and poor health promotion habits. Usually, these women wait until an acute episode to seek health care. Many may rely on home remedies or alternative medicine for health care. The fact remains that inadequate health care access results in needless suffering and often death.

Despite the reality that more women are caregivers to our country, they play a small role in public decision making regarding health care issues. Women have traditionally been a small percentage of physicians, legislators, and health care administrators. This trend is changing, however, as more women are entering male-dominated professions and being elected to public office. There are more women in Congress than ever before. Women should be encouraged by community health nurses to become more involved in increasing community awareness regarding women's health issues.

RESEARCH BRIEF

Wilcox, S., & Stefanick, M. (1999). Knowledge and perceived risk of major disease in middle-aged and older women. Health Psychology, 18(4), 346–353.

This study examined the perceived health risks of middle-aged and older women related to mortality risks, personal risk, control, and preventability of risk diseases. The sample consisted of 200 women from 41 to 95 years of age. One in two women will eventually die of heart disease or stroke, and one in twenty-five will die of breast cancer. Middle-aged women and older women were more likely to know the leading cause of mortality for men in their age group than for women. Only 34% of the older women in the study knew that coronary heart disease was the leading cause of death in older women. Women in both age groups overestimated a woman's risk of death from breast cancer and underestimated the risk from lung and colon cancer. The authors speculate that heart disease is known as a "man's disease" and breast cancer has received a great deal of media attention and is more closely identified as a "woman's disease." This has implications for health providers in the education of women about the need for heart disease screening and for taking action to reduce their risks for all diseases.

CASE STUDY

Frances Benton is a 68-year-old widow who has recently been referred to your community health clinic by Rachel Jackson, a concerned neighbor. According to Ms. Jackson, Mrs. Benton's husband died about 8 months ago. Mr. Benton had been Mrs. Benton's caretaker. The couple did not have children, and there are no close relatives. Mrs. Benton had fallen and sustained a hip fracture approximately 1 year ago and recently a cracked vertebra. She has begun to have lapses of memory and has lost her way home from the grocery store. Two days ago, Mrs. Benton was out in the yard with only her slip on, which is definitely out of character according to Ms. Jackson. The landlord stopped by several times to collect the rent but could not get Mrs. Benton to understand that she had not paid it in 3 months. He had spoken with Ms. Jackson and was planning to evict Ms. Benton.

1. What are your nursing diagnoses in this situation?

2. What secondary and tertiary preventive measures might be appropriate in working with Ms. Benton?

3. What community resources could you collaborate with to address the health risks for Mrs. Benton?

CONCLUSION

Community health nurses are invaluable in assisting women with health care needs in the community. They should be knowledgeable regarding the various health concerns that women face, such as violence, homelessness, incarceration, poverty, osteoporosis, and cancer, and be able to define these needs. They should be aware of the local resources that are available and be skilled in linking these resources with the clients and their communities. Finally, they should be able to evaluate the process, fill in the gaps, and provide continuity of care for the individual client and the community.

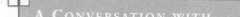

A CONVERSATION WITH...

While the education of girls and women is obviously desirable for its own sake, it is especially crucial to lowering birthrates because of the different possible futures it opens up.... By opening the doors of education and social participation for the world's women and children, we can not only help our human family to a better life, but reduce our pressure on the planet as well.

Source: Pope, C. (1999). Solving the population problem: The key is to improve the lives of women. *Sierra Magazine, 84*(5), 14–15.

CRITICAL THINKING ACTIVITIES

1. You are a rural community health nurse working on a mobile van visiting a large migrant community at a local farm. Selena King, a 16-year-old Hispanic female, comes into the van to have her blood pressure checked because she has been feeling tired and nauseated lately and is having difficulty working in the fields. She is also complaining of a coin-shaped rash on her arms, palms, and trunk. In completing your history, you find that she has not had any medical care since she was 8, when she had her appendix removed in Florida. Her blood pressure is 100/68 mm Hg. She cannot remember when her last menstrual period was, but she thinks it was 2 month ago. She is sexually active and uses condoms occasionally. She lives with her mother, four sisters, two brothers, and her father (who has forbidden her to see her boyfriend, Juan) in a travel trailer that they pull from town to town.

   - What are your nursing diagnoses in this situation?

   - How would you address the two dimensions of secondary prevention (diagnosis and treatment) of pregnancy and secondary syphilis?

   - What secondary and tertiary preventive measures might be appropriate in working with Miss King?

   - What resources could you as a community nurse tap to assist Miss King?

2. Mrs. Wise, a 67-year-old woman, is being discharged from the hospital after having surgery to repair a broken hip and bilateral wrist fractures. She will have bilateral casts for 8 weeks. She is a widow and has two sons who live within 2 miles of her. She lives alone. Her daughters-in-law will be the main caretakers. Both daughters-in-law work outside the home, neither have had any medical training, and they are afraid of assuming the health care of their mother-in-law. Mrs. Wise is reluctant to move in with her sons and would rather return to her small townhouse. The discharge diagnosis includes hip and wrist repair as a result of osteoporosis, diabetes, hypertension, and obesity.

   - What are your nursing diagnoses in this situation?

   - How would you address considerations of competence, time management, and supervision in planning the care of Mrs. Wise?

CRITICAL THINKING ACTIVITIES—CONT'D

- What resources could you as a community nurse use to assist this family in caring for Mrs. Wise and at the same time address Mrs. Wise's concerns regarding her independence?

3. Empowerment of women may well be seen in a depiction of the Greek Goddess Sarasvati (sa-RAS-vah-tee). She is the goddess of knowledge and is credited with the creation of the fruits of civilization, arts, and music. Her color and brightness represents the powerful, pure light of education, which destroys the darkness of ignorance. Sarasvati is depicted with four arms, showing that her power extends in all directions. In one of her hands, she holds a book (representing learning) and in another a strand of beads (representing spiritual knowledge). In the other hands, she holds and plays the vina, an Indian lute, representing the art of music (Waldherr, 1996).

- How does this depict our society of women in the United States today?

- Is education encouraged in women?

- What is spirituality, and how is it seen in our society? How is it seen in Sarasvati?

- What does music represent to Sarasvati or to the women of many other cultures and diversities?

- What is the darkness of ignorance?

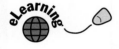

Explore Community Health Nursing on the web! To learn more about the topics in this chapter, use the passcode provided to access your exclusive web site:
http://communitynursing.jbpub.com
If you do not have a passcode, you can obtain one at this site.

REFERENCES

Allen, K., & Phillips, J. (1997). *Women's health across the lifespan: A comprehensive perspective.* Philadelphia: J. B. Lippincott.

American Cancer Society. (1995). *Cancer facts and figures.* Atlanta: Author.

American Medical Association (AMA). (1998). *Women's health overview:* www.ama-assn.org/insight/h_focus/wom_hlth/40-60.htm.

Benderly, B. (1997). *In her own right: The Institute of Medicine's guide to women's health issues.* Washington, DC: National Academy Press.

Bennett, M. (1987). Afro-American women, poverty and mental health: a social essay. *Women and Health Care, 12,* 213–228.

Biegel, D., Sales, E., & Schulz, R. (1991). *Family caregiving in chronic illness.* Thousand Oaks, CA: Sage Publications.

Center for Disease Control and Prevention (CDC). (1999, September 11). *Monthly Vital Statistics Report, 46, 1*(2), 2: www.cdc.gov/nchsww/datamu46_l52.pdf.

Deevey S., & Wall. L. (1992). How do lesbian women develop serenity? *Health Care Women International, 13,* 199–208.

Department of Health and Human Services (DHHS). (1991). *Healthy people 2000: National objectives for health promotion and disease prevention.* Washington, DC: U.S. Government Printing Office.

Division for the Advancement of Women. (1995, September). *The United Nations fourth world conference on women*: www.undp.org/fwcw//daw1.htm.

Fogel, C., & Woods, N. (1995). *Women's health care: A comprehensive handbook*. Thousand Oaks, CA: Sage Publications.

Garner, C. (1991). Midlife women's health. *NAACOG Clinical Issues, 2*, 473–481.

Giger, J., & Davidhizar, R. (1995). *Transcultural nursing: Assessment and intervention*. St Louis: Mosby.

Gilliard, D. K., & Beck, A. J. (1994, June). *Prisoners in 1993: Bureau of Justice statistics*. Washington, DC: U.S. Department of Justice.

Golub, S., & Freedman, R. (1985). *Health needs of women as they age*. New York: Haworth Press.

Hogan, S. (1990). Care for the caregiver: social policies to ease their burden. *Journal of Gerontological Nursing, 16*(5), 12–17.

IGC. www.igc.apc.org/justice/prisons/women/women-in-prison.html.

Lawton, M., Rajagopal, D., Brody, E., & Kleban, M. (1992). The dynamic of caregiving for a demented elder among black and white families. *Journal of Gerontology, 47*(4), S516–S164.

Leading causes of mortality and morbidity and contributing behaviors in the United States.(1997). In *United States adolescent health summary*: www.cdc.gov/nccdphp/dash/ahsumm/ussumm.htm.

Lipson. J., Dibble, S., & Minarik, P. (1996). *Culture & nursing care: A pocket guide*. San Francisco: UCSF Nursing Press.

Mark, D., Shaw, L., & DeLong, E. (1994). Absence of sex bias in the referral of patients for cardiac catheterization. *New England Journal of Medicine, 330*, 1101–1106.

McGinn, K. A., & Haylock, P. J. (1993). *Women's cancers*. Alameda, CA: Hunter House.

National Center for Health Statistics. (1993). *Health promotion and disease prevention: United States, 1990* (Series 10, No. 163, DHHS Publication No. 1850. Hyattsville, MD: Department of Health and Human Services.

Pasquale, S. A. (1994). Helping patient make informed contraceptive decisions. *Contemporary OB/GYN, 39*(10), 12–22.

Pollard, K, & Tordella, S.(1993). Women making gains among professionals. *Population Today, 21*, 1–2.

Phillips, J., Sexton, M., & Blackman, J. (1996). Demographic overview of women across the life span. In K. Allen & J. Phillips (Eds.), *Women's health across the lifespan*. Philadelphia, J. B, Lippincott.

Purnell, L., & Paulanka, B. (1998). *Transcultural health care: A culturally competent approach*. Philadelphia: F.A. Davis.

Riggs, J. (1991). The family caregiver support act. *Caring, 10*(12), 18–21.

Rosser, S. (1995). *Women's health—missing from U.S. medicine*. Bloomington: Indiana University Press.

Smith, P.A. (1995). Preventive Services. In D. P. Lemcke, J. Pattison, L. A. Marshall, & D. S. Cowley (Eds.), *Primary care of women* (p. 53). Norwalk, CT: Appleton & Lange.

Stevens, P., Tatum, N., & White, J. (1996). Optimal care for lesbian patients. *Patient Care, 30*(5), 121–134.

Taeuber, C. (1991). *Statistical handbook on women in America*. Phoenix: Oryx Press.

U.S. Census Bureau. (1997, June). National Center for Health Statistics: New report document trends in childbearing, reproductive health: www.cdc.gov/nchswww/releases/97facts/97sheets/nsfgfact.htm.

U.S. Census Bureau. (1999, April 29). National Center for Health Statistics: National vital statistics reports: www.cdc.gov/nchswww/data/nug47_18.pdf.

Waldherr, K. (1996). *The book of goddesses*. Hillsboro, OR: Beyond Words Publishing.

Wheeler, S. (September, 2000). Female prisoners in the United States. *Gender Policy Review*. Online: www.igc.org/igc/gateway/wnindex.html.

Williams R., & Thomas, D. (1997). Women's health. In J. Swanson & M. Nies (Eds.), *Community health nursing* (2nd ed.). Philadelphia: W. B. Saunders.

Wuest, J. (1993). Institutionalizing women's oppression: The inherent risk in health policy that fosters community participation. *Health Care Women International, 14*, 407–417.

Zeidenstein, L. (1990). Gynecological and childbearing needs of lesbians. *Journal of Nurse Midwifery, 35*, 10–18.

Chapter 33
Men's Health

A. Serdar Atav, Sharyn Janes,
and Joseph E. Farmer

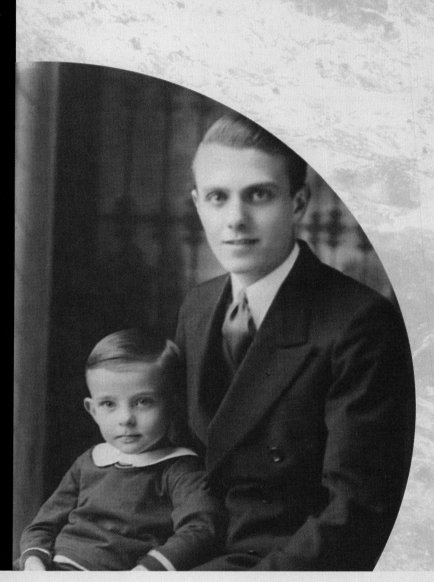

Historically, most research studies have been based on male subjects. In many Western cultures, years of a predominantly male workforce have resulted in health care systems and policies being established by men. Despite this dominance of men in health care systems, women still have longer life expectancies than men.

QUESTIONS TO CONSIDER

After reading this chapter, answer the following questions:

1. What are some of the major factors affecting men's health?
2. How are risk factors for illness or injury different for men compared with women?
3. How does the threat of testicular and prostate cancer affect the lives of young and middle-aged men?
4. What is the nurse's role in the treatment of erectile dysfunction?
5. What are some roles for the community health nurse in the promotion of men's health?

KEY TERMS

Erectile dysfunction	Health status	Socialization process	Viagra
Fertility	Homosexuality	Stress	Violence
Gender differences			

Most nursing students have at least been introduced to, if not completed a course on, women's health or women's issues, but health issues specifically concerning men are a neglected topic in nursing. The role of the community health nurse in improving the health of men is explored in this chapter.

Men's Health

The data on mortality rates by gender are clear—women live longer than men. Men are many times more likely to die of lung cancer, motor vehicle accidents, cirrhosis of the liver, heart disease, and acquired immunodeficiency syndrome (AIDS) than women. Suicide rates are three times higher for men. Possible factors involved in such **gender differences** in health are (1) genetic factors, (2) sociocultural factors, (3) environmental factors, and (4) behavioral factors.

Genetic Factors

Genetic factors related to gender influence a man's physiological and psychological well-being. According to the genetic approach, some gender differences are natural in origin. They are driven from instinctual, hormonal, structural, or neurological characteristics of the male gender (Sabo & Gordon, 1995). For example, gender differences in ischemic heart disease mortality may be a result of the protective effects of female sex hormones and men's tendency to accumulate fat in the upper abdomen (Fackelmann, 1998; Waldron, 1995). Similarly, women with cancer generally have a more optimistic prognosis, probably because of the role of female sex hormones (Adami, Bergstrom, Holmberg, Klareskog, Perrson, & Ponten, 1990). For as yet unknown reasons, girls with medulloblastoma, a common brain tumor in children, have a much better prognosis than boys (Weil, Lamborn, Edwards, & Wara, 1998). It is also argued that higher levels of testosterone contribute to men's predisposition to **violence** (Stillion, 1995). Some of the other physiological differences between men and women include the following (Tanne, 1997):

- *Men's brain cells die faster than women's as they age.*
- *There are structural differences between men and women in the mitral valve, which separates the left atrium of the heart from the left ventricle.*
- *Women's hearts beat more rapidly than men's hearts.*
- *Men have weaker immune systems than women.*

Sociocultural Factors

In many cultures, particularly Western cultures, the male **socialization process** has emphasized traits such as the following (Torres, 1998):

- *Assertiveness*
- *Preoccupation with achievement and success (individualism, status, aggression, toughness, and winning)*
- *Restricted emotionality and affectionate behavior*

- *Concerns about power and control*
- *Fear and bias related to **homosexuality***

As a result, most males tend to conform to these stereotyped gender expectations and behaviors, leading to definite health consequences. Some men may experience more frequent trauma because of their belief that taking physical risks is a sign of masculinity. Boys are socialized into competitive games at an early age and learn to endure physical punishment as part of having fun or as a prerequisite to becoming a man (Stillion, 1995). From Little League on, a boy is told to "act like a man." Hence, to admit to having pain or some other health problem may be seen as a confession of weakness. This male denial factor is pervasive and not related to occupation, age, race, or socioeconomic status (Male Health Center, 1998a). High death rates from coronary heart disease for men in the United States may be due in part to these stereotyped gender expectations, which increase the risk of the disease (Helman, 1994).

The lack of healthy emotional channels for men contributes to higher risks among men for suicide, heart disease, accidents, and violence. The traditional male socialization process has historically emphasized restricted emotionality and affectionate behavior. This traditional male gender role is inconsistent with the provision and receipt of social support, particularly emotional support that includes expressiveness and disclosure. Such characteristics may have adverse health consequences. The lack of expressiveness becomes especially significant in the way men deal with **stress** and depression. Most men tend not to cry and try to keep emotions hidden. They are far less likely to seek psychological counseling than are women. Along with other cultural messages that men need to be strong, powerful, and independent, men are taught not to react to physical, psychological, or spiritual pain. Some men are unwilling to seek health care simply because they fear the risk of appearing "unmanly" (Men's Health Network, 1998).

. . . .

I think we have a national crisis of boys in America. For some boys who are not allowed tears, they will cry with their fists or they will cry with bullets.

Dr. William Pollack,
Psychologist, Harvard Medical School, August 20, 1999

. . . .

The sociocultural differences between men and women must be considered when planning and developing intervention and prevention programs. Strategies that target the general population may not consider the diversity of expectations and behaviors of men. Although some publicly funded programs may attempt to target as many people as possible, programs with more specifically focused segments or populations may be more effective with men. The nurse must consider the vast number of socialization possibilities that exist within male societies. Health interventions directed toward men may be more effective when men are separated from women, divided into age-specific groups, or grouped into a larger audience. For example, instead of a smoking cessation program for all people, with an emphasis on the long-term effects of smoking, a program targeting men ages 15 to 25, with an emphasis on the sex appeal of nonsmokers, may be more effective.

Environmental Factors

Physical and occupational environments affect the **health status** of men. More men are employed than women, and male-dominated occupations such as mining, construction, and farming are often more hazardous. Accidents on the job are a major contributor to higher death rates among men. In addition, men in these types of occupations are more likely to be exposed to carcinogens and other toxins that are associated with higher rates of pneumoconiosis (black lung), asbestosis, leukemia, and cancer of the bladder. Men's greater exposure to occupational hazards account for about 5% to 10% of the gender difference in mortality (Waldron, 1995).

The high number of men in high-risk employment settings may be advantageous to community health nurses, who can use these environments to introduce men to health care. Prevention and screening programs in the workplace can be effective interventions for men who would not seek health care in other settings.

Behavioral Factors

Unlike genetic factors, behaviors such as diet, tobacco use, alcohol consumption, illicit drug use, lack of physical exercise, physical and sexual risk taking, and suicide and violence are controllable and subject to human influence and intervention. Individuals can make wiser choices such as always wearing their seatbelts; exercising and eating right; not using tobacco, drugs, or alcohol, or at least not driving while under the influence of alcohol or drugs; not bungee jumping; or not committing acts of violence against themselves or others. Partly as a result of the cultural expectations of society and the gender socialization process, men's behavior is consistently less healthy than that of women. As a result, behavior is the cause of the largest differences in mortality between men and women (Stillion, 1995).

Data in the United States indicate that men's diets have had higher ratios of saturated to polyunsaturated fat, which contribute to higher ischemic heart disease mortality among men. More males than females smoke cigarettes and drink heavily. Men's smoking habits account for as much as 90% of gender differences in cancer mortality and roughly one-third of gender differences in ischemic heart disease mortality. Similarly, men's drinking contributes to higher mortality in liver disease, accidents, suicide, and homicide (Waldron, 1995).

Diet

Obesity and consumption of fatty foods increase the risk of cardiovascular disease, which is a major killer for men. Men consume a large amount of fatty foods and are less likely than women to change their eating habits, even though more than 33% of men meet the definition of obesity (a body mass index [BMI] of 27.8 kg/m^2). Researchers suggest that low-fat diet programs for men should target work site and peer-group organizations and place emphasis on adapting usual recipes (Coakley, Rimm, Colditz, Kawachi, & Willett, 1998; Nguyen, Otis, & Potvin, 1996).

Tobacco

Gender differences in smoking prevalence have been decreasing for decades, but still more males than females smoke cigarettes. In 1994, 27.8% of males were smokers, compared with 23.3%

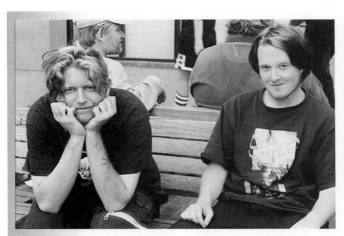

Attitudes about health change during adolescence, and teen males may have needs that go unmet.

CIGARETTE SMOKING IN ADULTS BY EDUCATION AND GENDER, 1994

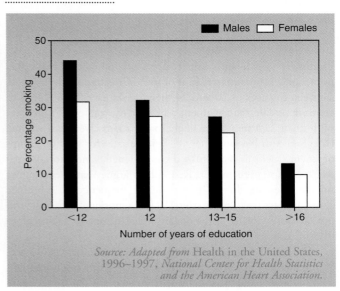

Source: Adapted from Health in the United States, 1996–1997, National Center for Health Statistics and the American Heart Association.

of females (American Heart Association, 1998). Smoking is positively correlated with men's higher mortality from bronchitis, emphysema, and asthma.

Men, especially rural men, are more likely to use smokeless (chewing) tobacco. Despite the general declining trends in the use of cigarettes, there has not been a decline in the use of smokeless tobacco. Smokeless tobacco use is associated with higher risks of cardiovascular disease and cancers of the oral cavity, as well as gum recession and nicotine addiction. Heavy marketing efforts by tobacco companies toward rural men might explain the slight increase in the use of smokeless tobacco (Nelson, Tomar, Mowery, & Siegel, 1996).

Alcohol

Alcohol abuse is well known for its devastating effects on physical and emotional health. Not including alcohol-related motor vehicle accidents, there were 20,000 alcohol-related deaths in 1995, and most of the victims were men. More men (68%) drink than women (55%), and men are five times more likely to drink heavily. Higher numbers of male drinkers contribute to males' higher mortality, related to chronic liver disease, cirrhosis of the liver, accidents, and homicide. In addition, male drivers have substantially higher risk of fatal motor vehicle accidents because they are more likely to have high blood alcohol levels (Waldron, 1995).

Alcohol use must be taken into consideration in developing strategies to prevent the transmission of sexually transmitted diseases (STDs), including human immunodeficiency virus (HIV), because alcohol consumption is related to risky sexual behavior. A number of studies have suggested that people who drink more heavily are more likely to have multiple partners, and among young men, consistent use of condoms decreases at higher levels of alcohol use (Graves, 1995). It is estimated that two-thirds of all alcoholics are men; more than 80% of those who have serious drug addictions are men; more than 80% of those who die of drug abuse are men; and 90% of those arrested for alcohol or drug abuse are men.

Suicide and Violence

Deaths by suicide and violence are a predominantly male phenomenon. Approximately four of five deaths by suicide are men. Between the ages of 20 and 24 men are six times more likely to commit suicide than women; and over the age of 85, men are more than 11 times more likely to kill themselves than women (Men's Health Network, 1998). Suicide rates for specific groups of men, such as veterans, divorced men, and homosexual teenagers, are even higher. Researchers argue that men's higher suicide rates are due to men's greater frequency of substance abuse, subjection to more stress, lack of emotional channels, and use of more violent, immediately lethal means of taking their lives in comparison with women.

The world of men is much more violent than that of women. White men are three times more likely to die in a homicide than white women; and African American men are five times more

likely to die in a homicide than black women (Stillion, 1995). The persons at greatest risk for violence victimization, as well as becoming the perpetrators of violence, are young males who are members of underrepresented ethnic groups and live in poor urban communities. In 1991, nearly half of all homicide victims were males 15 to 34 years of age. These young men risk injury to themselves, disrupted personal lives, damaging criminal records, extended imprisonment, and in some cases, capital punishment (DHHS, 1995a).

Much of the violent actions of men are directed at women. In the United States female murder victims are most often killed by their husbands, boyfriends, other male family members, or close male friends (Gerlock, 1997). Violence against women will not cease until greater emphasis is put on prevention and treatment programs for the men who perform the violent acts. The nursing literature that addresses the issue of working with men who batter women and children is almost nonexistent, yet nurses who work in hospitals and community settings deal with the results of domestic violence every day. Because nurses are on the front line, they are in the best position to intervene in ways that are sensitive to both the perpetrators and the victims of family violence. Nurses working in settings such as schools, churches, and work sites can conduct education programs to promote awareness of the potential for family violence (Rynerson & Fishel, 1998).

Healthy People 2010

The purpose of *Healthy People 2010* is to improve the health of Americans with specific objectives in many health-related areas. Although men are not specifically listed as a targeted group, several objectives do focus on either racial or ethnic groups of men. Selected objectives are listed in the following *Healthy People 2010* box.

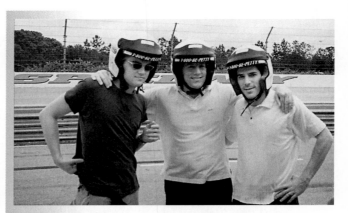

Young males are likely to be involved in risk-taking behavior. However, as role model Leonardo DiCaprio and friends demonstrate, risk can be decreased through the use of protective gear.

HEALTHY PEOPLE 2010

OBJECTIVES RELATED TO MEN'S HEALTH

Cancer

3.2 Reduce the lung cancer death rate.

3.7 Reduce the prostate cancer death rate.

3.10 Increase the proportion of physicians and dentists who counsel their at-risk patients about tobacco use cessation, physical activity, and cancer screening.

Family Planning

9.6 Increase male involvement in pregnancy prevention and family planning efforts.

Heart Disease and Stroke

Heart Disease

12.1 Reduce coronary heart disease deaths.

Stroke

12.7 Reduce stroke deaths.

Blood Pressure

12.8 Reduce the proportion of adults with high blood pressure.

HIV/AIDS

13.2 Reduce the number of new AIDS cases among adolescents and adult men who have sex with men.

13.3 Reduce the number of new AIDS cases among females and males who inject drugs.

13.4 Reduce the number of new AIDS cases among adolescent and adult men who have sex with men and inject drugs.

Injury and Violence Prevention

Unintentional Injury Prevention

15.15 Reduce deaths caused by motor vehicle crashes.

15.21 Increase the proportion of motorcyclists using helmets.

15.22 Increase use of helmets by bicyclists.

Violence and Abuse Prevention

15.32 Reduce homicides.

15.33 Reduce physical fighting among adolescents.

15.34 Reduce weapon carrying by adolescents on school property.

Mental Health and Mental Disorders

Mental Health Status Improvement

18.1 Reduce the suicide rate.

Occupational Safety and Health

20.1 Reduce deaths from work-related injuries.

Substance Abuse

Adverse Consequences of Substance Use and Abuse

26.1 Reduce deaths and injuries caused by alcohol- and drug-related motor vehicle crashes.

26.2 Reduce drug-induced deaths.

Substance Use and Abuse

26.12 Reduce average annual alcohol consumption.

26.13 Reduce steroid use among adolescents.

Tobacco Use

Tobacco Use in Population Groups

27.1 Reduce tobacco use by adults.

27.2 Reduce tobacco use by adolescents.

Source: DHHS, 2000.

Health Care System Utilization

Patterns of health care utilization by men are cited as an important contributor to the inferior health status of men. One-third of American men do not have a checkup every year. Nine million men have not seen a doctor in 5 years (Male Health Center, 1998a). Men visit doctors 25% less often than women. At the same time, men account for 66% of the clients admitted to emergency rooms (Men's Health Network, 1998). Men tend to have fewer contacts with the health care system, perhaps as a result of psychological and sociological factors such as a reluctance to admit that they need assistance. This situation is exacerbated by the fact that the American health care system tends to focus on health from an illness perspective, with relatively little attention paid to prevention. As a result, unlike women who have annual gynecological examinations that include screening for other conditions, men are less likely to enter the health care system for a physical examination on a routine basis. Moreover, although men come in contact with many health care professionals in a wide variety of settings, they have no specialist to whom they can go for their specific care needs. Men have to be to attended by generalists, such as family practitioners, or by other specialists such as urologists who also see women.

Strategies to improve men's utilization of preventive health care must target all ages. Men must establish a committed relationship with preventive health care as early as possible. For men to use preventive health care, programs that present health prevention as masculine and strengthening must be developed and implemented. The required school physical before participation in extracurricular activities may be used in the resocialization of men for the active and lifelong usage of preventive health care.

Ambulatory Care

Of the 860.9 million ambulatory care visits made to physician offices, hospital outpatient departments, and hospital emergency department in 1995, 353.8 million (41.1%) were made by men. This means that men made 153.3 million fewer trips to ambulatory care settings than women. Men have significantly lower

ANNUAL RATE OF AMBULATORY CARE VISITS BY CLIENT'S AGE AND GENDER

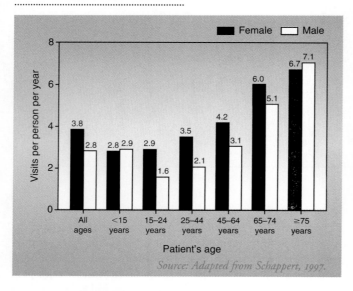

Source: Adapted from Schappert, 1997.

rates of visits to physician offices and hospital outpatient departments than women, but the visit rates to hospital emergency departments do not differ by sex. Overall, men made 2.8 visits to ambulatory care settings per person and women made 3.8 visits (Schappert, 1997). This difference is even greater for ages 15 to 24 and 25 to 44.

By age 75, men have had approximately 395 contacts with physicians, whereas women have had about 517 contacts. This discrepancy persists even when the contribution of pregnancy and birth control–related issues is not counted in women's contacts. The patterns in physician contacts indicate that, for all ages, the difference between men and women has been increasing. In 1989, physician contacts were 4.8 per person for men and 5.9 per person for women. By 1992, physician contacts were 5.1 for men and 6.6 for women. In 3 years, the difference in contacts went up by 0.5 visits. Men do not go to the doctor, partly because of fear, denial, embarrassment, and threatened masculinity (Male Health Center, 1998a). Although the total number of physician contacts is lower for men, men are seen more frequently than women for chronic diseases, such as heart and lung disease, which are more prevalent among men.

Hospital Care

Hospitalization rates and length of stays in hospitals vary by sex. Hospital discharge rates, the numbers used to determine usage, from short-stay hospitals are higher for women (138 per 1,000 women) than for men (96 per 1,000). However, in 1995, men had more days of hospital care (5.8 days on the average per person) than women (5 days) (Graves & Owings, 1997). When gynecological disorders in women and reproductive disorders in men are excluded, rates of hospitalization for men are about the same as for women. The lower rate of discharge and longer hospital stays may be due to the fact that when men are hospitalized their conditions are more severe.

Preventive Care

Men and women differ in their ability to seek preventive care for the early diagnosis of health care problems. Unlike women, who seek routine reproductive health screening, most men do not have routine checkups that would detect health problems at an early stage. Men are more likely to have examinations at the insistence of their employers, and they do not perceive that they need a regular source of care. More often than women, men perceive their health as very good or excellent and therefore may not think that they need to be involved in health promotion activities (Clark, 1999). Women are more likely than men to exhibit stronger health promotion behaviors in terms of blood pressure checks, dental flossing, diet, smoking, drinking, physical activity, weight, and hours of sleep. Men tend to view exercise as sufficient to compensate for unhealthy behaviors such as fatty diets. As a result, men are at greater risk for several of the top killers such as heart disease, cancer, suicide, accidents, and violence. Because most of these killers are preventable, changes in eating habits, workplace environments, and educational strategies are needed to improve preventive care for men.

Specific Male Health Issues

Prostate Cancer

The American Cancer Society lists prostate cancer as the second leading cause of cancer death in American men after lung cancer (Brock, 1997; Male Health Center, 1998b). Prostate cancer is most common in men older than 40, and the risk increases with each decade thereafter (Brock, 1997). Most often, prostate cancer is asymptomatic until the disease has progressed. Symptoms that may indicate prostate disease include the following (Male Health Center, 1998b):

- *Difficulty or pain with urination*
- *Painful ejaculation*
- *Blood in urine or semen*

Although prostate cancer is the second leading cause of cancer deaths in American men, how many prostate cancer prevention and awareness campaigns have you seen? Can the same be said for breast cancer? Consider the financial appropriations and expenditures for cancer in the United States detailed in Table 33-1.

Information about the necessity of digital rectal examinations beginning at age 40 for all men, with possible earlier intervention for those with signs and symptoms of problems or a positive family history, must be included and incorporated into health fairs and promotions. Information related to prostate-specific antigen (PSA) blood testing that is used in conjunction with the digital rectal examination should also be provided. In 1986, the U.S. Food and Drug Administration approved the PSA test for prostate cancer screening. Many physicians believe that the subsequent fall in prostate cancer mortality rates can be

FYI

Several high-profile men came forward in the 1990s to talk about their experiences with prostate cancer in an effort to remove the embarrassment surrounding the disease. As a result of the openness of men like former U.S. Senator and presidential candidate Bob Dole, professional golfer Arnold Palmer, and retired General H. Norman Schwarzkopf, many books and journal articles appeared and support groups surfaced all over the country.

attributed to early diagnosis with PSA testing (Feuer & Merrill, 1999). The importance of the procedure and information regarding signs, symptoms, and the screening process should be emphasized in promotions. Nurses should also include written information for distribution because some men are ill at ease discussing the procedure and testing in public.

The community health nurse can also organize targeted prostate-specific screenings, during which the men actually have the digital rectal examination and PSA blood tests. In a study that explored the relationship between attitudes toward digital rectal examinations and prostate screening among African American men, the results revealed that fear of the procedure did not prevent men from participating in the screening (Gelfand, Parzuchowski, Cort, & Powell, 1995).

Testicular Cancer

Testicular cancer accounts for only 1% of all cancers in men (National Cancer Institute, 1998; Walbrecker, 1995). However, testicular cancer is the most common form of cancer in men between the ages of 20 and 34 (Brock, Fox, Gosling, Haney, Kneebone, Nagy, & Qualitza, 1993; Clore, 1993; DHHS, 1995b; National Cancer Institute, 1998; Peate, 1997; Rosella, 1994; Walbrecker,

TABLE 33-1	**BREAST VERSUS PROSTATE CANCER EXPENDITURES**		
		BREAST	**PROSTATE**
National Cancer Institute research		$1.8 billion	$376 million
Department of Defense research		$455 million	$20 million
U.S. government:			
Per person diagnosed		$3,000	$250
Per death		$12,000	$2,000
Jaffe, 1997.			

1995). It is the second most common cancer for men between the ages of 35 and 39 and the third most common for men between the ages of 15 and 19 (National Cancer Institute, 1998). This type of cancer is 4.5 times more common among Caucasian men than African American men (DHHS, 1995b; National Cancer Institute, 1998), with rates for Hispanics/Latinos, Native Americans, and Asians falling somewhere in between (National Cancer Institute, 1998).

•••••••••••••••••••••••••••••••

I'm prouder of being a cancer survivor than I am of winning the Tour de France. If I never had cancer, I never would have won the Tour de France. I'm convinced of that. I wouldn't want to do it all over again, but I wouldn't change a thing.

Lance Armstrong,
winner of the Tour de France (21-day, 2287-mile bicycle race) and testicular cancer survivor (Montville, 1999)

•••••••••••••••••••••••••••••••

Epidemiological data show an increase in the incidence of testicular cancer over the past 20 years (Clore, 1993; Koshti-Richman, 1996). As recent as the early 1980s, testicular cancer was fatal (Brock et al., 1993) for 8 of 10 clients (Walbrecker, 1995). But today, because of advances in chemotherapy and improved surgical techniques (Brakey, 1994; Brock et al., 1993), testicular cancer is one of the most curable forms of cancer (Rosella, 1994). Testicular cancer has a nearly 100% cure rate with early detection and treatment (Brakey, 1994; Clore, 1993; Peate, 1997; Rosella, 1994; Walbrecker, 1995). This optimistic prognosis with early intervention makes testicular self-examination (TSE) a critical component of health teaching for young men (American Family Physician, 1999; Rosella, 1994; Walbrecker, 1995), especially because most cases of testicular cancer are found by the clients themselves (National Cancer Institute, 1998). Boys should begin TSE around age 13 and make it a lifelong practice because, although testicular cancer is most likely to occur before the age of 40, it can occur at any age. In fact, the incidence rises again after the age of 70 (Brakey, 1994).

The characteristics that put men at higher risk for testicular cancer include Caucasian race, young age, high socioeconomic status, or family history, as well as having a mother who took estrogen during her pregnancy (Brakey, 1994; Kinkade, 1999). Males with undescended testicles or late descending testicles (after age 6) have a 3 to 17 times higher than average risk for developing testicular cancer (National Cancer Institute, 1998; Walbrecker, 1995). Despite this information, the health education literature suggests that most of the men who are most susceptible to testicular cancer are unaware of the signs and symptoms of the disease and how to detect them (Rosella, 1994). Research has indicated that although information has been readily available to young women regarding breast self-examination (BSE) and the importance of regular Pap smears, the information related to TSE has not been as widely communicated (Turner, 1995; Walker, 1993).

Nurses are in the best position to provide young men with the information to learn the self-examination techniques needed for early detection and cure (Peate, 1997; Walbrecker, 1995). TSE education and screening programs can be set up in high schools and presented simultaneously with BSE and screening programs. Models can be used for practicing self-examination with lifelike lumps and abnormalities to teach young men what they should be looking for. Testicular examination and TSE education should be part of every routine physical examination for adolescent and young adult males. Instructions for self-examination of the testicles are given in Box 33-1.

The only way a positive diagnosis of testicular cancer can be made is through surgical removal (orchiectomy) of the affected testicle for direct examination (Henkel, 1996; Walbrecker, 1995). Because testicular cancer occurs most often in men of reproductive age, **fertility** is a major concern. Although sperm count may be lowered, a unilateral orchiectomy usually does not affect sexual function or fertility (Brakey, 1994; Henkel, 1996; Walbrecker, 1995). However, abnormalities in the remaining

---

BOX 33-1 TESTICULAR SELF-EXAMINATION

- Self-examination should be done once a month after a warm bath or shower because heat relaxes the scrotum and loosens the skin, making the testes easier to examine.

- Visually inspect the scrotum for any swelling or changes in color.

- Examine each testicle with both hands by placing the index and middle fingers under the testicle with the thumbs placed on top. Roll the testicle gently between the fingers and thumbs, feeling for any changes such as lumps, swelling, or painful spots.

- The first sign of testicular cancer is usually a hard, painless lump about the size of a pea. However, if there are any kinds of changes or abnormalities, immediately notify your health care provider, because only he or she can make a positive diagnosis.

Sources: Adapted from American Family Physician, 1999; Henkel, 1996; & Walbrecker, 1995.

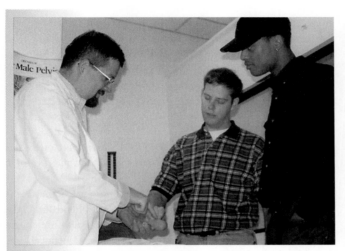

Chapter author, Joseph Farmer, uses a model to teach young men how to do a testicular self-examination.

testicle or the effects of radiation and chemotherapy may have adverse effects on sexual function and fertility (Brakey, 1994), although studies have shown that many men recover fertility within 2 to 3 years after chemotherapy (Henkel, 1996).

A CONVERSATION WITH . . .

I love my job. I absolutely love what I do. Cancer controls your life, and I didn't want cancer to take me off the ice.

Shock and fear are the first two things that you feel. Then you feel a feeling of anxious desperation. And then when the diagnosis was complete, and I heard there was a treatment, it was non-stop humor. My goal is to find a way to laugh every day.

For people with testicular cancer that are going through their treatments and challenges, feel fortunate that there is a treatment. Understand that it will be a hard episode in your life. Understand that the treatment will try to defeat you and damage your spirit. But you can fight back and win.

—Scott Hamilton,
Olympic Figure Skating Champion
and Testicular Cancer Survivor
Source: A chat with Scott Hamilton
(excerpts from a chat on ABC News:
http://vix.com/menmag/tcschotth.htm.)

Erectile Dysfunction (Impotence)

Many sexual topics are now discussed openly, but **erectile dysfunction** is still a subject that causes fear and anxiety for many men and women (Male Health Center, 1998c). Although a significant amount of scientific data is available about erectile dysfunction (also called *impotence*), large segments of the public, including health care professionals, are still uninformed, or even worse, misinformed. A lack of accurate information, as well as reluctance on the part of many health care providers to deal openly with sexual issues, has left many clients without a source of help for their sexual concerns. Improving both public and professional knowledge and attaining a comfort level in talking about erectile dysfunction will provide both men and their sexual partners with an avenue for obtaining needed information and effective treatment (NIH, 1992).

What Is Erectile Dysfunction?

Erectile dysfunction is the inability to achieve or maintain a penile erection sufficient for sexual intercourse. About 15 million American men suffer from erectile dysfunction, and the incidence increases with age. Approximately 5% of men experience erectile dysfunction by the age of 40, increasing to between 15% and 25% by the age of 65 (National Kidney and Urologic Disease Information Clearinghouse, 1998). Erectile dysfunction is often assumed to be a normal part of the aging process, but that assumption is incorrect (Male Health Center, 1998d; National Kidney and Urologic Diseases Clearinghouse, 1998; NIH, 1992). In fact, sex researchers Masters and Johnson discovered that although sexual activity slows down with advancing age, it does not end. Several reports indicate that most men and women between the ages of 50 and 60 are still interested in remaining sexually active (Male Health Center, 1998c, 1998d).

Causes

Most cases of erectile dysfunction have a physical cause such as disease, injury, or drug side effects. Diabetes mellitus, kidney disease, multiple sclerosis, atherosclerosis, chronic alcoholism, hypertension, and vascular disease account for approximately 70% of all cases of erectile dysfunction. Of men with diabetes mellitus, 35% to 50% experience erectile dysfunction (National Kidney and Urologic Diseases Information Clearinghouse, 1998; NIH, 1992). Various kinds of surgeries are also associated with increased incidence of erectile dysfunction. The most common are surgeries that can cause injury to nerves and arteries near the penis. These include surgeries for prostate, colon, rectal, and bladder cancers. Vascular surgery can also be high risk. Many common medications list erectile dysfunction as a side effect, including drugs used to treat hypertension, antihistamines, antidepressants, sedatives, tranquilizers, appetite suppressants, and pain medications (Male Health Center, 1998c; National Kidney and Urologic Disease Information Clearinghouse, 1998; NIH, 1992). Smoking has also been shown to have an adverse effect on

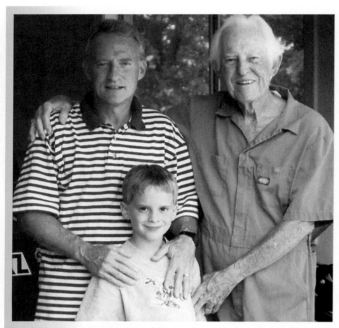

Men with at least two close relatives with prostate cancer have a very high risk of developing the disease before the age of 70. Men with a family history of prostate cancer should have PSA screening and prostate examinations between the ages of 50 and 70.

erectile function by increasing the effects of other risk factors such as vascular disease or hypertension. Vasectomy, however, has not been associated with increased risk for erectile dysfunction (NIH, 1992).

In 10% to 20% of cases of erectile dysfunction the cause is deemed to be psychological. Factors such as stress, anxiety, guilt, depression, low self-esteem, and fear of sexual failure can cause erectile dysfunction without the presence of any physical problems or can be secondary reactions to underlying physical causes (National Kidney and Urologic Disease Information Clearinghouse, 1998; NIH, 1992). Important facts that should be emphasized when counseling a man and his sexual partner about erectile dysfunction include the following (Male Health Center, 1998c):

- *Most men experience erectile dysfunction related to stress or alcohol at some time in their lives.*

- *Past sexual practices, including masturbation, do not cause erectile dysfunction.*

- *Physical disorders can directly affect sexual functioning.*

- *An occasional problem with erectile dysfunction does not mean a chronic problem will develop.*

- *A man can sabotage his ability to have an erection by worrying about it.*

Treatment

Treatment varies according to the severity and cause of the dysfunction. Health care providers start with the least invasive treatment and progress to more invasive treatments until erectile dysfunction is corrected. Reducing the dosage or eliminating drugs that may be causing erectile dysfunction is the first step. Psychotherapy and behavior modifications are next. Vacuum devices, oral drugs, drugs injected into the urethra, and finally surgically implanted penile devices or vascular surgery are offered as treatment if the problem persists (National Kidney and Urologic Disease Information Clearinghouse, 1998; NIH, 1992).

In 1998, a new "wonder drug" called *sildenafil citrate* (commonly known as **Viagra**) was approved by the U.S. Food and Drug Administration. Viagra is taken 1 hour before sexual intercourse and works by boosting the effects of nitric oxide, a chemical produced by the body to relax smooth muscle in the penis and allow increased blood flow during sexual stimulation. This drug does not trigger automatic erection as other drugs used to treat erectile dysfunction do, but rather just allows the man to respond to sexual stimulation (National Kidney and Urologic Disease Information Clearinghouse, 1998). The drug is very successful in treating many forms of erectile dysfunction, although some fear the drug may be overused by middle-aged and older men who may not actually suffer from erectile dysfunction but just want to "boost" their sex lives.

Role of the Community Health Nurse

The most important things the community health nurse can do for men with erectile dysfunction are to provide accurate and easily understandable information and to encourage the man and his sex partner to talk openly and comfortably about the problem. Including the man's sex partner in the discussion acknowledges his or her importance in the relationship. The partner may also have questions, doubts, and insecurities that need to be addressed. Many persons whose partners are impotent blame themselves for the problem. The partner may also feel hurt and angry because the male has withdrawn physically and emotionally. Understanding that he or she is not to blame can go a long way in enabling the partner to support the diagnosis and treatment (Male Health Center, 1998c). It is important for the nurse to be sensitive to the needs of clients whose values or sexual orientation may be different from the nurse. Not all partners of male clients will be their wives. In fact, some of the sex partners of male clients may also be male. Whatever the relationship of the partners, all couples should be treated with dignity and respect.

Cardiovascular Disease

Cardiovascular disease is the single greatest cause of death in men. Approximately 1 in 3 male deaths is related to cardiovascular disease. Similarly, more than one-third of men dying between the ages of 45 and 65 die of a heart attack. Cardiovascular disease is caused by the accumulation of fatty deposits within the artery wall that causes stiffness and reduced blood flow. When the brain interprets reduced blood flow as low blood pressure, it sends a signal to the heart to compensate. The heart works faster with less rest and increases the pressure on each contraction. Normal blood pressures for men range from 120/70 to 150/80 depending on age. With severe hardening of the arteries, blood pressure may increase to 200/100 mm Hg (Men's Health Network, 1998). Although there are many explanations for higher cardiovascular disease rates among men than women, research points to two major factors:

1. *Men's diets have higher ratios of saturated to polyunsaturated fat, which contributes to cardiovascular disease.*

2. *Men's sociocultural environments lead to higher levels of stress, which contributes to cardiovascular disease.*

Cardiovascular disease and hypertension can often be prevented by changes in behavior, including stopping smoking, increasing activity, and improving diet. Community health nurses can design educational programs that target men to promote behavior changes that reduce the risk of cardiovascular disease. These recommendations may include the following:

* *Losing weight*
* *Reducing salt intake*
* *Quitting smoking*
* *Eating foods rich in natural sources of fiber and antioxidant vitamins*
* *Exercising*
* *Relaxing*

RESEARCH BRIEF

Johnson, J. V., Stewart, W., Hall, E. H., Fredlund, P., & Theorell, T. (1996). Long-term psychosocial work environment and cardiovascular mortality among Swedish men. American Journal of Public Health, 86, 324–331.

A sample of 12,517 Swedish men were studied over 14 years to examine the effect of cumulative exposure to work organization (in terms of psychological demands, work control, and social support) on cardiovascular disease mortality. The study identified 521 deaths from cardiovascular disease. Using a nested case-control design, work environment scores were assigned to cases and controls by linking lifetime job histories with a job exposure matrix. Cardiovascular mortality risk in relation to work exposure after adjustment for age, year last employed, smoking, exercise, education, social class, nationality, and physical job demands was analyzed. The results of the study indicated that workers who had combined work exposure to low control and low support had higher risks for cardiovascular disease mortality.

In addition, consumption of moderate amounts of alcohol and sexual activity are associated with reduced risks of cardiovascular disease (Men's Health Network, 1998).

Selected At-Risk Populations
Men with HIV/AIDS

According to the Centers for Disease Control and Prevention (CDC, 1998a), by 1994 AIDS had become a leading cause of death in the United States for men between the ages of 25 and 44. With the introduction of new medications in recent years, AIDS-related death rates have steadily declined, but the incidence of new HIV cases continues to rise (CDC, 1998b). AIDS has historically been viewed in the United States as a disease targeting a specific population—homosexual men. Although the initial cases in the United States, Canada, Australia, and Western Europe were found among this population, this was not the case for the rest of the world. After two decades of the pandemic, many still view HIV/AIDS as something that will not affect them. As a result of this apathy, the safer sexual practices adopted in the homosexual communities have not been applied as readily in heterosexual communities. High-risk behaviors, such as alcohol and drug use and unprotected sex with numerous partners, continue to put heterosexual men at risk. Heterosexual transmission rates continue to escalate, especially in the African American and Hispanic communities, where 41% of all new reported cases are found (CDC, 1997).

The introduction of new medications has reduced the number of AIDS-related deaths, which can be interpreted to mean persons with HIV are living longer. What does this mean to younger men? An entire generation of sexually active men has never known of a world without HIV or AIDS. To some, this may be interpreted as, "Why bother to protect myself, because I can always take the medications." Some are applying safer sexual practices haphazardly, thus allowing the introduction of drug-resistant strains of HIV into their bodies. To others, especially an alarming number of young homosexual men, the principle of "I'd rather die young and beautiful" applies. Intervention and prevention programs must address these issues and concerns. The community health nurse's best option would include the education of young men who would act as role models for their peers.

What does the increase in HIV cases within the African American and Hispanic communities mean to the community health nurse? Intervention and prevention programs need to specifically target these communities. The church is an institution generally accepted as having a powerful influence within both of these communities. By securing the commitment from religious leaders and their congregations, the community health nurse can create positive change from within the system. Developing role models and implementing prevention programs that utilize members of the community results in much more effective outcomes.

For example, the community health nurse working within a community often develops a relationship with community

You are a nurse working in a community clinic. One of your clients is Rick Fernandez, a 34-year-old married man who complains about fever and swollen glands. Fearing the possibility of HIV, you ask Rick the typical textbook questions to assess his HIV risk behaviors: You ask if he uses intravenous drugs, if he has had any blood transfusions, if he has sex with men, and if he is homosexual. He responds with a no to all questions. Based on his replies, you do not pursue HIV testing. When he comes back a few months later with complaints of recurrent skin lesions, you again ask about his HIV risk behaviors and receive the same answers as before. Rick insists that he is a happily married man in a monogamous relationship and does not use any sort of drugs. Rick seems offended by your questions. You approach the physician and ask if he has considered testing Rick for HIV. The physician has assessed the risk behaviors and

concluded that Rick does not have any of the risk factors associated with HIV. When Rick returns to the clinic for a third visit, you are more assertive and convince Rick to have an HIV test. The test comes back positive. Rick reveals to the HIV counselor that he had been imprisoned a while back and that his only potential exposure to HIV might have been through another inmate who raped him.

1. What is your reaction to Rick's situation?
2. Do you feel that your personal beliefs and values influenced your reaction?
3. Why do you think Rick did not disclose the key information earlier?
4. What could you have done to obtain the accurate information?
5. What specific questions could you have asked Rick to obtain this information?

members. Once a trusting relationship has been established, the nurse can approach some of the unofficial leaders within the community to enlist their support and discuss strategies and objectives to decrease the epidemic of infection affecting the population. This needs to be done in a nonjudgmental manner, in which the nurse details the problems and possible solutions without passing blame or creating fear. By enlisting the members' support in the initial stages, the nurse can formulate plans and develop goals that are perceived as important to the community, thus securing support for the intervention.

Homosexual Men and Families

The special needs of homosexual men include more than just HIV/AIDS education. Homosexual men and their families exist in virtually every community, regardless of how restrictive or liberal the community proclaims to be. However, societal stigmatization of homosexuality forces many to remain "in the closet" (Giger & Davidhizar, 1995). Homosexual myths and stereotypes abound, particularly in cultures that value male dominance or masculinity. Homosexual men and their sexual practices run the entire spectrum, just as in the heterosexual community. Also, homosexual men may be married or have children, live alone or with a partner. Individuals define who makes up their family group, not nurses or institutions.

The community health nurse's role in interactions with any group of men is inclusion instead of exclusion. Nurses should ask questions in such a manner that the man does not feel obligated to give an answer he believes the nurse expects. When using such

items as risk assessments, questions should be phrased in a general manner. For example, the nurse should ask about "the number of sexual partners" instead of "the number of women." Nurses should maintain a nonjudgmental tone and manner throughout all interactions. Just as in any interaction, including the entire family whenever possible is recommended. By developing a trusting and honest relationship, the nurse can be instrumental in generating assistance and implementing change of unsafe or risky behaviors.

Community Health Nursing Roles

The community health nurse assumes a wide range of duties and responsibilities while providing health care to men. A typical week could include hundreds of miles traveled, diverse teaching methods and strategies, and numerous new encounters. Community health nursing roles may include client advocate, educator, and facilitator.

Client Advocate

As a client advocate, the role of the community health nurse includes interfacing with health care providers and health care agencies to support the best care for the client. For instance, a nurse realizes that a recently diagnosed HIV-positive man has been prescribed AZT alone, rather than the more effective cocktail combination medications. A proper assessment must be made to determine whether alternative medications could have been prescribed. With the permission of the client, the nurse can contact the appropriate health care provider and discuss the client's options with a nonthreatening and nonjudgmental stance to allow for future interactions. Any new information must be shared with the client.

Educator

The role of a health educator for men can often be challenging. Education can occur in any setting from the stockyards to the corporate boardroom. Safety issues, violence, diet, and physical exercise are examples of topics that may be addressed. The community health nurse must customize education efforts to the specific needs of the clients. The first step involves a correct assessment of the educational needs of the individuals. The nurse determines the level of the learners to ensure that the level of the educational program is neither too low nor too high for the specific group. Providing educational programs for men in their own environments requires versatility and flexibility.

Facilitator

The community health nurse as facilitator brings various people and groups together to talk about issues and needs. The most significant facilitator role involves helping people and groups of different views to reach a compromise so that they can find a common ground to solve problems and bring about positive changes to alleviate a specific community health problem. For instance, a community health nurse, as the facilitator, may initiate positive change through programs with specific targeted groups such as adolescent boys. This can be accomplished by teaching safer sexual practices to prevent STDs and teenage pregnancies by bringing together parents, school administrators, politicians, health care providers, and teens.

Men's Health Research Issues

Despite the advances in medical technology and research, men still continue to live an average of 7 years less than women. Although most medical research was historically based on men, men's health issues no longer dominate the research agenda because of recent federal mandates. Research on men's health must focus on the areas where prevention, early detection, and treatment efforts will significantly improve the quality of life of men across the life span. Table 33-2 includes some priority areas of research on men's health issues.

In addition, research studies must be more inclusive and utilize subjects that represent the diversity within the male population. Studies need to report findings based not only on middle-aged, middle class, Caucasian males, but also on other males representing various ethnic and socioeconomic groups.

TABLE 33-2	MEN'S HEALTH RESEARCH PRIORITIES

RESEARCH AREA	JUSTIFICATION FOR RESEARCH PRIORITY
Prostate cancer	The likelihood that a man will develop prostate cancer is 1 in 11; one-third of the cases are expected to die from the disease; the death rate for prostate cancer has grown at almost twice the death rate of breast cancer in the last decade.
Testicular cancer	It is one of the most common cancers in men aged 15–34, and, when detected early, has an 87% survival rate.
Lung disease	85% of the cases are expected to die from the disease.
Colon cancer	Nearly one-third of the cases are expected to die from the disease.
African American men	Highest incidence of prostate cancer in the United States.
Drunk driving and other alcohol-related problems	Men are seven times as likely as women to be arrested for drunk driving and three times as likely to be alcoholics.
Health promotion	Significant numbers of male related health problems such as prostate cancer, testicular cancer, infertility, and colon cancer, could be detected and treated if men's awareness of these problems was more pervasive. Women visit the doctor more often than men, enabling them to detect health problems in their early stages.

Adapted from 103d Congress H. B. Res. 209 As introduced in the house.

CONCLUSION

Men's health care is not easily defined as a single issue with a limited focus or target population. Although men constitute half the population, their needs and health system utilization vary greatly from those of women. Issues faced by men must be addressed to improve their overall health and decrease the variance in life expectancy between men and women.

The community health nurse can be instrumental in securing access to and promoting the utilization of health care by men. Health promotion and screening programs can be implemented with specifically targeted groups of men. The community health nurse also assumes the roles of client advocate, educator, and facilitator to secure the most advantageous outcomes for the improvement of men's health.

CRITICAL THINKING ACTIVITIES

1. *Smoking is a behavior issue that plays an important role in the reduction of the length and quality of life of men. As a community health nurse, what programs would you develop to improve this situation? What groups would you specifically target? How would you most effectively implement your plans?*

2. *Based on the information provided regarding men's utilization of preventive health care, what would be the most effective intervention(s) to ensure participation? Where should the intervention(s) be implemented? How would the intervention(s) be modified to address differences in age, religion, education, or socioeconomic status?*

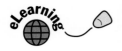

Explore Community Health Nursing on the web! To learn more about the topics in this chapter, use the passcode provided to access your exclusive web site: http://communitynursing.jbpub.com
If you do not have a passcode, you can obtain one at this site.

REFERENCES

Adami, H., Bergstrom, R., Holmberg, L., Klareskog, L., Perrson, I., & Ponten, J. (1990). The effect of female sex hormones on cancer survival: a register-based study in patients younger than 20 years at diagnosis. *The Journal of the American Medical Association, 263*(16), 2189–2193.

American Family Physician. (1999, May 1). Testicular cancer—What to look for. *American Family Physician, 59*(9), 2549–2550.

American Heart Association (AHA). (1998). *Risk Factors*: www.amhrt.org/Scientific/Hsstats98/08rskfct.html.

Brakey, M. R. (1994, September). Myths and facts . . . About testicular cancer. *Nursing, 24.*

Brock, D. L. (1997). Male genital cancers. In C. Varricchio (Ed.), *A cancer source book for nurses* (7th ed., pp. 327–334). Atlanta: American Cancer Society.

Brock, D., Fox, S., Gosling, G., Haney, L., Kneebone, P., Nagy, C., & Qualitza, B. (1993). Testicular cancer. *Seminars in Oncology Nursing, 9*(4), 224–236.

Centers for Disease Control and Prevention (CDC). (1998a). *Trends in the HIV/AIDS epidemic.* Washington, DC: Department of Health and Human Services.

Centers for Disease Control and Prevention (CDC). (1998b, April 24). Diagnosis and reporting of HIV and AIDS in states with integrated HIV and AIDS surveillance—United States, January 1994–June 1997. *Morbidity and Mortality Weekly Report*, pp. 309–315.

Centers for Disease Control and Prevention (CDC). (1997, February 28). Update: Trends in AIDS incidence, deaths, and prevalence—United States, 1996. *Morbidity and Mortality Weekly Report*, pp. 165–173.

Clark, M. J. (1999). *Nursing in the community* (3rd ed.). Stamford, CT: Appleton & Lange.

Clore, E. R. (1993). A guide for the testicular self-examination. *Journal of Pediatric Health Care, 7*(6), 264–268.

Coakley, E.H., Rimm, E. B., Colditz, G., Kawachi, I., & Willet, W. (1998). Predictors of weight change in men: Results from the Health Professionals Follow Up Study. *International Journal of Obesity, 22*, 89–96.

Fackelmann, K. (1998). An enzymatic sex difference. *Science News, 153*(13), 204.

Fareed, A. (1994). Equal rights for men. *Nursing Times, 90*(5), 26–29.

Feuer, E. J., & Merrill, R. M. (1999). Cancer surveillance series: Interpreting trends in prostate cancer—Part II: Cause of death misclassification and the recent rise and fall in prostate cancer mortality. *Journal of the National Cancer Institute, 91*(12), 1025–1032.

Gelfand, D. E., Parzuchowski, J., Cort, M., & Powell, I. (1995). Digital rectal examinations and prostate cancer screening: Attitudes of African American men. *Oncology Nursing Forum, 22*, 1253–1255.

Gerlock, A. A. (1997). New directions in the treatment of men who batter women. *Health Care for Women International, 18*, 481–493.

Giger, J., & Davidhizar, R. (1995). *Transcultural nursing: Assessment and intervention.* St Louis: Mosby.

Graves, E. J., & Owings, M. F. (1997). 1995 summary: National hospital discharge survey. *Advance Data Form Vital and Health Statistics,* p. 291.

Graves, K. L. (1995). Risky sexual behavior and alcohol use among young adults: Results from a national survey. *American Journal of Health Promotion, 10*(1), 27–36.

Helman, C. G. (1994). *Culture, health, and illness* (3rd ed.). London: Butterworth-Heinemann.

Henkel, J. (1996, January/February). Testicular cancer: Survival high with early treatment. *FDA Consumer:* www.vix.com.

Jaffe, H. (1997, September). Dying for dollars. *Men's Health,* p. 134.

Johnson, J. V., Stewart, W., Hall, E.H., Fredlund, P., & Theorell, T. (1996). Long-term psychological work environment and cardiovascular mortality among Swedish men. *American Journal of Public Health, 86*(3), 324–331.

Kinkade, S. (1999, May 1). Testicular cancer. *American Family Physician, 59*(9), 2539–2544.

Koshti-Richman, A. (1996). The role of nurses in promoting testicular self-examination. *Nursing Times, 92*(33), 40–41.

Male Health Center. (1998a). *Why men don't go to the doctor?* www.malehealthcenter.com.

Male Health Center. (1998b). *What do various symptoms mean?* www.malehealthcenter.com.

Male Health Center. (1998c). *How erections really happen*: www.malehealthcenter.com.

Male Health Center. (1998d). *Getting older and having sex*: www.malehealthcenter.com.

Men's Health Network. (1998). *National campaign to significantly improve male health and longevity*: www.menshealthnetwork.org.

Montville, L. (1999, August 9). Tour de Amerique. *Sports Illustrated, 91*(5), 68–72.

National Cancer Institute. (1998). *Screening for testicular cancer*: www.cancernet.nci.nih.gov.

National Institutes of Health (NIH). (1992, December 7–9). Impotence. *NIH Consensus Statement, 10*(4), 1–31: www.text.nlm.nih.gov.

National Kidney and Urologic Disease Information Clearinghouse. (1998). *Impotence*: www.niddk.nih.gov.

Nelson, D. E., Tomar, S. L., Mowery, P., & Siegel, P. Z. (1996). Trends in smokeless tobacco use among men in four states, 1988 through 1993. *American Journal of Public Health, 86*(9), 1300–1303.

Nguyen, M. N., Otis, J., & Potvin, L. (1996). Determinants of intention to adopt a low-fat diet in men 30 to 60 years old: Implications for heart health promotion. *American Journal of Health Promotion, 10*(3), 201–207.

Peate, I. (1997). Clinical. Testicular cancer. The importance of effective health education. *British Journal of Nursing, 6*(6), 311–316.

Rosella, J. D. (1994). Testicular cancer health education: An integrative review. *Journal of Advanced Nursing, 20*(4), 666–671.

Rynerson, B. C., & Fishel, A. H. (1998). Expressions of men who batter: Implications for nursing. *Journal of the American Psychiatric Nurses Association, 4*(2), 41–47.

Sabo, D., & Gordon, D. F. (1995). Rethinking men's health and illness. In D. Sabo & D. F. Gordon (Eds.), *Men's health and illness: Gender, power, and the body* (p. 21). London: Sage Publications.

Schappert, S. M. (1997). Ambulatory care visits to physician offices, hospital outpatient departments, and emergency departments: United States 1995. *Vital Health Statistics, 13*(129).

Stillion, J. (1995). Premature death among males. In D. Sabo & D. F. Gordon (Eds.), *Men's health and illness: Gender, power, and the body* (pp. 47–67). London: Sage Publications.

Tanne, J. H. (1997). Medicine's new motto: One sex does not fit all. *American Health For Women, 16*(5), 54–58.

Torres, J. B. (1998). Masculinity and gender roles among Puerto Rican men: Machismo on the US mainland. *American Journal of Orthopsychiatry, 68*(1), 16–26.

Turner, D. (1995). Testicular cancer and the value of self-examination. *Nursing Times, 91*(1), 30–31.

Department of Health and Human Services (DHHS). (1995a). Counseling to prevent youth violence. In *Guide to clinical preventive services: Report of the U. S. Preventive Services Task Force* (pp. 687–698). Washington, DC: U.S. Government Printing Office.

Department of Health and Human Services (DHHS). (1995b). Screening for testicular cancer. In *Guide to clinical preventive services: Report of the U. S. Preventive Services Task Force* (pp. 153–157). Washington, DC: U.S. Government Printing Office.

Department of Health and Human Services (DHHS). (1991). *Healthy people 2000: National health promotion and disease prevention objectives.* Washington, DC: U.S. Government Printing Office.

Walbrecker, J. (1995, January). Start talking about testicular cancer. *RN*, pp. 34–35.

Waldron, I. (1995). Contributions of changing gender differences in behavior and social roles to changing gender differences in mortality. In D. Sabo & D. F. Gordon (Eds.), *Men's health and illness: Gender, power, and the body* (pp. 22–35). London: Sage Publications.

Walker, R. (1993). Modeling and guided practice as components within a comprehensive testicular self-examination educational program for high school males. *Journal of Health Education, 24*(3), 162–168.

Weil, M. D., Lamborn, K, Edwards, M. S. B., & Wara, W. M. (1998). Influence of a child's sex on medulloblastoma outcome. *The Journal of the American Medical Association, 279*(18), 1474–1476.

Chapter 34
Children's Health

Harriet J. Kitzman, H. Lorrie Yoos,
Anne C. Klijanowicz

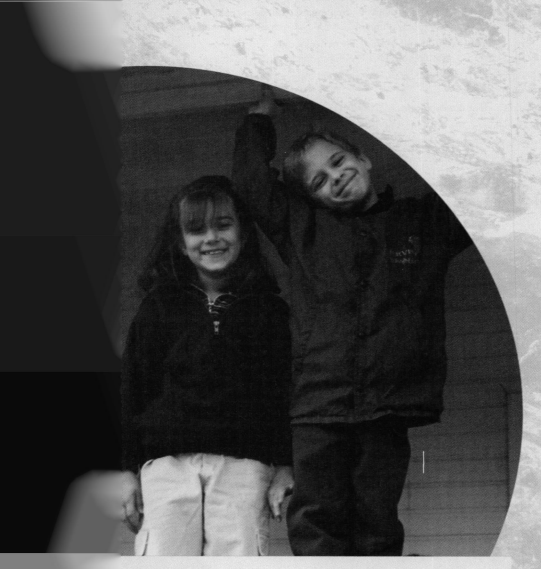

a-round o'roses
cket full of posies,
oo! A-tishoo!
fall down.

nglish children's rhyme which dates back to the Great Plagues
to the "rosy rash"; "posies" of herbs were kept in pockets as pro-
from the disease, and sneezing was often a final, fatal symp-
ith resulting death and "falling down."
Oxford Dictionary of Nursery Rhymes

QUESTIONS TO CONSIDER

After reading this chapter, answer the following questions:
  1. What is the significance of the infant mortality rate in the assessment of a community's health?
  2. What are three common health problems of children?
  3. How is chronic disease manifested in children?
  4. How are risk-taking behaviors of adolescents related to health?
  5. What are common behavioral problems that have health consequences during adolescence?
  6. What is the scope of maltreatment of children in the United States?
  7. What is the ecology of child health?
  8. What is the United Nations Rights of the Child Convention?
  9. What are delivery of care issues related to child health?
  10. How does the role of the community health nurse in child health differ from the acute care setting?

KEY TERMS

Asthma	Cancer	Neonatal mortality	Rights of children
Attention–deficit hyperactivity disorder (ADHD)	Cerebral palsy	Preterm delivery and low birth weight	Sudden infant death syndrome (SIDS)
	Congenital malformations		
	Growth failure		

Children, our greatest national resource, are one of the nation's most vulnerable groups. Despite having the most expensive health care system in the world, the health status of children in the United States still lags behind many countries on important health indicators such as low birth weight, preterm delivery, and infant mortality. Data on the specific indicators of well-being of the nation's children and on the leading causes of death for specific age cohorts are available from the Federal Interagency Forum on Child and Family Statistics and the Centers for Disease Control and Prevention (CDC).

In addition to those who die, a significant number of U.S. children have compromised health. For example, 19% of children in 1996 were rated by their parents as having less than very good or excellent health, up only slightly from 1984 (Federal Interagency Forum on Child and Family Statistics, 1999).

Although parents and society want the best for children and youth, many infants begin their life compromised by low birth weight and/or prematurity and are often cared for by parents who are significantly stressed by overwhelming, competing demands resulting from young age, work, illness, disability,

poverty, and isolation. They face day-to-day challenges as they attempt to nurture their children.

One of the most critical challenges of our times is to establish and maintain healthy physical and social environments for children. Communities are being challenged to support the nurturing role of parents. For generations, community health nurses have been central figures in the community's effort to protect the health of children and families (Deal, 1993; Kitzman, Cole, Yoos, & Olds, 1997). This chapter examines selected children's health problems, provides an ecological perspective of child health, explores societal responses to child needs in relation to community health nursing, and describes systems of care delivery that influence successful services in relation to children and their families.

• •

Children can infuse something special into our souls . . . it is a privilege to watch a child discover the world.
Arlene McFarland, RN, DNS, 1999

• •

Mothers and babies during the first half of the 20th century were at a greater risk for dying from acute infection.

Morbidity and Mortality Rates

One of the primary indicators of a nation's overall health status is its infant mortality rate. Despite the fact that the United States is one of the world's leaders in health care, its infant mortality rate, although improved between 1983 and 1994 (10.9 to 7.1 per 1,000 births), remains higher than many other industrial nations. Within the United States, infant mortality, like adult mortality, is related to socioeconomic status. The poor are more likely to die early than the more affluent.

• •

Remember the children behind the statistics. All over America, they are the small human tragedies who will determine the quality and safety and economic security of America's future, as much as your and my children will.
Marian Wright Edelman, *The Measure of Our Success: A Letter to My Children and Yours*, 1992

• •

Death rates for children ages 1 to 4 declined by almost half between 1980 and 1997 (64 to 36 per 100,000 children, respectively). Death rates for children ages 5 to 14 declined about a third (31 to 21 per 100,000), and those for adolescents ages 15 to 19 declined about 20% (89 to 79 per 100,000) (Federal Interagency Forum on Child and Family Statistics, 1999).

Depending on definition of terms, chronic illnesses and disabilities affect between 2% and 32% of the nation's children. Approximately 2% of children have conditions that lead to numerous limitations in daily activities and can be classified as severe, and approximately 9% of children experience conditions of moderate severity (Newacheck & Taylor, 1992). Among school-aged children 5 to 17 years old, approximately 12% have difficulty performing at least one daily activity, with learning being the most common difficulty (Federal Interagency Forum on Child and Family Statistics, 1999).

As treatment of childhood disease has improved over the past decades, so have survival rates, resulting in a population of children with severe chronic illness and disabilities who previously would not have survived to adulthood. Currently, 90% survive, and slow progress is expected for the future in further reducing the mortality rates in the chronically ill and disabled. Nevertheless, this leaves a significant population of children with complex, severe, and permanent impairments requiring specialized services.

Problems of Infancy, Childhood, and Adolescence

Preterm Delivery and Low Birth Weight

In industrialized countries where infectious and nutritional diseases have been largely eliminated, death in the first month of life (**neonatal mortality**) accounts for about three-fourths of all deaths occurring in those younger than 1 year of age. The most common causes of neonatal death are preterm delivery, low birth weight, and congenital malformations. About three-fourths of all neonatal deaths occur in infants weighing less than 2,500 g at birth, the World Health Organization's adopted definition of low birth weight. According to the 1999 National Center for Health Statistics report, the low birth weight rate in the United States (7.5% in 1997) differs by race and socioeconomic status. African Americans (13.1%) have rates that are more than double those for Caucasians (6.5%). Hispanic, Native American, and Asian American infants' birth weights are very close to those of Caucasians.

Preterm delivery is the primary cause of low birth weight. The cause of preterm delivery is thought to be multifaceted; however, it has eluded scientists. Although risk profiles for preterm delivery have been developed, the mechanism(s) by which risk factors affect preterm delivery has not been determined. Interventions, regardless of their nature, have been demonstrated to be of limited value (Goss, Lee, Koshar, Heilemann, & Stinson, 1997). Preterm delivery rates in the United States have not improved in the last 30 years; instead they have become worse. Similarly, low birth weight has remained largely unchanged during that time despite the fact that more than 85% of mothers currently receive care as early as the first trimester (Racine, Joyce, & Grossman, 1992).

The rates of multiple births increased 33% between 1980 and 1994 (currently 25.7 per 1,000 births), an increase believed to be a result of infertility treatments (National Center for Health Statistics, 1996). Twins and other multiples are more likely to be of low birth weight than singletons. Nevertheless, multiple births account for only a portion of low-birth-weight infants, and there remain significant opportunities for improvement in the low birth weight rate.

Limited progress was made toward meeting the *Healthy People 2000* objective for abstinence from tobacco and alcohol during pregnancy, despite their scientifically established detrimental effects on the fetus. Maternal smoking during pregnancy is associated with low birth weight. The rates of fetal alcohol syndrome are actually on the rise. *Healthy People 2010* has an objective related to smoking cessation during pregnancy. Although there are alcohol control objectives targeted to people of childbearing age, there are none that specifically address alcohol use and pregnancy (DHHS, 2000). Selected *Healthy People 2010* objectives appear in the box on p. 788.

Despite no improvement in the rates of low birth weight, the infant mortality rate has decreased dramatically over the past 30 years. This decrease is primarily due to improvements in technology and care available in neonatal intensive care units (Ahmann, 1996). Many more infants, particularly those of very low birth weight, are now surviving. The survivors are having a long-term impact on the demographics of the childhood population. Although infants weighing 500 to 1,000 g are now living, about 20% have serious handicaps, including cerebral palsy, mental retardation, deafness and blindness, and seizures. At least one-third have significant learning difficulties (Hack, Horbar, & Malloy, 1991), affecting the number of children requiring special education and other services. Those at highest risk for low birth weight (i.e., the poor and many African Americans) become increasingly vulnerable in childhood because of the combined impact of chronic disability and social disadvantage.

Until more is learned about the causes of **preterm delivery and low birth weight**, recommendations must follow what is known about factors associated with these conditions. Early and regular prenatal care and reduction in unhealthy habits such as cigarette smoking, drug and alcohol use, poor nutrition, and exposure to sexually transmitted diseases currently top the list of primary prevention strategy recommendations. Reduction in these unhealthy practices is among the goals of community health nursing practice with pregnant women; nurses working in homes and in the community are in an ideal position to give counsel about healthy practices to women who are planning to become or who are pregnant.

Injuries

Injuries kill more children than all diseases combined and are the leading cause of childhood morbidity and disability from year 1 through adolescence. Every year, approximately 25% of children in the United States have an injury for which they seek medical attention (Adams & Benson, 1993). Injuries in children generate more hospital days of care, cause a higher proportion of discharges to long-term care facilities, and result in a higher proportion who require home health care after hospital discharge than any disease.

Death rates for injury differ by age. Rates are high in infancy (26.7 per 100,000), gradually reducing to a low of 9.2 per 100,000 for those 5 to 9 years old and increasing to a high of 66.1 per 100,000 for those 15 to 19 years old. Although motor vehicle accidents and suffocation are the leading causes of death in infancy, motor vehicle accidents and firearms are the leading causes among adolescents. Death rates as a result of injuries also differ by race and socioeconomic status, with rates for African American children being nearly twice that for whites (Division of Injury Control, 1990).

As a society we have established multiple preventive strategies, with some strategies requiring more active participation than others. Legislation has made the environment safer, and less behavioral change in consumers is required to ensure children's protection. Product safety legislation has been effective. Legislation requiring safety caps on medication bottles, for example, has been instrumental in reducing poisoning. Legislation requiring seatbelt use, smoke detectors, and bike helmets have made specific preventive behaviors more difficult to avoid. Self-determined, preventive safety behaviors that are affected by beliefs and motivation, such as keeping household cleaners and irons out of reach, require more active decision making on the part of caregivers and are more difficult to change. Community health nurses, working in primary prevention of injuries, need to attend to the influence of health beliefs and social conditions of families when providing interventions (Russell, 1996). A nurse's recommendations need to take into consideration the parenting beliefs as well as the physical environment. The American Academy of Pediatrics (1997) recently published a comprehensive sourcebook on injury prevention and control for children and youth.

Although a safe environment is beneficial, caregiving activities that accommodate to the child's capacity are critical. Some children are more injury prone (e.g., those with hyperactivity and impulsivity) than are others and some mothers have greater capacity to respond to their children's supervision needs than do others. The community health nurse can assess the physical and social environment and the parent-child interaction and can work with the parent, helping the parent to understand the child's cognitive and physical capacities and to develop day-to-day practices that reduce risk of childhood injuries. See the following Research Brief for an example of an intervention.

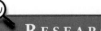

RESEARCH BRIEF

Kitzman, H., Olds, D. L., Henderson, C. R., Hanks, C., Cole, R., Tatebaum, R., McConnochie, K. M., Sidora, K., Luckey, D. W., Shaver, D., Engelhardt, K., James, D., & Barnard, K. (1997). *Effects of prenatal and infancy home visitation by nurses on pregnancy outcomes, childhood injuries and repeated childbearing.* Journal of the American Medical Association, 278, 644-652.

A randomized trial of a program of home visiting by nurses found that children of low-income, first-time mothers visited by nurses had fewer health care encounters for injuries and poisonings than those who were not visited, concluding that nurses can be instrumental in helping parents protect their child from harm.

Inadequate Nutrition, Obesity, and Eating Disorders

As a society, we have worked to eliminate hunger in children. Food is provided to low-income pregnant and breast-feeding mothers and their children up to age 5 through the Women, Infants and Children (WIC) Program. Women enrolled in WIC receive other related services, including education about nutritional requirements, prenatal care, and other preventive services. Many low-income children qualify for school breakfast and lunch programs. According to the U.S. Bureau of the Census, in 1997, less than 5% of children lived in households where there was moderate or severe hunger as a result of food insecurity (less than 1% with severe hunger) (Federal Interagency Forum on Child and Family Statistics, 1999).

Despite the availability of WIC and other supplements, many children simply do not have adequate amounts of nutritious food (Yoos, Kitzman, & Cole, 1998). Even though food is expected to be available to every child, the food intake of many children does not match their metabolic maintenance and growth needs. Reports of a recent survey by the U.S. Department of Agriculture's Center for Nutrition Policy and Promotion showed that most children (76% of ages 2 to 5, 88% of age 6 to 12, and 94% of ages 13 to 18) had a diet that was either poor or needed improvement.

Grocery stores carry a wide range of foods, making adequate nutrition for children and youth at all ages possible at any time with limited work required for preparation. In most metropolitan areas, prepared food can be purchased 24 hours a day. Yet failure to thrive, undernourishment, and obesity continue to be problems for many young children.

The cause of **growth failure** is sometimes difficult to determine. In the past, failure to thrive was classified as organic or nonorganic. In recent years, there has been an increased appreciation of the multidimensional nature of the problem. Intense interventions with families in the home often are required as part of the diagnostic and treatment process. These interventions are aimed at providing adequate nutrition, understanding and enhancing the quality of parent-child interaction, and developing strategies whereby the methods of feeding match the biological, social, and emotional needs of the child. The community health nurse who visits in the home and has a therapeutic relationship with the parent is a critical member of the diagnostic and treatment team.

Many adolescents (rates range from 0.1% to 3%) are afflicted with anorexia nervosa, a disease associated with limited food intake and inadequate nutrition (Coupey, 1998). Anorexia nervosa is a disease that primarily afflicts middle and upper socioeconomic adolescent girls older than 14. Its cause remains unclear. Although often attributed to psychological and psychosocial factors, physiological origins continue to be investigated. Diagnostic criteria include refusal to maintain body weight, fear of gaining weight, amenorrhea, and disturbance in the way body weight and shape is experienced. There are two types of anorexia nervosa: restricting type and binge-eating/purging type. This is a serious, potentially life-threatening syndrome and may require extensive treatment.

Although failure to thrive and anorexia nervosa persist, obesity in childhood and adolescence is increasing, placing many children at risk for chronic illness in adulthood. The third National Health and Nutrition Examination Survey found 20% to 27% of children (depending on age group) meet the criteria for obesity. It is the most common nutritional disorder of youth. Many genetic and environmental factors influence the development of obesity. Of the environmental influences, unlimited access to unhealthy foods, facilitated by the lack of norms for specific mealtimes, and a sedentary lifestyle with limited exercise represent the primary factors. Although the relationship is not strong, obesity during the school-age years does appear to increase the child's risk for obesity in adulthood, with approximately 40% of obese children remaining obese as adults (The Third National Health and Nutritional Examination Survey 1988–1994, 2000).

The community health nurse can use multiple strategies in working with parents and children, beginning with counseling related to breast-feeding and infant feeding and continuing through the establishment of healthy food and feeding practices that are age appropriate. A comprehensive understanding of nutritional needs and growth and development challenges is required. The reader is referred to pediatric and growth and development texts for that information.

One of the most central assessment activities of the community health nurse is regularly and systematically plotting the child's weight and height on a growth chart. The graph of growth changes is an invaluable first screen in discovering problems and in assessing response to interventions. When the quality of the diet is evaluated, 1-day dietary recall and a diary of all food taken for each day of a week are very informative to both the community health nurse and the primary care team and often are enlightening to the parent. Nutritional counseling needs to start with an adequate assessment of current practices and cultural values related to food. Because foods are prepared in multiple ways in different cultures,

care needs to be taken to evaluate the nutritional quality of the foods rather than the types of dishes being served.

••••••••••••••••••••••••••••••

There is no finer investment for any country than putting milk into babies.

Winston Churchill

••••••••••••••••••••••••••••••••

Communicable Diseases

One of public health's most successful programs has been immunizations. Progress continues to be made in the development of vaccines for the more severe communicable diseases, sparing children from death and the ravaging effects of many of the complications of these diseases. For example, smallpox has been eliminated worldwide, and polio has been dramatically constrained.

Although immunization clinics were a common method of distributing vaccines in the past, today the responsibility for immunizing children is often assumed by the primary care provider. In 1997, 85% of children younger than 18 had health insurance coverage, making immunizations theoretically available to most children through health insurance. Schedules for immunizations are recommended with the first agents given in early infancy. For the child to be protected, it is important to give the appropriate number of doses. New immunizing agents are currently under development, making it vital for professionals to keep up to date on the most recent recommendations. Because recommendations for immunizing agents are undergoing change, the current recommendations are not included here. The CDC is an up-to-date source for recommended immunization schedules.

Immunization rates are considered an important indicator of the adequacy of health care for children and of the level of protection a community enjoys from preventable communicable diseases. Despite high rates of health insurance, in 1997, only 76% of children 19 to 35 months of age had received the key recommended vaccinations. Factors other than health care availability often stand in the way of universal vaccine coverage. The community health nurse is in a key position within the community to identify barriers to care, educate families regarding immunizations, and facilitate health care visits for immunization.

Viral gastrointestinal and respiratory infections remain common, particularly among infants and young children, resulting in frequent illness days and challenges for working parents who try to find quality care for sick children. Young children in organized child care tend to have greater exposure to these common infections, thus increasing the scope of the problem. Most of these infections are self-limiting in healthy children but may be serious in premature infants and children with chronic illness.

Sudden Infant Death Syndrome

Sudden, unexpected, and unexplained death during the first year of life is referred to as **sudden infant death syndrome (SIDS)**. It is the leading cause of infant death after the postneonatal period and most often occurs when the child is between 1 and 5 months of age. Although the cause is not known, male preterm and low-birth-weight infants, infants living in low socioeconomic households, and infants whose mothers smoke are more likely to die from SIDS.

A link between sleeping position and SIDS has been found: Infants who sleep in the prone position are more at risk for SIDS. A 1992 statement issued by the American Academy of Pediatrics (AAP) advised the supine position for sleeping and avoidance of soft materials such as pillows and quilts that might trap exhaled air and promote rebreathing. As for all children, a smoke-free environment is recommended.

There are undoubtedly numerous causes of SIDS. Abnormal control of heart rate or respirations is one of the factors associated with sudden death. Some infants with idiopathic apnea of infancy (AOI) who exhibit apnea during sleep, an episode of apnea while awake, or color change during sleep succumb to unexpected death. Thus, apnea episodes should be reported and evaluated. Home cardiorespiratory monitoring, medication, careful parent teaching of interventions for apnea events, and parent support may be required.

Parents of infants who die from SIDS have special needs, and community health nurses often are involved in their support during the grieving process. The National SIDS Resource Center has made important information available to parents and professionals alike.

Growth and Development in the Presence of Chronic Illness

Although the presence of a chronic illness does not imply developmental problems, the limitations imposed by chronic illness and disabilities place children at risk for a wide range of developmental lags as they confront their ever-expanding worlds. The goal of care for the chronically ill and disabled child is to minimize the biological manifestations of the illness or disability on health and development, avoid complications, and reduce further disease. Outcomes can be improved by careful periodic assessments and early, individualized treatment by a multidisciplinary team of which nurses are critical members. The family's responsiveness to the child as well as responsiveness of the broader environment contribute to the outcomes (McGrath & Sullivan, 1999); thus, they are among the factors that need to be considered in any assessment and plan.

Children with chronic illnesses and disabilities and their families have a broad range of health, education, and supportive service needs. Their primary and specialty health care needs often include a range of nutritional, physical, occupational, speech and hearing, respiratory, and other therapies. Because of the issues they face, including uncertain prognosis and ambiguity, families and children often benefit from a range of preventive mental health services. The costs of missed work and added expenses associated with frequent long-distance travel to obtain specialty services, and costs associated with day-to-day in-home care should not be underestimated.

Unlike common chronic illnesses of adulthood, with the exception of **asthma,** there are few common, severe disabling conditions in childhood. Most life-threatening and severe diseases are rare, leaving an insufficient client population base to develop extensive categorical services locally. Because families with a chronically ill or disabled child have needs in common, regardless of the diagnosis, community-based services that meet the generic needs of children and families have gradually been developed (Perrin, 1997).

Every domain of family life is affected when a child is chronically ill or disabled (Miles, Holditch-Davis, Burchenal, & Nelson, 1999). Health professionals increasingly appreciate the significant physical, psychological, social, and emotional burden that families experience. Significant improvements in child and family functioning have been demonstrated as a result of carefully crafted, innovative programs.

Families are very active partners of professionals in the treatment of their children with chronic illness and disability. Many have become important advocates for the services needed and active supporters of one another. Because many of the families are coping with rare diseases, feelings of isolation are common. Parents are reaching out to other parents of children with chronic illness and disability, providing information, understanding, and support. Community health nurses are helping them with this networking process. In addition, families who are sharing the same experiences are increasingly connecting through the Internet.

Asthma

In the United States, asthma is the major cause of morbidity in children. This chronic condition affects 5.8% of children in the United States and is responsible for 25% of days missed from school. There has been an increase in the prevalence and in the severity of asthma during the past 20 years, with hospitalizations for asthma on the rise. From 1980 to 1993, the death rate for children ages 5 to 14 years nearly doubled (CDC, 1996). Although medications and therapeutic regimens to control the disease have improved, this disease continues to have devastating effects on the lives of large numbers of children and their families. The prevalence and severity of the disease is greater in African American children living in poverty and in crowded conditions (Yoos & McMullen, 1998).

Viral respiratory infections as well as exposure to specific allergens, such as cigarette and other smoke, dust mites, molds, cockroaches, and pet dander, often provoke this disease. Asthma education programs have been developed that are aimed at increasing adherence to prescribed medical regimens and reducing exposure to allergens (Yoos, McMullen, Bezek, Hondors, Berry, Herendeen, MacMaster, & Schwartzberg, 1997). These programs have had varying degrees of success. One of the explanations for limited adherence to regimens is that the disease produces intermittent symptoms. It is difficult for families to maintain regular day-to-day prevention practices during asymptomatic times.

CASE STUDY

Ben is a 16-year-old, Hispanic male with severe asthma. Originally diagnosed at 6 months of age, Ben's asthma has escalated in severity over the past 3 years. He has experienced multiple emergency department visits and hospitalizations, often requiring intensive care.

Ben's parents are divorced. He lives with his father but often spends time at his mother's home or at his maternal grandmother's residence. Ben has experienced many school absences throughout this academic year as a result of the persistent nature of his symptoms and frequent need for hospitalization. He thinks his grades are suffering because of his absences. Ben's usual asthma triggers include dust, cigarette smoke, upper respiratory infection, and weather change.

Ben is currently being discharged after a 3-day hospitalization for an asthma exacerbation. One week before admission, Ben began to experience nasal congestion and cough. On the day of admission, he developed labored breathing and wheezing despite increased use of his albuterol inhaler. In the emergency department, Ben did not respond to continuous albuterol nebulizer treatments and was transferred to the pediatric intensive care unit. His condition gradually improved with supportive medical therapy. Because of Ben's anxiety associated with his asthma attacks, the psychiatry service was consulted and relaxation therapy was initiated.

At the time of discharge Ben was feeling well, with peak flow readings of 560 before and after albuterol treatments. Chest examination at discharge revealed an occasional expiratory wheeze but was otherwise clear to auscultation. His discharge medications included the following: prednisone 30 mg/day orally; fluticasone (Flovent) twice daily; nedocromil (Tilade) MDI 2 puffs twice daily; albuterol MDI 2 puffs every 6 hours, increasing to 2 puffs every 4 hours for cough or wheeze. A community health nursing referral was initiated.

1. What lifestyle changes might you recommend to Ben and his family for avoiding his asthma triggers? Be sensitive to his family situation and needs and consider cultural influences.

2. Education about asthma and its management is an essential part of your care. Develop a teaching plan for Ben and his family including learning objectives, content, and appropriate teaching strategies.

3. His father is very concerned about Ben's absences from school and the work that he has missed. What options might you consider for approaching this problem? How might you work with school personnel to help Ben remain in school?

4. Community-based, comprehensive service programs are needed to provide the full continuum of required services to asthmatic children and their families. Describe the role of the community health nurse in advocating for and developing such services. What resources are available in your community?

Because of the continued advancement of asthma therapy, like in other conditions, it is important for those providing care to be current in their understanding of the disease and its treatment. The community health nurse is in an ideal position to understand the day-to-day concerns of the family with a child with asthma and to facilitate their understanding of and adherence to the environmental and pharmacological regimen.

Cancer

The approximate overall incidence of malignancy in children younger than 15 years of age is 14 per 100,000 per year. Incidence for nearly all types varies worldwide. Among the common sites of childhood **cancer** are blood and bone marrow, bone, lymph nodes, brain, central nervous system, kidneys, and soft tissue. Although the disease may present itself as a mass or symptoms related to a mass, the symptoms are often nonspecific. Among the symptoms related directly to tumors are unexplained bleeding, bruising, or petechiae; headaches and vomiting; bony pain; limping; paleness; hematuria; and unexplained endocrine symptoms. There also may be signs of obstruction. Among the nonspecific symptoms are weight loss, failure to thrive, diarrhea, malaise, and low-grade fevers. Children with unexplained signs and symptoms should be referred promptly for an evaluation.

After diagnosis, state-of-the-art treatment can be provided in specialty cancer treatment centers where nurses are employed as members of multidisciplinary teams. The treatment is based on the type and extent of the cancer. Among the multiple treatments are surgery, chemotherapy and radiation therapy, and biological response modifiers. Bone marrow transplantation may also be used. The community health nurse may provide care to the child and family in consort with a long-distance, specialty cancer treatment center. Parents, of course, struggle with not only the illness of the child and the threats to the child's survival, but also the threat to long-term health and development caused by the toxic treatments provided. With new treatments, survival rates for children with cancer have improved, and the disease is considered a chronic illness.

Cerebral Palsy

Central nervous system damage or insult in the early periods of brain development (prenatally or within the first years of life) can result in nonprogressive disorders that cause abnormal movement and posture; these are referred to as **cerebral palsy**. The causes of cerebral palsy differ and include developmental anomalies, perinatal trauma, congenital infections, and perinatal period metabolic disorders. Cerebral palsy also has very different manifestations. Based on motor dysfunction, the four types of cerebral palsy are spastic, dyskinesia, ataxia, and mixed. The degree of dysfunction ranges from mild to severe.

In the United States, the incidence of cerebral palsy has remained relatively steady. Approximately 1.8 per 1,000 children younger than 18 are affected. Severe cases of cerebral palsy are usually diagnosed within the first 6 months of life, with parents often expressing concerns about lack of developmental progress. Often, moderate and mild spastic hemiplegia are not diagnosed until the second year. Delay in meeting developmental milestones as well as abnormal tone (either low or high) are among the presenting problems. Specific signs of neurological dysfunction that raise concerns include scissoring of the legs, abnormal crawling, and abnormal reflexes.

Maintaining mobility, maximizing joint range of motion, and developing optimal muscle control and balance are among the treatment goals for infants with cerebral palsy. Because of the variation in manifestations as well as the specific needs of families, treatment of the infant and toddler with cerebral palsy is individualized. It usually involves physical and occupational therapy. Diverse physical therapy programs have been developed for children with cerebral palsy, often requiring tremendous effort on the part of parents. The community health nurse practicing in homes and in child care and other community settings may be the first to listen to the parents' emerging concerns or observe signs of dysfunction. Support during diagnosis and treatment is important. It may be some time before the full extent of the disability will become evident. Care during the preschool and school-age period involves optimizing function.

Congenital Malformations

The community health nurse may encounter any of a large number of rare, **congenital malformations** and abnormality syndromes. The severity of these conditions ranges from very minor, circumscribed abnormalities to very severe, complex, multisystem malformations. Refer to current pediatric and pediatric nursing texts for more details.

Attention-Deficit Hyperactivity Disorder

A behavioral syndrome, **attention-deficit hyperactivity disorder (ADHD)** is thought to have its origins in biological variations in central nervous system development. Prevalence rates in elementary grades range from 3% to 10%, with the condition being more prevalent in males (Wender, 1998). Inattention, overactivity, and impulsiveness are among the behaviors exhibited. Although first appearing in childhood, symptom manifestation differs by age. Symptoms, however, persist through adolescence and adulthood. These behaviors, associated with lack of success in school, often are attributed to a learning disability.

Although some persons diagnosed with ADHD do indeed have a learning disability, it is not a symptom of the disease. Currently, it is thought that ADHD may be overdiagnosed. The use of methylphenidate (Ritalin), a common medication used to treat ADHD, increased nearly sixfold from 1990 to 1995 according to the U.S. Drug Enforcement Administration. ADHD is a complex disease requiring careful attention to accurate diagnosis, pharmacological treatment, environmental management, and counseling. Community health nurses working in schools, homes, and programs in the community are in ideal positions to assess children within the context of their day-to-day physical and social environments and to develop modifications in those environments that help align the environmental demands with the capacity of the child and family.

Behavioral Problems

Children develop a range of behaviors as they learn to accommodate to the demands of society. Many problematic behaviors have their origin in the impulsivity of young children, which makes it difficult for them to resist temptation, work toward distant goals, control emotions, and wait for their need to be fulfilled. As children work toward learning self-control, these behaviors are at times problematic. With the support of nurtur-

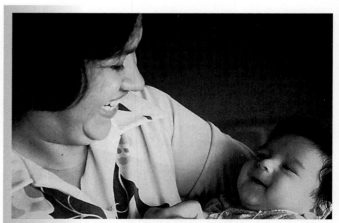

The health of an infant is greatly influenced by the ability of the mother to meet the infant's security needs.

ing parents, most of the common behavior problems of early childhood subside as the child develops self-control and self-regulating processes. In conjunction with those in the family's supportive network, health and social service professionals can help parents anticipate and respond to problematic but developmentally appropriate behaviors. As soon as problems such as aggression, sadness, and self-destructive behaviors are evident, however, a careful evaluation is warranted, because early intervention can reduce the risk of later parent-child interactional problems and more serious child psychological and antisocial behavioral problems.

Risk-Taking Behaviors of Adolescents

A variety of conflicts emerge with physical puberty, and adolescence is considered an age when many individuals become more vulnerable to risky behaviors and reckless deviance. There are multiple theories about the source of the conflicts that emerge during adolescence. One of the most noted is the "lack of fit between human organisms shaped by evolutionary forces that act very slowly and are difficult to change and opportunities for action determined by social conditions that change relatively quickly" (Csikszentmihalyi, 1998, p. 7). This theory suggests that as a society we are uncertain about the readiness of adolescents for contemporary adult roles. The desires that are genetically based in the adolescent do not match the opportunities provided by the culture. Anxiety that emerges in the adolescent is expressed in conflicts associated with taking responsibility, sexuality and intimacy, control and power, and interaction with adult role models (Csikszentmihalyi, 1998).

I am not young enough to know everything.

Oscar Wilde

The complexity of adolescent risk behaviors needs to be acknowledged because no single intervention is likely to be successful for all. Findings of recent research suggest that self-concept is important in the early stages of development of risky behaviors, as well as being the structure through which these behaviors continue and become enduring aspects of the self (Stein, Roeser, & Markus, 1998). These findings support the emphasis of recent adolescent programs on the development of self-esteem.

Regardless of origin, it is important to note that adolescents use a wide range of methods to manage their changing bodies and roles, some carrying more health risk than others. Nevertheless, experimentation with smoking, alcohol, illegal drugs, and other risk behaviors are serious matters. Communities are challenged to develop environments where youth can mature to adulthood without unnecessary risks. Community centers, sports programs, and volunteer programs are among the many approaches used.

Smoking

Despite extensive public health campaigns designed to reduce adolescent smoking, the rates remain high, placing yet another generation at risk for smoking-related chronic diseases in adulthood. Chemical dependency on nicotine is established easily. Approximately 50% of those who smoke half a pack of cigarettes a day in high school will have great difficulty stopping (MacKenzie & Kipke, 1998). Surveys in 1996 found that 22% of seniors smoked daily. Only 10% of adult smokers begin after age 20 and only 40% begin after age 14 (MacKenzie & Kipke, 1998). These statistics form the basis for the extensive public health efforts to cut the sale of cigarettes to minors and encourage adolescents not to smoke. In addition, for some cultural groups, cigarette use ushers in the subsequent use of alcohol and other drugs, making it particularly important to stop the introduction to smoking.

Substance Use

The United States leads the industrialized nations in its high teen alcohol and drug abuse rates. Alcohol remains the most popular drug, with 80% of adolescents having tried it by their 18th birthday and 51% of high school seniors having used it in the previous month (MacKenzie & Kipke, 1998). White males have higher rates of use than do African American males and higher rates than their female counterparts.

Although the use of other drugs is lower, drug use continues to place adolescents at risk. For example, prevalence rates of marijuana use by high school seniors in 1996 was 36%; cocaine use was 7%, and amphetamines and other stimulants use was 15% (MacKenzie & Kipke, 1998). Although rates were somewhat lower in 1998, use of illicit drugs remains a significant problem.

Sexual Activity

Unintended pregnancy, sexually transmitted disease, and pregnancy compromised by sexually transmitted disease are among the problems encountered by adolescents who engage in unprotected sex (Institute of Medicine, 1995). Recent surveys indicate that approximately half of all high school students have had sexual intercourse at some time. An estimated 12% of all adolescent females 15 to 19 years of age become pregnant each year, with half of these pregnancies carried to term (Gold & Gladstein, 1998). It is difficult to determine the number of pregnancies that are welcomed versus the number that are intended because many adolescents do not have intercourse with the intent of becoming pregnant but know that it could happen, do nothing to prevent it, and welcome it when it occurs. The intention of having a child in adolescence differs by culture and socioeconomic status, with some groups accepting parenthood earlier than others.

The risk of contracting a sexually transmitted disease increases with each additional sexual partner and with the addition of their partners' partners, over a lifetime of sexual activity. Many adolescents do not feel vulnerable, expecting any sexually transmitted disease to be treated successfully if they become infected. Nevertheless, some infections, if undetected and left untreated, and others for which there is no cure, result in chronic infection, infertility, and pregnancies compromised by preterm labor or neonatal infection. Strains of at least one sexually transmitted disease, human papillomavirus (HPV), have been associated with cervical dysplasia. Human immunodeficiency virus (HIV) infection and acquired immunodeficiency syndrome (AIDS) increasingly involve adolescents who engage in unprotected sex. Because there may be as much as a 10-year latency period between development of the HIV infection and development of AIDS, many people become infected during adolescence but are not aware of their infection.

Public health campaigns have been developed to encourage delaying the introduction of sexual intercourse in adolescence, to encourage the use of condoms for protection from disease and pregnancy, and to encourage the use of other forms of birth control. Nevertheless, evidence suggests that many adolescents have significant deficits and inaccuracies in knowledge related to sexual risk and its prevention. In addition, knowledge of contraception and condom use does not ensure their actual use because behavior does not always follow information. This makes it important to understand the motivation of the adolescent when providing preventive service. Communities and health care providers continue to struggle to find effective prevention strategies.

Violence

A major source of morbidity and mortality in the United States today is adolescent peer violence. Peer violence may be considered an epidemic and most often involves people who know one another. Complex factors contribute to peer violence. Inflicted injury most commonly occurs as a result of a fight among classmates and peers. A number of intervention programs have been developed, including those that teach conflict resolution.

Homicide is the second leading cause of death for older adolescents and young adults, leading to debate about society's responsibility in regulating exposure to violence and accessibility of handguns. Recent outbreaks of violence in schools and other public places that have resulted in deaths have raised the level of concern for violence and increased government awareness that violence is an important public health problem.

Primary prevention strategies for violence are recommended to begin at birth and continue throughout childhood. Avoidance of guns, television violence, and exposure to neighborhood and family violence is appropriate for all ages. In addition, there are recommended strategies that are age specific. Prevention for children from birth to 4 years old involves helping parents establish effective parenting practice with behavioral management skills that do not involve corporal punishment. Children 5 to 12 years old risk exposure to bullying and fighting in school. Because bullies and their victims are both at risk for poor performance and long-term relationships, identification of these practices as important is recommended. Although this behavior has often been overlooked in the past, it is now taken seriously. Henry J. Kaiser Family Foundation and Children Now (a nonpartisan, independent advocacy group for children) recently published information and tips for talking with children about violence.

Adolescents who are not in school, are using drugs, and are involved in fights are at particularly high risk for violence. Adolescents who are trying to use nonviolent techniques should be supported to continue and those engaged in combative behavior should be encouraged to become involved in a conflict resolution program.

The potential negative impact of domestic violence among adults in the household on children of all ages needs to be an ongoing concern. Not only do children risk injury themselves, but they also risk the emotional trauma associated with seeing the abuse (Eisenstat & Bancroft, 1999). Because more than 90% of domestic violence includes women being abused by men, children often see the abuse of their mother. Clinical issues related to domestic violence are complex and not easily resolved. The community health nurse needs to be open to the possibility and willing to address the problem as it emerges.

Delinquency

The number of youth ages 12 to 17 who have been identified as perpetrators of serious violent crimes had decreased from 52 crimes per 1,000 in 1993 to 31 crimes per 1,000 in 1997. Similarly, youth have been less likely to be the victims of crime (rates were 44 per 1,000 in 1993 versus 27 per 1,000 in 1993) (Federal Interagency Forum on Child and Family Statistics, 1999). The reason for the decrease is not known.

Although federal, state, and local governments have funded numerous primary prevention programs that target youth groups, the degree to which they are efficacious is not known. From a community health perspective, statistics suggest that there may be duplication and overlap of services to prevent delinquency on one hand and services that are too limited in scope to be effective on the other. Services that are broad-based, responding to the psychological needs of individual youth while simultaneously creating a positive environment within which youth can thrive, appear to be more effective than services that speak to only the youth or the environment.

Suicide

Suicide rates for males increased more than fivefold between 1950 and 1990. The rate in 1990 for males 15 to 19 was 18.8 per 100,000 and for females 3.7 per 100,000 persons (National Center for Health Statistics, 1996). When there is a handgun in the house, the teen is six times more likely to commit suicide, perhaps because it facilitates one to act impulsively. Community health nurses who work with children and youth need to be continuously conscious of suicide potential and able to detect early signs of problems for which suicide is the end outcome. A public health and educational campaign of the Educational Fund to End Handgun Violence has developed a program, Hands Without Guns, for youth.

Child Maltreatment

It is estimated that nearly 1 in 20 children is a victim of physical abuse. Of those who die from maltreatment (estimated at more than 2,000 children in the United States annually), 48% are a result of abuse, 37% of neglect, and the remainder from the combination (Lung & Daro, 1996). Of the injury-related deaths to infants in 1995, 761 were deemed unintentional, 311 were homicide, and 57 were undetermined (National Center for Health Statistics, 1996). The number of children identified as experiencing harm from neglect, physical abuse, emotional abuse, and sexual abuse continues to increase (Sedlak & Proadhurst, 1996). Because of the increasing awareness of the phenomenon and mandated reporting, it is unclear whether the real extent of child maltreatment has increased or whether our methods to identify it have improved. Nevertheless, the number of reports has increased each year since the Child Protective Service (CPS) was established.

Children younger than 3 years of age are more likely than older children to be identified as abused or neglected. Parents at increased risk to maltreat their children include those who are living in stressful situations, have poor parenting skills, are substance abusing, and have been maltreated themselves as children.

It has been hard to determine rates of maltreatment in children with disabilities because of the difficulty many children have in communicating their experience (Reichert & Krugman, 1997). Children with mild and moderate disabilities do appear to be at greater risk for physical and sexual abuse. Their needs and their behaviors often make parenting particularly challenging. In addition, it is often difficult to know what can be expected of the child with mild or moderate disabilities and parents at times expect behaviors that do not match the child's abilities. When children are severely disabled and expectations are clearer, it is believed that parents tend to accommodate and the children do not appear to be at greater risk for maltreatment.

It has been estimated that as many as 1 in 10 children before age 18 have been exposed to some form of sexual abuse, probably the most underdiagnosed of all types of maltreatment. The child knows the offender in approximately 90% of the cases, and offenders are predominantly male. Family risk factors for sexual abuse include poor relationships between parents and with the child, the presence of a nonbiologically related male in the house, and parental alcohol and drug abuse.

Impact of Maltreatment

The physical, emotional, and psychological damage to the child from maltreatment is determined by multiple factors, including developmental stage at time of maltreatment, the severity and duration of the abuse, and the relationship of the perpetrator to the victim. Child maltreatment occurs across social, ethnic, geographic, cultural, and economic boundaries; however, because it often occurs in the context of poverty, substance abuse, and family stress, it is difficult to determine the independent impact of the maltreatment on the negative outcomes in the child. For children with chronic illness or disability, it is particularly difficult to determine the added contribution of maltreatment to their behavioral and physical functioning over and above the disability. Nevertheless, there is substantial evidence of a relationship between maltreatment and such outcomes as later school failure, relationship disorders, substance abuse, and arrests.

Government Involvement

The extent of government involvement in the lives of families where children are maltreated is controversial. Although there is general agreement that there should be involvement when there is high risk of immediate serious injuries or death, there is less agreement about involvement with emotional and physical neglect, even when these may have significant long-term consequences. In the United States, cases of suspected child abuse and neglect are reported to governmental child protective agencies.

There is an ongoing need for a system that is both balanced and flexible in its protection of children. Individual child tragedies, with the associated media attention, far too often have driven case decisions and reform, upsetting the balance between protecting the child and maintaining the family on behalf of the child (Larner, Stevenson, & Behrman, 1998). Removing a child from home and parents is a serious act with significant long-term consequences for the child and the family.

A very important role for the community health nurse in child maltreatment is in primary prevention. By providing information, guidance, and support, the nurse helps parents develop the competencies necessary to care for their children. The nurse also helps parents define and identify methods to meet their own needs, whether they are for socioemotional or cognitive fulfillment or for material resources. Because parents are helped to meet their own needs, they are more able to provide care to their children.

Nurses who care for families with children also are responsible for early detection of child maltreatment. They, as well as other professionals, are required by law to report to the appropriate state agency any case of suspected abuse and neglect. Thus, they need to be well prepared to identify signs and symptoms of all kinds of maltreatment and to act as an advocate for the child as well as for the parent. It needs to be recognized that, regardless of the sensitivity exhibited by officials investigating a report of suspected child abuse and neglect, the experience is stressful for the parents and ultimately the family.

Children need to be protected from abuse while abusive parents or caregivers obtain the services necessary to meet their needs (these include parenting skills; financial, job, and housing support; and psychiatric services). Thus, when situations of immediate risk come to the attention of authorities, children are removed from the home until the family situation can be stabilized. Very often, it is the community health nurse who supports the family, provides many if not all of the necessary educational and counseling services, and acts as a case manager as families work to prepare themselves for the retention of, or return to, custody of their children.

A voluntary program of home visiting for families at risk for maltreatment (Wallach & Lister, 1995) has been recommended as a primary prevention strategy by the U.S. Advisory Board on Child Abuse and Neglect. There is now evidence that some home visiting programs are effective in reducing the incidence of maltreatment (Olds & Kitzman, 1993). As secondary prevention strategies, intensive family preservation programs have been developed for those facing serious and immediate threats, with the short-term goal of keeping the child in the home or returning him to the home soon. These intensive programs have low caseloads (two to six families), 24-hour availability, and intensive contact.

....

The undeniable fact is that our children's future is shaped both by the values of their parents and the policies of our nation.
    Putting Children and Families First: A Challenge for our Church, Nation, and World. National Conference of Catholic Bishops—Pastoral Letter, November, 1991

....

The Ecology of Child Health

Children reside in multiple contexts, and their health is affected by each of these settings. The theory of human ecology emphasizes the importance of social contexts on child development (Bronfenbrenner, 1979). The structural characteristics and interrelations of families, social networks, schools, neighborhoods, communities, and culture affect the day-to-day life experiences of the child. Although families are the closest to and have the greatest impact on young children, the nurturing that families can provide depends on their social and physical environmental context.

Poverty

Although the overall poverty rate for children younger than 6 years of age decreased more than 10% between 1993 and 1996, poverty still places a significant proportion of our children at risk for poor health and developmental outcomes (Aber, Bennett, Conley, & Li, 1997; National Center for Children in Poverty, 1998). The most recent drop in rate can be attributed to improvements in rates of full-time employment. The Earned Income Tax Credit has also been effective in helping move some families out of poverty. There are important differences in poverty rates by states, with the rates for some states (e.g., Louisiana, Mississippi) being more than three times higher than for other states (e.g., Utah, New Hampshire).

In 1996, among children younger than 6 years of age, 11% were living in extreme poverty, an additional 12% were living in less severe poverty, and an additional 20% were living near

> **A CONVERSATION WITH . . .**
>
> *Too many young people—of all colors, and all walks of life—are growing up today unable to handle life in hard places, without hope, without adequate attention, and without steady internal compasses to navigate the morally polluted seas they must face on the journey to adulthood.*
>
> *As a result, we are on the verge of losing two generations of Black children and youths to drugs, violence, too-early parenthood, poor health and education, unemployment, family disintegration— and to the spiritual and physical poverty that both breeds and is bred by them. Millions of Latino, Native American, and other minority children face similar threats. And millions of white children of all classes, like too many minority children, are drowning in the meaninglessness of a culture that rewards greed and guile and tells them life is about getting rather than giving.*
>
> **—Marian Wright Edelman**
> Source: Edelman, 1992.

poverty (defined as combined family income between 100% and 185% of the federal poverty line). In 1997, African American and Hispanic children younger than 6 years of age were much more likely than white children to be living in poverty (37% and 36%, respectively, versus 11%) (Federal Interagency Forum on Child and Family Statistics, 1999).

The risks of being poor increases with single parenthood, low educational attainment, part-time employment or unemployment, and low wages (National Center for Children in Poverty, 1998). In mother-only families, 55% of children younger than 6 years of age lived in poverty, in contrast to 12% of two-parent families. The educational level of parents was a strong predictor of family income. The poverty rate was 62% among children younger than 6 when neither parent had a high school education.

Effects of Poverty on Children

Poverty increases the barriers to a healthy environment. The negative influences of poverty on child health and development have been well established. Neonatal and postneonatal mortality rates are higher in children living in poverty. Poor children also are at greater risk for accidents, maltreatment, developmental delays, and some diseases.

Poverty varies in severity and in duration. For some children, poverty is transitory and sporadic, whereas for others, it is persistent. The relative impact of the severity and duration of poverty on child outcomes has not been determined. Persistent poverty may have greater negative consequences on the child's expectations for the future than intense poverty of short duration.

Although children are at higher risk for adverse outcomes when they are persistently very poor, there is no consensus about how the experiences of poverty work to negatively influence child health and development. Income poverty directly affects the resources of the family and in many ways defines the social context into which the child is born and lives. Social context affects the risk of low birth weight and gestational age of infants, which in turn makes the children more vulnerable to cognitive, physical, and mental health problems. It also affects children's social environment, the quality of their physical environment, the physical care they receive, the quality of their interaction with caregivers (including their stimulation), discipline and expectations, and the social and educational resources available to them in the community (Aber, Brooks-Gunn, & Maynard, 1995).

The social context in which youth develop affects their risk for developing maladaptive behaviors. Teens living in poverty are three times more likely than those not living to poverty to drop out of school. High school dropout rates continue to be high, particularly among ethnic minorities, with 27% of Hispanics dropping out of school in 1993. Youth who drop out of school are more likely to be unemployed and subsequently be in trouble with the law.

It is important to note that many children who live in poverty succeed and even excel in education, employment, and family and community life. These children are often referred to as *resilient*. Community health nurses, as well as other important people in their lives, can help create the environment within which children can develop the psychological resources necessary for future health.

Environmental Hazards
Playgrounds

The availability and quality of playgrounds and recreational areas for children of all ages differs by location, with some neighborhoods having much better developed and safer facilities than others. Developmental capacity, as well as presence or absence of disability, is important when developing a safe playground. Nurses often provide consultation to community groups in the development of play areas.

Environmental Smoke

More than 40% of children are exposed to environmental tobacco smoke or secondhand smoke. This environmental pollutant places a large proportion of our children at increased risk for impairment in lung growth, middle ear infection, higher incidence of respiratory infections, and exacerbation of symptoms of asthma. The recent attempts to eliminate smoking in many closed public places have been helpful in reducing unwanted exposure. Community health nurses can provide information to parents about the risks of secondhand smoke to children and can support parents as they participate in programs to stop smoking.

Toxins

Although the toxicity of some hazards, such as lead, diazinon, and mercury, is now well accepted, the long-term risks to development associated with other chemicals is not well known. For example, the impact of chemicals used on lawns in children's playgrounds and to clean and disinfect the home often is not fully known. The most common form of birth defect is cognitive development deficits. The causes of many are unknown, but scientists have speculated that many birth defects may be associated with environmental toxicants during the prenatal period (Dietrich, 1999).

An important exposure to toxins occurs during the preconception and intrauterine periods. Among the well-established toxins are lead, alcohol, drugs, and tobacco. There now is significant evidence that these substances can have a profound effect on the neurodevelopmental integrity of the infant and child. Public health warnings urging women to avoid these substances during pregnancy are backed by a substantial body of research.

Infants and children have different kinds of exposure to environmental toxins than do adults. They tend to be in the same room for longer periods and to be in different parts of the room than adults. For example, infants spend the majority of the time in a crib and toddlers/preschoolers spend nearly half their time in their bedroom. Also, because small particles in the air may be distributed in layers, air near the floor where the infants and young toddlers play may be more toxic than air at the level of the room where adults inhale. Similarly, chemicals and pesticides on treated carpets are more accessible to creeping infants and exploring toddlers than they are for adults. Some children spend considerable time using potentially toxic art and craft supplies.

In addition to differential exposure, the internal biological mechanisms of young children make them more vulnerable to toxins. Because of developmental differences, infants and children breathe or ingest, process, and excrete toxic substances from the air, water, and food differently than do adults. The growth and maturation of the organs make them more susceptible to harmful substances. For example, a 2-year-old child will absorb about five times as much of the ingested lead as will an adult (Rout & Holmes, 1991), making occupational limits that are set for adults many times higher than are safe for children.

Lead is an environmental toxin that has been attacked through public health measures after empirical research found the deleterious impact of lead poisoning on the long-term intellectual capacity of children. Significant legislation to reduce this environmental hazard has been enacted. Aggressive legislation has been effective in reducing lead in gasoline and paint and in elimination of lead in older homes, thus reducing the incidence of lead in the environment. Although lead poisoning in children has been reduced dramatically, some children continue to be at risk. At the level of the individual child, health care providers currently incorporate risk assessment and early detection as tools against this devastating disease that has reduced the intellectual potential of many children. Health care providers can complete risk assessments, however, only when children seek service. Therefore, it is

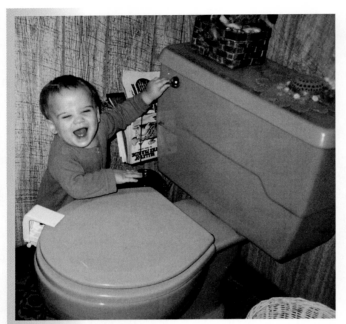

Creating a healthy environment is critical to raising a healthy child. This toilet has a safety latch to prevent accidents.

BOX 34-1 UNITED NATIONS CONVENTION ON THE RIGHTS OF THE CHILD

Children have the right:

- To live with protection from torture, economic and sexual exploitation, and abuse and neglect
- To freedom of expression and their own identity
- To remain or be reunited with parents (unless it is not in their best interests)
- To a reasonable standard of living, health and basic services, opportunities for education and personal development, compassion, respect for their diversity
- To adequate resources

Source: Freeman, 1996a.

important that the community health nurse recognize conditions that place the child at risk and ensure that the child seeks care and is tested and treated if necessary. Some families need to be moved to different housing while their house is being deleaded.

Overall, environmental hazards produce unique risks for children because of their developmental demands. Thus, constant vigilance is required. Continued research is needed to understand the potential toxicity of old and new environmental agents. With evidence of their toxicity, policy makers supported by health care providers, teachers, community members, and families can support laws and regulations necessary to reduce environmental risks. There remains, however, significant responsibility on the part of parents and caregivers to continuously monitor and avoid environments that may be harmful to children.

One of the most critical challenges of our times is to establish and maintain healthy physical and social environments for children. Because community health nurses work within the community, they often are the first to be aware of a hazard and the first to make the hazard known to others. They may act as advocates for the families and problem solvers with community planners and community service providers.

Social Responses to the Needs of Children

Rights of Children

Children are the most vulnerable group in society. They do not have the political power that other potentially vulnerable groups

have (e.g., disabled, seniors, ethnic minorities). To ensure that children do not suffer unduly, adults must assume responsibility. The United Nations Convention of the Rights of the Child has provided some guidance about **rights of children** through its convention report (Box 34-1).

As a society, we have placed the primary responsibility for assuring that the rights of individual children are respected with parents. The community, however, is increasingly held responsible for creating an environment that supports parents as they care for their children and for acting as a safety net for children whose parents are unable to meet their children's basic needs.

There is increasing consensus among those advocating for children that as a society we should strive for children to be conceived by parents who have established their physical and emotional readiness to protect the fetus during pregnancy and to provide care for their child after birth.

Respecting the rights of children is a societal responsibility and is shared by all. The need for a broad community approach to the development of optimal nurturing of our youngest children is found in the following statement by David Hamburg (1994), President of the Carnegie Corporation. (The assumptions underlying this quote are the same for all children and youth.)

> If some traditional sources of stability and support have become weakened by enormous historical changes, then how can young children's development best be nurtured? The pivotal institutions are the family, the health care system, the emerging child care system, religious institutions, community organizations, and the media.

Family Context

Human infants grow and develop in a social environment where they are protected and cared for by others. Increasingly, grandparents and extended family live at distances and are unable to provide help to parents. It is useful for parents, with the help of communities, to have established supportive informal (friends and relatives) and formal (service providers) social networks as they face the challenges of parenthood. Community health nurses hold important responsibilities in helping communities and families create a context where these social networks can thrive.

In addition to information that comes from direct contact with others, there are many sources of information for parents including books, television, and the Internet. The support obtained from discussing this information with peers, as well as professionals, however, should not be underestimated.

Home visiting programs are an important source of support for families, particularly those with children at high risk because of physical or social condition (Kang, Barnard, Hammond, Oshio, Spencer, Thibodeaux, & Williams, 1995). Most of the primary prevention home visiting programs begin during pregnancy or early infancy and continue until the child is between 1 and 3 years of age. More than half a million children currently are enrolled in home visiting programs. The goals of the programs include the promotion of effective parenting practices, the prevention of child maltreatment, the promotion of healthy child development, and the improvement in the mothers' lives (Gomby, Culross, & Behrman, 1999). Because of the positive impact of some of these programs, there is renewed interest in home visiting as a support to young families, and new funding streams are increasingly becoming available.

Child Care

There has been a dramatic, steady increase in the number of women working. This trend is expected to continue with welfare to work initiatives. The demand for child-care vouchers is growing as welfare loads decline (National Center for Children in Poverty, 1999). The proportion of married women with children younger than 6 years of age in the United States who work has increased from approximately 10% in 1948 and 30% in 1970 to 60% in 1994. Day care is rapidly becoming the norm for children, and securing a quality child-care arrangement is an important challenge for parents (Hofferth, 1996).

Who cares for children when their mothers work? For children younger than 5 years of age whose mothers were in the workforce in 1993, parents or relatives cared for 47%, center-based programs cared for 30%, family child care cared for 17%, and in-home sitters cared for 5% (West, Wright, & Hausken, 1995). Children increasingly are entering formal, center-based day care and at earlier ages.

There are five major challenges facing dual-earner parents and single-parent families related to the care of their children. First, the time available to share activities with children is constrained. Second, the energy necessary to be emotionally involved with the children may be limited. Third, monitoring and supervision of children's activities is difficult. Fourth, in an attempt to meet the children's need, the parent's own needs for friendships, diversion, recreation, and relaxation may be difficult to meet, leaving them more vulnerable to the first three chal-

lenges. Fifth, the challenge may leave questions about competency that in turn threatens the maternal self-concept. It is argued by many, however, that low-income women face the same challenges as do middle-income women but also have the added burden of meeting the challenges with fewer resources, for example, less reliable transportation and more chronic illness.

Each age group of children provides a new set of challenges to working parents who use child care and a new set of potential risks to the child. Because of the developmental needs for attachment, particular attention has been given to children younger than 1 year of age (Broom, 1998). Yet in 1994, more than half of all infants were cared for by someone other than their parents on a regular basis.

The consequences for children of poor mothers entering the workforce are not known. There is fear by some that the children's basic needs for food, shelter, and protection will not be met. If adequate, nurturing child care is not available, women, already stressed by social conditions, may need to leave their children in conditions that do not support optimal development. There is also concern than children will be denied access to health care because they will not be eligible for Medicaid (Larner,

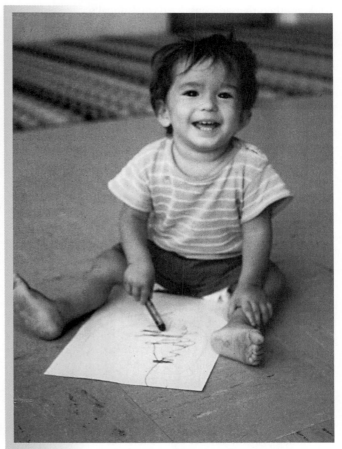

As children grow, they need a stimulating environment for optimal development.

Terman, & Behrman, 1997). The developmental consequences for infants and young children are unclear. Among mothers who have been receiving welfare, research to date suggests that maternal employment may influence positive child development and not be harmful in school-age children (Larner, Terman, & Behrman, 1997).

Choice of child care is one of the most important decisions parents make. Community health nurses involved with children need to become familiar with the resources available in the community and the financing of child care. In addition to providing information about characteristics of quality child care, nurses direct parents to resources and assist them in problem solving as they make their decisions about child care. Community health nurses are also an important resource for child care providers who struggle with developing a safe and nurturing environment, particularly when children become ill.

Child-care financing has fluctuated widely in the United States because there has not been a broad-based purpose or approach. Funding has been provided to meet immediate crises but has not been sustained, resulting in a collection of funding streams rather than a coherent system (Cohen, 1995). In some situations, child-care services have been considered custodial care, while at others they are considered educational services. Increased public support for direct child-care service subsidies has emerged with subsequent changes in the tax code and entitlements (Cohen, 1995). There is increased recognition by industry of the importance of family life to employees and some companies are offering daycare for children as a support to employees.

Systems of Care for Children and Families

Financial Support: Welfare to Work Programs

Although Americans have valued the protection of children, the Aid to Families with Dependent Children (AFDC) program increasingly has been seen as a system that simply does not work and also is inconsistent with American values that stress individual work and self-sufficiency (Payne, 1998). Originally passed in 1935, the AFDC program guaranteed cash assistance for poor single-parent families and enabled mothers to remain at home with their children. In recent years, many social scientists have charged that the AFDC program traps families in dependency and poverty and results in families being negatively stereotyped. With the passage of the Personal Responsibility and Work Opportunity Reconciliation Act in 1996, welfare was reconstructed in an attempt to discourage out-of-wedlock parenting and encourage mothers to work. It is not known how the stress imposed on poor women with limited social resources will affect the quality of their parenting. Although many experts believe that the negative impact of family stress associated with the mother working out of the home will be more than offset by the advantages gained in the self-worth

that comes from self-sufficiency, others are less certain. Experience to date is too limited to draw conclusions

Primary Health Care

One of the primary goals in health care is consistent health care providers who work in partnership with parents on behalf of the health of the child. The health care provider would know the child and family and have a comprehensive record of health assets, problems, and current therapeutic regimen. Ideally, primary care services are proactive and anticipatory. Preventive strategies, such as immunizations and safety counseling, necessary for the child's optimal growth, development, and protection should be included. The services also need to be reactive to health problems, based on the needs identified through health supervision and those expressed by the family. Services extend, through referral and consultation, to other specialty and supportive services. The community health nurse is an active partner of the primary care provider in the care of many children who are at risk because of physical, developmental, or social conditions. There is increasing recognition that for many families needs extend beyond a traditional primary care system. A more integrated system of health and social services is emerging. Managed care provides new opportunities for health care systems and communities together to develop a more comprehensive approach to the health needs of children. The approaches to managed care differ, and it is important for the community health nurse to understand how services are integrated in the community being served.

School Health Services and School-Based Primary Care

There was early recognition in the United States that the health of children affects their ability to attend school and to be ready to learn. School health services were built on that understanding. By the early 1900s, health and social services had become important components of the educational experience for children. The 1994 Joint Statement on School Health, presented by the secretaries of the Department of Education and the Department of Health and Human Services, provided a renewed focus on the interactive nature of health and education (Riley & Shalala, 1994). (See chapter 39.)

While school health in the early part of the 20th century focused primarily on communicable disease control, health education, emergency services, and screening, some primary care services began to be introduced into the schools by 1960. School nurse practitioners joined the schools in Denver in 1969 and began providing primary care services. Since the 1980s, health clinics have been established in many schools, introduced primarily to make it easy for youth to receive primary health care services. School-based clinics provide a range of diagnostic and treatment services, primarily to adolescents. Funding for school-based clinics have ranged from private foundations to public funds. For more information on the role of the community health nurse in the school, see chapter 39.

Home Care

With the survival of more children with complex diseases and disabilities, greater demands have been placed on the health care system to meet basic nursing needs, needs that more appropriately are met in the home than in the hospital. Home care has replaced hospitalization for care of many children with complex care needs. Nurses in the community often direct or provide around-the-clock care to children on ventilators and other life-saving technologies. They rapidly become partners with parents as they plan to meet the needs of the children.

Services for Children: Early Intervention

The basis for health is formed in the early years. Early intervention recognizes that education in infancy and early childhood can enhance the functioning of some children with disabilities and developmental delays. This position has evolved over a period of years following extensive research that has demonstrated the impact of environments on subsequent functioning of children at risk for developmental delays. In the late 1970s, children with disabilities between the ages of 6 and 18 had a right to education as a result of the Education for All Handicapped Children Act of 1975. The 1986 amendments to that act, often referred to as *Early Intervention,* mandated services for children 3, 4, and 5 years of age with disabilities. It also established a system of services that would benefit children with disabilities from birth to age 3 and their families. It is designed to provide a coordinated payment system, facilitating and enabling states to develop statewide, comprehensive, coordinated, multidisciplinary, interagency programs of early intervention services for infants and toddlers with disabilities and their families (Ruppert, 1997).

In 1991, through grants to states to plan and deliver services, the Individuals with Disabilities Act made coordinated intervention services available to infants and toddlers with disabilities who are or are at risk of becoming developmentally delayed. Services include "(1) early identification, screening, and assessment services, (2) medical services only for diagnostic or evaluation purposes, (3) health services necessary to enable the infant or toddler to benefit from the other early intervention services, (4) family training, counseling, and home visits, (5) special instruction, (6) speech pathology and audiology, (7) occupational and physical therapy, (8) psychological services, and (9) case management" (Ruppert, 1997). Early intervention in its ideal form also includes education for family life, pre-conception counseling, education and support for healthy behaviors during pregnancy, and identification and treatment of infants at risk for developmental delays. Participation of parents is considered central, with some services being provided in the home and others being center based.

Services for Children with Special Health Care Needs

Originally established in 1935, Title V of the Social Security Act was designed as a means for states to develop public health programs that serve children with special health care needs. Originally referred to as the *State Crippled Children's Services Program,* several legislation amendments have resulted in the current State Programs for Children with Special Health Care Needs. Its current mission includes: "1) the provision and promotion of family-centered, community-based, coordinated care for children with special health care needs; 2) the development of community-based systems of services for these children and their families; and 3) the provision of rehabilitation services for blind and disabled children who meet certain eligibility requirements" (Wallace & Gittler, 1998).

In the past, many services have been organized around specific diseases. Professionals, expert in the diagnosis and treatment of single or closely related conditions, have produced important condition-specific therapies. As special services have developed, eligibility for coverage has been determined by diagnostic labels. These diagnostic labels also determined eligibility for other benefits, including Social Security Supplemental Security Income, which provides supplements to poor and low-income blind and disabled children. A recent decision by the U.S. Supreme Court has resulted in a change by requiring children's functioning, as well as severity of specific diagnosis, to be considered in determining eligibility for services and benefits. The future of generic and specialized health and supportive services for children with chronic illnesses and disabilities and their families will depend on the future financing of health and social services.

Many children have chronic illnesses and disabilities, such as ADHD, that can interfere with progress in education. Public Law No. 94-142 (Education for All Handicapped Children; later referred to as the Individuals with Disabilities Act [IDEA]), passed in 1975, mandated all states to provide a free, appropriate public education to all students with disabilities. IDEA includes protections regarding special education eligibility, parental rights, a requirement for least restrictive environment for the child, the provision of related services, and individualized education programs.

When regular education is unable to accommodate the educational needs of the child because of persistent and substantial individual differences, the student is considered "disabled" from an educational perspective. Special needs may be physical, cognitive, behavioral, or a combination thereof. More than 10% of children are found to have a disability, and learning disabilities account for about half of all disabilities.

Children often have co-morbidities as well as different strengths and weaknesses, making their educational needs different. Recommendations for a specific set of services by disability category have been judged to be inappropriate. Therefore, individual plans appropriate to the child's needs are considered optimal. School administrators and teachers look to the nurse for consultation and support in their daily work with students and with the establishment of individual plans for the child. This is particularly important for children with multiple physical and behavioral disabilities.

As children with chronic illnesses and disabilities have been mainstreamed into regular classrooms for the child to be in the least restrictive environment, they have brought with them a host of special needs, including gastrostomy tube feedings, catheterizations, special medications, and related therapies. Although supervision of these procedures generally has been considered the province of the school nurse, staffing often leads to procedures being carried out by teachers or teacher's aides with limited supervision.

Transitioning Children to Adult Services

Many children with severe diseases, such as cystic fibrosis and sickle cell anemia, are now surviving into adulthood, leaving professionals and society in general with questions relating to their intimate relationships, employment, independence in living, and health services. Many medical care and supportive services have eligibility requirements that are age-based, leaving those reaching adulthood abruptly uncovered. Public Law No. 94-142 and IDEA do address the need for preparation for adult services, including planning with interagency links for supported employment, independent living, and so on, based on the needs of the client. The community health nurse often is the professional who identifies the gaps in services for individuals no longer eligible for children's services but who have extensive prevention as well as health promotional needs as they strive for adult independence.

A Look to the Future of Children's Health

When comparing the mortality and morbidity rates for infants and children in the United States with those of other industrialized countries, it is apparent that there is considerable opportunity for improvement in the United States. If, as a society, we are to succeed in lowering these rates, ongoing consideration needs to be given to programs and policies that have the potential to support parents in providing care to their children. The direct health and human services that are offered to families with children, whether those children be healthy or with significant chronic illness and/or disability, need to be sufficiently coordinated to ensure that families receive the needed services. The number of children with complex chronic illness calls for continued effort on the part of health and human services to integrate services in a way that will respond to their needs. The ultimate goal is to support every parent and child so that the child can achieve to his or her potential and unnecessary future costs associated with preventable health and behavioral problems can be avoided.

HEALTHY PEOPLE 2010

OBJECTIVES RELATED TO CHILDREN'S HEALTH

Immunization and Infectious Diseases

Vaccination Coverage and Strategies

14.22 Achieve and maintain effective vaccination coverage levels for universally recommended vaccines among young children.

Injury and Violence Prevention

Unintentional Injury Prevention

15.20 Increase use of child restraints.

Violence and Abuse Prevention

15.33 Reduce maltreatment and maltreatment fatalities of children.

Maternal, Infant, and Child Health

Fetal, Infant, and Child Death

16.1 Reduce the rate of child death.

Mental Health and Mental Disorders

Treatment Expansion

18.7 Increase the proportion of children with mental health problems who receive treatment.

Vision and Hearing

Vision

28.2 Increase the proportion of preschool children aged 5 years and younger who receive vision screening.

Hearing

28.12 Reduce otitis media in children and adults.

Source: DHHS, 2000.

CONCLUSION

Nurses working in the community have a unique opportunity to visit families in their homes and community and observe as parents go about their day-to-day activities, struggling to do the best for their children, often in the face of tremendous adversity. Because of their perspectives and the information they have available to them, nurses become critical members of community effort of planning for services for children and families. Finally, in providing direct care, nurses can individualize services to the needs of the family being cared for and the health and human resources available in the community.

CRITICAL THINKING ACTIVITIES

1. Is it necessary for prospective parents to be prepared for pregnancy and parenthood?

2. The United Nations Convention on the Rights of the Child suggests that a woman planning on becoming pregnant should be in a state of optimal health. She should schedule a pre-conception health examination (including a review of nutritional status); have a plan for regular prenatal care with early detection and treatment of complication and have a plan for managing day-to-day demands during pregnancy; be free from infections and chemical agents that may affect the sperm, ovum, and fetus; be emotionally, psychologically, and economically committed to being a parent; be socially connected with a supportive network and living in a community that values the rights of children.

- Are these suggested conditions feasible?

- What are the social implications of these recommendations?

- Do these recommendations conflict with the rights of individuals as they have been operationalized?

- What is the role of the community health nurse in education and advocacy regarding the bases for these recommended conditions?

- What role should nurses play when working with families who do not meet these conditions?

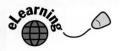

Explore Community Health Nursing on the web! To learn more about the topics in this chapter, use the passcode provided to access your exclusive web site:
http://communitynursing.jbpub.com
If you do not have a passcode, you can obtain one at this site.

REFERENCES

Aber, J. L., Bennett, N. G., Conley, D. C., & Li, J. (1997). The effects of poverty on child health and development. *Annual Review of Public Health*, *8*, 463–483.

Aber, J. L, Brooks-Gunn, J., & Maynard, R. A. (1995). Effects of welfare reform on teenage parents and their children. *The Future of Children*, *5*, 53–71.

Adams, P., & Benson, V. (1993). *Vital health stat 10, 1991*. Hyattsville, MD: National Center for Health Statistics.

Ahmann, E. (1996). Profile of the high-risk premature infant. In E. Ahmann (Ed.), *Home care for the high-risk infant* (pp. 1–16). Gaithersburg, MD: Aspen Publishers.

American Academy of Pediatrics. (1997). *Injury prevention and control for children and youth*. Elk Grove Village, IL: Author.

Bronfenbrenner, U. (1979). *The ecology of human development: Experiments by nature and design*. Cambridge, MA: Harvard University Press.

Broom, B. L. (1998). Parental sensitivity to infants and toddlers in dual-earner and single-earner families. *Nursing Research, 47*(3), 162–170.

Centers for Disease Control and Prevention (CDC). (1994). Program for the prevention of suicide among adolescents and young adults. *Morbidity and Mortality Weekly Report, 43* (RR6), 1–7.

Centers for Disease Control and Prevention (CDC). (1996). Asthma mortality and hospitalization among children and young adults—United States, 1980–1993. *Journal of the American Medical Association, 275*, 1535–1536.

Children Now. (1998). *Right time, Right place: Managed care & early childhood development*. Oakland, CA: Author.

Children's Defense Fund. (1994). *The state of America's children yearbook*. Washington, DC: Author.

Cohen, A. (1995). A brief history of federal financing for child care in the United States. *The Future of Children, 6*, 26–40.

Coupey, S. (1998). Anorexia nervosa. In S. Friedman, M. Fisher, S. Schonberg, & E. Alderman (Eds.), *Comprehensive adolescent health care* (pp. 247–262). St. Louis: Mosby.

Csikszentmihalyi, M. (1998). Evolution of adolescent behavior. In S. Friedman, M. Fisher, S. Schonberg, & E. Alderman (Eds.), *Comprehensive adolescent health care*. St. Louis: Mosby.

Deal, L. W. (1993). The effectiveness of community health nursing interventions: A literature review. *Public Health Nursing, 11*, 315–323.

Dietrich, K. (1999). Environmental toxicants and child development. In H. Tager-Flusberg (Ed.), *Neurodevelopmental disorders*. Cambridge, MA: The MIT Press.

Division of Injury Control, Centers for Disease Control and Prevention. (1990). Childhood injuries in the United States. *American Journal of Diseases of Children, 144*, 627–649.

Edelman, M. W. (1992). *The measure of our success: A letter to my children and yours*. Boston: Beacon Press.

Eisenstat, S., & Bancroft, L. (1999). Domestic violence. *The New England Journal of Medicine, 341*, 886–892.

Federal Interagency Forum on Child and Family Statistics. (1999). America's children: Key national indicators of well-being. Washington, DC: U.S. Government Printing Office.

Freeman, M. (1996). *Children's rights: A comparative perspective*. Brookfield, VT: Dartmouth.

Freeman, M. (1996b). Introduction: Children as persons. In M. Freeman (Ed.), *Children's rights: A comparative perspective*. Brookfield, VT: Dartmouth.

GAO report to congressional requesters. At-risk and delinquent youth. (GAO/HEHS-96-34). Washington, DC: U.S. Government Printing Office.

Gold, M. A., & Gladstein, J. (1998). Epidemiology of mortalities and morbidities in adolescents. In S. Friedman, M. Fisher, S. Schonberg, & E. Alderman (Eds.), *Comprehensive adolescent health care*. St Louis: Mosby.

Gomby, D., Culross, P., & Behrman, R. (1999). Home visiting: Recent program evaluations—Analysis and recommendations. *The Future of Children, 9*, 4–26.

Goss, G. L., Lee, K., Koshar, J., Heilemann, M. S., & Stinson, J. (1997). More does not mean better: Prenatal visits and pregnancy outcome in the Hispanic population. *Public Health Nursing, 14*, 183–188.

Hack, M., Horbar, J. D., & Malloy, M. H., et al. (1991). Very low birth weight outcomes of the National Institutes of Child Health Neonatal Network. *Pediatrics, 87*, 587–597.

Hamburg, D. (1994). *Starting points: Meeting the needs of our youngest children*. New York: Carnegie Corporation of New York.

Hofferth, S. (1996). Child care in the United States today. *The Future of Children, 6*, 41–61.

Institute of Medicine. (1995). *The best intentions: Unintended pregnancy and the well-being of children and families*. Washington, DC: National Academic Press.

Kang, R., Barnard, K., Hammond, M., Oshio, S., Spencer, C., Thibodeaux, B., & Williams, J. (1995). Preterm infant follow-up project: A multi-site field experiment of hospital and home intervention programs for mothers and preterm infants. *Public Health Nursing, 22*, 171–180.

Kitzman, H., Olds, D. L., Henderson, C. R., Hanks, C., Cole, R., Tatebaum, R., McConnochie, K. M., Sidora, K., Luckey, D. W., Shaver, D., Engelhardt, K., James, D., & Barnard, K. (1997). Effects of prenatal and infancy home visitation by nurses on pregnancy outcomes, childhood injuries and repeated childbearing. *Journal of the American Medical Association, 278*, 644-652.

Kitzman H. Cole, R., Yoos, H. L., & Olds, D. (1997). Challenges experienced by home visitors: A qualitative study of program implementation. *Journal of Community Psychology, 25*, 95-109.

Larner, M., Stevenson, J., & Behrman, R. (1998). Protecting children from abuse and neglect: Analysis and recommendations. *The Future of Children, 8*, 4–22.

Larner, M., Terman, D., & Behrman, R. (1997). Welfare to work: Analysis and recommendations. *The Future of Children, 7*, 4–19.

Lung, C. T., & Daro, D. (1996, April). *Current trends in child abuse reporting and fatalities: The results of the 1995 annual fifty states survey* (Working Paper No. 808). Chicago, IL: National Committee to Prevent Child Abuse.

MacKenzie, R., & Kipke, M. (1998). Substance use and abuse. In S. Friedman, M. Fisher, S. Schonberg, & E. Aderman (Eds.), *Comprehensive adolescent health care.* St Louis: Mosby.

McGrath, M. M., & Sullivan, M. C. (1999). Medical and ecological factors in estimating motor outcomes of preschool children. *Research in Nursing and Health, 22*(2), 155–167.

Miles, M., Holditch-Davis, D., Burchenal, P., & Nelson, D. (1999). Distress and growth outcomes in mothers of medically fragile infants. *Nursing Research, 48*, 129–140.

National Center for Children in Poverty. (1998). *Young child poverty in the States—Wide variation and significant change* (Research Brief 1). New York: Columbia School of Public Health.

National Center for Children in Poverty. (1999). Demand for child care vouchers grows as welfare loads decline. *News and Issues, 9*, 5.

National Center for Health Statistics. (1996). Epidemiology and health promotion from data compiled by the Division of Vital Statistics. U.S. Bureau of Census population file RESD9795. Washington, DC: U.S. Government Printing Office.

Newacheck, P., & Taylor, W. (1992). Childhood chronic illness: Prevalence, severity, and impact. *American Journal of Public Health, 3*, 364–371.

Olds, D. L., & Kitzman, H. (1993) Review of research on home visiting for pregnant women and parents of young children. *The Future of Children, 3*, 53–92.

Payne, J. (1998). *Overcoming welfare.* New York: Basic Books.

Perrin, J. (1997). Systems of care for children and adolescents with chronic illness. In H. Wallace, R. Biehl, J. MacQueen, & J. Blackman (Eds.), *Children with disabilities and chronic illness* (pp. 156–161). St. Louis: Mosby.

Racine, A. D., Joyce, T. J., & Grossman, M. (1992). Effectiveness of health care services for pregnant women and infants. *The Future of Children, 2*, 40–57.

Reichert, S., & Krugman, R. D. (1997). Child abuse, neglect, and disabled children. In H. Wallace, R. Biehl, J. MacQueen, & J. Blackman (Eds.), *Children with disabilities and chronic illness* (pp. 137–143). St. Louis: Mosby.

Riley, R. W., & Shalala, D. E. (1994). *Joint statement on school health.* Washington, DC, U.S. Departments of Education and Health and Human Services.

Rout, U. K., & Holmes, R. S. (1991). Postnatal development of mouse alcohol dehydrogenases: Agarose isoelectric focusing analysis of the liver, kidney, stomach, and ocular isozymes. *Biology of the Neonate, 59*, 93–97.

Ruppert, E. (1997). Early intervention. In H. Wallace, R. Biehl, J. MacQueen, & J. Blackman (Eds.), *Children with disabilities and chronic illness* (pp. 338–345). St. Louis: Mosby.

Russell, K. M. (1996). Health beliefs and social influence in home safety practices of mothers with preschool children. *Image: The Journal of Nursing Scholarship, 28*, 59–64.

Sedlak, A. J., & Proadhurst, D. D. (1996). *The third national study of child abuse and neglect.* Washington, DC: Department of Health and Human Services.

Stein, K., Roeser, R., & Markus, H. (1998). Self-schemas and possible selves as predictors and outcomes of risky behaviors in adolescents. *Nursing Research, 47*, 97–106.

Wallace, H., & Gittler, J. (1998). Federal legislation for children with special health care needs and their families: Past, present, and future. In H. Wallace, R. Biehl, J. MacQueen, & J. Blackman (Eds.), *Children with disabilities and chronic illness.* St. Louis: Mosby.

Wallach, V. A., & Lister, L. (1995). Stages in the delivery of home-based services to parents at risk of child abuse: A healthy start experience. *Scholarly Inquiry for Nursing Practice: An International Journal, 9*, 159–173.

Wegman, M. E. (1993) Annual summary of vital statistics—1992. *Pediatrics, 92*, 743–54.

Wender, E. (1998). Attention-deficit hyperactivity disorder. In S. Friedman, M. Fisher, S. Schonberg, & E. Alderman (Eds.), *Comprehensive adolescent health care* (pp. 967–972). St. Louis: Mosby.

Vital Statistics of the United States. (1997). *Mortality Detail, 1994.* Washington, DC: National Center for Health Statistics.

West, J., Wright, D., & Hausken, E. G. (1995). *Child care and early education program participation of infants, toddlers, and preschoolers.* Washington, DC: U.S. Department of Education.

Yoos, H. L., Kitzman, H., & Cole, R. (1998). Family routines and the feeding process. In D. Kessler & P. Dawson (Eds.), *Failure to thrive and pediatric undernutrition: A transdisciplinary approach* (pp. 377–387). Baltimore: Paul H. Brookes Publisher.

Yoos, H. L., & McMullen, A. (1996). Illness narratives of children with asthma. *Pediatric Nursing, 22*, 285–290.

Yoos, H. L., & McMullen, A. (1998). Risk factors for Asthma. Unpublished, University of Rochester.

Yoos, H. L., McMullen, A., Bezek, S., Hondors, C., Berry, S., Herendeen, N., MacMaster, K., & Schwartzberg, M. (1997). An asthma management program for urban minority children. *Journal of Pediatric Health Care, 11*, 66–74.

Chapter 35

Elder Health

Virginia Lee Cora

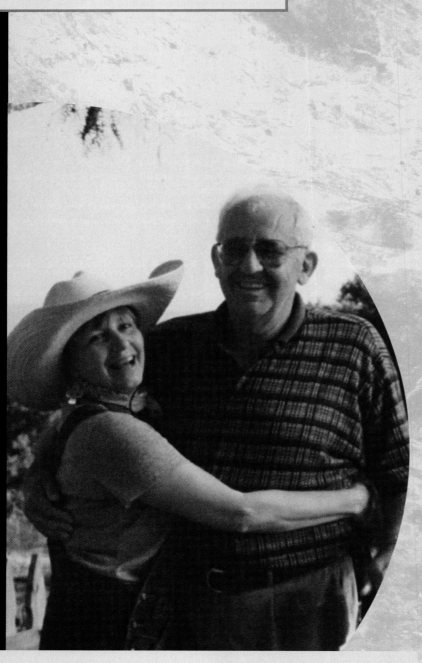

As community health nurses stand at the dawn of a new century, more than one-third of our nation's citizens are elderly. How can we prepare for the future of a generation of more than 76 million whose numbers, demands, expectations, and diversity have no precedent?

CHAPTER FOCUS

Aging
  Aging Terminology
  Gerontological Nursing
  Aging and Health

Nursing of Elders
  Elders in the Community
  Elders in the Family
  Elders as Individuals

Preventive Health Care
  Sensory Integrity
  Nutrition and Sleep
  Elimination

  Mobility and Communication
  Cognition and Affect
  Employment and Retirement:
  Thermal Regulation and Skin Integrity
  Comfort and Spirituality

Special Elder Health Issues
  Immunizations
  Medications
  Chemical Abuse
  Ethical Dilemmas

  Healthy People 2010: Objectives Related to
  Older Adults

QUESTIONS TO CONSIDER

After reading this chapter, answer the following questions:
  1. What are the various meanings of *aging*?
  2. What is gerontological nursing?
  3. What are the major health concerns of the aging population?
  4. How are ideas and misconceptions about aging related to the care of elders?
  5. What are the major preventive health issues of the elderly?
  6. What are specific intervention strategies for the community health nurse in promoting the health of elders?
  7. What are special health considerations that the community health nurse should be aware of in caring for the elder?
  8. What ethical issues are involved when working with the elderly?

KEY TERMS

Ageism
Aging
Activity of daily living
  (ADL)
Advance directives
Alzheimer's disease
Cohort
Confusion

Delirium
Dementia
Depression
Elder abuse
Geriatrics
Gerontology
Instrumental activity of
  daily living (IADL)

Life expectancy
Life review
Life span
Longevity
Orthostatic
  hypotension
Osteoporosis

Presbycusis
Presbyopia
Primary aging
Polypharmacy
Respite care
Secondary aging
Senescence

In caring for elders, we cannot look to the past for direction, for never have so many people lived this long and in such good health. We cannot expect our current ways of thinking about aging and models of caring for the elderly population to provide us with much guidance. Such ways of thinking are outdated in our quest for more progressive attitudes about aging and health. As nurses work with ever increasing numbers of elderly persons in a variety of settings, we must develop improved ways of promoting independence, dignity, and self-care among our older clients. Most of our investments in health care for elders have been in institution-based secondary and tertiary prevention strategies, with little attention to preventive, holistic "aging-in-place" centered care. In the future, home- and community-based alternatives will become the norm for health care of elders, and nurses will provide the leadership to promote maximum levels of independence and the highest possible quality of life for elders and their families.

Grow old along with me. The best is yet to be!

Rabbi Ben Ezra

Aging

Elders differ from middle and young adults in many ways. Persons 80 years old obviously are not the same as persons 20 or 50 years old. Aging is the sum of all the changes that normally occur in a person with the passage of time; life and aging begin at conception and end at death. Aging is a natural, lifelong, and total process that varies among individuals and within various domains and organ systems of each individual. Aging is *universal*—it occurs at different rates and degrees; *progressive*—it interferes with lifestyle; *decremental*—it has a general gradual decline; and *intrinsic*—it is unmodifiable.

Primary aging is "a biologic process whose first cause apparently is rooted in heredity" (Busse & Blazer, 1980, p. 4). Secondary aging is "the defects and disability whose first cause comes from hostile factors in the environment, particularly trauma and disease" (Busse & Blazer, 1980, p. 4). Although health care providers may have little impact on *primary aging*, they can have a significant impact on *secondary aging* by altering risk factors associated with lifestyle, safety, and the like. Nurses can identify genetic predispositions in family health histories, use data from screening tests, and teach appropriate lifestyle changes (e.g., healthy diet, regular exercise, weight management, pollution reduction). For example, for an elder with heart disease in both parents and a sibling, total cholesterol levels greater than 240, and low-density lipoprotein (LDL) levels greater than 160, the nurse can encourage a low-fat diet and exercise; the primary care provider may prescribe hypolipidemic agents.

I'm not afraid of growing old, because I am. That's just a fact of life. I'm not out to "arrest" life, the way some people do. I'm living with it, and that's a part of your journey, that's part of who you are. You carry it with you.

Robert Redford, actor, age 60,
May 1998

Aging Terminology

In working with elderly populations, community health nurses must differentiate among several age-related terms: age, life span, life expectancy, longevity, senescence, and cohort. Age, of course, is the length of time a person has existed. **Life span** is the maximum potential for survival of a particular species. The maximum duration of existence for a human being is 115 to 120 years. **Life expectancy** ("expected life") is the average observed years of life of a species from birth to death or at any stated age. For example, the life expectancy of a child born today is 75 years; the life expectancy of an 85-year-old is 6 more years. Living most of the potential human life span is a relatively contemporary phenomenon. The life expectancy during the Stone Age was 15 years; in the time of Hippocrates (460-377 BC), it was about 18 years; in the time of George Washington (1732-1799), it was 30 years; in the time of Florence Nightingale (1820-1910), it was 50 years; in 2000, it is 75 years. **Longevity** ("long life") usually is the expected length of an individual's life, based on the lives of their immediate family members. **Senescence** ("grown old") is the last stage of a lifelong process of aging. This period culminates in changes in behavior with decreased powers of survival and adjustment (Comfort, 1990). In the United States, old age, or senescence, was designated by the 1935 Social Security act as being over age 65. **Cohort,** a term derived from the Roman military unit, is a group of people who share a particular age, historical moment, or geographical area (e.g., born between 1900 and 1920, Depression era, or urban ghetto). Cohorts tend to develop similar attitudes and values because they share experiences of a certain period (e.g., frugalness may be seen in many elders who survived the Great Depression).

Language used to designate elderly persons is more poorly differentiated than it is for children. It is inexact to lump together all individuals ages 65 to 120 years simply as old. Elders usually are persons age 65 years or older. They often are referred to as pre-old, ages 55 to 64 years; young-old, ages 65 to 74 years; middle-old, ages 75 to 84 years; and old-old, ages 85 and older.

Geriatrics (*geras,* "old age," *iatros,* "physician") is a medical term for the branch of health science concerned with the diseases and problems of old age. **Gerontology** (*geron,* "old man," *logos,* "word") is a sociological term for the study of old age and aging. It is a multidisciplinary, applied science that can be examined from several perspectives: myths and folk wisdom, efforts to prolong life, demographics, and scientific inquiry (Ebersole & Hess,

1998). Gerontology has no core, unifying theory of aging. Instead, there are biological theories at the molecular, cellular, and system levels; psychological theories of the life span; and sociological theories of elders as social beings (see appendix A).

* *

To learn from the old, we must love them, not just in the abstract, but in the flesh, beside us in our homes, businesses, churches and schools. We must work together as a people to build the kinds of rituals, communities, institutions, and language that allow us to love and care for one another.

Mary Pipher, 1999

* *

Gerontological Nursing

Although elderly populations in poorhouses and rural settings were the focus of nurses in the 1800s and early 1900s (Burnside, 1988), the evolution of a nursing specialty concerned with older people is a recent phenomenon (Box 35-1). Gerontological nursing, the nursing of the aged, began evolving as an area of practice in the early 1960s. The standards and scope of gerontological nursing practice are well defined by the American Nurses Association (see appendix B). *Gerontic nursing* also is a nursing term coined by Gunter and Estes (1979) to define "a health service for the aged." Because most elders live in the community, especially in rural settings, as opposed to being in institutions, the needs of elders have been a focus of community health nurses throughout their history.

BOX 35-1 EVOLUTION OF GERONTOLOGICAL NURSING

THE AMERICAN NURSES ASSOCIATION (ANA)

1966	Established a Division of Geriatric Nursing Practice
1968	Developed the first standards of geriatric nursing practice
1973	Established certification in geriatric nursing as generalists (1974), nurse practitioners (1976), and clinical nurse specialists (1989)
1981	Developed the first statement of the scope of gerontological nursing practice
1983	The National Conference of Gerontological Nurse Practitioners (NCGNP)
1984	Creation of the National Gerontological Nursing Association (NGNA)
1985	Creation of Canadian Gerontological Nursing Association (CGNA)
1986	Creation of the National Association of Directors of Nursing administration in Long-Term Care (NADONA/LTC)

Aging and Health

With this country's many advantages, Americans are able to live long enough to grow old. As community health nurses we must examine our own attitudes and values about aging and elderly people to gain holistic, realistic views and provide age-appropriate care for this elderly population.

Aging does not equal health. The changes associated with normal aging are differentiated from the changes associated with health problems. For example, a 65-year-old may be confined to bed with end-stage rheumatoid arthritis while an 85-year-old may run a 26-mile marathon.

Aging changes are both relative and absolute. For example, the individual who has poor eye-hand coordination as a young adult will have poorer eye-hand coordination as an elder than his or her peers, a *relative* change. A person with a 10% reduction in vital capacity of the lungs has an *absolute* change. The principal of individual variation is that the best predictor of a person's current performance is that person's previous performance. Elders should not be judged by the average age-related decline seen in cross-sectional studies (Kane, Ouslander, & Abrass, 1999).

Aging is a comprehensive process. It is not only a series of biological changes; it also is a complex series of psychosocial, socioeconomic, and spiritual changes that influence and are influenced by the elders, their families, communities, and society. Any changes that affect one domain simultaneously affect all other domains.

Old age is a time of continued growth, development, and fulfillment (i.e., achieving self-actualization or ego integrity). This culmination of the life cycle is a balance of both gains and losses of the processes of change. As with other transitional periods of life, old age is a time of holding on and letting go. Some performance may be enhanced with aging. For example, with greater wisdom, perspective, and problem-solving skills, cognitive function may improve.

The elderly population is heterogeneous and diverse. Human beings tend to be more homogeneous (similar) at birth and become quite heterogeneous (different) in old age. As with other age or ethnic groups, we must avoid simplistic generalizations and neither romanticize elders nor stereotype or stigmatize them. Rather, we must balance their positive aspects with their negatives to accept them as they are with specific health problems countered by many real strengths.

Elders are tough. Very few elders are frail; a great majority are hardy, vigorous, and active through the very end of their lives. They are not *victims* of aging processes, but rather *survivors* of life's experiences as part of family systems within their environment. They usually appreciate direct, factual information rather than ambiguous indirect statements.

....

You don't get old from calendar years. You get old from inactivity.
Jack LaLanne

....

Nursing of Elders

The "age wave" is coming, and society will need well-educated and experienced nurses to meet the challenge of providing care for this ever-increasing, complex segment of the population. To provide holistic care, community health nurses will need to consider these elders within the context of their community, their family, and themselves.

Elders in the Community

The status and roles of elderly people in the community are influenced by the values placed on aging by society. In some cultures, elders and their collective wisdom are held in very high esteem; in other cultures, old age exemplifies loss of productivity with subsequent loss of status and stigmatization. **Ageism** is the systematic stereotyping of and discrimination against people because they are old (Butler & Lewis, 1998). Learned at an early age, these prejudices may surface in younger people's negative beliefs about older people, as well as from the elders' beliefs about themselves. These views can influence the outcomes of health care. For example, elders may be viewed as too old for surgical interventions when most tolerate surgery well. Demented elders may be seen as not needing analgesics or comfort measures when

in pain. Nurses need to listen for ageism in themselves and others, then confront it as they would racism or sexism in any age group through the education about the realities of old age, both positive and negative.

Demography of Elders

The aging population is growing by both absolute and relative numbers (U.S. Bureau of the Census, 1991). In 1900, persons 65 and older numbered 3 million, or 3% of the American population. With a 10-fold rise, they currently make up 32 million, or 12% of the total population, the "graying of America." In 2010, the "age wave" will hit as the first of the Boomers turns 65 years of age. In 2050, they will be 20% of the population and number 80 million. Elders are 6% of the world population. The old-old, age 85 and older, are the fastest growing segment of the population, projected to grow from 50,000 now to 1 million in 2050. Most older men (74%) are married, and many older women (40%) are not. The elderly population in this country is becoming more racially, ethnically, and culturally diverse than ever before: 87% are Caucasian, 7.7% are African American, 3.4% are Hispanic, 1.4% are Asian/Pacific Islanders, and 0.4% are Native American. By 2050, African American elders will increase to 12%, Hispanics will grow eightfold, and Asian and Native American groups will increase significantly. Cultural and ethnic differences in aging and health are reflected in the life expectancy of men and women. For example, the life expectancies of white men and women are 73 and 80 years, respectively; life expectancies of black men and women are 65 and 74 years, respectively. Elders of various cultural groups may have different responses to health problems, modifiable risk factors, and health promotion activities like education. Community health nurses need to determine the values of elderly populations within their local area and how these cultural differences affect health care. For example, elderly family members may be immigrants to this country. They may not understand or speak English; they may not be literate in any language. These individuals may delay seeking health care because of fear of the system.

The distribution of the elderly population is four to one in rural settings compared with urban settings. Rural elders are the oldest old, are poorer, and have more chronic illness, compounded by greater problems with access, transportation, and inadequate health care facilities. In 1990, nine states had more than 1 million elders: California, Florida, New York, Pennsylvania, Texas, Illinois, Ohio, Michigan, and New Jersey. The largest percentage of the oldest old are clustered in five farm states: Iowa, South Dakota, Nebraska, North Dakota, and Kansas.

Currently, the median annual income of elderly men is approximately $15,000; for elderly women, it is approximately $8,500. Only 11% are below the poverty line, but 27% are near poor. Women make up 74% of poor elders; African Americans account for 24% of these poor. The major source of income for elders is the federal Social Security program; more than half have pensions and 19% have private pensions. Eight percent receive public assistance, 6% receive food stamps, and 12% have Medicaid. The education of elders is improving from a median level of 9 years in 1970 to 12 years in 1990, but currently, only 55% have a high school education and 13% have completed college. As many as 50% to 80% of elders have inadequate *functional health literacy;* that is, they are unable to read prescription bottle labels, comprehend health literature and appointment slips, complete health insurance forms, follow diagnostic test instructions, and so on (Williams, Parker, Baker, Parikh, Pitkin, Coates, Nurss, 1995).

Twenty-one million households are headed by elders, 78% are owners and 22% are renters. Approximately 15% of elderly men and 79% of elderly women live alone, primarily because women tend to live longer than men. Because of their economic status, disabilities, or social needs, many elders resort to a wide variety of living arrangements, including senior housing units, home sharing, home equity conversion, group homes, "granny flats," and others. Although only about 5% of elders age 65 years live in nursing homes, about 20% of elders age 85 years are in these facilities, with many more women and Caucasians comprising this population than men or other ethnic groups. A growing number and variety of alternative housing arrangements for frail and/or demented elders are emerging. These newer services include adult day-care centers, personal care homes, and assisted living facilities.

With regard to health care access, the elderly population account for 36% of America's health care expenditures: $72 billion from Medicare, $20 billion from Medicaid, and $10 billion from other sources. Health care consumes up to 20% of the income of elders, an average of $1,500 out-of-pocket expenses annually. Although only 12% of the total population, older adults account for 37% of hospital stays and 47% of hospital days. Most of these hospital expenditures are made in the last 6 months of life. Individual, family, cultural, and health provider beliefs and values all may influence choices for health care during this period. For example, family members may refuse to "give up" on an elder and want every medical intervention to be done for a terminal illness, whereas the elder may believe "the only cure for old age is death" and resist further care, even pain management.

Healthy People 2010 *for Older Adults*

For the elderly population, *Healthy People 2010* goals are to maintain their health and functional independence and compress morbidity and dependence into the shortest possible time. Objectives related to improvements in nutrition, reductions in tobacco use, weight control, physical activity, immunizations, and health care visits are focused on all age groups. Community health nurses can help address the need for more health educa-

tion and programs for older adults. For example, only 30% of elders participate in moderate physical activity (e.g., walking, gardening), and less than 10% in vigorous physical activity; only 10% have had the pneumococcal vaccine, and less than 20% get annual influenza vaccine. All these problems can be addressed during clinic and home visits or other contacts with elders. Selected objectives for older adults are summarized in the *Healthy People 2010* box on p. 798. Some of the programs and organizations concerned with improving the health and living situation of elders are suggested in Box 35-2.

Elders in the Family

As the basic social unit mediating between the individual person and the whole of society, the family is the focus of intervention for elders in the community. One definition of family is that a family is "a social system of multiple, interdependent generations of persons who identify each other as being related by birth, marriage, adoption, or mutual consent, as being committed to one another over time, and as having common properties, rights, and responsibilities" (Cora, 1985). By helping families maintain positive attitudes toward aging, nurses can assist elders to look forward to and take advantage of their long and active lives. Elders can give their children one final gift: a positive model of old age.

Aging Families

Aging families are assessed according to their structure, functions, or development, or as systems that encompass all of these attributes. No matter the setting, elders should be approached as members of multigenerational families.

The structural approach to aging families is demonstrated by the family genogram, including at least three generations. Even when elders live alone, their families influence their needs, behaviors, and health care. When assessing elders' families, community health nurses need to develop brief genograms of immediate, distant, and extended family members to help explain their behaviors and understand their meanings as well as to establish support systems for frail or demented elders. Nurses may need to help contact these family members or create surrogate families to assist with care.

The functional approach to aging families describes activities to meet the sexual, economic, reproductive, and educational needs of aging family members and provides a convenient checklist for identifying functional and dysfunctional family relationships (see Duvall in Box 35-3). However, in modern societies, the state has assumed many responsibilities for functions that previously were within the family. Care of elders may be added to the list of services performed by the state in the form of elder care centers, residential centers, and nursing homes. Examining the functional tasks of aging families is helpful for nurses when assessing their patterns of control and levels of involvement with their elders. For example, when helping adult children adjust to

HEALTHY PEOPLE 2010

OBJECTIVES RELATED TO OLDER ADULTS

Cancer

3.13   Increase the proportion of women aged 40 years and older who have received a mammogram within the preceding 2 years.

Heart Disease and Stroke

Heart Disease

12.6   Reduce hospitalization of older adults with heart failure as the principal diagnosis.

Immunization and Infectious Diseases

14.29   Increase the proportion of adults who are vaccinated annually against influenza and ever vaccinated against pneumococcal disease.

Injury and Violence Prevention

Unintentional Injury Prevention

15.27   Reduce deaths from falls.

15.28   Reduce hip fractures among older adults.

Medical Product Safety

17.3   Increase the proportion of primary care providers, pharmacists, and other health care professionals who routinely review with their patients aged 65 and older and patients with chronic illnesses or disabilities all new prescribed and over-the-counter medicines.

Vision and Hearing

Vision

28.6   Reduce visual impairment due to glaucoma.

28.7   Reduce visual impairment due to cataract.

Hearing

28.14   Increase the proportion of persons who have had a hearing examination on schedule.

28.15   Increase the number of persons who are referred by their primary care physician for hearing evaluation and treatment.

Source: DHHS, 2000.

---

familial roles and responsibilities as caregivers, knowledge of family tasks may assist nurses to support family members and prevent burnout from overtaxing the system.

The developmental approach emphasizes the synchronization of several dimensions of time: individual time, family time, and historical time (Erikson, 1963). Individual time is the chronological movement of a person over a lifetime. Family time is the timing of epoch events in the family that involve birth, death, and transitions of persons from one role to another. Historical time is the chronology of a society over an extended period, such as decades or centuries. Elders nearing the end of their individual time are experiencing role changes that involve the transition of power from themselves to younger family members. These changes become important events in the evolving of family time, but also must be interpreted in the context of the historical moment of the society of which they are a part (Erikson, 1963). (See Carter and McGoldrick in Box 35-3.)

Family Caregivers

As part of the intergenerational family life process, family members accept familial responsibility in times of crisis. More than 23% of American households include at least one caregiver, of whom more than 76% are caring for a relative or friend who is at least 50 years old (AARP, 1997). The average age of caregivers is 46 years. These individuals often represent the "sandwich generation," adults who may be both raising children and caring for elders—often while working outside the home; however, 12% of caregivers are elders age 65 and older. More than 73% of the caregivers are female; two-thirds are working. The average Amer-

> ### BOX 35-2 LEGISLATION, PROGRAMS, AND ORGANIZATIONS CONCERNED WITH OLDER ADULTS
>
> #### FEDERAL PROGRAMS
>
> - Social Security Act of 1935: Social Security Administration (SSA), Old Age, Survivors, and Disability Insurance (OASDI), Social Security (SS), Supplemental Security Income (SSI)
>
> - Older Americans Act (OAA) of 1965: Administered by Department of Health and Human Services (DHHS) Administration on Aging (AOA)
>
> - State and area agencies on aging, multipurpose senior centers (social, recreational, educational, and nutritional services for senior citizens), senior employment and volunteer programs (ACTION: Foster Grandparents, RSVP, Senior Companions), senior nutrition programs, health education and prevention activities, senior transportation services, in-home health care. National Aging Information Center (202-619-7501). Eldercare Locator (800-677-1116).
>
> - Research on Aging Act of 1974: Created the National Institute on Aging (NIA) within National Institutes of Health. Publishes a resource guide for older Americans (Age Pages)
>
> - Health Care Financing Administration (HCFA): Administers Medicare and Medicaid insurance programs
>
> - Department of Agriculture: Offers food and nutrition programs including food stamps
>
> - Department of Veterans Affairs: Provides services and benefits to veterans
>
> - Department of Housing and Urban Development: Offers low-cost public housing for elders
>
> - Department of Treasury Internal Revenue Service (IRS): Offers assistance with income tax problems and filing
>
> - Department of Interior: Access to federal park system, Gold age Passports (free), Golden Eagle Passports (low-cost)
>
> #### NATIONAL PRIVATE AND VOLUNTARY NONPROFIT ORGANIZATIONS
>
> - National Council on Aging (NCOA): Established in 1950 as a national resource for information, consultation; sponsors publications, special programs, advocacy activities, research, training, Health Promotion Institute
>
> - American Association of Retired Persons (AARP): Founded in 1958 by Dr. Ethel Percy Andrus, founder (also National Retired Teachers association); 30 million members; 4,000 local chapters; largest nonprofit, nonpartisan membership organization in the world; purpose is to enhance quality of life for older persons; promote independence, dignity, and purpose for older persons; provide leadership in determining the role of older persons in society; and improve the image of aging. Members 50+. *Modern Maturity* magazine, AARP News Bulletin. Tax assistance, health insurance, mail order drugs, information.
>
> - National Eldercare Institute on Health Promotion
>
> - Andrus Foundation on gerontological research
>
> - American Society on Aging (ASA): Enhance knowledge and skills of those working with older adults and their families
>
> - Gerontological Society of America (GSA): Multidisciplinary professional and scientific organization for those working in the field of gerontology.
>
> - Gray Panthers: Founded in 1970 by Maggie Kuhn (1905-1995) as an intergenerational activist group dedicated to social change. "Speak your mind. Even if your voice shakes, well-aimed slingshots can topple giants. . . . The best age to be is the age you are."

ican woman will spend 16 years caring for children and 17 years caring for elderly relatives. A majority of the care recipients are female relatives. Twenty-one percent of caregivers live in the same household as the recipient and 94% live within 2 hours' commuting distance. The average time of care provided is 18 hours per week, but 57% provide 40 or more hours of weekly care. While the average outlay for caregiving expenditures is $171 per month, the average for high-intensity caregivers is $357 a month. Most caregivers provide assistance with at least one **instrumental activity of daily living (IADL)** (e.g., telephon-ing, shopping, transportation, medications, money, food preparation, housekeeping, and laundry), about half assist with one **activity of daily living (ADL)** (e.g., bathing, dressing, toileting, transfer, continence, and feeding), and a third help with at least three ADLs. Most view caregiving as having some impact on family life, leisure time, work life, and personal finances. They also see caregiving as an overall positive experience (AARP, 1997).

Community health nurses need to assess caregivers for their *competence* (i.e., caregiving knowledge, skills, confidence, and

BOX 35-3 CHECKLISTS OF AGING FAMILY TASKS AND PROCESSES

Duvall's (1977) family developmental tasks for elderly family members:

- Do the elders have satisfactory living arrangements for their current situation?

- Have the elders established comfortable routines for their old age?

- Are the elders adjusting to their retirement income?

- Is the family helping safeguard the elders' physical and mental health?

- Are the elderly couple maintaining love, sex, and marital relations?

- Are the elders remaining in touch with other family members?

- Are the elders keeping active and involved with family and community?

- Are the elders and family finding meaning in the elders' life?

- Are the elders and family finding meaning in the elders' death?

Carter and McGoldrick's (1980) family life cycle of aging families:

Primary emotional transition:

- Are the elders and family members accepting their shifting generational roles?

Second-order changes in family status required to proceed developmentally:

- Are the elders maintaining their own and/or the couple's functioning and interests in face of physiological decline? Are they exploring new familial and social role options?

- Are the elders providing support for a more central role for the middle generation?

- Is the family making room in the system for the wisdom and experience of the elders, supporting the older generation without over functioning for them?

- Are the elders dealing with loss of spouse, siblings, and other peers and preparation for own death? Is there life review of elders and integration of the family?

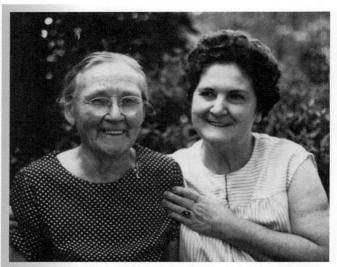

More women than men survive, and the very old are often cared for by their elder children.

objectivity), *burden* (number of hours of caregiving per day/week, nature of tasks to be completed), and *burnout* (psychological stress related to the nature of the illness and the necessary care and support system). Because many caregivers are elderly themselves, their own health issues need to be addressed, especially if they too are frail. When problems are identified, caregivers may need to expand their support systems through family, friends, or community agencies (e.g., home health social services, area agencies on aging, religious groups). Caregivers may need assistance to manage financial and legal concerns, or they may benefit from participation in caregiver groups for their educational and social support. They usually need to increase their access to resources and may need respite services for relief of stress.

A respite ("look back") is an interval of rest; **respite care** provides family members temporary relief of caregiving responsibilities for elders. The availability of these services varies widely in rural and urban areas and different regions of the country. They may be offered in the home by other family members, religious organizations, or federal or state programs; they may be offered in institutional settings by adult day-care centers, assisted living facilities, or nursing homes. Social workers may be helpful in locating respite services in various communities, or the community health nurse may need to help create opportunities for respite for overburdened caregivers.

Elder Abuse, Exploitation, and Neglect

With most caregiving for elders occurring in homes, community health nurses must be aware of the potential for abusive, dysfunctional family relationships. More than 1 million elderly women are victims of abuse each year. They often fail to report maltreatment because of shame, fear of retaliation, or previous unsatisfactory experiences with police, district attorneys, or social workers who lacked sensitivity to the concerns and needs of older people. As a form of domestic violence, **elder abuse** or maltreatment is defined as the willful infliction of physical pain, injury, or debilitating mental anguish, unreasonable confinement, or willful deprivation by a caregiver of services that are necessary to maintain physical and mental health (O'Malley, 1987). *Elder neglect* refers to elderly persons who are either living alone and not able to provide for themselves the services that are necessary to maintain physical and mental health or are not receiving necessary services from responsible caretakers (O'Malley, 1987). Types of elder maltreatment are described in Table 35-1. Maltreatment occurs with 5% to 10% of elders, typically by family members. The most frequently abused, exploited, and neglected elders are those with functional disabilities who are frail, confused, and dependent; are older than 70, female, and of minority status; and have poor social networks. The abuse often is invisible—it is repeated, not reported. Adult protective service laws require mandatory (46 states) or voluntary (4 states) reporting of suspected abuse or neglect.

Nurses who encounter elders in the community have opportunities to assist with both primary prevention and secondary prevention of elder maltreatment. The goals of primary prevention are to support caregivers and reduce the potential for abuse. The goals of secondary prevention are early case finding of abuse and crisis intervention, referral, and follow-up with the elders

TABLE 35-1 **TYPES OF ELDER MALTREATMENT**

TYPES	BEHAVIORS OF ABUSERS AND/OR ELDERS
ABUSE	
Physical or sexual	Slapping, pushing, restraining, molesting
Psychological	Threats, intimidation
Exploitation	Misappropriation of funds or property
Medical	Withholding necessary medications, treatments, or assistive devices
NEGLECT	
Passive	Unintentional lack of caregiving because of lack of knowledge and/or skills
Active	Abandonment or intentional failure to provide caregiving
Self-neglect	Intentional or unintentional lack of attention to self-care

and family caregivers. Techniques for interventions in the maltreatment of elders are summarized in Box 35-4.

Elders as Individuals

The goals of health care for individual elders are to maximize independence and to minimize dependence. For nurses working directly with elders in the community, the focus of intervention is on health promotion and primary prevention to maintain autonomy of the elders as members of family systems within their environment. Health care providers need to focus on the elders' abilities, what's left to build on, rather than disabilities, what's lost. The ability to function depends on individual characteristics and the setting/environment. The health care providers' role is to enhance coping ability by careful clinical assessment and management of remediable problems and facilitating changes in the environment to maximize function in the face of those problems that remain (Kane, Ouslander, & Abrass, 1999).

Elders usually exhibit multiple health problems with complex interactions. Health care interventions often require multidisciplinary approaches. Nurses work in collaboration with primary care providers (e.g., physicians, nurse practitioners, physician assistants), therapists (e.g., physical, occupational, speech therapists), pharmacists, social workers, psychologists, and many others. Health care for these elders must consider the issues of access, quality, and cost.

In the community, providers of health care become integral to the elder's environment. Nurses may be viewed as friendly visitors or surrogate family members rather than as health care providers. We must be aware of factors that foster dependency, including our own attitudes and behaviors. The aversion to risk of health care providers, families, and the elders themselves can bias thinking toward conservative interventions without consideration of quality of life issues (Kane, Ouslander, & Abrass, 1999). For example, fear of falling in an elder may suggest using a wheelchair with further deconditioning rather than emphasizing walking to strengthen muscles and improve balance and gait. Nurses can help keep elders as active and healthy as possible, encourage their independence, and support their health decisions.

Chronic Illness

The cost of surviving the acute illnesses and injuries of young and middle ages are the chronic illnesses of old age. Approximately 85% of elders have at least one chronic disease; 30% of the aged have three or more chronic conditions (Reuben, Yoshikawa, & Besdine, 1996). There is an increase in functional disabilities with 20% of elders being dependent in at least one ADL. The causes of morbidity and mortality in elders are summarized in Table 35-2. With the focus of nursing for health promotion being on self-care, a universal prescription for every age, including elders, is reduction of health risks. In the United States, there is ample evidence that at the start of the 21st century, we are living better, as well as longer. The disability rate,

FYI

Elders Have Their Own Dreams

John Glenn, Osceola McCarty, and Lillian Carter are well-known public figures who pursued their dreams throughout their lives. Each took different paths toward realizing their dreams as they grew older.

John Glenn took his first ride in space in 1962, becoming the first man to orbit the earth. Thirty-six years later, he became the oldest person in space when at the age of 77, he returned as part of the crew of the Discovery. When Glenn went into space in 1962 as a young man, the thought of sending a 77-year-old into orbit seemed unthinkable; today it is not only possible but expected. Glenn states, "Just because we grow older, doesn't mean we give up our dreams."

Ms. Osceola McCarty never set out to get attention. McCarty, a tiny 87-year-old woman, washed clothes all her life. She lived a simple life, never married, and never had children, yet amazingly she was able to amass a small fortune of $250,000. When she donated $150,000 to the University of Southern Mississippi to fund scholarships for African American students, she was surprised at the reaction. Her generosity so touched people the world over that she became a cultural heroine: She shared the spotlight with Oprah Winfrey and Jesse Jackson and received the Presidential Citizen's Medal from President Bill Clinton. She simply said, "If you can help somebody, help them." She dreamed of a future in nursing but was forced to drop out of school in the sixth grade. The USM College of Nursing made her an honorary graduate of its nursing program in 1996.

Lillian Carter, mother of President Jimmy Carter, was a retired RN at the age of 68 when she joined the Peace Corps and served as a nurse in Bombay, India, for 2 years.

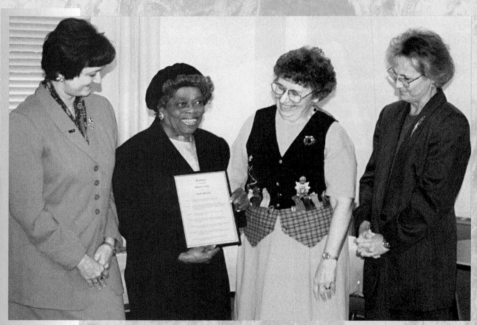

Ms. Osceola McCarty with her "honorary nurse" certificate from the Mississippi Nurses Association.

Contributed by Karen Saucier Lundy.

Continued

FYI—CONT'D

Miss Lillian Sees Leprosy for the First Time

When I nursed in a clinic near Bombay,
A small girl, shielding all her leprous sores,
Crept inside the door. I moved away,
But then the doctor called, "You take this case!"
First I found a mask, and put it on,
Quickly gave the child a shot and then,
Not well, I slipped away to be alone
and scrubbed my entire body red and raw.
I faced her treatment every week with dread
and loathing—of the chore, not the child.
As time passed, I was less afraid,
and managed not to turn my face away.
Her spirit bloomed as sores began to fade.
She'd raise her anxious, searching eyes to mine
To show she trusted me. We'd smile and say
a few Marathi words, then reach and hold
Each other's hands. and then love grew between
Us, so that, later, when I kissed her lips
I didn't feel unclean.

By Jimmy Carter
Source: Carter, 1995.
Used with permission.

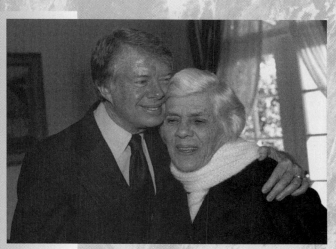

Mrs. Lillian Carter greets her son, President Jimmy Carter, in 1977, upon her return from India, where she spent 2 years working as a nurse in the Peace Corps.

BOX 35-4 TECHNIQUES FOR INTERVENTION IN THE MALTREATMENT OF ELDERS

PRIMARY PREVENTION

- Be aware of the risk factors for potentially abusive situations—in both elders and caregivers (e.g., frailty, confusion, dependence, functional disabilities, age 70+ years, female, minority status, poor social networks).

- Provide anticipatory guidance to help families plan for future needs of frail and/or demented elders.

- Broaden support systems for families with dependent elders by involving other family and friends in caregiving activities.

- Teach families stress management techniques and provide information about caregiving and local resources (e.g., caregiver classes, support groups, respite and day care, financial aid, counseling).

SECONDARY PREVENTION

- Observe for physical injuries (e.g., bruises, lacerations, burns, fractures, pressure sores, malnu-

trition, poor hygiene, dehydration, recurring injuries) and/or psychological damage (e.g., unusual fears, caregiver not letting elder be alone with providers).

- Ask direct questions while alone with the elder: "Has anyone tried to hurt you or make you do things you didn't want to do?"

- Do a complete physical examination, including the skin, head, neck, breasts, abdomen, genitals, and rectum.

- Document findings with the elder's own words, detailed descriptions, and, if possible, photographs of injuries.

- Assess the severity and frequency of the abuse and the safety of the elder. Report findings to adult protective services. If potentially lethal, make immediate referrals (call the police).

- Provide follow up with the elder and family, because many abusive situations are repetitive.

TABLE 35-2   **MORBIDITY AND MORTALITY IN ELDERS**

MORBIDITY: INCIDENCE OF *CHRONIC DISEASES* OF PERSONS AGED 65+ YEARS

Arthritis	47%	Orthopedic impairments	17%
Hypertension	37%	Sinusitis	15%
Heart disease	32%	Diabetes	10%
Hearing impairments	29%	Visual impairments	10%

MORTALITY: CAUSES OF *DEATH* IN PERSONS AGED 65+ YEARS

CAUSE	RATE*	RISK FACTORS	RISK REDUCTION
Heart disease	217.3	Smoking, hypertension, hypercholesterolemia	Take aspirin, estrogen, low-fat diet, exercise
Cancer	104.7	Tobacco use, radiation	Screen breast, colon, skin, prostate, uterus, mouth
Stroke	46.4	Hypertension, tobacco	Aspirin, smoking cessation
Lung disease (COPD, pneumonia/influenza)	20.6	Tobacco use, allergies	Immunization, smoking cessation
Diabetes	9.6	Screen, diet, exercise	
Accidents/falls	8.7	Weakness, imbalance, polypharmacy	Exercise, drug review, home and community safety
Kidney disease	6.1	Hypertension, diabetes	Treat infections
Liver disease	3.4	Avoid toxic substances,	ETOH; immunization

*Rate per 10,000 population.
Adapted from Kane, Ouslander, & Abrass, 1999.

although high for elders, has been falling steadily since the early 1980s. There is a shrinking percentage of elders older than 65 who have hypertension, arteriosclerosis, and dementia. All of this is most likely the result of improved treatment of disease and the acceleration of studies in the science of aging. A growing body of knowledge confirms that chronic illness and disability are not an inevitable consequence of aging as we have been led to believe. Those individuals who suffer the most and the longest from disabilities are often the victims of unhealthy lifestyle choices, such as smoking, obesity, sedentary lifestyle, or poor adaptation to stress. There is convincing evidence that the way we age is more dependent on how we live than who our parents are.

Assessment of Elders

Nurses in community health emphasize wellness with the goal of maintaining optimal function, physically, mentally, socially, and spiritually so as to be as independent as possible for as long as possible. The four primary domains of geriatric assessment to accomplish this goal are functional ability, physical health, mental health, and socioenvironmental factors.

Functional assessment

As a measure of physical and mental abilities to manage ADLs, functional assessment is an important parameter for determining an elder's ability for self-care at home. (See appendix C.) In addition to self-reports by the elder and family members, the ability to perform the ADLs also needs to be observed by the nurse by having the elder perform as many of these activities as possible (e.g., putting on a button shirt, getting on the toilet, picking up a penny). (See appendix D.)

Physical assessment

In the physical assessment of elders, emphasis is placed on areas that most impact functional ability (e.g., vision, hearing, strength). The health history for older adults must include frequent inquiries about exercise, nutrition, medications, substance use (tobacco, alcohol, caffeine), incontinence, memory and depression, social activities, and isolation. In addition to the usual height, weight, and vital signs, blood pressure needs to be checked sitting, lying, and standing for **orthostatic hypotension**, a common problem in elders. Along with the usual adult physical examination, vision and hearing, mouth, skin, breasts (women), prostate (men), and feet need to be checked regularly in elders. Diagnostic screening tests performed by primary care providers for asymptomatic, low-risk older adults usually include cholesterol every 5 years, clinical breast examination and mammography every 1 to 2 years, sigmoidoscopy every 3 to 5 years, and digital rectal examination and fecal occult blood testing (FOBT) annually. Complete blood count, urinalysis, thyroid

Clinical Pearls for the Community Health Nurse

- *Ten pennies make one dime.* Loss of independence in elders may be the result of many subtle changes accumulated over time rather than sudden, dramatic events. Look for multiple simple interventions (the pennies) to support existing strengths and maximize function (the dime). For example, correcting poor vision, losing a few pounds of excess weight, and strengthening deconditioned extremities through a walking program may enable elders threatened with impending relocation to become more mobile and remain in their own homes living independently.

- *Never ask an elder's age.* Rather than ask elders their ages, ask when they were born to identify their cohort and the rich information this fact provides about the physical, psychological, and social factors that have influenced their lives. For example, to know a man is 91 identifies him as old-old; to know he was born in 1909 places him at the depth of the Great Depression during his early adulthood while trying to establish work and family roles.

- *Listen to be heard.* Community health nurses usually are younger than their elderly clients. There is a tendency for nurses to "preach" about health care and for elders to "turn off" these young "know-it-alls." After all, they are the survivors of many hardships in their life experience. If you are talking more than 50% of the time, you are not listening. To avoid this common pitfall, each nurse needs to center the self to focus on the elder; ask clarifying questions, then listen to the elder's answers; reinforce positive aspects of the situa-

tion and support the elder's control, then listen to the elder's concerns; verify understandings, then listen to the elder's responses; reinforce outcomes and enable maximum autonomy, and, yes, *LISTEN* to the elder! Then you just may hear each other.

- *To hydrate elders, encourage them to drink fluids in small, frequent amounts:* a 4- to 6-oz. glass of juice offered every 1 to 2 hours, or a 1-pint, covered plastic mug sipped frequently between breakfast and lunch, refilled, and consumed again between lunch and supper. Avoid fluids after the evening meal to reduce nocturia.

- *Be realistic about weight management goals for elders.* Rather than using ideal body weight (IBW), ask about the usual body weight (UBW) at about age 30 to 50 to establish more individualized goals for gaining or losing weight.

- *For health teaching with elders, remember the four S's:* Start small and stay simple. Take more time, break content into smaller units, present one idea at a time, be concrete (not abstract), increase repetitions (three to seven times), and use more than one modality (visual, verbal, and written).

- *Be aware of bowel function.* Any time an elder presents with anorexia, nausea and vomiting, constipation, abdominal pain, loose stool, fecal incontinence, urinary retention or incontinence, delirium, fever, arrhythmia, or tachypnea, inquire about the last bowel movement and check for a fecal impaction.

- *Teach elders to use it or lose it.* "The right amount of exercise in old age is 'more than yesterday.' If you don't do it today, you can't do it tomorrow" (Ham & Sloane, 1997).

screen are done periodically depending on the situation. Pap smears usually are not indicated after age 70 or after a hysterectomy. The normal values on diagnostic laboratory tests and other physical findings may differ between younger and older adults. For example, uric acid and alkaline phosphatase increase slightly with age; the erythrocyte sedimentation rate (ESR) and C-reactive protein increase significantly with age.

Mental assessment

The assessment of mental health in elders is focused on memory and mood. The Folstein, Folstein, and McHugh (1975) Mini-Mental State Examination (MMSE) is an 11-item instrument designed to screen five areas of cognitive functioning: orienta-

tion, registration, attention and calculation, recall, and language and praxis. Scores may be adjusted for educational and visual deficits, but generally a score of 24 to 30 indicates no cognitive impairment, 18 to 23 is *mild impairment*, and 0 to 17 is severe impairment (see appendix E).

The 30-item Yesavage and Brink (1983) Geriatric Depression Scale is used to screen for depression in elders with intact cognition or only mild cognitive impairment (see appendix F). The 15-item short form is used for initial screening, and if depression is indicated by missing 5 or more items, the remaining 15 items are administered. Depression is suspected if the elder misses 11 or more items on the full instrument (sensitivity, 84%; specificity, 95%). Elders with significant mental/emotional impairments are referred to their primary care provider for further evaluation and treatment.

Socioenvironmental assessment

Socioenvironmental factors are assessed to identify family and living situations, social support systems, financial status, and environmental hazards. A home safety checklist may be administered on the initial visit and periodically thereafter to monitor for the hazards contributing to accidents, falls, and injuries in elders (see appendix G). A community assessment can be completed as described elsewhere in this text.

Interpreting assessment data

In analyzing the findings of geriatric assessments, nurses must remember that the effects of normal aging are being redefined continuously. The presentation of signs and symptoms of illnesses in older adults may be atypical. They may underreport or overreport symptoms of illnesses or have multiple, nonspecific complaints that require explication. Older adults may have a lessened tolerance for stress, yet have difficulty communicating their health needs. The focus of this chapter is on maintaining abilities for a vigorous old age through health promotion and environmental management and preventing disabilities through disease prevention in elders.

Preventive Health Care

In providing preventive health care for elders in the community, nurses can use 16 verbs that represent basic functions. These eight verb sets are easily understood by elders and their families. How well does the elder:

- *see* and *hear*
- *think* and *feel*
- *eat* and *sleep*
- *work* and *play*
- *eliminate* **bladder** and **bowel**
- **heat/cool** and **touch/feel**
- *walk* and *talk*
- *hurt* and *believe?*

Sensory Integrity

The elderly person depends on accurate perception of environmental information from all of the senses to maintain independence. Interventions to maximize perception are essential for successful living alone or with the family. In addition to regular assessment of vision and hearing, the community health nurse needs to be aware of the potential for sensory overload or sensory isolation in elders.

Vision

Normal aging is associated with increasing impairment of vision, most commonly a progressive farsightedness called **presbyopia.**

In addition, four major ocular diseases are commonly seen in elders ages 75 to 85: cataracts (46%), macular degeneration (28%), glaucoma (7%), and diabetic retinopathy (7%) (Kane, Ouslander, & Abrass, 1999). Approximately 92% of elders older than 65 wear eyeglasses; however, the vision of only 65% of those older than 85 are corrected well enough to be able to recognize a friend across the street or read newsprint. Yellowing of the lens reduces color clarity, so reds, oranges, and yellows are seen more clearly than greens, blues, and purples. Decreased lens elasticity and pupil size (miosis) decrease accommodation and contribute to central ("tunnel") vision, and night blindness. Diminished lacrimation may cause xerophthalmia ("dry eyes"). Loss of skin elasticity may result in entropion (inversion) or ectropion (eversion) of the eyelids, which are associated with conjunctivitis and blindness.

Visual acuity should be assessed annually. Individuals with scores greater than 20/40 are referred to an ophthalmologist. Correction typically involves magnification with bifocal glasses. Other interventions to improve function in visually impaired elders are summarized in Box 35-5.

Auditory

Because of its implications for social interactions and safety, hearing is an essential component of sensory integrity. Hearing

---

BOX 35-5 TECHNIQUES FOR VISUALLY IMPAIRED ELDERS

- Increase background color contrast; use warm tones.
- Increase light intensity, but avoid or reduce glare by using blinds, unwaxed floors, and so on.
- Check corrective glasses daily for cleanliness and fit; use magnifying lenses.
- Simplify and unclutter the environment; check for safety hazards (e.g., throw rugs).
- Caution about altered perception when using uneven surfaces (e.g., stairs, escalators, ramps).
- Avoid night driving; assess driving ability every year.
- Increase print size, use large print books.
- Consult the local library for the Library of Congress directory of publishers of large type books, talking books, and catalogues of visual aids, appliances, and computer training.
- Check radio reading services that offer the weather, news, sports, and readings of interest.
- Have annual visual acuity screening; refer to an ophthalmologist as indicated.

impairment is the most common sensory problem experienced by elders. It occurs in 25% to 30% of people older than 60, especially males. It is the most poorly recognized and undercorrected sensory deficit. Only 25% of those who might benefit from a hearing aid actually use one (Reuben, Yoshikawa, & Besdine, 1996). The most common impairment of aging is **presbycusis**, a gradual, progressive bilateral sensorineural hearing loss of predominately higher frequencies and impairment of speech discrimination (especially the consonants *f, s, th, h,* and *sh*). Hearing sensitivity may be assessed with the simple whisper test: Whisper random numbers about 12 inches from each ear while covering the opposite ear. Those with hearing deficits require referral to a audiologist for amplification with a hearing aid or assistive listening device such as the "pocketalker." Techniques to improve communication with hearing impaired elders are summarized in Box 35-6.

Because of the increased viscosity of cerumen and coarseness of hairs lining the auditory canal, another common problem that can affect hearing in elders is cerumen impaction. A simple intervention is to soften the ear wax daily for 3 to 4 days with a ceruminolytic agent (e.g., Cerumenex, Debrox), then irrigate with warm water until the wax is removed (see package instructions). The client should be referred to a primary care provider if the impaction is not resolved.

Nutrition and Sleep

In every culture, meals have great social significance as well as nutritional value. Changes in appetite and weight may be the first indicators of altered health status. A balance of activity and rest are important for feelings of well-being. Therefore, nutrition and sleep are functions to be assessed thoroughly and often in elderly individuals.

Nutrition

Of community dwelling elders, 15% to 50% are believed to have poor nutrition or be malnourished. Because of this major health problem, the Nutrition Screening Initiative (1992), a coalition of the American Academy of Family Physicians, the American Dietetic Association, and the National Council on Aging, was developed to identify nutritional problems, improve nutrition, and improve delivery of nutrition programs. Common factors associated with malnutrition in community-dwelling elders include physical illness, medications, lack of hydration, social isolation, oral health problems, limited mobility, lack of transportation, limited vision, poverty, dementia, depression, and alcoholism.

The nutritional needs of elders change significantly with advanced age. For example, calorie requirements progressively decrease, about one-third from a lowered metabolic rate and two-thirds from reduced physical activity. There is a decrease in the acuity and differentiation of taste (dysgeusia) and smell (anosmia), which contributes to anorexia and malnutrition. With loss of salty and sweet tastes, foods taste more bitter and sour. Less volume and acidity of salivation contributes to xerostomia ("dry mouth"), dysphagia ("difficult swallowing"), and difficulty digesting starches. Loss of gingiva and wearing down of teeth contributes to gingivitis, loss of teeth, ill-fitting dentures, and potential mouth ulcers. Thinning of the esophageal wall and relaxed cardiac sphincter contribute to early satiety (feeling of fullness) and dyspepsia (acid indigestion/heartburn), as does less mucin, decreased gastric juices (HCl, enzymes) and slower peristalsis in the stomach. Thinning of the intestinal wall and slower peristalsis in the colon contributes to increased flatulence, polyps, and diverticula. As with other age groups, the nutritional requirements for elders differ in some categories (Table 35-3). The health problems and associated nutritional deficits of elders are summarized in Table 35-4.

Changes in weight may be early indicators of multiple health problems in older adults (e.g., depression, congestive heart failure, diabetes). Height and weight should be measured

---

BOX 35-6 TECHNIQUES FOR HEARING IMPAIRED ELDERS

- Minimize background noise (e.g., turn off or down the television or radio).
- Stand within 2 to 3 feet of the person.
- Speak face-to-face, on the same level, and toward the best ear.
- Speak at a normal level or slightly louder volume—do *not* shout (it distorts sound).
- Speak a little more slowly in a clear, slightly lower pitched voice.
- Get the person's attention; call his or her name first.
- Use short, simple sentences; pause at the end of each sentence (e.g., "Ms. Smith, here is a glass of water").
- Repeat by paraphrasing the message in a different way.
- Provide extra time for responses and give visual clues or transitional sentences to preface a message (e.g., pointing to the door, "It's time for lunch"); avoid appearing frustrated.
- Write down key words if the person can read.
- Have the person repeat to be certain the message was understood.
- Be sure hearing aids are worn, functioning (check batteries), and fit properly.
- Inspect ears at least every 3 months for impacted cerumen.

TABLE 35-3 NUTRITIONAL REQUIREMENTS OF ELDERS

MACRONUTRIENTS

Protein	1.0-1.25 g/kg/day
Calories	1,800-2,100 kcal/day
Water	2 L/day; 30 ml/kg/day
Sodium	Minimum, 0.5 g/day; maximum, 2.4 g/day
Sodium chloride	Minimum, 1.3 g/day; maximum, 6.0 g/day
Dietary fiber	Typical 8-17 g/day; ideal 20-35 g/day

MICRONUTRIENTS

Vitamins	
Water-soluble (B and C)	Become deficient over weeks to months
Fat-soluble (A, D, E, and K)	Become deficient over many months to years
Minerals	
Calcium	1,200-1,500 mg/day
Zinc	12-15 mg/day

Source: Adapted from Reuben, Yoshikawa, & Besdine, 1996, pp. 145-148.

BOX 35-7 FORMULAS FOR CALCULATING THE NUTRITIONAL STATUS OF ELDERS

World Health Organization calorie estimates for adults over age 60 years:

Women $(10.5) \times$ (weight in kilograms) $+ 596$

Men $(13.5) \times$ (weight in kilograms) $+ 487$

Harris-Benedict equations for estimating resting calorie requirements:

Women $= 655 + (9.6)$(Weight in kg) $+ (1.7)$(Height in cm) $- (4.7)$(Age in yr)

Men $= 66 + (13.7)$(Weight in kg) $+ (5.0)$(Height in cm) $- (6.8)$(Age in yr)

where kg $=$ *Weight in pounds* $\times 0.45$
cm $=$ *Height in inches* $\times 0.39$

Body mass index $= \dfrac{\text{Weight in kilograms}}{(\text{Height in meters})\,2}$ **OR**

$\dfrac{\text{Weight in pounds}}{(\text{Height in inches})\,2} \times 703.1$

M $=$ Height in inches $\times 0.025$

Percentage of weight change $=$

$\dfrac{\text{Usual/previous weight} - \text{Actual/current weight}}{\text{Usual/previous weight}} \times 100$

Importance of weight change:

Time Interval	Significant	Severe
1 week	1%-2%	>2%
1 month	5%	>5%
3 months	7.5%	>7.5%
6 months	10%	>10%

and the body mass index (BMI; 24 to 25 is ideal in elders) should be calculated with the initial assessment of the elder's nutritional status, then, on every visit, the client's weight should be rechecked and the percentage of change calculated. The client should be referred to the primary care provider if the percentage of change is significant or severe. The formulas for calculating the caloric needs and BMI and the standards for estimating the significance of weight change over time are in Box 35-7.

The community health nurse can begin the nutritional assessment with a 3-day diet recall and calorie count. Consider *financial* (fixed income, buying habits), *physical* (transportation, limited mobility, poor vision), and *personal barriers* (food prepa-

TABLE 35-4 HEALTH PROBLEMS AND NUTRITIONAL DEFICITS OF ELDERS

HEALTH PROBLEM	NUTRITIONAL DEFICIENCY
Resistance to infection	Protein, calories
Poor wound healing and skin friability	Vitamins A, B_6, D, E; selenium; zinc; copper, iron
Osteopenia	Protein, zinc, vitamins C and E
Anemia	Calcium, vitamins D and K, estrogen*
Cardiovascular diseases	Iron, folate, vitamin B_{12}
Cataracts, age-associated macular degeneration	Folate, Vitamins E, B_{12}; excess fat
Constipation	Zinc; selenium; vitamins A, C, E
	Water, dietary fiber

Source: Adapted from Reuben, Yoshikawa, & Besdine, 1996, p. 145.

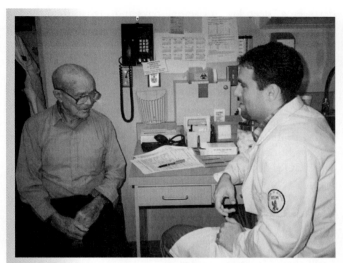

Elders are living longer than in generations past and are healthier than their predecessors.

ration, preferences, eating problems, medications). Oral assessment includes checking for ill-fitting dentures, lost teeth, periodontal disease, and the last dental visit.

The goals for nutrition are to assist elders to plan and provide a well-balanced diet with a variety of foods from each food group and maintain a desirable weight. They need to be encouraged to eat low-fat, high-fiber foods and avoid fried, fatty, concentrated sweet, and salty foods.

Nutritional services may start with shopping assistance, which can be provided by family, friends, religious groups, senior centers, and local homemaker services. Grocery stores may offer senior parking and electric shopping carts. Community services include aggregate meal sites in senior centers, Meals on Wheels, area agencies on aging, and county extension services.

For elders with limited income, stretching money to purchase both food and medications can be a challenge. They may buy easy-to-prepare "empty calorie" foods (concentrated sweets or salty snacks) rather than foods for a balanced diet. The nurse can suggest a variety of foods that will not break the budget, including dried legumes, beans, whole cereal grains, poultry, fish, dried fortified milk, less expensive cuts of meat, low-fat cheeses, yogurt, and dried instant breakfast.

The goal of weight management is to help elders approach an ideal body weight (IBW) for their age, sex, and body frame. These individuals may be involuntarily gaining or losing weight and need to stabilize their weight, or they may have a long history of being seriously overweight or underweight and now are experiencing health problems. Techniques for maintaining or improving the nutritional status of elders are suggested in Box 35-8.

Underweight

For elders who are malnourished or underweight (BMI less than 20 or more than 10% *below* IBW), the goal is to increase the calorie

---

BOX 35-8 TECHNIQUES TO MAINTAIN OR IMPROVE THE NUTRITIONAL STATUS OF ELDERS

- Maintain a vigilant watch on weight changes, gains or losses, in elders. Weigh at least once month if stable; weigh daily or weekly if significant or severe changes.
- Stimulate appetite and taste by having an attractive presentation with different textures and aromas, seasonings, switching from item to item, appropriate texture (soft for edentulous persons), oral hygiene, and appetite stimulation with a small glass of wine.
- Suggest moister, softer foods, smaller, unhurried meals, and artificial sweeteners and flavor extracts to stimulate taste.
- Use dental hygiene before and after meals; visit the dentist annually to retain natural teeth.
- Recommend a well-balanced, low-fat, low-salt, high-fiber diet, possibly with blander foods; increase fluid intake; emphasize the importance of calcium-rich foods for this age group.
- Use nutritional supplements (e.g., Ensure with Fiber, Resource Plus, Carnation Instant Breakfast) offered after or between meals two or three times daily.
- Check medications for drugs that cause anorexia and avoid drugs such as cyproheptadine (Periactin), which develop rapid tolerance and have high anticholinergic side effects in elders.
- Recommend smoke alarms because of lessened sense of smell.
- Weigh malnourished persons at least weekly.

---

intake, including daily multivitamin with mineral supplementation. Loss of smell affects taste and enjoyment; loss of appetite may be from loneliness and depression. The nurse calculates the caloric needs based on the desired weight for these elders. For example, if an 83-year-old frail man's current weight is 130 pounds; his height is 5 feet, 11 inches; and his usual body weight is 160 pounds, his caloric needs are between 1,460 (World Health Organization [WHO] formula) and 2,160 calories (estimated formula) per day.

Overweight

For elders who are obese or overweight (BMI greater than 29 or more than 20% *above* IBW), the weight management goals are to decrease calories and increase activity levels. Diets to promote weight loss generally limit intake to 1,500 to 1,800 calories per day (including daily multivitamin with mineral supplementation) with adjustments for age, sex, and body frame. The lifestyle adjustments required for weight loss are difficult to accomplish and maintain at any age, and no less so in elders. In addition to reducing amounts or eliminating certain types of foods, elders must incorporate exercise into daily routines to compensate for their reduced metabolism and achieve their weight loss goals. They are especially prone to fads and gimmicks rather than adjustment of eating and exercise patterns. Appetite suppressants should be avoided because they generally are ineffective and may have serious side effects in elders. To assist with weight loss, many nutritionally sound, holistic commercial weight loss programs (e.g., Weight Watchers) are available. Public television may offer low-impact exercise programs, such as chair aerobics. Community and religious groups also may offer weight loss and exercise programs, or the nurse can facilitate the formation of a neighborhood weight loss group. Whatever the approach, overweight elders often need weight loss programs that are relatively inexpensive, easily accessible, age appropriate, and socially supportive. Obese persons on weight loss diets also need to be weighed weekly.

Hydration

Often overlooked as part of nutrition, adequate hydration is a key factor to prevent dehydration, soften stools, increase salivation and expectoration, maintain skin and renal function, and aid in absorption of medications and high-fiber foods. Elders usually require at least 12 quarts or 1,500 ml of fluids per day, especially water. For diabetic or overweight elders or those who dislike the taste of water, sugar-free liquids (e.g., Crystal Light, Sugar Free Kool-Aid) can be encouraged.

As with infants, elders are particularly vulnerable to variations in fluid volume (overhydration or underhydration) because of their decreased cardiovascular and renal reserves. Signs of dehydration include weight loss; concentrated urine, decreased output; elevated temperature; sunken eyeballs; dry, parched, coated tongue; pallor, poor skin turgor, and dry mucous membranes. A weight loss of 2% to 4% is mild, 5% to 9% is moderate, and 10% or more is severe dehydration with danger of circulatory collapse and death. These individuals require immediate referral to their primary care provider for careful rehydration.

Sleep

Adequate periods of sleep and rest are essential for the restoration of energy in all living beings. Elderly persons commonly experience changes in both sleep pattern and sleep structure. These changes can result in initial insomnia (disturbances, difficulty falling asleep), interim insomnia (frequent awakenings), and terminal insomnia (earlier morning awakenings), or hypersomnolence (excessive sleep).

Community health nurses can prevent or intervene in many of these problems by thorough assessments of patterns of activity and rest. Consider the nature of the sleep problem by determining its onset and duration (i.e., acute, transient, or chronic [>3 weeks]). A sleep history can be obtained by having the el-

der keep a "sleep log" for several days and nights; then the log can be analyzed for patterns of wakefulness and sleep: total sleep time, total time in bed, sleep problems, day problems that interfere with sleep. The nurse should inquire about recent changes in behavior or performance and evaluate the use of caffeine (e.g., coffee, tea, cola), xanthine (e.g., chocolate), nicotine, alcohol, and medications that interfere with sleep (prescription and over-the-counter [OTC] drugs). The nurse should consider health problems that may interfere with sleep, especially pain (e.g., arthritis, heart failure, chronic obstructive pulmonary disease [COPD], gastroesophageal reflux disease [GERD], diabetes, anxiety, depression, dementia, nocturnal myoclonus, sleep apnea). Finally, the nurse should teach the client good sleep hygiene (Box 35-9).

....

I still climb Mount Everest just as often as I used to. I play polo just as often as I used to. But to walk down to the hardware store I find a little bit more difficult.
From an interview with Theodor S. Geisel, "Dr. Seuss," in the *New York Times Book Review*. Cited in *Seuss–isms: Wise and Witty Prescriptions for Living from the Good Doctor*, New York: Random House, 1997

....

Elimination

Problems with elimination can have devastating consequences for elders. Fear of "accidents" may contribute to social withdrawal and isolation. An inability to control the bladder or the bowels is a major precipitant to institutionalization. Therefore, nurses must take every opportunity to maintain elimination patterns in older adults.

Urinary Elimination

Although aging alone does not cause urinary incontinence, several age-related changes and health problems can contribute to its development (e.g., childbirth, menopause, prostate surgery, stroke). Urinary incontinence is the involuntary loss of urine severe enough to have social or hygienic consequences. The prevalence is 15% to 30% in elderly community-dwelling men and women, respectively (Reuben, Yoshikawa, & Besdine, 1996). Stress, urge, and overflow incontinence are caused by failure to store urine or empty the bladder. Functional incontinence is caused by an inability to toilet efficiently. A neurogenic bladder usually is associated with urinary retention; it often requires an indwelling catheter or intermittent catheterizations and is managed on an individual basis. As much as 80% of incontinence can be eliminated with bladder rehabilitation programs.

To assess the nature of urinary incontinence, the nurse must determine previous patterns of urination and daily activities. The nurse should ask the elder to record fluid intake and voiding patterns for at least 3 days to establish the current schedule of urination. In collaboration with the primary care provider, the nurse should determine cause, duration, and degree of incontinence. Common factors associated with this problem include medications, caffeine, and fecal impactions. For frail or confused elders, it is especially helpful to observe the level of function for toileting activities (e.g., walking, dressing, transfers, hygiene). When establishing realistic goals for urinary continence, the nurse should consider the anticipated cooperation of the elder

---

BOX 35-9 TECHNIQUES FOR SLEEP HYGIENE

- Standardize bedtime and rising time. Go to bed at the same time each night and get out of bed at the same time each morning regardless of sleep during the night. Avoid drastic shifts in sleep-wake cycle.
- Minimize daytime napping to 30 to 60 minutes in early afternoon.
- Encourage daily exercise and both daytime and evening activities with adequate exposure to bright light during the day.
- Avoid large meals and fluids within 4 hours of bedtime. Eliminate or limit caffeine, xanthines, nicotine, and alcohol, especially within 4 hours of bedtime. Avoid diuretics within 8 hours of bedtime.
- Engage in bedtime rituals (e.g., personal hygiene, toileting, relaxation activities, prayer, meditation).
- If in pain, provide comfort measures (e.g., acetaminophen 500 mg, one to two tablets HS if indicated).
- If hungry, have a light bedtime snack with milk (contains tryptophan).
- Wear comfortable sleep clothes and keep bedroom cool, clean, and quiet, with only a night light if desired. Use the bedroom only for sleep and sex (not for reading, watching television, eating, or working)
- If unable to sleep within 30 minutes, go to another room and engage in restful activities (reading, soft music, hobbies); avoid active television. Return to bed only when sleepy.
- Avoid over-the-counter drugs for sleep (especially diphenhydramine [Benadryl], which interrupts the sleep cycle, can be cumulative, and may cause delirium in elders). Avoid regular use of hypnotics (they cause interruption of sleep cycle, tolerance, and habituation); limit to three times per week.
- Consult with primary care provider concerning health problems and medications that interfere with sleep.

---

and family for bladder rehabilitation activities (e.g., total continence, daytime continence with nighttime padding).

Treatments for urinary incontinence include pelvic muscle rehabilitation (Kegel exercises, biofeedback, vaginal weight training, pelvic floor electrical stimulation), behavioral therapies (bladder training, toileting assistance), medications (oxybutynin, estrogen), and surgeries (AHCPR, 1996). Techniques for urinary incontinence in elders are summarized in Box 35-10. By working on bladder rehabilitation with these elders, their caregivers, and primary care providers, community health nurses often can prevent or minimize this condition with significant impact on overall functioning and quality of life.

Fecal Elimination

Bowel elimination has significant implications for elders' comfort and quality of life. Bowel regularity and fecal continence take on enormous significance for some elders. Common problems include diarrhea, fecal incontinence, and constipation.

Diarrhea

For diarrhea in elders, the criterion is the volume of stool per day, rather than the number or consistency of stools, which may be altered with changes in food or fluid intake but still may be within normal limits. Diarrhea can be infectious or noninfectious and is a significant cause of morbidity and mortality among those elders who are frail and more susceptible to fluid and electrolyte imbalances. This condition is prevented by scrupulous food preparation and storage, frequent handwashing, and avoidance of fecal contamination and polypharmacy. Initial assessments include onset, volume, number, consistency of stools; duration (acute versus chronic); the presence of bright red blood in the stool (hematochezia) or black, tarry stool (melena); the presence of other symptoms (e.g., abdominal cramping or distension, lassitude, thirst, nausea, vomiting, fever, malaise); diet; and medications. The nurse should evaluate the elder's general appearance, vital signs, and weight and perform an abdominal examination for pain or tenderness.

Although common diarrhea often is treated in the home (Box 35-11), any condition lasting more than 24 hours in elders should be referred to their primary care provider for evaluation and possible rehydration. The protocol for chronic diarrhea, often a part of an irritable bowel syndrome, is developed in collaboration with the primary care provider and usually includes a high-fiber diet, possibly with a bulking agent (e.g., methylcellulose or psyllium hydrophilic mucilloid [Citrucel or Metamucil]) or loperamide (Imodium A-D).

Constipation

For elders, the most common bowel problem is constipation, a difficulty in passing stools or incomplete or infrequent passage of hard stools (usually less than three per week). The usual causes of small, hard, or infrequent stools are poor bowel habits, including a lack of dietary fiber, poor fluid intake, inadequate exercise, psychological factors, and medications, often with inappropriate use

BOX 35-10 TECHNIQUES FOR BLADDER REHABILITATION IN ELDERS WITH URINARY INCONTINENCE

- Explain the nature of urinary incontinence and establish mutual goals to encourage participation and cooperation in bladder rehabilitation activities.

- Provide adequate fluid intake, at least 1,500 ml/day, to dilute urine and minimize bladder and skin irritation and odor.

- Check for medications that precipitate incontinence (e.g., diuretics) and give them early in the day. Check caffeine use (e.g., coffee, tea, colas) and reduce or eliminate (switch to decaffeinated beverages).

- When usual voiding times have been established, prompt the elder to toilet 2 hours before these times, usually hourly at first, then every 2 hours, and finally every 3 hours if tolerated. Encourage the elder to void before meals, after naps, before bed, and before any special activities, such as walks or outings. Advance times only when the elder is successful during shorter periods of continence for several days.

- Encourage the elder to empty the bladder completely at each voiding by leaning forward and gently pushing down with abdominal muscles (Crede maneuver).

- Observe the amounts of urine voided (i.e., bladder capacity). If the quantity is very large, schedule more frequent visits to the toilet; or if it is very small, schedule less frequent voiding.

- For women with stress incontinence, teach Kegel exercises to help recondition pelvic muscle and improve sphincter control. With the woman on the toilet, instruct her to stop the flow of urine for a few seconds; repeat several times. When she has learned to interrupt her flow of urine, have her execute the same contractions while sitting in a chair, starting with 5 repetitions and advancing to 10 repetitions held for 5 seconds, with each set done four or more times a day. An alternate activity is to contract and relax successively the urethral, vaginal, and rectal sphincter muscles in the same manner described above.

- For urge incontinence, once on the commode, teach elders to hold back the urine as long as possible by tightening the pelvic musculature.

- If elders are confused, demented, or demonstrate anxious behavior, check them frequently for the need to void. During activities, place elders nearest the bathroom and remove barriers in their path.

- Encourage the elder and family to use incontinence pads (*not* diapers!), such as Attends or Depends, to promote dryness until continence is reestablished. These products are not much more bulky than regular underwear and can be worn with confidence under everyday clothing. If skin breakdown is a problem, coat the perineum with a thin layer of petroleum or zinc oxide ointment (e.g., Vaseline, A&D Ointment, or Desitin).

- Monitor rehabilitation activities daily and evaluate them at least weekly until a voiding pattern is established. Check for dryness and odor, use of toilet for voiding, skin integrity, and self-concept. Encourage the elder frequently, praise successes, reinforce teaching frequently, and do not permit discouragement when accidents occur. Reconditioning of the bladder may require several weeks, but with patience and persistence it usually is successful.

BOX 35-11 TECHNIQUES FOR COMMON DIARRHEA IN ELDERS

- Place the bowel at rest for 36 to 72 hours. Give clear liquids for the first 12 to 24 hours, full liquids or soft diet for next 24 to 48 hours, then regular diet as tolerated. Maintain adequate hydration (1,500 to 2,000 ml/day).

- Give an over-the-counter antidiarrheal agent:
  - Absorbent agents (Kaopectate) 15 to 30 ml every 4 to 6 hours prn loose stool × 24 hr OR

  - Bismuth subsalicylate (Pepto-Bismol) 15 to 30 ml every 4 to 6 hours prn loose stool × 24 hr OR

  - Opioid (Imodium AD) two 2-mg tables initially, then one tablet prn loose stool × 24 hr (maximum, 16 mg/day).

- Teach elder to avoid irritating foods.

- If not improved in 24 hours, refer to primary care provider for prompt evaluation.

of laxatives. Common complications are fecal impaction and fecal incontinence.

To assess the nature of constipation, the nurse must determine previous patterns of previous bowel habits and daily activity patterns. The nurse should ask the elder to record food and fluid intake (noting dietary fiber and free water) and bowel movements (frequency, timing, difficulty) for at least 3 days. The elder's general physical and mental condition should be evaluated, and if the client is frail or confused, the nurse should observe the level of function for toileting activities (e.g., walking, dressing, transfers, hygiene). The nurse must consider possible associated factors (e.g., medications, fecal impactions, illnesses) and make referral to primary care provider if indicated. When setting goals for bowel elimination, the nurse should consider anticipated cooperation of the elder and family for bowel rehabilitation activities. By working with these elders, their caregivers, and primary care providers, community health nurses often can prevent and intervene with a bowel rehabilitation including a high-fiber diet, adequate fluids, daily exercise, and elimination of laxatives (Box 35-12).

BOX 35-12 TECHNIQUES FOR BOWEL REHABILITATION IN ELDERS WITH CONSTIPATION

- Explain the nature of constipation and establish mutual goals to encourage participation and cooperation in bowel rehabilitation activities.

- Encourage a high-fiber diet that adds bulk to stool. This diet usually starts with high-fiber cereals (i.e., more than 10 gm of dietary fiber per serving, such as All Bran, Bran Buds, 100% Bran, or Fiber One), and/or supplemental wheat bran (miller's bran) 1 to 4 tablespoons per day added to moist foods (e.g., cereals, grits, oatmeal, cream of wheat, applesauce, soup, cottage cheese, ice cream). Vegetables and fruits also add bulk to stools (e.g., at least 5 servings per day of green leafy vegetables, raw fruits, vegetables).

- Provide adequate fluids to make the stool softer and easier to pass. Include at least $1/2$ to 2 quarts (1,500 to 2,000 ml) of fluids per day, unless contraindicated (see Hydration, p. 810).

- Encourage exercise daily to promote circulation to the bowel and stimulate evacuation. For example, walk at least 1 mile per day, ride a stationary bicycle or swim for at least 30 minutes per day, unless contraindicated (see Critical Thinking Activities).

- Establish a regular evacuation time to correspond with daily activities or family lifestyle patterns. Defecation is a learned, conditioned response that generally occurs at the same time each day. Most elders prefer an early morning time for bowel evacuation, but if scheduling of family activities in the morning precludes sufficient time for bowel hygiene, an evening bowel program is recommended (i.e., after supper and before bathing).

- Start the bowel program with a clean bowel (i.e., give a laxative or enema if necessary). For 3 consecutive days, insert a bisacodyl (Dulcolax) suppository into the rectum approximately 30 minutes before the established evacuation time. Wait 30 minutes, then assist the elder to the toilet with a book or magazine to promote relaxation. Another approach is to use 1 to 3 tablespoons of an osmotic agent (lactulose or sorbitol) daily for 3 to 5 days to get a bowel pattern established. Stool softeners (e.g., docusate [Colace, Dialose]) generally are ineffective for constipation in elders.

- Absolutely avoid laxatives, especially the long-term use of stimulant laxatives with phenolphthalein (i.e., Correctol, Ex-Lax, Feen-a-Ment) because of their blunting of natural evacuation and purging of the bowel. A daily bowel movement is not necessary, but avoid going for more than 3 days without defecation. If no BM occurs in 2 days, use a bisacodyl (Dulcolax) suppository. If no BM occurs in 3 days, use a phosphate (Fleets) enema. If the enema is not successful, use 1 ounce (30 ml) of Milk of Magnesia to get the bowels restarted. Daily osmotic agents may be needed; consult primary caregiver

- Observe the consistency of stools (i.e., normal, soft, hard, or watery). If stools are hard or painful, increase the water intake. If stools are small or scant, increase the bulk with dietary fiber. Recommend a stool softener, such as docusate (e.g., Colase, Dialose) only if needed because of hemorrhoids or other rectal problems.

- Monitor rehabilitation activities daily and evaluate them at least weekly until a bowel pattern is established. Check for constipation, use of the toilet for defecation, fecal impaction, skin integrity, and self-concept. If relapses occur, restart the program with suppositories for 3 days. Encourage the elder frequently, praise successes, reinforce teaching frequently, and do not permit discouragement when accidents occur. Reconditioning of the bowel may require several weeks to overcome years of poor bowel habits, but with patience and persistence it usually is successful.

Mobility and Communication

The ability to move about the environment is crucial for independent living. The ability to communicate one's thoughts and feelings to others is essential for well-being. Therefore, nurses must take an active role in maintenance of mobility and communication in elderly individuals striving to remain in the community.

Mobility

Adequate mobility is critical for elders to maintain their functional independence. Even brief periods of immobility can lead to rapid deconditioning and loss of flexibility and strength in elders increasing the risk of falls and injury. Conversely, daily exercise helps the elder to prevent diseases (e.g., osteoporosis, arterial/venous insufficiency, gastrointestinal stasis, musculoskeletal stiffness, coronary heart disease, obesity, stroke, depression, anxiety, dementia); improve sleep, mobility, strength, flexibility, and mood; increase life expectancy; and improve quality of life. Community health nurses can encourage elders to exercise individually, with families, or in groups.

BOX 35-13 TECHNIQUES FOR EXERCISE AND MOBILITY IN ELDERS

- Explain to the elder and family the benefits of an exercise program, and set mutual, realistic goals to encourage participation and cooperation in physical rehabilitation activities. It is important to emphasize functional independence rather than an arbitrary physical goal (e.g., the ability to walk to the bathroom unassisted rather than to walk 100 feet).

- Maximize visual and hearing functions by referral to an ophthalmologist and/or otologist and wearing corrective glasses and/or hearing aids (see Sensory Integrity, p. 806).

- In collaboration with the primary care provider, evaluate medication regime for drugs that alter cardiovascular function, impair central nervous system function, interact, and polypharmacy, and simplify the drug regime by eliminating all nonessential drugs.

- Check footwear for proper fit and condition. Athletic shoes with shock absorbent soles and good support are ideal for an exercise program; shoes with Velcro closures are more easily managed by elders with hand problems. Check clothing for comfort and fit. Athletic apparel (e.g., cotton fleece or windbreakers) is designed for maximum movement, comfort, and convenience, if acceptable to the elder.

- In collaboration with the primary care provider, refer to a physical therapist or rehabilitation facility for correction of major physical decrements (i.e., stroke, arthritis).

- Provide for gait retraining through a program of physical exercise, basically walking outside or at a covered mall for at least 30 to 60 minutes per day for at least 5 to 6 days per week. *Start low, go slow* with regular, low impact, unstressed, but progressive exercise. Begin with a distance the elder can manage (e.g., 100 feet or $1/4$ mile); increase the distance at weekly intervals until the elder is walking 1 to 2 miles, then gradually increase the speed until a comfortable cadence is achieved (i.e., mild perspiration, increased respiratory and pulse rate). Alternatively, use stationary exercise machines, bicycling, swimming, or low impact aerobic, strengthening, flexibility programs (Tai Chi, YMCA/YWCA, fitness centers, community parks, senior programs, senior Olympics). Exercise is better maintained if done with a partner (spouse, friend) at the same time every day.

- Use assistive devices (e.g., straight cane, four-pronged cane, or walker) for balance and support, and/or support stockings for venous return. Check these devices for proper fit and safety, including nonskid tips on canes and walkers.

- Use mild analgesics for relief of soreness, aches, and pains. Acetaminophen, one or two 500-mg tablets for up to four times a day, is recommend over aspirin or ibuprofen, which have increased side effects in elders. Taking analgesics 30 minutes before exercise may minimize discomforts from deconditioning.

- Encourage the use of adaptive behaviors (e.g., rising slowly, using rails or furniture for balance) to minimize the risk of falls and, when appropriate, teach techniques for falling and getting up after a fall to minimize complications.

- Avoid physical restraints that actually increase, rather than decrease, falls injuries, and compound immobility.

- Monitor the exercise program daily and evaluate at least weekly for improvement in muscle strength, flexibility, and gait stability. Check for orthostatic hypotension, falls, pain, motivation, and self-concept. Encourage elders frequently, praise successes, reinforce teaching frequently, and do not permit discouragement when problems occur. Reconditioning of muscles may require several weeks or months, but with patience and persistence some progress will be made.

Impaired mobility in elders usually involves multiple factors, including an initial physical deficit (i.e., fractured hip or degenerative joint disease), compounded by a sedentary lifestyle, deconditioning, inadequate daily exercise patterns, sensory impairment (i.e., vision and hearing), confusion, inappropriate medications, improper assistive devices, and/or environmental hazards. To assess the mobility of elders, the nurse must determine previous types and levels of exercise and daily activity patterns, any history of activity-related injuries and falls, and possible associated factors influencing mobility (e.g., medications, confusion, illnesses). The nurse should then evaluate the elder's general physical and mental condition, food and fluid intake, environmental safety, and availability of assistive devices and observe the level of function for physical activities (e.g., posture, gait, balance, strength, endurance). When establishing a program for exercise or physical rehabilitation, the nurse should consider the anticipated cooperation of the elder and family for physical activities and address the physical deficits as well as contributing factors (Box 35-13).

Falls

Accidents are the fifth leading cause of death among elders, and falls account for two-thirds of these deaths. Seventy percent of fall injuries are in persons older than 75; 50% of those hospitalized do not survive for 1 year. Fear of falling further inhibits many elders from performing activities that would prevent falls (e.g., exercise) and contributes to functional decline, depression, helplessness, and social isolation. Falls result from environmental hazards, deconditioning, sensory deficits, and impaired central processing. The best prevention for falls is a combination of rehabilitative, environmental, and behavioral strategies. For example, correcting vision, using assistive devices, installing bathroom grab bars, and initiating a progressive exercise program that emphasizes conditioning of the lower extremities all help reduce the occurrence of falls.

Osteoporosis

A multifactorial disease of increased skeletal fragility, **osteoporosis** places elders at risk of fractures during activities of daily living. Postmenopausal women are affected initially, but men also are subject to senile bone loss. With a bone mineral density more than 2.5 standard deviations below young normals, the vertebral bodies, proximal femur, and distal radius are common fracture sites. In collaboration with primary care providers, community health nurses can assist with preventive strategies for osteoporosis (Box 35-14).

Communication

Other than slower speech, verbal communication usually is unaffected by aging. The most common causes of language disorders in elders are strokes and dementia resulting in some form of aphasia. Strategies for improving communication are summarized in Box 35-15.

BOX 35-14 PREVENTION OF OSTEOPOROSIS IN ELDERS

- Establish a daily exercise program.
- Encourage dietary intake of calcium (1,200 to 1,500 mg/day) with dairy products (milk, cheese, yogurt) and/or calcium supplementation 500 mg tid with meals (e.g., Tums 500, Oscal).
- Encourage dietary intake of vitamin D (400 to 800 IU/day) and/or supplementation with multivitamin with minerals once or twice daily.
- In collaboration with primary care provider, consider estrogen replacement therapy, selective estrogen receptor modulators, or bone density enhancers.
- On sunny days, try to sit outside for 2 to 3 hours (avoiding 11 AM to 2 PM) to enhance vitamin D intake.

Cognition and Affect

Because people are sentient beings, attention, memory, and emotion are integral with personal identity, environmental adaptation, and quality of life. Changes in cognitive abilities may be stereotyped as "senility" and either minimized or maximized by elders and family members. Altered mood and emotional responses may further confound the situation. Impaired cognition and affect may exhaust family resources and precipitate relocation from the home to a long-term care facility. Therefore, nurses can assist elders to remain independent in their own environments by being sensitive to cognitive and affective changes.

BOX 35-15 TECHNIQUES FOR SPEECH IMPAIRED ELDERS

- Reduce environmental distractions (radios, television) before engaging the elder in conversation.
- Gain the elder's attention and maintain eye contact.
- Speak slowly and use a simple vocabulary with short sentences; ask simple yes/no questions.
- If the elder does not respond, repeat the question with the same wording.
- Encourage the elder to say one word at a time; if unable to say a word, substitute another word.
- Praise successes. If unable to complete a thought, avoid appearing frustrated; take a break, then try again.

Cognition

Cognitive functioning changes very little with normal aging. Intelligence is unchanged, and with the wisdom gathered from life experience, problem solving often is improved. Memory involves pattern recognition and is declarative (factual, "what") and procedural (process, "how"). With diminished attention and immediate recall, elders may have some declarative memory loss (forgetfulness), but procedural memory usually is not affected. Learning, which depends on memory, also is undisturbed but is slower. Performance may be slower but often is more precise.

Confusion is a common problem in some elders and may result from alterations in sensory or central processing. The most common causes of confusion are delirium, dementia, and depression.

Delirium

Acute confusional state (**delirium**) is a physiological state that usually is reversible and is characterized as an altered level of consciousness, disorganized thinking (incoherent speech, repetitive speech and behavior), with a rapid onset and fluctuating course; it is often worse at night and has an underlying medical cause (e.g., pneumonia, urinary tract infection, fecal impaction, septicemia). Prevention involves adequate oxygenation, hydration, nutrition, elimination, sensory stimulation, exercise, and avoidance of certain medications.

Dementia

Age-associated memory impairment is the mild, gradual deterioration in memory performance, speed of cognitive processing, and executive functions that accompanies normal aging and does not interfere with activities or relationships. **Dementia** is "a syndrome of progressive decline that relentlessly erodes intellectual abilities, causing cognitive function deterioration leading to impairment of social and occupational functioning" (AHCPR, 1996, p. 1). Dementia occurs in 5% of persons age 65, a rate that doubles every 5 years after age 65, and affects almost 50% of persons 85 or older. This cognitive impairment is irreversible, has an insidious onset, and is stable over time, with progressive amnesia (loss of memory), aphasia (loss of language), agnosia (loss of object recognition), apraxia (loss of motor function), and loss of executive function (abstract thinking and complex behavior). **Alzheimer's disease** is a cortical degeneration that accounts for 80% of dementia. Most elders with mild or moderate dementia live at home and are cared for by family members. Community health nurses can assist with early case finding and referral to a primary care provider or specialist (geriatrician, neuropsychologist, or psychiatrist). Assessment includes elimination of reversible causes (e.g., drugs, depression, delirium, thyroid dysfunction, vitamin B_{12} deficiency). Cognitive functioning is screened with mental status examinations, which test orientation, memory, attention, language, and praxis.

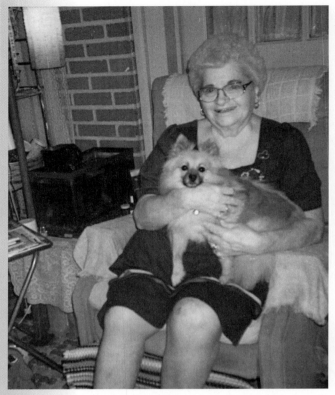

Pets are often very important to elders who live alone.

The basic principles for working with elders who have cognitive deficits are to *simplify the environment*, *provide structure* for daily activities, *minimize changes* in that structure, and when changes are necessary, *prepare for changes* well in advance. The goals of cognitive behavioral programs are to help elders maintain their highest level of function, enable them to continue living at home, and offer support to caregivers. These programs are based on strengths, areas of deficit, and realistic goals for their living situations. Strategies for the management of dementia are summarized in Box 35-16.

Affect

Self-concept evolves from what persons think and feel about themselves, what they think and feel about others, and what they think and feel others think and feel about them (Satir, 1964). Assurance of personal worth is based on feeling valued, useful, and competent. Old age is accompanied by many epoch events—retirement, altered health, relocation of home, deaths of family and friends, and finally one's own transition from life to death. With the frequent, multiple losses associated with old age, elders may experience feelings of powerlessness, hopelessness, and spiritual distress. These feelings may result in anxiety, fear, and anger or depression.

BOX 35-16 STRATEGIES FOR MANAGEMENT OF DEMENTIA IN ELDERS

- Structure time/place. Use daily and weekly schedules that provide consistency, predictability, and repetition. Structure and simplify activities of daily living, family activities, specific tasks, and the environment to maximize ability with less clutter, complexity, and hurry. For example, activities are done in the same order and at the same times and places each day (e.g., arise at 7:00, breakfast at 7:30); certain activities are done on the same days of the week every week (e.g., bathe on Tuesday and Saturday, laundry on Monday).

- Anticipate change. Known events, such as holidays and family gatherings, are anticipated several weeks in advance, mentioning every day the names of people who will be involved and using photos, stories, or other aids to familiarize the elder with the anticipated situation. Persons with cognitive deficits can learn, but the key is repetition—as many as 7 × 7 times!

- Modify the environment. Reorganize the elder's living situation to compensate for sensory and functional impairments. Use memory aids (e.g., clocks, calendars, simple written cues) for orientation and identification of items and places. Keep the environment as simple and uncluttered as possible. Avoid situations that stress intellectual capabilities. For those with early dementia, newspapers, television, telephone calls, and e-mail may be helpful. For those with severe dementia, security devices and electronic monitoring may be indicated. Recommend identification jewelry, photo ID, and current photos; suggest Medialert or the Alzheimer's Association Safe Return Program (800-272-3900).

- Manage problem behaviors. Analyze each behavioral problem in three parts:

  A **A**ntecedents (what happens before to trigger or cause the behavior)

  B **B**ehavior (what specific actions can be seen and described)

  C **C**onsequences (what happens after or because of the behavior)

- Develop a plan to either avoid or prevent problem behaviors by changing either the antecedents or the consequences of the behavior. Avoid catastrophic reactions by minimizing the common antecedents (too much too fast, fatigue).

- Support caregivers. Because persons with dementia may not be able to change as a result of their illness, the caregivers have to be the ones to change. Altering problem behaviors is not easy, and not every attempt will be successful. If the plan isn't working, look at the situation again and try another approach. Be flexible and willing to try new approaches as the elder changes over time. Reward successes, no matter how small. Remember to laugh.

- Provide information and referral: Contact the Alzheimer's Association (919 North Michigan Ave., Suite 1000, Chicago, IL 60611; 800-272-3900), Alzheimer's Disease Education and Referral (ADEAR), area Agency on Aging, community mental health centers, and/or Internet groups.

- Community-based care: adult day centers, home health agencies.

- Caregiver burden: caregivers classes, support groups, respite care.

- Long-term care: personal care/assisted living homes, skilled care nursing homes.

Depression

The most common disturbance of mood experienced by elders is **depression**. Prevalence varies by setting: 5% to 20% in community-dwelling elders, 25% in hospitalized elders, and 40% in nursing home residents (AHCPR, 1993). Its presentation may differ from younger populations, with somatic complaints being more likely in elders than emotional statements about guilt, anger, or depressed mood. The cause may be exogenous (situational), resulting from poor finances, disability, bereavement, loneliness, or social isolation; or endogenous (biochemical), resulting from physical illnesses, pain, or medications; or both. Among community-dwelling elders, depression can be clinical (1%) or subsyndromal (15%) (Reuben, Yoshikwa, & Besdine, 1996).

The assessment of depression in elders requires information from the elder and family members. New physical complaints or exacerbations of previous pain, gastrointestinal symptoms, cardiovascular symptoms, preoccupation with poor health or physical limitations, diminished interest in pleasurable activities, sleep disturbances, fatigue, poor concentration, patchy memory loss, and expressions of negativism should be noted. The Geriatric Depression Scale should be administered and the elder referred to a primary care provider as indicated by assessments. In collaboration with the primary care provider, the nurse should

BOX 35-17 STRATEGIES FOR MANAGEMENT OF DEPRESSION IN ELDERS

- Offer unconditional positive regard for the changes of aging and altered function.
- Emphasize with the elder and family that depression is very manageable and reversible; offer hope.
- Encourage the elder to maintain control over self and the situation by offering choices for simple decision making.
- Assist the elder to identify positive aspects of the situation and opportunities for gains as well as losses.
- In collaboration with primary care provider, encourage the use of medications, psychotherapy, and exercise to treat the depression.

BOX 35-18 STRATEGIES FOR PREVENTION OF SUICIDE IN ELDERS AT RISK

- Reduce the immediate danger of self-harm by removing hazardous articles.
- Refer any potentially suicidal elder promptly to their primary care provider (same day). Provide a constant companion (family, friend) in route.
- Extract a promise from the elder not to attempt suicide before the agreed intervention (e.g., clinic visit, your next visit).
- Mobilize resources by restoring a sense of control, reconnecting the elder with significant others, and developing lifelines of support systems and community resources.
- Follow up with regular calls on the elder and maintenance of support systems.

check for physical problems and medications that cause depression. Interventions for depression are summarized in Box 35-17.

Suicide among elders

With the prevalence of depression among elders, it is not surprising that they have the highest suicide rate of any demographic group. Suicides among elders are characterized by physical illnesses and functional losses rather than the problems with employment, finances, and family relations that are more common among younger adults. Completed suicides more often are by men (60%); attempted suicides more often are by women (75%). The methods include guns, hanging, drug overdose, and cutting or slashing. Threats are real, and first attempts usually are successful. Half to two-thirds of victims see primary care providers in the month before the suicide; 10% to 40% have seen providers within 1 week of their death (Reuben, Yoshikawa, & Besdine, 1996). These visits represent a cry for help and provide a window of opportunity to intervene. More insidious sui-

CASE STUDY

Martha Miller is a 72-year-old widow who has lived alone for 12 years. She has four grown children, two who live in a nearby town and two who live in a distant state. Mrs. Miller has a history of coronary artery disease and hypertension that is controlled with medication. She is unemployed and living on social security and a small pension from her deceased husband. Two weeks ago, Mrs. Miller was involved in a collision while making a left turn at an intersection near her home. She was not injured except for some bruising of her right arm and shoulder. She was evaluated by her family physician immediately after the accident and sent home with instructions to rest and take Tylenol for any discomfort. However, her car, which she had recently purchased, was sent to the garage for exten-

sive repairs. Since the accident, Mrs. Miller has not left the house and calls one of her children every day crying. She is not eating or sleeping well and says she is not able to live alone any longer. One of her children calls the agency where you work to ask for assistance and you are sent to assess Mrs. Miller in home and make a recommendation for action.

1. What kind of information are you seeking regarding Mrs. Miller's condition?

2. What kind of assessment data would you collect?

3. Can you think of any specific assessment tools that might be appropriate to use in this situation?

4. Just from the information you have received before your visit, what do you think might be some issues Mrs. Miller is dealing with?

cide activities used by elders include a refusal to eat, take medications, or follow simple safety procedures and the overuse of alcohol and drugs.

Nurses must consider the potential for suicide in any elders who are depressed or exhibit negativism and hopelessness. Elders fear loneliness, abandonment, loss of control, and pain, but they do not always fear death. Incidence of suicide is higher among elders who are white, male, Protestant, or widowed; they often live alone, have financial problems, have a history of alcoholism, and have poor health, especially a recent diagnosis of terminal illness. The nurse must not hesitate to inquire about suicidal fantasies and ideation. Such questions do not increase the likelihood of suicidal behavior. If these thoughts are present, the nurse should ask directly about plans, method, and means. Behavioral clues such as getting personal affairs in order, giving away possessions, making wills and funeral arrangements, self-neglect, erratic behavior, suspiciousness, hoarding of pills, and personality changes must be attended. Community health nurses have unique opportunities for suicide prevention through early case finding and enrichment of resources and support systems (Box 35-18).

Employment and Retirement

Approximately 12% of older adults are employed or actively seeking employment, 7% men and 5% women, with an increasing trend toward women working in their later years. Of these working elders, more than 50% work part-time (often without benefits) and 24% are self-employed (U.S. Bureau of the Census, 1991). With a life expectancy of 20 years at age 65, transition from work into retirement, a 20th century phenomenon, is the major normative event of the second half of life. Issues for retirement planning include financial security; role restructuring; location; new or part-time careers; educational, recreational, and leisure activities; and relationships with family and friends. With the loss of a formal work role and more leisure time, many elders enjoy volunteering with community agencies or programs such as the Retired Senior Volunteer Program (RSVP) through the local area agency on aging. They also pursue lifelong learning through community education programs through schools (including high school equivalency programs), colleges, and universities, and Elderhostel programs throughout the world. Travel around the country or abroad also may be an option.

By being aware of the meanings of *work* and *play* for elders, community health nurses can be alert for the problems that may arise during these transition periods. For those who are able to redefine themselves with meaningful activities, the latter stages of life can be times for achieving ego integrity (Erikson, 1963) and self-actualization (Maslow, 1968) through lifelong learning and creativity. For those who are unable to make these transitions, old age may become a time of loneliness, hopelessness, and boredom. Quality of life rather than quantity of life becomes the issue. Mastery of the past is the basis for adaptation to the present and hope for the future. Family, friends, and faith are integral with self-concept and spirituality.

Nurses can help alert elders to the characteristics and normality of aging and the **life review** process to find purpose in life (Ebersole & Hess, 1998). Interventions to facilitate these transitions are summarized in Box 35-19. For frail and/or demented elders, programs are needed to combat the plagues of loneliness, boredom, and helplessness in nursing homes by using companionship, variety, and helpfulness. The integration of resident animals, abundant plants, children, and community activities into this environment makes it a more human habitat. For example, a nursing home may adopt suitable dogs and cats from animal shelters, sponsor a scout troop, offer their meeting rooms for local gardener groups, and provide summer day camps for children.

Sexuality

Aging is no deterrent to the need for love and belongingness. The desire for intimacy usually is with one's own generation (spouse, partner, friend), rather than with previous generations (parents) or subsequent generations (children). Elders in any community

---

BOX 35-19 STRATEGIES FOR LATE LIFE TRANSITIONS

- Encourage spontaneous reminiscence and life review that provide opportunities for elders and their families to recapture events in their lives, for elders to create material and/or symbolic legacies, and for families to develop their family and cultural heritage.

- Facilitate connections between past hopes, present events, and future expectations. Support the elder's spiritual belief system. Confront conflicts and anxiety regarding death, guilt, and dependency; instill a sense of hope.

- Use an eclectic approach with counseling, coaching, and listening based on individual situations. Be a dependable confidant, and be aware that life review may be carried out sporadically over several months or years.

- Recommend motivation and remotivation, purpose in life, or validation therapies for frail and/or demented elders.

- Avoid stereotyping and premature closures by elders, families, and caregivers, including nurses.

- Suggest age-appropriate social, recreational, and diversional activities with family and peers to establish support systems and prevent social isolation (e.g., volunteerism, educational programs, 50 Plus, RSVP, civic and religious groups, senior citizens centers).

BOX 35-20 SAFETY PRECAUTIONS FOR ELDERS

- Check to see that stairs are well lighted, free of clutter, and have nonskid surface and handrails.
- Check bathrooms for handrails, nonslip adhesive surfaces in tubs/showers, nonslip flooring.
- Provide rooms with adequate, nonglare lighting; eliminate clutter and throw rugs, casters on chairs, dangling cords, waxed floors. Avoid sedation with narcotics and sedatives. Use carbon monoxide and smoke detectors.
- Provide for easy access to the local emergency system, including telephone numbers. If frail and/or homebound, suggest "Friendly Caller" or lifeline services.
- Encourage defensive driving; suggest the local AARP mature/defensive driving program.
- Recommend identification jewelry (i.e., bracelet or necklace) and current photo identification.
- When accidents occur, investigate for specific information on location, time, environmental factors, and intervene to prevent their recurrence.

setting need social interactions with their peers. Their sexual expressions may take a variety of forms, including touching, holding, kissing, fondling, petting, and intercourse, and as with other age groups, these expressions may be heterosexual or homosexual. For older adults living with children or in institutions, nurses may need to facilitate their needs for privacy and intimacy. For those with no spouse or partner, masturbation or fantasy may be alternatives. As with any age group, sexually active elders are at risk for sexually transmitted diseases (STDs), including human immunodeficiency virus (HIV) and acquired immunodeficiency syndrome (AIDS). The PLISSIT model (Permission, Limited Information, Specific Suggestions, Intensive Therapy) is helpful for assessing and intervening in sexual problems with elders (Annon, 1976). For example, nurses can support the sexuality of elders indirectly by saying gently that romance does not end at a certain age and wonder if the person has any questions or concerns in this area (get permission to discuss sexuality). If men indicate a problem, the nurse should ask them more directly, but tactfully, if they are having problems with erections or intercourse; if women indicate a problem, the nurse should ask about lubrication; both should be asked about satisfaction and what they want to do about it. The nurse should provide limited information and make specific suggestions for simple problems (e.g., mild analgesia and alternate positions for painful joints), then make referrals to a primary care provider for intensive therapy as indicated.

Safety and Security

As an aspect of work and play, safety for elders is concerned with accidental injuries in the home and community, especially from falls, fires, and motor vehicle accidents. Older adults with generalized weakness, slow reaction time, unstable gait, visual changes, hearing loss, and multiple medications are at greater risk for accidents and crime. Unfortunately, their vulnerability makes them frequent targets of purse snatchings, pickpocketing, fraud (e.g., fraudulent claims, confidence games, medical quackery), theft, vandalism, and harassment. Community health nurses need to assess home safety to eliminate hazards (see Appendix G), teach elders and caregivers basic safety measures, and advocate for greater safety in the community. Safety precautions for elders are summarized in Box 35-20.

Thermal Regulation and Skin Integrity

With less efficient thermal regulation, elders are at higher risk for health problems during temperature extremes. As the largest organ in the body, the skin of elderly people undergoes many age-related changes and is subject to serious complications. Nurses are at the forefront of preventive health care for both thermal regulation and skin integrity.

Thermal Regulation

Internal body temperature is a balance of cellular metabolism, muscle activity, and heat loss by radiation, convection, and evaporation through the skin (Ebersole & Hess, 1998). The ability to feel heat and cold is impaired in elders, and their return to core body temperature in response to heating or cooling is twice as long as in their youth. Drugs such as sedative-hypnotics, phenothiazines, and alcohol may further impair thermoregulatory mechanisms (Reuben, Yoshikawa, & Besdine, 1996). Fear of costly utility bills may decrease their use of air conditioning or heating systems during extreme temperatures. These factors place community-dwelling elders at high risk for hypothermia and hyperthermia during very hot and cold weather. Community health nurses can help prevent life-threatening emergencies by encouraging elders and families to check homes for insulation and caulking to maintain heat and cool. Assistance with fuel costs, which is available in most states, also may be needed. Nurses can help establish "buddy" systems among family, friends, and neighbors for daily checks on elders during weather extremes. A low threshold of suspicion should be used for referrals of at-risk elders to primary care providers or emergency care centers.

Hypothermia

Elders produce less heat per kilogram of body weight. They usually have decreased muscle mass and subcutaneous fat, reduced muscle activity, and less efficient shivering. Their vasoconstriction response of the skin arterioles to cooling is diminished, so heat within the body is not conserved. They are less able to discriminate temperature differences and may have delayed perception of being cold. These age-related changes contribute to an increased risk of hypothermia in elders when indoor temperatures are below 65°F. Symptoms of hypothermia include a body temperature of 95°F (96°F rectal) or below, cold to touch, absent shivering and piloerection, slow capillary refill, pallor or cyanosis, bradypnea, arrhythmia and bradycardia, hypotension, slurred speech, and lethargy. Treatment requires slow warming and may require hospitalization for metabolic imbalances if cooling is prolonged or extreme. See Box 35-21 for techniques to prevent hypothermia.

Hyperthermia

The vasodilation response of the arterioles to heating is diminished in elders so that heat is not delivered to the skin for dissipation. A greater threshold temperature is needed to initiate perspiration and less sweat is produced in response to heating. Elders also are less sensitive to thirst. Individuals with cardiovascular and peripheral vascular diseases, diabetes, and infections, as well as those taking certain medications (e.g., anticholinergics, antihistamines, diuretics, β-blockers, antidepressants, antiparkinsonian drugs), are at risk for hyperthermia. The three types of hyperthermic emergencies are heat syncope, heat exhaustion, and heat stroke. Symptoms include increased body temperature (especially 105°F and above), flushed skin, tachypnea, tachycardia, headache, weakness, and seizures. Suggested techniques to prevent hyperthermia in elders are listed in Box 35-21.

Skin Integrity

With increased elasticity and decreased surface acidity, dryness of the epidermis (xerosis), thinning of the dermis, and loss of subcutaneous fat, skin integrity is an ever-present potential problem in this age group. Skin also has strong symbolic significance and influence on self-esteem. Some elders feel "untouchable" as they experience the wrinkling associated with aging. Gentle touch on the hand, arm, or shoulder helps establish contact with many elders. Nurses need to inspect the skin during any clinical encounter or procedure to check for the many skin disorders of elders (e.g., pruritus [itching], urticaria, intertrigo, seborrheic dermatitis and keratosis, rosacea, psoriasis); several skin cancers are common in elders (e.g., actinic keratoses [precancerous], basal cell and squamous cell carcinomas, melanomas). The nurse should check skin lesions for the ABCD of cancers: Asymmetry, irregular Boarder, multiple Colors, Diameter greater than 1 cm; positive findings should be reported to the primary care provider. Lacerations (especially skin tears), abrasions, and pressure ulcers also are common. Maintenance of skin integrity can be accomplished by limiting bathing (i.e., two to three times a week in warm weather, once or twice a week in cold weather), liberally using emollients (e.g., Eucerin lotion, Vaseline ointment), and avoiding direct sun exposure (i.e., wearing protective clothing or sunscreens). Bath oils should be avoided because they may exacerbate skin problems and increase the risk of falls; water softeners and perineal wipes often are too harsh for the thin skin of elders and should be avoided.

Pressure ulcers

Maintenance of skin integrity and prevention of pressure ulcers requires ever-present vigilance of elders, family caregivers, and nurses in the community. As with other age groups, skin problems are prevented with adequate nutrition and avoidance of pressure, friction, shear, and moisture (AHCPR, 1992). Individuals most at risk are immobile, incontinent, malnourished, frail, or confused. With elders who are confined to bed or wheelchairs, the most common sites of pressure ulcers are the ischium (24%), sacrum (23%), trochanters (15%), heels (35%), and malleolus (7%). Community health nurses can help prevent these painful, costly, and life-threatening complications by being systematic, comprehensive, and routine about skin care. Two instruments often used for assessment of risk factors are the Braden Scale for predicting pressure sore risk and the Norton Risk Assessment

BOX 35-22 TECHNIQUES TO PREVENT PRESSURE ULCERS IN ELDERS

- Teach elders and family members to inspect the skin daily, especially the sacrum, hips, and heels. Use a hand mirror for pressure sites not easily seen. Nurses directly observe the skin of vulnerable elders on *every* visit.

- Improve skin tolerance to pressure by cleansing vulnerable areas with mild soap; avoid hot water and excessive friction. Treat dry skin with moisturizers or emollients. Avoid massage over bony prominences.

- Minimize exposure to moisture. Check persons with incontinence at least every 2 hours, clean the skin, and change clothing or pads immediately. Use topical moisture barriers if necessary.

- While in bed, absolutely reposition the elder every 2 hours (post a schedule); use positioning devices (i.e., pillows, foam wedges) at no more than 30 degrees lateral inclined position; avoid trochanters. Use pressure-reducing devices such as 4-inch dense foam mattresses. Use the lowest degree of head elevation (30 degrees maximum) and limit time of head elevation. Keep the heels off the bed —*no doughnuts.*

- While in a chair or wheelchair, absolutely reposition every hour. Consider postural alignment, weight distribution, balance, and stability. Use pressure-reducing devices, such as a 4-inch dense foam cushion—*not a doughnut.*

- Use lifting devices (i.e., trapeze, bed linens) to avoid friction and shear.

Scale. Techniques to prevent pressure ulcers in elders are listed in Box 35-22.

Comfort and Spirituality

Elders may not complain of discomfort or pain; health care providers may treat it inadequately; and poorly managed pain may aggravate other health problems. With all the age, health, and lifestyle changes experienced by elders, an intact spiritual belief system is essential. Comfort and spirituality conclude this section on preventive health care.

Comfort

Altered proprioception is more common in elders with increased light touch and pain thresholds. Maintaining comfort and managing pain, both acute and chronic, are essential to keep elders mobile and fully involved in their daily activities. Community health nurses need to assess comfort levels frequently using standard pain scales for persistent problems. Gentle massage, warm (*not* hot) baths, and fragrances are just a few of the techniques that may be helpful for common discomforts. In collaboration with the primary care provider, regular use of analgesics may be helpful to raise the pain threshold and improve comfort and mobility (e.g., acetaminophen 500 mg one to two tablets four times daily as needed discomfort). Nurses must be vigilant for overuse of OTC nonsteroidal antiinflammatory drugs (NSAIDs, e.g., aspirin, ibuprofen, naproxen), which can lead to gastrointestinal bleeding in elders, and they must be cautious with narcotic and sedative drugs, which can contribute to delirium and falls in this age group.

Spirituality

With the experiences of aging and changes in health status, many elders and families are faced with the need to discover a continuing purpose in the elder's life, find new meanings in their existence, and prepare for their transcendence from life to death. As they approach the end of their lives, elders may contemplate their movement from the concrete reality of their physical existence toward more abstract, metaphorical conceptualizations of their oneness with God, a divine being, or a higher power. Spirituality, the essence of the soul, may be integral with elders' beliefs, hope, energy, creativity, acceptance of life and death, and transcendence (Ebersole & Hess, 1998). As with other age groups, nurses assess the spiritual health of elders by inquiring discretely about their spiritual perspectives and religious commitments. Observations include their ability to discover continuing meaning and purpose in life, give and receive love, have hope, be creative, and share humor. The goals of spiritual care are to preserve the elders' unique beliefs and values and support their religious practices. Nurses may need to help elders make contact with religious advisors (e.g., minister, priest, rabbi, shaman) and use religious articles (e.g., Bible, Koran, crucifix, medals, prayer shawls, incense). They may need to have privacy for prayer and meditation or may want to sing hymns, read or write poetry, or offer other forms of self-expression. Elders may ask the nurse to share in these practices, as is appropriate for the situation. Other spiritual issues, life review, and advance directives are discussed elsewhere in this chapter. However elders express their spirituality, it is important that nurses recognize these needs and assist with their being met.

Special Elder Health Issues

Community health nurses must consider special issues in the elderly population. Comprehensive health care for elders includes immunizations, medication review, chemical abuse, and ethical dilemmas.

Immunizations

Pneumonia and influenza combined are a leading cause of death in the United States. Elders with chronic illnesses are at the highest risk for these respiratory illnesses. In the elderly population, immunizations usually are limited to three vaccines: influenza, pneumococcal, and tetanus/diphtheria. For elders who travel to foreign countries, other immunizations may be indicated. Elders should be referred to their local health department immunization clinic for information about the requirements for specific countries.

Medications

Elders purchase 40% of all prescription drugs (most commonly cardiovascular, anti-infective, antipsychotic, antidepressant, and diuretic agents) and 40% of OTC medicines (mostly analgesics, laxatives, and antacids). An average of five prescription drugs and three OTC drugs are taken by 90% of elders (Ebersole & Hess, 1998). Because aging changes affect the absorption, distribution, metabolism, and elimination of pharmacological agents, elders are more prone to drug interactions, adverse reactions, and toxicities.

Polypharmacy (many drugs) is a multifactorial problem that results from a "pill-oriented" society, elders' beliefs about health care and their various acute and chronic health problems, the prescribing practices of primary care providers, and the use of multiple primary and specialty providers. Problems of adherence to drug regimes occur with 25% to 50% of medications, including underuse, overuse, and misuse; many of these errors contribute to unnecessary hospitalizations (Ebersole & Hess, 1998). Medicare does not fund prescription drugs; Medicaid limits recipients to five prescriptions per month; some insurance plans may offer assistance with drugs. Because of their expense, elders may not fill prescriptions or may discontinue medications or decrease dosages and/or frequencies to stretch their medicines.

Community health nurses must be attentive for errors of omission (e.g., unfilled prescriptions, skipped doses, discontinuing medicines) and errors of commission (e.g., self-medication by increasing or decreasing dosages, changing times, using another person's drugs, taking OTC drugs). Nursing interventions for drug therapies are summarized in Box 35-23.

BOX 35-23 STRATEGIES TO IMPROVE MEDICATION USE BY ELDERS

- Obtain a medication history and consider the ability of elders to manage their medications, including financial status (purchase), environmental situation (storage), educational level (literacy), cognitive status (memory), visual acuity (reading labels), functional status (opening containers), and drug allergies.

- Remind elders to bring their medicines to each clinic visit; do a drug review ("brown bag check") for correct medications, dosages, instructions, refills, and their drug knowledge.

- Check medications frequently during home visits, including their storage and the disposition of old medications.

- In collaboration with primary care providers, simplify drug regimes and eliminate all unnecessary drugs, both prescribed and over-the-counter. Use once or twice daily dosing whenever possible.

- Teach elders and family members about all medications and prepare a written schedule, including each drug name and strength, size/color, frequency (specific times), purpose, and important side effects.

- Encourage elders to purchase all medications through the same pharmacy to check for drug allergies and interactions.

- Encourage elders to take medications at the same times and place every day with 4 to 6 ounces of water. Use memory aids to assist with adherence to drug regimes (e.g., written lists, medication calendars, pill boxes).

- Store all medicines together in a safe dry place, in their original containers, and out of the reach of small children.

- Remind elders to take a sufficient supply of all medicines when traveling away from home.

- If elders have memory problems, functional impairments, or complicated drug regimes, suggest the use of medication boxes pre-filled by the elder or caregiver either daily or weekly.

- If elders have arthritic problems, suggest easy-opening containers; if they have visual problems, use large print for labels; if they have swallowing problems, use liquid forms. Caution against crushing tablets or emptying capsules into food or fluid before checking with a pharmacist.

- Monitor elders continually for efficacy and side effects of medications. Use the abnormal involuntary movement scale (AIMS) to monitor drugs (especially antipsychotics) with extrapyramidal side effects such as tremors, akinesia, akathisia, and rigidity (tardive dyskinesia).

Chemical Abuse

Among elders, chemical abuse include all of the psychoactive chemicals used by younger populations, with alcohol being the substance that is most commonly abused. Alcoholism is estimated to affect 10% to 15% of community-dwelling elders. With their decreased tolerance to alcohol combined with normal aging changes and use of multiple prescription and OTC drugs, elders are at higher risk for falls, accidents, and burns. Nurses in the community can help identify these individuals by noting changes in behavior (e.g., anxiety, memory loss, depression, blackouts, confusion), health status (e.g., weight loss), hygiene, falls, and injuries. Elders can be screened with the TWEACK test (Reuben, Yoshikawa, & Besdine, 1996):

Tolerance	*How many drinks before you feel effects of alcohol?*
Worry	*Have you ever felt worried by criticism of your drinking?*
Eye opener	*Have you ever taken a morning eye opener?*
Amnesia	*Are there times after drinking when you can't remember what you did?*
Cut down	*Have you ever felt the need to cut down on drinking?*
Drin**K**ing	*How many drinks before you fall asleep or pass out?*

Those elders and families found to have alcohol problems are referred to their primary care providers, community mental health centers, Alcoholics Anonymous, or other local agencies for treatment of chemical abuse. Because denial of alcohol abuse is so prevalent and the necessary lifestyle changes are so difficult to maintain, recovery often is a long, irregular process. Nurses need to persist in their support, referral, and follow-up for these individuals and their families.

Other substances abused by elders include nicotine, caffeine, prescription and OTC drugs, illicit street drugs, and food. Assessments and interventions for these chemicals are similar to those for younger populations.

· ·

All We Need To Know

All we need to know is that we're needed.
All we have to feel is we're worthwhile.
It's not very difficult; indeed, it's
Something you can do with just your smile.

All we ask from you is some attention.
Notice us! We're special. If you please,
Pardon us, if now and then we mention
We would like a tender loving squeeze.

Old and gray, we wait. And don't forget that
Inside us, the child is waiting, too.
Help us feel important.
You can bet that
Then we'll want to be our best for you!

Ellen Johnston-Hale, age 83

· ·

Ethical Dilemmas

Because community health nurses become so involved with elderly people in their own environment, they often encounter ethical dilemmas and end-of-life issues. All too often there is no simple, easy, "right" answer to these complex situations—if there were, the dilemma would not exist. Usually, the choice is between two or more "bad" options. Beware of simple solutions for these usually ignore the complex nature of dilemmas. For example, when a frail, demented elder is anorexic, losing weight, and at risk for complications, one option is to insert an enteral feeding tube—which may improve nutrition, but also may prolong the person's suffering and dying and may be against his or her wishes for end-of-life care.

In American society, critical values in most ethical dilemmas concern autonomy (freedom of choice), nonmaleficence or beneficence (do no harm/do good), and distributive justice (use of resources). Because elders consume large amounts of health care resources, ethical conflicts occur around the issues of old versus young and quantity of life (adding years to live) versus quality of life (adding life to years). For many elders, the finality of death must be weighed against dependence, pain, abandonment, and loneliness. Clarification of beliefs and values of the elder, the family, and the health care providers may offer insights

RESEARCH BRIEF

Gloth, F. M., Tobin, J. D., Sherman, S. S., & Hollis, B. W. (1991). Is the recommended daily allowance for vitamin D too low for the homebound elderly? Journal of the American Geriatrics Society, 39, 137–141.

The recommended daily allowance (RDA) for vitamin D is 200 IU for adults. Although there is inadequate research on the specific requirements for elders older than 65, there is evidence that homebound and institution-bound elders are at special risk for vitamin D deficiency. Symptoms of vitamin D deficiency include weakness, pain, and bone loss, which can lead to osteoporosis and spontaneous fractures, all devastating conditions for elders. These symptoms compound the hardships already suffered by many older persons whose health is already impaired. The body's main source of vitamin D is direct exposure to the sun's ultraviolet rays. Approximately 5% of the U.S. population age 65 and older is in nursing homes. In addition, many older people in poor health at home tend to stay indoors and therefore are not exposed to sunlight. Recommendations of the study include encouraging all elders to sit outside on sunny days for 2 to 3 hours to enhance their vitamin D intake.

into these perspectives and facilitate satisfactory resolution of these conflicts.

Advance directives can help clarify elders' desire for health care interventions in the event of life-threatening situations. Nurses can encourage elders and families to discuss end-of-life issues (e.g., cardiopulmonary resuscitation, hospitalization, antibiotics, intravenous and enteral feedings) while elders are relatively young, healthy, and competent to express their wishes. The elder can complete a living will and/or durable power of attorney for health care in accordance with state statutes to assist family members to implement these wishes. In elders, intellectual competence for informed consent can be determined with the FMMSE (see appendix E).

For elders who have no advance directives and are very frail or demented, nurses can anticipate the occurrence of end-of-life issues. Nurses should take the initiative to approach families about these decisions *early*, encourage them to talk with extended family members as appropriate, and consider what the elders would prefer if they were able to express their wishes. Consider criteria for decision making (e.g., reversibility or irreversibility of the condition), communicate with the primary care provider, and document decisions appropriately. If elders are able to participate in these decisions, the nurse should encourage them to do so. Supporting the spiritual integrity of all concerned helps sort out the issues and maintain positive attitudes and behaviors.

CONCLUSION

With the "graying of America," elders are integral with the delivery of community health care. These older adults were socialized in a reactive health care system that focused on illness. Until recently, they have not been especially proactive or focused wellness or prevention. Community health nurses in 21st century can help elders by the three A's: awareness, assessment, and advocacy. Nurses can help elders practice health promotion and primary disease prevention through good nu-

trition, regular exercise, family and community involvement, stress management, anticipatory guidance, and safety checks. Secondary prevention requires self-monitoring activities (e.g., breast or testicular self-examinations), periodic screening, regular physical and oral health examinations, and adherence to therapeutic regimens. By working collaboratively with primary care providers, nurses can improve the health and quality of life of older adults—and help celebrate the joy of aging.

CRITICAL THINKING ACTIVITIES

1. After reading the following, what are some ways that community health nurses can help "reconnect" elders with other clients in the health care delivery system? Identify settings where health promotion interventions might be created to meet this need.

On the need to reconnect with elders . . .

A great deal of America's social sickness comes from age segregation . . . . We segregate the old for many reasons: prejudice, ignorance and a lack of good alternatives . . . If we aren't around dying people, we don't have to think about dying . . . and, the more involved we are with the old, the more pain we feel at their suffering . . . The old often save the young. And the young save the old . . . If 10 people ages 2 to 80 are grouped together, they will fall into a natural hierarchy that nurtures and teaches them all . . . the incredible calculus of old age—that as more is taken, there is more love for what remains.

Mary Pipher (1999, March 19-21). The new generation gap: For the nations health, we need to reconnect young and old. *USA Weekend*, p. 12.

2. Using photographs, assist an elderly client with visualizing independence in his or her life today. How can photographs throughout our lives assist in maximizing our ability to care for ourselves and promote our autonomy? Think of times in your own life when you were dependent and had limitations. What kinds of images helped improve your confidence in becoming self-sufficient again?

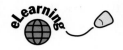 **Explore Community Health Nursing on the web!** To learn more about the topics in this chapter, use the passcode provided to access your exclusive web site:
http://communitynursing.jbpub.com
If you do not have a passcode, you can obtain one at this site.

REFERENCES

Agency for Health Care Policy and Research (AHCPR). (1992). *Pressure ulcers in adults: Prediction and prevention*. Rockville, MD: U.S. Government Printing Office.

Agency for Health Care Policy and Research (AHCPR). (1993). *Depression in primary care*. Rockville, MD: U.S. Government Printing Office.

Agency for Health Care Policy and Research (AHCPR). (1996a). *Recognition and initial treatment of Alzheimer's disease and related dementias*. Rockville, MD: U.S. Government Printing Office.

Agency for Health Care Policy and Research (AHCPR). (1996b). *Managing acute and chronic urinary incontinence*. Rockville, MD: U.S. Government Printing Office.

American Association for World Health. (1999). *Healthy aging, healthy living—Start now! Resource booklet*. Washington, DC: Author.

American Association of Retired Persons (AARP) and National Alliance for Caregiving. (1997). *Family caregiving in the U.S.: Findings from a national survey*. D16474 Washington, DC: AARP.

American College of Physicians. (1994). *Guide for adult immunization* (3rd ed.). Philadelphia: Author.

Anderson, K., & Anderson, L. (1994). *Mosby's pocket dictionary of medicine, nursing, & allied health* (2nd ed.). St. Louis: Mosby.

Annon, J. (1976). The PLISSIT model: A proposed conceptual scheme for behavioral treatment of sexual problems. *Journal of Sex Education and Therapy*, January, pp. 18–20.

Bellack, P., & Edlund, B. (1992). *Nursing assessment and diagnosis* (2nd ed.). Boston: Jones and Bartlett.

Burnside, I. (1988). *Nursing and the aged: A self-care approach* (2nd ed.). New York: McGraw-Hill.

Burnside, I., & Haight, B. (1994). Reminiscence and life review: Therapeutic interventions for older people. *Nurse Practitioner*, *19*(4), 55-61.

Butler, R., & Lewis, M. (1998). *Aging and mental health* (5th ed.) Boston: Allyn & Bacon.

Busse, E., & Blazer, D. (1980). *Geriatric psychiatry*. Washington, DC: American Psychiatric Press.

Carter, E., & McGoldrick, M. (1980). *The family life cycle: A framework for family therapy* (pp. 3-20). New York: Gardner.

Carter, Jimmy. (1995). *Always a reckoning*. New York: Random House.

Cora, V. L. (1985). *Family life process of intergenerational families with functionally dependent elders*. Dissertation. University of Alabama at Birmingham.

Comfort, A. (1990). *Say yes to old age: Developing a positive attitude toward aging*. New York: Crown.

Duvall, E. M. (1977). *Marriage and family development*. Philadelphia: J. B. Lippincott.

Ebersole, P., & Hess, P. (1998). *Toward healthy aging: Human needs and nursing response* (5th ed.). St. Louis: Mosby.

Erikson, E. (1963). *Childhood and society*. New York: Norton.

Folstein, M., Folstein, S., & McHugh, P. (1975). Mini-mental state: A practical method for grading the cognitive state of patients for the clinician. *Journal of Psychiatric Research*, *12*, 189-198.

Gunter, L., & Estes, C. (1979). *Education for gerontic nursing*. New York: Springer.

Ham, R., & Sloane, P. (1997). *Primary care geriatrics: A case-based approach* (2nd ed.) St. Louis: Mosby.

Health People 2000: The nation's health. (pp. 23-26, 588-591).

Kane, R., Ouslander, J., & Abrass, I. (1999). *Essentials of clinical geriatrics* (4th ed.). New York: McGraw-Hill.

Katz, S., Ford, A., Moskowitz, R., et al. (1963). Studies of illness in the aged. The index of ADL. *Journal of the American Medical Association*, *185*, 914.

Lawton, M., & Brody, E. (1969). Assessment of older people: Self maintaining and instrumental activities of daily living. *Gerontologist*, *9*, 179–186.

Lueckenotte, A. G. (1996). *Gerontologic nursing*. St. Louis: Mosby.

Maslow, A. (1968). *Toward a psychology of being* (2nd ed.). Princeton, NJ: Van Nostrand.

National Center for Health Statistics, Centers for Disease Control and Prevention. (1994). *Health United States, 1993* (U.S. Public Health Service, DHHS Publication No. 94-1232). Washington, DC: U.S. Government Printing Office.

Nutrition Screening Initiative. (1992). *Consensus conference.* Washington, DC:

O'Malley, R. (1987). *Inadequate care of the elderly: A health care perspective on abuse and neglect.* New York: Springer.

Reuben, D., Yoshikawa, T., & Besdine, R. (1996). *Geriatrics review syllabus; a core curriculum in geriatric medicine* (3rd ed.). Dubuque, IA: Kendall/Hunt.

Satir, V. (1964). *Conjunct family therapy: a guide to theory and technique.* Palo Alto, CA: Science & Behavioral Books.

Staab, A., & Lyles, M. (1990). *Manual of geriatric nursing.* Glenview, IL: Scott, Foresman/Little, Brown.

U.S. Bureau of the Census. (1991). *Statistical abstract of the United States: 1993* (112th ed.). Washington, DC: U.S. Government Printing Office.

United States Public Health Service (USPHS). (1994). *Clinician's handbook of preventive services: Put prevention into practice.* Washington, DC: Department of Health and Human Services.

Williams, M., Parker, R., Baker, D., Parikh, N. S., Pitkin, K., Coates, W. C., & Nurss, J. R. (1995). Inadequate functional health literacy among patients at two public hospitals. *JAMA, 274,* 1677-1720.

Yesavage, J., & Brink, T. (1983). Development and validation of a geriatric depression screening scale: A preliminary report. *Journal of Psychiatric Research, 17,* 37-49.

APPENDIX A

SELECTED THEORIES OF AGING

BIOLOGIC THEORIES

Molecular Theories

Gene: Selected genes become active in later life, causing the organism to fail to survive
Error, error catastrophe:
  Somatic mutation
  Transcription
Programmed, programmed senescence
Run-out-of-program

System Level Theories

Neuroendocrine control (pacemakers)
Immunological/autoimmune

Cellular Theories

Free radical, antioxidants
Cross-link/connective tissue
Clinker
Wear-and-tear

PSYCHOLOGICAL THEORIES

Maslow's hierarchy of human needs
Jung's individualism
Course of human life
Erikson's (1963) eight stages of life:
Sense of ego integrity versus sense of despair
Peck (1968):
Ego differentiation versus work-role preoccupation
Body transcendence versus body preoccupation
Ego transcendence versus ego preoccupation
Feil (1982): resolution of the past versus vegetation
Butler's (1963) life review
Levinson's (1977) Seasons of Life
Lowenthal's (1973) life transitions
Havighurst's (1974) developmental tasks:
Establishing satisfactory living arrangements
Adjusting to retirement and reduced income
Adjusting to decreasing physical strength and health
Establishing an explicit affiliation with one's age group

Meeting civic and social obligations

Adjusting to death of spouse

Psychosocial theories of aging:

Interpersonal, disengagement, continuity, activity (life review, reminiscence)

SOCIOLOGICAL THEORIES

Cummings & Henry (1961): Disengagement

Lemon (1972): Activity

Havighurst (1963): Continuity

Age stratification

Person-environment fit

Sociological aging life course, life transitions, status and role changes, social supports

APPENDIX B

ANA Standards of Gerontological Nursing Practice

STANDARDS OF CLINICAL GERONTOLOGICAL NURSING CARE

Standard I. Assessment

The gerontological nurse collects client health data.

Information obtained from the aging person, significant others, and the interdisciplinary team and nursing judgment based on knowledge of gerontological nursing are used to develop the comprehensive care plan. Interviewing, functional assessment, environmental assessment, physical assessment, and review of health records enhance the nurse's ability to make sound clinical judgments. Assessment is culturally and ethnically appropriate.

Standard II. Diagnosis

The gerontological nurse analyzes the assessment data in determining diagnosis.

The gerontological nurse evaluates health assessment data to identify the aging person's state of health and well-being, and treatment of and responses to illness, aging, and reduced activity. Each person responds to aging in a unique way. Nursing diagnoses form the basis for nursing interventions.

Standard III. Outcome Identification

The gerontological nurse identifies expected outcomes individualized to the client.

The ultimate goals of providing gerontological nursing care are to influence health outcomes and im-

prove the aging person's health status. Outcomes often focus on maximizing the aging person's state of well-being, functional status, and quality of life.

Standard IV. Planning

The gerontological nurse develops a plan of care that prescribes interventions to attain expected outcomes.

A plan of care is used to structure and guide therapeutic interventions and achieve expected outcomes. It is developed in conjunction with the aging person and significant others.

Standard V. Implementation

The gerontological nurse implements the interventions identified in the care plan.

The gerontological nurse implements a care plan in collaboration with the aging person, significant others, and the interdisciplinary team. The gerontological nurse provides culturally competent direct and indirect care, using concepts of health promotion, illness prevention, health maintenance, rehabilitation, restoration, and palliation. The nurse educates and counsels the aging person and significant others involved in that person's care. In addition, the gerontological nurse supervises and evaluates both formal and informal caregivers to ensure that their care is supportive and ethical and demonstrates respect for the aging person's dignity. Gerontological nurses select interventions according to their level of practice.

Standard VI. Evaluation

The gerontological nurse evaluates the aging person's progress toward attainment of expected outcomes.

Nursing practice is a dynamic process. The gerontological nurse continually evaluates the aging person's responses to therapeutic interventions. Collection of new data, revision of the database, alteration of nursing diagnoses, and modification of the care plan are often required. The effectiveness of nursing care depends on ongoing evaluation.

STANDARDS OF PROFESSIONAL GERONTOLOGICAL NURSING PERFORMANCE

Standard I. Quality of Care

The gerontological nurse systematically evaluates the quality of care and effectiveness of nursing practice.

The dynamic nature of geriatric care and the growing body of gerontological nursing knowledge and research provide both the impetus and the means for gerontological nurses to improve the quality of client care.

Standard II. Performance Appraisal

The gerontological nurse evaluates his or her won nursing practice in relation to professional practice standards and relevant statutes and regulations.

The gerontological nurse is accountable to the public for providing competent clinical care and has an inherent responsibility to practice according to standards established by the profession and by regulatory bodies.

Standard III. Education

The gerontological nurse acquires and maintains current knowledge in nursing practice.

Scientific, cultural, societal, and political changes require a continuing commitment form the gerontological nurse to pursue knowledge, to enhance nursing expertise and advance the profession. Formal education, continuing education, certification, and experiential learning are some of the means for professional growth.

Standard IV. Collegiality

The gerontological nurse contributes to the professional development of peers, colleagues, and others.

The gerontological nurse is responsible for sharing knowledge, research, and clinical information with colleagues and others through formal and informal teaching methods and collaborative educational programs.

Standard V. Ethics

The gerontological nurse's decisions and actions on behalf of clients are determined in an ethical manner

The gerontological nurse is responsible for providing nursing services and health care that are responsive to the public's trust and client's rights. Co-workers and other formal and informal care providers must also be prepared to provide the care needed and desired by the aging person and to render services in an appropriate setting. Special ethical concerns in gerontological nursing care include informed consent; emergency interventions; nutrition and hydration of the terminally ill; pain management; need for self-determination by the aging person; treatment termination; quality-of-life issues; confidentiality; surrogate decision making; nontraditional treatment modalities; fair distribution of scarce resources; and economic decision making.

Standard VI. Collaboration

The gerontological nurse collaborates with the aging person, significant others, and health care providers in providing client care.

The complex nature of comprehensive care for aging persons and their significant others requires expertise from a number of different health care providers. Collaboration between consumers and providers is optimal for planning, implementing, and evaluation care. Meetings of the interdisciplinary team provide a forum to evaluate the effectiveness of the care plan and make necessary adjustments.

Standard VII. Research

The gerontological nurse uses research findings in practice.

Gerontological nurses are responsible for improving nursing practice and the future health care for aging persons by participating in research. At the basic level of practice, the gerontological nurse uses research findings to improve clinical care and identifies clinical problems for study.

Standard VIII. Resource Utilization

The gerontological nurse considers factors related to safety, effectiveness, and cost in planning and delivering client care.

The aging person is entitled to health care that is safe, effective, and affordable. Treatment decisions must maximize resources and maintain quality of care.

Source: American Nurses Association (ANA). (1995). Scope and standards of gerontological nursing practice. *Washington DC: Author.*

APPENDIX C

ACTIVITIES OF DAILY LIVING AND INSTRUMENTAL ACTIVITIES OF DAILY LIVING

	INDEPENDENT	ASSISTED	DEPENDENT		INDEPENDENT	ASSISTED	DEPENDENT
Bathing	0	1	2	Telephoning	0	1	2
Dressing	0	1	2	Shopping	0	1	2
Toileting	0	1	2	Transporting	0	1	2
Transfer	0	1	2	Medicating	0	1	2
Continence	0	1	2	Handling money	0	1	2
Feeding	0	1	2	*Preparing food	0	1	2
				*Housekeeping	0	1	2
				*Laundry	0	1	2

ADL Score (0–12) _____   IADL Score (0–16)_____   Total Score (0–28)_____

0	Independent	0	Independent	0	Independent
1–6	Assisted	1–8	Assisted	1–14	Assisted
7–12	Dependent	7–16	Dependent	15–28	Dependent

Source: Adapted from Katz, 1963, and Lawton & Brody, 1969 (alternate scoring).

APPENDIX D

TINETTI FALL ASSESSMENT SCALE

BALANCE:	(SEATED IN HARD, ARMLESS CHAIR)	SCORING
Sitting balance	leans or slides in chair	5 0
	steady, safe	5 1_____
Arises	unable without help	5 0
	able, uses arms to help	5 1
	able without using arms	5 2_____

Attempts to rise	unable without help	5 0
	able, requires .1 attempt	5 1
	able to rise, 1 attempt	5 2_____
Immediate standing	balance (1st 5 sec)	
	unsteady (staggers, moves feet, trunk sway)	5 0
	steady but uses walker or other support	5 1
	narrow stance without other support	5 2_____

Standing balance	unsteady	5 0
	steady but wide stance and uses other support	5 1
	narrow stance without support	5 2_____
Nudged	begins to fall	5 0
	staggers, grabs, catches self	5 1
	steady	5 2_____
Eyes closed	unsteady	5 0
	steady	5 1_____
Turning 360°	discontinuous steps	5 0
	continuous steps	5 1
	unsteady (grabs, staggers)	5 0
	steady	5

1_____

Sitting down	unsafe (misjudged distance, falls into chair)	5 0
	uses arms or not a smooth motion	5 1
	safe, smooth motion	5

2_____

Balance Score: _____/16

Gait:	(stands, walks about 10 ft at usual pace, then back at rapid, but safe pace with aids)	Scoring
Initiation of gate	any hesitancy or multiple attempts to start	5 0
	no hesitancy	5 1_____

Step length and height

right swing foot	does not pass left stance foot with step	5 0
	passes left stance foot	5 1
	right foot does not clear floor completely	5 0
	right foot completely clears floor	5 1

left swing foot	does not pass right stance foot with step	5 0
	passes right stance foot	5 1
	left foot doesn't clear floor completely	5 0
	left foot completely clears floor	5 1_____
Step symmetry	right & left step length not equal (estimate)	5 0
	right & left step appear equal	5 1_____
Step continuity	stopping or discontinuity between steps	5 0
	steps appear continuous	5 1_____
Path	marked deviation	5 0
	mild/moderate deviation or uses walking aid	5 1
	straight without walking aid	5 2_____
Trunk	marked sway or uses walking aid	5 0
	no sway but flexion of knees or back or spread arms out while walking	5 1
	no sway, no flexion, no use of arms, and no use of walking aid	5 2_____
Walking time	heels apart	5 0
	heels almost touching while walking	5 1_____

Gait Score: _____/12

Balance 1 Gait Score: Score _____/28

Key to Risk for Falls:	Score
low	25-28
moderate	19-24
high	0-18

APPENDIX E

Mini-Mental State Exam

FOLSTEIN MINI-MENTAL STATE EXAM

Highest school grade completed _____

Maximum	Score	Orientation
5	_____	What is the (year), (season), (date), (day), (month)?
5	_____	Where are we: (state, city), (county), (facility), (floor)?

Registration

| 3 | _____ | Name 3 objects: 1 second to say each; ask person all three objects after they are said. Give 1 point for each correct answer. Then repeat objects until all three are learned Count trials and record: _____ |

| 5 | _____ | **Attention and Calculation**
Serial 7s. One point for each
correct. Stop after 5 answers.
93 86 79 72 65. alternatively,
spell "world" backwards:
D L R O W | 3 | _____ | Follow a 3-stage command:
"Take this paper in your right
hand, fold it in half, and put
it on the table." |

Attention and Calculation

5 _____ Serial 7s. One point for each correct. Stop after 5 answers. 93 86 79 72 65. alternatively, spell "world" backwards: D L R O W

Recall

3 _____ Ask for three objects repeated above. Give 1 point for each correct answer.

Language and Praxis

2 _____ Name a pencil and a watch.

1 _____ Repeat the following phrase: "No ifs, ands, or butts."

3 _____ Follow a 3-stage command: "Take this paper in your right hand, fold it in half, and put it on the table."

1 _____ Read and obey the following command:

CLOSE YOUR EYES

1 _____ Write a sentence:

1 _____ Copy this design:

30

Key to FMMSE Scores

no cognitive impairment	24-30
mild cognitive impairment	18-23
severe cognitive impairment	0-17

Source: Folstein, Folstein, & McHugh, 1975.

APPENDIX F

GERIATRIC DEPRESSION SCALE

Mood Scale

1.	ARE YOU BASICALLY SATISFIED WITH YOUR LIFE?	yes	NO
2.	HAVE YOU DROPPED MANY OF YOUR ACTIVITIES AND INTERESTS?	YES	no
3.	DO YOU FEEL THAT YOUR LIFE IS EMPTY?	YES	no
4.	DO YOU OFTEN GET BORED?	YES	no
5.	Are you hopeful about the future?	yes	NO
6.	Are you bothered by thoughts that you just can't get out of your head?	YES	no
7.	ARE YOU IN GOOD SPIRITS MOST OF THE TIME?	yes	NO
8.	ARE YOU AFRAID THAT SOMETHING BAD IS GOING TO HAPPEN TO YOU?	YES	no
9.	DO YOU FEEL HAPPY MOST OF THE TIME?	yes	NO
10.	DO YOU OFTEN FEEL HELPLESS?	YES	no
11.	Do you often get restless and fidgety?	YES	no
12.	Do you prefer to stay home at night rather than go out and do new things?	YES	no
13.	Do you frequently worry about the future?	YES	no
14.	DO YOU FEEL THAT YOU HAVE MORE PROBLEMS WITH MEMORY THAN MOST?	YES	no
15.	DO YOU THINK IT IS WONDERFUL TO BE ALIVE NOW?	yes	NO
16.	Do you often feel downhearted and blue?	YES	no
17.	DO YOU FEEL PRETTY WORTHLESS THE WAY YOU ARE NOW?	YES	no
18.	Do you worry a lot about the past?	YES	no
19.	Do you find life very exciting?	yes	NO
20.	Is it hard for you to get started on new projects?	YES	no

21. DO YOU FEEL FULL OF ENERGY?	yes	NO
22. DO YOU FEEL THAT YOUR SITUATION IS HOPELESS?	YES	no
23. DO YOU THINK THAT MOST PERSONS YOUR AGE ARE BETTER OFF THAN YOU ARE?	YES	no
24. Do you frequently get upset over little things?	YES	no
25. Do you frequently feel like crying?	YES	no
26. Do you have trouble concentrating?	YES	no
27. Do you enjoy getting up in the morning?	yes	NO
28. Do you prefer to avoid social gatherings?	YES	no
29. Is it easy for you to make decisions?	yes	NO
30. Is your mind as clear as it used to be?	yes	NO

Score   Circled capitalized answers   _____
               Crossed out lowercase answers   _____
               Total   15 or 30

Key to Scoring	GDS
No depression	0–4 capitalized on 15-item screen
Mild depression	5–10 capitalized on 30-item scale
Severe depression	11–30 capitalized on 30 item scale

Directions for Scoring: This scale is intended to be administered orally to the elderly person in a quiet, private setting. Circle the capitalized *answer* if the elder answers the question with the capitalized response. Draw a line through the lower case *answer* if the elder answers with the lower case response.

   Score 1 point for each circled capitalized answer.

   Score 0 for each lower case answer.

For screening purposes, use the 15 short-form *questions* which are capitalized. If the elder scores more than 5 points, administer the full 30-item scale.

Interpretation: A score of 5 or more capitalized responses on the 15-item screen is suggestive of depression and indicates the need to administer the full scale. a score of 0-10 is   Normal range; a score of 11 or more capitalized responses on the 30-item scale is positive for depression.

   According to Yersavage and Brink (1983), a cut-off score of 11 has a sensitivity of 84% and a specificity of 95%. A cut-off score of 14 has a sensitivity of 80% and a specificity of 100%.

Source: Yesavage & Brink, 1983.

APPENDIX G

HOME SAFETY CHECKLIST

HOME INTERIOR

Floors: clean, clutter-free, rugs anchored and in good repair (no scatter rugs), surface smooth and nonskid wax;

Electrical appliances: cords in good repair and out of traffic lanes

Lighting: adequate not-glare lighting; stairs illuminated; night lights where needed

Temperature: range 70-75°F; adequate heating, cooling, and ventilation; insulation; fireplace/heaters with protective screens

Furniture: sturdy, good repair

Stairs: sturdy railings; nonskid steps; uncluttered

Organization: uncluttered, navigable traffic lanes

COMMUNICATION

Lock/unlock door; reach light switches

Emergency telephone numbers posted, legible (fire, ambulance, doctor, family)

If no telephone, life line, neighbor, "buddy," or other means to summon help

Smoke alarms available with working batteries

KITCHEN

Food: adequate supply, fresh

Stove: free of grease and flammables, backing soda or fire extinguisher

Refrigerator: cooling effectively, food available and fresh

Sink: draining properly, hot (check temperature) and cold water; dishes washed

Cleaning supplies: stored separately and clearly marked

Garbage: taken out; regular pick up

Ladder or step stool: sturdy with handle

BATHROOM

Handrails for tub and toilet

Skid-proof mats for tub and/or shower

Nonskid rug on floor

Electrical outlets safe distance from tub

MEDICATIONS

Stored safely; current; disposal of old medicines

Current list with times, dosage, description, purpose

OUTSIDE

Walks, driveways, and stairs: smooth surfaces in good repair (no raised or uneven places); edges painted or clearly visible; handrails secure

Doors and windows: panes and screens in good repair

Fire escape or alternate exit from house

Source: Adapted from Burnside, 1988.

Chapter 36

Mental Health in the Community

Sarah Steen Lauterbach

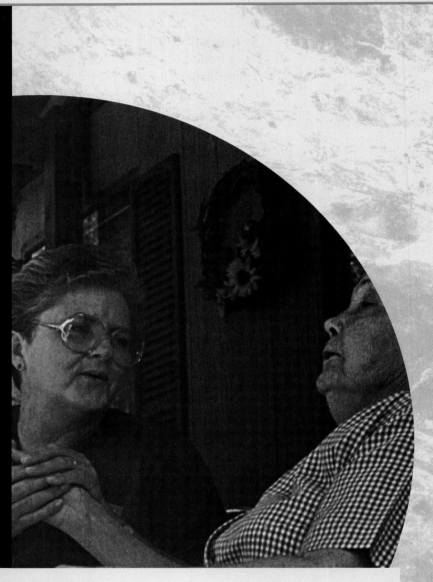

Much madness is divinist sense
To a discerning eye;
Much sense the starkest madness.
'Tis the majority
In this, as all, prevails.
Assent, and you are sane;
Demur, — you're straightway dangerous,
And handled with a chain.

Emily Dickinson

QUESTIONS TO CONSIDER

After reading this chapter, answer the following questions:
1. What is the definition of *mental health in the community*?
2. What is the history of community mental health nursing?
3. What is the current mental health status of Americans?
4. What are some of the conceptual and theoretical frameworks for psychiatric-mental health nursing?
5. What are some of the models for psychiatric-mental health nursing practice?
6. What will psychiatric-mental health nursing practice be like in the future?

KEY TERMS

Advocacy	Phenomena of	Prevention	Seriously mentally ill
Community Mental	concern	Psychiatric-mental	Universal human
Health Centers (CMHCs)	Phenomenology	health nursing	experiences

The idea of mental health is embedded within the contexts of culture, the tenor of the times, knowledge, and science. This chapter examines the American public's mental health using current information—demographic, population, and epidemiological data. Where population and numerical data are useful, it is also important to use a qualitative, humanistic perspective lens for assessing and understanding mental health. Conceptual frameworks, interdisciplinary theory, nursing theory, and models for community mental health nursing practice are particularly useful in providing an understanding of current psychiatric-mental health nursing care.

The central context for defining the scope of mental health nursing has been focused on knowledge and science underpinning the discipline as well as nursing's historic role in social activism. Of particular importance is **psychiatric-mental health nursing**'s focus on facilitating and using therapeutic relationships with persons, families, groups, and populations at risk. Hildegard Peplau, a psychiatric nursing scholar, was one of the first grand nursing theorists. She ushered in the focus on interpersonal relationships and theory underpinning nursing, which became a major focus of the nursing discipline throughout the 1960s to 1980s. The multiple theoretical perspectives that nursing uses contribute to its unique role, which are discussed later, and underpin its potential role in promoting, treating, and restoring the mental health of the public.

A discussion of **phenomenology**, which focuses on identifying and discovering meanings in human experiences to understand lived experience, is proposed as an appropriate underpinning philosophy for psychiatric-mental health nursing practice. The traditional role of public health nursing as advocate is especially appropriate today within the practice domain of psychiatric-mental health nursing.

Finally, public health policy needs to be inclusive of mental health, and psychiatric-mental health programs need to be mainstreamed into the health care system. Currently, a private system exists that provides services to persons with insurance and third-party reimbursement. However, the public system consists of community mental health services and provides treatment services to the seriously mentally ill population.

Textual contributions from creative writers and artists are included and discussed as reflective of classic struggles humans have faced in living with problems of mental health. Mental health phenomena are discussed as needing attention, perhaps better informed by using a phenomenological perspective to promote understanding of meanings of many common, **universal human experiences.** Creative artists and writers contribute to understanding experiences of living and coping with mental illness and threats to mental health.

. . . .

No temper could be more cheerful than hers, or possess, to a greater degree, that sanguine expectation of happiness which is happiness itself.

Jane Austen, 1775–1817

. . . .

NURSING SCHOLARSHIP BRIEF

"Out of the Box"

Nurse researcher and scholar, Patricia L. Munhall, ARNP, EdD, FAAN, PsyA, was an invited keynote speaker for the Nursing Research Conference in Biloxi, Mississippi, sponsored by Gamma Lambda Chapter Sigma Theta Tau International of The University of Southern Mississippi, November 12–13, 1998. The address titled, "Out of the Box," challenged nurses and researchers to question assumptions and preunderstandings in nursing and education that inhibit thinking, behaving, and creative nursing action. She states in an editorial in *Image, the Journal of Nursing Scholarship,* that "Boxes are useful for storage and keepsakes. Out of the box is going off the block. Staying in the box is standing still, stripped of awe" (Munhall, 1998, p. 203)

Definitions of Mental Health

Definitions of mental health in literature range from a focus on the absence of disease to the attainment of one's potential. The definition provided by *Healthy People 2000* "refers to an individual's ability to negotiate the daily challenges and social interactions of life, without experiencing undue emotional or behavioral incapacity" (DHHS, 1990). Missing in this definition is the human expectation and experience of living happily, as well as functionally, mentally healthy.

Concepts of mental health and illness have changed drastically over the last few centuries. In the 15th century the mentally ill were thought to be witches "possessed" by demons. Some cultures historically regard persons with psychiatric conditions as worthy of great respect, as having uncanny abilities and visionaries. At one time, mental illness was thought to be caused by a lesion or physical injury to the brain. If no objective injury or lesion was found, mental illness was thought to be a defect in morality and character.

. . . .

Everything has been figured out, except how to live.

Jean Paul Sartre, 1905–1980

. . . .

Since the early 1900s, identifying the mentally ill has been the focus of psychiatry. Great efforts were made toward the diagnosis and treatment of specific mental disorders and conditions. The development of the *Diagnostic and Statistical Manuals* (DSM) by the American Psychiatric Association (APA) since the 1950s (APA, 1980, 1987, 1992) has contributed to differentiation and research. Designated as "the decade of the brain," the focus of research in the 1990s has contributed to a fuller understanding of biological determinants of behavior (Hedaya, 1996). The major psychiatric milestones of the 20th century included the development of the diagnostic manual and assessment procedures; psychotherapy, including psychoanalysis; developmental theories; behavioral, cognitive, and psychological foci for psychotherapy, including crisis intervention, short-term, group, family, and long-term therapy; psychopharmacology; and knowledge concerning the biological determinants of behavior.

The definition of *mental health* is still in need of our attention and continued thinking in nursing. Many believe that the focus on biology has obscured, once again, the understanding of mental illness or mental health. The view of mental health in this chapter encompasses the notion that *mental health* involves connection of body, mind, and spirit, mental and physical wholesomeness. The concept of "balance" is common in holistic literature. Mental health is further viewed as involving a process through which a (w)holistic balance between mind, body, and spirit (of individuals, families, groups, and the public) is pursued through meaningful life activities. The mentally healthy person seeks experiences that promote well-being, productivity, and happiness as fully as possible given the particular situational contexts and limitations.

This notion of health is very similar to the aim of phenomenological inquiry. The ultimate aim of phenomenology is to assist persons, through understanding, to "become fully human." Nursing has historically embraced a role with caring that has focused on maximizing human potential. A focus on maintaining harmony and balance is needed in many areas of human endeavor and experience: in meaningful work, occupation or pursuit; in relationships with loved ones, significant others, and in social relationships, friendships, and work relationships; in meaningful relaxation, leisure, balanced nutrition, and fitness activities; and in having a respect and responsibility for the planet and world.

Mental illness or dysfunction, although it exists more in vulnerable population groups, is not wholly a respecter of vulnerability. There have been and currently are many gifted as well as ordinary people who have periodic mental health issues and conditions. The arts and sciences are filled with examples of brilliant and revolutionary contributions from people who had mental health problems. For example, the symbolist artist Edvard Munch, born in 1863, was an alcoholic and experienced depression throughout his life. His work focuses on themes of life and death and his experience with mental illness. The lithograph *The Scream* is one of his most important and popularized pieces. Of particular interest are three other works, *Anxiety, The Sick Child,* and *Death in the Sick Room.* As a young child, Munch experienced the death of his mother, and when he was 14, his sister died. *Death in the Sickroom* depicts the family scene years earlier. The following quote by Munch illustrates this anguish:

> I was born dying . . . Sickness, insanity, and death were the malevolent angels that guarded my cradle and have followed me through my life ever since.

> I must retain my physical weaknesses; they are an integral part of me. I don't want to get rid of illness, however unsympathetically I may depict it in my art.

History of Community Mental Health

In the United States today, the public community mental health program is the primary model of care for people with serious mental illness. Begun in 1963, President John Kennedy raised awareness and attention to mental health with the Community Mental Health Centers Act. Federal funds were committed for the construction and staffing of **community mental health centers (CMHCs)**, using the catchment area concept, which distributed mental health services throughout states all over the country. Today these programs provide access to a range of services that before this legislation were nonexistent.

Community mental health development has been closely associated with legislation. Box 36-1 describes the major mental health legislative efforts and its influence on the development of mental health services. Understanding that community mental health as a humanitarian reform is seen when considering the early reform history of mental health. It is still in need of reform today.

· ·

Mental illness is the last great stigma of the 20th century. Most people treat someone with a mental illness as if it's their fault or as if they can just snap out of it.

Tipper Gore, June 18, 1999

· ·

Early Humanitarian Reform

Early treatment for people with mental illness was both cruel and inhumane. In 1843, Dorothea Dix, a school teacher, started the reform movement for the treatment of criminals, the mentally ill, and later, victims of the Civil War. Her work led to the establishment of asylums dedicated to humane treatment for the mentally ill. States built institutions for housing and treating persons with severe mental disorders. Intended as a humane movement, the large numbers of patients, combined with little knowledge and information about either cause or cure of mental illness, the establishment of asylums was, in retrospect, anything but humane. Within a few years, these large state institutions

BOX 36-1 MENTAL HEALTH LEGISLATION AND ITS INFLUENCE ON MENTAL HEALTH SERVICES

1935   *Social Security Act*
        Shifted care for ill people from state to federal government.

1943   *National Institute for Mental Health*
        Established as one of the Institutes of Health, where funds for research and development were committed to mental health.

1955   *Mental Health Study*
        Established Joint Commission on Mental Illness & Health.
        Led to the transformation of state hospitals to establishment of CMHCs.

1963   *Community Mental Health Centers Act*
        Marked beginning of CMHCs and deinstitutionalization of large psychiatric hospitals.

1960s   *Funds were committed from federal government for grants for education for mental health disciplines, including nursing; stipends were made available for traineeships for undergraduate and graduate nursing students; gradually these were less frequent and finally were no longer available.*

1975   *Developmental Disabilities Act*
        Addressed rights of developmental disabilities and provided for similar actions for individuals with mental disorders.

1977   *President's Commission on Mental Health*
        Reinforced importance of community-based services, protection of human rights, and national health insurance for mentally ill persons.

1978   *Omnibus Reconciliation Act*
        Rescinded much of the 1977 commission's provisions and shifted funds for all health programs from federal to state governments in the form of block grants.

1986   *Protection and Advocacy for Mentally Ill Individuals Act*
        Legislated advocacy programs for mentally ill persons.

1990   *Americans with Disabilities Act*
        Prohibited discrimination and promoted employment opportunities for people with disabilities, including mental disorders.

Source: Adapted from Stanhope & Lancaster, 1996.

provided the only mental health treatment and grew to be overcrowded. Patients were not discharged to families in communities that had no treatment services. Psychiatric treatment was limited to somatic therapies and did very little to handle difficult symptoms. The asylum population continued to grow as new people were admitted and the long-term residential population grew. It was not uncommon for "backward" patients to have stays of 20 to 40 years.

Community Mental Health Reform

The community mental health centers movement, a century after Dorothea Dix's reform efforts, was another mental health reform movement. Some progress had been made in mental health science and treatment. The development of psychopharmacology was a milestone in treatment reform. Previously untreatable conditions were opened to the possibility of treatment. Since the early 1900s, psychotherapy had also been the focus of scholarship from several disciplines, including psychiatry, psychology, social work, and nursing. Psychotherapies that developed included long- and short-term and crisis intervention with individuals, groups, and families.

The community mental health centers movement was short lived as the ideal solution to mental health care. Currently, large numbers of clients discharged from the state institutions and those who would have required institutional care in years past are residing in communities. A large number of the homeless population in urban centers are chronically mentally ill. They continue to have exacerbating mental conditions and experience environmental stresses, including the stress of meeting basic needs. This group of homeless, chronically mentally ill is especially vulnerable.

As individuals were discharged from state mental institutions, private fee-for-service psychiatric services sprang up quickly in communities all over the country. Although care and a full range of treatment services are now more easily accessible within the community, there is inequity in access as a result of economic issues. Often, the families of the **seriously mentally ill** are unable to do what is necessary to ensure continuity of care or to get any care.

The goals and dreams of young mental health professionals of the community mental health movement showed great promise but have never been realized fully. The inequity in access and economics of mental health care and physical care continues to dominate the environment of mental health care. Within most communities, supportive services have been developed, primarily by the consumer movement, to meet particular support needs of the general population. Box 36-2 identifies vulnerable populations who are in need of preventive,

---

BOX 36-2   VULNERABLE POPULATIONS

- Young and old
- Experiencing developmental transitions— adolescents, with young families
- Experiencing work and vocational problems and transitions
- Unemployed
- Part of the growing aggregate of the very old, older than 85, elderly
- Living in poverty
- Single parents of young children
- Adolescent parents
- Grandparents in parenting roles because adult children are suffering with dysfunction
- Uneducated
- Isolated and marginalized
- Dealing with learning and attention deficits, have disabilities
- Living as minority populations
- Depressed
- Angry
- Acutely or chronically ill
- Have histories of incarceration
- Have been victims of human and environmental abuse
- Victims of oppressive political systems
- Seeking asylum
- Experiencing stress, crisis, and change

BOX 36-3   SUPPORT GROUPS

- Compassionate Friends: focus on death, bereavement and loss (spouses, sudden infant death syndrome, perinatal, sibling)
- Cancer Support: focuses on variety of phenomena, including breast cancer and ostomy
- Caregivers Support Group: for caregivers of elderly, cancer, mentally ill
- Infertility Support: for couples experiencing infertility
- Parents without Partners
- Suicide Survivors
- Addictions Anonymous: for alcohol, gambling, exercise, shopping, food
- Smoking Cessation: including smokeless tobacco
- Families of Murdered Victims
- Families of Seriously Mentally Ill
- Medication follow-up and education: for clients and families
- Parenting Groups: for parents of adolescents, learning disabilities, autism, incarcerated
- Grandparenting
- Homeless Mothers
- Diabetes Education
- Alzheimer's Family Support: including Parkinson's
- Fibromyalgia Support
- Cardiac: Mended Hearts
- Organ Donor Group Support: families of donors and recipients of organs
- Physical Disabilities Support
- Homeless Mothers and Families Support

---

health promotion, and specialized treatment. Box 36-3 provides a listing of support services and groups available in many communities.

Beginning with the consumer movement of the 1970s, the groups focusing on support and psychoeducational issues with particular conditions have grown. These groups are available to the public, are listed in the telephone directories, and are advertised in varying community bulletin boards.

There is a growing need for identifying areas in need of care and attention, such as recent experiences of community loss, stress, and crisis experienced in the bombing of the federal building in

Oklahoma City in 1996. The 1998 Pearl, Mississippi, and 1999 Columbine high school shootings demonstrate that there is a growing need for both crisis and preventive intervention with adolescents and in schools. There is also need for more humanitarian reform involving economics and equity of mental health care.

Mental health programs offer many services to the seriously mentally ill population. Box 36-4 provides a listing of examples of mental health services available in a community mental health center in Mississippi.

Increasingly, community programs are being called to provide consultation to schools and communities in dealing with sensitive issues needing professional mental health attention.

BOX 36-4 COMMUNITY MENTAL HEALTH SERVICES

SERVICES

- Seriously mentally ill day treatment
- Acute partial hospitalization for seriously mentally ill
- Children's services
- Adult day care
- Day Treatment Club House: for those with chronic conditions who live in the community
- Alcohol and chemical addictions programs
- Outpatient follow-up
- Group living

POSSIBLE TREATMENT MODALITIES AVAILABLE IN THESE PROGRAMS

- Resocialization, remotivation, and life skills assistance
- Social services
- Psychological services, including testing
- Medical services management and referral
- Psychopharmacological management
- Occupational therapy
- Recreational therapy
- Group, family therapy, and individual therapy
- Outreach and home visiting
- 12-step program
- Vocational rehabilitation
- Psychotherapy, long and short term

The *Healthy People 2000* priority areas are listed in Box 36-5 on p. 843. Even though mental health and mental disorders are listed separately, it is clear that mental health underpins many other priority areas, such as those listed in preventive services and health promotion.

Inpatient services for the seriously mentally ill are still provided by the state hospital system. Clients experiencing acute problems or acute exacerbations of chronic conditions are usually housed within jails in holding facilities, which usually have consultative psychiatric services. Despite attempts to build in continuity and access to care, there are needed reforms in all systems that use holding rather than inpatient treatment facilities. Inpatient services for the private system exist within relative geographic access in most communities. However, as cost containment measures have been instituted, inpatient care is often too brief. Insurance and economics are currently the greatest barriers to access to comprehensive, appropriate, and timely care in both the private and public systems.

The Art and Science of Mental Health Nursing
History of Psychiatric-Mental Health Nursing

. . . .

As a nurse, I try to do for them what they would do for themselves if they had the strength, the will, and the knowledge that a nurse has. And I try to do it in such a way that I don't make them dependent on me, any more than is necessary.
Interview with Virginia Henderson in Baer, 1990

. . . .

The role of nursing, defined by Henderson, is relevant to the role of nursing in mental health. Box 36-6 identifies important events in the history of psychiatric nursing. Peplau, considered the founder of psychiatric nursing, and later Travelbee further proposed that the context and development of the nurse-client relationship underpinned the professional nursing role. At a specially convened memorial service at the 1999 International Council of Nurses in London, the contributions of Hildegard Peplau were acknowledged. Psychiatric nurses from around the world gave tribute to their "formidable" leader, who has been lovingly referred to as the "mother of psychiatric nursing." Historically, nursing has been a profession that, in response to societal need, developed and was shaped by social, political, and economic forces within society. To study nursing history is to study the story of women who were the social activists of their time. To understand the unique position and role of psychiatric-mental health nursing today especially, as cost cutting and economics have shaped staffing patterns and care, one determines

BOX 36-5

PRIORITY AREAS
Health Promotion

1. Physical Activity and Fitness
2. Nutrition
3. Tobacco
4. Alcohol and Other Drugs
5. Family Planning
6. Mental Health and Mental Disorders
7. Violent and Abusive Behavior
8. Educational and Community-Based Programs

Health Protection

9. Unintentional Injuries
10. Occupational Safety and Health
11. Environmental Health
12. Food and Drug Safety
13. Oral Health

Preventive Services

14. Maternal and Infant Health
15. Heart Disease and Stroke
16. Cancer
17. Diabetes and Chronic Disabling Conditions
18. HIV Infection
19. Sexually Transmitted Diseases
20. Immunization and Infectious Diseases
21. Clinical Preventive Services

Surveillance and Data Systems

22. Surveillance and Data Systems

Age-Related Objectives

Children

Adolescents and Young Adults

Adults

Older Adults

Source: DHHS, 1990.

that nursing *must* find a better way to participate in social policy and health planning. Even though the American Nurses Association has been involved in health care reform, reform is still needed. One only needs to look at the plight of private, inpatient nursing staffing and roles to know that nursing still suffers from its political and social power base. The early nursing leaders were involved with social reform movements and human rights and advocated for the poor and politically powerless. In addition, they knew the critical importance of social support. Nurses must learn to care for each other and the profession or else caring for others will continue to suffer (Lauterbach & Becker, 1996).

The community mental health (CMH) movement of the 1960s provided nursing an opportunity for **advocacy** and social reform. Concurrent with the Civil Rights movement, the movement heightened awareness and articulated rights of persons suf-

fering with mental illness. Furthermore, at the 100th International Congress for Nursing in London (July 1999), human abuse was discussed as a global concern in the etiology of mental illness. This community mental health movement is discussed in detail in a later section; it remains, along with our growing population of incarcerated people, an example of needed research regarding **prevention** and rehabilitation reform. Short lived because of cuts in federal funding, community mental health care and other mental health services, developed in the 1960s and early 1970s, became a focus for partisan politics in the 1980s. This, along with business and cost containment in the health care market, has a formidable role in health care policy. The business of care, exemplified in its language, has replaced humanistic health care language and health policy in the 1980s and 1990s. Insurers and providers are primarily looking for behavioral and objective outcomes of care.

BOX 36-6 IMPORTANT EVENTS IN PSYCHIATRIC NURSING HISTORY, 1773–1955

1773   *First mental hospital in the United States established in Williamsburg, Virginia*

1846   *First use of the term* psychiatry *by physicians attempting to upgrade the status of their work with the mentally ill*

1882   *First school for psychiatric nurses (or mental nurses) established at the McLean Asylum in Somerville, Massachusetts*

1913   *Johns Hopkins Hospital included psychiatric nursing in the course of study for general nurses*

1920   *Publication of the first psychiatric nursing textbook,* Nursing Mental Diseases, *by Harriet Bailey*

1946   *Passage of the National Mental Health Act, which established the National Institutes of Mental Health (NIMH)*

1948   *Publication of the Brown Report, which recommended that psychiatric nursing be included in general nursing education*

1952   *Publication of* Interpersonal Relations in Nursing *by nurse theorist Hildegard Peplau*

1955   *National League for Nursing made psychiatric nursing a requirement for accreditation of basic nursing programs*

Source: Adapted from Frisch & Frisch, 1998.

BOX 36-7 PSYCHIATRIC MENTAL HEALTH NURSING: AREAS OF PRACTICE

BASIC-LEVEL FUNCTIONS

- Health promotion and health maintenance
- Intake screening and evaluation
- Case management
- Milieu management and therapy
- Self-care activities
- Psychobiological interventions
- Health teaching
- Crisis intervention
- Counseling and therapeutic relationships
- Home visiting
- Community action
- Advocacy

ADVANCED-LEVEL FUNCTIONS

- Psychotherapy
- Psychobiological interventions
- Medication management and prescriptive authority (in most states)
- Clinical supervision/consultation
- Consultation/liaison building

Source: Adapted from ANA, 1994.

There is particular need for documenting qualitative experiences with treatment and health services, which are legitimate, sought-after outcomes of treatment. As growing dissent is articulated regarding the quality and access to care provided by managed care and health maintenance organizations, it is anticipated that an informed, educated American consumer, the "customers," or "health care recipients," will begin finding a voice. Increasingly, nursing research efforts are being focused on the qualitative aspects of mental illness; hopefully, research focusing on qualitative outcomes of treatment will follow.

To address the current state of the art, science, and spirit of psychiatric-mental health nursing, particular attention will be given to nursing within the community context. The potential role of psychiatric-mental health nursing mandates that mental health care and services be integrated *within* the health care system. Ideally, the role encompasses routine as well as specialty and advanced care, alongside a full range of primary, secondary, and tertiary care. There is potential for nursing to be involved in all levels of prevention and promotion of mental health, especially in advocacy for the inclusion of mental health care in community health care and mental health promotion and education. Box 36-7 identifies basic and advanced levels of practice for psychiatric-mental health nursing. These are discussed later as the role of the nurse is fully articulated.

There is a particular need for psychiatric-mental health nursing to promote personal and professional health and well-being. The idea that caring for self underpins caring for others is the central thesis in Lauterbach and Becker's work (1996) on caring for self. There is a growing recognition of the need for reflective education (Schon, 1983, 1990), and this is being articulated as being critical to professional nursing practice (Lauterbach & Becker, 1996). The use of reflection in nursing practice offers an opportunity to care for the profession or group as well as for the public.

Current Assessment of Mental Health Status

In 1978, the President's Commission on Mental Health estimated that nearly 15% of the population needed some type of mental health services at any given time. Furthermore, it was estimated that 25% of the population have what are considered mild forms of disorder, such as anxiety or depression. These are conservative figures, and when compared with recent epidemiological data (Tsuang, Tohen, & Zahner, 1995) and the 1996 progress review of *Healthy People 2000* (DHHS, 1996), they are further obscured. Recent estimates are summarized in the progress review in the *Healthy People 2010* box on p. 846. In addition, the box on p. 847 presents the highlights of the *Healthy People 2000* progress review. The *Healthy People 2010* box on p. 848 identifies follow-up needed at this particular time. It is clear from reviewing these boxes that much more attention, research, and funding is needed in the mental health arena.

Incidence and Prevalence of Psychiatric Conditions

Two of the most important issues in population assessment are the need for mental health care and the extent of unmet need. Descriptive population demographics reveal some general trends in incidence and prevalence and services used for treatment. The National Reporting Program of the National Institute of Mental Health (NIMH) found that there was a drop in inpatient census from 471,451 in 1969 to 214,065 in 1981. This period coincided with the beginning of the deinstitutionalization process brought about by the development of CMHCs, which increased access to mental health services to the public. Not until the late 1970s did deinstitutionalization noticeably change the pattern of public services.

Initial reports from the NIMH Epidemiological Catchment Area (ECA) program established under Jimmy Carter's Presidential Commission on Mental Health in 1978 have been useful in estimating prevalence of mental health disorders within the general population. The establishment of DSM, which correlated with the World Health Organization (WHO) publication of International Classification of Diseases (ICD), has been one of the most important contributions of the DSM-III epidemiological study. Data from this program estimates that approximately 32% of adults in the United States report symptoms meeting criteria for one or more psychiatric disorders during their lifetime. Illness was distributed differently between genders, with 36% of men meeting criteria for an addictive or mental disorder and 30% of women meeting criteria for psychiatric diagnosis of disorder. Men and women had similar rates for an active disorder, with 20% having had symptoms within the last year. These population figures show differences from Leighton, Harding, Macklin, MacMillan, and Leighton's 1963 study.

Age cohorts between 18 and 44 years have the highest lifetime rates of disorder. This study also showed that for persons 65 and older, only 21% met criteria for any lifetime disorder and that this group also had lower prevalence rates. Higher lifetime (38%) and active (26%) rates occurred for African Americans than for whites (32%) and Hispanics (33%). Persons who did not finish high school had an increased risk (36%) compared with graduates (30%). Those who are financially dependent had a rate of 47%; those not dependent had a rate of 31%. Although the highest rates occurred among men who were not working (48%), men in unskilled jobs had high rates (40%) of mental disorder. Only small differences were noted between urban and rural sites. Forty-four percent of persons separated or divorced and 52% of persons who were unmarried and cohabited had experienced mental disorder in their lifetime (Tsuang, Tohen, & Zahner, 1995, pp. 141–145). Findings from these studies confirm the findings of an earlier study relating to the relationship between social class and mental illness (Hollingshead & Redlich, 1954).

Pattern of Use of Psychiatric–Mental Health Services

According to Tsuang, Tohen, and Zahner (1995, p. 202), mental health services data show that the burden of mental disorders in the population is large. Even with only 1 in 5 individuals with a diagnosable disorder using services in 1 year, the cost of treatment is large. The human costs are exorbitant when the ability to have a quality, meaningful, and productive life is considered.

Mental health services comprise a very large portion of the health care budget. It was estimated that in 1988, the total costs to society (including costs relating to accidents, crime, and other problems associated with mental disorders) were $273.3 billion. Given that approximately 14% of the population has no health insurance and a large portion are uninsured, 18% have no mental health coverage (Tsuang, Tohen, & Zahner, 1995, p. 203). Insurance plans typically require the covered individual seeking mental health services to pay a larger co-payment and perhaps a higher deductible than for physical health services.

HEALTHY PEOPLE 2010

OBJECTIVES RELATED TO MENTAL HEALTH AND MENTAL DISORDERS

Mental Health Status Improvement

18.1   Reduce the suicide rate.

18.2   Reduce the rate of suicide attempts by adolescents.

18.3   Reduce the proportion of homeless adults who have serious mental illness (SMI).

18.4   Increase the proportion of persons with serious mental illnesses who are employed.

18.5   Reduce the relapse rates for persons with eating disorders, including anorexia nervosa and bulimia nervosa.

Treatment Expansion

18.6   Increase the number of persons seen in primary health care who receive mental health screening and assessment.

18.7   Increase the proportion of children with mental health problems who receive treatment.

18.8   Increase the proportion of juvenile justice facilities that screen new admissions for mental health problems.

18.9   Increase the proportion of adults with mental disorders who receive treatment.

18.10   Increase the proportion of persons with co-occurring substance abuse and mental disorders who receive treatment for both disorders.

18.11   Increase the proportion of local governments with community-based jail diversion programs for adults with serious mental illnesses.

State Activities

18.12   Increase the number of states and the District of Columbia that track consumers' satisfaction with the mental health services they receive.

18.13   Increase the number of states, territories, and the District of Columbia with an operational mental health plan that addresses cultural competence.

18.14   Increase the number of states, territories, and the District of Columbia with an operational mental health plan that addresses mental health crisis interventions, ongoing screening, and treatment services for elderly persons.

Source: DHHS, 2000.

HEALTHY PEOPLE 2010

HIGHLIGHTS OF *HEALTHY PEOPLE 2000* PROGRESS REVIEW

During their lifetime, 22% of adult Americans have some form of diagnosable mental disorder.

The prevalence of depression is much higher for women than for men.

The disabling conditions arising from depression can now be treated more successfully, thus enhancing the quality of life for individuals.

Recent studies have documented the phenomenon of co-morbidity of depression, that is, its etiological association with smoking, alcohol abuse, or drug abuse in some clients. Recognition of these linkages can provide the basis for more effective treatment.

Continuing public stigmatization of mental disorders creates one of the greatest barriers to obtaining mental health care.

Too few primary care providers are trained to recognize depression and the variety of disabilities associated with it.

Five states have legislated parity in insurance benefits for treatment of mental disorders and physical illnesses.

The provision of mental health services in schools provides an opportunity for early intervention. For example, the city of Baltimore through collaboration with local universities is able to offer the services of full-time mental health professionals in more than 60 of its public schools.

Sixty-three percent of people with health insurance coverage are enrolled in managed health care plans for mental health care services. A relative few companies predominate in this $2 billion business.

Cost-shifting from private to public mental health services is occurring as service limits in insurance plans are reached.

Source: Adapted from DHHS, 1996.

HEALTHY PEOPLE 2010

FOLLOW-UP PROPOSED BY *HEALTHY PEOPLE 2000* PROGRESS REVIEW

Conduct more rigorous studies on the cost-effectiveness of preventive intervention and mental health treatment to document the long-term benefits of these services.

Promote early access to mental health diagnostic services for children.

Seek to enhance communication between mental health and primary care providers so that concepts of mental health are integrated in the overall health assessment of individuals of all ages.

Promote activities that foster the training and continuing education of primary care providers in the recognition of symptoms of depression and other mental and emotional disorders with their resulting disabilities.

Place greater emphasis on the provision of mental health care services in a variety of community settings, including schools and workplaces.

Expand the base of knowledge about the influence of differences in age, race, sex, and culture on the prevention and treatment of mental disorders.

Promote antistigma campaigns stressing the value and successes of early interventions. Using celebrities in such campaigns can raise the visibility of both the problem and available solutions.

Stress the importance of early interventions, as in Head Start and childhood immunization programs, as strong determinants of positive mental health at later stages of life.

Evaluate mental health services targeted to children and their families with mental disorders, such as a conduct disorder or depression, to ensure that service designs effectively meet their needs.

Apply findings from studies of the co-morbidity of depression to mitigate substance abuse, smoking, and alcohol abuse, beginning with adolescents.

In planning for *Healthy People 2010,* provide for broad participation of consumer groups from the outset and ensure that new objectives for mental health take account of the full spectrum of acute, intermediate, and long-term/chronic care needs.

Source: Adapted from DHHS, pp. 1–4.

The aforementioned studies reveal that approximately 14% to 18% of the respondents reported at least one admission for general medical conditions during the year prior to the ECA interview. On the other hand, 2% to 6% reported an inpatient admission for mental health. Analysis of the 1980 data has projected estimates of services used for 1 year by combining the ECA and a follow-up interview, the Diagnostic Interview Schedule (DIS), 1 year later. Analysis of this data suggests that the 1-year prevalence of DSM-III covered by the DIS was 28.1% (Tsuang, Tohen, & Zahner, 1995, p. 202), or about 44.7 million people older than 18. Statistics for general problems (e.g., anxiety, depression) are underreported.

NURSING SCHOLARSHIP BRIEF

Pursuit of the Ordinary: Short-Term Inpatient Treatment

Goren's (1997) article discusses the tension that often exists between administrative mandates to reduce costs through shortened inpatient stays and the staff's commitment to the philosophy, treatment, and milieu organization of extended inpatient care. Effective short-term care needs a radically altered culture and treatment model from the traditional model.

We are more alike, my friends,
than we are unalike.
We are more alike, my friends,
than we are unalike.

Maya Angelou

Individuals and Population Groups Needing Psychiatric-Mental Health Services

Mental health and mental disorders are included in *Healthy People 2000* as part of health promotion. The *Healthy People 2010* boxes discussed earlier identify mental health problems and populations in need. The *Healthy People 2000* 1996 review report refers to an increasing problem of drug and alcohol use among teens, but it seems to be more serious than even the statistics show. Parents with young teens are aware of this growing population of youth who are encountering very serious substance use, including cigarettes, smokeless tobacco, an incredible variety of inhalants, abuse of prescription "pills," and daily and large quantities of marijuana use, coupled with alcohol. In addition, the epidemics of rape, violence, legal entanglements, and pregnancy among junior and senior high school students is, from the perspective of the youth, much greater than statistics demonstrate. The pattern of misuse and abuse that is reflected in the aforementioned behaviors, along with a recognition that problems with anxiety, depression, and attention to school and learning warrant careful investigation, research, and concurrent social action. Many of the behaviors are seen by professionals as attempts to self-medicate. However, research is needed to identify factors that are associated with and contribute to "using" behaviors. We need to understand more about these human phenomena.

There are a growing number of individuals and populations at risk in need of primary mental health nursing as well as specialized psychiatric-mental health care. This reflects the growing consumer and public recognition that specialized support is need to cope with particular human phenomena and experiences. Box 36-8 lists common, universal human experiences that are often in need of special support and crisis or continuing care. The potential direction and roles for psychiatric-mental health nursing will focus on assisting persons and groups in handling living through difficult human experience.

As a focal phenomenon, changes in the American family warrant particular attention. A growing number of children grow up in single-parent homes, usually with the father absent. There are changes in the structure and function of families. Single parents and working women are growing aggregates. This combined with poverty serves to compound vulnerability.

RESEARCH BRIEF

Beck, C. (1998). The effects of postpartum depression on child development; a meta-analysis. Archives of Psychiatric Nursing, 12(1), 12–20.

The adverse, short-term effects of postpartum depression on maternal-infant interaction has been documented, but are there long-term sequelae for children of these women? This meta-analysis was to determine the magnitude of cognitive and emotional development of children older than 1 year of age. Nine studies were examined and indicated that postpartum depression had a small but significant effect. The strength of the effect seems to have weakened as the child grew older. An earlier meta-analysis by the same researcher found that postpartum depression displayed a moderate to large adverse effect on infants' behavior. Implications for future research as well as the cautioned use of meta-analyses of research using linear thinking, was discussed.

The growing elderly population with cognitive impairments, institutionalized elders, and those with Alzheimer's and their families further reflect the concept of compounding vulnerability. More work, more research, and more preventive efforts are needed for serious mental health conditions and diagnoses, such as schizophrenia, which involve exacerbations of acute symptoms of distress and disturbance. This population represents a large

BOX 36-8 COMMON HUMAN EXPERIENCES

- Loss, death, separation
- Crisis
- Relationships with significant others—family, friends, work, society
- Anxiety
- Sadness, depression, and mood conditions
- Developmental eras and transitions—individual, family, group, societal
- Illness—acute and chronic
- Stress and coping
- Coping with change

RESEARCH BRIEF

Co-Occuring Addictive and Mental Disorders

El-Mallakh (1998) examined national co-morbidity surveys of epidemiological research, which indicate that 51% of individuals with a serious psychiatric disorder are also dependent on or addicted to illicit drugs. However, only 50% of these clients received treatment for both co-occurring conditions. El-Mallakh's article provides a historical overview of treatment philosophies and approaches to treatment. It also describes current models and outcome data regarding efficacy of treatment. Recommendations were made to include effective treatment models into nursing practices.

number of persons and families who experience periods of acute exacerbation of chronic illness. Other chronic illnesses, such as diabetes, have patterns involving crisis and management and need psychiatric-mental health nursing attention.

Ethics of Psychiatric-Mental Health Services

Inequity that exists around mental health care impoverishes a group of people who are already at risk. Furthermore, cost of services is a factor in access and serves to compound risk in an already vulnerable population. This is in direct conflict with prevention concepts and health promotion, which require delicate timing and appropriate intervention within the least restrictive environment. The right to fair and equal mental health treatment is a human rights issue. Interestingly, the community mental health movement was concurrent with the Civil Rights movement and was just about as successful. Where civil rights and care are much improved today, there is great need for equity and mainstreaming of mental health services into the health care system of services.

Mental health problems, in contrast to physical health problems, are often very complex, involving an interaction of many factors, including heredity, cultural, social class, living conditions, lifestyle, family relationships, occupation, and economic and political factors. There are often unrecognized mental health issues surrounding and involved with physical health and illness conditions that, if treated along with the physical illness, would promote a healthier adjustment. The separation of mental health services from other health services creates problems of access to treatment. Problems occur both for those with major or chronic and debilitating mental health conditions and for those who have symptoms that, if treated appropriately at the time, would contribute to the recovery, health, and well-being of the person.

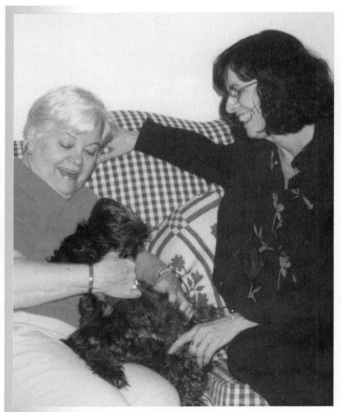

Dr. Sarah Steen Lauterbach, chapter author, in encounter with elder client.

Psychiatric-Mental Health Nursing's Unique Perspective on the Public's Health

The focus on nursing's unique role in health care has also continued to be articulated within the role of psychiatric mental health nursing. Dialogs about nursing have traditionally centered around the contributions from natural science. Increasingly, this dialog is including contributions and knowledge coming from the qualitative, human science tradition. The development of a trajectory of research from the other side of the research paradigm is seen in an increase in reports of qualitative research in scholarly journals. Psychiatric-mental health nursing journals increasingly include qualitative research. In the future, research will look to triangulated methodologies that include both paradigms, quantitative and qualitative.

The development of qualitative nursing research has much to offer nursing, but especially psychiatric-mental health nursing. It will help in understanding the person with a condition and the nurse providing care. Each qualitative research perspective has unique contributions: Phenomenology facilitates in understanding meanings surrounding mental health conditions; grounded theory leads to identifying and understanding basic social processes and social interaction theory as it relates to human experience; ethnography offers to understand the culture and meanings surrounding a condition and the care system; philosophical inquiry and critical social theory aim to provide a fuller understanding of the social and philosophical contexts surrounding mental health issues; historical inquiry looks at past practice as it relates to current and future issues surrounding nursing and practice.

In addition to the particular perspectives that scholarship and research have provided nursing, throughout its history, nursing has through its particular focus and proximity to life and people, provided a unique contribution in promoting the health and well-being of all people—through professional nursing's involvement with persons, regardless of life station, through its special attention to persons, groups, communities, and nations at risk or vulnerable and forgotten people, through commitment to care and service. It is through nursing's conceptualizations about the nature of human experience, of the reality of people's experience throughout the world, that nursing serves a necessary and critical service. It is through its temporality and role in relationships with people and communities that nursing has a particular vantage for understanding people, their unique as well as individual differences, along with their common and shared needs, hopes, and dreams.

Psychiatric-Mental Health Nursing's Roles and Phenomena of Concern

The preceding discussion is particularly important in understanding the complexities of the art and science of psychiatric-mental health nursing care. The American Nurses Association (ANA, 1994a) identified a list of actual or potential mental health problems presented in Box 36-9 that comprise phenomena of psychiatric-mental health nursing's concern. These include phenomena presented earlier as universal human experiences in need of attention, care, and research. Basic-level functions of the psychiatric-mental health nursing presented previously are inclusive of both prevention and promotion activities as well as treatment and intervention activities. Advanced-level functions further delineate the specialty and therapist role of the advanced-practice psychiatric-mental health nurse.

The psychiatric-mental health nursing role includes health promotion, health maintenance, health teaching, community action, and advocacy; however, this area comprises one of the greatest needs in community mental health program development. Currently, nurses in practice within community programs function primarily as managers of care, overseeing care, adminis-

---

BOX 36-9 PSYCHIATRIC-MENTAL HEALTH NURSING'S PHENOMENA OF CONCERN

Actual or potential mental health problems of clients pertaining to the following:

- The maintenance of optimal health and well-being and the prevention of psychobiological illness
- Self-care limitations or impaired functioning related to mental and emotional distress
- Deficits in the functioning of significant biological, emotional, and cognitive systems
- Emotional stress or crisis components of illness, pain, and disability
- Self-concept changes, developmental issues, and life process changes
- Problems related to emotions such as anxiety, anger, sadness, loneliness, and grief
- Physical symptoms that occur along with altered psychological functioning
- Alterations in thinking, perceiving, symbolizing, communicating, and decision making
- Difficulties in relating to others
- Behaviors and mental states that indicate the client is a danger to self or others or has a severe disability
- Interpersonal, systemic, sociocultural, spiritual, or environmental circumstances or events that affect the mental and emotional well-being of the individual, family, or community
- Symptom management, side effects/toxicities associated with psychopharmacological intervention and other aspects of the treatment regimen

Source: ANA, 1994.

---

tering medication, and maintaining records. Community action and advocacy activities are often limited. Some nurses are involved in developing and maintaining the therapeutic milieu, but staffing issues are prevalent throughout the private and public programs.

Missing from the list of functions is the nurse's key role in providing continuity of care. The nurse's unique role and position with persons and groups over time provide opportunities for support and intervention that others on the treatment team simply do not have. In addition, the commitment to using strengths of people and active involvement of those cared for place nursing in a key position.

Since the beginning of modern nursing, the concept of *prevention as intervention* has been a key concept of public health care. The unique vantage provided by the nursing perspective, nursing presence, and the temporality of this role is often underused in therapeutic relationships with individuals, groups, and communities. This is an area in need of attention in both public and private programs.

The psychiatric-mental health nurse of the 21st century has assumed more coordinating, collaborative, and case management activities than ever before. At the same time, the role encompasses direct service and therapeutic interventions with individual and groups within services and programs that are located at a variety of locations, within community agencies, and the home. The role of nursing in the public's mental health needs continued assessment and evaluation.

In primary mental health care environments, the basic-level psychiatric-mental health nurses are key professionals who are ideally positioned to assume a variety of roles in multiple settings ranging from acute inpatient to community settings. They are often the only member of the health care team who has knowledge to monitor general health as well as mental health needs and care. They are prepared in early identification of problems, including preventive intervention, primary prevention, and health promotion. They possess skills in assessment, social intervention, and psychoeducational processes connected with understanding illness and experience of mental illness, and also have knowledge of symptom management, pharmacology, and rehabilitation. The advanced-practice psychiatric-mental health nurse is prepared to manage the care of persons, including monitoring medications.

Guiding Conceptual and Theoretical Frameworks for Mental Health Nursing

The purposes of theory are description, explanation, prediction, and control of human phenomena. In addition, nursing theory serves the purpose of providing understanding of human experience and phenomena. Nursing, as a practice discipline, until the last 40 years, operated based on theories related to a biological model of health. It also used interdisciplinary theory. In addition, the use of practice experience as described in the discussion of "tacit understanding" provided a basis for nursing intervention. Nurses have always borrowed and "cut and pasted" theory, sometimes without enough concern for the relevance or "fit." Increasingly, with the development of qualitative research that focuses on developing theory and quantitative research, which requires a theoretical structure, clarity and operationalization of concepts, mid-level nursing theory is being developed. The 1960s and 1970s were the decades for development of nursing grand conceptual models (Table 36-1). In addition, the development of doctoral programs in nursing have provided impetus for theory analysis, theory derivation, and theory construction. Advanced-level psychiatric-mental health nurses involved with theory development can be seen in dissertations and writings

TABLE 36-1	**GRAND NURSING THEORIES**	
AUTHOR	**DATE**	**PUBLICATION**
Peplau	1952	*Interpersonal Relations in Nursing*
Orlando	1961	*The Dynamic Nurse-Patient Relationship*
Wiedenbach	1964	*Clinical Nursing: A Helping Art*
Henderson	1966	*The Nature of Nursing*
Levine	1967	*The Four Conservation Principles of Nursing*
Ujhely	1968	*Determinants of the Nurse-Patient Relationship*
Rogers	1970	*An Introduction to the Theoretical Basis of Nursing*
King	1971	*Toward a Theory of Nursing*
Orem	1971	*Nursing: Concepts of Practice*
Travelbee	1971	*Interpersonal Aspects of Nursing*
Neuman	1974	*The Betty Neuman Health-Care Systems Model*
Roy	1976	*Introduction to Nursing: An Adaptation Model*
Newman	1979	*Toward a Theory of Health*
Johnson	1980	*The Behavioral System Model for Nursing*
Parse	1981	*Man-Living-Health*
Watson	1985	*Nursing: Human Science and Human Care*
Newman	1986	*Health as Expanding Consciousness*

Source: Walker & Avant, 1988.

of several qualitative nurse researchers, including Becker (1991), Hutchinson (1986), Lauterbach (1992, 1996), Swanson-Kaufmann (1983), and Swanson (1993). Aguilera's (1994) classic nursing text is in its seventh edition and is almost universally used in nursing education curriculums that teach crisis intervention. Aguilera's model of crisis intervention assesses the presence of balancing factors.

Of particular importance in psychiatric nursing is the work of Hildegard Peplau (1952), which was published in the classic text *Interpersonal Relations in Nursing*. This work articulated the focus for nursing work as being the nurse-client relationship. Orlando's 1961 text, *The Dynamic Nurse-Patient Relationship*, also focused on the therapeutic relationship. Ten years later, Joyce Travelbee's (1971) text focused on describing the process of developing relationships with clients. These theorists' writings in particular have been useful not only for psychiatric-mental health nursing, but proposed that the therapeutic relationship is the central context for practice.

More recently, writings from psychiatric-mental health nurses such as Boyd (1988), Lauterbach and Becker (1996), Munhall (1994), Munhall and Boyd (1993) and others also embrace the philosophy of phenomenology. Jean Watson's writings and contributions identify caring as the central focus of nursing. There is need for continuing theory development in psychiatric-mental health nursing. Researchers and scholars such as Janice Morse and her colleagues' (1998) symposium on the Comfort Project and other qualitative nurse researchers show potential for theory development.

....

Millions of nurses throughout the world hold the key to an acceptance and expansion of primary health care because they work closely with people . . .
      Dr. Halfdan Mahler, Director-General of World Health
      Organization, at the time of the Alma Ata Declaration

....

Models for Psychiatric–Mental Health Nursing Practice

The writings of educator John Dewey in the early 1900s, who was a friend and colleague of Isabel Stewart, then Chair of the Department of Nursing at Teachers College, Columbia University, are informative. The 1938 writings of Horace Mann (Cremin, 1957) are appropriate considering his views on the value of universal education as the "great equalizer" of human conditions, the "balance wheel of the social machinery," and the creator of wealth undreamed of. He believed that poverty would disappear as an educated public discovered new "treasures of natural and material wealth." Horace Mann also stated that "a nation cannot remain ignorant and free." Education is the key to an informed public and underpins psychiatric-mental health nursing practice at all levels.

Public Health Model

The traditional public health model includes all levels of prevention: primary, secondary, and tertiary. It has been a viable model for psychiatric-mental health nursing practice. Central to this model is the critical role of public education. This model uses concepts of mental health and illness, epidemiology, and population-focused statistics in assessing mental health needs as well as risks. Population statistics, when combined with knowledge of mental health issues, are useful in identifying populations vulnerable to experiencing dysfunction.

Currently, the major thrust of American mental health care is toward secondary prevention efforts, providing treatment and minimizing disability. There is a need for research and funding in all areas of prevention, but particularly within primary prevention. The following primary prevention activities are in need of public policy inquiry and research: mental health promotion and dysfunction prevention; holistic, meaningful, mind-body wellness activities; personal and community education; acquisition of effective coping skills; wholesome early attachments and healthy lifelong relationships; facilitating environments conducive to meaningful work and mental and physical health; and finally, self-empowerment. There is need for a large-scale community studies of stress and crisis conditions.

Secondary prevention activities are the major thrust of care and include early diagnosis and intervention, accessible services, and

RESEARCH BRIEF

Moore, S. (1997). A phenomenological study of meaning in life in suicidal older adults. Archives of Psychiatric Nursing, 11(1), 29–36.

This hermeneutical phenomenological study was to explore how older suicidal adults experienced meaning in their lives. Using Van Manen's (1990) method, 11 participants between the ages of 64 and 92 were interviewed about their subjective experiences of feeling suicidal. Three main themes emerged as characteristic of the experiences and life worlds of the participants. These themes centered around: Psychache, described as current emotional suffering; the feeling that Nobody cares; and Powerlessness. The sensitive research into the qualitative experience of elders' experiences of suicidality has many practice implications. In the words of the researcher, "Nurses have long espoused an ideological commitment to health. This commitment must go beyond ideology and take action on promoting strategies that will allow older persons to develop and main caring connections and meaningful roles within society (p. 35).

timely, appropriate treatment. One of the most important contributions of the community mental health movement of the 1960s and since has been the development of crisis intervention services. This, combined with the consumer movement of the 1970s, has made a significant contribution to support services for individuals and communities. Still, major primary prevention work is needed to address the conditions and environments that create and perpetuate interpersonal crises. Situational crises, which are superimposed on predicted developmental crises, further create risk, but with proper attention, they can be addressed. Consumer involvement has been helpful in the development of suicide prevention programs, services for rape crisis and victim recovery, and other phenomena needing support and therapeutic intervention. However, more research into crisis prevention, intervention, and impact of crises on life is needed. The phenomenon of human abuse and violence needs to be researched and better understood. Where treatment usually is focused on the victim, more work is needed in addressing the treatment and rehabilitation of the perpetrator, facilitating a violence-free environment. Phenomena need to be reconceptualized and investigated as a community and social phenomenon as well as an individual phenomenon.

Tertiary care has been the focus of community mental health programs and currently provides most of the care for the seriously mentally ill public, including state hospitalization. The community mental health care system includes a range of community-based services addressing a full range of needs and particular groups needing care. These programs address ongoing and acute exacerbations of conditions and chronic care. Activities aimed at rehabilitation and reducing the discomfort and suffering associated with particular mental health problems need research.

Community studies of health have provided information that is potentially useful in articulating nursing's future role in community mental health. Early studies such as Hollingshead and Redlich's (1958) associated social class and mental health. Studies that also show the promise of stress and education are Folkman and Lazarus' analysis of coping in a middle-aged community (1980). Antonovsky's (1979, 1987) work on health focuses on "salutogenesis," the origins of health, and "what healthy people have in common." This mid-level theory, along with Selye's (1956, 1974) classic work on the biological model of stress and the work of Benson (1975, 1984), have contributed much. The value of theories such as these combines the idea of the connection between mental and physical health and a sociological model for conceptualizing stress.

Primary Care Model

Since the beginning of modern nursing, nursing has offered two different perspectives for the focus of care: caring for the individual and caring for the needs of populations. There is often tension between these two different perspectives. This is especially true for psychiatric-mental health nursing, where the individual often is seen as the identified client but in reality reflects dysfunction within a family, community, or larger social system. Taking the example of the state of the mental health care system

FYI

Primary Mental Health Care: A Model for Psychiatric–Mental Health Nursing

Haber and Billings (1995) state that primary care is increasingly becoming synonymous with the provision of health care. In addition to discussing roles of basic and advanced level nursing practice in primary mental health care, these authors state that anxiety disorders, depression, and substance abuse are among the most commonly misdiagnosed categories in primary mental health care practice. In addition, they propose that the boundaries of mental health care delivery must be redefined and expanded from a specialty focus to a primary mental health care model. Furthermore, they state that nurses are beginning to find their niche in nontraditional settings.

within the nation, there is dichotomization, stigma, and economic differences within systems providing physical care and mental health care. Privatization of mental health care, reimbursement differences between physical and mental care, and the current contrast with public mental health care's focus on tertiary care are reflective of sentiment and thinking in a society that values economics and physical care over mental health.

Nursing has traditionally been able to provide care to both individuals and groups, using both paradigms for providing care: the public health model and person-focused or family-centered model. Nurses have seen the need for the current "illness care" system to be transformed into a "health care" system.

Primary health care is increasingly being viewed as synonymous with provision of health care (Haber, 1995). If this concept is to be fully actualized, then primary care will necessarily have to include mental health care. Whether this is to be fully realized is doubtful. Rather than be a reactive profession, nursing needs to take a position for advocating planned change, advocating for the right for each citizen to have responsive, quality mental health care alongside responsive quality health care. Access to the health care system needs to include both.

Primary Mental Health Care Model

Increasingly, the discussion of a primary mental health care model is being proposed as a model for delivering community-based, comprehensive psychiatric-mental health nursing (Haber, 1995). It has the potential to integrate the two traditional models of care and posits nursing in a key role meeting needs of both individuals and communities. There is need for continued dialog between psychiatric nurses themselves, represented by the Coalition of Psychiatric Nursing Organizations (COPNO), including the ANA Council on Psychiatric Mental Health Nursing, the American Psychiatric Nursing Association (APNA), the Association of Child and Adolescent Psychiatric Nurses, and the Society for the Education and Research in Psychiatric Nursing (SERPN). Even though many nurses belong to more than one organization, there is need for uniting as a body, a process that has been under way.

More recently, SERPN advocates for nursing to continue to articulate the role of advanced-practice nurses in psychiatric-mental health care to include flexibility and an ability to perform a variety of tasks and roles. This should include generalized care (provided by the primary care focus) and also provide psychiatric nursing's tradition of specialty care (including psychotherapy with individuals, families, and groups, and consultation).

Primary care roles need to be conceptualized to include providing psychiatric-mental health care within front-line health care and should include more than case management of the large population of psychiatric clients receiving tertiary and chronic psychiatric-mental health care.

Person-Focused Model of Practice and Nursing's Therapeutic Use of Self

This model is not necessarily an exclusive model of practice but can be operationalized within practice models described earlier. The focus of care is on developing therapeutic relationships with recipients of care, whether the recipient is an individual, family, group, or community. Within this context, nursing knowledge of theory and processes of care, including assessment, planning, therapeutic interventions, and relationship-building skills, are key. In addition, the nurse as the facilitator of healing and mental health, as the therapeutic instrument of care, is critical. In no area of nursing is the health and philosophy of the nurse more critical than in mental health. Within the community context, where social supports available for nurses, such as exists within institutions, may be more elusive, it is imperative that the nurse's development, health, and clinical and caring experience be respected. Thus, caring for self and each other operationalizes the use of systems theory, as is described in the later discussion of conceptual frameworks of psychiatric-mental health nursing community care. We need more attention to developing systems of support in nursing in psychiatric-mental health nursing. Nursing roles and functions within case management, coordination of care, collaboration, and providing continuity of care can be seen as part of this person-centered model of care.

• •

I always said that mental health got what was left over after everybody else in the health field got what they wanted.
Rosalyn Carter, who as first lady served as co-chair of the President's Commission on Mental Health and championed the rights of those with mental illness

• •

Phenomenology as a Philosophical Perspective for Psychiatric-Mental Health Nursing

• •

We do not see things as they are, we see them as we are.
Talmud

• •

Phenomenology, which focuses on human lived experience, provides a valuable perspective in thinking about the nurse-client relationship, about our being instruments of care, about facilitating therapeutic environments. Lived experience for nurses is what we live through, not what we think about it. Perception is key. Paying attention to experience, increasing awareness of meanings within experience, is what is meant when describing a *wide-awakedness.* Knowing one's self is as important as knowing the client. Phenomenology offers an increasing understanding of self and others. Phenomenology as a philosophy for nursing is increasingly seen in nursing scholarly literature. It has potential to offer us new understandings when, according to Munhall (1994, p. 23), it calls us to do the following:

• *Listen to the experience.*
• *Feel the experience.*
• *Be unknowing.*
• *Become the experience.*
• *Raise our consciousness. The ordinary now becomes wondrous and extraordinary.*
• *Feel amazed.*
• *Feel puzzled.*
• *Begin to understand differences as "real".*

• •

Time present and time past are contained in time future
And time future contained in time past.
T. S. Eliot, 1936

• •

The Future of Psychiatric–Mental Health Nursing Practice

Current psychiatric-mental health nursing practice operates within the managed care, cost containment drive behind health care. A growing number of persons, groups, and communities are not receiving care, do not have basic needs met, and are being lost between services and programs. Preventive care, although identified in *Healthy People 2000* as being targeted (Table 36-2), is still in need of development. Psychiatric-mental health nurses need to be in integrated into primary health care environments and in community-based programs, such as in schools,

RESEARCH BRIEF

Hayne, Y., & Yonge, O. (1997). The lifeworld of the chronic mentally ill: Analysis of 40 written personal accounts. Archives of Psychiatric Nursing, 11(6), 314–324.

In this study, hermeneutic phenomenology was used to investigate descriptions of chronic mental illness as it is lived rather than how it might be conceptualized. The disclosure of meanings was sought through using the work of Van Manen (1990) to look at the four existential lifeworlds of human beings: corporeality (lived body), relationality (lived human relation), spatiality (lived space), and temporality (lived time). Insight and understanding of personal accounts of the lifeworlds of chronic mentally ill persons is key in selecting a more benevolent direction for nursing care, in caring for individuals and groups and for pursuing advocacy roles and informing general as well as psychiatric-mental health care.

day-care programs, parenting programs, and self-help and support programs. Most importantly, there is need for psychiatric-mental health advocacy in the area of health policy and health care planning. Increasingly, communities are experiencing acts of violence. Grandparents are parenting their dysfunctional adult children's children. The future looks bleak as the future grandparents are today's dysfunctional adults. Within this day of information and technology, the growing Third World vulnerable populations, within the larger affluent American society, are cause for concern. Unless we support and care for all our population's needs, health and human rights, including shelter, nutrition, and meaningful life, the health and happiness of the public is threatened. Caring comprehensively for a multicultural population and world is key.

TABLE 36-2   PROBLEMS AND POPULATIONS TARGETED IN NATIONAL HEALTH OBJECTIVES FOR MENTAL HEALTH

PROBLEM	TARGET POPULATION
Persistent mental disorders	Children
	Adolescents
	Adults
Adverse health effects from stress	Adults
Injurious suicide attempts	Adolescents
Suicide	Adolescents
	Adult and elderly men
	Native Americans and Alaska natives in reservation states
Maltreatment	Children and youth age 18 and younger
Assault injuries	Children aged 12 and older
	Adults
Physical abuse	Women
Rape and attempted rape	Women and adolescents age 12 and older
Homicide	Children age 3 and younger
	Spouses
	African American men and women
	Hispanic American men
	Native Americans and Alaska natives in reservation states

Source: Adapted from DHHS, 1990.

CONCLUSION

"There, but by the grace of God, go I" is an apt phrase for thinking about mental health and illness. Isolation and stigma that surround mental health has in the past sur-

rounded other conditions. Cancer was in years past such a dreaded and stigmatized disease. Education and knowledge along with progress in making scientific advances and successful treatment contribute to increased awareness and understanding.

It was not until the 1950s, with the advent of psychopharmacology, that symptoms were treated successfully. The reliance on somatic therapies, such as hydrotherapy, insulin shock, and physical restraints before the psychopharmacological agents, further produced fear and stigma. The newer developments with antipsychotics and antidepressive agents have greatly enhanced treatment of serious episodes and acute exacerbations of chronic conditions. With knowledge has come greater openness and acceptance. Although we have come a long way, we still have a long way to go in meeting the public's mental health needs. Psychiatric-mental health nursing must continue a commitment to social reform. Of all specialties, we offer to guide the world in becoming more aware of meanings of human experiences. Through our interventions in the planning and policy arena and in our daily interactions with clients, families, communities, and colleagues, we hope to enable all people to live as fully as possible—in the words of one young man, "to live life out" as meaningfully, productively, healthfully, and happily as possible.

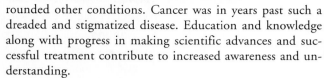

RESEARCH BRIEF

Psychobiology and Psychopharmacotherapy of Unipolar Depression: A Review

O'Toole and Johnson's (1997) article is focused on how psychopharmacology has informed the biological perspective of major depression. Included is a brief historical review of psychopharmacology used in treatment of depression, as well as its neuroendocrine and neurochemical effects. It discusses the use of four classes of antidepressants: monoamine oxidase inhibitors, tricyclic antidepressants, atypical antidepressants, and selective serotonin reuptake inhibitors. There is a need for advanced practice nurses to become and remain knowledgeable of current research findings related to psychobiology and psychopharmacology.

CRITICAL THINKING ACTIVITIES

1. Consider what is it like to experience the following:
   - Serious mental illness, such as schizophrenia, mania, or depression
   - Paranoid feelings, to the degree that you know that if you do not take medication, you will get sicker and sicker
   - Feeling that the medication dulls your attention, which helps you stay vigilant; feeling that something bad will happen if you let down your guard
2. What is it like to experience the following?
   - Having no one who you feel understands you and likes you just the way you are
   - Having no friends
   - Experiencing your little brother's death after he was sick so long with leukemia
   - Watching your dad begin to drink heavily in the evenings
   - Feeling fat, even though you only ate lettuce today, weigh 105 and are 5 feet, 7 inches tall
   - Wanting and feeling very independent but still being told by your parents what time you must come in

CRITICAL THINKING ACTIVITIES—CONT'D

3. What is it like to experience the following?
   - Wanting your parents to stop fighting
   - Wanting your parents to get back together even though you remember how awful it was before they separated
   - Being devastated when your dad moved out
   - Living with your mom, who works too hard and still does not have enough money even though she gets some child support
   - Visiting your dad, who has forgotten what it is like to have anyone, much less a child, around

4. What is it like to experience the following?
   - Being so depressed that you simply are too tired to get out of bed
   - Feeling that you have nothing to live for
   - Feeling that the world and your family would be better off if you just died
   - Being 17 and suddenly discovering that you had lost all your dreams and goals

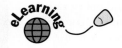

Explore Community Health Nursing on the web! To learn more about the topics in this chapter, use the passcode provided to access your exclusive web site:
http://communitynursing.jbpub.com
If you do not have a passcode, you can obtain one at this site.

REFERENCES

Antonovsky, A. (1979). *Health, stress, and coping.* San Francisco: Jossey-Bass.

Antonovsky, A. (1987). *Unraveling the mystery of health: How people manage stress and stay well.* San Francisco: Jossey-Bass.

Aguilera, D. (1994). *Crisis intervention: Theory and methodology.* St. Louis: Mosby.

American Nurses Association (ANA). (1994a). *A statement on psychiatric-mental health clinical nursing practice and standards of psychiatric-mental health clinical nursing practice.* Washington, DC: American Nurses Publishing.

American Nurses Association (ANA). (1994b). *Scope and standards of advanced practice registered nursing.* Washington, DC: American Nurses Publishing.

American Nurses Association (ANA). (1994c). *Psychiatric mental health nursing psychopharmacology project.* Washington, DC: American Nurses Publishing.

American Psychiatric Association (APA). (1980). *Diagnostic and statistical manual of mental disorders* (3rd ed.). Washington, DC: Author.

American Psychiatric Association (APA). (1987). *Diagnostic and statistical manual of mental disorders (3rd ed., rev.)* Washington, DC: Author.

American Psychiatric Association (APA). (1992). *Diagnostic and statistical manual of mental disorders* (4th ed.) Washington, DC: Author.

Angelou, M. (1971). *Just give me a cool drink of water 'fore i die: The poetry of Maya Angelou.* New York: Random House.

Angelou, M. (1993). *Wouldn't take nothing for my journey now.* New York: Random House.

Baer, E. (1990). *Editor's notes. Nursing in America: A history of social reform, a video documentary.* New York: National League for Nursing Press.

Beck, C. (1998). The effects of postpartum depression on child development; a meta-analysis. *Archives of Psychiatric Nursing, 12*(1), 12–20.

Becker, P. (1991). *Perspectives of ethical care: A grounded theory approach.* Ann Arbor, MI: University Microfilms International Dissertation Service.

Benson, H. (1984). *Beyond the Relaxation Response.* New York: Times Books.

Benson, H. (1975). *The relaxation response.* New York: Avon Books.

Boyd, C. (1988). Phenomenology: A foundation for nursing curriculum. In *Curriculum revolution: Mandate for change*. New York: National League for Nursing Press.

Caplan, G. (1964). *Principles of preventive psychiatry*. New York: Basic Books.

Cremin, L. (1957). *The republic and the school: Horace Mann on the education of free man*. New York: Teachers College University Press.

Department of Health and Human Services (DHHS). (1996, July). *Progress review: Mental health and mental disorders*: http://odphp.osophs.gov/pubs/hp2000/progrvw/mentalprog.htm.

Department of Health and Human Services (DHHS). (2000). *Healthy People 2000: Conference edition*. Washington, DC: U.S. Government Printing Office.

Department of Health and Human Services (DHHS). (1978). *Women's Worlds: NIMH supported research on women*. Washington, DC: U.S. Government Printing Office.

Department of Health, Education, & Welfare. (1978). *Women's worlds: NIMH supported research on women*. Washington, DC: U.S. Government Printing Office.

Dewey, J. (1938). *Education and experience*. New York: Collier Books.

Donahue, M. (1989). *Nursing: the finest art*. St. Louis: Mosby.

El-Mallakh, P. (1998). Treatment models for clients with co-occurring addictive and mental disorders. *Archives of Psychiatric Nursing, 12*(2), 71–80.

Folkman, S., & Lazarus, R. (1980). An analysis of coping in a middle-aged community sample. *Journal of Health and Social Behavior, 21*(3), 219–239.

Frisch, H., & Frisch, L. (1998). *Psychiatric mental health nursing*. Albany, NY: Delmar.

Goren, S. (1997). Pursuit of the ordinary: Short-term inpatient treatment. *Archives of Psychiatric Nursing, 11*(2), 82–88.

Haber, J., & Billings, C. (1995). Primary mental health care: a model for psychiatric-mental health nursing. *Journal of the American Psychiatric Nurses Association, 1*(5), 154–163.

Hayne, Y., & Yonge, O. (1997). The lifeworld of the chronic mentally ill: Analysis of 40 written personal accounts. *Archives of Psychiatric Nursing, 11*(6), 314–324.

Hedaya, R. (1996). *Understanding biological psychiatry*. New York: W. W. Norton & Company.

Henderson, V. (1966a). *The nature of nursing*. New York: Macmillan.

Henderson, V. (1966b). *The nature of nursing: Reflections after 25 Years*. New York: National League for Nursing Press.

Hollingshead, A., & Redlich, F. (1958). *Social class and mental disorder*. New York: Wiley.

Hutchinson, S. (1986). Grounded theory: The method. In P. Munhall & C. Oiler (Eds.), *Nursing research: A qualitative perspective*. New York: National League for Nursing Press.

Lauterbach, S. (1995). (Issue Ed.) The experience of loss. *Holistic Nursing Practice, 9*(3).

Lauterbach, S. (1992). *In another world: A phenomenological perspective and discovery of meaning in mothers' experience of death of a wished-for baby*. Ann Arbor, MI, University Microfilms International Dissertation Service.

Lauterbach, S., & Becker, P. (1996). Caring for self: Becoming a self-reflective nurse. *Holistic Nursing Practice, 10*(2), 57–68.

Leighton, A. (1982). *Caring for mentally ill people: Psychological and social barriers in historical context*. Cambridge, UK: Cambridge University Press.

Leighton, D., Harding, J., Macklin, D., MacMillan, A., & Leighton, A. (1963). *The character of danger: Psychiatric symptoms in selected communities*. New York: Basic Books.

May, R. (1961). *Existential psychology*. New York: Random House.

Moore, S. (1997). A phenomenological study of meaning in life in suicidal older adults. *Archives of Psychiatric Nursing, 11*(1), 29–36.

Morse, J. (1997, December 1–6). *The comfort project*. Presentation at 75th Anniversary Sigma Theta Tau Conference, Indianapolis.

Munhall, P. (1998). Editorial—Out of the box. *Image: The Journal of Nursing Scholarship, 29*(3), 203.

Munhall, P. (1994). *Revisioning Phenomenology: Nursing and Health Science Research*. New York: National League for Nursing Press.

Munhall, P., & Boyd, C. (1993). *Nursing research: A qualitative perspective*. New York: National League for Nursing Press.

Nightingale, F. (1859). *Notes on nursing: What it is and what it is not*. New York: Dover Publications.

O'Toole, S., & Johnson, D. (1997). Psychobiology and psychopharmacotherapy of unipolar major depression: a review. *Archives of Psychiatric Nursing, 11*(6), 303–313.

Peplau, H. (1952). *Interpersonal relations in nursing*. New York: G. P. Putnam's Sons.

President's Commission on Mental Health. (1978). *Report to the President from the President's Commission on Mental Health*. Stock # 040-000-00390, Vol. 1. Washington, DC: US Government Printing Office.

Schon, D. (1983). *The reflective practitioner*. New York: Basic Books.

Schon, D. (1990). *Educating the reflective practitioner*. San Francisco: Jossey-Bass.

Selye, H. (1974). *Stress without distress*. New York: Signet.

Selye, H. (1956). *The stress of life*. New York: McGraw-Hill.

Sills, G. (1999, May/June). Obituary: Hildegard E. Peplau, 89, nursing scholar, educator, and leader. *The American Nurse*.

Stanhope, M., & Lancaster, J. (1996). *Community health nursing.* St. Louis: Mosby.

Swanson, K. (1993). Nursing as informed caring for the wellbeing of others. *Image: The Journal of Nursing Scholarship, 45*(4), 352–357.

Swanson-Kaufmann, K. (1983). *The unborn one: A profile of the human experience of Miscarriage.* Ann Arbor, MI: University Microfilms International Dissertation Service.

Todd, M., & Higginson, T. (1982). *Collected poems of Emily Dickinson.* New York: Random House. (Originally published in 1890.)

Travelbee, J. (1971). *Interpersonal aspects of nursing.* (2nd ed.). Philadelphia: F.A. Davis.

Tsuang, M., Tohen, M., & Zahner, G. (1995). *Textbook in psychiatric epidemiology.* New York: John Wiley and Sons.

Walker, L., & Avant, K. (1988). *Strategies for theory construction in nursing* (2nd ed.). Norwalk, CT: Appleton & Lange.

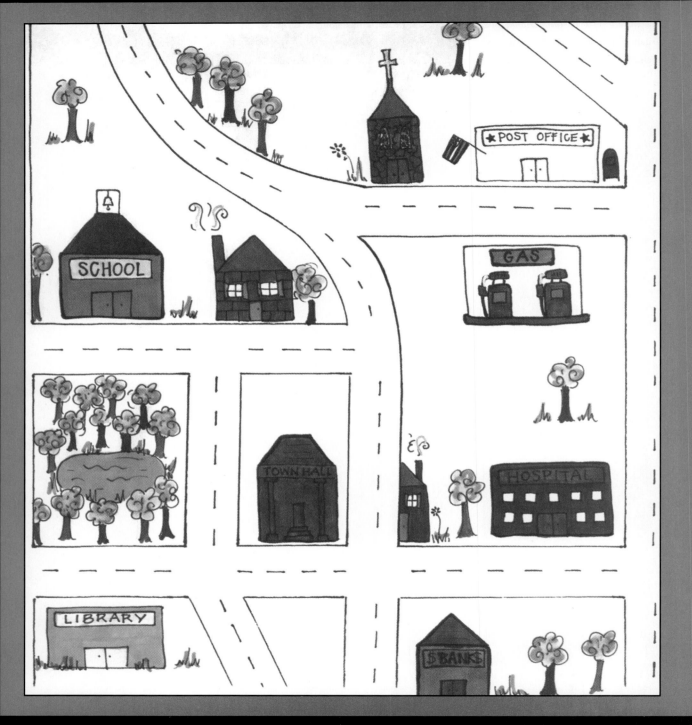

PART THREE

Diversity in Community Health Nursing Roles

Community health nursing may offer nurses more diversity than most any other specialty because of the focus on population groups rather than on individual clients. Community health nursing roles are unique in their diversity because of the *nature of their implementation*, not simply because of the *setting* where the care occurs. Community health nursing has always embraced a variety of roles due to the diversity and complexity of public health problems. Because the focus of the care is on the group or population, community health nurses are involved in the identification of populations at risk for illness or disability. Community health nurses assist communities, groups, and populations, such as schools and churches, in the prevention of health problems through self-care and accountability. For example, a public health nurse may administer immunizations to preschool children in a day care to prevent and control communicable diseases in the community at large. Although the focus of these roles remains health promotion and protection, specializations such as occupational health nursing, school nursing, public health nursing, advanced practice, home health, and the care of faith communities through health ministries have emerged as challenging career opportunities for community health nurses.

Unit VIII

Community Health Nurse Roles

Chapter 37

Public Health Nursing: Pioneers of Health Care Reform

Kaye W. Bender and Marla E. Salmon

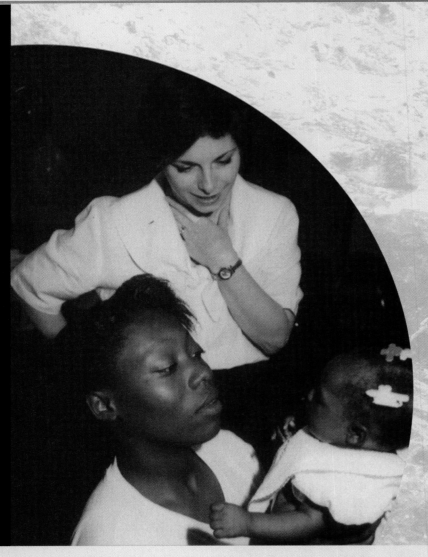

*When **Florence Nightingale** founded modern nursing, the relationship between the environment and the health of the individual was a cornerstone. Nightingale's text **Notes on Nursing** described the nurse's role in altering the client's immediate environment through ventilation and heating, cleanliness of housing, modification of noise, provision of light, and proper preparation and availability of food. These factors were found by Nightingale to be of importance to the health and well-being of individuals and therefore relevant to nursing intervention. The public health nurse role emerged from these early links between health and the environmental conditions under which we live.*

CHAPTER FOCUS

History of Public Health Nursing
Early Health Care Reform
The Later Years

Public Health Nursing Philosophy
Institute of Medicine Study
Conceptual Basis for Public Health Nursing Practice

Definition and Development of Public Health Nursing
Essential Public Health Services
Activities for Essential Services

The Year 2000 and Beyond: Challenges for Public Health Nursing

QUESTIONS TO CONSIDER

After reading this chapter, answer the following questions:

1. What were the early public health reform efforts?
2. Who were the early public health nursing leaders?
3. What were the primary contributions of public health nurses during the early part of the 20th century?
4. What are characteristics of nursing from the 1960s through the 1980s?
5. What is the role and focus of public health nursing practice?
6. What is the significance of the Institute of Medicine report of 1988?
7. How are conceptual models used in public health nursing?
8. What is the Construct for Public Health Nursing, and what is its usefulness in present public health nursing practice?
9. What is meant by *essential public health services*?
10. What is the future of public health nursing in the 21st century?

KEY TERMS

Commonwealth Fund
Conceptual model
Construct for Public
  Health Nursing: A
  Framework for the
  Future

Essential public health
  services
Florence
  Nightingale
Hospital and
  Reconstruction
  Act of 1946

Institute of Medicine
  Study of 1988
Lillian Wald
Mary D. Osborne
Medicare
Milbank Report
Notes on Nursing

Salk vaccine
Social Security
  Act of 1935

History of Public Health Nursing

There have been public health problems in the United States since colonization, but it was not until after the Civil War that concerted efforts were made to improve morbidity and mortality and to control infectious diseases. Poverty, unsanitary living conditions, rampant spread of communicable diseases, natural disasters such as floods, malnutrition, and lack of health care were contributing factors to morbidity and mortality. Public health nursing pioneers emerged as public health efforts began, the most notable being **Lillian Wald,** who is recognized as the leader of public health nursing in the United States. Wald was the first to use the term *public health nurse* to describe visiting nurses who provided direct care to the sick in their homes. These nurses also taught basic hygiene, sanitation, care of children, and proper care and preparation of food. Public health nurses proved versatile; their skills seemed endless, with a mission to prevent disease, promote health, and to provide care; their communities truly became their workplace as they became involved in health concerns associated with access to health care, labor movements, maternal and child health, reproductive health, mental health, prison reform, and school health.

Early Health Care Reform

Organized public health efforts were initiated across the country in the late 1800s and early 1900s. This early health care reform movement was aimed at improving the health status of all citizens. Leading causes of death were tuberculosis, pneumonia and influenza, diarrhea, malaria, heart and cerebrovascular diseases, and infectious diseases in early infancy; complicating factors were the deplorable living conditions and malnutrition of many citizens. Most notable among the early public health nursing activities were services to river travelers in the south and seaports along the nation's coasts and preventive health services to immigrants in large eastern seaboard cities.

Many of the early efforts to establish public health nursing occurred as a result of collaborative agreements between municipalities and the American Red Cross. It was not uncommon for public health nurses to be assigned to posts in geographical areas other than the ones in which they lived at the time of their employment. One such early pioneer in was **Mary D. Osborne,** who came to a rural southern state to work toward the improvement of infant mortality. Her philosophy of public health nursing is reflected in her writings, in which she described qualities she deemed essential for public health nurses of the time, "nurses chosen for public health needed vision, a great desire to do community work, the ability to work up resources at hand, the adaptability to meet situations as they arose, and most of all infinite patience with people they serve" (Mississippi Department of Archives, 1920–1980); these qualities are as essential today for public health nurses as they were in Osborne's time. Osborne received national and international recognition in 1929 for her work in forging a strong network of public health nurses and for their accomplishments in lowering maternal and infant mortality through improved midwifery practice.

The Great Depression is remembered today as one of the most dramatic times in U.S. history, and most states felt the difficult economic effects of the early 1930s. Public health and public health nursing struggled through this era; however, federal initiatives through Roosevelt's New Deal programs and private entities such as the **Commonwealth Fund** provided funding to expand public health nursing services. The hope was to place one public health nurse in each county in many of the states. Immunization efforts against smallpox, diphtheria, and typhoid were one of the special initiatives with the expanded public health nursing workforce. New initiatives were integrated with previously established activities centered around communicable diseases, perinatal and infant care and midwifery supervision, and tuberculosis control. Their place of service delivery was literally all places in their community as public health nurses made home visits, school visits, and often set up clinic sites in rural churches or under shade trees.

The public health nurse was equipped with a large brown leather bag to carry essential items such as needles, syringes, a Sterno stove, and matches to set up clinic sites. A black nursing bag was added to provide a mechanism for carrying needed items for home visits. To get where they needed to be, the nurses might travel down muddy paths by riding a mule, borrowing a horse and buggy, or walking lengthy distances; and sometimes a boat might be the mode of transportation. An automobile was a luxury item and a prized possession when available.

Early Health Outcomes

The dramatic results of this health care movement are noted in mortality and morbidity statistics from 1926 to 1936, with reductions in typhoid fever, diphtheria, pulmonary tuberculosis, pellagra, puerperal septicemia, and eclampsia. One state health official gave much credit to public health nursing by noting that the public health nursing service had come to be recognized as a vital part of an efficient public health administration.

Syphilis had been recognized for several years as a major source of morbidity and mortality. Several boards of health participated with the United States Public Health Service (USPHS) in major studies in the 1930s and 1940s to develop means to conquer the disease. Public health nurses were recognized by the USPHS project director as the chief means to find cases, access medical care for treatment, provide education, find contacts, and follow up on lapsed cases.

Despite interferences of World War II, public health nurses continued to receive education in prevention and treatment of disease processes, including tuberculosis, vaccine-preventable diseases, maternal and child health, and syphilis. Remarkable advances in medical prevention and diagnostic and treatment measures such as the introduction of penicillin were changing public health service delivery and opening new challenges for public health nurses. After World War II, social and economic changes in the states (e.g., improved housing and transportation, movement from farms to towns, expansion of industry) also brought challenges for public health nursing. A public health nurse was employed to institute industrial nursing, which would focus on disease prevention, improvements of hazardous work conditions, promotion of personal health (including nutrition), and first aid.

The country had experienced cyclic polio epidemics since 1934, but disaster struck with the most virulent and widespread epidemic in 1951–1952. Public health nurses made home visits to assist in rehabilitative measures for persons affected with this crippling disease. Regional orthopedic clinics were manned by public health nurses to support access to medical care and set up client treatment plans. With the availability of the injectable **Salk vaccine** in 1955, public health nurses set up mass immunization sites, while using needles and syringes that required sterilization between each use. These efforts prevented the occurrence of any further polio epidemics.

Health care reform was again under way as federal funds were made available through the **Hospital and Reconstruction Act in 1946.** The increased availability of local hospitals resulted in more physician-attended births, another significant contribution to lower maternal and infant mortality rates. A dilemma resulted, however, as newly constructed hospitals, expanding industry, and public health were competing for the short supply of nurses in the country. Concerns such as the turnover of nursing personnel, the below-average ratio of public health nurse to population, inadequate salaries, and increased responsibilities caused by a shortage of medical directors in county health departments were prevalent. During this era, public health nursing services shifted significantly from the community to the clinic, rendering the large brown bag used to set up outlying clinics extinct. A shift from family health to more technical, disease-oriented services occurred as a result of limited medical coverage and increased demands for nursing services.

The individual states, along with the rest of the nation, were flourishing economically as the 1960s began. Tuberculosis and several other infectious diseases were no longer the leading causes of death. Typhoid fever, diphtheria, malaria, smallpox, and pellagra had been leading causes of death in 1930–1931; by 1959–1960, only a few deaths were reported from these diseases. Heart disease, circulatory diseases, cancer, accidents, and diabetes were reported as the leading causes of death.

Changes in morbidity and mortality required evaluation by public health, and consequently, new strategies and public health programs were needed to continue the public health mission. Public health nursing established chronic illness objectives to identify cases and treat diabetic and hypertensive clients. Nursing interventions included referrals to local physicians to initiate treatment plans, nutrition and general health education, administration of medication, and teaching administration of insulin. In addition, new vaccines to prevent measles and rubella were integrated into routine immunization standards.

Tuberculosis, although no longer a leading cause of death, remained a public morbidity threat. Medications and treatment modalities had greatly advanced, however. Recognizing the value of early detection of persons susceptible to tuberculosis and providing prophylactic treatment, public health nurses accepted the challenge of a major initiative by boards of health to eradicate tuberculosis. Public health nurses identified contacts to active cases and others determined to be infected, coordinated medical evaluations, initiated plans of care for further diagnostic measures, and administered INH medication.

Landmark federal legislation in 1965 transformed health care with an amendment to the **Social Security Act of 1935,** establishing **Medicare,** a health insurance plan for people 65 years and older and for those with long-term disabilities. Many boards of health supported expanded efforts to meet the federal conditions of participation and, over a 4- to 5-year period, implemented certified home health services. Educational opportunities provided public health nurses with knowledge and skills to provide skilled rehabilitative nursing care to persons who were essentially confined to their homes. Public health nurses had been providing home nursing services on a limited basis since the 1920s, but this would be the first reimbursement established for direct nursing services.

Another new federal initiative for public health nursing by the mid 1960s was family planning. The objective was aimed at lowering maternal and infant mortality rates and improving the general health of women and children, primary interests of public health nurses since the 1920s. Public health nurses promoted family planning, taught contraceptive methods, and were key in identifying those women at highest risk and need for such services.

The quantity and variance of public health nursing activities continued to increase. The number of public health nursing visits increased in the areas of communicable disease, maternal and child health, school health, tuberculosis control, sexually transmitted disease, home health, mental health, accident prevention, and chronic disease. Particularly in the southern states, the work of public health nurses in all health programs was perhaps the greatest force in delivering health services to all citizens.

The Later Years

Social and political unrest begun in the 1960s continued into the 1970s, and simultaneously the nation was faced with inflation. Travel budgets were cut; public health nursing activities were again evaluated and were relocated from the field to the clinic setting. Continued vigilance in protecting the public's health was in order, and public health nursing rose to the occasion. Increased teen pregnancy rates, a higher incidence of premature births in poorer women, and frequent pregnancies were the focus for public health nursing interventions. More intense family planning initiatives and high-risk tracking systems were implemented to reduce unintended pregnancies and ensure quality, continuous care. In addition, public health nurses supported program implementations to improve nutrition to mothers and children and newborn screening with follow-up for select genetic diseases.

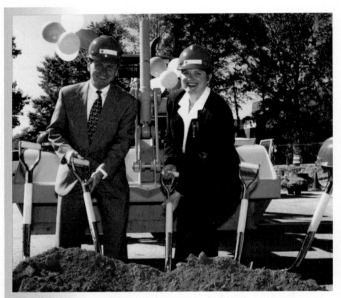

At the September 1999 groundbreaking for the Nell Hodgson Woodruff School of Nursing of Emory University's new building, James Curran, MD, MPH, dean of the Rollins School of Public Health, and Marla Salmon, ScD, RN, FAAN, dean of the School of Nursing, and chapter author, broke ground together. The new building is being built directly next to the School of Public Health building. Drs. Curran and Salmon hold joint faculty appointments in each other's schools, concrete evidence of a collaboration and partnership between the two schools.

Public health was confronted in the 1970s with increasing demands for services and a limited availability of physicians. Federal funds were made available to provide education to expand the scope of nursing in primary care. Many nurse practice acts were revised by legislation to allow for the expanded role of public health nurses. Boards of health, recognizing the value of this level of practitioner in public health, selected public health nurses to return to school with primary areas of study in maternal and child health. This proved to be an added advantage as nurses returned to more client- and family-centered care, which had been the traditional philosophy of public health nursing.

Public health nurses of the 1980s and 1990s have continued to provide an array of public health services to the general public, to medically underserved populations, and to culturally diverse populations. Their workplace remains the same as they provide services in individual homes, schools, industry, jails and prisons, and the county health departments; and their mission, to prevent disease and to promote health, remains constant. With today's national and state focus on health care reform, public health nurses are positioned to assist both communities and individuals within to bridge the transitions of health care. Their versatile skills include assessing the health status of communities, translating and interpreting among health care disciplines, promoting and teaching health, delivering primary community-based health care, and sustaining measures to control communicable disease.

History reveals that health care reform is a continuous process, not a new phenomenon. The elements currently influencing health care reform are both old and new—tremendous technology advances, explosive and diverse population growth, political changes, an array of extreme social problems, escalating health care costs, access to care, financing for acute care rather than preventive health, and the need to encourage individual responsibility for health.

Public Health Nursing Philosophy

Fundamental to the philosophy of public health nursing are holistic beliefs about humanity, health, and nursing. Public health nursing has been defined as "the practice of promoting and protecting the health of populations using knowledge from nursing, social, and public health sciences" (APHA, 1996).

Public health nursing practice is a systematic process that accomplishes the following:

1. *The health and health care needs of a population are assessed to identify subpopulations, families, and individuals who would benefit from health promotion or who are at increased risk of illness, injury, disability, or premature death.*

2. *A plan for intervention is developed with the community to meet identified needs that take into account available resources and the range of activities that contribute to health and the prevention of illness, disability and premature death.*

3. *A plan is implemented effectively, efficiently, and equitably.*

4. *Evaluations are conducted to determine the extent to which the interventions have an impact on the health status of individuals and the population.*

5. *The results of the process are used to influence and direct the current delivery of care, deployment of health resources, and the development of local, regional, state, and national health policy and research to promote health and prevent disease.*

This systematic process is based on and is consistent with (1) community strengths, needs, and expectations; (2) current scientific knowledge; (3) available resources; (4) accepted criteria and standards of nursing practice; (5) agency purpose, philosophy, and objectives; and (6) the participation, cooperation, and understanding of the population. Other services and organizations in the community are considered, and planning is coordinated to maximize the effective use of resources and enhance outcomes. The philosophy of public health nursing is based on the belief that clients (individuals, families, groups, or communities) have the right to quality health care that is available, accessible, and acceptable and that will include them in the planning of their health care.

Institute of Medicine Study

Recognizing that organized public health efforts had been vital to ensuring the health of the nation, the **Institute of Medicine** completed a 2-year study of the future of public health in 1988. During that 2-year period, the committee members interviewed an array of public health workers, policy makers, members of the general public, and public health academicians. The study's final recommendations have become a cornerstone for guiding public health's organizational development. Those recommendations included a description of the mission of public health.

. . . .

Public health's mission is to fulfill society's interest in assuring conditions in which people can be healthy.

Institute of Medicine, 1988

. . . .

This mission statement said succinctly what public health nurses had been practicing for many years. With the goal of improving the health of the public as a whole, public health nurses systematically provide nursing interventions at both the individual and community levels. These interventions vary with the changing health status of the citizens of the country. In the early years when living conditions and crowded housing created opportunities for diseases to spread, public health nurses provided assessment, treatment, and education on tuberculosis, sexually transmitted diseases, and general personal hygiene. In these later years, as lifestyles and personal health habit choices are significant to the causes of morbidity and mortality, public health nurses have added education about the prevention of tobacco use, exercise benefits, and domestic violence to their menu of interventions. The role of ensuring that the public remains as healthy as possible is shared between government and the private sector. The Institute of Medicine described government's role in ensuring the public's health as follows:

- Assessment: *Public health agencies systematically collect, analyze, and publish information on the health status of the community.*
- Policy development: *Public health agencies promote the use of scientific knowledge as the basis for formulating public policy about health.*
- Assurance: *Public health agencies assure that services that are needed to ensure the health of the public are in place and are of high quality.*

Several levels of responsibility were attached to these roles. Local, state, and federal governments were all challenged with their respective responsibilities in ensuring the health of the public. Special linkages to environmental health, mental health, and the care of the indigent were also described in the study.

Public health nurses have the potential to develop roles in all of the areas described in the IOM report. Although the most commonly defined role of the public health nurse has been that of providing services to control communicable diseases, there are numerous other roles for public health nurses. At the beginning of the 21st century, public health nurses are working in epidemiology, policy development, administration, specialized research areas, and nurse-managed projects aimed at improving the health of special populations.

Conceptual Basis for Public Health Nursing Practice

The new millennium has brought forth countless predictions about the nature of tomorrow's health care delivery system. These scenarios range from visions of health care being delivered through primarily technological means as part of the many services provided by one of a few large health-related corporations to more humanistic portrayals of high-touch, community-based programs that reflect the unique nature of where people live and work. What is common to almost all scenarios is that they seem to ignore two very important factors: the changing social context worldwide and the ongoing role of government in the protection and assurance of the health of the public.

Clearly, it is difficult to predict what the world will be like over the next two to three decades; however, there are some crucial themes that will undoubtedly play major roles in shaping the health of all people. The first of these is globalization and the resulting interconnectedness of all people. Through increasingly interlaced economies, markets, and the media, it is now virtually impossible to remain unaffected by what is happening in other countries and cultures. In addition, travel, migration, and the forced movement of masses of people by political and natural disasters have mixed peoples together in ways never before seen. Communities based on shared culture and history are disappearing rapidly. The global disruption of people and communities, coupled with the rise in religious fundamentalism and nationalism worldwide, promises a highly unstable and challenging future for the health of all people.

Global changes of the magnitude described here place heavy burdens on individuals, communities, and governments. The United States is not immune to these changes and is already struggling to address these at all levels. Rising violence of all types and growing gang membership; increasing diversity in language, culture, and race; and growing separation between the rich and the poor are challenging every social institution and community. In the face of these enormous challenges, it is difficult to imagine any health care system without considering how governments at all levels will work to ensure that the health of the public is protected.

It is in the context of ensuring the health of the public that the future of public health nursing will emerge. We will now look at those key themes that are critical to the creation of the future roles of public health nurses and propose the application of a fundamental **conceptual model** in the development of future public health nursing interventions.

When one examines most every health systems scenario for the 21st century, there is an implicit assumption that the system of health care will be deeply embedded in the marketplace and governed by the principles of competition and a market economy. Often accompanying this assumption is the belief that the market has the ability in and of itself to deal with the problems of access and quality that plague our system. There is a view that the more troubling issues of equity and social justice—who receives care and in what ways—will be solved by letting the market do its work. As noted financier George Soros has observed, there are inherent dangers in this optimistic view of relying heavily on the marketplace to address these crucial issues (Soros, 1997). Our economy has as its fundamental purposes the creation of goods, services, and profit, based on willingness and ability to pay. Unfortunately, when health services become a commodity, not everyone can afford them or pay for them.

Faced with the reality that large sectors of the American population are denied access to reasonable health care is neither in the interest of these individuals, nor does it work to the benefit of the overall public. The failure or inability of the marketplace to address public health needs—whether in provision of health care, protection of the environment, or containing and preventing disease and injury—is where much of public health's future lies. It is comforting to know that this mandate of acting in the overall interest of the public has been in existence for well over a century. The historic **Milbank Report** on Higher Education for Public Health offered a timeless definition of public health:

> Public health is the effort organized by society to protect, promote and restore the people's health. The programs, services, and institutions involved emphasize the prevention of disease and the health needs of the population as a whole. Public health activities change with changing technology and social values, but the goals remain the same: to reduce the amount of disease, premature death and the disease-produced discomfort and disability (Milbank Memorial Fund Commission, 1976, p. 3).

The history of public health nursing clearly illustrates both the changing nature and timelessness of ensuring the health of the people. For more than 100 years, public health nurses have filled multiple roles and created an endless variety of strategies, interventions, and programs to fulfill their mission. It is in both the constancy of the mission and flexibility of its means that public health nursing will find its future (Salmon, 1993).

What this means in practical terms is that public health nursing needs to clearly understand the impact of the changing society on health and the forces that are at work either enhancing or eroding the health of the people. To do this, public health nurses need an overall operating framework that encompasses public health values, health determinants, practice priorities, types of interventions, and an understanding of the interplay of these at all levels. The model presented in this chapter is "**Construct for Public Health Nursing: A Framework for the Future**" (White, 1982).

In 1982, the Construct for Public Health Nursing first appeared in *Nursing Outlook*. The purpose of the construct or model was to provide a systematic model through which public health nursing could be both understood and practiced. Since that time, the model has been incorporated into both education and practice through its adoption in curricula, incorporation in a variety of texts and articles, and extensive use in the creation of public health nursing programs at a variety of levels.

This model is particularly useful as public health nursing grapples with understanding and shaping the health of the public in the 21st century. The model itself is built on the premise that the fundamental difference between public health nursing and all other nursing rests in its commitment to the health of the public. This notion of the public good is understood to be both the ethical base for public health nursing practice and the consequences of fundamentally social and political processes. As a result, the model depicts a practice that is both based on explicit valuing of the public good and a "form follows function" approach to actual interventions. The values of public health nursing are interlaced in the circular depiction of the public health nursing process: assessing, diagnosing, planning, implementing, and evaluating. In other words, each of those actions is based on the primacy of the public's health and good.

· ·

The Profession of Public Health Nursing

Public health nursing it's time to celebrate;
Mankind's woes we seek to alleviate.
One hundred years old in nineteen hundred ninety-three,
The wonders unfold as you review its history.

Some note its origin with Phoebe,
Paul's friend at the start of Christianity.
In the USA we herald Lillian Wald's establishment.
For the most vulnerable, she began the Henry Street Settlement.

No transportation, health care unaffordable,
Chronic disease, and living conditions unsuitable—
Public health nurses concerned today
With the same health issues of yesterday.

The home, the school, the factory, the jail,
Caring for the sick, promoting good health for the well.
The grimaces, the smiles of all the faces
The fields of public health nursing are all places.

Communicable disease has taken its toll,
Wretching each community's heart and soul.
Measles, cholera, polio and TB—
New to the scene are HIV and Hepatitis B.

Evaluation, investigation, and collaboration,
A loving hand and much determination.
Public health nurses possess great versatility;
Their mission is to lower morbidity, lower mortality.

Immunizations public health nurses have given,
Education is provided to all who will listen.
Public health nursing, a challenge you see,
To help a community be disease free.

Skilled care to the homebound for rehabilitation,
Also often preventing institutionalization.
Public health nursing, an opportunity you see,
To help many stay home with their family.

Mothers and babies public health nurses nourish,
What joy is felt when these infants flourish.
Public health nursing, a belief you see,
That each life improved may be.

The community, the family, the individual, too,
Benefit greatly from all these nurses do.
Public health nursing, a career you see,
That makes a great difference, don't you agree?

by Margaret Morton

· ·

CONSTRUCT FOR PUBLIC HEALTH NURSING MODEL.

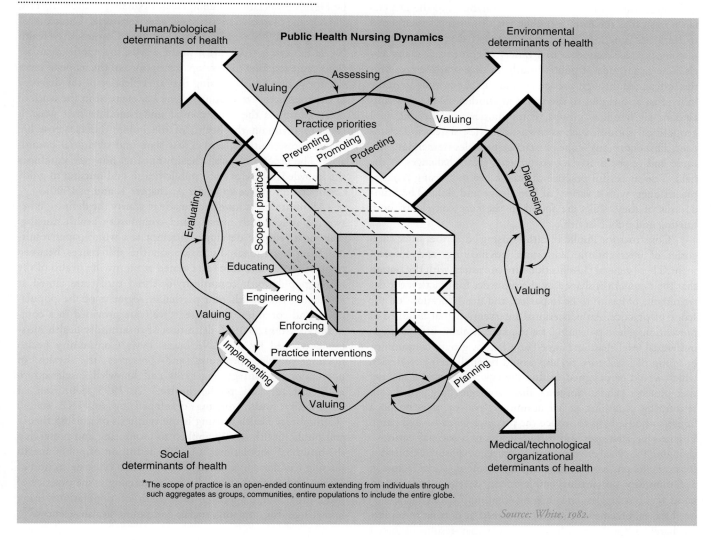

*The scope of practice is an open-ended continuum extending from individuals through such aggregates as groups, communities, entire populations to include the entire globe.

Source: White, 1982.

This notion of valuing the public's good does not sit easy with most health professionals, whose ethics are grounded in advocacy for individual clients. It is for this reason that the explicit delineation of public health values is critical to the successful future practice of public health nursing. Most of our health care system has been built on the notion of serving individuals—very little consideration has been given to the impact on the well-being of the public.

In the model, the health of the public is seen as being impacted by four determinants of health: social, human-biological, environmental, and medical/technological/organizational. The first three are fairly well understood—it is the fourth that continues to be less a part of most practitioner's concept of health determinants. Another way of describing these determinants is that they are *made up* of the technology, organization, and policies relating to health care delivery. It is the content and organization of health care itself. This determinant has shown itself to be an ex-

tremely important point of consideration during this last decade of "health care reform," which has focused entirely on this factor.

In understanding the determinants of health and their dynamics, public health nursing has the knowledge on which to target interventions. In other words, public health nursing practice is fundamentally focused on impacting determinants of health as the primary mechanism for enhancing and protecting the health of people.

The practice of public health nursing that is described in the model has three priorities: prevention, protection, and health promotion. Understood as somewhat overlapping concepts, each is given its own prominence because of the importance of considering all three in actual practice. These priorities serve to focus the ways in which public health nurses interface with health determinants. The message in all three of these priorities is that early intervention is always most desirable, with prevention being the primary goal.

When one considers the mandate of ensuring the health of the public, the nature of health determinants, and the utilitarian notion that the form of public health nursing is sharpened to fulfill its function, it becomes apparent that public health nursing practice can occur in a variety of contexts at many levels. The magnitude of public health nursing practice possibilities is depicted through a scope of practice that extends from the individual at one end to the world at another. Along this continuum sit families, groups, communities, populations, and geopolitical entities, such as towns, counties, states, and countries. This enormous scope of practice provides tremendous latitude and opportunity; it also presents great challenges to the field. The successful practice of public health nursing requires practitioners with a variety of knowledge and skills. The foundations of these skills are found in the core content of both nursing and public health.

"Construct for Public Health Nursing" describes three categories of interventions: education, engineering, and enforcement. These general classifications are consistent with the notion that their content is shaped by the priorities for practice, the determinants of health to be impacted, and their "location" on the scope of practice. An educational intervention that is aimed at prevention of lead poisoning, for example, is quite different at an individual level than one aimed at a family, group, community, or group of legislators. So also would be engineering strategies, which would be designed to alter the environment in a manner that protects people. Some of these strategies might focus on retrofitting plumbing at a community level or working on a house-to-house basis to reduce the presence of lead-based paint. Engineering strategies also include those of a societal nature—changing the social environment to prevent exposures. Consider, for example, preventing crime through changing social factors in a community—increasing employment, developing neighborhood watch strategies, encouraging community policing, and so on. Last, enforcement strategies are aimed at putting into place mechanisms for "compelling" behavior that results in better health. Laws that require motorcycle helmets are one such example. Enforcement strategies can also be used on an individual level, such an individually observed therapy for high-risk clients with drug-resistant tuberculosis.

The underlying theme throughout this model is that actions are guided by commitment, context, clear priorities, public health values, flexibility, and the melding of nursing and public health knowledge and skills. This means that public health nursing is really a practice that is shaped by intent, not by convention. The intent, of course, is serving the public's health.

Definition and Development of Public Health Nursing

There are four organizations that work together to develop policy and practice-related guidelines for public health nursing. Those organizations, collectively called the *QUAD Council,* include the American Nurses Association's Council on Commu-

nity, Primary, and Long-Term Care (ANA); the American Public Health Association's Public Health Nursing Section (APHA, PHN); the Association of State and Territorial Directors of Nursing (ASTDN); and the Association of Community Health Nurse Educators (ACHNE). In the 1990s, these four organizations came together to develop descriptions of the scope of practice for public health nursing that are reflective of the diversity of the roles across the country. One key element in the work of these groups is the fundamental understanding that what it takes to maintain the health of the public differs across life spans, across cultures, and across state and territorial boundaries. The process of public health nursing, however, combines the knowledge base of both public health and nursing to guide the intervention (see appendix A, chapter 1, and p. 1000).

Many attempts have been made to clarify the definition between public health nursing and community health nursing. The most recently developed attempt is a white paper resulting from a national discussion on the differences between population-focused care (care aimed at improving health of the whole population), community-oriented care (care aimed at improving the health of a particular segment of the population), and community-centered care (care provided in a community setting). A 1986 definition of community health nursing developed by the ANA states that "Community health nursing practice promotes and preserves the health of populations by integrating skills and knowledge relevant to both nursing and public health." A 1995 definition of community health nursing developed by ACHNE stated: "Community health nursing is the synthesis of nursing theory and public health theory applied to promoting and preserving the health of populations." A 1996 definition of public health nursing was developed by the Public Health Nursing section of APHA and states that "public health nursing is the practice of promoting and protecting the health of populations using knowledge from nursing, social, and public health sciences."

Essential Public Health Services

A public health functions steering committee made additional attempts to describe public health in a document published in 1994. This document describes the **essential public health services** as follows:

- *Monitor the health status of the population.*
- *Diagnose and investigate community health problems and health hazards.*
- *Inform, educate, and empower the people about health issues.*
- *Mobilize community partnerships to identify and solve health problems.*
- *Develop policies and plans that support individual and community health efforts.*
- *Enforce laws and regulations that protect health and ensure safety.*

**ASTDN PUBLIC HEALTH NURSING PRACTICE MODEL:
ESSENTIAL PUBLIC HEALTH SERVICES AND PUBLIC HEALTH NURSING, 1999.**

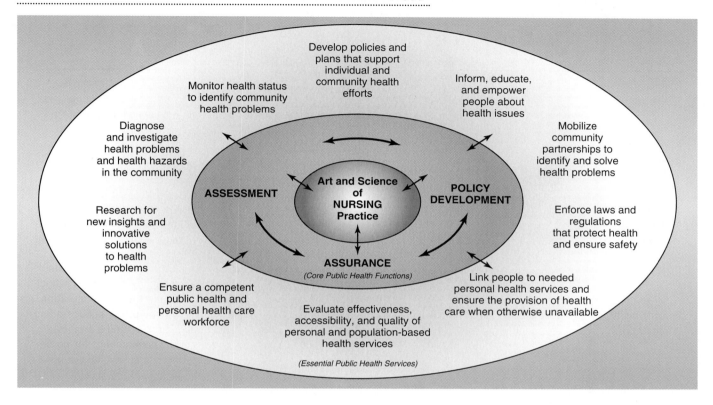

- *Link people to needed personal health services.*
- *Ensure a competent public health and personal health care workforce.*
- *Evaluate effectiveness, accessibility, and quality of personal and population-based health services.*
- *Research for new insights and innovative solutions to health problems.*

Activities for Essential Services

In an attempt to provide practice guidance to public health nurses in official governmental agencies, the directors of public health nursing throughout the country developed examples of nursing activities for each essential service (Table 37-1).

The Year 2000 and Beyond: Challenges for Public Health Nursing

The year 2000 brought to the nation, and to public health nursing, myriad challenges. This new century will bring an era of tremendous technological advances in health care, exciting

worldwide political changes, and explosive, diverse population growth. As a nation, we will reach that milestone with a greater interest in personal health than has ever been demonstrated, but with also a greater health debt and a greater problem with access to care than has ever been measured. Public health nursing is no doubt destined to continue to play a vital part in the evolution of the health care system as we continue in this new century. There are three major areas that will affect these changes: personal responsibility in health promotion and disease prevention, international health, and biological and chemical terrorism. If the nation and the states are to adequately address the escalating costs of health care, the individual must be a key factor in the design of a new system of care. To this end, public health nurses are the best equipped to deal with these changes.

Adequate attention to the health and related socioeconomic problems in this country will require community level interest and intervention. The public health nurse will be called on to once again mobilize communities to meet the needs of their citizens for the improvement of society as a whole. In empowering the community to act, the public health nurse will be challenged to develop a greater understanding of the significant effect that culture has on the individual's response to health promotion, intervention, and education. The explosive population growth and

TABLE 37-1 **ASTDN** PUBLIC HEALTH NURSING PRACTICE MODEL:
ESSENTIAL PUBLIC HEALTH SERVICES AND PUBLIC HEALTH NURSING, 1999.

ESSENTIAL SERVICE	PUBLIC HEALTH NURSING ACTIVITIES	EXAMPLE
Monitor health status.	Community assessment	A public health nurse asked a civic group and local health providers to participate in a study of major risk factors for disability in their community. As a result, the community developed a walking trail and wrote a federal grant for a health center.
Diagnose health hazards.	Disease case identification	Public health nurses provided tuberculosis skin testing to a plant's workers. As a result, two cases of tuberculosis were identified early and contacts were placed on preventive therapy.
Inform and educate public.	Community education	Public health nurses provided classes to local community group on prevention of disease transmission in day-care centers.
Mobilize community partnerships.	Community organization	A public health nurses called a community meeting to discuss accident prevention. As a result of several meetings, the community raised funds for streetlights.
Develop policies.	Advocate for funding	Public health nurses organized efforts to secure funding for a school nurse in a community with high teen pregnancy rates, high school dropout rates, and increased drug use among the teen population.
Enforce health regulations.	Implementation of health regulations	After hearing a complaint from a member of the public about finding needles and syringes in a public garbage area behind a medical clinic, the public health nurse assessed the complainant for potential blood and body fluid exposure testing and contacted the appropriate authorities to work with the local clinic to develop proper disposal policies.
Link people to services.	Provision of health services	In an underserved area, public health nurses provide prenatal care to women and then refer them to a nearby physician for delivery.
Ensure competency.	Participation in organized educational sessions	Public health nurses attend a workshop on the new treatment for HIV-infected individuals.
Evaluate effectiveness.	Participation in research	Public health nurses collaborate with a local university on a study to determine the effectiveness of a new home visiting program for preterm babies.
Research for new ideas.	Implementation of new strategies	Public health nurses test a new health education model for reducing youth tobacco use.

the resultant migration of families will result in a variety of cultures to be served, even in rural communities.

The greatest number of elderly ever seen in this country will emerge as the typical client as the baby boomers reach retirement age. This phenomenon will occur as the workforce is getting smaller and more diversified, thereby creating a need to evaluate the role of the public health nurse. Health promotion and disease prevention activities will be primary among the services offered by the public health nurse. The created health care system will place greater emphasis on what public health nurses have known all along, that prevention is more cost-effective than technological intervention.

This millennium should be an exciting one for public health nurses. The challenges will be great, but the opportunity to practice traditional public health nursing will also be more available than it has been since its inception.

As public health nurses consider the future for their practice, there are a number of questions that surface over and over again. The framework provided by the Construct for Public Health Nursing is useful in helping public health nurses address these, given both the rapidity and magnitude of changes that we are encountering. *As clinical services seem to be moving out of health departments, what will public health nurses' role be in the future?* Clinical services should be understood as a strategy for providing needed services when they are otherwise not available. These services need to be seen as a way of ensuring health, not an end unto themselves. Public health nurses offer a tremendous breadth and depth of skills that are important to almost *any* public health intervention. When public health and public health nursing are understood through the frameworks of core functions and models like the Construct for Public Health Nursing, future roles are envisioned based on their utility, not their history.

Is it possible to be a public health nurse in a managed care setting? There is no question that the skills that public health nurses bring to managed care are extremely useful and needed, but the important distinction is the purposes for which these skills are used. The organizational values of public health and the mandate of ensuring the health of the public reside in the public sector; it is that sector alone that has this responsibility. Public health nurses can and do practice in a variety of settings, some of which focus on the health of populations. Their practice may be one of community health, but it lacks the essential public nature of public health.

Should public health nurses practice in the private sector? Having public health nurses practicing in the private sector benefits everyone. The skills certainly benefit clients, and the overall values and commitments help pave the way for networking and partnerships between the public and private sectors. It is important for these individual nurses to understand that there are some critical differences between the public and private sectors in their values, priorities, and "bottom lines."

What are the biggest challenges that public health nursing faces? Perhaps the most significant challenge facing public health nursing and public health in general is finding ways to address the broader issues of equity and social justice that are currently so much a part of the health "equation." As long as there are such huge inequities—disparities between the "haves" and "have nots"—the major health problems that we see today will only continue. Public health nurses must view their practice as going beyond the narrow boundaries of health services if they are to truly enhance the health of the people.

CONCLUSION

Shakespeare's *The Tempest* contains a sage observation: "The past is prologue. The future is yours and mine to dispatch." So it is with public health nursing. Our history is our prologue, our foundation. Our future is what we create within the framework of what we value, what we understand, what we know, and what we can do. When one considers the work of Lillian Wald, which included her own "hands on" reaching out to destitute individuals and families and helping create the League of Nations and the United States Children's Bureau, it is clear that our foundation can provide us with the inspiration and wisdom that we need to move forward. There are no promises for public health nursing in the 21st century. There is only the ironic assurance that within the significant challenges that will confront societies around the world will be opportunities for public health nurses. The ways in which we define ourselves and our practice will either limit or enable our abilities to take hold of these opportunities. In the final analysis, public health nursing in the future will be what we make it.

CASE STUDY

Case Presentation: *Staphylococcus* Food Poisoning in a University Cafeteria

Stephanie is a 19-year-old white female who is a sophomore at a local university. She lives on campus in one of the dormitories. After dinner one evening, she became ill with nausea, vomiting, diarrhea, and abdominal cramps. Five other women who live in Stephanie's building became ill that same evening with similar symptoms. When others in the dorm became aware of the symptoms, most of the women thought that there was a gastrointestinal virus that was making the women ill. None of these six women became ill enough to seek medical attention. That same evening Mary, a 20-year-old African American female who lives on campus in another dormitory, also became ill with nausea, vomiting, and severe abdominal cramps. Mary was not able to get the vomiting under control, so her roommate brought her to the local hos-pital emergency department. Mary was hospitalized and placed on replacement intravenous fluids and medication for nausea and diarrhea. The hospital, which serves the university town, is relatively small, and the staff soon became aware that nine individuals, all students from the university, had been admitted with the same symptoms within a period of approximately 6 hours that evening. The hospital staff notified the campus clinic physician. He verified that he had treated eight students that same evening for nausea, vomiting, and abdominal cramps. He notified the local county health department that he suspected a food-borne illness outbreak. The public health nurses organized the follow-up of the problem utilizing the core functions of public health and the definition of public health nursing.

1. Discuss the activities that the public health nurse might conduct in this follow-up.

2. Identify the core functions and essential services that are described in this case.

QUESTIONS TO CONSIDER

After reading this chapter, answer the following questions:
1. What is home health?
2. How is a home visit conducted?
3. What are the stages of a home visit?
4. What are the advantages of a home visit?
5. How effective are home visits in improving health for populations?
6. What factors have contributed to the increased growth in home health care in the past 30 years?
7. What is a typical home health client like as far as diagnosis and age?
8. What are common reimbursement sources for home health services?
9. How does home health nursing differ from other health care settings?
10. How are technologies being used in home care?
11. What is hospice, and how does it differ from home health?
12. What is the future of home care nursing?

KEY TERMS

Behavioral distractions	Environmental distractions	Hospice	Palliative care
Capitated rate	Fee-for-service rate	Informal caregivers	Plan of care
Conditions of participation (COP)	Home health care	Nurse-initiated distractions	Skilled nurse visits (SNVs)
Disease state management	Home health care nurses		Visiting nurse

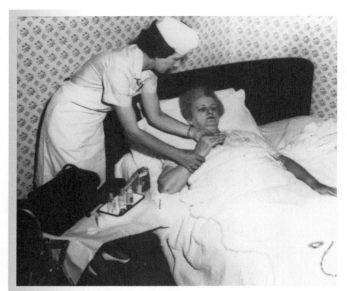

The acceleration of home health nursing came during the 1960s, when Medicare approved home health visits for reimbursement.

Community health nursing roles during the latter part of the 19th century and throughout the 20th century have always had the home as a common setting for practice. One specialized role that emerged was that of the **visiting nurse,** organized by visiting nurse associations funded by philanthropic donations. Physicians often made home visits as well. Box 38-1 identifies milestones in the historical development of health care at home.

The evolution of home care in the United States resulted from social, economic, technological, demographic, and political forces that continue to shape our health care delivery system (NAHC, 1999). By the end of World War II, the physician shortage and the continued explosion of medical technology in the hospital brought many physicians into hospitals, and physician home visiting became a thing of the past (Hafkenschiel, 1990). By the early 1960s, home care was primarily provided by public health and visiting nurses, who assessed clients, provided the necessary services, and managed the therapeutic plan of care. Public health nurses focused on prevention and education; visiting nurses provided sick care in the home. By 1963, according to NAHC (1999), the number of home health agencies, primarily private philanthropic organizations, had grown to 1,100. The services involved a variety of professional disciplines, including skilled nursing. Nurses who make home visits today are employed by a variety of agencies, and roles can encompass elements of the visiting nurse (sickness care) and public health nurse (health promotion, case finding, disease prevention and education). However, in the current reimbursement driven health care system, most nurses who visit clients at home tend to specialize in home health services, with an emphasis on illness care and posthospital follow-up, or public health services, which deliver care in the home for prevention and health education. The role of the home care nurse is increasingly more important as a specialty within community-based health care. Home health nurses may be employed by home health agencies, hospices, hospitals, public health departments, or clinics. Public health nurses may see clients at home through the auspices of the state health department, a local hospital, or a rural clinic. In this chapter, these various roles and

---

BOX 38-1 MILESTONES IN THE HISTORY OF HOME HEALTH NURSING

1800–1900	*Most individual care was given at home. Sources of care varied but most care was provided by small, mostly voluntary philanthropically financed organizations.*
	Visiting nurses were viewed as the solution to warding off infectious diseases born by the poor and immigrants that threatened urban life.
1877	*Precursor of modern home health nursing, visiting nursing, was first established in the United States at the New York City Mission in the women's branch.*
	First home health nurse, Frances Root, visited the sick poor for the New York City Mission. Root graduated in the first nursing class of Bellevue Hospital in 1874.
1912	*The American Red Cross established a rural visiting nurse service for the "sick country person" nationwide. Following the war, the need was so tremendous that the Red Cross could not keep up with the chapter's demands for nurses.*
	Three thousand visiting nurses were working on behalf of 810 associations and agencies.
	Metropolitan Life Insurance made visiting nurse services available to 90% of its 10.5 million policyholders in the United States and Canada, creating the first nationwide system of insurance payment for home-based care.
1920s	*Marked distinction between public health nurses, with a focus on health promotion and prevention, and visiting nurses, with an emphasis on bedside care for the sick occurred during this era.*

BOX 38-1 MILESTONES IN THE HISTORY OF HOME HEALTH NURSING—CONT'D

1947	Montefiore Hospital in the Bronx, New York, started the first hospital-based home care program, offering medical nursing and social services to its clients.
1965	Medicare legislation was enacted to meet the home care needs for the elderly. Approximately 1,275 organizations were initially certified and were limited to nonprofit home care agencies and health departments.
	Medicaid, a state medical assistance program for the poor, was established. Services were expanded to include therapists, aides, homemakers, social workers, and nutritionists.
	The Older Americans Act was initiated to help maintain and support older persons in their homes and communities. Home care entered its current period of rapid growth.
1967	Medicare certified agencies reached 1,753. Home health expenditures amounted to less than 1% of the total Medicare budget.
1970s	Health policy providers saw home care as a cost-containment measure and as an alternative to institutional care.
	Consumers expressed great acceptance for home care when available as an alternative to institutional care.
1973	Home health Medicare benefits were extended to the younger disabled population.
1980	Medicare-certified agencies reached 2,924.
	The percentage of Medicare clients discharged to home health care increased from 9.1% in 1981 to 17.9% in 1985.
	Government expense on home-based services totaled $4.5 billion, while an estimated 2–4 times this amount was spent by families for privately purchased home-based care.
1981	Proprietary agencies were admitted to the Medicare program.
1982	The National Association for Home Care (NAHC) was founded.
1983	Medicare added hospice benefits.
	Diagnosis-related groups (DRGs) and the prospective payment system (PPS) implemented by the federal government results in shorter hospitalization incentives and the discharge of sicker clients to the home setting.
1986	The growth of Medicare-certified home care agencies leveled off at around 5,900 as a result of increasing Medicare requirements and unreliable payment policies.
1987	Approximately 2.5% of the U.S. population received home care services.
	A coalition of U.S. congressmen, consumer groups, and the NAHC filed a lawsuit against the Health Care Finance Administration that resulted in a rewrite of the Medicare home care payment policies. This rewrite allowed the program for the first time to provide beneficiaries with the level and type of services that Congress originally intended.
1997	The Federal Bureau of Labor Statistics declared home care as the fastest growing segment of health care and the second fastest growing industry.
	An estimated 20,215 home care organizations provide service to more than 7 million Americans with acute, long-term, or terminal health conditions.
	Congress passed the Balanced Budget Act (BBA) of 1997, which resulted from the rapid growth of the home care industry and the increasing concern and incidence of fraud and abuse in health care; an interim payment system (IPS) for home health services was created as a new reimbursement mechanism.
1998	The BBA of 1997 took effect. This change in the reimbursement mechanism for home care services resulted in sweeping changes. Home care agencies were reimbursed by the Medicare program by an aggregate per beneficiary payment limit. This was an interim step toward a prospective payment system similar to the DRG system used in the acute care setting.
2000	Prospective payment system (PPS) implemented.

practice environments are described in the context of the emerging community-based health care system.

The Home Visiting Process

One has only to look around any local hospital to see that it would seem to be much more efficient for clients to come to the nurse and other health care providers, where resources are plentiful. Certainly, one of the primary reasons that hospitals were first developed in the Middle Ages was so that caregivers could see more clients and watch them throughout the day and night. Yet there are very good reasons for seeing clients in their own homes. Box 38-2 lists common purposes of home visiting; Box 38-3 details the stages of the home visit, with information about the sequential steps in the home visiting process; and Box 38-4 provides information about differences between the home setting and the acute care setting. Box 38-5 provides hints on communicating effectively in the home setting.

Advantages of Home Visits

Community health nursing is holistic. Seeing clients in the artificial and controlled environment of a hospital reveals little to the nurse about the family's health influences and ability to carry out the plan of care (Allen, 1991). In the home, the nurse gets the complete picture, including environmental factors that affect health, social and psychological influences, relationships between and among family members, and the interaction of the client with family and social networks. In a hospital, clients are separated from the context of their everyday lives: health care providers control

their every movement (including self-regulated body functions), they wear institutional clothes, and care is organized around physician and nurse schedules. Such separation of the client from the context of their lives makes it easier for nurses in the hospital to focus only on the biomedical aspects of disease (Liaschenko, 1994). This is not the case in the home, where illness is but one aspect of the totality of the client's living experience (Coffman, 1997). Hazards and resources are quickly evident and allow a more realistic plan of care to be established, which promotes the achievement of mutually set health strategies and goals. In addition, on a home visit, the nurse can see firsthand how well the client can perform self-care and can make a more accurate evaluation of medical and nursing interventions. Such information can provide the nurse with valuable indicators in the evaluation of the effects of therapeutic interventions, as compared with the limited time and artificial constraints of the clinic or hospital environment (Liepert, 1996). Consider the following example:

> A community health nurse is following a child with high blood lead levels. During a follow-up visit to the clinic, the mother was distracted and kept looking at her watch while the nurse explained how important it was to keep the child from coming in contact with leaded paint. The child failed to keep an appointment with a university clinic for a chelation treatment. The community health nurse could not reach the mother because the phone had been disconnected. On a home visit, the nurse found out that the father had been injured while working at his car repair service shop, located on the same lot as their mobile home. He had taken a temporary job while he recovered from the back injury, on an "as-needed"

BOX 38-2 PURPOSES OF HOME VISITS

CASEFINDING
- Public health and protection
- Abuse, neglect cases
- Communicable disease
- School-related health conditions

ILLNESS PREVENTION
AND HEALTH PROMOTION
- Prenatal and well baby care
- Child development
- Elder care

CARE OF THE SICK
AND TERMINALLY ILL
- Home health
- Hospice

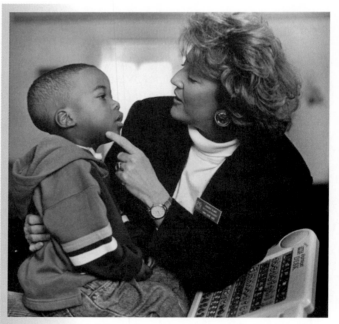

Home health visits take an average of 45 to 60 minutes to complete.

BOX 38-3 FROM BEGINNING TO END . . . CONDUCTING A SUCCESSFUL HOME VISIT

PREVISIT/PLANNING STAGE

- Determine which clients need to be seen.
- Prioritize the scheduled visits based on client need, distance between visits, laboratory work, and coordination with other professionals and physician.
- Review the chart, orders, client diagnosis, goals of care, and reasons for the home visit.
- Telephone the client for validation of scheduled visit; ask client about specific needs, such as supplies, and any special hazards, such as pets or environmental concerns; caregiver schedule.
- Secure directions to the home.
- Conduct inventory of bag, needed equipment and supplies for clients, and educational materials.
- Review safety considerations, such as timing of visit, environmental assessment.

IMPLEMENTING THE VISIT

- Initiate the visit: introduction and identification of nurse to client, brief social phase to establish rapport.
- Practice appropriate hygienic practices before client assessment.
- Review plans for visit with client.
- Determine expectations of client regarding home visits.
- Conduct assessment: environment, client, medication, nutrition, functional abilities and limitations, psychosocial issues, and evaluation of previous visit intervention effectiveness.
- Modify the plan of care based on client need and situational dictates.
- Perform nursing interventions.
- Deal with distractions: environmental, behavioral, and nurse initiated.

EVALUATING THE VISIT

- Evaluate effectiveness of interventions based on established short-term (response during visit) and long-term outcome criteria (effects of intervention at subsequent visits or other client contact).
- Evaluate as to primary, secondary, tertiary interventions.
- Evaluate conduct of visit: availability of appropriate supplies, preparation of nurse for visit.

DOCUMENTATION

- Document based on established outcome criteria and agency requirements.
- Validate diagnoses and additional health needs based on visit.
- Evaluate goals and objectives.
- Review actions taken, response of client, and outcome of interventions (short and long term).
- Record both objective (nurse-based) and subjective (client-based) data.
- As appropriate, use federal agency reimbursement guidelines, such as Medicare, for progress documentation and certification/recertification requirements.

TERMINATION

- Termination begins with the first visit as nurse prepares the client for time-limited nature of home visiting.
- Review goal attainment with client/family and make recommendations and referrals as necessary for continued health care issues.
- Develop strategies for appropriate closure with clients who die, refuse visits, or are terminated because of nonreimburseable services.

basis for a local garage, and used his own tow truck for jobs. He was on call 24 hours a day. Because of his business, many old cars were all over the yard, explaining a potential source for the lead poisoning in the child. Also, his injury had kept him from repairing the family car, so the only transportation was the tow truck. The community health nurse was able to access information from one home visit that would lead to a more appropriate plan on intervention for this family.

Other advantages include the comfort of being seen in one's own home, rather than having to obtain transportation to a health care facility. Transportation can be an obstacle for many clients, including those who do not have access to a private car or mass transit, are unable to drive, or are confined to their homes. Another advantage is that clients are able to exercise more autonomy on their own turf, which allows the nurse to promote a sense of empowerment in the client and family (Ruetter & Ford, 1996). The client becomes part of the interdisciplinary team, rather than a dependent, passive recipient of care. As such, effective community health nurses can use this as

BOX 38-4 CHALLENGES IN HOME SETTINGS

Control belongs to the client *because care is being provided in his/her home.*

A feeling of isolation and lack of support *often results from the nature of the home setting.*

There are no nurses or other team members in the next room to confirm an assessment or to distinguish an abnormal finding.

The home environment and family support system *are unpredictable and not always conducive to optimal care.*

Dealing with multiproblem families *is difficult emotionally for the nurse, especially in the home setting where family dynamics and interactions are more intense and visible.*

Difficulty in communicating with the various team members *can be a stressor.*

The volume of documentation *required can be difficult as a result of the variety and demands of various funding sources and standards.*

Frustrations with the system *are a common concern. There is often difficulty explaining Medicare or Medicaid's ever-changing requirements to clients and families, as well as to other providers.*

Complex case loads *that encompass all age groups with diverse problems are common home care. The skills and knowledge required is broad, requiring the nurse to become a strong generalist.*

Concern for personal safety *is an issue as violence has increased in all delivery settings.*

Home Call: Mother and Child

There's so little here: one table,
not laden, one blind
shut. One bulb
hung straight down. One woman,
not well (that look
of someone who won't talk
because they've been beaten
so the bruises don't show), and one
boy, dancing over, no
diaper, eager for the coin
of candy you lay in his
hand. He leans into your
yellow dress, reaching up,
a tendril attaching, lifting
out of the dark, unfurling
his last leaf. She watches him
watch you,
you with a house
she imagines half glass, where light
pours in, and everything
is already paid for: your
dress, the shine of health you wear
as though you own it, the look
of wealth, and (this too is
visible) the knowhow
to make the right phone calls,
calls to those, who, when you call,
will do what you say, pay
what you tell them, when
and to whom. You, she imagines,
who have at least two
of everything, you lift her son
to your yellow breast, that
well lighted place, where the air's
clean, and you don't
hate yourself, waiting in line
to pay for a sack of potatoes
you can't afford, She watches him
cling to you, she waits to see
what you will do; you who
have things, you who can
do things, you who can do
what you choose to, you
who can do something for them,
if you choose to, a little something
or nothing.

by Marilyn Krysl
Source: Krysl, M., *Midwife and other poems on caring.*
New York: National League for Nursing, pp. 11–12.

a way to increase the client's ability for self-care and enhance the sense of accomplishment in meeting health goals for self and family.

Home visits often take place over long periods, which afford the nurse ample opportunities for developing the authentic trust relationship necessary for a true collaborative partnership to develop between nurse and client. A result is that clients are often more willing to share sensitive and more intimate issues in the home setting, which allows the nurse to gain insight into complex interpersonal influences (Stulginsky, 1993a, 1993b).

Effectiveness of Home Visits

Research from a variety of studies indicates that successful home visiting programs have resulted in improved health outcomes. But how effective are home visits, such as those that are preventive in nature, in the long run? In a recent research study, prenatal and early childhood home visits by nurses reduced subsequent antisocial behavior and experimentation with drugs in adolescents born into high-risk families. The study, which evaluated the effects of home visits by nurses over the course of 15 years to low-income, unmarried women, found long-term benefits that included fewer episodes of children running away from home, arrests and convictions, and drug abuse when compared with similar groups of women who received prenatal and well-child care in a clinic. The adolescent children of these mothers also had fewer sexual partners and smoked and drank less (Olds & Kitzman, 1993).

Other research has revealed that successful home visiting programs should be broad in focus (e.g., improved pregnancy outcome versus hypertension management during pregnancy), which may contribute the most lasting effects in health status. Also, home visits that occur over time and in greater frequency accomplish more in terms of improved health status for the clients than single visits (Barkauskas, 1983). Home visiting to targeted high-risk groups who have complex and multiple needs have been linked with more significant changes in health status than those at medium or low risk (Byrd, 1998; Deal, 1994; Olds & Kitzman, 1993). Numerous studies have demonstrated that home visiting by nurses to pregnant and postpartum women and their infants reduces risk factors that result in preterm births, abuse and neglect, and maternal health problems. In addition, home visits improve healthy behaviors and are cost-effective (Gomby, Larson, Lewit, & Behrman, 1993; Olds, 1992; Olds, Henderson, Phelps, Kitzman, & Hanks, 1993).

Home health visits have been linked with fewer hospital readmissions, fewer emergency department visits, and cost savings when compared with acute care. A study of clients with congestive heart failure who were visited by home health nurses linked fewer hospital admissions, from 3.2 admissions per year to 1.2 admissions per year, with home health visits. The length of stay decreased from 26 days per year to 6 days per year (Kornowski, Zeeli, Averbuch, & Finkelstein, 1995).

Schoen and Anderson (1998), in their extensive review of the effectiveness of home visiting programs, found that the most successful programs have the following elements:

- *A focus on families in greater need of services rather than universal programs*
- *Interventions that begin in pregnancy and continue through the second to fifth years of life*
- *Flexibility and family specificity regarding duration and frequency of visits, according to the family's need and risk level*
- *Active promotion of positive health-related behaviors*
- *Use of a broad, multiproblem focus to address the full complement of family needs*
- *Assistance to family with reduction of stress by improving social and physical environment*
- *Use of nurses and professionals specifically trained in home visiting*

Challenges of Home Visits

Ironically, many of the aspects of home visiting that make it more advantageous for the nurse and client than the hospital environment also contribute to the challenges of home visiting. Because the nurse is more independent and less tied to the physical constraints of the agency, professional isolation can be a problem, especially for a novice nurse. In the clinic or hospital, help or consultation with other professionals is only a few steps away. For the home visiting nurse, that becomes more difficult and can be a source of considerable anxiety. With advanced technology, such as laptop computers, pagers, and cellular phones, the nurse must use different strategies for connecting with other professionals.

The intimacy of the home visit can create boundary issues for the nurse and the client. For example, the boundary between professional distance and social intimacy because of the informality of the home is a constant challenge for the community health nurse. Certainly, there is a certain amount of socialization that occurs in all home visits as the nurse maintains therapeutic rapport and extends courtesy to her client hosts. Nurses also may find themselves disclosing more about themselves than they would in a hospital setting. Such self-disclosure must be monitored carefully so that the client-nurse relationship remains therapeutic. For example, a nurse's concern about her own child's illness might be mentioned in casual comments and then become a significant source of anxiety for the elder client who becomes overly worried about the child's well-being.

The nurse must also deal with the challenge that providing care may actually increase a person's feelings of vulnerability, simply by being seen at home by a nurse. The client may perceive that by accepting the nurse's help, his or her own ability to give self-care is inadequate. In their ethnographic study, Magilvy, Brown, and Dydyn (1988) found that home health clients often expressed concerns about relying on a home health nurse as a sign of vulnerability. They expressed a need to maintain their independence and mobility and saw the nurse as a reminder of their dependency or reliance on outside help. Therefore, the nurse must constantly promote the collaborative nature of the client-nurse relationship and frequently praise the client for efforts to improve health, no matter how small or insignificant the changes might be. Nurses accustomed to using "take charge" skills such as are rewarded in the hospital often find that they may lead to failure in the home setting (Coffman, 1997; Liaschenko, 1994).

In the home setting, the client has the right to self-determination and can reject or accept the therapeutic interventions offered by the nurse. This important aspect of autonomy cannot be overemphasized when in the client's home. The nurse must remember that true collaboration means that the nurse and client set goals, develop strategies, and evaluate outcomes of care together, no matter how difficult that may be for the nurse who has been taught that "the nurse always knows best" (Zerwekh, 1997). For example, a prenatal client may refuse to stop smoking during pregnancy, expressing to the nurse that she is too nervous because her mother-in-law has moved in with the family. The nurse may be able to provide the client with assistance in reducing the number of cigarettes smoked per day.

Successive approximations in the attainment of client goals means that progress is measured in small increments, rather than in the dramatic turnaround of the acute care setting (Stulginsky, 1993a). For many nurses, this is perhaps the most difficult challenge of all, especially for nurses who have primary experience in the hospital specialty units, such as the trauma department or intensive care unit. The community health nurse cannot solve all of the client's problems during home visiting, nor should such attempts be made. Only those health problems that are amenable to therapeutic nursing interventions and that are mutually agreed on by the client and nurse should be the focus during home visits. For example, the client with diabetes may not be able to eliminate sugar from her coffee and tea but over time has discontinued using sugar with her cereal.

Another challenge that often emerges is when the nurse faces the immediate pressing demands of the family and a different, preset agenda determined by the agency, usually as a result of funding source policy (Cowley, 1995). Usually, the funding source states a specified number of visits or a specified time frame for the care (e.g., 60 days). The dilemma occurs for the community nurse when the client needs additional care but not specifically at the skilled level. The client may express the need for more assistance in learning to exercise with the artificial hip appliance. The nurse could refer the client to local support groups and community senior centers that offer specialized exercise classes. Community health nurses may be some of the most creative nurses out there as they struggle to find myriad ways of meeting client needs when conventional reimbursement sources end. Consulting with other team members and using support groups provide resources and support in these complex and frustrating situations, which are becoming all too common in the managed care arena.

Distractions in the Home Environment

Conducting a visit in the home, as compared with the nurse-controlled environment of the hospital, is unique in that the nurse must compete with many distractions. Although the distractions that nurses encounter on home visits may seem on the surface negative and interfere with the plan of care, Pruitt, Keller, and Hale (1987) contend that distractions can also provide valuable information about the client's world. Distractions can generally be classified as environmental, behavioral, or nurse-initiated.

Environmental distractions take the form of excessive stimuli, such as television and radio, children playing and making noise, phone calls, traffic, or construction noise. Other environmental sources of distraction may come from crowded or cluttered living conditions; the nurse almost always faces less than ideal living conditions on home visits. Nurses have their own picture of what an ideal living environment should look like, and such values influence the way distractions affect assessment and interventions. For example, the nurse may find a cluttered home a sign of a client's depression or disinterest in a healthy environment. By remaining open to other explanations, the nurse may discover that the client feels comforted by the various objects, furniture, and photos. How we "clutter" our homes has much to do with what is important to us—and to our clients—and thus this can be a valuable way for us to learn about the client's values. How we "use" our space, no matter how large or how small, reflects our values and lifestyles (Pruitt, Keller, & Hale, 1987). Noticing how the furniture is arranged, the number and kinds of photographs around the home, and the kinds of objects displayed can help nurses understand a client's family circle and ties as well as those things that bring the client joy. The "doggie smell" and dog hair throughout the house may be what makes an elderly woman's house a home. Elders often have cluttered homes because they have accumulated the memories and possessions of a lifetime; they also may place furniture close together to make it easier to hear conversations. The nurse learns to minimize distractions, for example, by asking to turn down or "mute" the television or avoiding visiting when the client is most likely to be watching favorite television programs. If interruptions become a problem, observing how the client reacts can provide the nurse with clues to how much of a threat the distraction is to the client's health (Pruitt, Keller, & Hale, 1987). One solution in visiting a pregnant women with a 3-year-old who may be distracting her is to have the child draw a picture for the nurse. Such a strategy can provide the nurse with ample time to perform assessment tasks with the mother. In a multiperson household where privacy is premium, often retreating to a back room or even outside to a porch is all that is necessary for a few moments of distraction-free assessment time. Balancing courtesy with objectives for the visit becomes a skill that requires tact, humor, and creativity.

Another distraction is **behavioral distraction**. The client may exhibit behaviors that distract the nurse from the plan of care and goals of the home visit. Clients may avoid talking about health problems for a variety of reasons and may instead engage in social communication. Clients may have very real concerns that are not consistent with what the nurse sees as priority problems (Pruitt, Keller, & Hale, 1987). By examining such avoidance, the nurse may find that these concerns should be addressed first. For example, a nurse who is seeing an older woman with diabetes may find that the client refuses to discuss her daily blood sugars, but instead wants to talk about an auto accident that occurred the night before near the client's home. Upon closer examination, the nurse finds that the accident has claimed the life of an elderly woman only casually known to the client, and the client then remarks, "It isn't too much longer that I will be able to drive, and then what will I do?" The client was exposing her feelings of vulnerability about losing her mobility and independence. Other behaviors that may hinder the goals of the home visit include blocking or silence in response to inquiries related to health status. The nurse must use appropriate therapeutic communication techniques, as well as exhibit patience, to provide optimal comfort for the client in the home environment.

BOX 38-5 SECRETS OF PROFESSIONAL CONVERSATION: THE HOME VISIT

1. *Break the ice with a warm topic.* Try opening with a cliché such as the weather, pets, sports, children, yard flowers, garden, or any subject that interests *most* people. This often establishes initial a conversational bond that helps make the transition to other more sensitive topics easier. Example: "How has all this rain lately affected your garden?" or while pointing to pictures in home, ask "Are these your children?"

2. *If you are extremely uncomfortable or have a sense of unidentified anxiety, explore possible source with the client.* Often, nurses can sense nonverbal conflict in the home, with the client, or with the family. By acknowledging that this is valuable information can be elicited from the client. Example: "Things seem a little unsettled today. Do you want to talk about anything before we get started with your assessment?"

3. *Pick up the pace by asking open-ended questions.* This forces discussion because questions can't be answered with a simple yes or no. Answers will be longer so you will be able to notice other things that are being said to keep the conversation going. Example: "Why do you like living out in the country? What do you think about the new road going through town? What if . . . ?"

4. *Show sincere interest.* Listening is a skill that must be practiced daily. This means make good eye contact. When the client is speaking, our tendency is to spend that time planning what we will say next. This is not only discourteous and nontherapeutic, but causes us to miss important information. Flatter your client/family with sincere comments: All people crave appreciation. Make sure you *individualize* compliments with details, such as commenting on how much more energetic your client is or noting that a young mother is attending to her new baby's cries very well. Listening is an excellent way to demonstrate your respect for your client! Example: Instead of rehearsing your next line, focus on your *genuine* response to what he/she is saying. Challenge yourself to come up with questions about the points the person has raised.

5. *Develop a broad outlook.* Avoid using the word *I* too often. Watch the great conversationalists—Oprah Winfrey, Jane Pauley, Barbara Walters,

Katie Couric, or Larry King—they seldom mention themselves, know a little bit about a lot of subjects, and demonstrate a curiosity about a broad range of topics. Example: Read the local newspaper daily and try to listen to at least one news show every other day. This ensures that you will expand your consciousness about community and national issue that concern your clients. Read a variety of opinions about a wide range of issues. Challenge yourself to think about things in new ways.

6. *Avoid judging others in advance (i.e., "prejudice").* Try to suspend judgment about your client. Coming to conclusions about people before you have even entered their homes, based on what you have read in their chart or know about their income, shuts down your curiosity and prevents you from learning what you need to know about their health status. Example: In a home visit with a new mother who consistently misses clinic appointments, keep an open mind and ask her about other aspects of her life. Listen to her accounts of how her life has changed since giving birth.

7. *Quote your client when possible.* A very flattering and confirming strategy to promote your client's self-confidence is to use actual quotes from previous conversations (either from the same visit or previous visits, which means you have to really listen!) to illustrate health information. Example: "Since you mentioned last visit that you felt a 'bit better when I am able to cook my own breakfast,' I think that taking care of yourself as much as possible really makes a difference."

8. *End a conversation gracefully.* Breaking away from a conversation in the home can often be more difficult than starting one. After we "connect" with someone, most of us are hesitate to interrupt when you need to move on to other topics or to end the visit. The reality is that there will eventually come a point in any conversation when you will have to end it. Prepare when you enter the home to end the conversation. Example: Prepare an exit early on in a polite and friendly way. "I have so enjoyed our visit, but I must get going in order to see my other clients," or, "I see from the clock that it is near lunch and I know you must be hungry."

Source: Adapted from King, L. (1994). How to talk to anyone, anytime, anywhere: The secrets of good conversation. *New York: Crown.*

Nurse-initiated distractions can evolve from prejudices, fears, preoccupation with the tasks of home visiting, and reactions to lifestyles and living conditions different from the nurse's own. This "baggage" that all nurses carry with them on home visits should be carefully acknowledged and examined to prevent negative effects on nurse-client interactions. Nurses may fear home visiting because of safety concerns, concerns over being alone without colleagues for support and consultation, and fears of being rejected by the client. Practicing nursing in the uncontrolled environment of a client's home can threaten even the most secure nurse in terms of autonomy and control. Other distractions that are common are talking on the phone with the home office or other health care professionals or making arrangements for other clients while in the client's home. The nurse must be aware of how such distractions influence the nurse-client relationship. While in the home, the client should remain the focus as much as possible. By being preoccupied with staying on schedule, tasks, and documentation of the visit, the effectiveness of home visiting can be seriously threatened.

The nurse may also become frustrated with clients who are labeled as noncompliant or seem to have contributed in some way to their health problems, such as emphysema in a smoker or liver cancer in an alcoholic. Understanding that these feelings are shared at one time or another by most nurses can be the first step to prevent effects on care. Talking with colleagues and having open dialog with other professionals in similar settings can help nurses understand not only the source of these distractions but helpful ways that others have used to minimize their effects on client care (Pruitt, Keller, & Hale, 1987).

Home Health Nursing

Home health care refers to the delivery of health services in the home setting for purposes of restoring or maintaining the health of individuals and families. Managed care and technological advances and research have all contributed to the movement from the hospital to the home as a diverse and dynamic service delivery setting for care (NAHC, 1999). Providing home care services to some 7 million individuals who require health care, home health care nursing is the choice for many community health nurses who are attracted by the autonomy, flexibility, and challenge of caring for persons in their own home. Home health care nursing, according to the American Nurses Association (ANA, 1999), is a synthesis of community health nursing and selected technical skills from other nursing specialties. It involves the same primary preventive focus on care of population aggregates of the community health nurses and the secondary and tertiary prevention foci on the care of individuals in collaboration with the family and caregivers. **Home health care nurses** provide care to a broad spectrum of ages and clinical diagnoses (Rice, 1996).

Home health care should be holistic and focused on the individual client, integrating family and caregivers, environmen-

tal and community resources to promote optimal health for the client confined to the home. See Boxes 38-6 and 38-7 for a look at a typical home health nurse's day and client load.

Annual expenditures for home health care were close to $42 million for 1998. Almost any care that can now be provided in the hospital can also take place in the home, which has created numerous practice opportunities for home health nurses. Home care services are provided to persons with acute care needs, long-term health conditions, permanent disabilities, or terminal illnesses (NAHC, 1999).

According to the Department of Health and Human Services, home health care is that component of the continuum of comprehensive health care whereby health services are provided to individuals and families in their places of residence for the purpose of promoting, maintaining, or restoring health, or of maximizing the level of independence while minimizing the effects of disability and illness, including terminal illness (Warhola, 1980). The appropriate services to meet the needs of the individual client and family are planned, coordinated, and made available by providers organized for the delivery of home care through the use of employed staff, contractual arrangements, or a combination of the two patterns.

Changes in the health care system and advances in technology and information challenge nurses to redefine the terms *home* and *care* (Frantz, 1997). Clarke and Cody (1994) challenged nurses to rethink the central concepts of nursing: person, environment, health, and nursing. In the home, boundaries between nurse and family as caregivers become blurred, each providing essential care to the client. The home has long been considered the private domain of the family—it is increasingly becoming the "employment setting" for the home

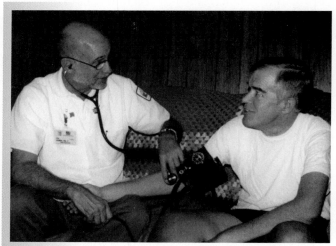

Home health nurse Jim Jones, RN, conducts a physical assessment.

BOX 38-6 SUMMARY DESCRIPTION OF CLIENTS IN SAMPLE HOME HEALTH DAILY NURSING SCHEDULE

On each skilled nursing visit:

1. Wash hands.
2. Set up equipment.
3. Obtain complete assessment with review of systems. DOCUMENT.
4. Contact physician with assessment results, if indicated. DOCUMENT.
5. Ask the client or caregiver to recall previous instruction, making corrections if needed. DOCUMENT.
6. Perform procedures; wash hands. Note response to care. DOCUMENT.
7. Instruct client/caregiver from plan of care. Note response to instruction. Review as needed. DOCUMENT.
8. Schedule next visit with the client/caregiver.
9. Clean equipment; wash hands.

Ms. Lottie AAA. Hx: 74 y/o with a longstanding history of osteoarthritis, using a walker for mobility in her small rural home. She has a recent diagnosis of type II DM. The physician has requested daily SNVs to instruct her in blood glucose monitoring, diabetic diet, and medication regimen after the initiation of an oral hypoglycemic agent. She lives alone but receives assistance from her many children and grandchildren in the community.

Mr. Ali BBB. Hx: 81 y/o with CHF for several years and is particularly forgetful since the death of his wife last year. His physician has requested SNVs because he has had two recent hospitalizations with exacerbations of his disease. Although he lives alone, his daughter drops by each morning at 09:00 to offer help. The nursing visit is set so that instruction can be given to both.

Mr. Carlo CCC. Hx: 26 y/o with paraplegia and development of a stage II sacral ulcer. He has a roommate who helps with shopping and some activities of daily living. He previously spent most of his day in the wheelchair but has begun to take rest periods midmorning, midafternoon, and early evening. He is pleased with the air cushion for his wheelchair and the gel overlay for his bed.

Ms. Helaria DDD. Hx: 78 y/o with recent onset of idiopathic HTN. She lives with her elderly husband and a very active dog, Maggie. Her children have hired a caregiver for ADLs and housekeeping. The physician has ordered BP assessments 2–3 times a week for 3 weeks to assess the effects of her new medication, quinapril HCl. Systolic pressure at 160 or greater and diastolic pressure at 94 or greater are to be reported. One dosage adjustment has been made, and she has been normotensive on the last two visits. Visit times are varied to give the physician an across the day view.

Mr. Paul EEE. Hx: 34 y/o with congenital lower extremity malformation, type I DM, and open wounds on both lower limbs. He helps his elderly father with financial matters and record keeping. The client meticulously records his wound progress and e-mails any concerns to the nurse and physician. He provides wound care to the areas he can reach, and the nurse performs care to the area outside his reach. He is well educated about his health conditions. He depends on home health aides for most of his personal care. A supervised home health aide visit is planned.

Key for Abbreviations: ADLs, *activities of daily living;* BP, *blood pressure;* CHF, *congestive heart failure;* DM, *diabetes mellitus;* HTN, *hypertension;* Hx, *history;* SNVs, *skilled nursing visits;* y/o, *year old.*

Contributed by: Jim Jones, RN, C, Case Manager Home Health Nurse, South Mississippi Home Health, Hattiesburg, Mississippi.

health nurse, where nurse and client needs intersect. In the hospital, there are often dramatic changes from illness to health; in the community home setting, the changes are subtle as a chronic disease state emerges as the dominant mode of health and illness. The physician remains the center authority in the hospital; in the home, autonomy of the family and client are vi-

tal and requires a collaborative effort between caregivers and health providers.

Standards of Home Health Nursing

The ANA has endorsed the Standards of Home Health Nursing as the basis for home health nursing practice and are found in

BOX 38-7 SAMPLE HOME HEALTH DAILY NURSING SCHEDULE*

◆ 07:00   Get ready for the day:

✔ **Call office, check overnight voice mail for schedule changes or additions.**

[Night on call nurses may have taken calls that require schedule change, such as notification that a patient had entered the hospital for an emergent condition.]

✔ **Organize client visits by priority.**

[Some patient's require a timed visit due to needed lab studies or the presence of a caregiver to receive instruction.]

✔ **Review notebook to see that all education materials, plans of care, directions, and documentation forms are available.**

[Many forms are needed during the course of any day. They include but are not limited to; nurses notes, lab request forms, verbal order confirmation forms, OASIS forms, telephone contact notes, discharge summaries, and transfer forms.]

✔ **Check nursing bag and automobile to see that all needed supplies are available for assessment and procedures.**

◆ 07:30   Turn on pager and cell phone, grab the lunch cooler. You need to travel about 30 minutes to the outlying community to see your first two clients.

◆ 08:00   Arrive at Ms. Lottie AAA. Utilize her slow response to the door bell to open nurse's note and review the plan of care. Ms. AAA is now testing her blood glucose with minimal prompting. She is praised for her performance and correct entry of the WNL results. Her meal plans for the day are reviewed, and suggestions are made. Instruction on signs and symptoms of hyperglycemia/hypoglycemia is given with handouts of this in pictorial and text form. She is reminded to fast for tomorrow's visit. The visit has lasted an hour and you will travel back toward town to see your next client.

◆ 09:15   Arrive at Mr. Ali BBB. His daughter greets you at the door with his daily wt. record and the information that he has gained 3 pounds overnight. He is SOB, resp. 34, pulse is 100, BP is 150/92 mm Hg, temp. 98.3°F. His 14:00 dose of furosemide is in the mediplanner for the past 2 days. Ausc. of his lung fields, posterior, indicate fine crackles in the lower lobes bilaterally, and the mid lobe on the right. Physician contact is made, and furosemide is given IV as ordered. He admits to forgetting medications that don't come at meal

times. Instruction is given to move the 14:00 dose to noon, and his daughter will call after lunch as a reminder on medications. Signs and symptoms that require contact with the nurse/physician are reiterated. Now vital signs indicate resp. at 26, pulse 92, and BP 132/84. He has voided twice. Arrangements are made to return later in the afternoon for reassessment. A call is placed to the office to move an afternoon visit to tomorrow and the other patient is notified. You have spent an hour and a 15 minutes here and now you travel back into town for your remaining clients.

◆ 10:50   Arrive at Mr. Carlo CCC. You arrive at his home 15 minutes after the scheduled time with sincere apologies. The old dressing is removed, and the wound is gently cleaned with normal saline. The 0.5-cm measurement reveals that healing is rapidly occurring. Skin preps are applied to the intact skin, a hydrocolloid dressing is placed, and the edges are secured with tape. You continue discharge planning because the wound is nearly healed. A review of pressure relief measures and self-inspection using a mirror are discussed. He is eager to return to a more regular routine, and you encourage his plans. His roommate offers coffee, which you graciously decline. Your 40-minute visit is ended with travel a short distance to the next client.

◆ 11:40   Arrive at Ms. Helaria DDD. Maggie, an energetic poodle, has loudly announced your arrival, and she meets you at the door before the bell is rung. You are led to the bedroom for her positional BP checks, but extracting Maggie from Ms. Helaria's lap is a problem. This accomplished, you find her sitting BP is 138/82, standing BP is 128/80, and supine BP is 144/88. She denies headache, dizziness, back pain, fatigue, dry mouth, or GI upset. She is still unclear about taking the medication because she feels "just fine." You repeat the silent threat of HTN, and the need to take her medication as ordered. She agrees and promises to call if any side effects are noted. At 12:10 you are ready to travel toward the next client, with a pull over for lunch.

◆ 12:15   After your fruit and cheese, you check your voice mail for any messages that may affect your afternoon travel.

◆ 12:50   Arrive at Mr. Paul EEE. The door is open when you arrive, and he calls out to "come on back." The aide has arrived just before you and is performing his routine care. You check the aide worksheet and note that the POC isn't being followed. You provide the needed supervision and document your findings. Before care can begin, a trip back to the car is needed to bring in sterile syringes. His self wound care is observed along with the wound characteristics noted. The distal

BOX 38-7 SAMPLE HOME HEALTH DAILY
NURSING SCHEDULE*—CONT'D

wound is irrigated with $^1/_2$ H_2O_2/$^1/_2$ normal saline using an 18-gauge blunt needle. The wound is rinsed with normal saline, and packed with NS moistened gauze packing, covered with gauze sponges, and wrapped with roll gauze. Tape is applied to secure the dressing. Your pager goes off and requires a brief call to one of the clients with medication instruction. Your visit, with interruptions, has lasted an hour and 10 minutes.

♦ 14:15   Arrive at Mr. Ali BBB. He reports voiding several times since you left. You note that there is no apparent SOB, resp. is 22, pulse is 80, BP is 132/82, and temp. is 98.8°F. His lungs have only faint scattered crackles in the bases. Instruction is given again regarding which high potassium foods to include in his diet. He has several bananas on hand and eats one while you talk. His daughter is called at home and reminded to call the agency if signs and symptoms indicate a fluid increase. This visit is over after 30 minutes, and you leave to return to the office.

♦ 15:05   Arrive at the office. Submit notes, verbal order, and check voice mail for tomorrow's assignments and schedule. Load supplies, and return any calls. Make a note in your daily planner about the in-service on laptop use in the home for next Wednesday. Check the on call schedule and leave a report for the night nurse should Mr. BBB call with continuing problems.

♦ 15:30   GO HOME. (Your own!)

Key for Abbreviations: Ausc., *auscultation;* BP, *blood pressure;* GI, *gastrointestinal;* H_2O_2, hydrogen peroxide; *HTN,* hypertension; *IV,* intravenous; *NS,* normal saline; *POC,* plan of care; *resp.,* respirations; *SOB,* shortness of breath; *temp.,* temperature; *WNL,* within normal limits; *wt.,* weight;

Refer to corresponding Box 38-6 for a summary description of each client.
Contributed by: Jim Jones, RN, BEd, Case Manager Home Health Nurse, South Mississippi Home Health, Hattiesburg, Mississippi.

Box 38-8. These standards, similar to other nursing practice standards, use the nursing process and identify two levels of nursing practice: the generalist and the specialist to detail the role and function of the home health nurse. Generalist roles include direct care provider, educator, resource manager, collaborator, and supervisor of ancillary personnel. The nurse as specialist has a master's degree and serves as consultant, administrator, researcher, and clinical specialist. The nurse in the specialist role may develop and evaluate agency policy, perform staff development, and be responsible for organizing and managing interdisciplinary staffing services. The ANA offers certification in home health nursing through the American Nurses Credentialing Center. Certification as a generalist in home health requires the following:

* *Active RN (registered nurse) license in the United States*
* *Baccalaureate or higher degree in nursing*
* *A minimum of 2 years of practice as an RN*
* *A minimum of 2,000 hours of practice as an RN in home health nursing during the past 2 years*
* *Current practice as an RN in a home health nursing setting for a minimum of 8 hours per week*

The nurse in home health nursing must have excellent critical thinking and decision-making skills. In the home health setting, the nurse practices autonomously and without the support of a peer group. In addition, giving care in the home of the client necessitates a sensitivity for the client's environment and culture to a much greater degree than other practice settings. Current advances in technology and pharmacology have resulted in the need for the home care nurse to be increasingly more competent in infusion therapies and complex wound therapies.

The Medicare Era

With the enactment of Medicare in 1965, significant growth and change throughout the U.S. health care system created a broad spectrum of health services for the elderly population. Medicare made home care services, primarily **skilled nursing visits (SNVs)** and curative or restorative therapy, available for all persons older than 65. These services were extended to the disabled population in 1973, and hospice services were added in 1983. **Hospice** services provide **palliative care** and supportive social, emotional, and spiritual services to the terminally ill and their families (NAHC, 1999). There were 9,655 Medicare-certified agencies in the United States in 1998 that provided home health services (NAHC, 1999). The total national expenditure for health care was approximately $1.147 billion in 1998, with a slowing down of growth for an average annual growth rate of 5.3%. The slowed growth trend is attributed to the influence of managed care and an overall low inflation rate for the economy. Approximately 62% of total personal care, which is a subset of health care as goods and services used by individuals, went to hospitals and physicians, whereas only 3% was spent on home care (NAHC, 1999). Medicare is the largest single payer of health care services in the home.

Certainly, one of the primary benefits of health care in the home is that it is significantly less expensive than in the hospital. Home health care can reduce per client expenditures, as well as

BOX 38-8 ANA STANDARDS OF HOME HEALTH NURSING PRACTICE

STANDARD I: ORGANIZATION OF HOME HEALTH SERVICES

All home health services are planned, organized, and directed by a master's-prepared professional nurse with experience in community health and administration.

STANDARD II: THEORY

The nurse applies theoretical concepts as a basis for decisions in practice.

STANDARD III: DATA COLLECTION

The nurse continuously collects and records data that are comprehensive, accurate, and systematic.

STANDARD IV: DIAGNOSIS

The nurse uses health assessment data to determine nursing diagnoses.

STANDARD V: PLANNING

The nurse develops care plans that establish goals. The care plan is based on nursing diagnoses and incorporates therapeutic, preventive, and rehabilitative nursing actions.

STANDARD VI: INTERVENTION

The nurse, guided by the care plan, intervenes to provide comfort; to restore, improve, promote health; to prevent complications and sequelae of illness, and to effect rehabilitation.

STANDARD VII: EVALUATION

The nurse continually evaluates the client's and family's responses to interventions to determine progress toward goal attainment and to revise the database, nursing diagnoses, and plan of care.

STANDARD VIII: CONTINUITY OF CARE

The nurse is responsible for the client's appropriate and uninterrupted care along the health care continuum and therefore uses discharge planning, case management, and coordination of community resources.

STANDARD IX: INTERDISCIPLINARY COLLABORATION

The nurse initiates and maintains a liaison relationship with all appropriate health care providers to assure that all efforts effectively complement one another.

STANDARD X: PROFESSIONAL DEVELOPMENT

The nurse assumes responsibility for professional development and contributes to the professional growth of others.

STANDARD XI: RESEARCH

The nurse participates in research activities that contribute to the profession's continuing development of knowledge of home health care.

STANDARD XII: ETHICS

The nurse uses the code for nurses established by the American Nurses Association as a guide for ethical decision making in practice.

Source: ANA, 1999.

---

reduce the number and length of hospitalization episodes. For example, an average Medicare charge on a per-day basis for hospital care in 1995 was $1910 compared with $402 for a skilled nursing facility and only $84 for a home health charge per visit (NAHC, 1999).

Nearly half the clients who receive home health care are older than 65, and the amount of home health they use tends to increase with age. Approximately 40% of the clients have one or more functional limitations. The most common single diagnos-

tic category for home health services is for diseases and conditions associated with the circulatory system. Cancer, diabetes, and hypertension are also common causes for home health care (NAHC, 1999). The services focus on assisting the client to reach or maintain an optimal state of health, independence, and comfort in their home setting. Box 38-9 lists the most common diseases and disorders seen in the home health client.

Persons who most need home health care require assistance in activities of daily living (National Institute on Disability and

Rehabilitation Research, 1996). **Informal caregivers**, such as family members, friends, and others who provide services on an unpaid basis, provide the bulk of home care with guidance and support from home health professionals.

The provision of care in the client's place of residence contributes to the unique nature of this part of the health care delivery system. Home care represents a cost-effective and satisfying means of meeting the client's health care needs (Shamansky, 1988). Many factors have contributed significantly to the growth of the home care industry in recent years, including the aging of the population, advances in technology, shorter inpatient hospital stays, and the increasing availability of outpatient services. According to Maraldo (1989, p. 303), "Home care is most suited to become the centerpiece of a new health care delivery system, because survey after survey demonstrates that consumers prefer home care to other types of care." Many complex therapies previously administered only in hospital intensive care units are now safe and available in the home setting. Intravenous (IV) therapy has become

common in the home setting, infusing antibiotics, chemotherapy, analgesics, total parenteral nutrition (TPN), and blood products (Sheldon & Bender, 1994). Pediatric hospitalizations have dropped by 46% in the years 1971 to 1993 as more procedures and treatments have been done outpatient and in the home. Pediatric postoperative recovery often occurs in the home (Dougherty, 1998). The ability to provide sophisticated pain control and other comfort measures to the terminally ill, along with an increased understanding and recognition of the importance of preserving dignity in the dying process, have contributed to the growth of hospice services. Often, with the provision of an intermittent skilled service, along with the assistance of the home health aide for personal care and exercise therapy, the client is able to remain in the comforts of his or her own home rather than requiring institutional care (Milone-Nuzzo, 1998). (See Box 38-10.)

Types of Home Health Agencies

Home health agency structures vary depending on the type of organization and corporate structure. These differences impact the entity's obligations to local, state, and federal law and

Public/Governmental Agencies: *A public or governmental agency is an agency operated by a state or local government. Examples are state-operated health departments and county hospitals.*

Nonprofit Agencies: *A private, nongovernmental agency exempt from federal income tax. These agencies are often supported, in part, by private contributions or other philanthropic sources, such as foundations. Examples include Visiting Nurse Associations and Easter Seal Societies, as well as nonprofit hospitals.*

Proprietary Agencies: *A private, profit-making agency or profit-making hospitals.*

Institution-Based Agencies: *An institution-based agency can be propriety, nonprofit, official, or voluntary and operates within the organizational structure of a hospital or HMO. The nature of the home health agency will be dictated by the type of hospital structure.*

Source: Home Health Agency (HHA). (1998). Med-Manual 2180. Citations and Description, State Operations Manual (HCFA Publication No. 7). Washington, DC: U.S. Government Printing Office.

regulations. The structure also determines the agency's tax obligation. Agencies are classified as official, nonprofit, proprietary, and institution-based. Box 38-11 describes the various classifications of agencies.

Official agencies are publicly funded units in state or local health departments and supported by taxes. These agencies provide home health services through legislative statutes. Home health services when offered through official agencies may be provided by community health nurses who also function in various other roles, such as in health promotion and communicable disease prevention. Medicare, Medicaid, and private insurance companies reimburse for home health services. Such reimbursement formulas are often complex. Because of the proliferation of private agencies as well as reevaluation of priorities for public health for disease prevention, most public health services that provide home health are located in underserved and isolated areas.

Nonprofit home health agencies are made up of voluntary agencies, as well as private, nonprofit agencies. Voluntary agencies are supported by charities such as United Way or private endowments. The earliest Visiting Nurse Associations are examples of voluntary agencies. This type of agency is privately owned and exempt from federal income tax. These agencies do not receive any state or local tax revenues. Certain nonprofit hospitals may also have home health agencies as part of their community services. These types of agencies are usually governed by boards of director composed of representatives from the community from which they serve. With the increase in numbers of for-profit private agencies, the numbers of these agencies have declined in recent years. Service is provided by the client's need for home health rather than by ability to pay.

Proprietary agencies include private, profit-making agencies or profit-making hospitals. These agencies receive the largest percentage of their revenue through third-party payers. Because of a highly competitive, managed care market, many proprietary agencies are now part of national health care organizational chains managed through corporate headquarters. Another trend is the development of alliances among home health care agencies and other agencies that become contracting partners in networks. Proprietary agencies make up approximately 43% of all Medicare-certified agencies.

Institution-based agencies emerged in the 1970s as hospitals began providing a greater emphasis on continuity of care. As the high cost of hospitalization and movement with diagnosis-related groups (DRGs) to earlier discharges, hospitals developed their own home health agencies with their inpatient population as the major source of referrals to home health. Clients have the advantage of staying within the same system and greater ease of movement between and among services. These agencies are second only to proprietary agencies in total number of Medicare-certified agencies in the United States, making up around 27% of agencies.

Home Health Care Documentation

Before the advent of Medicare and federal reimbursement of home health services, home health care was paid for by clients, primarily through donations and philanthropic organizations. Today, Medicare and Medicaid make up the principal funding sources for home health. Part A (hospital insurance) and Part B (supplemental medical insurance) of Medicare include coverage for home health services. Because Medicare and Medicaid together finance more than 75% of home health services, the discussion of financing and documentation of care is directed primarily toward meeting Medicare requirements. Medicaid, as a state-administered program, provides a range of home care benefits that vary widely from state to state. Private, third-party health insurance also provides some reimbursement for home health services.

Because of the reimbursement policies of the Medicare program, accurate and appropriate documentation by the home health nurse is critical for current and future reimbursement of the agency and maintenance of certification of the agency. Documentation activities affect the home health to a much greater degree than in perhaps any other setting (Rice, 1996). Documentation requirements are defined in the Medicare Condition of Participation (COP). These documentation requirements have a direct impact on reimbursement for the home health agency. Basically, documentation requirements for home health care are more stringent than for other health care settings. Each professional note of documentation must demonstrate a skilled level of care and must be inclusive of all care rendered. The professional nurse is responsible for documenting the supervision of the licensed practice nurse (LPN) as well as the home health aide.

As Lovejoy (1997) states, "Because visits and supplies translate to dollars and cents, nurses enter the front-line of reimbursement responsibility when moving from hospital or other settings to home care" (p. 12).

Disease state management (DSM) is an emerging approach to population disease managed care that considers all elements of home health care in an integrated fashion, rather than each one separately as in present outcome management (Schaffer & Behrendt, 1998). Clinical pathways are outcome driven with specific time frames of expected courses of recovery. The home health nurse participates in controlling the timing and coordination of the practice patterns to achieve the desired outcome set for the client. Because multiple providers and team members from different practice settings are involved, they each share in the responsibility and accountability of outcomes.

DSM provides a standardization of approach to clients within a population defined by a particular disease they all have in common (Hickey, 1998). Disease management improves the health of certain client populations while cutting the costs to the health care delivery system. Although DSM is not managed care, it is associated with managed care as an effective way to reduce total costs of care. DSM has been most effective when applied to chronic disease management. Many managed plans are implementing DSM, which standardizes care in all settings, including the home.

Martin (1998) provides this example of how DSM works. Consider the population of diabetics and the role played by the examination of feet. Diabetes is an expensive disease, and amputations are common, costly outcomes of poorly managed diabetes. The question for a facility might be asked: "Do we have more diabetic amputations in our home health agency than the national average?" A benchmark, such as a state or national statistic, is always used as the basis for DSM. If the answer is yes, an examination begins with a review of all clients with diabetes in that agency. Charts are reviewed, and how clients with diabetes are cared for are analyzed, from the physician to the home health nurse to the family caregiver to the client himself or herself. Through such an analysis, it is discovered that observation of the feet, while widely known to be a part of the assessment of a diabetic, has not been consistently examined by all caregivers. Research directs this intervention, based on the knowledge that

routine observation of the feet provides opportunity to not only detect early signs of poor circulation, but gives the client a chance to learn what to look for in a self-examination. If the caregivers conduct these assessments, along with the home health client, fewer amputations should occur. A new policy is implemented: "At every client encounter, examine the feet of diabetic clients and at that time, teach them to do the exam themselves." This policy is shared with everyone who has any contact with the client. A year later, amputation rates are again examined. A predicable change should have occurred: There should be a decline in the amputation rate. This example shows that other populations with chronic conditions, such as asthma, hypertension, and sinusitis, can benefit from the application of DSM (Hickey, 1998).

The challenges of DSM are related to the expense of implementing such an approach. When DSM is applied to a population, there will be additional time and visits on the front end, client education programs will be necessary and additional staff may need to be hired to manage the information system. Clients are managed by protocol and are given the information they (and their caregivers) need in a standardized format at every encounter. Support is provided so that clients can manage their chronic disease. All members of the health care team must be involved, from the pharmacist to the social worker. There is a heavy emphasis on teaching clients why, when, and how to take medications and how to manage the plan of care. Community organizations, such as the American Lung Association, are used for support and educational resources.

Clinical practice guidelines are now available for the most commonly seen chronic diseases in the population (Schwartz, 1997). Disease management programs will continue to grow in the future as outcomes research and database integration provide a continuum of care from hospital to home (Remington, 1997). See Box 38-12 for DSM concepts and guidelines. See Box 38-13 for proper documentation language.

Financial Reimbursement for Home Health Services

Medicare

The federal government, through the Health Care Finance Administration (HCFA), contracts with regional insurance companies or fiscal intermediaries to provide reimbursement for home care services. To qualify for Medicare benefits for their client population, home health agencies must follow the federal regulatory requirements called **conditions of participation (COP)**. The COP for home health agencies and hospice services define the requirements that an agency must meet to participate in the Medicare program. The COPs are detailed and prescriptive. Requirements related to organizational structure, clients' rights, and the covered disciplines, which include skilled nursing, physical therapy, speech therapy, occupational therapy, home health

BOX 38-12 DISEASE STATE MANAGEMENT CONCEPTS

COORDINATION OF PRIMARY AND SPECIALTY CARE

1. Referrals are coordinated from one provider to another.
2. Client is treated by the most appropriate caregiver in the most appropriate setting.

PRACTICE GUIDELINES

1. Optimal approach to client care is established.
2. Providers are educated to follow the established practice guidelines given the clients' individual needs.
3. Client care and cost-effective treatment are enhanced.
4. Clients achieve optimal outcomes.

CLIENT EDUCATION AND EMPOWERMENT

1. Clients are educated in appropriate self-care.
2. Health awareness is increased, and complications are decreased.

PREVENTIVE CARE AND WELLNESS

1. Individuals at risk for a given disease are targeted.
2. Individuals are taught wellness and prevention strategies.
3. Future complications and costs are minimized.

BOX 38-13 CHOOSING THE RIGHT WORDS: DOCUMENTATION AND LANGUAGE IN HOME HEALTH NURSING

KEY WORDS TO USE

Unstable	Does not comprehend
Deteriorating	New problem
Change in	Leaving
Improving	Remaining at
Taught	Deterioration in
Assessed	Complains of
Instructed	Needs assistance with
Observed	Unable to perform
Evaluated	Specific limitations
Comprehends	Remains

WORDS TO AVOID

No change	Reinforced
Doing well	Chronic
No problems	Reviewed
No complaints	Reinstructed
Condition stable	Monitored
(unless at discharge)	Generalized weakness
Appears	

Source: North Mississippi Medical Center Home Health. (1999). Tupelo, MS.

aides, and medical social services, are all specified in the COP. The COP also address the specific skilled services that each of these disciplines can provide, training requirements for aides, and other requirements that the agency must abide by to become an approved provider of Medicare home care or hospice services. The standards set forth in the COP not only stipulate what agencies must do to qualify for Medicare but also form the basis for evaluation of the quality of the services provided. Each agency must incorporate these requirements in their policies and procedures. The home health agency must follow these policies and procedures with absolute compliance to the regulations to ensure Medicare reimbursement of visits.

Under the current Medicare program, home health services are reimbursed on a cost basis. Essentially, this means that the Medicare program will reimburse a home health agency for the expenses it incurs related to the provision of home health services to its beneficiaries. Expenses are considered allowable, ones that the Medicare program will pay for, as long as they can be considered "reasonable and necessary" to providing client care. Examples of allowable expenses are salaries for professional and support staff, nursing supplies (e.g., gloves), certain medical supplies, computer hardware and software, clerical and office supplies, and advertising costs related to recruitment of staff. Advertising costs related to increasing the agency's client referrals or increasing the use of home health services are not allowable expenses to the Medicare program.

As previously discussed, documentation requirements and record-keeping standards must be adhered to strictly and are primary responsibilities of the home health care nurse. This is required to ensure reimbursement for the expenses that are incurred by the agency in the process of providing services to its clients. The visit and progress notes completed by the direct care staff are essential to justifying the need for the services rendered. Each visit made by the agency must be considered "reasonable and necessary" to the plan of treatment established by the physician in order for Medicare to reimburse its expense. The fiscal intermediaries for Medicare are responsible for reviewing a portion

BOX 38-14 GENERAL QUESTIONS TO GUIDE THE NURSE IN DOCUMENTATION OF HOMEBOUND STATUS

- How often does the client leave home for social reasons?
- How long does he or she stay gone?
- How taxing or difficult is it for the client to leave home?
- What kind of assistive devises are used when the client leaves home?

Source: Denise Pugh, RN, MSN, North Mississippi Medical Center Home Health, Tupelo, MS.

of the agency's clinical documentation on an ongoing basis. This is done to ascertain that the services provided by the agency were appropriately ordered by the physician, were reasonable and necessary, and met the qualifying and coverage criteria for payment.

Agencies are responsible for filing detailed cost reports. These cost reports identify expenses made by the agency in providing direct care of the client, which include the total number of visits made per discipline, total number of Medicare clients, and indirect care such as administration and other overhead expenses. This cost report is used to determine the reimbursement the agency will receive and establish that the costs incurred were under the cost limits established by Medicare. Payment can and will be denied without proper legal documentation by the health care team.

The COPs require that the client meet several qualifying criteria to receive covered services by the Medicare program. These qualifying criteria for home health services are that the client be (1) under the care of a physician, (2) essentially confined to the home, and (3) require skilled services of a registered nurse, physical therapist, or speech pathologist on an intermittent basis. See Box 38-14 for general questions that can guide the nurse in the documentation of homebound status.

The physician must certify that the client is essentially homebound and establish an individual plan of care (POC) for the client. The POC is established by the physician in collaboration with the home health team and must be updated as changes occur in the client's condition or at least every 62 days. The nurse plays a key role in establishing the POC for both home care and hospice. The nurse collaborates with the physician and with other health team members to establish the appropriate POC for the client. The POC is based on the client's health history and a current comprehensive assessment of the client's physical, psychological, social, and spiritual needs. The nurse's knowledge of the resources available in the community is very important to establish the plan that will optimally meet the client's needs. Box 38-15 summarizes the concepts of Medicare criteria for home health clients.

FYI

How is home health paid for?
- *Medicare*
- *Medicaid*
- *Private insurance*
- *Payment by individual or "out of pocket"*

BOX 38-15 SUMMARY OF MEDICARE CRITERIA FOR HOME HEALTH CLIENTS

QUALIFYING CRITERIA FOR A MEDICARE BENEFICIARY TO RECEIVE HOME HEALTH SERVICES
- Essentially confined to the home
- Under a plan of care established by a physician
- In need of intermittent skilled nursing, physical, or speech therapy

COVERED SERVICES FOR HOME HEALTH
- Skilled nursing
- Physical therapy
- Speech therapy
- Occupational therapy
- Home health aide
- Medical social services

QUALIFYING CRITERIA FOR A MEDICARE BENEFICIARY TO RECEIVE HOSPICE SERVICES
- A life expectancy of 6 months or less
- Seeking palliative treatment only

HOSPICE INTERDISCIPLINARY TEAM
- Registered nurse
- Physician
- Pastoral/counselor
- Medical social services

TABLE 38-1   **A COMPARISON OF MEDICARE AND MEDICAID IN HOME HEALTH REIMBURSEMENT**

MEDICARE (TITLE XVIII)	MEDICAID (TITLE XIX)
Age 65 and older or disabled	Income-based eligibility
Homebound status	Homebound status not always required
Intermittent service	Intermittent service
Skilled service	Skilled service not always required
Restorative services	Custodial and maintenance services
Physician certification required	Physician certification required
Medical, therapy, or social service	State option: medical, therapist, or social service
Provides rental and purchase payments	Provides purchase payments
Reimbursement: "reasonable cost"	Reimbursement: maximum allowed, determined by state

Medicaid

Medicaid is authorized by Title XIX of the Social Security Act and provides health services to low-income persons. As a source of reimbursement for home health services, Medicaid is federally aided but state operated and state administered. Each state determines program eligibility, benefits covered, and the rates of payment for providers. Clinical guidelines for Medicaid reimbursement basically follow those of the Medicare program. Medicaid covers home health services, including skilled and unskilled services. If a client qualifies for both Medicare and Medicaid, Medicare is often the primary reimbursement source. A comparison of Medicare and Medicaid benefits are detailed in Table 38-1.

Private Insurance

For a growing number of home health clients, private insurance as a third-party payer in the private sector provides reimbursement for home health care services. Three major types of organizations provide this type of reimbursement: indemnity insurance companies that pay a percentage of billed charges, nonprofit Blue Cross and Blue Shield, and health maintenance organizations (HMOs). As more managed care networks emerge as reimbursement mechanisms, HMOs are growing in number and scope in comprehensive health care services. The services provided in the private sector vary by payer, but most often, the documentation and clinical guidelines follow Medicare standards for reimbursement (MacLaren, 1994).

Payment by Individual

Individuals who do not have health insurance, those who do not meet their insurance coverage requirements, or those who do not qualify for federal assistance may pay the established charges by the agency or be allowed to pay on a sliding scale based on income. Clients who no longer qualify for Medicare or Medicaid may also desire home health care services and continue to pay after certification has expired. Each agency has its own regulations and policies concerning both payments by individual and medically indigent care, which may be provided at no charge.

Quality Assurance and Public Accountability

Regulation and Licensure

In addition to Medicare requirements, most states require that home health and hospice agencies be licensed to operate within their state. Agencies operating in states that require licensure must abide by the state's minimum standards for licensure, in addition to the regulations included in the COPs. The HCFA, under the direction of the Department of Health and Human Services, contracts with state licensing and certification authorities to provide survey and audit services for the purposes of certifying home care agencies to participate in the Medicare program. Survey are performed at regular intervals, such as every 2 to 3 years, to determine eligibility for renewal of licensure. These surveys may be conducted more often for new providers or providers that had deficiencies on their previous evaluations. These surveys involve record reviews, staff and client interviews, and home visits. The purpose of the survey process is to ascertain that all regulations are being met in providing home care services to the Medicare and Medicaid beneficiaries. State authorities are responsible for responding to and investigating any complaints lodged against the agency and initiating any action indicated through the appropriate regulatory body.

Accreditation

Accreditation of agencies is another aspect of quality assurance, but unlike state licensure, it is not required for Medicare or Medicaid participation. Accreditation is a demonstration of a commitment to providing a high standard of excellence in the delivery of care. Some third-party payers, such as managed care networks or insurance companies, may require accreditation. To meet the stringent standards of accreditation, an agency must demonstrate team effort from all involved in the delivery of care (Lovejoy, 1997). There are three nationally recognized organizations which provide voluntary accreditation for home health agencies: The Joint Commission's Home Care Accreditation Program (JCHCA), The Community Health Accreditation Pro-

CASE STUDY

Mrs. Ollie Mae Thompson is a 68-year-old woman. Her referral diagnosis is congestive heart failure. She was discharged from Baxterville General Hospital after a 5-day stay. She lives with her 75-year-old sister in a two-bedroom house in a small rural community. Upon arrival at the home, the health nurse finds Mrs. Thompson lying in bed. Her sister is watching television in the living room. During the visit, Mrs. Thompson relates the history of her illness. About a month ago, she noticed swelling in her feet and legs and extreme shortness of breath while picking tomatoes from her garden. She had to rest after picking only a small bucket of tomatoes. She also noticed that she had to stop midway between the house and the mailbox to catch her breath. Mrs. Thompson recalled that she had to use two or more pillows in order to breathe easy enough to sleep. She began awakening during the night with shortness of breath and had to sit up in the bedside chair to "get her breath back again" before going back to sleep. She also reported getting up several times a night to urinate, which was a change in her usual habits. She grew increasingly more concerned about herself when she became so fatigued that she neglected her garden crops.

The nurse, when conducting a medication review, found that Mrs. Thompson had been taking digoxin following a myocardial infarction 9 months earlier. Immediately before the present symptoms began, Mrs. Thompson has discontinued taking the digoxin because "I felt fine and didn't think I needed it anymore."

Mrs. Thompson's present medications are as follows: digoxin 0.25 mg/day, furosemide (Lasix) 40 mg/day, and KCl 20% tsp per day in juice. She re-

ports that she is taking the "heart pill" but has stopped the "fluid pill" because it makes her have to urinate frequently and getting up makes her dizzy. She took the "other liquid" for about 2 days but has since quit taking it "because it makes the juice taste funny." Since discharge from the hospital, she has required assistance with self-care and is using a wheelchair for most ambulation. She spends much of her day in bed, because "I feel so weak, I can't stand for very long." Her physician told her to "cut down on her salt," and she was given a diet sheet in the hospital, which she misplaced before reading it. She has a return appointment to see her physician in 2 weeks.

Her breakfast today consisted of two fried eggs, two pork sausage patties, two slices of toast with butter and jelly, and two cups of regular coffee. She is complaining of shortness of breath and is expressing frustration that "I will never be able to grow my own vegetables again." Her legs are extremely swollen with 3+ pitting edema; they are cool to the touch. She does not have socks on. She reports that she is concerned about her sister's "back problems" and that she fears relying on her too much for care such as bathing and ambulating. Her vital signs are as follows: blood pressure, 140/90 mm Hg; pulse, 54 beats/min; and respiratory rate, 24 breaths/min.

1. Based on the preceding information, is Mrs. Thompson homebound?
2. Identify two nursing goals for Mrs. Thompson.
3. What action would you take regarding Mrs. Thompson's physical findings?
4. Identify one nursing goal related to Mrs. Thompson's caregiver.
5. What further information would you want about Mrs. Thompson?

gram (CHAP), a subsidiary of the National League for Nursing (NLN), and the National Home Caring Council.

Managed Care and Home Health

Managed care has become the dominant pattern of organizational reimbursement in the United States. As a result, most persons in the United States with private health insurance are in some type of managed care arrangement or network. A majority of states are in some form of Medicaid managed care program (Children's Defense Fund, 1998). Managed care will influence

nursing practice as agencies respond to strong incentives to lower costs. As has been discussed, nursing interventions and their effectiveness will be measured against client outcomes and client satisfaction of care. Home health nurses will continue to focus on the family as caregiver, with a greater emphasis on teaching the family/caregiver more effective ways of caring for the client. With increasing responsibilities resting with the caregiver, more efficient use of the nurses' time can occur resulting in shorter illness episodes. All home health nurses must be effective case managers to ensure that the highest quality care is delivered in the shortest time possible (Peters & Eigsti, 1991).

RESEARCH BRIEF

Ettinger, B. (1998). Disease management: Maintaining skeletal health among postmenopausal women. American Journal of Managed Care, 4(3), 387–396.

Although disease management is often considered oriented toward treatment, the emerging paradigm for prevention of osteoporotic fractures in postmenopausal women is changing. Conventional wisdom backed by previous research has considered menopausal women to have little opportunity for building bone resulting from calcium loss of aging. With diagnostic procedures, such as bone densitometry, and recently developed drugs, such as biphosphonates and deselective estrogen receptor modulators, there is increasing optimism that bone mass can be regained. Even when treatment is begun in women in their 60s and 70s, fractures can be prevented through increased bone building interventions. Implications for home health nurses are to educate older women about the use of such pharmacological agents, weight-bearing exercises, calcium intake, and the need for bone density screening tests.

A CONVERSATION WITH...

You have to be prepared for anything in home health. Home health nurses use the nursing process just like other nurses; one difference is that they begin the assessment when they pull into the driveway or yard. The nurse may see a 2-month-old for an evaluation for failure to thrive at 8:00 AM, a 10-year-old for post-appendectomy nonhealing surgical wound care at 9:30 AM, and a 101-year-old for catheter care at 10:45 AM. I believe that more than any other nursing care, the art and science of nursing must hold hands in home health. You must know how to administer a high-powered antibiotic IV, know the science and possess the skill it calls for to do it properly. And at the same time, the home health nurse must use the art of caring when a client hammers a nail into his wall for you to hang that IV on when the medical equipment company fails to deliver the IV pole on time. The true art is to use the client's nail and tell him how important he is in the delivery of his care.

—Ilene Purvis Bloxsom, RN, BSN,
Home Health Nurse

The Balanced Budget Act of 1997 mandated that the HCFA be prepared to implement a prospective payment system (PPS) for home health by federal fiscal year 2000. A prospective payment system for home health is anticipated to be similar to the methodology used for hospitals since 1981 and for skilled nursing facilities beginning in 1998. In 1981, hospital reimbursement by the Medicare program changed from a cost-based reimbursement system to a prospective payment system using DRGs as the basis for reimbursement. Skilled nursing facility reimbursement is a prospective rate varied by a "case-mix adjuster." This case-mix adjuster is determined from information collected in a standardized data collection tool designed to measure clients' need for additional care and services. Managed health care plans, such as HMOs, preferred provider organizations (PPOs), and networks, are providing home care services as part of their health plans at an increasing rate.

Managed care plans generally reimburse home health agencies based on a fee-for-service or capitated rate methodology. A **fee-for-service rate** is generally based on a per visit or hourly rate for each discipline. A **capitated rate** is generally awarded based on a population or group of "lives" for which the agency is paid a "per member per month" rate. Reimbursement of this nature requires that the agency make an estimation of the anticipated needs of the population to determine if the arrangement is financially feasible.

As the focus in managed care shifts to outcomes of care, research linking outcomes to care delivery has resulted in Medicare's OASIS: Standardized Outcome and Assessment Information Set for Home Health Care. Shaughnessy (1996) developed the OASIS instrument as a data set with the following categories of items: demographics and client history, living arrangements, supportive assistance, body systems, activities of daily living/independent activities of daily living (ADL/IADL), medications, equipment management, and emergent care. Data are collected upon admission to the home health agency, at a specified time during care, and upon discharge of home health services. OASIS is used to measure outcomes of care based on the home health interventions provided. The instrument is mandated by Medicare and the condition of participation for certified home health agencies. These data are being used by the HCFA to provide information about the population of Medicare and Medicaid clients receiving home health care and their clinical outcomes.

Interdisciplinary Team Approach in Home Health

Collaboration in home health is mandatory in home health nursing. Medicare requires an interdisciplinary team approach in order for agencies to be Medicare certified. A collaborative approach is clearly evident in the definitions and standards of home health nursing. Collaboration is necessary to ensure the continuity of care as the client moves from hospital to home. *Discharge* has traditionally referred to the client's exit from the hospital to the home; in today's fluid health care system, clients are transitioned in and out of different realms of agency service necessitating complex professional referrals. To be in legal compliance with federal regulatory statutes, the physician must certify the plan of treatment for the client. In most instances, it becomes the responsibility of other team members to evaluate the client's status and response to treatment and then with the physician modify the plan of treatment accordingly. The nurse serves as manager or coordinator of care for this interdisciplinary team effort. To function in this role, the nurse must have a clear understanding of the roles of the other team members, and a working knowledge of community resources. Traditionally, the roles and functions of the home care nurse have been that of direct care provider, educator, and case manager or coordinator of care. Direct care activities or skills include assessments, performing procedures and treatments, and client and family teaching. Indirect care includes ancillary personnel supervision, referrals, consultation, and team conferences. The nurse assesses and identifies the problems and needs. Referrals to other disciplines and community agencies may be needed and this care is coordinated by the nurse under the direction of the physician. For example, if a nurse identifies a home health client who is having financial difficulty with out-of-pocket deductibles for necessary equipment, a referral to a social worker would be appropriate.

Within an interdisciplinary model, the unit of care should be the family, and nursing care is designed and provided within the context of the community in which the client lives. The home care nurse cares for clients across the life span with multiple medical diagnoses and responses to illness. Health promotion and disease prevention are the focus of care (Brown, 1998). The nurse develops a POC under the direction of a physician with the assistance of a multidisciplinary team, which becomes the home health care team and may include social workers, therapists, chaplains, nutritionists, and others as appropriate. The client also participates in developing their plan of care, and evaluating, along with the team, the outcomes of care. The nurse and team members plan their visit schedule around client preferences, other discipline visits, physician appointments, and geographic areas. Appropriate planning by all disciplines before the visit is essential. This includes laboratory work or any supplies needed along with the activities of the visit that center around the goals set for the client in the previously established POC. Some agencies have care maps or critical paths that define the day-to-day activities and outcomes to be met during each visit. Others use goals established on admission and modify them as appropriate. Detailed descriptions of member roles of the home health care interdisciplinary team can be found in Box 38-16.

BOX 38-16 MEMBERS OF THE HOME HEALTH CARE INTERDISCIPLINARY TEAM

- *Home health nurse* is the traditional provider of care in the home. Home health nurses provide skilled nursing services and coordinate care within the interdisciplinary team.

- *Physician* refers clients for home care services and approves the plan of care.

- *Home health aides* provide personal care that includes activities such as bathing, shaving, and skin and nail care. The home health aide also performs basic tasks that include things such as emptying urinary drainage bags, taking vital signs, assisting with ambulation and performing exercises assigned, and light homemaking activities such as preparing a meal, changing linens, cleaning room, and laundry.

- *Physical therapists* provide evaluation of the client's rehabilitation needs and potential, which may include areas such as range of motion, strength, balance and coordination, gait analysis, muscle tone, pain, endurance, equipment needs, and home safety. The physical therapist then develops and implements the treatment plan that includes teaching the client and family the home therapy regime and establishing a maintenance therapy program.

- *Speech therapists* provide services related to the evaluation of rehabilitation needs and potential in clients with speech and language disorders and swallowing disorders. The speech therapist develops and implements a restorative treatment program involving the client and family.

- *Occupational therapists* focus on evaluation and treatment of the client's upper extremities by assisting to restore muscle strength and mobility for functional skills. The program established is designed to restore physical function and sensory-integrative function or develop compensatory techniques. Vocational and prevocational assessment and training, as well as design and fitting of orthotic and self-help devices, are also provided by the occupational therapist.

- *Medical social workers* provide assessment of the social and emotional factors related to the client's illness and plan of treatment. This includes assessment of the relationship of the client's medical/nursing requirements to the home situation, financial resources, and community resources. The Medical social worker may provide counseling for the client related to areas such as depression, addictions, reaction/adjustment to illness, and strengthening family support systems. Counseling for the client's family may be necessary to treat the client's illness/injury in resolving family problems that are obstructing or preventing the client's treatment.

Role of Family Caregivers in Home Health

As community health nurses have long been aware, home health nurses contribute less to the well-being of a home health client than the more significant influence of family caregivers. Informal caregiving provided by family caregivers is an integral part of our health care system. Among people 45 and older, approximately 2 in 5 report some experience with long-term care in their families. As the population ages, the demand for informal, family caregivers will escalate over the next 30 years (ANA, 1995). Home health clients would be unable to stay in their homes even to be the recipient of home health nursing care were it not for the family members and other caregivers who dedicate themselves to their care. Community health nurses have traditionally been family-oriented when conducting home visits. One only has to look at our legacy of Lillian Wald and the Henry Street nurses to see the foundation of family-oriented care. Only when the family becomes recognized as the unit of service within the context of the larger community can significant, long-lasting change occur. With the ever-present influence of Medicare and other funding sources, nurses often focus their care efforts on providing only those services that are reimbursable in the home setting (Kenyon, Smith, Hefty, Bell, McNeil, & Maraus, 1990). The individual ill client has steadily become the focus in home care, with the family and other caregivers fading to a contextual backdrop (Bradley, 1996).

Recent research has revealed that the family caregivers of home health clients often have unmet health needs and that the role of caregiver is associated with high stress and increased illness when compared with similar populations. The role is often unpaid and associated with isolation and selfless dedication to the health

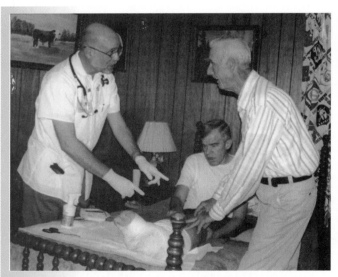

Home health nurses work with the family caregiver to implement the plan of care.

of the home health client (Levine, 1999). Quite often, these caregivers are the only other adult in the home and, as such, have little choice about being the one responsible for the household and ill client. Many studies report that family caregivers tend to be female and themselves in late adulthood (see Bull, 1990; Pruchno & Potashnik, 1989; Kiecolt-Glaser, Glaser, Shuttleworth, Dyer, Ogrocki, & Speicher, 1987). The community health nurse must strive to consider these caregivers in the assessment of the environment and resources, because if the family caregiver has unmet health needs, eventually his or her caretaking abilities will be affected. Zelwesky and Deitrick (1987) go so far as to state, "Accurate needs assessment of the client and his or her family may prevent family burn-out, extend care-giving abilities, conserve family resources, and delay or prevent institutionalization." (p. 77). In her 1996 study, Bradley contends that although prevention activities are not covered by Medicare in home health, "We depend on the family care giver to provide needed care to many of our clients. If the care givers become ill, their caregiving ability decreases. The likelihood of our losing the original home health client to nursing home care or hospitalization increases when we do not promote the family care giver's health" (p. 287). So although not a financial gain in the short term, there may be significant long-term financial benefits in caring for the ones who care for our clients day in and day out. The home health nurse must assess the role of the family caregiver in the context of how well the client functions in the home environment (Levine, 1999). Supporting the caregiver may mean little more than listening carefully to his or her needs regarding personal health status and providing suggestions for health promotion and time management apart from the client. Support groups for caregivers can also provide valuable resources that ultimately strengthen the care provided to the client. The home health nurse has many opportunities to praise the caregiver and remind him or her of the need to pay attention to self for the sake of the client. Day-care programs and respite care can provide needed breaks for the family caregiver and should be encouraged by the home health nurse. As the need for informal caregiving increases in the future, home health nurses will need to become more involved in the promotion of local, state, and national health care policy development related to the support of family caregivers as a health care resource (ANA, 1995).

Legal and Ethical Issues in Home Health

Home health nurses are confronted with legal and ethical issues related to nursing practice daily. Complex family situations create daily dilemmas for the home health nurse, such as questions regarding caretaking abilities of the family caregivers, financial constraints, and respect for autonomous decision making with the vulnerable client. In the home, nurses are often caring for clients over a long period, as compared with the acute care setting, and as a result, they face boundary issues related to processionals and self-responsibility for care.

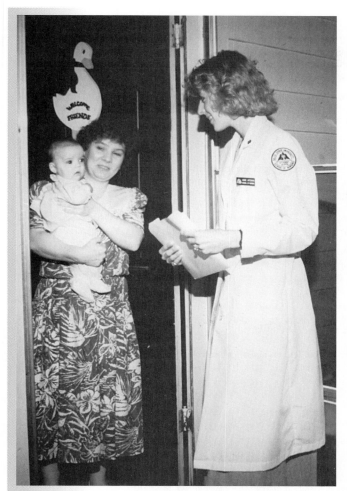

Home health nurses see a variety of clients with diverse health care needs.

One source of ethical dilemma in health care is in providing necessary nursing care for identified client needs when financial reimbursement is no longer available. Agency policy may include options for temporary services or the nurse must assist the client and family in making alternative plans for care. Clients noncompliance with the treatment plan are constant, and ethical issues related to use of resources can be sources of significant ethical conflict. Reporting abusive, neglectful, and unsafe conditions, care, or practices may often be necessary as a legal and ethical mandatory practice. Knowing a client's rights and responsibilities, as well as the rights and limitations of the home health care nurse, is a critical component of home health care nursing practice. Referral to social work, support groups, and appropriate agencies are often the appropriate response. Lovejoy (1997) recommends the creation of agency support groups for home health care nurses and other professionals. A support group can provide needed discussion and conflict resolution in the environment of shared experiences with others. Lovejoy

(1997) makes the following recommendations in the creation of an efficient support group in home health:

- *A clinical nurse specialist should facilitate and coordinate the support group. This clinical nurse specialist should have experience in leading support groups and ideally should have experience in the field as a home health staff nurse.*
- *Support group meetings should not be mandatory. Nurses should be encouraged to attend meetings but never required to attend.*
- *Support groups should have a mix of new and experienced nurses. All other health professionals should be encouraged to be a part of the group as well.*

The support group should be sponsored by the agency, be a part of the formal organizational structure, and have rules and bylaws as appropriate. If the group is informal, minimal rules should relate to frequency of meetings, commitment of members, confidentiality issues, and termination of membership.

An effective support group should help make members feel better about themselves and their abilities and more at ease in the complex home environment. One unexpected benefit of the support group in home health agencies is that members often are able to see co-workers in a new light and learn to trust them as resources. Home care is often a lonely profession without the benefit of working closely with colleagues on a daily basis. The support group, along with modern telecommunication strategies, can bridge the isolation of "nursing on the road" (Lovejoy, 1997).

Home Care Bill of Rights

Medicare-certified agencies are required to provide home health clients with a written bill of rights before the initiation of service. Each home health client is required to be informed of his or her right for health care treatment, and this must be documented in the client's permanent record. To assist home health provider agencies with this requirement, the National Association of Home Care has developed a Home Care Bill of Rights. This document provides the client with details of what can be expected from home care agencies in the delivery of their care. Agencies often use a modified form of the NAHC Bill of Rights.

Advance Medical Directives

Home health nurses must also be involved in the requirements for informed decision making as specified in the Home Care Bill of Rights related to treatment options and refusal when the client is unable to make decisions and communicate those decisions to the health care provider. The advance medical directive is a document that describes client intent and wishes regarding various types of medical treatment in selected situations. Medical directives were developed in the early part of the 1990s in response to increased technology in the treatment of acute and chronic illnesses and the increased awareness by the consumer population of the need to make informed decisions regarding

HOME HEALTH BILL OF RIGHTS.

SOUTH MISSISSIPPI HOME HEALTH, INC.
BILL OF RIGHTS & RESPONSIBILITIES

Each patient referred to South Mississippi Home Health, Inc. (henceforth referred to as SMHH) has the right to be informed in writing of his or her rights and responsibilities prior to care being rendered. The patient's family or guardian may exercise the patient's rights when the patient has been judged incompetent. SMHH has an obligation to protect and promote the rights of their patients.

Quality of Care

Patients have the right:
- to have a relationship with SMHH that is based on honesty, ethical standards of conduct, and compliance with state and federal laws;
- to be assured of service without regard to age, race, religious preference, sex, marital status, national origin, handicapping condition or whether or not he has executed an advance directive;
- to expect kindness, consideration, and respect;
- to discuss problems regarding services by calling locally _____;
- to voice a formal complaint with SMHH by calling Corporate headquarters at _____ , and requesting the Patient Rights Coordinator;
  - to know about the disposition of such complaints;
  - to voice their grievances without fear of discrimination or reprisal; and
- to know the state's home health hotline;
- the purpose of the hotline is to receive complaints or questions about home health agencies.

Decision Making

Patients have the right:
- to be notified in writing of the care that is to be furnished and the proposed frequency of the visits;
- to participate in the planning of the care and in any changes;
- to accept or refuse services or request a change in home health care provider without fear of reprisal or discrimination;
- to make advance directives concerning his care; and
- to refuse to participate in experimental research.

Privacy

Patients have the right:
- to expect confidentiality; and
- to expect SMHH to release information only as required by law or authorized by the patient.

Financial Information

Patients have the right:
- to be informed of the extent to which payment may be expected from Medicare, Medicaid or any other payer known to SMHH;
- to be informed of the charges that will not be covered by Medicare;
- to be informed of the charges for which the patient may be liable;
- to be notified of any changes in the above, orally and in writing, within thirty working days.

South Mississippi Home Health Policy:

South Mississippi Home Health, Inc. nurses, aides and therapists are CPR certified. It is the policy of this company that, in the event of a cardiac arrest and in the absence of a Do Not Resuscitate order from your physician, CPR efforts will be initiated.

SMHH will comply with a patient's advance directives in providing care, to the extent allowed by State law. However, SMHH respects the right of our employees not to implement your advance directive due to personal convictions. In this case, SMHH will make every effort to comply with your advance directive or transfer you to another provider. SMHH may discharge or refer the patient to another source of care if the patient's inability or refusal to comply with the plan of care compromises SMHH's commitment to quality care.

Patients have the right:
- to know SMHH policies which apply to his/her conduct.
  A patient and/or his family shall be responsible for:
  a. cooperation with SMHH staff in the plan of care.
  b. providing SMHH personnel with accurate information as to the symptoms and condition as well as compliance with the prescribed plan of care.
- to be given notice of the reason for transfer or discharge from SMHH, which may be any of the following:
  a. Goals have been met.
  b. Requires a different level of care.
  c. Refuses the continuation of care.
  d. Ill will on the part of the patient and/or family toward SMHH.
  e. Danger to SMHH staff.
  f. Noncompliance with Bill of Rights and Responsibilities.
  g. Noncompliance with Patient Account Policies.
  h. Unsigned physician's Plan of Care.

RESEARCH BRIEF

Twohy, K. M., & Rief, L. (1997). What do public health nurses really do during prenatal home appointments? Public Health Nursing, 14(6), 324–331.

This research study used a descriptive design to identify and describe the nursing interventions and activities used by public health nurses in home-based delivery of care to high-risk prenatal clients. Fourteen home appointments by nine public health nurses were audio taped, transcribed, and coded using the Nursing Interventions Classification (NIC) as the coding scheme. Seven interventions accounted for nearly 83% of the nursing care during the home visits. Those seven interventions were active listening, childbirth preparation, family integrity promotion (childbearing), parent education (childbearing family), prenatal care, self-esteem enhancement, and support system enhancement. Weak relationships were found between the interventions and the written care plan, the interventions identified in the coded transcriptions, and the chart documentation of the events of the home visit. Many interventions or activities were not part of the written nursing care plan. Implications are for further study to clarify what constitutes a nursing intervention, to clarify the need to formalize psychosocial activities as nursing actions, and to examine the usefulness of the nursing care plan. Because the nursing care plan should give direction to care, it should be relevant to care and consulted before and updated after each home visit. Further research needs to be conducted regarding the actual use of the nursing care plan and for what purpose it is written.

RESEARCH BRIEF

Anderson, M., Pena, R., & Helms, L. (1998). Home care utilization by congestive heart failure patients: A pilot study. Public Health Nursing, 15(2), 146–162.

This study was conducted to determine norms of resource utilization for client with congestive heart failure (CHF) who are admitted and discharged from a not-for-profit home health agency (HHA). Forty agency records were retrospectively reviewed using the resource utilization inventory to collect the characteristics and resource utilization of the sample group. The CHF clients were older than most home care clients and had chronic health problems. Because of these chronic health problems, more than half the study population had caregivers so that the clients could remain in their own homes. Most clients clearly demonstrated the need for skilled nursing or home health aide visits after being hospitalized for an acute CHF episode. Less than half the study group was discharged from the HHA as improved and often were discharged to another health care facility. These results provide a beginning direction for profiling the CHF client's consumption of resources for setting prospective payment reimbursement rates. Home health care costs have increased more than any other health care service covered by Medicare, and new payment methods are being considered. A prospective payment system would replace the per visit rate paid to home care agencies by Medicare. To remain viable under a new payment system, HHAs will need information about resource utilization of various diagnoses in order to demonstrate effective client care.

treatment options and the refusal of medical interventions. There are two types of advance medical directives: living wills and health care proxies, also known as *durable power of attorney.* Either type of directive specifically addresses the client's desire for health care or refusal in the event of becoming incapacitated and unable to make decisions. The living will documents a client's decision to decline life-prolonging interventions if that client becomes terminally ill. A health care proxy, or durable power of attorney, specifies the name of a person who will make health care decisions if the client becomes incapacitated and cannot make them. The client maintains the right to change any of these documents at any time. Each state differs in laws and regulation in the implementation of advance directives, and the home health nurse must remain informed to such statutes.

Information and Technology in Home Health
Communication and Data Management

Home health care nurses depend on the use of information technology in clinical practice. There is continued demand for and improvement in the information systems available for use in the home. Chapter 14 provides a detailed look at how technology is changing the way client care is being delivered in all settings. As health care becomes more mobile, remote points of access within a safe and secure infrastructure will become the norm (Nugent, 1999). Computerized records and care planning tools, such as critical pathways, are helping the home care nurses achieve greater time and client management. Many home health nurses now practice almost exclusively from home and use laptop computers to document visits. Although working from home does not allow for the camaraderie of team communication that occurs in other settings, it does provide many nurses with more work flexibility (Neal, 1997). With tools to manage this information, many health care organizations have decision-support systems that would benefit the management of client care in the home by issuing reminders, offering a menu of options, or linking the nurse to important educational tools and information needed. As improvements in health networks continue, the nurse can access test results from the laboratory, and information from other providers involved in the coordination of care in the home. Electronic commerce may replace traditional home health methods of communicating with partners in health care, especially as disease management programs continue to grow. Security programs within the organization should protect the confidentiality of individually identifiable health care information. This includes training, security audits, and policies regarding access to different types of information.

Health care information systems of the 21st century should guide quality improvement efforts, improve the coordination of care, advance evidence-based health care practice, and support continued research. Because the health care industry is so fragmented, it will be important to work toward data sharing as is common now in so many nonhealth industries. Although all health care organizations collect information, it is uncommon for this to be brought together in a way that can shed light on how variations in the process of care affect outcomes. Information on the experiences and perspectives of clients and the health care team can now be collected with available computer systems. Information on health care outcomes is becoming standard practice in most home care settings (President's Advisory Commission on Consumer Protection and Quality in the Health Care Industry, 1998).

Delivery of Care

Home care nursing must redefine the assessment parameters that are critical to be performed in person and those than can be done through technology such as telenursing. We must also redefine "touch." Do we touch a client physically, as in palpation, or do we also use the term generically, in that we can touch a client with a few therapeutic words over the phone, television, or computer (Frantz, 1997)? The home care nurse can now deliver care and information through a lens, a screen, or a telephone into the home. Home telenursing can never replace in-person home health care; however, the appropriate mix of in-person and electronic visitation, along with the appropriate level of providers to accomplish both, will provide better and more holistic care for the home client and family. Telenursing technology can assist the home care nurse in managing the plan of care remotely to capture vital signs and teach clients and their families self-care management.

Laptop-based medical management systems have been used in the home setting for monitoring wound care and linking the home health nurses to physician consultation. This allows the

RESEARCH BRIEF

Jerant, A.F., Schlachta L., Epperly, T.D., Barnes-Camp, J. (1998). Back to the future: The telemedicine house call. *Family Practice Management, 5,* 18–22, 25–26, 28.

The Center for Total Access at the Department of Defense Southeast Telemedicine Testbed at Fort Gordon, Augusta, Georgia, in clinical partnership with Eisenhower Army Medical Center and its regional hospitals, has ongoing research trials of telenursing applications. Telenursing is the use of telemedicine technology to deliver nursing care. The word *telemedicine* comes from the Latin word *tele,* meaning "distance," and *mederi,* meaning "healing." Telenurses "visit" clients at home using telemedicine technology developed by the Eisenhower Army Medical Center, the Georgia Institute of Technology, and the Medical College of Georgia. A real-time connection over the local cable network allows audio and video contact and measurement of physiological parameters in the client's home. The system, called the Electronic Housecall, includes blood pressure cuff, oxygen saturation monitor, temperature probe, three-lead electrocardiogram monitor, and stethoscope. Clients with common chronic conditions, such as diabetes, heart disease, asthma, and chronic obstructive pulmonary disease, are the target population for study. Findings are that these frequent electronic home visits result in fewer expensive emergency department encounters and inpatient admissions. Home telenursing enables closer monitoring so that problems are identified and acted on before they escalate into crises.

physician consultants to view client wounds from a live video image. The traditional method in the home requires the nurse to take Polaroid photographs of wounds and forward them to physicians for review. Using the telemedicine system, visiting nurses dial the physician, forward the image in real time, and decisions regarding treatment protocols are exchanged between the providers and client (Kincade, 1997).

As home telemedicine and telenursing systems mature, physical therapy can be administered, nutrition counseling conducted, and occupational therapy supervised. As computer ownership and use in the home become as common as television use, e-mail can be used to communicate with clients and clients can report directly to health care providers. Successful programs have used e-mail to remind clients about medication dosing and educational information for postsurgery clients on a daily basis (Jerant, 1999). Client access to the Internet is becoming more common. Such systems will allow nurses aides to

RESEARCH BRIEF

Johnson, B., Wheeler, L., & Deuser, J. (1997). Kaiser Permanente Medical Center's Pilot Tele-home health project. Telemed Today, 5, 16–18.

The home health department at Kaiser Permanente Medical Center in Sacramento, California, followed 100 clients who had chronic obstructive pulmonary disease, cardiac disease, stroke, and wounds requiring regular nursing care with home telemedicine visits by nurses, while another 100 clients received traditional home visits in person and occasional phone calls. Telemedicine units, which work via phone lines and were approved by the U.S. Food and Drug Administration (FDA), provide interactive video conferencing as well as heart and breathing sounds monitoring with an integrated electronic stethoscope. The home units cost approximately $5,000, while the central monitoring station costs approximately $7,500. Client satisfaction with telemedicine visits and the in-person home visits were both rated high, with no difference in the two groups. Care delivery cost savings of 33% to 50% were estimated for the telemedicine group.

conduct physical home visits and be supervised by nurses at an agency or at home (Schlachta, 1996). The home care industry will use these technologies to track client outcomes, reduce service redundancy, and supplement care provided by visiting nurses and other disciplines.

• •

Healing a person does not always mean curing a disease.

Dr. Dame Cicely Saunders,
founder of St Christopher Hospice in London

• •

Hospice Care in the Home

Hospice services for the terminally ill became covered expenses under Medicare in 1983. Hospice nursing provides palliative nursing care for terminally ill clients and their families, with an emphasis on physical, psychosocial, emotional, and spiritual needs. Palliative care is comfort-oriented care and refers to interventions that alleviate or lessen the severity of disease or illness without curing. The goal of the hospice program for home care is to improve the quality of life for people who are no longer able to benefit from curative interventions, with an emphasis on treating the symptoms of the disease to promote comfort. The word *hospice* comes from Latin *hospitium,* meaning "guesthouse." Hospice is holistic in nature and views dying as a normal part of living. Through hospice care in the home, the client can live in dignity and comfort in the context of home and family. Hospice care is primarily provided at home, although facilities also exist that provide these services in an inpatient setting while still offering support for families in a homelike environment. Clients in long-term care facilities can also receive hospice services with the facility considered by Medicare as the place of residence of the client (Brooks, 1997). Medicare can pay for bereavement counseling for as long as a year after the loved one's death. Clients who most often benefit from hospice care and are most commonly seen in hospice care are individuals with cancer, acquired immunodeficiency syndrome (AIDS), end-stage lung or heart disease, and those with chronic diseases. Many HMOs and insurance companies also cover hospice services for their clients. Thirty-six states now offer hospice coverage under their Medicaid programs. Although each hospice service has individual policies concerning payment for care, a common principle of hospice care is to offer services based on a need rather than the ability to pay. For this reason, hospice services may often rely more than other home health services grants and voluntary donations (Hospice Foundation of America, 1999).

For hospice services, the physician must certify that the client has a life expectancy of 6 months or less and is seeking palliative treatment only. Hospice clients must be recertified every 60 days. Clients and family are encouraged to be involved in all decisions about caregiving and medical interventions. Admission to a hospice should not be viewed as a failure of other therapies. Rather, a more holistic approach would suggest that previous treatments had become inappropriate and referral to a hospice as movement into another model of more appropriate therapy for terminal care (Hospice Foundation of America, 1999).

The nurse has traditionally cared for the dying and the bereaved, whether on the battlefield or in the trauma unit or in the home—so how is hospice different? Hospice emerged as an organized movement in England with the founding of the first hospice at St. Christopher in London in 1950 by Dr. Dame Cicely Saunders. Dr. Saunders defined hospice care as "hospice is not a place to go to die, but rather a concept of care based on the promise that when medical science can no longer add days to life, more life will be added to each day." She inspired the hospice movement in the United States with the first home care hospice services founded by Wald in 1974 in Connecticut (Box 38-17).

FYI

In 1998, hospices served nearly 540,000 clients throughout the United States.

Source: National Hospice Association, 1999.

BOX 38-17 FLORENCE WALD, RN, FOUNDER OF U.S. HOSPICE HOME CARE

Florence Wald introduced America to the hospice tradition by founding the first home care hospice program in the United States in New Haven, Connecticut, in 1974. Ms. Wald, at age 81, was inducted into the National Women's Hall of Fame in July 1998 in recognition of her work to bring care for the terminally ill through palliative and psychological care. Wald believed that although medical science has given doctors new ways to understand and control disease, "their focus on the patient as a human being was being eroded."

Source: Associated Press. (1998, July 14). Wald among inductees in Women's Hall of Fame.

BOX 38-18 HOSPICE PHILOSOPHY: ONE AGENCY'S COMMITMENT

Hospice affirms life. Hospice exists to provide support and care for persons in the last phases of incurable disease so that they might live as fully and comfortably as possible. Hospice recognizes dying as a normal process whether or not resulting from a disease. Hospice exists in the hope and belief that, through appropriate care and the promotion of a caring community sensitive to their needs, clients and families may be free to attain a degree of mental and spiritual preparation for death that is satisfactory to them.

North Mississippi Medical Center Home Health Services. (1999). Hospice Philosophy.

The hospice movement was strongly influenced by the research of Dr. Elisabeth Kubler-Ross, who conceptualized death as the final stage of growth as contrasted with the prevailing fear of death and the dying process as failure on the part of the medical system (Kubler-Ross, 1969, 1975). Over the past 30 years, with the prolongation of life, advanced technology, and a growing recognition that dying and terminally ill clients require a special kind of care, hospice as a community health nursing specialty has grown. Thousands of persons with life-limiting diseases have relied on hospice services for comfort, dignity, and compassion at the end of life. Medicare hospice care for the terminally ill in the home generally cost significantly less than care for clients in the standard Medicare program. Reasons include less technology used in the care of the client and family and friends provide most of the day care at home. Although hospice care does not provide 24-hour-a-day care in the home, hospice staff members are usually on call 24 hours a day. Volunteers make up an integral part of hospice care and are required to be a part of Medicare-certified hospice service. Inpatient respite care is available for the family, which provides family caregivers periodic relief. A written POC is also required. Medicare mandates that four core services be provided directly by the hospice: nursing, medical, social work, and counseling (Wilson, 1993). Services provided by hospice are as follows:

- *Nursing service on an intermittent basis*
- *Physician services*
- *Drugs for pain relief*
- *Physical, occupational, and speech therapy*
- *Home health aides*
- *Medical supplies*
- *Spiritual and pastoral services*

- *Continuous care during a crisis*
- *Bereavement services for the family, up to a year following death*

Hospice provides coordinated services for the family of the client with a terminal illness. Hospice, as a specialized kind of home health care, is designed to provide comfort and support to clients and families in the final stages of terminal illness. Goals center on providing care in which clients can spend their last days with dignity, at home or in a homelike setting, surrounded by family members and loved ones. Comfort involves physical and spiritual comfort and emotional support of the client, family, and caregivers (Waters, 1996). See Box 38-18 for a sample agency hospice philosophy.

. . . .

I look up in the night sky. Is anything more certain that in all those vast times and spaces, if I were allowed to search them, I should nowhere find her face, her voice, her touch? She died. She is dead. Is the word so difficult to learn?

C.S. Lewis

. . . .

Hospice Care for Children

Although hospice services have traditionally been associated with adults, recognition has grown among health care professionals that children with terminal illnesses can also benefit from hospice care (Martinson, 1993). The epidemic of children with AIDS has prompted the development of pediatric hospice services for children with life-limiting illnesses (Oleske & Czarniecki, 1999). The first hospice home for children, The Helen House, was established in 1982 in the United Kingdom. By 1993, only 1% of U.S. hospice clients were children. Palliative care for children with terminal diseases, such as AIDS and cancer, can ensure the child's comfort through the course of their illness. Oleske and Czarniecki (1999) advocate that children with a life-limiting illnesses, regardless of diagnosis, socioeconomic status, or geographic location, should receive a continuum of palliative care and have access to hospice services that enhance life and ease the burden of dying. They contend that "children should know, in an age appropriate way, that death is near but that it will not be painful, not faced alone, but rather in the company of those they love" (Oleske & Czarniecki, 1999, p. 1291). Opportunities for hospice nursing with children will most likely increase in the future.

Nurses who work in hospice care have specialized training in grief and bereavement management. Although spiritual care has been a major component of nursing practice since its inception, nurses are often uncomfortable with spiritual components related to death (Brant, 1998). Hospice nurses must be especially comfortable in their skills related to the spiritual needs of their clients. Holistic nursing care for the hospice client means assessing for suffering in the spiritual realm, because the total person is incomplete without such consideration. Providing spiritual care does not mean that hospice nurses must hold the same beliefs of those for whom they care (Brant, 1998). Hospice nurses who provide palliative care approach clients with a nonjudgmental, listening ear. Nurses provide spiritual care by assisting clients in their final days in their search for meaning of past, present, and future events. They attempt to make sense of their life experiences and nurses, in the holistic tradition, must be involved in this healing aspect of this last stage of life.

Nurses as team members in hospice care are often the ones with the prolonged, close contact with clients and family members and as such can provide comprehensive information about the well-being of the family and caregivers to the physician and other members of the hospice team.

Knowing in Nursing

I stepped outside of myself so that I could know
So that I could know the meaning of the earth
Its green springs and quiet winter nights.
So that I could know the depths
of the great, blue ocean
A place from which we all came.

I stepped outside of myself so that I could know
that there was more than the moon,
and the sun, and the stars...
And that when I looked upon the earth
so that I could know the meaning of life and
appreciate its continuance in death.

I stepped outside of myself so that I could know
how to raise my arms in loving, caring ways
And say to those who would listen
Let me share myself with you and all that I know...

by Robyn Rice, RN, MSN

Ethical issues have special considerations for hospice workers. Working with families during a family member's eminent death brings challenges related to professional boundaries, family responsibilities, and complex decisions about care. The threat of legalized suicide is of concern to all nurses but is an especially significant issue in the field of hospice nursing. Legalized suicide and euthanasia practices threaten the natural cycle of dying and the final stage of growth (Brant, 1998). Providing appropriate, holistic, and comforting end of life care, as larger numbers of the baby boom generation age, will continue to emerge as critical professional issues for home health nurses who specialize in hospice care (Brant, 1998).

Hospice does not speed up nor slow down the dying process. It does not prolong life and it does not hasten death.
National Hospice Foundation

Other future issues for hospice nursing care include the expansion of community-based residential hospice care facilities, which include respite care, home care, acute inpatient care, and expanded bereavement counseling for families. With the growing number of elders, adults with AIDS, and children with prolonged terminal illnesses, hospice services will be challenged to provide myriad home- and community-based services for families caring for the terminally ill. Humane care for the dying strains families who are already overburdened with dual career demands and child care. Such facilities can provide nurse managed, holistic care for the terminally ill in a noninstitutional, natural environment more conducive in the promotion of health in the final stage of life (Barant, 1998; Wilson, 1993).

We need to continue to educate nurses in the art of palliative care, emphasizing holistic care that encompasses the mind, body and spirit. Total suffering encompasses all three of these components, and end-of-life care must include the same. We can instill hope that goes beyond the grave.
Jeannine M. Brant, RN, MS, AOCN,
oncology clinical nurse specialist
Saint Vincent Hospital and Health Center, Billings, Montana

Life Goes On

I felt like a rainbow covered with dirt in this room.
I couldn't bear seeing
my uncle and aunt washed
with sad feelings.
My grandpa's hand had no life to it.
Though life went on and the
trees kept swaying.

I wondered what would life
be like without his hand to
cross my hair.
My rainbow just did not shine that day.
The wind took over everything.
I love the wind.
It changed everything in that room.
It made me feel like a hundred
butterflies had flown from his
chest.
His stuck together lips and
hard breathing harmed me.
I couldn't stand there.
Water was pulled from my eyes.
Our hands parted and I
kissed him and walked into
reality.

Alexandra Zacharias, age 10,
on the occasion of the death of her grandfather
Source: *The Educational Forum*, 55(3), Spring, 1991.

....

The Future of Health Care in the Home

As the home health industry continues to evolve, the home care nurse will require advanced clinical skills in community health nursing, as well as an understanding of data management and information technology systems. Knowledge of case management concepts to reach positive clinical and financial outcomes by using resources more effectively will be required. Case managers within home care will have clinical nursing expertise and a sense of measuring nursing impact on specific client populations, such as those with heart disease or cancer. These case managers will be increasingly required in home health nursing practice to possess problem-solving and decision-making skills that require negotiation, and a strong sense of client collaboration. Principles of managed care and practicing in coalitions are important skills for all health care workers, but especially for those who work in the home health field (Frantz, 1997). The opportunity for professional growth in home care nursing is endless. A challenge to provide clients and their caregivers the best of home care continues to be a challenge with the myriad changes in health care today. Growth in information systems and decision-making technology are offering business solutions to home health care. These advances enhance the practice of home care nursing by offering additional resources to manage client care to achieve quantifiable positive health outcomes.

Advanced practice nurses and nurse specialists will become required roles on the interdisciplinary team that offer direction, education, and support (Nemcek & Egan, 1997). As advanced practice nurses assume service privileges in acute care facilities, it is expected that they will eventually demand the ability to discharge clients to home health. Home health nurses will be increasingly accountable for not only client outcomes but will be called on to use business skills, such as cost-benefit analysis, to objectively support the total cost of care. The planning for care based on expected outcomes and participating in policy-making decisions that involve nursing practice will be an expectation of all staff home health nurses (Blaha, 1998).

CONCLUSION

The origins of home visiting began with organized health care. In a managed care environment where the most efficient and effective delivery setting is chosen, nurses will find the home setting a likely practice environment. Community health nursing will continue to include the home as a viable and attractive setting for practice in sickness and in health. See Box 38-19 for some nurses' thoughts about being home health nurses.

BOX 38-19 THOUGHTS ON BEING A HOME HEALTH NURSE . . . FROM THE FIELD

"Probably the best part of the job is being on your own and being able to spend quality time with clients who really believe you can help them."

"There have been so many good memories and experiences—all of my clients are very special, they are like family. I really get to know them, their families, their fears, and their dreams. Home health is very rewarding."

"After working for many years in intensive care, I had grown weary of less and less time getting to

know my patients as I was getting better and better managing the machines that really cared for them. In home health, each day I am doing exactly what I went into nursing for–helping people feel better, using the skills I have worked so hard to develop."

"One of the more memorable home visits was the time the client's pigs got out of the pen and the physical therapist and I had to chase the pigs before we could attend to the client's needs."

CRITICAL THINKING ACTIVITIES

1. Read the poem *Home Call: Mother and Child* by Marilyn Krysl on p. 886.
   - How does the mother perceive the nurse in terms of power?
   - Do the status differences in the nurse and the mother affect the outcome of this home visit as intervention?
   - How could the nurse be culturally sensitive in this situation while educating the mother about appropriate child care?
   - How is power represented in this poem?
   - Identify one appropriate nursing intervention in the described home visit.
2. The following questions are common ones that students nurses ask about home visiting. As you read this chapter, reflect on your own responses to the questions.
   - What do clients in the home think of student nurses caring for them, especially if an instructor is not present?
   - What if the client or family member asks me a question that I don't know?
   - What will I be expected to do as far as skills in the home setting?
   - What about safety issues?
   - What do I do if a client "codes" while I am there?
   - Are there specific legal implications that I should be aware of in the home setting?

CRITICAL THINKING ACTIVITIES—CONT'D

3. Home health care is one of the fastest growing nursing roles in health care today. Managed care has created incentives for hospitals to limit acute care episodes and client admissions. Clients continue to be discharged earlier than ever after surgery, childbirth, and acute episodes of chronic diseases. More and more "high-tech" health care can be replicated in the home, such as chemotherapy, IV therapy, and assisted ventilation. With this likely to continue as all health agencies struggle to contain costs, consider the following opinions about home health nursing. Respond to each statement and document your agreement or disagreement with the opinion.

- Home health nursing is more accurately described as "hospital care at home."

- Home health nursing is a new emerging specialty in preventive acute care and is not really a community health role or a hospital role.

- Home health nurses are generalists who can provide health promotion services to well clients, such as newly discharged mothers and babies, as well as newly discharged post–heart transplant clients with complex intravenous immuno-suppressive drug therapy.

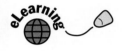

Explore Community Health Nursing on the web! To learn more about the topics in this chapter, use the passcode provided to access your exclusive web site:
http://communitynursing.jbpub.com
If you do not have a passcode, you can obtain one at this site.

REFERENCES

Allen, C. E. (1991). Holistic concepts and the professionalization of public health nursing. *Public Health Nursing, 8*(2), 74–80.

American Nurses Association (ANA). (1999). *Standards of home health nursing practice.* Washington, DC: Author.

American Nurses Association (ANA). (1995). *Position statement: Informal caregiving.* Washington, DC: Author.

Anderson, M., Pena, R., & Helms, L. (1998). Home care utilization by congestive heart failure patients: A pilot study. *Public Health Nursing 15*(2), 146–162.

Barkauskas, V. H. (1983). Effectiveness of public health nurse home visits to primarous mothers and their infants. *American Journal of Public Health 73*(5), 573–580.

Blaha, A. (1997). The current and future national voice for home healthcare nursing. *Home Healthcare Nurse, 15*(12), 873.

Bradley, P. J. (1996). Home healthcare nurses should regain their family focus. *Home Healthcare Nurse, 14*(4), 281–288.

Brant, J. (1998). The art of palliative care: Living with hope, dying with dignity. *Oncology Nursing Forum, 25*(6), 995–1004.

Brooks, S. (1997). Of hope and hospice. *Contemporary Longterm Care, 20*(7), 56–61.

Brown, D. (1998). Home care nursing as a philosophy of care. *Home Healthcare Nurse, 16*(3), 164–165.

Byrd, M. E. (1998). Long-term maternal-child home visiting. *Public Health Nursing, 15*(4), 235–242.

Bull, M. J. (1990). Factors influencing family care giver burden and health. Western Journal of *Nursing Research, 12,* 758–776.

Children's Defense Fund. (1998) *The state of America's children yearbook 1998.* Washington, DC: Author.

Clarke, P., & Cody, W. (1994). Nursing theory-based practice in the home and community: The crux of professional nursing education. *Advances in Nursing Science, 17,* 41–53.

Coffman, S. (1997). Home-care nurses as strangers in the family. *Western Journal of Nursing Research, 19*(1), 82–96.

Cowley, S. (1995). In health visiting: a routine visit is one that has passed. *Journal of Advanced Nursing, 22,* 276–284.

Deal, L. W. (1994). The effectiveness of community health nursing interventions: A literature review. *Public Health Nursing, 11,* 315–323.

Dougherty, G. (1998). When should a child be in the hospital?: A. Frederick North, Jr, M.D. Revisited. *Pediatrics, 101*(1), 19–25.

Franz, A. (1997). Prognosis: Home care nursing. *Home Healthcare Nurse, 15*(12), 876–877.

Gomby, D. S., Larson, J. D., Lewit, J., & Behrman, R. (1993). Home visiting analysis and recommendations. *The Future of Children, 3*, 6–22.

Hafkenschiel, J. H. (1990). Home care past and future. *HMQ*, Third Quarter.

Hickey, M. (1998, July). Disease management improves patient care, cuts costs. *Physicians Management*, p. 214.

Hospice Foundation of America. (1999). "*What is Hospice?*": http://hospicefoundation.htm.

Jerant, A. (1999). Home telemedicine: Merging the old and new ways. *American Family Physician, 60*(4), 1096–1098.

Jerant, A. F., Schlachta, L., Epperly, T. D., Barnes-Camp, J. (1998). Back to the future: The telemedicine house call. *Family Practice Management, 5*, 18–22, 25–26, 28.

Keeling, B. (1978, March). Making the most of the first home visit. *Nursing, 78*, 24–28.

Kenyon, V., Smith, E. Hefty, L. V., Bell, M. L., McNeil, J., & Maraus, T. (1990). Clinical competencies for public health nursing. *Public Health Nursing, 7*, 33–39.

Kiecolt-Glaser, J. K., Glaser, R., Shuttleworth, E. C., Dyer C. S., Ogrocki, B. S., & Speicher, C. E. (1987). Chronic stress and immunity in family care givers of Alzheimer's disease victims. *Psychosomatic Medicine, 49*, 523–535.

Kincade, K. (1997). Growing home-care business benefits from telemedicine TLC. *Telemedicine*, p. 4.

Kornowski, R., Zeeli, D., Averbuch, M., & Finkelstein, A. (1995). Intensive home care surveillance prevents hospitalization and improved morbidity rates among elderly patients with congestive heart failure. *American Heart Journal, 4*, 762–766.

Kubler-Ross, E. (1975). *Death: The final stage of growth.* New York: Simon and Schuster.

Kubler-Ross, E. (1969). *On death and dying: what the dying have to teach doctors, nurses, clergy and their own families.* New York: Macmillan.

Levine, C. (1999). Home sweet hospital: The nature and limits of private responsibilities for home health care. *Journal of Aging and Health Care, 11*(2), 341–360.

Liaschenko, J. (1994). The moral geography of home care. *Advances in Nursing Science, 17*, 16–26.

Liepert, B. D. (1996). The value of community health nursing: A phenomenological study of the perceptions of the community health nurses. *Public Health Nursing, 13*, 50–57.

Lovejoy, D. (1997). *Making the transition to home health nursing.* New York: Springer.

MacLaren, E. (1994). Basics of managed care. *NurseWeek*, pp. 10–11.

Magilvy, J. K. Brown, N. J., & Dydyn, J. (1988). The experience of home health care: Perceptions of older adults. *Public Health Nursing, 5*(3), 140–145.

Maraldo, P. (1989). Home care should be the heart of a nursing sponsored national health plan. *Nursing and Health Care, 10*(6), 301–306.

Martinson, I. M. (1993). Hospice care for children: past, present and future. *Journal of Pediatric Oncology Nursing, 10*, 93–98.

Milone-Nuzzo, P. (1998). Beyond venipuncture as the qualifying service for Medicare: Seeing the forest for the trees, *Home Healthcare Nurse, 16*(3), 177–183.

National Association of Home Care (NAHC). (1999). *Basic statistics about home care.* Washington, DC: Author.

National Institute on Disability and Rehabilitation Research and Training Center. (1996, November), *U.S. Department of Education Disability Statistics Abstract* (Number 17). University of California, San Francisco.

Neal, L. (1977). Current clinical practice of home care nursing. *Home Healthcare Nurse, 15*(12), 881–882.

Nugent, D. (1999). Providing solutions for the growing trend toward home health care. *Health Management Technology, 20*(8), 28–31.

Olds, D. L. (1992). Home visitation program for pregnant women and parents of young children. *American Journal of Diseases of Children, 146*, 704–708.

Olds, D. L., Henderson, C. R., Phelps, C., Kitzman, H., & Hanks, C. (1993). Effect of prenatal and infancy nurse home visitation on government spending. *Medical Care, 31*, 155–174.

Olds, D. L., & Kitzman, H. (1993). Review of research on home visiting for pregnant women and parents of young children. *The Future of Children, 3*(3), 53–92.

Oleske, J., & Czarniecki, L. (1999). Continuum of palliative care: Lessons from caring for children infected with HIV-1. *Lancet, 354*(9186), 1287–1891.

Peters, D., & Eigsti, D. (1991). Utilizing outcomes in home care. *Caring, 10*, 44–51.

Pruchno, R. A., & Potashnik, S. L. (1989). Caregiving spouses: Physical and mental health in perspective. *Journal of the American Geriatric Society, 37*, 697–705.

Pruitt, R. H., Keller, L. S., & Hale, S. L. (1987). Mastering the distractions that mar home visits. *Nursing and Health Care, 8*, 344–347.

Remington, L. (1997). Disease management programs. *The Remington Report, 5*(4), 1.

Rice, R. (1999). A little art in home care: Poetry and storytelling for the soul. *Geriatric Nursing, 20*(3), 165–166.

Rice, R. (1996). *Home health nursing: concepts and application* (2nd ed.). St. Louis: Mosby.

Ruetter, L. I., & Ford, J. S. (1996). Perceptions of public health nursing: Views from the field. *Journal of Advanced Nursing, 24*, 7–15.

Schaffer, C., & Behrendt, D. (1997). Disease state management across the continuum: Bettering lives, providing value. *The Remington Report, 5*(4), 20–23.

Schoen, M. A., & Koenig, R. J. (1997). Home health care nursing: past and present–Part I. *Medical-Surgical Nursing 6*(4), 230–232.

Schoen, S., & Anderson, S. (1998). The role of home visitation programs in improving health outcomes for children and families. *Pediatrics, 101*(3), 486–490.

Schwartz, R. (1977). News from Washington. *The Remington Report,* 5 (4), 12-13.

Shamansky, S. (1988, June). Providing home care services in a for-profit environment, *Nursing Clinics of North America, 23*(2), 387–398.

Shaughnessy P. W. (1996, June 14). *Using outcomes to build a continuous quality improvement program for home care.* 11th National Nursing Symposium on Home Health Care, University of Michigan School of Nursing, Ann Arbor, MI.

Sheldon, P., & Bender, M. (1994, September). High-technology in home care, *Nursing Clinics of North America 29*(3), 508–519.

South Mississippi Home Health Orientation Manual for Registered Nurses.(1996). Hattiesburg, MS: Author.

Stulginsky, M. M. (1993a). Nurses' home health experience. Part 1: The practice setting. *Nursing and Health Care, 14*, 402–407.

Stulginsky, M. M. (1993b). Nurses home health experience. Part 2: The unique demands of home visits. *Nursing and Health Care, 14*, 476–485.

The President's Advisory Commission on Consumer Protection and Quality in the Health Care Industry. (1998). *Quality First: Better Health Care For All Americans*. Washington, DC: U.S. Government Printing Office.

Twohy, K. M., & Reif, L. (1997). What do public health nurses really do during prenatal home appointments? *Public Health Nursing, 14*(6), 324–331.

Warhola, C. (1980). *Planning for home health services: A resource handbook*. DHSS Pub. No. (NRA) 80-14017. Washington, DC: Public Health Service. Department of Health and Human Services.

Waters, K. (1996). Hospice: Comforting the dying patient. In R. Stone (Ed.), *Gerontology Manual*. Tacoma, WA: University of Puget Sound.

Wilson, S. (1993). Hospice and Medicare benefits: Overview, issues, and implications. *Journal of Holistic Nursing, 11*(4), 356–368.

Zelwesky, M. G., & Deitrick, E. P. (1987). Rx for care givers: Respite care. *Journal of Community Health Nursing, 4*, 77–84.

Zerwekh, J. V. (1997, Spring). Making the connection during home visits: Narratives of expert nurses. *International Journal of Human Caring, 1*(1), 325–333.

Chapter 39
School Health Nursing
Frances R. Martin and Ann Elizabeth Kaiser Brown

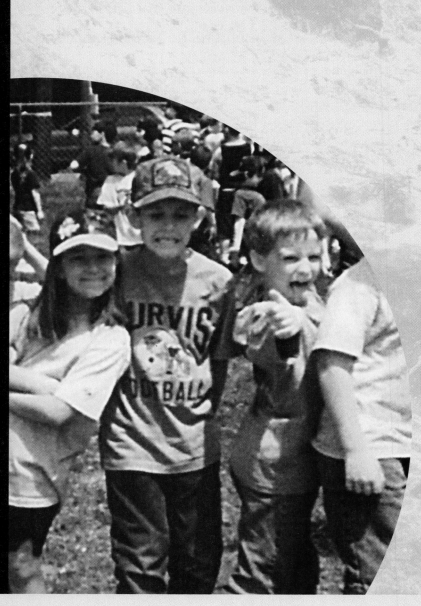

School nursing is a specialized practice of professional nursing that advances the well-being, academic success, and life-long achievement of students. To that end, school nurses facilitate positive student responses to normal development, promote health and safety, intervene with actual and potential health problems, provide case management services, and actively collaborate with others to build student and family capacity for adaptation, self management, self-advocacy, and learning (NASN, 1999).

CHAPTER FOCUS

History of School Health Nursing
Origins
Evolution
Federal Mandates

School Health Nursing Today
Goals 2000
Education's Expectations of the School Nurse

Education and Credentials
Entry-Level Education
Continuing Professional Education
Credentialing

School Health Nursing Practice

Healthy People 2010
Role Definition
Role Within the Profession
At-Risk Populations
Case Finding
Nurse as Team Member

Practice Issues
Legal-Ethical Considerations
Documentation
Delegation
Supervision and Accountability
Funding
School Violence

Community Issues
School-Linked Health Services
Collaboration
Resources

Innovations
School-Based Clinics and Primary Care
Increased Role of the Media
Technology

Healthy People 2010: Objectives Related to School Health

QUESTIONS TO CONSIDER

After reading this chapter, answer the following questions:

1. What is school nursing?
2. What services are typically offered as school health services?
3. Who was the first school nurse in the United States?
4. What role did Lillian Wald play in the development of school nursing?
5. What is a school nurse practitioner?
6. What are the major federal programs which relate to school health?
7. What is the relationship between educational goals and school nurse goals?
8. What are educational requirements of the school nurse?
9. What kinds of health issues do school nurses deal with?
10. What kinds of roles do school nurses play?
11. What are current practice issues in school nursing?
12. What are community issues related to school health?
13. What is a school-based clinic?

KEY TERMS

Delegation
Health-related services
IDEA, 1991
Inclusion ("mainstreaming")

Individual educational plan
Individual health plan
Individualized family service plan

Medically fragile child (special education)
School health
School health services
School nursing

School-based clinic (SBC)
School-based services
Unlicensed assistive personnel

Effective school nurses are "bilingual"; they speak both "education" as well as "health" (Costante, 1996). Current school nursing practice seeks to be as comprehensive as possible while providing episodic or emergency health care, monitoring health status, identifying problems that may affect educational achievement, developing health care plans, and administering medications. In addition, health education and staff training, program development, and family outreach are part of expected practice (Passarelli, 1996). School nurses often must also find resources to implement needed programs or services.

How can school nurses make a difference with societal problems affecting children? The school nurse must accept the educational agenda. This includes meeting health-related educational needs of staff and students, helping students obtain and maintain high test scores, and socializing children within a safe environment. Presently, however, the limited resources have been prioritized and given to meeting the needs of at-risk students, such as those with poor achievement, or chronic diseases (e.g., human immunodeficiency virus/acquired immunodeficiency syndrome [HIV/AIDS], severe asthma, seizures).

The school setting is the workplace of nearly 20% of the U.S. population (children and adults). Fifty million young people attend more than 110,000 schools across the nation. Many of these children come to school with learning disabilities.

Case Study: "A Day in the Life of a School Nurse" on p. 921 demonstrates the multiple roles of a school nurse: health care provider, case finder, planner of health care, health educator to parents as well as school staff and students, communicator, child and family advocate, home visitor, and investigator.

Statistics and trends show that "a choice is at hand: invest now in children's physical and emotional health to create tomorrow's healthy citizens, or pay ten-fold down the road" (NCSBN, 1990). In 1990, there were more than 30,000 cases of measles, mumps, and whooping cough, all preventable diseases. Only 67% of all American children are immunized before the age of 2 years (Annie E. Casey Foundation, 1999). Half of adolescents between the ages of 15 and 19 are sexually active (CDC, 1997). Homicide and suicide are the second and third most common causes of death in teenagers (following motor vehicle accidents). Two million new cases of child abuse are reported to authorities every year. In 1991, nearly 60% of children in urban areas were in poverty. According to the NCES (National Center for Educational Statistics, 1993), a survey of teachers showed that teachers of elementary children perceived poverty as a serious educational threat for 21% of students. Even for high school students, 16% were in poverty and suffered educationally as a result. There is a natural relationship between schools and health care services (Chauvin & Davis, 1994).

The National Longitudinal Study of Healthy Adolescents (NLSHA) highlighted the importance of a child feeling "connected" to the school for greater school success (Resnick, Bearman, Blum, Blum, Bauman, Harris, Jones, Tabor, Beuhring, Sieving, Shew, Ireland, Bearinger, & Udry, 1997). Students at risk, such

FYI

A survey of 1,546 school districts with an identifiable school health program showed that in only 60% of these was "nursing" listed as the major field of the person in charge of school nursing.

as technologically dependent children, may experience stigma from other children in the classroom because of their disability. Helping the child with socialization is an important part of the school nurse role.

Immigration numbers have increased in the United States. Unlike previous immigrants who came from countries where education was valued, immigrant children today often come from countries where survival takes precedence over education (New Faces, 1991). Language barriers have implications for health access, learning, and socialization. This group is at risk for poor physical and mental health and also have challenges to their learning ability.

Many children currently in schools do not constitute an at-risk population but still can be healthier with school nurse intervention. Obesity, depression, poor dental health, and lack of personal hygiene are concerns of the nurse as well as of a teacher or a coach. Establishing healthy habits and behaviors in childhood sets a foundation for a lifetime of improved health.

Health-related problems surrounding vision and hearing impairment, chronic illness, substance use and abuse, teen pregnancy and sexually transmitted diseases (STDs), injuries, and violence make demands on school nurses. However, school nurses also promote preventive efforts such as the school's nutritional services, health education, and student access to school health services in order to reduce long-term health risks (Igoe & Giordano, 1992). A healthy school environment, free of communicable disease, risks for injury, substance use, or violence, is promoted by the school nurse.

School health typically refers to (1) health assessment, (2) health-promotion and prevention activities, (3) case management, and (4) policy development. For many educators, school health has the limited meaning of complying with state laws regarding immunizations, and record keeping around various health screens (vision/hearing/scoliosis/lice). Yet the literature supports the view that a direct link exists between health and academic performance (Boyer, 1991).

The U.S. Secretaries of Education and of Health and Human Services recognize this link. They issued a joint statement supporting comprehensive school health programs, which underscores the two worlds in which school nurses provide services. Support is given to school-based centers to promote better access to health care (see p. 922).

School health services (Passarelli, 1996) may consist of basic health, expanded health, or comprehensive health ser-

A Day in the Life of a School Nurse

Pleasantville Elementary School, early September: The school nurse, Ms. Davis, RN, plans to do the first grade vision screening today, but first she will see the children who are waiting outside her clinic office door. First in line is Jason. Jason's mother wants him to be "checked out for chicken pox." Jason's cousin, Tommy, a second grader, now has chicken pox.

The school secretary knocks on the door. She has Mrs. Perez, who is visibly upset, and her three children with her. "We have a problem," says the secretary. "These children, ages 8, 6, and 5 years old, have not had any shots since their birth in Mexico. School policy will not allow me to register them. I told the mother that you could help them."

In the hallway sits 8-year-old Shelly Strong. Mr. Bullen, her teacher, is concerned because Shelly says she has asthma and needs a "breathing treatment." This is Mr. Bullen's first year to teach school. He is not sure what Shelly is talking about and says that he never has seen a breathing machine like the one Shelly brought to school in her backpack today.

Out in the hall, 9-year-old Steven (who is taking Ritalin for ADHD) and Hiram (who has a physical disability and uses crutches) are yelling and shoving each other. Both 9-year-olds have a history of poor anger control. Mr. Bullen assists Ms. Davis in breaking up the fist fight. Their teacher, Mrs. Adams, has become very frustrated with their behavior.

Ms. Davis seems to be in control of the situation. She has learned to be flexible with her schedule and to prioritize her nursing duties. Ms. Davis assesses Shelly's respiratory condition. Shelly has the signed papers from her mother and the physician giving permission for the inhalation treatment. The school nurse documents her condition and begins Shelly's treatment. She also records the time of treatment and the amount of albuterol as prescribed by her physician. She calls Mrs. Strong, Shelly's mother, at work and sets up an appointment for that afternoon to discuss Shelly's emer-

gency care plan for future asthma attacks. Ms. Davis informs Mr. Bullen of the meeting and requests his presence. She makes a note to schedule a staff in-service on asthma: its signs, symptoms, medications, and treatments.

Ms. Davis assesses Jason for chicken pox and finds him presently free of eruptions. She sends him back to class with an excuse, then records the office visit in a nurse's note for the day. She schedules herself to check Jason in 1 week, because he has been exposed to herpes zoster and has not had chicken pox.

Ms. Davis has not forgotten about the Perez family. She discusses the immunization schedule with the mother. She teaches her about the diseases covered by the immunizations, reviews their medical records and a brief medical history for each child, then prepares the correct immunizations for each one. Ms. Davis administers the immunizations and discusses possible side effects with the mother. Ms. Davis gives the mother and the school secretary the proper paperwork for the children to be registered in school that day.

Mrs. Perez speaks mostly Spanish. Ms. Davis has been taking Spanish night classes at a local college to communicate with the growing Spanish population in her area. Mrs. Perez requests information on applying for Medicaid. Ms. Davis sets up an appointment with the Medicaid office for Mrs. Perez to discuss this and draws a map for the mother. Ms. Davis asks if she can visit with her and the children at home to assess for other needs. The mother agrees.

Shelly's treatment has been completed. Ms. Davis assesses her respiratory condition and allows her to return to Mr. Bullen's class. Ms. Davis then schedules an appointment with Mrs. Adams (Steven and Hiram's teacher). She wants to share some resource materials on behavior management that are now available. Also, she wants to discuss Steven's medication dosage and classroom behavior. Ms. Davis then makes a referral to the school psychologist regarding the repeat incident between the two boys. She schedules time on her calendar for classroom education regarding children with disabilities in grades K–6. By 10 AM she is ready to begin calling on her first class for vision screening.

vices. Funding often determines the extent of services offered. The emphasis at present from the federal government is on comprehensive, rather than basic, school health services. The Centers for Disease Control and Prevention (CDC) proposes a comprehensive school health model that includes eight components: (1) health education, (2) health services, (3) nutrition services, (4) physical education, (5) a healthy school environment, (6) counseling and social services, (7) health

JOINT STATEMENT ON SCHOOL HEALTH.

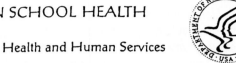

JOINT STATEMENT ON SCHOOL HEALTH
by
The Secretaries of Education and Health and Human Services

Health and education are joined in fundamental ways with each other and with the destinies of the Nation's children. Because of our national leadership responsibilities for education and health, we have initiated unprecedented cooperative efforts between our Departments. In support of comprehensive school health programs, we affirm the following:

■ *America's children face many compelling educational and health and developmental challenges that affect their lives and their futures.*

These challenges include poor levels of achievement; unacceptably high drop-out rates; low literacy; violence; drug abuse; preventable injuries; physical and mental illness; developmental disabilities; and sexual activity resulting in sexually transmitted diseases, including HIV, and unintended pregnancy. These facts demand a reassessment of the contributions of education and health programs in safeguarding our children's present lives and preparing them for productive, responsible, and fulfilling futures.

■ *To help children meet these challenges, education and health must be linked in partnership.*

Schools are the only public institutions that touch nearly every young person in this country. Schools have a unique opportunity to affect the lives of children and their families, but they cannot address all of our children's needs alone. Health, education, and human service programs must be integrated, and schools must have the support of public and private health care providers, communities, and families.

■ *School health programs support the education process, integrate services for disadvantaged and disabled children, and improve children's health prospects.*

Through school health programs, children and their families can develop the knowledge, attitudes, beliefs, and behaviors necessary to remain healthy and perform well in school. These learning environments enhance safety, nutrition, and disease prevention; encourage exercise and fitness; support healthy physical, mental, and emotional development; promote abstinence and prevent sexual behaviors that result in HIV infection, other sexually transmitted diseases, and unintended teenage pregnancy; discourage use of illegal drugs, alcohol, and tobacco; and help young people develop problem-solving and decision-making skills.

■ *Reforms in health care and in education offer opportunities to forge the partnerships needed for our children in the 1990s.*

The benefits of integrated health and education services can be achieved by working together to create a "seamless" network of services, both through the school setting and through linkages with other community resources.

■ *GOALS 2000 and HEALTHY PEOPLE 2000 provide complementary visions that, together, can support our joint efforts in pursuit of a healthier, better educated Nation for the next century.*

GOALS 2000 challenges us to ensure that all children arrive at school ready to learn; to increase the high school graduation rate; to achieve basic subject matter competencies; to achieve universal adult literacy; and to ensure that school environments are safe, disciplined, and drug free. HEALTHY PEOPLE 2000 challenges us to increase the span of healthy life for the American people, to reduce and finally to eliminate health disparities among population groups, and to ensure access to services for all Americans.

In support of GOALS 2000 and HEALTHY PEOPLE 2000, we have established the Interagency Committee on School Health co-chaired by the Assistant Secretary for Elementary and Secondary Education and the Assistant Secretary for Health, and we have convened the National Coordinating Committee on School Health to bring together representatives of major national education and health organizations to work with us.

We call upon professionals in the fields of education and health and concerned citizens across the Nation to join with us in a renewed effort and a reaffirmation of our mutual responsibility to our Nation's children.

Richard W. Riley
Secretary of Education

Donna E. Shalala
Secretary of Health and Human Services

promotion for staff, and (8) family/community involvement. However, at the local school district level, the principal may choose to implement only the basic school health services (screening, immunizations, and first aid) or the expanded model (which includes health education and a healthy school environment).

History of School Health Nursing

Origins

School nursing grew out of a need identified by a school official in England around 1891. Without immunizations or antibiotics, children were losing school time to "minor ailments and infectious troubles" (Oda, 1981). A lack of parental support for education was pervasive; poorer families often used children as breadwinners or as baby-sitters for younger siblings. A school official and a nurse were concerned that some children's education was being hampered by absenteeism due to poor health, so the school official asked the nurse to visit the children at home. This was the beginning of school health nursing.

Around the same time (1902) in the United States, Lillian Wald became concerned about the education and general welfare of tenement children in New York. In particular, the health and education status of tenement children excluded from school due to illness or disabilities distressed Wald. At Wald's suggestion, Lina Rogers Struthers, the first school nurse in America, was hired by the Board of Education. Her task was to treat children in the school, if possible, or visit homes to monitor environmental conditions in need of attention (Pollitt, 1994).

Wald worked out of her home, known as the Henry Street Settlement. Wald's lifetime efforts brought nurses into the New York schools. Even though she was a nurse, she addressed social problems such as child labor. She established the first neighborhood playgrounds, centers, youth clubs, vocational classes, and foster homes. With remarkable foresight, Wald was the forerunner of comprehensive school health services: special education classes began with her development of the first ungraded classrooms for "defectives," or children with disabilities.

Evolution

School nurses were most associated during the first half of the 20th century as the person at school who made sure immunizations were up to date, who identified health problems (e.g., communicable diseases, vision and hearing deficits, mobility disorders), who took care of emergencies, and who trained and counseled students and teachers regarding health-related matters.

In the early 1960s, a new role, nurse practitioner as primary care provider, was proposed. Begun in collaboration with medicine and nursing at the University of Colorado, the vision was to address two issues simultaneously: access to care and preparation of providers to meet health needs of children. Dr. Loretta Ford and Dr. Henry Silver, among others, focused the nurse practi-

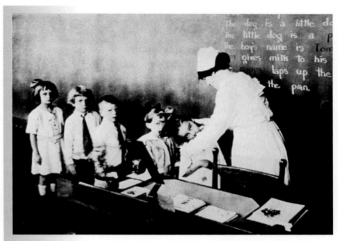

Early school nurses screened for hearing, vision, and orthopedic problems.

tioner role on school health nursing in 1969 with the School Nurse Practitioner (SNP) Program.

The school nurse practitioner role is one that provides primary care in schools, while also receiving financial support through partnerships with managed care models and third party reimbursements to school-based clinics. There is also a possibility of client-generated revenue at such clinics (Urbinati, Steele, Harter, & Harrell, 1996).

Changes in funding and in public expectations of government agencies in the late 1970s produced school health services that were episodic and uncoordinated. Parents and educators disagreed about teaching sensitive and value-laden material. To some parents, school health services became synonymous with sex education, a controversial stance. Schools began to decline as centers for dispensing preventive health care for children. As technology-dependent students required more time from both teachers and the school nurse, school nurses assumed increased responsibility for meeting complicated health needs of disabled and chronically ill students, who began attending regular classrooms.

Federal Mandates

In 1973, Section 504 of the Rehabilitation Act required that disabled students receive "free and appropriate education," which includes specially designed instruction, and related services such as transportation assistance. The school nurse was seen as a necessary part of "special education" at schools medically fragile children attended. Teachers had grave concerns about teaching children with chronic medical conditions such as cerebral palsy, seizure disorders, mental retardation, and emotional problems.

The 1975, Public Law No. 94-142 (the Education for All Handicapped Children Act) initiated a further broadening of "free and appropriate education" by bringing children with various disabilities into the regular classroom setting. Called inclusion (or *mainstreaming*), this legislation mandated appropriate in-class support to students with various educational risks or disabilities, for the maximum extent possible during the school day (National Association of State Boards of Education, 1992). The school nurse was expected to train staff on the care of children with disorders such as spina bifida, asthma, and attention-deficit hyperactivity disorder (ADHD).

In 1978, Congress passed the Health Education Act (PL 95-561). This act proposed comprehensive school health services in least restrictive environments (generally outside the home). Subsequent state court cases have given legal weight to allowing severely disabled students to enter public schools in record numbers.

In 1979, the Department of Health, Education and Welfare established an Office of Comprehensive School Health to implement comprehensive school health services to disabled students in least restrictive environments, as proposed by the Health Education Act. School services were extended to the preschool years (Head Start) and were expanded to include nutrition. Since then, the Department of Agriculture has assumed a role in school nutrition.

Two years later (1981), the Office of Comprehensive School Health was abolished. In 1983, school health was placed with the USPHS in the Department of Maternal-Child Health. Funding was not sufficient to meet increased demands of chronically ill children on the school budgets. Funding for school health nursing came under multiple agencies.

In 1988, Congress authorized the Office of School Health in the Department of Education. It was now no longer with health-related departments. Since that time, as many as 300 federal agencies related to child health, school health, and the environment have taken an interest in the school child. These include the CDC, Health Resources Services Administration (in the Department of Health and Human Services), the Department of Agriculture, and physical fitness or environmental agencies.

Initial legislation in 1975 (PL 94-142) has been modified through **IDEA (Individuals with Disabilities Education Act)** legislation of 1991. Federal legislation (PL 99-457) mandated specific conditions for which care from birth to 21 years of age was mandated. Thirteen conditions that are included in the IDEA (1991) legislation include autism, developmental delay, deafness, hearing impairment, visual impairment, blindness, multiple disabilities, orthopedic impairment, mental retardation, special learning disabilities, serious emotional disturbances, traumatic brain injury, and other health impairments. For summary of federal mandates, see Box 39-1.

Coordination of services and funding are major issues for school health nursing (personal communication, J. Igoe, April 1999). Yet responsibility for student outcomes remains vaguely defined. The CDC (Division of Adolescent and School Health [DASH]) participates in chronic disease prevention through health education.

BOX 39-1 SELECTED FEDERAL MANDATES RELATED TO SCHOOL HEALTH

1973	*Section 504, Rehabilitation Act*
1975	*Education for all Handicapped Children Act (PL 94-142)*
1978	*Health Education Act (PL 95-561)*
1979	*Office of Comprehensive School Health*
1988	*Office of School Health (Health, Education, and Welfare)*
1990	*Birth to Twenty-One legislation (PL 99-457)*
1991	*IDEA (Individuals with Disabilities Education Act)*

School Health Nursing Today

School nurses have always provided nursing services in non-health, non-nursing settings. Client outcomes in school nursing are measured in educational terms (school attendance and test scores) rather than morbidity.

Landmark research conducted during the 1980s by Judith Igoe and colleagues in Colorado highlighted the great potential for impact on school health when adequately prepared school nurses were used in the schools. This federally funded research addressed issues such as shifting student needs, volatile societal expectations, unpredictable legislation, and funding. They even suggested a new paradigm for delivering health services: the school-based clinic. Their work gave a broader context for school health nursing both within and outside the school.

Goals 2000

National Education Goals (1991), written by governors in the Bush administration as a "striking vision for our schools," contains references to health in relation to the education of children. Examples of goals for early childhood include Goal 1, "Every parent will be the child's first teacher," and "All children will start school ready to learn: with proper nutrition and health care."

Other health-related 2000 goals include the following:

* *Goal 1.3: Increase to at least 30% the proportion of people aged 6 and older who engage regularly, or daily, in light to moderate physical activity at least 30 minutes per day.*

* *Goal 1: Every school will be free of drugs, alcohol, and violence.*

* *Goal 2: The nation must reduce its dropout rate; 90% high school completion is a goal.*

Having qualified nurses in schools has been shown to decrease absenteeism (National Health Policy Forum, 1992), an important outcome measure for schools. Absenteeism may be an indication of family problems, lack of resources or medical access, or abuse and neglect.

RESEARCH BRIEF

Swanson, N., & Leonard, B. (1994). Identifying potential dropouts through school health records. Journal of School Nursing, 10(2), 22–26, 46.

Lack of basic health information and lack of routine screening and follow-up of identified problems, in combination with poor attendance, seemed to be strong predictors of students at risk for dropping out of an inner-city high school in the Midwest. The mean number of visits to the health office for those who dropped out of school was less than it was for those who stayed in school ($p = < .001$).

Education's Expectations of the School Nurse

Educators and school administrators measure school success, in large part, on the student's successful completion of each year, and then of the entire K–12 curriculum. Costante (1996) says, "Health-related activities that affect daily attendance are perhaps the hallmark of school nursing services" (p. 5). Teachers find that students who are not distracted by unmet health needs, such as decreased hearing ability, adolescent pregnancy, or emotional distress, are more motivated and attentive in class.

For many years, principals of each school district have viewed the school nurse as their employee (Zimmerman, Wagoner, & Kelly, 1996). Meeting health service needs in an educational setting often poses a dilemma, not because the needs are questioned or the benefits disputed, but because the responsibility and priorities for service are poorly defined.

School administrators have multiple constituents, and practice in a more political arena than nurses often do. Health issues may be surrounded by conflicting values. Administrators face social mores which vary greatly even within the same geographic area, in terms of cultural, religious, and even language differences. One principal stated, "If I make even one parent unhappy, it may cost me my job."

Since "mainstreaming" came to school in 1975, school resources have been stretched to cover special health needs of disabled or chronically ill students. Services to just one child with disabilities in Alabama can run as high as $30,000 to $35,000 per year (*USA Today*, 1999), compared with $15,000 per year to educate a nondisabled child. Efforts to cut their budgets have at times made schools cut nurse positions and replace them with health aides. In a *USA Today* editorial, Ornstein (1997) states, "The disappearance of school nurses leaves a hole in health care. Cost of care can be a deterrent, but costs come in more ways than expenditure of money. Insurance alone will not ensure that children get regular preventive attention that is both sensible and cost effective for the child and society" (p. 15a).

School nursing services, although valued by schools, have not been funded widely by those outside education. However, in 1994, 25 state governments invested $12 million of their Maternal and Child Health block grant dollars and $22.3 million of general fund dollars in school-based health centers, increases of 45% and 140%, respectively, over the preceding 2 years (Making the Grade, 1995, p. 1). Health care reform dialog and new national emphasis on primary care and preventive services have encouraged school administrators who value school nursing services yet must also fund them.

Through NASN (National Association of School Nurses) and establishment of the National School Health/Education Coalition (1991), school nursing is again gaining in professional status and accountability. However, school nurses must still communicate the difference between their clinical judgment, acquired by years of education and experience, and the training for health tasks which secretaries and/or health aides receive. Otherwise, budgetary constraints could continue to cut nursing positions in the school system.

Education and Credentials

Entry-Level Education

The appropriate level of educational preparation for school nurses remains controversial. Passarelli (1994) says that "the level of knowledge, skill, and decision-making demand competencies acquired in a baccalaureate program" (p. 14), and, in time, "master's level preparation will be increasingly needed" (p. 17). A survey of school nurse administrators (Oda, 1993) resulted in disparate answers concerning an essential curriculum for school nurses, but their answers included the usual pediatric content (child growth and development), as well as education law, computer skills, and interdisciplinary team and case management skills. The NASN recommends that courses in special education, the family, community health nursing, and health counseling and education also be included.

Passarelli (1994) proposed that academic institutions design graduate level and practitioner programs that respond to the broad scope of school nursing. An NASN strategic goal for 1994 to 1997 was "to pursue and advocate for greater access to graduate, undergraduate, and practitioner programs by influencing higher education to provide appropriate professional content to a larger school nurse enrollment" (p. 9).

Currently, there are insufficient numbers of educationally prepared nurses, much less practitioners, to meet the needs. "If school-based clinics were to be established for 5% of the 80,000 public schools, this would create an immediate demand for 4,000 Nurse Practitioners" (Passarelli, 1994, p. 16).

Continuing Professional Education

Continuing education offerings specific to school health may be hard to find outside the school system. Literature reviews and professional organizations offer support and continued competence in a changing field of care. Nurses could encourage use of staff development days for their own continuing education.

Continuing professional education is crucial due to a changing societal and political climate, the advances in technology, and the need to update clinical skills. Continuing education related to management, supervision, and delegation are relevant and essential. Topics of specific interest to school nurses include (1) being able to identify the administrator's expectations regarding level of care, (2) allocating time to developing relationships so critical to meeting many client needs, and (3) avoiding the burnout that characterizes the careers of many motivated nurses (IDEA Book). Other topics of interest include (4) health assessment skills, (5) legal issues related to school health, (6) supervision and delegation issues, (7) pharmacology, and (8) political skills.

Credentialing

Every state requires that school nurses have an active nursing license to practice. Some State Departments of Education offer and/or require school nurse certification. Twenty-three of fifty states require specialized readiness for the practice of nursing in schools (Proctor, Lordi, & Zaiger, 1993). Some states require a teaching certificate of the school nurse.

Presently, there is an increased interest in specialization among nurses. Registered nurses may sit for a School Nurse Certification examination through the American Nurses' Credentialing Center (ANCC); there were 155 certified school nurses in 1999. Master's-prepared nurse practitioners can pursue a primary, clinician tract, or a managerial tract. For the primary care role, certification as a School Nurse Practitioner (SNP) is available; in 1998, there were only two nurses who took the School Nurse Practitioner Certification examination (ANCC). However, in 1998, 367 nurses took the Pediatric Nurse Practitioner examination, and 4,669 took the Family Nurse Practitioner examination (ANCC, 1999). School nurse specialists are educationally prepared to evaluate and care for medically fragile children, as well as to provide education services to families of children at risk, and health promotion to all students and staff.

School Health Nursing Practice

The experience of school health officials and school nurses is that health problems exist everywhere, but the nature of these health problems varies by geographic area, economic status, and gender. The National Longitudinal Study of Healthy Adolescents (NLHSA) underscores differences (Blum & Rinehart, 1997) among the 20,000 surveyed teens and families:

- *Of the 49% of high school students who had experienced sexual intercourse, teens living in the south, teens in rural areas, and teens whose parents were on welfare were most likely to be experienced.*

- *Among teens in the northeast, white teens were at greater risk for cigarette and alcohol use, whereas teens on welfare were at greater risk for marijuana use.*

- *Rural welfare recipient teens were at greater risk for emotional distress than urban or suburban teens.*

- *Substance use and abuse were reported to be a greater problem for teens living in the suburbs than for urban youths, according to this study (1997).*

It is therefore difficult to proscribe one set of health promotion guidelines for all school nurses and school districts in the United States.

Healthy People 2010

Although no single plan of action can be applied to all schools, a body of problems common to school-aged and adolescent youth has been identified in *Healthy People 2010* (DHHS, 2000). These common problems include health problems or communicable disease, sensory screening, injury prevention, sexual activity, mental health, substance abuse, violence, and school dropout. School-based clinics have been shown to be effective primary care providers of services to school children and youth, families, and their communities (Igoe & Giordano, 1992). School-based and school-linked clinics are providing such services in a number of states (National Health Policy Forum, 1992). In addition, school nurses participate in screening of dental, vision, hearing, and growth and development status.

Unintended injuries from motor vehicle accidents, and falls or drowning account for 40% of deaths among 5- to 24-year-olds (DASH, 1999). The 1997 Youth Risk Behavior Surveillance System (YRBSS) data showed that 20% of students (and 31.3% of African American students) have rarely or never worn seat belts as passengers. In the preceding 30 days, 37% of students had ridden with a driver who had been drinking alcohol.

Health education is one strategy to meet the *Healthy People 2010* goals. Many school nurses work with teachers, coaches, or the health educator (if there is one) to plan educa-

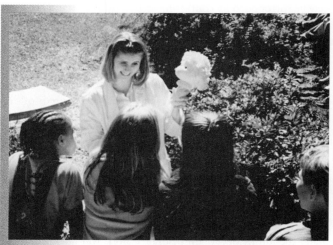

School nurses use creativity in teaching children about good health choices.

HEALTHY PEOPLE 2010

OBJECTIVES RELATED TO SCHOOL HEALTH

Disability and Secondary Conditions

6.9 Increase the proportion of children and youth with disabilities who spend at least 80% of their time in regular education programs.

Educational and Community-Based Programs

School Setting

7.1 Increase high school completion.

7.2 Increase the proportion of middle, junior high, and senior high schools that provide comprehensive school health education to prevent health problems in the following areas: violence; suicide; tobacco use and addiction, alcohol and other drug use; unintended pregnancy; HIV/AIDS and STD infection; unhealthy dietary patterns; inadequate physical activity; and environmental health.

7.3 Increase the proportion of college and university students who receive information from their institution on each of the six priority health-risk behavior areas.

7.4 Increase the proportion of the nation's elementary, middle, junior high, and senior high schools that have a nurse-to-student ratio of at least 1:750.

Injury and Violence Prevention

Unintentional Injury Prevention

15.31 Increase the proportion of public and private schools that require use of appropriate head, face, eye, and mouth protection for students participating in school-sponsored physical activities.

Violence and Abuse Prevention

15.39 Reduce weapon carrying by adolescents on school property.

Physical Activity and Fitness

Physical Activity in Children and Adolescents

22.8 Increase the proportion of the nation's public and private schools that require daily physical education for all students.

22.9 Increase the proportion of adolescents who participate in daily school physical education.

Tobacco Use

Exposure to Secondhand Smoke

27.11 Increase smoke-free and tobacco-free environments in schools, including all school facilities, property, vehicles, and school events.

Source: DHHS, 2000.

---

tional programs. The CDC reports a 37% reduction in onset of smoking among seventh grade students in one program (1999). However, coordinated health education is not the norm; and some risk behaviors have worsened from 1991 to 1997: tobacco use is up (from 27.5% to 36.4%), and marijuana use is up (from 14.7% to 26.2%). Peer pressure has significant impact on youth behavior: The data show that when teenagers band together on prevention issues such as not drinking and driving, lifestyles are modified much more successfully than with a course on driving sober.

School nurses can assist in bettering these numbers through health education. High school students have been surveyed a number of times regarding health topics of interest to them. These consistently include acne, sex education, depression, obesity, or getting along with parents. Role-playing is a useful tool for interpersonal relationship building.

Every year, approximately 3 million adolescents become infected with an STD, and almost a million become pregnant (CDC, 1999). Between 1991 and 1997, a drop in current sexual activity (from 37.5% to 34.8%) was reported.

Exercise, fitness activities, and good nutrition clearly affect physical and mental health of children. Yet daily participation in high school physical education classes dropped from 42% in 1991 to 27% in 1997. Almost three-fourths of young people do not eat the recommended number of servings of fruits and vegetables (CDC, 1999).

School nurses are often called upon when child abuse is suspected. They have a great challenge and opportunity to assist families in addressing this problem. Home visits are best for assessment of parent-child relations (in the student's natural environment, rather than at a teacher conference).

Role Definition

A yet-unresolved issue in school health service delivery is the ambiguity of school nursing practice. "School nursing is at once the best and least understood form of practice on the part of the lay public and nursing professionals," wrote Oda in 1979. This is still largely true.

Igoe (1990) coined the term *boundary dwellers* to describe school nurses. For some school nurses, there commonly is a perceived competition between two priorities: health and education. What may be prudent healthwise (doing physical exams or screening routines) may at times be disruptive because class time is lost.

Role confusion, which characterizes school nursing, is being addressed by the National Association of School Nurses (NASN). The school nurse role is often defined for nurses by school administrators, and others, who may not clearly understand the nursing role. The Roles and Standards for School Nursing Practice (1983) are intended to guide school nurses, who typically practice alone in an educational setting.

The NASN (1993) illustrates comprehensive school nursing practice as spokes in a role "umbrella" (see the following figure).

Provider of Health Care

Screening for communicable diseases (e.g., lice, fever) and for developmental disorders (e.g., deficits in vision, hearing; scoliosis; emotional distress) is a large component of nursing practice. Immunization surveillance is another important duty. Adequate clinical knowledge is critical and requires frequent updating. The scope of clinical knowledge required ranges from wellness to developmental delay and other special needs of children and their families.

Some states write guidelines specific to their school nurse needs. One such publication is the *Communicable Diseases/Conditions and Return to School Guidelines* (1998), prepared by the Division of Epidemiology/Office of Community Health Services, Mississippi State Department of Health.

SCHOOL NURSING ROLES.
....

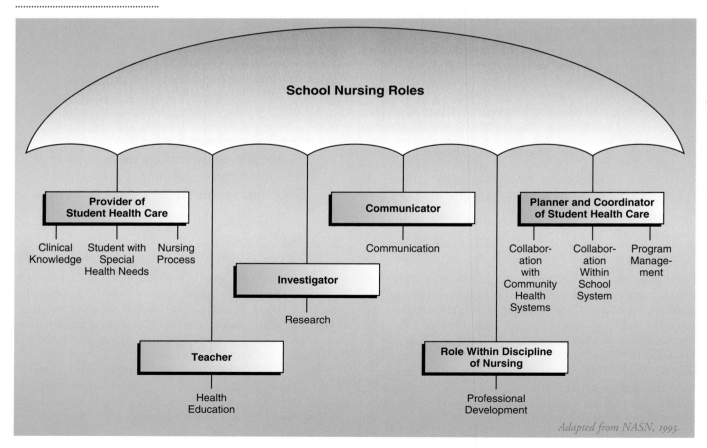

Adapted from NASN, 1993.

TABLE 39-1	HEALTH SERVICES PROVIDED IN SCHOOLS

TYPE OF SERVICE	% DISTRICTS OFFERING
Administration of first aid	98.7
Administration of medication	97.1
Screens (height/weight, sensory)	86.8
Abuse evaluation/follow-up	82.8
Emotional/behaviors	80.0
Monitoring of vital signs	77.7
Cleaning/changing of dressings	76.8
Health component of IEP	75.6
Case management	58.1
Nutritional counseling	57.5
Mental health counseling	56.2
Cardiovascular screenings	49.6
Complex nursing to at-risk students	49.6
Employee wellness	48.6
Fitness screenings	45.2
Urinary catheterizations	40.2
Health risk appraisals	35.7

Source: A Closer Look, *1995.*

Nurses can provide health services for school staff. Educational personnel often have chronic, stable medical conditions. School nurses are concerned for the health of the bus driver and the cafeteria worker as well as the health of teachers and students.

Familiarity with theory can guide decision making by the school nurse. Besides nursing theory, such theories include change theory, developmental theory, management theory, role theory, and systems theory. School nurses, like all other nurses, use the nursing process as the framework for all assessment, diagnosis, planning, intervention, and evaluation activities. A partial list of school health services is provided in Table 39-1.

Communicator

The following parent's story illustrates the importance of communication with parents:

> I was adamant that our daughter would have at least one setting where she was treated as a "typical" kid. Because she has spina bifida, we see a lot of specialists. I wanted her child care program to be a place where we could escape the disability focus. So when the program director asked me to sign an information request form so she could get a copy of Karen's records, I refused. I wanted the child care staff to treat Karen just like all the other children.
>
> A few months later, Karen's teacher again asked if I would be willing to share information from the IFSP (Individualized Family Service Plan). She explained that it would help her develop better lesson plans if she knew more about what Karen could do, and the skills we were working on. It was the first time I realized that Karen's special needs could be incorpo-

rated into the games and activities that happened in her school day. A little reluctant, I gave my permission.

> Now, I wish that at the very beginning, the Director had explained why it was important for them to have the IFSP and other information. You can't blame a parent for wanting to protect their child's (and their own) privacy. I remember being offended when asked to release Karen's records, and I am sure other parents feel that way (Notes from Home, 1997, p. 7).

Health, welfare, and social services for students are often complex, fragmented, or even unavailable. Good written and verbal communication skills are needed in order for the school nurse to work efficiently with the learners (students), teachers, parents, and the medical community.

School nurses who can identify problems and recommend solutions in terms that evoke policy responses are desperately needed. To date, this fourth component of school health (policy development) is lagging behind the other three. Communicating the problems, as well as the positive contributions that school nurses make to the school's mission, is an important part of nursing activities, often directly affecting funding for school nurse positions.

Student health has been shown to have "peace dividends" (intangible, but real, rewards), but cost containment is a byword of current policy activities. A long-term investment in health makes sense; but immediate needs with potential for quick success may receive greater attention from policy makers. Unless the school nurse's voice is heard loud and clear, policies may not reflect school health as a priority.

Many school nurses provide health education inside and outside the classroom, with individuals, with groups, and with families. Good communication skills help get important messages across to the children, school staff, and the community.

Planner and Coordinator of Student Health Care

Case management is a demanding component of school health services. Children with complex health problems may require home visits and referrals to medical services or resource agencies such as the Health Department. One individual responsible to coordinate this activity is the school nurse.

The school nurse must be self-motivated, organized and flexible, while performing multiple activities. Many times, the school nurse is assessing rapidly changing situations, planning with teachers for addressing behavioral and emotional problems, evaluating the student and sometimes the family, or coordinating care with a physician. School nurses must also be ready to deal with unforeseen events (e.g., emergencies) in the midst of everything else.

Monitoring school health through record keeping and tracking is a part of coordinating services. The area of sexual health is often an area of discomfort in terms of documentation. A sensitive school nurse "will have her finger on the pulse of the school and be sensitive to school politics" (Proctor & Lordi, 1993, p. 58).

Teacher

School nurses serve as teachers to students as well as to school staff, to parents as well as to community agencies. Staff consultation regarding individual students is a major component of the school nurse activity (Anderson, 1994). Teachers and staff are open to assistance with behavioral problems, conflict resolution, and student performance in general. School nurses may also be asked to provide training on how to render first aid or handle emergency situations (e.g., injuries, fighting).

Students with disabilities and their parents may need individualized education provided by the school nurse. However, it is not only the chronically ill or at-risk students who need the teaching role of the nurse; all students benefit by receiving specific health-related information about nutrition, maintaining a safe environment, and proper rest and exercise.

Investigator

Currently, there are very little meaningful data on school health nursing services. In the past, outcome parameters have included (1) number of teen pregnancies, (2) degree of substance abuse, (3) school attendance, and (4) dropout rates.

School nurses collect data from health records, home visits, and teacher conferences. These data have been used to demonstrate improved school performance in a child receiving glasses following a vision screening, for example.

School nurses may note an increased number of obese children during a weight screening. The school nurse may recommend, then implement, a weight-management intervention for such an aggregate group, often in conjunction with nutrition and physical fitness school personnel.

School health records maintained by school nurses were used by Swanson and Leonard (1994) to provide (with 85% accuracy) an estimate of actual dropout rates. Students who dropped out of school used school health services less than those who did not drop out and who received follow-up on identified health problems. Capturing the cost-benefit data of health services validates the benefits of having qualified nurses to provide such services. Studies that demonstrate the need for programs, or the impact of school nurses on absenteeism, for example, speak to educational leaders.

Utilization of the school as a research site is on the rise (Puskar, Weaver, & DeBlassio, 1994). A national survey to identify nursing interventions used in school settings (Cavendish, Lunney, Luise, & Richardson, 1999) found that there were 60 core interventions with school children. These interventions covered a wide range of nursing diagnoses. Their research supports the need for consistent language to document school nurse activities.

Role Within the Profession

The school nurse is a member of a profession now seriously committed to looking at school health. The American Nurses Association has established a Nursing Center for School Health, in

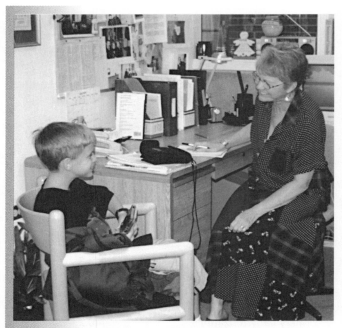

School nurse seeing student in office.

collaboration with the National Nursing Coalition for School Health. In 1990, more than 50 organizations participated to form the National Health and Education Consortium (NHEC), which was formed to bridge the health and education fields (Passarelli, 1994). NHEC conducts research and develops policy to promote the education of children.

Even in systems employing more than one nurse, school nurses often work alone. Remaining an active member of the profession is important for the professional development of school nurses. "Obsolescence and isolation are therefore ever-present dangers; thus the necessity of involvement in professional school nurse organizations and for continuing education becomes most important" (NASN Standards 10, p. 55).

At-Risk Populations

The **medically fragile child** is a child with chronic illnesses, one who is dependent on technology, or one with developmental delays. Because of advancing medical technologies that have allowed tiny premature infants or children born to mothers with conditions such as AIDS, fetal alcohol syndrome, or substance abuse to survive, increasing numbers of medically fragile children are attending school across the country. In fact, 10% to 15% of school-aged children within the United States have a chronic health problem; 10% of these are complex and severe illnesses such as asthma, abuse or neglect, leukemia, hemophilia, mobility problems, and seizure disorders (Passarelli, 1994). Poverty may influence a child's ability to learn. When compounded with a chronic illness, these children constitute an at-risk population. The school nurse is involved in both the health needs of the child and the training of teachers and staff who care for this student.

Health-related services is a term used to describe distinct needs of medically fragile students: the child with tracheostomy equipment needs extra physical space, as will a child in a wheelchair. Other children may require medication administration for asthma, seizures, diabetes mellitus, ADHD, hemophilia, or other chronic illnesses such as HIV. Children using inhalers and oxygen may be common in regular classrooms.

At times, children in schools may need technology (e.g., catheters, respirators, gastrostomies) for survival. School personnel may be asked to perform tasks such as suctioning children with tracheostomies, providing parenteral nutrition in gastrostomies, and performing catheterization. Medication administration and emergency measures are often required as well.

An **individualized educational plan (IEP)** is written for at-risk students in regular classrooms. The IEP is an educational plan tailored to each child's unique needs to assist each child in meeting educational needs. IEPs may be written for exceptionally bright, as well as at-risk, children.

Individualized health care plans (IHPs) are plans of care used in the educational setting to identify, communicate, and document an individual student's health care needs. IHPs are the health-related component of the IEP. IHPs are based on the nursing process and are required by law to be written by a health team (Grabeel, 1996). Each child's IHP contains medical data, as well as plans for medication administration and emergency care (e.g., bee stings or anaphylaxis). Emergency care plans for IHPs must be written by a nurse. Emergency care plans anticipate injuries on the school grounds, exacerbation of chronic disease, and needed resources for health care.

The IHP is equivalent to the nursing care plan but is often implemented by non-nurses. The IHP is used along with the IEP to plan educational goals and activities.

For the medically fragile child, a multidisciplinary team writes an IHP. The school nurse is part of this team, which may consist of administrator, teachers, a local physician, social worker, speech pathologist, nutritionist, or occupational/physical therapists, and parents.

The composition of the team is determined by district administration. An educational coordinator is responsible for the child's assessment, training, and monitoring. Input from parents or guardians is critical for optimal educational placement.

Case Finding

Early intervention programs to identify children from birth to 3 years of age who have disabilities may utilize schools to conduct screening. Input from primary physicians becomes part of the **individualized family service plan (IFSP)**. The IFSP is designed to assist in fostering the optimal development of children with disabilities from birth to 3 years of age.

All school personnel assist with identification of children and youth at risk for physical, emotional, or educational problems. The school nurse has a health perspective that can supplement the observations of teachers and staff, but teachers play a crucial role in assessing student health needs. Observation of children in the hallway, in the lunchroom, or on the playground provides teachers and school nurses with tips on physical, nutritional, or emotional needs.

Planned screening by the school nurse for developmental progress or vision, hearing, and dental screening are also important components in case finding. Review of attendance records is another form of case finding. Students who miss more than 10 days of school may need a home visit and/or family assessment, because high-risk families sometimes are unable to manage the tasks of getting their students off to school.

When a physician identifies a special need, referral to the school system may be less efficient. Hospital discharge planning may not include consideration of school needs. It may take months between the time a need is identified, the school is notified, and the child is actually enrolled in the school. This is particularly true for children experiencing the life changes that occur from a motor vehicle accident or other major trauma events. A school nurse is a key contact for health care providers in the community.

Collaboration with the community health care providers requires case management, which begins with identifying the child's health care needs. The school nurse has all parents complete an emergency information card that includes the name of child's health care provider (if any), as well as where the parent can usually be found during the day. If a student needs referral to a health care provider, parental permission is required to discuss the case with the provider.

Good documentation of the reason for referral, and requests for feedback, improve coordination of care with key contacts in the medical community. Some school nurses produce a newsletter with the goal of keeping community resource persons informed about school health.

Nurse as Team Member

A model of nursing services proposed by the School Nurse Organization of Minnesota (SNOM) captures the complexity of school nursing. Nursing services to children from birth to 21 years include case management, health assessment, disease-prevention activities, nursing care, policy development, and health promotion. In addition to this load, many school nurses collaborate with managed care organizations or private providers and with public health agencies.

Roles are fluid. Collaboration is the key to building an effective team. Schools operate under three levels of rules and regulations, as well as under parental and business community expectations (Bridging the Gap, 1992). Educators often feel they are "under siege" just to educate.

The entire school community is the school nurse's client. School nurses work with families, with access health services, and with the environment in which learning activities occur. The health of the greater community is important to school nurses. Issues of concern to school nurses are similar to those of public

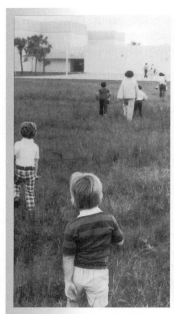
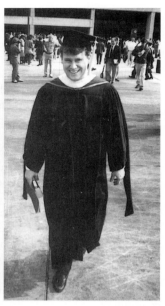

School health is important from entry into kindergarten through college graduation.

health nurses. Bachman (1995) says that "as the school nurse role expands to accommodate the multiple needs of a diverse client population, a wide variety of collaborative practitioners is essential to the school setting" (p. 22).

Practice Issues

School nursing practice involves well children as well as the chronically ill child. Certain physical morbidities (e.g., childhood diseases, blindness) have steadily decreased as a result of immunization programs, vision and hearing screening, and nutritional improvement. Other morbidities have increased as very tiny infants now survive into childhood, and the severely injured child may go to school despite the disabilities.

"Social" morbidities are also on the rise. Schools feel the effects that social conditions place on their children, problems such as poverty, single parenthood, homelessness, and child abuse. Day care needs and the problems for children who are latch-key kids are often encountered by working parents. "Substance-abusing students, pregnant and parenting teens, and chronically ill students may not be able to progress as expected, or to graduate, without assistance from a school health

SCHOOL NURSING SERVICES IN THE GREATER SCHOOL COMMUNITY.

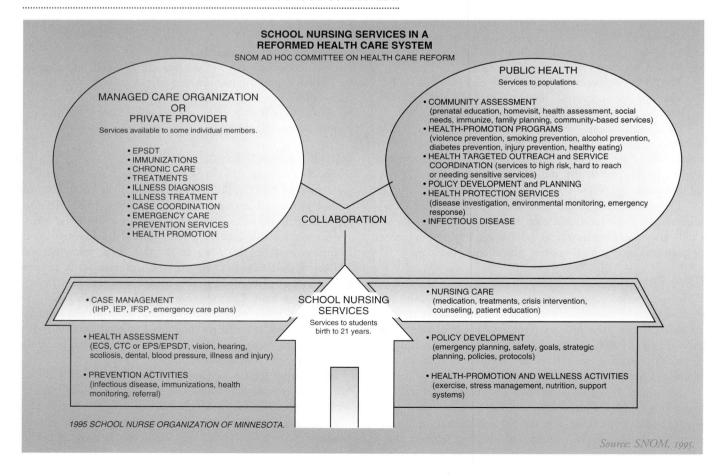

SCHOOL NURSING SERVICES IN A
REFORMED HEALTH CARE SYSTEM
SNOM AD HOC COMMITTEE ON HEALTH CARE REFORM

**MANAGED CARE ORGANIZATION
OR
PRIVATE PROVIDER**
Services available to some individual members.

- EPSDT
- IMMUNIZATIONS
- CHRONIC CARE
- TREATMENTS
- ILLNESS DIAGNOSIS
- ILLNESS TREATMENT
- CASE COORDINATION
- EMERGENCY CARE
- PREVENTION SERVICES
- HEALTH PROMOTION

PUBLIC HEALTH
Services to populations.

- COMMUNITY ASSESSMENT
  (prenatal education, homevisit, health assessment, social needs, immunize, family planning, community-based services)
- HEALTH-PROMOTION PROGRAMS
  (violence prevention, smoking prevention, alcohol prevention, diabetes prevention, injury prevention, healthy eating)
- HEALTH TARGETED OUTREACH and SERVICE COORDINATION (services to high risk, hard to reach or needing sensitive services)
- POLICY DEVELOPMENT and PLANNING
- HEALTH PROTECTION SERVICES
  (disease investigation, environmental monitoring, emergency response)
- INFECTIOUS DISEASE

COLLABORATION

SCHOOL NURSING SERVICES
Services to students birth to 21 years.

- CASE MANAGEMENT
  (IHP, IEP, IFSP, emergency care plans)
- HEALTH ASSESSMENT
  (ECS, CTC or EPS/EPSDT, vision, hearing, scoliosis, dental, blood pressure, illness and injury)
- PREVENTION ACTIVITIES
  (infectious disease, immunizations, health monitoring, referral)

- NURSING CARE
  (medication, treatments, crisis intervention, counseling, patient education)
- POLICY DEVELOPMENT
  (emergency planning, safety, goals, strategic planning, policies, protocols)
- HEALTH-PROMOTION AND WELLNESS ACTIVITIES
  (exercise, stress management, nutrition, support systems)

1995 SCHOOL NURSE ORGANIZATION OF MINNESOTA.

Source: SNOM, 1995.

professional. Many disabled students cannot attend school without nursing support" (Costante,1996, p. 4).

Legal-Ethical Considerations

Legal issues abound in school nursing. Laws provide guidance in the areas of medication administration, student confidentiality and parental consent, delegation, documentation, supervision of unlicensed personnel, child abuse and neglect, and malpractice issues.

Each school nurse practices under that state's Nurse Practice Act. In addition, there are many state and federal laws designed to protect the rights of children. These laws affect the nature of health care services that can be provided for school children. Such laws vary greatly from state to state. School health services may be mandated in some states, but only recommended in others. A few states have no policy on school health. School nurses must be familiar with the laws in their state, because these laws are foundational in development of school health programs and the provision of school health services.

School districts should have health policies that follow state and federal guidelines, especially when dealing with medical emergencies when a parent or guardian is not available to give consent. Parental consent is usually required for health services to children. These services include health screening for psychological or learning disabilities, administration of medication or immunization, medical treatments, and human sexuality or drug education classes.

Medication administration is a common legal concern. Often, children need medications, particularly for seizures, asthma, ADHD, or otitis media. School personnel may be leery about taking on the responsibility for medication administration but may be asked to administer these in the absence of the school nurse. They have a right to be concerned (Gelfman & Schwab, 1991). School administrators, faculty, and staff are becoming more aware of the legal liability of medication administration.

Nursing practice standards apply to documentation, even though the nurse works in an educational setting (Proctor, Lordi, & Zaiger, 1993). In any type of documentation, it is important that the nurse demonstrate use of the nursing process. Schools themselves may also have documentation requirements, which vary from school to school. Many school districts carry liability insurance on school nurses. However, school nurses should carry their own liability insurance as well (NASN, 1992).

Examples of ethical dilemmas include "the right of a school district to cut staff which include care-givers for severely disabled students, versus the child's right to safe, adequate and competent care; the refusal of a school district to implement DNR (do not resuscitate) orders for a medically-fragile child, versus the right of parents as guardians to forego extraordinary procedures to prolong life; the right of the school to exclude a child with chronic head lice, versus the need of the child to return to school for so-cial and educational reasons. Advance directives (e.g., DNR orders) raise serious ethical concerns for parents or guardians of a medically fragile child, as well as for teachers and other school personnel (Grant, Cureton, & Yahiro, 1998). Although any group of school nurses could list ethical concerns in school nursing, little discussion centers around this arena (Proctor, 1998).

Confidentiality is another legal-ethical issue in school health. School-aged children may have STDs, be medically neglected, or be abused. Sexuality, mental health, and substance abuse commonly involve ethical decisions. All school personnel must know the law regarding reporting of neglect or suspected abuse in minors; they look to the school nurse for direction.

Confidentiality of information may be breached, as in lunchroom conversations between staff and volunteers, for example. Confidentiality of medical records is of concern to parents as well as nurses and staff. School health records are protected by the Family Education Rights and Privacy Act (FERPA) of 1974, which gives parents the right to review and appeal records about their child and prohibits release of student records without authorization.

Documentation

Documentation (also called *charting* in acute care settings) is the only solid evidence that the nursing process was applied and the standard of care was met. Although malpractice suits against school nurses are rare, increasing complexity of care and public expectations of health care providers may increase legal exposure without adequate documentation. Most courts associate inadequate documentation with inadequate health care or no care. Lack of documentation may also indicate that the nurse did not use the appropriate assessment, intervention, or evaluation techniques in giving care.

In the past, student health documentation took three major forms: (1) information kept on cards (including immunization data, vision and hearing screening, and other examinations mandated by the law); (2) daily logs, or records of visits to the health office; or (3) more detailed medical records for chronically ill students. Presently, computer programs are designed for school health documentation. These programs help control access according to security clearance given to the person logging on to the system. These computerized records could decrease legal risks associated with handwritten documentation.

Delegation

Delegation is a legal issue in that it involves transferring authority to perform a selected nursing task to a competent, unlicensed individual in selected situations (NCSBN, 1990). Delegation is also "the transfer of responsibility for the performance of an activity from one individual to another while retaining accountability for the outcome" (ANA, 1992).

Delegation of nursing activities may only be done as prescribed by state law (Panettieri & Schwab, 1996). In an attempt to address shared concerns regarding liability and training needs, the American Federation of Teachers (AFL-CIO) issued a resource manual in 1992 for teachers and paraprofessionals. AFL-CIO supports the role of nurses as staff trainers, in addition to supervisors of complex medical care. The manual seeks to answer questions such as "Who should be providing health care in schools?" and "Who should be supervising this care?" The AFL-CIO views school nurses as key players in school health, who contribute to the creation of healthy environments in which students can learn (Novello, DeGraw, & Kleinman, 1992).

The NASN recommends that the school nurse to pupil ratio be 1:750. In 1995–1996, Southeastern United States data show the ratio of school nurses to pupils averages 1:3,190 students (Clemen, 1997). Many school district administrators who do not have the adequate ratio of school nurses to students may delegate or assign health-related activities to faculty and staff. Teachers, teachers assistants, secretaries, and others are often assigned duties such as medication administration, first aid, or notification of parents when a child becomes ill. These staff members are also called *unlicensed personnel* (working with, or in the absence of, the school nurse). The school nurse must know state and federal law before agreeing to accept responsibility for these staff members' actions.

An **unlicensed assistive person** (also variously called a *health para-professional* or *health aide*) is an individual who is trained to function as an assistant to the licensed registered nurse in the provision of client care activities as delegated by the nurse (NCSBN, 1990). These individuals have had specific training by a nurse regarding tasks delegated to them, such as catheterizing, suctioning, or gastrostomy feedings.

A curriculum for basic training of school health para-professionals is available from the School Health Resources Services Project ASSIST. Other training aids related to medication administration or specified medical procedures are available from the NASN, and occasionally from state nurses' associations. Reference books (Agins, 1997) and video training programs (Learner Managed Designs, Inc.) are also available.

Supervision and Accountability

Supervision issues arise daily. Some school nurses practice alone in their school settings and may be accountable to the school administration. Others work out of school health units in Public Health Departments. The nurse must be able to determine and articulate which decisions regarding health care rest with school administration and which rest with nurse practice laws. There is sometimes a fine line required of the school nurse.

Accountability involves meeting deadlines, following through with commitments, and providing competent nursing care. The

FYI

More than 52 million children attend schools in the United States. It is estimated that 10% to 20% have chronic, social, emotional, and/or health problems.

Source: National center at ANF addresses school nurse issues, American Nurse, May/June, 1998, p. 7.

CASE STUDY

Teachers Challenge Ruling on Medical Procedure

Teachers at the Burkett Center for the Multi-handicapped in Birmingham, Alabama, appealed a state ruling that forces them to perform medical procedures on their students. They argued that because they must handle complicated medical procedures for students in their classrooms, they were violating state nursing codes. They were also concerned that their liability insurance would not cover them if something went wrong. Among the procedures the teachers were required to perform were catheterization, tube feeding, suctioning, and certain blood tests.

The circuit court judge ruled that while they were in college they should have known they would have to perform medical procedures at work. He also said that the state nursing code exempts the "gratuitous nursing for the sick by friends or members of the family" and that due to the close nature of teacher and student work, the teachers are friends. The president of the county Federation of Teachers points out that if teachers are "friends" of the students, why do they have to get written permission to do such things as take them on field trips? If teachers are "friends," why are they paid employees? "Our teachers want to educate rather than medicate."

Source: Teachers Challenge Ruling on Medical Procedure, 1993.

nurse is always accountable to follow mandates of the state nurse practice act. School nurses are also bound by local school board policies for students and staff. Being accountable involves risks. School nurses should request and welcome performance evaluations from peers.

Funding

Funding needs are dependent on a multitude of variables and cannot be assumed to be equal across regions. Nurse staffing and funding should be based on student and program needs, not on enrollment numbers. Common factors influencing funding needs may include socioeconomic variations, the number of special need students, the complexity of the families and diversity of cultural needs, the number of sites being served by each nurse, and the distance between schools. School nurses are in an excellent position to conduct a student-faculty needs assessment to determine the needs of their individual district.

There must be adequate pay to keep nurses (and other providers) in the workplace where they are needed. One of the greatest challenges facing school nurses today is to be creative in finding sources of funding to carry out their missions. According to the National School Boards Association, special education expenditures nationwide rose from $11.8 billion in 1982 to $32 billion by 1994. Initially, the federal government promised to pay 40% of the cost of special education (1991) but as of 1993–1994 was only paying 7.1%. State and local governments have had to pick up the rest. Managed care and soaring health care costs require justification of all health expenditures.

Creative fee structures have been used, including managed care (Igoe & Giordano, 1992), business-school partnerships (Bishop, 1991), and Medicaid (NASSNC, 1993). SNOM has proposed that local school districts become direct providers of medically delegated functions for student who have an IEP in place and who are eligible for funding under Medical Assistance. In addition to obtaining funds for students with special needs, SNOM has assisted local school districts to access federal funds for immunizations, Mantoux testing, and for Early Periodic Screening and Developmental Testing (EPSDT) (SNOM, 1995). Chauvin and Davis (1994) reported an EPSDT model for funding preventive services in schools.

Typical sources of funding for school-based programs serving indigent children (IDEA Book, 1996) were (1) federal grants (usually Public Health Service Act sections 329, 330, or 340); (2) state block grants, especially for maternal-child health; (3) local government funds; (4) grants from national or local foundations or local hospitals; and (5) Medicaid reimbursement (primarily EPSDT).

Large businesses often contract out ("outsource") their employee health to agencies better equipped to provide them. This gives responsibility and leadership for the service to persons best prepared to provide them. Contracting out of school health services may be an option for departments of education. Naturally, such services would also report to the principal and the board of education. School nurses and the public health department are well prepared to provide school health services to students as well as to staff and families.

Business involvement in school health services has been used to assist with funding of comprehensive health services. The "Cities in Schools" model is one example of a program developed to connect appropriate human services with youth at risk for dropping out of school. A hospital on the Mississippi Gulf Coast has helped schools set up six school-based, nurse-run clinics to provide health services (Clemen, 1997).

School Violence

Violence in schools has sent ripples through the nation, as when two young men opened fire in 1998 on children obeying a fire alarm (killing five persons) in a Jonesboro, Arkansas, school; or in 1997, when school shootings resulted in deaths in Paducah, Kentucky, and Pearl, Mississippi. The death of 15 persons at the hand of two high school students in Littleton, Colorado, in 1999 has created greater community outcry for a solution to this problem. Violence is a challenge to all school personnel and their communities.

••••••••••••••••••••••••••

A clinician specializing in children would not have difficulty finding the kinds of mental and emotional disturbances present in a child preparing to murder. The masks of children are very transparent, though understandably not to busy or untrained parents and teachers who are emotionally invested in not seeing problems in the children they care for.
                    Peter Loffredo, *New York Times,* March 26, 1998
                    An editorial after the Jonesboro shooting

••••••••••••••••••••••••••

Community Issues
School-Linked Health Services

School-based services are services delivered on the school grounds. *School-linked services,* on the other hand, may be delivered across the street or across town and are initiated by school personnel. The definition of eligible services varies greatly from state to state. The school-based clinic offers primary care to students, their families, and school personnel. All the aforementioned are considered *school-health linkages.*

In some communities, there are persons who believe that schools should provide only education, while health and social agencies should provide health and social services. Parental involvement and community linkages are crucial for success in each local school-health linkage. Unless the community is involved in planning and supporting the services, one single component of the program, such as birth control education, can derail an entire program.

Collaboration

The trend toward delivery of health care in a community setting amounts to a paradigm shift for providers and consumers alike. Service through collaboration will become the norm, not the exception. The 1993 State Adolescent Health Coordinators Conference underlined the need for collaboration as a strategy for fostering healthy children. Parents, teachers, health care providers, mental health services, social workers, and physical fitness and nutrition agencies all have vested interest in the health of children.

Interdisciplinary practice is a term used in academia, but seldom do students practice with other disciplines before graduation. Thus, after graduation, interdisciplinary practice is seldom implemented. It will increasingly be required. Education majors, particularly those going into educational administration, may welcome interdisciplinary practice with schools of nursing preparing school nurses. Partnerships are no longer a wonderful idea, but an idea whose time has definitely come.

Resources

The School Health Resource Services (SHRS), from the Office of School Health, University of Colorado Health Sciences Center, provides a school health reference collection. Timely updates, linkages with programs already in operation in schools and communities across the United States, "starter kits" for specific topics in school health, information links with other projects, and bibliographic services for drawing together educational and health databases are available.

Innovations

Expanding technology, changing disease trajectories, and increased accountability for client outcomes contribute to the need for visionary innovations for school health services. Policy makers report that poor health and poor health utilization is exacerbated by a number of system factors: inadequate number of public health providers, inaccessible hours of operation, and fragmented delivery of care (Schlitt, 1991). For young people needing care, lack of transportation, lack of information, and lack of money are formidable access issues. School-based clinics have helped meet these needs (Passarelli, 1994). One teacher explained the benefit to children and families of their school-based clinic:

> A lot of our kids are here without shots, without the appropriate care that they need because their parents can't reach the services - they don't have transportation or the motivation of getting up and going across town. Whereas at the school, the teachers can make sure the kids get the services. If health care providers can't get the kids to the health centers, then bring the health centers to the kids (IDEA Book, 1996, p. 4).

School-Based Clinics and Primary Care

Because children spend a lot of time in schools and many of them need health care that they are not receiving, the concept of a clinic offering primary care with proximity to the school has

been adopted by many states. *Primary care* includes preventive services (e.g., immunization, physicals) and management of minor injury or chronic illness.

The school-based clinic (SBC) movement began in the late 1960s in west Dallas. Staffed with nurse practitioners, part-time physicians, and social workers, the SBC provided primary care. Funding was separate from the education budget, and included both private and public funds (Urbinati, Steele, Harter, & Harrell, 1996). The movement has grown and gained acceptance as a means to address access to care issues.

••••••••••••••••••••••••••••••

Health services need to be where students can trip over them. Adolescents do not carry an appointment book, and school is the only place they're required to spend their time.
P. Porter, Medical Director for School-Based Adolescent Health Care Program, Robert Wood Johnson Foundation.

••••••••••••••••••••••••••••••

In the past 25 years, changes have taken place surrounding access to care: a change in focus and a change in setting. There is an increasing emphasis on primary prevention and wellness (rather than a focus on illness cure) and a shift to the community, doctor's office, or home (rather than the hospital) for provision of health care.

Key reasons for promoting SBCs are accessibility, availability, and appropriateness of services to the school population (Passarelli, 1992). "Schools are a natural locus for community-based family health care," say Igoe and Giordano (1992). "Aggressive health education programs may decrease consumer passivity . . . by placing more responsibility on the individual. The

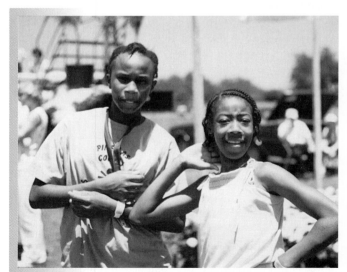

Playground safety is a constant health concern in schools.

need for quality, affordable health programs in or near schools is evident" (p. 18).

There are currently more than 500 SBCs in elementary, middle, and high schools in the United States (GAO, 1995), and the number is growing. School-based primary care to technologically dependent students promotes seamless and nonduplicated health services to a very needy population.

School nurse practitioners do not replace the school nurses. However, some school nurses have concerns about their role when a school-based clinic is operative at their school. Nurse practitioners knowledgeable about chronic illness in children have a valuable role in SBCs. Main issues of concern to school nurses are (1) that clinic staff will take on all the nurse's responsibilities and (2) that there will be confusion among students and staff over the different roles. At one site, the concerns became a grievance (IDEA Book, 1996, p. 49). Clinic nurses covered by the community health center's liability insurance were legally able to provide more services than school nurses, and school nurses were worried about their own liability.

Four decades of research regarding alternatives to the traditional model of health care delivery have shown the value of community-based health care, using qualified personnel. Witness the rise in home health care, industrial nursing, and school health services. School-based or school-linked clinics are an obvious school-health linkage.

SBCs may be portable in some geographic areas. For other communities, access to care might mean mobile clinics, like the old bookmobiles that went where the kids were. In rural states, physicians and nurse practitioners may schedule travel to provide predictable in-school opportunities for checkups and immunizations (particularly for preschool).

. . . .

You have brains in your head.
You have feet in your shoes.
You can steer yourself
Any direction you choose.

Dr. Seuss

. . . .

Increased Role of the Media

The print media is an untapped source for developing school-health linkages and for advertising school health nursing. The media is looking for news to provide to the public: newsletters, data from successful programs like the CDC's "Closer Look," coverage of regional meetings, and family training centers. School nurses should step up and speak out! Television programming can be very effective in portraying health providers at work (as in the show *ER*). School health professionals should receive training in using this resource.

Technology

Information technology is becoming critical to group work, data management, and research. In a 1998 survey of computer technology in school nursing, Smith, Cureton, Hooper, and Deamer found a strong desire among school nurses for more access to computers as a means for record maintenance, access, and information retrieval. The surveyed nurses indicated the need for preservice education and continued funding for computer knowledge.

Various automated and other formats have been proposed to facilitate the large amount of record keeping that constitutes a school nurse's activities (Sedlacek & Bergren, 1993). Given sufficient precautions, computerized record keeping may alleviate many of the concerns regarding paper: document loss, breach of confidentiality, or failure to provide access to information needed by various school personnel.

Examples of computerized resources include the following:

- *Dyn-o-mite/dyn-o-log*
- *Snap-log: school nurses assistance program*
- *Patient Medical Records, INC (uses SOAP format)*
- *The School Nurse's Source Book on Individualized Healthcare Plans (Excel)*
- *Drug Guide on-line*
- *School Healthcare—ON:LINE!! From Medical and Educational Software, Inc.*
- *Web links to sites for medical professionals, such as www.cdc.gov and www.usinternet.com/users/bergren*
- *Healthmaster (Sedlacek & Bergren, 1993, p. 8)*

Increased telecommunication facilities are an innovation for education as well as for practice. Net linkages with students in the classroom may provide diagnosis, therapy, and health education. The emphasis is on assisting the learner, by whatever method.

CONCLUSION

This chapter has highlighted the historical journey of school nursing and education. School districts face overwhelming constraints and competing demands. They need the invaluable assistance of school nurses to help them meet their agendas of improving test scores and literacy, as well as overall health. A flow of research questions and answers is a vision for school health nursing in the 21st century.

Significant factors that influence public and private schools as well as school nursing include the following:

- *Societal and cultural context of school health nursing*
- *Federal mandates*
- *Educational preparation of school nurses and SNPs*

- *At-risk children in school*
- *Legal-ethical considerations*
- *School violence*
- *School-based health centers for primary care*
- *Increased role of the media*
- *Technology*

A paradigm shift is required of both providers and consumers: Nursing is not just for the acute care setting, but also for the community. Far-reaching media and exploding technology could help change the public perception of school nursing in the next millennium.

CRITICAL THINKING ACTIVITIES

1. Juan, a 10-year-old boy, has spina bifida and hydrocephalus. As a result, he has limited bowel function, wears a brace for severe curvature of the spine, and uses a wheelchair for mobility. In addition, Juan has only one kidney and wears a urine collection bag under his clothing. This appliance requires frequent emptying during the school day. He takes several medications to prevent infection and promote waste elimination. Juan lives in a single-parent family with his mother and two brothers. His extended family of aunts, uncles, and cousins is 200 miles away in another state. As a community health nurse, discuss four health outcomes that you and his family would plan for Juan's care. Give the rationale for each one.

2. Danielle, a 15-year-old student, recently learned that she is 3 months' pregnant. When she informed her mother, Danielle was "thrown out" of the house and is now staying with her 28-year-old boyfriend. Danielle has been absent from school four times in the last 2 weeks. Select nursing interventions at the primary, secondary, and tertiary levels for Danielle. Include holistic interventions.

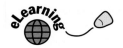 Explore Community Health Nursing on the web! To learn more about the topics in this chapter, use the passcode provided to access your exclusive web site: http://communitynursing.jbpub.com
If you do not have a passcode, you can obtain one at this site.

Distance learning technology is available for continuing education and should be seized as a means to meet a critical need for continuing education of school nurses. The Internet is increasingly a source of information and assistance.

REFERENCES

A closer look: A report of selected findings from the National School Health Survey, 1993–94. (1995). Office of School Health, University of Colorado Health Sciences Center.

Agins, A. (1997). *Teachers' drug reference: A guide to medical conditions and drugs commonly used in school-aged children.* Technomic Publishing.

Anderson, J. (1994). The changing role of school nurses: one state's experience. *Journal of School Nursing, 10*(3), 22–26.

Annie E. Casey Foundation. (1999). *1999 KIDS COUNT.* Baltimore: Annie E. Casey Foundation.

Bachman, B. (1995). A University's response to a need for school nurse education. *Journal of School Nursing, 11*(3), 20–23.

Bishop, S. (1991). Creating partnership: A hospital-based newsletter for teachers. *Journal of School Health, 61*(8), 361–362.

Blum, R., & Rinehart, P. (1997). *Reducing the risk: Connections that make a difference in the lives of youth.* Minneapolis: Division of General Pediatrics and Adolescent Health, University of Minnesota.

Boyer, E. (1991). *Ready to learn: A mandate for the nation.* The Carnegie Foundation, Princeton University Press.

Bridging the gap: Education primer for health professionals. (1992). National Health/Education Consortium.

Cavendish, R., Lunney, M., Luise, B., & Richardson, K. (1999). National survey to identify the nursing interventions used in school settings. *Journal of School Nursing, 15*(2), 14–21.

Centers for Disease Control and Prevention (CDC). (1997). *Youth risk behavior surveillance system.* Atlanta: U.S. Government Printing Office.

Chauvin, V., & Davis, C. (1994). EPSDT model training program. *Journal of School Nursing, 10*(2), 6–9.

Clemen, P. (1997). Status of school health services in Mississippi: Executive summary. *The HPER Journal, 14*(2), 19–21.

Costante, C. (1996). Supporting student success: School nurses make a difference. *Journal of School Nursing, 12*(3), 4–6.

Department of Health and Human Services (DHHS). (2000). *Healthy People 2010: Conference Edition.* Washington, DC: U.S. Government Printing Office.

Gelfman, M. & Schwab, N. (1991). School Health services and educational records: Conflicts in the law. *West's Education Law Reporter, 64*(2), 319–338.

Grabeel, J. (1996). Nursing practice management: IHPs revisited. *Journal of School Nursing, 12* (4), 28–29.

Grant, L., Cureton, V., & Yahiro, M. (1998). Advance directives and do not resuscitate orders: Nurses' knowledge and the level of practice in school settings. *Journal of School Nursing, 14*(2), 4–13.

Idea Book. (1996). *Linking community health centers with school serving low-income children.* Washington, DC: Health Resources and Services Administration.

Igoe, J. (1990). School nursing and school health. In J. Natapoff & R. Wieczorek (Eds), *Maternal-child policy: A nursing perspective* (pp. 153–188). New York: Springer

Igoe, J. (1980). What is school nursing? A plea for more standardized roles. *MCN, 5*, 307–311.

Igoe, J., & Campos, E. (1991). Report of a national survey of school nurse supervisors. *School Nurse, 7*(2), 8–10, 12, 14, 16, 18–20.

Igoe, J., & Giordano, B. (1992). *Expanding school health services to serve families in the 21ˢᵗ century.* Washington, DC: American Nurses Publishing.

Making the Grade National Program Office. (1995). The George Washington University.

National Association of State School Nurse Consultants (NASSNC). (1993). Medicaid reimbursement school nursing services. *Journal of School Nursing, 9*(3), 37–39.

National Council of State Boards of Nursing (NCSBN). (1990). *Delegation: Concepts and decision-making process.* Chicago, IL: Author.

National Health Policy Forum. (1992). *Creating a vision for child health: School-based clinics confront access, training, coordination and funding issues* (Issue Brief No. 598) (pp. 1–12). Roundtable discussion at George Washington University, Washington, DC.

New faces at school: How changing demographics reshape American education. (1991). *Education of the Handicapped, 17*(16 Supplement), 1–4.

Notes from home: Parents want to know why. (1997). *Child Care Plus, 7*(2).

Novello, A., DeGraw, C., & Kleinman, D. (1992). Healthy children ready to learn: An essential collaboration between health and education. *Public Health Reports, 107,* 3–15.

Oda, D. (1979). School nursing: Current observations and future projections. *Journal of School Health, 49,* 437–439.

Oda, D. (1981). A viewpoint on school nursing. *American Journal of Nursing, 9,* 674–678.

Oda, D. (1993). Nurse administrators' views of professional preparation in school nursing. *Journal of School Health, 63,* 229–231.

Ornstein, N. (1997, September 16). Editorial. *USA Today,* p. 15A.

Passarelli, C. (1992). Case management of chronic health conditions of school-aged youth. In H. Wallace, K. Patrick, G. Parcel, & J. Igoe (Eds.), *Principles and practices of student health: vol. 2, School Health* (pp. 350–359). Oakland, CA: Third Party Publishing.

Passarelli, C. (1994). School nursing: Trends for the future. *Journal of School Nursing, 10*(2), 10–21.

Passarelli, C. (1996). School nursing services: Exploring national issues and priorities. *Journal of School Nursing, 12*(3), 24–36.

Panettieri, M., & Schwab, N. (1996). Delegation and supervision in school settings: Standards, Issues and guidelines for practice (Part 2). *Journal of School Nursing, 12*(2), 19–26.

Pollitt, P. (1994). Lina Rogers Struthers: The first school nurse. *Journal of School Nursing, 10*(1), 34–36.

Proctor, S. (1998). School nurses and ethical dilemmas: Are schools short on ethics? *Journal of School Nursing, 14*(2), 3.

Proctor, S., Lordi, S., & Zaiger, D. (1993). *School nursing practice: Roles and standards of school nursing practice.* Scarborough, ME: National Association of School Nurses.

Puskar, K., Weaver, P., & DeBlassio, K. (1994). Nursing research in a school setting. *Journal of School Nursing, 10*(4), 8–14.

Resnick, M., Bearman, P. S., Blum, P. S., Blum, R. W., Bauman, K. E., Harris, K. M., Jones, J., Tabor, J., Beuhring T, Sieving R., E., Shew, M., Ireland M., Bearinger, L. H., & Udry, J. R. (1997). Protecting adolescents from harm: Findings from the National Longitudinal Study on Adolescent Health. *Journal of the American Medical Association, 278*(10), 823–832.

Schlitt, J. (1991). *Bringing health to school: Policy implications for southern states.* Southern Legislative Conference, Governors' Association.

School Nurse Organization of Minnesota (SNOM). (1995). *Role for school nursing: A vision statement.* Ad Hoc Task Force on Health Care Reform.

Schwab, N., & Haas, M. (1995). Delegation and supervision in school settings: Standards, Issues and guidelines for practice. Part 1. *Journal of School Nursing, 11*(1), 26–35.

Sedlacek, K., & Bergren, M. (1993). Computer use in the health office. *Journal of School Nursing, 9*(2), 6–8.

Smith, C., Cureton, V., Hooper, C., & Deamer, P. (1998). A survey of computer technology utilization school nursing. *Journal of School Nursing, 14*(2), 27–34.

Swanson, N., & Leonard, B. (1994). Identifying potential dropouts through school health records. *Journal of School Nursing, 10*(2), 22–26, 46.

Urbinati. D., Steele, P., Harter, B., & Harrell, D. (1996). The evolution of the School NP: Past, present, and future. *Journal of School Nursing, 12*(2), 6–9.

Zimmerman, B., Wagoner, E., & Kelly, L. (1996). A study of role ambiguity and role strain among school nurses. *Journal of School Nursing, 12*(4), 12–18.

Chapter 40
Occupational Health Nursing
Bonnie Rogers

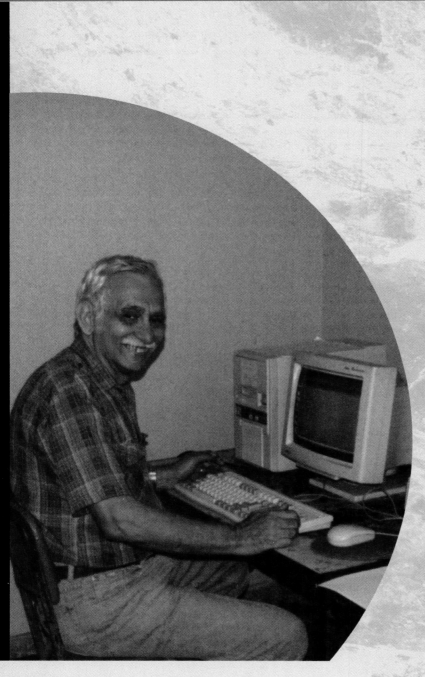

It is neither wealth nor splendor but tranquility and occupation which gives happiness.

Thomas Jefferson

QUESTIONS TO CONSIDER

After reading this chapter, answer the following questions:

1. What is occupational health nursing, and how does it relate to community health?
2. Why has the practice of occupational health nursing changed so dramatically over time?
3. What are the work and workplace hazards that result in illness, injury, and loss of life to the worker?
4. How have these hazards changed over the years, and what is the role of the occupational health nurse in dealing with work related illness and injuries?
5. What are the major laws governing occupational safety and health, and how have they impacted the workers and the role of the occupational health nurse?
6. What are the five models for worksite primary health care management in occupational health care?
7. How can the goal to provide quality, accessible, and cost-effective care be reached?
8. What is the critical link between occupational health nursing and environmental health?
9. Why will the occupational health nurses need additional competencies in environmental health in the coming years and what "competencies" will be needed?

KEY TERMS

American Association of Occupational Health Nurses

Ergonomics

National Institute of Occupational Safety and Health (NIOSH)

Occupational health nurse case manager

Occupational health nurse clinician

Occupational health nurse consultant

Occupational health nurse coordinator

Occupational health nurse corporate director

Occupational health nurse educator

Occupational health nurse health promotion specialist

Occupational health nurse manager

Occupational health nurse practitioner

Occupational health nurse researcher

Occupational health nursing

Occupational Safety and Health Act of 1970

Worker/workplace surveillance

TABLE 40-1   **CIVILIAN LABOR FORCE, UNITED STATES, BY INDUSTRY**

INDUSTRY	WORKFORCE SIZE (IN MILLIONS)
Agriculture	3.1
Mining	0.7
Construction	7.2
Manufacturing	19.6
Transportation and public utilities	8.5
Wholesale and retail trade	24.8
Finance, insurance, real estate	8.0
Services	41.8
Public administration	5.8
TOTAL	119.3*

Because of rounding, the sum of the components does not add up to the total. Source: Bureau of Labor Statistics, U.S. Department of Labor, 1994.

Work is generally considered one of life's worthwhile and exciting experiences. Most adults spend approximately one-fourth to one-third of their time at work, which becomes an integral part of their life. Work can be viewed as a source of strength helping people build lives and communities. Americans work in a wide range of industries and jobs, which are displayed in Tables 40-1 and 40-2.

TABLE 40-2   **LABOR FORCE BY JOB**

OCCUPATIONAL CATEGORY	NUMBER OF WORKERS (IN MILLIONS)
Executive, administrative, and managerial workers	15.4
Professional workers	16.9
Technicians and related support workers	4.0
Sales workers	14.2
Administrative support workers, including clerical workers	18.6
Precision production, craft, and repair workers	13.3
Operators, fabricators, and laborers	17.0
Service workers	16.5
Farming, forestry, and fishing industry workers	3.3
TOTAL	119.3*

Because of rounding, the sum of the components does not add up to the total. Source: Bureau of Labor Statistics, U.S. Department of Labor, 1994.

BOX 40-1   **CATEGORIES OF WORK-RELATED HAZARDS**

Biological/infectious hazards: *infectious/biological agents, such as bacteria, viruses, fungi, or parasites, that may be transmitted via contact with infected clients or contaminated body secretions/fluids to other individuals*

Chemical hazards: *various forms of chemicals, including medications, solutions, gases, vapors, aerosols, and particulate matter, that are potentially toxic or irritating to the body system*

Environmental/mechanical hazards: *factors encountered in the work environment that cause or potentiate accidents, injuries, strain, or discomfort (e.g., unsafe/inadequate equipment or lifting devices, slippery floors, work station deficiencies)*

Physical hazards: *agents within the work environment, such as radiation, electricity, extreme temperatures, and noise, that can cause tissue trauma*

Psychosocial hazards: *factors and situations encountered or associated with one's job or work environment that create or potentiate stress, emotional strain, and/or interpersonal problems*

Source: Rogers, 1994.

Although most workers may never face any serious adverse health effects from workplace exposures, all types of work have hazards (Box 40-1). These hazards can have short- and long-term health consequences, and every effort must be made to prevent and control work-related illness and injury. Thus, the necessity to provide occupational health and safety services to prevent and manage occupational health illness and injuries is paramount in this mission. This chapter provides an overview of the practice of occupational health nursing, with emphasis on the scope of practice. Examples of work-related illnesses and injuries and a discussion of governmental and professional influences are also provided.

History of Occupational Health Nursing

Occupational health nursing, then called *industrial nursing,* began in the latter half of the 19th century in Norwich, England, when Phillipa Fowerday was hired by the J. & J. Coleman Company in 1878. Her work in the mustard company was primarily to work in the dispensary and provide home care services to employees and their families (Godfrey, 1978). Although the company provided acute and tertiary care services for employees, the belief was that preventive care was better than cure in terms of healthy and quality living. Nurses were soon employed by other companies to provide health care services for employees who became ill and injured at work as well as health education services related to sanitation and hygiene, particularly given the high rates of tuberculosis at the time (Slaney, 1984).

In the United States, industrial or occupational health nursing, as it is now called, began in the late 19th century. In 1888, it is reported that a group of Pennsylvania coal mining companies hired Betty Moulder, a graduate of Philadelphia Blockley Hospital School of Nursing, to provide nursing care for ill and injured workers and their families (AAIN, 1976; McGrath, 1945; Wright, 1919). However, little more is known about her or the services she provided. In 1895, Ada Mayo Stewart, who is often credited as being the first industrial nurse, was hired by the Vermont Marble Company. She had previously worked as a district nurse in several cities. During her tenure, she visited sick employees in their homes, provided emergency care, taught healthy living habits, taught mothers about child care, and gave speeches on health and hygiene to school children. In this era, there was much ethnic diversity, and Ada Stewart incorporated cultural customs and methods of caring for the sick and their families into her practice. She was later joined by a second nurse, her sister Harriet, who provided health care to employees in the west and central sections of the state (Felton, 1985; Rogers, 1994).

In the early 1900s, industrial health services proliferated rapidly across the country as it became apparent that nursing care related to worksite health issues could have a positive impact on productivity, could decrease illness and injury, and could reduce absenteeism. Working conditions in many factories were harsh and unrelenting, as the industrial ethic often placed the importance of profit above human rights. This type of ethic was not supported by the public, and the advent of worker's compensation (discussed later) came to being.

In 1913, the first organized effort in American industrial nursing began in New England with the establishment of the first industrial nurse registry and the formation of the New England Industrial Nurses' Association in 1918. In 1917, Boston University's College of Business Administration offered the first specialty education course for industrial nurses that focused on industrial health issues and economics. This was followed in the 1920s by several colleges and universities offering short courses in industrial hygiene in which industrial nurses participated (Godfrey, 1978). The advent of World War II in the 1940s supported industrial growth and the concomitant demand for nursing services, with a reported 4,000 nurses employed in industrial health (Brown, 1981). With a viable group of nurses in need of professional support, the American Association of Industrial Nurses (AAIN) was created in 1942, with Catherine Dempsey as the first president. The purposes of AAIN were to improve industrial nursing practice, provide education, and increase interdisciplinary work (AAIN, 1976).

In the 1960s and 1970s, occupational health and safety became a public issue, with particular concern focused on mining accidents, cave-ins, and black lung disease, as well as the need for professional education and hiring in several disciplines. As a result, several laws were enacted to protect the health and safety of workers (e.g., Federal Coal Mine Safety and Health Act, 1969; Toxic Substances Control Act, 1976). The **Occupational Safety and Health** (OSH) **Act of 1970** was the first comprehensive law promulgated to ensure safe and healthful working conditions.

As the occupational health nurse's scope of practice broadened considerably, AAIN changed its name to the **American Association of Occupational Health Nurses** in 1977, with a current membership of approximately 13,000 occupational health nurses. The 1980s brought more role expansion into health promotion, management, policy development, research, and entrepreneurism. Several standards were promulgated to protect workers from unwarranted exposures (e.g., Hazard Communication Standard, 1983), and in 1988, the Occupational Safety and Health Administration (OSHA) hired the first occupational health nurse consultant to provide technical assistance in standards development, field consultation, and occupational health nursing expertise. In 1993, the Office of Occupational Health Nursing was established within the agency.

In 1990, AAOHN published its first occupational health nursing research priorities, updated in 1999, which provide the direction for occupational health nursing research (Box 40-2) (AAOHN, 1999; Rogers, Agnew, & Pompeii, 1999).

The priorities will be used to target grant funding by AAOHN for occupational health nursing research. In 1996, the first National Occupational Research Agenda (NORA) was developed, spearheaded by **National Institute of Occupational Safety and Health** (NIOSH) in partnership with more than 500 groups and individuals. NORA has identified 21 research priorities for occupational health and safety for which its funding is targeted. NORA priorities (CDC, 1999) are listed in Box 40-3.

Definition

In today's work environment, the delivery and management of occupational health services and programs is provided primarily by occupational and environmental health nurses. Collaboration with and referral to related occupational health and safety disciplines to resolve occupational health problems are essential to the practice. By definition, occupational and environmental health nursing is the specialty practice that focuses on the promotion, prevention, and restoration of health within the context of a safe and healthy environment. It includes the prevention of adverse health effects from occupational and environmental hazards. It provides for and delivers occupational and environmental health and safety services to workers, worker populations, and community groups. Occupational and environmental health nursing is an autonomous specialty, and nurses make independent nursing judgments in providing health care services (AAOHN, 1999).

BOX 40-2 RESEARCH PRIORITIES IN OCCUPATIONAL HEALTH NURSING

1. Effectiveness of primary health care delivery at the worksite
2. Effectiveness of health-promotion nursing intervention strategies
3. Methods for handling complex ethical issues related to occupational health
4. Strategies that minimize work-related adverse health outcomes (e.g., respiratory disease)
5. Health effects resulting from chemical exposures in the workplace
6. Occupational hazards of health care workers (e.g., latex allergy, blood-borne pathogens)
7. Factors that influence workers rehabilitation and return to work
8. Effectiveness of ergonomic strategies to reduce worker injury and illness
9. Effectiveness of case management approaches in occupational illness/injury
10. Evaluation of critical pathways to effectively improve worker health and safety and to enhance maximum recovery and safe return to work
11. Effects of shift work on worker health and safety
12. Strategies for increasing compliance with or motivating workers to use personal protective equipment

BOX 40-3 NATIONAL OCCUPATIONAL RESEARCH AGENDA PRIORITY RESEARCH AREAS

CATEGORY	AREAS
Disease and injury	Allergic and irritant dermatitis
	Asthma and chronic obstructive pulmonary disease
	Fertility and pregnancy abnormalities
	Hearing loss
	Infectious diseases
	Low back disorders
	Musculoskeletal disorders of upper extremities
	Traumatic injuries
Work environment and workforce	Indoor environment
	Mixed exposures
	Emerging technologies
	Organization of work
	Special populations at risk
Research tools and approaches	Cancer research methods
	Control technology and personal protective equipment
	Surveillance research methods
	Exposure assessment methods
	Risk assessment methods research
	Intervention effectiveness research
	Health services research
	Social and economic consequences of workplace illness and injury

Source: CDC, 1999.

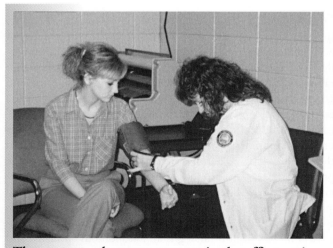

The nurse conducts assessments in the office setting.

Work and Workplace Hazards

Workers are exposed to many workplace hazards that result in illness and injury. There are about 138 million workers in the United States (Bureau of Labor Statistics, 1999). Each day, an average of 137 individuals die from work-related diseases, and an additional 16 die from injuries on the job. Every 5 seconds, a worker is in-

TABLE 40-3	NONFATAL OCCUPATIONAL INJURY INCIDENCE RATES IN THE UNITED STATES BY INDUSTRY, PRIVATE SECTOR

WORK-RELATED NONFATAL INJURIES (PER 100 FULL-TIME WORKERS)	
Construction	12.9
Agriculture	11.0
Manufacturing	10.8
Transportation/public utilities	8.8
Wholesale/retail trade	8.2
Mining	7.0
Services	6.8
Finance, insurance, realty	2.7
AVERAGE	8.3

Source: Bureau of Labor Statistics, U.S. Department of Labor, 1993.

TABLE 40-4	NEW CASES OF REPORTED OCCUPATIONAL ILLNESS IN THE UNITED STATES, BY CATEGORY OF ILLNESS, PRIVATE SECTOR

CATEGORY OF ILLNESS	NUMBER*	PERCENTAGE
Disorders associated with repeated trauma	459,300	61
Skin diseases or disorders	120,800	16
Disorders caused by physical agents	37,400	5
Respiratory conditions caused by toxic agents	36,900	5
Poisoning	13,400	2
Dust diseases of the lung	4,800	1
All other occupational illnesses	759,400	100

*Excludes farms with fewer than 11 employees.
Source: Bureau of Labor Statistics, U.S. Department of Labor, 1993.

jured; every 10 seconds, a worker is temporarily or permanently disabled. NIOSH estimates that at least 10 million injuries occur on the job each year, approximately 3 million of which are severe, and every workday more than 10,000 people sustain injuries that result in lost work time. Table 40-3 shows the highest work-related injuries by specific industry. In 1994, occupational injuries alone cost $121 billion in lost wages and productivity, administrative expenses, health care, and other costs. This figure does not include the cost of occupational illnesses.

Construction has the highest injury rate in the private sector compared with the whole (12.9 versus 8.3 per 100 workers). Lumber and wood products manufacturing have more worker injuries than other goods producers, and trucking and warehousing have the highest injury rates in the service sector. Mining injuries, including those involving oil and gas exploration, declined in the mid-1980s but remain high. Nearly half of the 170,000 disabling farm injuries each year result in permanent impairment, costing an estimated $2.5 billion in hospital and rehabilitation expenses. Reports of injuries among nursing home workers and other personal caregivers have increased, with back injuries accounting for more than 40% of these reports. An estimated 2.4 million eye injuries occur in the workplace each year, resulting from exposure to chemical, radiation, physical, and biological sources, with more than 60% of workers who experience

FYI

Back injuries are the most prevalent and most costly injury in the occupation of nursing.

eye injuries not wearing eye protection at the time of injury (Bureau of Labor Statistics, 1995).

Illnesses are much more difficult to capture because of the often long latency period between initial workplace exposure and disease occurrence and the lack of recognition on the part of the clinician that the disease manifestations are work related. Thus, the relative incidence and prevalence of occupational illness may be grossly underreported. What this means is that diseases such as skin disorders, which may be more easily recognized, are more likely to be reported (Table 40-4) and treated.

This may give a misleading representation of both the magnitude and severity of work-related illness. Let's examine the eight groups of occupational diseases/injuries as targeted in the NORA priorities (DHHS, 1996).

Allergic and Irritant Dermatitis

In the workplace, the skin is an important route of exposure to chemicals and other contaminants. According to the U.S. Bureau of Labor Statistics, occupational skin diseases—mostly in the form of allergic and irritant (contact) dermatitis—are the second most common type of occupational disease. From 1983 to 1994, the rate of occupational skin diseases increased from 64 to 81 cases per 100,000 workers. In 1994, approximately 66,000 cases of occupational skin diseases were reported, accounting for approximately 13% of all occupational disease. Moreover, occupational skin diseases are believed to be severely underreported, such that the true rate of new cases may be many-fold higher than documented. Estimated total annual costs, including lost workdays and loss of productivity associated with occupational skin diseases, may reach $1 billion annually. Workers' compensation claim rates for occupational skin diseases vary by state and range from 12 to 108 per 100,000 workers per year. Self-reported occupational dermatitis prevalence in the 1988 National Health Interview Survey was nearly 2% (1,700 cases per 100,000 workers).

Irritant contact dermatitis is the most common occupational skin disease, usually resulting from toxic reactions to chemical irritants such as solvents and cutting fluids. Allergic dermatitis is estimated to constitute approximately 20% to 24% of all contact dermatitis; it is caused by a wide variety of substances such as latex and some pesticides that trigger an allergic (delayed hypersensitivity) reaction. Contact urticaria (hives occurring soon after an allergen or irritant contacts the skin) is considered here also because it may evolve into contact dermatitis. A number of substances may cause both irritant and allergic dermatitis as well as contact urticaria. For example, latex, which has been reported to cause skin disorders in up to 10% of exposed health care workers, most commonly causes irritant dermatitis; however, it also results in allergic contact dermatitis and, least commonly, contact urticaria.

Because the prognosis of occupational irritant and allergic dermatitis is poor, prevention is imperative. Clients with occupational contact dermatitis often develop chronic skin disease. With thousands of potentially harmful chemicals being introduced into the workplace each year and with the threat of rapidly emerging skin diseases such as latex allergy, interventions need to be developed to reduce irritant and allergic contact dermatitis.

Asthma and Chronic Obstructive Pulmonary Disease

Asthma and chronic obstructive pulmonary disease (COPD—primarily chronic bronchitis and emphysema) are diseases of the lung airways. More than 20 million U.S. workers are potentially exposed to occupational agents capable of causing these diseases, including nearly 9 million workers occupationally exposed to known sensitizers such as toluene diisocyanate CTDI, a major ingredient in polyurethane manufacture, and irritants, such as ammonia, used in the manufacture of dyes, chemicals, plastics, and explosives (Levy & Wegman, 1995). Occupational asthma is now the most common occupational respiratory disease diagnosis among clients examined in occupational medicine clinics.

Asthma and COPD accounted for nearly 18 million physician visits in 1985 and an estimated 800,000 hospital admissions in 1987. In 1992, asthma and COPD caused nearly 92,000 deaths in the United States, making airway diseases the fourth leading cause of death overall. Mortality from asthma and COPD is increasing annually. Estimated yearly costs for occupational asthma are approximately $400 million. NIOSH reports that asthma currently affects more than 10 million individuals in the United States and is increasing in prevalence. Recent evidence suggests that as many as 28% of adult asthma cases may

be attributable to work settings. In addition to those who develop occupational asthma as a result of workplace exposure to sensitizers or irritants, many workers are unaware that preexisting asthma may be worsened by the work environment. Each year, the number of asthma cases is increasing, and major new problem areas are emerging. For example, as a result of increased use of protective gloves, due to the introduction of universal precautions and the OSHA regulations on blood-borne pathogens, latex allergies have become a major problem for health care workers. A significant number of these workers (2.5% in one study) have developed latex-related asthma.

Morbidity from occupational asthma is preventable. Early diagnosis holds substantial promise for effective intervention. Complete resolution of symptoms and pulmonary function abnormalities is most likely when an affected individual's exposure is terminated early in the course of the illness, so early diagnosis holds substantial promise for effective intervention.

The relationship of COPD to workplace exposures is also well documented in studies of several occupational agents (e.g., coal dust, grain dust, cotton dust). Investigations of the health consequences of particulate exposure in the general environment, where exposures are at a far lower level than in the workplace, also suggest that COPD resulting from generally dusty conditions may be an important cause of preventable disease and death. Those with lung disease from other causes are especially vulnerable to occupational respiratory hazards. Although cigarettes remain the primary cause of pulmonary diseases in the United States, many occupational and environmental exposures, both by themselves or in combination with smoking, are known to cause COPD. One estimate of the proportion of COPD attributable to occupational exposure in the general population is 14%.

Fertility and Pregnancy Abnormalities

Disorders of reproduction include birth defects, developmental disorders, spontaneous abortion, low birth weight, preterm birth, and various other disorders affecting offspring; they also include reduced fertility, impotence, and menstrual disorders. Infertility is currently estimated to affect more than 2 million American couples. One in twelve couples finds themselves unable to conceive after 1 year of unprotected intercourse. Although not all infertile couples seek treatment, it is estimated that approximately $1 billion was spent in 1987 on health care related to infertility. In 1991, physician visits for infertility services numbered 1.7 million. Although numerous occupational exposures have been demonstrated to impair fertility (e.g., lead, some pesticides, solvents), the overall contribution of occupational exposures to male and female infertility is unknown. Moreover, observed global trends in men's decreasing sperm counts have increased concerns about the role of chemicals encountered at work and in the environment at large.

Birth defects are the leading cause of infant mortality in the United States, accounting for 20% of infant deaths (more than

8,000) each year. Every year, approximately 120,000 babies are born in the United States with a major birth defect—about 3 per 100 live births. The 1992 costs for 17 of the most clinically important structural birth defects and for cerebral palsy were estimated to be approximately $8 billion. Neural tube defects, which include spina bifida and anencephaly, affect 4,000 pregnancies each year, with each new case of spina bifida having a discounted lifetime cost of $294,000 (1992 dollars). Of all children in the United States, 17% have some type of developmental disability. The major developmental disabilities of mental retardation, cerebral palsy, hearing impairment, and vision impairment affect approximately 2% of all school-age children.

Most birth defects and developmental disabilities are of unknown cause. The overall contribution of workplace exposures to reproductive disorders and congenital abnormalities is not known. Although some specific reproductive hazards have been identified in humans, most of the more than 1,000 workplace chemicals that have shown abnormal reproductive effects in animals have not been studied in humans. In addition, most of the 4 million other chemical mixtures in commercial use remain untested. Substances and activities that upset the normal hormonal activity of the reproductive system (e.g., shift work or pesticides that possess estrogenic activity) also need evaluation. Similarly, the effects of physical factors such as prolonged standing, reaching or lifting, or the interactive effects of workplace stressors and exposures on pregnancy and fertility have not been rigorously investigated.

Although the total number of workers potentially exposed to reproductive hazards is difficult to estimate, three-fourths of employed women and an even greater proportion of employed men are of reproductive age. More than half of U.S. children are born to working mothers. The vast number of workers of reproductive age together with the substantial number of workplace chemical, physical, and biological agents suggest that a considerable number of workers are potentially at risk for adverse reproductive outcomes.

Although the causes of reproductive disorders and adverse pregnancy outcomes are poorly defined, lost productivity and deep suffering by affected individuals and families are evident. The contribution that may be made by occupational factors is largely unexplored, because the reproductive health of workers has only recently emerged as a serious focus of scientific investigation. Identifying reproductive hazards in the workplace has the potential for significantly reducing the multibillion-dollar costs and alleviating the personal suffering associated with disorders of reproduction.

Hearing Loss

Occupational hearing loss is the most common occupational disease in the United States. It is so common that it is often accepted as a normal consequence of employment. More than 30 million workers are exposed to hazardous noise, and an additional 9 million are at risk from other ototraumatic agents. Occupational hearing loss knows no boundaries with respect to industries. Any worker, young or old, male or female, risks hearing loss when exposed to ototraumatic agents. Once the loss is acquired, it is irreversible.

Although noise-induced occupational hearing loss is the most common occupational disease and is the second most commonly self-reported occupational illness or injury, it has not been possible to create a sense of urgency about this problem. Efforts to prevent occupational hearing loss have been hindered because the problem is insidious and occurs without pain or obvious physical abnormalities in affected workers.

Problems created by occupational hearing loss include (1) reduced quality of life because of social isolation and unrelenting tinnitus (ringing in the ears); (2) impaired communication with family members, the public, and co-workers; (3) diminished ability to monitor the work environment (e.g., warning signals, equipment sounds); (4) lost productivity and increased accidents resulting from impaired communication and isolation; and (5) expenses for workers' compensation and hearing aids.

Infectious Diseases

Infections acquired in the work setting are diverse, with many different modes of transmission. Of particular concern are infectious diseases transmitted by humans (e.g., from client to worker, from worker to worker) in a variety or work settings. Blood-borne and airborne pathogens represent a significant class of exposures for the 6 million U.S. health care workers. Occupational transmission of blood-borne pathogens (including hepatitis B and C viruses and the human immunodeficiency virus [HIV]) occurs primarily by means of needlestick injuries but also through exposures to the eyes or mucous membranes. The risk of hepatitis B virus infection following a single needlestick injury with a contaminated needle varies from 2% to more than 40%, depending on the antigen status of the source individual. Similarly, the risk of hepatitis C virus transmission also depends on the status of the source and ranges from 3.3% to 10%. Before widespread use of hepatitis B virus vaccine, approximately 8,700 acute cases of hepatitis B virus infection were reported among health care workers each year. Although the incidence of occupational hepatitis C virus infection among these workers is unknown, antibody to hepatitis C virus (evidence of previous infection) is found in 1% of hospital-based health care workers.

Transmission of tuberculosis (TB) within health care settings, especially multidrug-resistant TB, has re-emerged as a major public health problem. Since 1989, outbreaks of this type of TB have been reported in 14 hospitals, and at least 17 workers have developed active drug-resistant TB. In addition, among workers of health care, social service, and corrections facilities who work with populations at increased risk of TB, hundreds have experienced tuberculin skin test conversions. Reliable data are lacking on the extent of possible work-related TB transmission among other groups of workers at risk for exposure. Some cases of influenza and other communicable respiratory infections are surely the result of exposure to infected persons at work. These are not generally considered occupational diseases, and the proportion acquired at work from co-workers, customers, clients, and the general public is unknown. The cost of lost work time and decreased productivity is likely to be substantial.

Low Back Disorders

Low back pain is one of the oldest and most common occupational health problems reported. Approximately 80% of workers will experience low back pain sometime during their active working life, and 11% of Americans report reduced functional ability. In 1993, back disorders accounted for 27% of all nonfatal occupational injuries and illnesses involving days away from work in the United States. The economic costs of low back disorders are staggering. In a recent study, the average cost of a workers' compensation claim for a low back disorder was $8,300, which was more than twice the average cost of $4,075 for all compensable claims combined. Estimates of the total cost of low back pain to society in 1990 were between $50 billion and $100 billion per year, with a significant share (approximately $11 billion) borne by the workers' compensation system.

As many as 30% of American workers are employed in jobs that routinely require them to perform activities that may increase their risk of developing low back disorders. For example, female nursing aides and licensed practical nurses were about 2.5 times more likely to experience a work-related low back disorder than all other female workers. Male construction laborers, carpenters, and truck and tractor operators were nearly two times more likely to experience a low back disorder than all other male workers.

The diagnosis of low back pain is primarily made by history and physical examination. The possibility of work-related origin must be explored in detail. Occupational factors often associated with the occurrence of low back pain include heavy physical work, static work postures, frequent bending and twisting, lifting, pushing and pulling, repetitive work, and vibrations.

In general, individuals with low back pain recover from an acute episode in a few days to a few weeks, requiring little treatment. Modifying work activities or work restriction may be needed short term. However, if indicated, employees with this problem may need to be placed in new jobs, even though this is not usual.

Prevention of work-related low back pain is key and involves several measures. These measures include a work process that is ergonomically sound, optimal work levels, good work organization to reduce repetitive loading and fatigue, and training and education of workers, managers, health care providers, and union representatives about disease etiology and control and prevention strategies.

Despite the overwhelming statistics on the magnitude of the problem, more complete information is needed to assess how changes implemented to reduce the physical demands of jobs will affect workplace safety and productivity in the future. A tremendous opportunity exists for prevention efforts to reduce the prevalence and costs of low back disorders.

Musculoskeletal Disorders of the Upper Extremities

Musculoskeletal disorders of the neck and upper extremities from work factors affect employees in every type of workplace and include such diverse workers as food processors, automobile and electronics assemblers, carpenters, office data entry workers, grocery store cashiers, and garment workers. The highest rates of these disorders occur in the industries with a substantial amount of repetitive, forceful work. Musculoskeletal disorders affect the soft tissues of the neck, shoulder, elbow, hand, wrist, and fingers. These include the nerves (e.g., carpal tunnel syndrome), tendons (e.g., tenosynovitis, peritendinitis, epicondylitis), and muscles (e.g., tension neck syndrome). The costs associated with these disorders are high, with more than $2.1 billion in workers' compensation costs and $90 billion in indirect costs (hiring, training, overtime, and administrative costs) incurred annually for these musculoskeletal disorders.

In 1994, 332,000 musculoskeletal disorders caused by repeated trauma were reported in U.S. workplaces. This figure represents nearly 65% of all illness cases reported to the Bureau of Labor Statistics—an increase of nearly 10% compared with 1993 figures and more than 15% relative to 1992 figures.

The most commonly reported musculoskeletal disorders of the upper extremities affect the hand-wrist region. In 1993, carpal tunnel syndrome, the most widely recognized condition, occurred at a rate of 5.2 per 10,000 full-time workers. This syndrome required the longest recuperation period of all conditions resulting in lost workdays, with a median 30 days away from work.

Traumatic Injuries
Fatal Occupational Injuries

From 1980 through 1992, more than 77,000 workers died as a result of work-related injuries. This means that an average of 16 workers die every day from injuries sustained at work. The leading causes of occupational injury fatalities over this 13-year period were motor vehicles, machines, homicides, falls, electrocutions, and falling objects. There were four industries—mining, construction, transportation, and agriculture—with occupational injury fatality rates that were notably and consistently higher than all other industries. Motor vehicle–related deaths in the transportation sector, machine-related deaths in agriculture, electrocutions and fatal falls in construction, homicide in retail trade and public administration, and deaths due to falling objects in mining and logging appear to be important because of particularly high rates of death from injury.

Nonfatal Occupational Injuries

In 1994, 6.3 million workers sustained job-related injuries that resulted in lost work time, medical treatment other than first aid, loss of consciousness, restriction of work or motion, or transfer to another job. The leading causes of nonfatal occupational injuries involving time away from work in 1993 were overexertion, contact with objects or equipment, and falls to the same level. Industries experiencing the largest number of serious nonfatal injuries include eating and drinking establishments, hospitals, and grocery stores. Industries facing higher risks of serious nonfatal injuries are concentrated in the manufacturing sector and include workers in shipbuilding, wooden building and mobile home manufacture, foundries, special products sawmills, and meat packing plants.

Clearly, work-related injuries and fatalities result from multiple causes, affect different segments of the working population and occur in myriad occupational and industrial settings. The total cost of work-related injuries and fatalities to industry and to society at large has not been fully recognized, but it is estimated to be greater than $121 billion annually.

Work/Workplace Change

The U.S. workplace is rapidly changing and becoming more diverse. Jobs in our economy continue to shift from manufacturing to services, with the service sector now employing 70% of all workers. Major changes are also occurring in the way work is organized. Longer hours, compressed work weeks, shift work, reduced job security, and part-time and temporary work are realities of the modern workplace. New chemicals, materials, processes, and equipment (e.g., latex gloves in health care, fermentation processes in biotechnology) are developed and marketed at an ever-accelerating pace. The workforce is also changing. As the U.S. workforce grows to approximately 147 million by the year 2005, it will become older and more racially diverse. By the year 2005, population diversity will represent approximately 28% and women approximately 48% of the workforce. These changes are accompanied by new issues, such as potential language barriers and women's health issues. Although much has been accomplished in controlling work-related illness and injury and reducing workplace fatalities, more needs to be done to ensure that worksites are safe and healthy for America's workforce (DHHS, 1996).

Healthy People 2010 outlines objectives related to reducing work-related risk and injury, improving worker health, supporting research, and increasing efforts in training and education of occupational health and safety professionals (see the following box for selected *Healthy People 2010* objectives).

Occupational Health Nursing Practice

The practice of occupational health nursing, previously defined, has changed dramatically over time, with increasing emphasis on autonomous decision making, independent practice, prevention and health promotion, analytical and investigative skills, management, and policy development (Rogers, 1994). This evolu-

tion is a result of the need to better deal with issues of changing workforce hazards, necessity for cost containment, and increased efforts to promote health and productivity at work.

The specialty practice has always been closely linked to public health nursing, which provides the practice underpinnings from a synthesis of the public health and nursing sciences directed at population health improvement (Rogers, 1994). Thus, familiarity with the definition of public health nursing is also important. The American Public Health Association (APHA), Public Health Nursing Section (1996) has defined public health nursing as follows:

> Public health nursing is the practice of promoting and protecting the health of populations using knowledge from nursing, social, and public health sciences. Public health nursing practice is a systematic process by which:
>
> 1. *The health and health care needs of a population are assessed in order to identify sub-populations, families, and individuals who would benefit from health promotion or who are at risk of illness, injury, disability, or premature death.*
>
> 2. *A plan for intervention is developed with the community to meet identified needs that takes into account available resources, the range of activities that contribute to health and the prevention of illness, injury, disability, and premature death.*
>
> 3. *The plan is implemented effectively, efficiently, and equitably.*
>
> 4. *Evaluations are conducted to determine the extent to which the interventions have an impact on the health status of individuals and the population.*
>
> 5. *The results of the process are used to influence and direct delivery of care, deployment of health resources, and the development of local, regional, state, and national health policy and research to promote health and prevent disease.*

Occupational health nursing practice is guided by the *Standards of Occupational Health Nursing Practice* (AAOHN, 1999), which are developed and published by the American Association of Occupational Health Nurses. The professional standards provide the framework for evaluating the practice and a mechanism through which accountability with the public is maintained. Standard elements are shown in Box 40-4.

AAOHN also establishes the *Code of Ethics with Interpretive Statements* for occupational health nurses which acts as a guide for the professional occupational heath nurse to maintain and pursue professionally ethical behavior in providing occupational health services. The *Code of Ethics* (AAOHN, 1996) is shown in Box 40-5.

To apply practice skills, occupational health nursing practice also requires more specific knowledge in fields nurses have some understanding of, including business and management, legal-regulatory fields, and behavioral sciences. In addition, it is essential that nurses be knowledgeable about the occupational health sciences, including industrial hygiene, toxicology, safety, and ergonomics (Rogers, 1994). A brief description of each of these occupational health science areas is provided.

By definition, industrial hygiene includes the anticipation, recognition, evaluation, and control of occupational hazards, arising in or from the workplace, which may cause sickness,

HEALTHY PEOPLE 2010

OBJECTIVES RELATED TO OCCUPATIONAL SAFETY AND HEALTH

Occupational Safety and Health

20.1   Reduce deaths from work-related injuries.

20.2   Reduce work-related injuries resulting in medical treatment, lost time from work, or restricted work activity.

20.3   Reduce the rate of injury and illness cases involving days away from work due to overexertion or repetitive motion.

20.4   Reduce Pneumoconiosis deaths.

20.5   Reduce deaths from work-related homicides.

20.6   Reduce work-related assault.

20.7   Reduce the number of persons who have elevated blood lead concentrations from work exposures.

20.8   Reduce occupational skin diseases or disorders among full-time workers.

20.9   Increase the proportion of worksites employing 50 or more persons that provide programs to prevent or reduce employee stress.

20.10   Reduce occupational needlestick injuries among health care workers.

20.11   Reduce new cases of work-related noise-induced hearing loss.

Source: DHHS, 2000.

---

impaired health and well-being or significant discomfort and inefficiency among workers or community citizens (AIHA, 1976). This is done through identifying and quantifying exposures, through sampling techniques, and through implementation and evaluation of control strategies to mitigate exposures.

Toxicology is the study of harmful effects of chemicals on biological systems. In the occupational setting, toxicology is primarily concerned with evaluating human health effects posed by workplace chemical exposures, including dusts, gases, fumes, mists, and vapors. This involves the recognition of routes of exposure, the relativity of these exposures to acute and latent health effects such as burns or cancer, and dose-response relationships.

Safety in the workplace is everyone's responsibility, and the safety is concerned with the design and implementation of strategies to prevent and control workplace exposures that result in injury or death.

The term **ergonomics** is derived from two Greek words *ergos* meaning "work" and *nomos* meaning "laws"; thus, the laws of work. The National Safety Council offers a simple but consistent definition: "Ergonomics is the science of designing the job and the workplace to fit the worker. The goal of ergonomics is to allow work to be done without undue stress." Within the framework of

FYI

With 879 fatalities, truck drivers suffered more workplace deaths in 1998 than any other profession.

Source: National Safety Council, 1999.

FYI

Women are more likely to be murdered at work than to die in a traffic accident. Of the 482 women killed on the job in 1998, 34% were murdered.

Source: National Safety Council, 1999.

BOX 40-4 AMERICAN ASSOCIATION OF OCCUPATIONAL HEALTH NURSES STANDARDS OF OCCUPATIONAL AND ENVIRONMENTAL HEALTH NURSING PRACTICE*

STANDARD I

Assessment

The occupational health nurse systematically assesses the health status of the client, workforce, and environment.

STANDARD II

Diagnosis

The occupational health nurse analyzes health data of the individual, workforce, and environment collected to formulate diagnoses for intervention planning.

STANDARD III

Outcome Identification

The occupational health nurse identifies a specific expected outcomes plan based on diagnosis.

STANDARD IV

Planning

The occupational health nurse develops a goal-directed plan of care that is comprehensive and that formulates interventions for each level of prevention and for therapeutic modalities to achieve desired outcomes.

STANDARD V

Implementation

The occupational health nurse implements interventions to promote health, prevent illness and injury, and facilitate rehabilitation, guided by the plan of care.

STANDARD VI

Evaluation

The occupational health nurse, reflecting best practice standards, systematically and continuously evaluates responses to interventions and progress toward the achievement of desired outcomes.

STANDARD VII

Resource Management

Based on corporate goals and objectives, number of clients, clients' health needs, specific health haz-ards, and associated costs, the occupational health nurse collaborates with management to provide resources that support an occupational health program that meets the needs of the workforce.

STANDARD VIII

Professional Development

To enhance professional growth and maintain professional competency, the occupational health nurse assumes responsibility for professional development and continuing education. Overall evaluation is accomplished through ongoing self-evaluation and analysis of data from quality improvement/assurance mechanisms.

STANDARD IX

Collaboration

To promote employee health and safety, and a safe and healthful work environment, and to provide effective and efficient health care services, the occupational health nurse collaborates with employees, management, other health care providers, professionals, and community representatives in assessing, planning, implementing, and evaluating care and services.

STANDARD X

Research

Through essential research, the occupational health nurse is committed to and contributes to the scientific base in occupational health nursing to improve and advance the practice and uses research findings in practice.

STANDARD XI

Ethics

As a client advocate for accessible, equitable, and quality health care services, including a safe and healthful work environment, the occupational health nurse uses an ethical framework, which provides parameters for ethical judgments, as a guide for decision making in practice.

*Note: This reflects only the category headings. Refer to source for entire document.
Source: AAOHN, 1999.

BOX 40-5 AAOHN *Code of Ethics*

- The occupational health nurse provides health care in the work environment with regard for human dignity and client rights, unrestricted by considerations of social or economic status, personal attributes, or the nature of the health status.

- The occupational health nurse promotes collaboration with other health professionals and community health agencies to meet the health needs of the workforce.

- The occupational health nurse maintains individual competence in health nursing practice, based on scientific knowledge, and recognizes and accepts responsibility for individual judgments and actions, while complying with appropriate laws and regulations (local, state, and federal) that have an impact on the delivery of occupational health services.

- The occupational health nurse participates, as appropriate, in activities such as research that contribute to the ongoing development of the profession's body of knowledge while protecting the rights of subjects.

- The occupational health nurse strives to safeguard the employee's right to privacy by protecting confidential information and releasing information only upon written consent of the employee or as required or permitted by law.

- The occupational health nurse strives to provide quality care and to safeguard clients from unethical and illegal actions.

- The occupational health nurse, licensed to provide health care services, accepts obligations to society as a professional and responsible member of the community.

Source: AAOHN, 1996.

RESEARCH BRIEF

Conrad, K. M., Furner, S. E., & Qian, Y. (1999). Occupational hazard exposure and at risk drinking. American Association of Occupational Health Nurses Journal, 47(1), 9–16.

This research study examined associations between workers' reported exposure to occupational hazards and their risk for alcohol use. The sample was drawn from the National Health Interview Survey (NHIS) and included 15,907 working adults. *Occupational hazard exposures* were defined as chemical or biological substances, physical hazards, injury risk, and mental stress. *At-risk drinking* was defined as binge drinking and driving while drinking. Of the workers in the sample, 60% reported exposure to one or more occupational hazards, 31% of the sample reported binge drinking, and 15% drove after drinking too much. In a multivariate analysis that controlled for background of the subjects, workers who reported occupational hazard exposure were 1.2 to 1.4 times more likely to engage in binge drinking than workers without exposures. Similar results were found for drinking and driving and occupational exposure. All multivariate statistical analyses were statistically significant. Findings suggest that workers who perceive themselves as being at risk for occupational hazards are at greater risk for binge drinking and driving after drinking. Occupational nurses can lead workplace initiatives to reduce occupational risk exposures and, at the same time, reduce risks for workers at risk for alcohol consumption.

these definitions, the goal remains the same, that is, to match job demands and requirements to the abilities and capabilities of the worker (Sluchak, 1992). However, note that ergonomics is concerned with matching work and job design to fit the capabilities of most people by adapting the product to fit the user rather than vice versa.

Scope of Practice

The scope of occupational health nursing practice as depicted in the figure on p. 955 is broad and dynamic and includes the following areas (Rogers & Cox, 1998).

Worker/workplace assessment and surveillance focus on identification of potential worker health problems and determination of worker health status. This is accomplished through knowledge of worker jobs and their demands, work processes and related hazards, and working conditions and exposures. Expert occupational health history taking is essential, as are appropriate assessments that help match the job to the worker. In addition to general health information, the history must include an examination of all previous jobs and exposures that may indicate potential interactions (e.g., smoking, antineoplastic agent exposure). An example of an occupational health history form is shown in Box 40-6.

In addition, preplacement examinations to evaluate health status related to the work and gather baseline data, periodic examinations to determine any adverse work-related health effects, return to work evaluations to make certain the employee is fit for duty, screenings to detect health problems, and surveillance activities to monitor health status are needed.

SCOPE OF OCCUPATIONAL HEALTH NURSING PRACTICE.

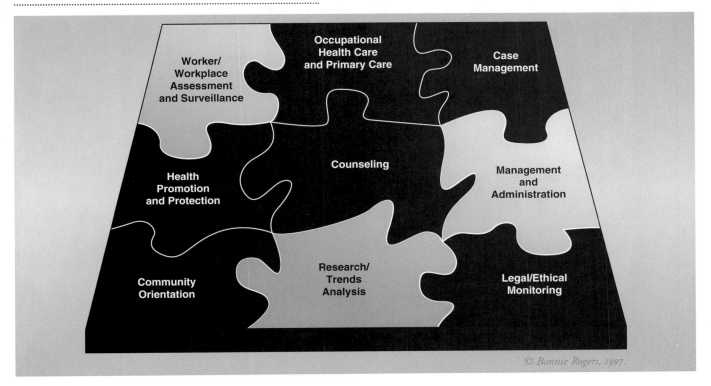

Worker/
Workplace
Assessment
and Surveillance

Occupational
Health Care
and Primary Care

Case
Management

Health
Promotion
and Protection

Counseling

Management
and
Administration

Community
Orientation

Research/
Trends
Analysis

Legal/Ethical
Monitoring

© Bonnie Rogers, 1997.

The workplace also needs to be assessed and monitored to identify potential unhealthy working conditions. A collaborative walk-through assessment provides for observation of the workforce doing the work, observation of the work processes for each specific job, and observation of the working conditions and work milieu. Box 40-7 provides elements in the conduct of a worksite assessment.

The occupational health nurse should be knowledgeable about all work/work processes, the total work environment, and workforce characteristics so that hazards and potential interventions can be adequately identified. In addition, knowledge of the corporate culture and mission related to occupational health and safety, as well as policies, staffing, and programmatic initiatives, will provide a sense about the relative importance of occupational health and safety at the worksite. The occupational health nurse will also want to know the most common illnesses and injuries at the worksite so that appropriate health care interventions can be made. These data will also provide information for problem solving, research, and determination of cost-effective health care delivery strategies.

During assessment and surveillance activities, preventive and corrective strategies such as engineering, work practice, administrative, and personal protective controls can be discussed

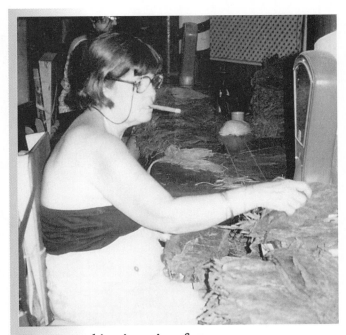

Woman working in a cigar factory.

BOX 40-6 OCCUPATIONAL AND ENVIRONMENTAL HEALTH HISTORY FORM

Work History

1. List your current and past longest-held jobs, including the military.

Company	Dates employed	Job title	Known exposures
_____	_____	_____	_____
_____	_____	_____	_____
_____	_____	_____	_____
_____	_____	_____	_____
_____	_____	_____	_____

2. Do you work full-time?   No ____   Yes ____   How many hours per week? ____
3. Do you work part-time?   No ____   Yes ____   How many hours per week? ____
4. Please describe any health problems or injuries that you have experienced in connection with your present or last jobs:

5. Have you ever had to change jobs due to health problems or injuries?
   If so, have any of your co-workers experienced similar problems?

6. In what type of business do you work currently?

7. Describe your work:

8. Have you had any current or past exposure (through breathing or touching) to any of the following?

___ acids	___ carbon	___ dichlorobenzene	___ manganese	___ pesticides	___ toluene
___ alcohols	___ tetrachloride	___ ethylene dibromide	___ mercury	___ phenol	___ TDI or MDI
___ alkalis	chlorinated	___ ethylene dichloride	___ methylene	___ phosgene	___ trichloroethylene
___ ammonia	___ naphthalenes	___ fiberglass	___ chloride	___ radiation	___ trinitrotoluene
___ arsenic	___ chloroform	___ halothane	___ nickel	___ rock dust	___ vibration
___ asbestos	___ chloropurine	___ heat (severe)	___ noise (loud)	___ silica powder	___ vinyl chloride
___ benzene	___ chromates	___ isocyanates	___ PBBs	___ solvents	___ welding fumes
___ beryllium	___ coal dust	___ ketones	___ PCBs	___ stryrene	___ x-rays
___ cadmium	___ cold (severe)	___ lead	___ perchloroethylene	___ talc	

9. Did you receive any safety training about these agents?

10. Are you involved in any work processes, such as grinding, welding, soldering, or polishing, that create dust or fumes?

11. Did you use any of the following personal protective equipment when exposed?

___ respirator	___ gloves	___ earplugs or muffs	___ safety shoes
___ shield	___ sleeves	___ glasses or goggles	___ boots
___ welding mask	___ coveralls		

BOX 40-6 OCCUPATIONAL AND ENVIRONMENTAL HEALTH HISTORY FORM—CONT'D

12. Is your work environment generally clean? Describe:

13. What ventilation systems are used in your workspace?

14. Do the ventilation systems seem to work? Are you aware of any chemical odors in your environment?

15. Where do you eat, smoke, and take your breaks when you are on the job?

16. Do you use a uniform or have clothing that you wear to work only?

17. How is this laundered?

18. How often do you wash your hands at work, and how do you wash them?

19. Do you shower before leaving the worksite?

20. Do you have any physical symptoms associated with work?

21. Are other workers similarly affected?

22. Do you have any home exposures (e.g., pesticides, household cleaners), hobbies, or community exposures (e.g., live near waste site, landfill)? Please describe:

---

as approaches to reduce risk and minimize health problems. Occupational health nurses critically analyze each job task to detect task situations that place employees at risk. They also note work-related risk factors, such as bending or twisting, that may also compromise the worker. The occupational health nurse is usually the first person to receive a complaint and must be prepared to recognize potential exposures and initiate exposure monitoring usually performed by an industrial hygienist.

Occupational health and primary care for both occupational and nonoccupational illness and injury is provided in most worksites by the occupational health nurse within the context of a collaborative multidisciplinary approach. Direct care is provided for emergency or urgent illness and injury (e.g., burns, head injuries), work-related acute illness and injury (e.g., back strain), minor health problems (e.g., headaches, lacerations), health care monitoring (e.g., high blood pressure), and preventive health care (e.g., immunizations, breast cancer screening). Also included here are mandatory or special programs such as hearing conservation, travel health, or drug and alcohol testing.

Case management is an integral component of occupational health care management involving conditions that may be occupational in origin (e.g., from an exposure) or nonoccupational in origin (e.g., cardiovascular disease). Coordination and management of cost-effective quality health care services from the onset of illness or injury to the return to work or optimal recovery are key. Early intervention and evaluation of outcomes, including cost savings, are essential components that provide for immediate problem identification and engage the worker in care planning from the beginning of the illness/injury to recovery. Early intervention helps prevent fragmented and delayed care by engaging appropriate health care providers at the beginning of care rather than later after complications may have developed. Case management requires knowledge of all factors that have an impact on worker health, including financial, spiritual, and cultural issues, and intense follow-up.

Health promotion/health protection activities are directed toward enhancing health and increasing the level of well-being toward optimal health. Activities are implemented at individual, group, and population levels through educational, behavioral, and environmental levels. Health protection is best described as preventive health behaviors designed to guard or defend an individual or group against specific illness or injury. Health protection is best achieved through a total range of prevention efforts incorporating primary, secondary, and tertiary prevention strategies. Primary, secondary, and tertiary prevention strategies, such as improved personal protective equipment, screening and surveillance activities, and return-to-work or cardiac rehabilitation programs, are used to reduce risks and restore health. Imple-

menting a concept of health that is integrated into the business structure will be key to a healthy environment. This means that health and safety must be a priority in terms of program planning and resource allocation.

Counseling is provided about health with regard to prevention and management of occupational illness and injury, work-related stress, productivity issues, family, conflicts, finances, personal issues, interorganizational relationships, and other areas. Knowing risk factors about employees such as recurrent absenteeism, substance abuse, social withdrawal, or changes in mood or appearance is critical for successful interventions, including referrals. The occupational health nurse is in the best position to provide counseling services to the worker because he or she is the health care provider most available to the employee. Some issues may interfere with the worker's ability to work or perform the job, and the employee will probably benefit from some form of intervention, such as listening, supporting, or referral.

The occupational health nurse should have specific counseling knowledge and skills such as problem recognition; building a supportive, trusting and confidential relationship; crisis intervention approaches; and knowledge about community resources for referral to effectively assist the employee and in some cases the family.

Management and administration, including the development of health policy, is a major role that focuses on ensuring effective occupational health and safety programs and services. Defining a corporate culture that is supportive of a healthy work environment is necessary for an effective occupational health and safety program. Increasingly, the occupational health nurse is assuming a major role in the management and administration of the occupational health unit and in policy-making decisions to ensure effective occupational health and safety programs and services for workers. At the unit level, the occupational health nurse manager is responsible for the overall operational management of the occupational health service, including program planning, organization, staffing, budget development and management, service coordination, and evaluation. Strategic or long-range planning shapes the future of the company and is key to the long-term success and growth of the occupational health program. Engaged in the strategic planning process, the occupational health nurse can use valuable expertise to set forth new ideas and positions and engage in policy development about furthering the occupational health and safety program within the context of the business mission. Understanding the business mission, the needs of the organization, and resource consumption variables is vital to a successful program. Keeping the workforce healthy and productive within the context of the cost containment is a major objective.

Community orientation emphasizes the development of partnerships and collaboration in the delivery of workplace health care. If used, services provided by voluntary or governmental agencies, such as parenting programs, cardiac or drug rehabilitation services, or home health care, can be cost beneficial to both the employee and employer. The occupational health nurse can help the industry create a health partnership with the community by working together on programs. Providing or sponsoring health fairs for workers, their families, and the community is another example of successful partnerships. Use of community programs and development of referral networks will aid the occupational health and safety program.

Research and trend analysis is necessary to improve and foster the health and well-being of the worker and workforce, to improve working conditions by eliminating or minimizing hazards, and to build a body of occupational health nursing knowledge. Research and practice go hand in hand with the mission to improve and foster the health and well-being of the worker and workforce and to improve working conditions, eliminating or minimizing potential or actual hazards. For example, understanding the effects of toxic exposures, designing strategies to prevent work-related accident/injuries or illnesses, evaluating the cost-effectiveness of health interventions, and understanding human behavior and motivation related to health promotion activities are important occupational health nursing investigations. Occupational health nursing research is essential in both preventive health management and control of workplace hazards.

Legal-ethical monitoring is paramount to ensure a safe and healthful work environment consistent with the OSH Act, related standards, and the Nurse Practice Acts. The occupational health nurse must be aware of occupational health and safety statutes and recommend programs and strategies to comply with mandated requirements. The nurse also should work to influence or help develop legislation such as confidentiality of employee health records protection or legislation specific to worker/workplace health protection.

Ethical issues abound in the work environment, and the occupational health nurse is faced with many challenges in ethical decision making. Issues related to confidentiality of employee health records, hazardous exposures, truth telling, inappropriate screening of employees, discrimination, and professional incompetence or illegal practice are but a few of these ethical challenges. As mentioned, the AAOHN *Code of Ethics* will help guide practice and acts as a framework for implementation of values related to occupational health and safety. The nurse is obligated to always act in the best interest of the worker and provide effective leadership skills in ethical health care. In this role, the occupational health nurse not only brings a special expertise to occupational health dilemmas but also structures the issues so that sound and deliberate decisions are made using a reasoned approach.

Occupational Health Nursing Roles

Occupational health nursing roles have expanded enormously (Rogers & Cox, 1998) to match the increased scope of practice. AAOHN (1999) describes the varied roles of occupational health nurses (see the figure on p. 960):

The **occupational health nurse clinician** provides direct care for both occupational and nonoccupational illness and injuries using established protocols; performs health assessments, screenings, surveillance and counseling; and conducts workplace walk-throughs/assessments and exposure follow-up.

The **occupational health nurse case manager** coordinates health care services for the employee from the onset of injury or illness to a safe return to work or an optimal alternative. Quality outcome-focused care is delivered in a cost-effective manner.

The **occupational health nurse coordinator** functions as the single occupational health nurse for a company responsible for the occupational and environmental health and safety services. The occupational health nurse coordinator conducts needs assessments of the client population and worksite and develops programs designed to address these needs. Evaluation is a component of the process.

The **occupational health nurse health-promotion specialist** has primary responsibility for the overall management of the health-promotion program. This includes the development of a comprehensive program that meets the needs of the workforce population within the context of supporting organizational business objectives for a healthy workforce and work environment. These initiatives might include exercise, nutrition, or smoking cessation programs.

The **occupational health nurse manager** is responsible for setting occupational health unit policy and directing, administering, and evaluating an occupational and environmental health and safety service. This includes the operational management of the occupational health unit, financial management consistent with organizational goals and objectives, and quality improvement of occupational health services.

The **occupational health nurse practitioner** uses independent and collaborative critical judgments in conducting health assessments, making differential diagnoses, promoting optimal health, and providing pharmacological and nonpharmacological treatments in the direct management of acute and chronic illness and injuries within the scope of state regulations. Services may range from preplacement physical examinations to comprehensive primary care for employees and their families.

The **occupational health nurse corporate director** functions as a policy maker at the corporate level and develops and directs the overall occupational and environmental health and safety programs in consultation with other health and safety specialists and corporate management. This individual also evaluates quantitative outcomes of occupational and environmental health and safety programs using cost-benefit analysis, engages in strategic planning and trend analysis in occupational and environmental health, and provides vision for the direction of the occupational health and safety program.

The **occupational health nurse consultant** provides advice for developing occupational and environmental health and safety services and for structuring the delivery of services, including managed care and case management. In addition, this individual consults about specific services such as hazard analysis, disability management review, hearing conservation, regulatory programming, and health promotion.

OCCUPATIONAL HEALTH NURSING ROLES.

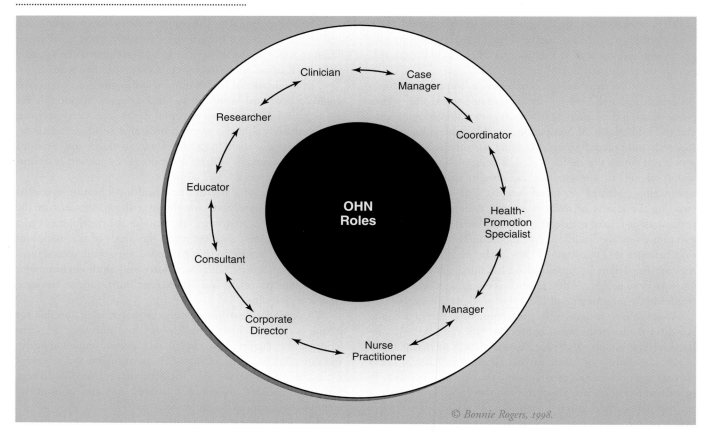

© Bonnie Rogers, 1998.

The **occupational health nurse educator** plans curricula appropriate to various levels of educational preparation and has responsibilities for occupational and environmental health nursing curricula and clinical experiences in college or university academic education, continuing professional education, or unit staff development programs. Evaluation is a continuous process.

The **occupational health nurse researcher** develops researchable questions, designs studies, conducts research, writes grants, and disseminates research findings to improve practice and build knowledge in the discipline.

These roles are multi-integrated, meaning that occupational health nurses often act in many capacities at the same time.

Within the knowledge context for role implementation, occupational health nurses must have a lifelong knowledge base in the public health and occupational health sciences (e.g., epidemiology, toxicology, industrial hygiene, safety/ergonomics), environmental health, business and economics, social and behavioral sciences, and legal and ethical parameters of practice.

It is important to recognize that in order to implement the roles effectively, occupational health nurses must work within an interdisciplinary framework with other health disciplines, typically the industrial hygienist, safety specialist, and occupational medicine physician. These fields are briefly described in Box 40-8.

Governmental Influence

Although occupational health nursing practice is governed by state nursing practice acts, other federal and state laws impact the practice as well. The major law governing occupational safety and health is the Occupational Safety and Health Act of 1970. This law was enacted to "assure so far as possible every man and woman in the Nation safe and healthful working conditions and to preserve our human resources." The Act is administered by OSHA within the Department of Labor (although states may administer their own programs with OSHA approval) to do the following:

- *Encourage employers and employees to reduce workplace hazards and to implement new or improve existing safety and health programs*
- *Provide for research in occupational safety and health to develop innovative ways of dealing with occupational safety and health problems*
- *Establish separate but dependent responsibilities and rights for employers and employees for the achievement of better safety and health conditions*
- *Maintain a reporting and record-keeping system to monitor job-related illnesses and injuries*

BOX 40-8 INTERDISCIPLINARY FIELDS OF PRACTICE SPECIFIC TO OCCUPATIONAL HEALTH NURSING

OCCUPATIONAL MEDICINE

The assessment, maintenance, restoration, and improvement of the health of the worker through the principles of preventative medicine, and promotion of worker health and productivity

INDUSTRIAL HYGIENE

The science devoted to the anticipation, recognition, evaluation, and control of environmental factors and stresses associated with work and work operations

SAFETY

The design and implementation of strategies aimed at preventing and controlling workplace exposure that result in unnecessary injuries and death

ERGONOMICS

The study of humans at work and the evaluation of the stresses that occur in the work environment and the ability of people to cope with these stresses so that the job demands are matched with human capabilities

---

* *Establish training programs to increase the number and competence or occupational safety and health personnel*
* *Develop mandatory job safety and health standards and enforce them effectively*
* *Provide for the development, analysis, evaluation, and approval of state occupational safety and health programs*

Within the legislation for the OSH Act, several bodies were created to help carry out the mandates of the Act. OSHA is the agency responsible to set and enforce the rules and regulations of the Act and standards the Agency develops. The NIOSH conducts research and training and makes recommendations for the prevention and control of work-related illnesses and injuries. NIOSH funds education and research centers that provide academic, research, and continuing education training for occupational safety and health professionals.

The Occupational Safety and Health Review Commission is a quasi-judicial body charged with reviewing on disputes, forwarded to it by the Department of Labor, regarding OSHA inspections.

The National Advising Committee on Occupational Safety and Health is a consumer and professionally appointed group that makes occupational and safety recommendations to OSHA and the NIOSH. The agency also promulgates numerous standards to eliminate or reduce risks (e.g., Blood-Borne Pathogens Standard, Hazardous Communication Standard, Lead Standard, Asbestos Standard). Occupational health and safety standards related to specific exposures have a health/medical component that generally addresses preplacement, surveillance, and monitoring activities. In most companies, the occupational health nurse manages implementation of these standards to ensure that employees are monitored appropriately for any adverse work-related health effects.

For example, the Blood-Borne Pathogens Standard (29CFR 1910.1030), established by OSHA in 1992, was designed to eliminate or minimize blood and body fluid exposure. The standard requires the employer to develop and implement an exposure control plan as follows:

* *It must be written and accessible to employees.*
* *Documentation of exposure determination must be included.*
* *A method for implementing the exposure control plan, including methods of compliance, employee education and training, description of the hepatitis B vaccination program and postexposure follow-up procedures, and record-keeping and communication procedures, must be provided.*
* *A procedure must be established for evaluating exposure incidents.*

The occupational health nurse assists management in developing an effective program consistent with the standard's elements. Occupational health nurses also serve as consultants to assist in establishing methods of compliance, such as engineering and work practice controls.

The occupational health nurse is usually the person responsible for the development and implementation of the hepatitis B vaccination program and postexposure follow-up. The standard requires that the hepatitis B vaccine be offered, at no expense, to all exposed employees. If the employee chooses not to accept the offer of the hepatitis B vaccination, he or she must sign a mandatory declination statement. The postexposure evaluation and follow-up is critical to employee safety and health; therefore, the most important component of effective postexposure evaluation is the method for reporting exposures. Exposures must be reported and acted upon immediately. Counseling the employee about the risk of infection, importance of early testing to determine whether transmission has occurred, and recommendations for postexposure prophylaxis and prevention of transmission of disease is essential and should occur over several sessions.

Employee education and training is also provided by the occupational health nurse. Information about the hazards of blood-borne pathogens and methods to prevent transmission to workers may be introduced at employed orientation. These programs are an ideal time to introduce the method for and importance of appropriate reporting of exposures. The occupational health nurses plays an active role in partnering with OSHA and the employer to reduce morbidity and mortality associated with exposures to blood-borne pathogens (BBP), such as hepatitis B and HIV. Occupational health nurses participate in all aspects of compliance with the BBP Standard, beginning with development and implementing an exposure control plan and ending with maintaining the health and training records for the appropriate number of years.

Within the OSH Act, the general duty clause states that employers are required to furnish all employees "employment and a place of employment which are free from recognized hazards that are causing or likely to cause death or serious physical harm." If a specific hazard is not covered by a standard, the general duty clause can be invoked. OSHA also provides consultative services to identify and correct hazards, provide technical assistance, and provide education and training for health and safety personnel. Occupational health nurses must be fully cognizant of all occupational health and safety laws, standards, and the regulatory implications in the workplace.

In addition, the OSH Act requires most employers with 11 or more employees to prepare and maintain records of work-related illnesses and injuries. There are detailed rules and regulations regarding what constitutes a recordable event and how these events are to be recorded. In most instances in which there is an occupational health nurse, he or she is usually delegated this responsibility. Data are recorded on logs that are analyzed in aggregate form (by OSHA and the Bureau of Labor Statistics) to identify companies with high-risk illnesses and injuries that may need enforcement and consultation efforts.

In addition to the OSH Act, examples of other pertinent laws affecting health and safety at the worksite include the following:

- American with Disabilities Act of 1990 (ADA): *This act is intended to prevent discrimination against persons with disabilities. Under Title I of the Act, persons with disabilities are entitled to equal employment opportunities with regard to their disability. Health assessments can be performed only after an offer of employment has been made, and applicants can be evaluated only in terms of their ability to perform essential job functions. In some situations, reasonable accommodations must be made by the employer for the disabled person to perform the work. The occupational health nurse may be actively involved in developing and implementing the company's ADA policy. This is done through the appropriate conduct of health examinations, review of job functions to determine job suitability, and recommendations for job accommodations.*

- The Family Medical Leave Act: *This act requires employers with 50 or more employees to provide a maximum of 12 weeks unpaid job-related leave in a 12-month period to eligible employees. The occupational health nurse has the responsibility to educate eligible employees about what constitutes an eligible leave of absence and counsel the employee regarding health issues.*

- Workers' Compensation: *The workers' compensation system in each state and the District of Columbia is designed to cover monetary loss as a result of work-related injuries, including salary; medical, hospital, or funeral expenses; and dependent support in case of occupational death. In turn, there is no employer negligence or fault, safe-guarding the employer from legal action. Federal civilian employees are covered by federal statutes.*

The occupational health nurse often manages worker compensation claims, ensuring that injured workers are medically treated and managed. In addition, the occupational health nurse monitors the employee's return to work, cautioning against reinjury, but getting the employee back to functional work in a reasonable period.

Professionalism in Occupational Health Nursing

The professional society in occupational health nursing is the American Association of Occupational Health Nurses (AAOHN). AAOHN does the following (AAOHN, 1999):

- *Promotes the health and safety of workers*
- *Defines the scope of practice and sets the standards of occupational health nursing practice*
- *Develops the* Code of Ethics *for occupational health nurses with interpretive statements*
- *Promotes and provides continuing education in the specialty*
- *Advances the profession through supporting research*
- *Responds to and influences public policy issues related to occupational health and safety*

The official journal is the *AAOHN Journal.*

Education and Certification

One must be a registered nurse to gain entry into professional occupational health nursing practice. Most companies prefer to hire occupational nurses with previous experience in occupational health, public health, or emergency care. A baccalaureate in nursing is the preferred degree (AAOHN, 1996). As stated, specialty academic education in occupational health and safety is generally offered at the graduate level (master's and doctoral) through NIOSH-funded Occupational Safety and Health Education and Research Centers (Table 40-5).

These centers provide academic, research, continuing education, and outreach programs. Grants support training and education of occupational health and safety professionals, including occupational health nurses, industrial hygienists, physicians, and safety specialists. In addition, a nurse practitioner option in occupational health is also offered. Doctoral-level education prepares nurses as scientists in occupational health and safety research.

Certification in occupational health nursing is conducted by the American Board for Occupational Health Nursing. Certification is met through educational qualifications, experience, continuing education, and examination.

TABLE 40-5 NATIONAL INSTITUTES FOR OCCUPATIONAL SAFETY AND HEALTH EDUCATION AND RESEARCH CENTERS

Alabama Educational Resource Center
University of Alabama at Birmingham
School of Public Health
Birmingham, AL 32594-0008
205-934-7032

California Educational Resource Center, Northern
University of California, Berkeley
School of Public Health
322 Warren
Berkeley, CA 94720
510-642-0761

California Educational Resource Center, Southern
University of Southern California
Institute of Safety and Systems Management
University Park
Los Angeles, CA 90089-0021
213-740-4038

Cincinnati Educational Resource Center
University of Cincinnati
Department of Environmental Health
3223 Eden Avenue
Cincinnati, OH 45267-0056
513-558-5701

Harvard Educational Resource Center
Harvard School of Public Health
Department of Environmental Health
665 Huntington Avenue
Boston, MA 02115
617-432-3325

Illinois Educational Resource Center
University of Illinois at Chicago
School of Public Health
PO Box 6998, M/C 922
Chicago, IL 60680
312-996-7887

Johns Hopkins Educational Resource Center
Johns Hopkins University
School of Hygiene and Public Health
615 North Wolfe Street
Baltimore, MD 21205
301-955-3602

Michigan Educational Resource Center
University of Michigan
School of Public Health
Department of Environmental and Industrial Health
Ann Arbor, MI 48109
313-936-0735

Minnesota Educational Resource Center
University of Minnesota
School of Public Health
1158 Mayo Memorial Building
420 Delaware Street, SE
Minneapolis, MN 55455
612-626-0900

New York/New Jersey Educational Resource Center
Department of Community Medicine
Mt. Sinai School of Medicine
PO Box 1057
10 E 102nd Street
New York, NY 10029
212-966-5001

North Carolina Educational Resource Center
University of North Carolina
School of Public Health
Rosenau Hall, CB #7400
Chapel Hill, NC 27599-7410
919-966-5001

Texas Educational Resource Center
The University of Texas Health Science Center at Houston
School of Public Health
PO Box 20186
Houston, TX 77225
713-792-4638

Utah Educational Resource Center
University of Utah
Rocky Mountain Center for Occupational and Environmental Health
Building 512
Salt Lake City, UT 84112
801-581-8719

Washington Educational Resource Center
University of Washington
Department of Environmental Health, SC-34
Seattle, WA 98195
206-543-6991

It is important to note that as the occupational health nurse professionally progresses, the use of technology, in addition to print materials, may be the preferred approach to seek state-of-the-art information.

Nurse-Managed Models in Occupational Health

In 1993, an initiative of the American Nurses Association and the American Association of Occupational Health Nurses about cost-effective health care services resulted in the publication *Innovations at the Worksite* (Burgel, 1993). This document addresses five models of worksite primary health care managed and delivered by occupational health nurses as cost-effective health care providers. These models apply principles of health promotion and risk reduction through continuing integration of these strategies in practice. The goal is to provide quality, accessible, and cost-effective care. Following are brief descriptions of each model.

Model 1: One-Nurse Unit, On-Site

This model may be the best choice for companies with limited resources, few workplace hazards, or a small workforce. The nurse acts as the in-house expert on health-related issues and develops a network of quality, community-based referrals for services not provided in-house.

Model 2: Multiple Nurses, On-Site

This model is ideal for medium to large employers. Essential services are offered on-site in a nurse-managed care center. The focus is on primary care as well as work-related illnesses and injuries.

Model 3: Consortium Model—Company Coalitions

This model is designed for groups of small employers to provide services in a centralized, nurse-managed, free-standing clinic. Essential services are provided on-site during expanded hours of service, with a local hospital providing services during off hours through a preferred provider arrangement.

Model 4: Large Employers with Outreach to Small Employers

This model is best for a large employer with on-site services (as in model 2) that provides services to neighboring small employers through a contractual arrangement.

Model 5: Occupational Health Nurse Consultant

This model focuses on providing services by an occupational health nurse acting as consultant to small employers in geographically scattered locations. The occupational health nurse consultant is on-site at each employer location on a periodic basis, providing some direct services and coordinating other services through a local hospital and nearby specialty providers.

In all of these models, a basic set of services is provided (e.g., direct care, health surveillance, regulatory compliance, case management, health promotion), either directly or by contracted arrangements. However, depending on the model, services may be modified to reflect the need.

Future Expansions

Environmental Health

More than ever before, the importance of integrating environmental health into occupational health nursing practice is well recognized. Environmental health can be defined as the interaction between individual and environmental agents, which may affect health states. The workplace is included because this is the place in which many of the most significant hazards occur. Environmental health has been a concept central to general nursing practice since its beginning. Since that time, the nursing profession has recognized that health is affected by many variables and has engaged a holistic approach to nursing care. Florence Nightingale viewed the environment as a fundamental aspect of nursing practice, and her interventions focused on modifying the environment as a primary means of promoting health. She cited five essential points in securing the health of individuals: pure air, pure water, efficient drainage, cleanliness, and light (Nightingale, 1869). Nightingale believed that the nurse was responsible for identifying any conditions that could affect the health of individuals and populations, such as ventilation, noise, heat, cold, and cleanliness, and responsible for developing ways to alter the environment so that health and healing could flourish. Environmental health is a natural extension of occupational health nurses to identify environmental health hazards, explore their interaction, and work with members of the interdisciplinary team, management, workers, and communities to reduce environmental and occupational health risk (Rogers & Cox, 1998).

The Institute of Medicine issued a report describing the importance of this integration and citing the important link between occupational health nursing and environmental health, which is supported by the professional organization AAOHN (AAOHN, 1998). Occupational health nurses therefore need additional competencies in environmental health, including the following:

- *Understanding the interaction of environmental agents, such as lead and waste products, with human systems, and related signs and symptoms of disease*
- *Developing prevention, protection, and control strategies for environmental health problems, such as indoor air pollution, and using environmental health resources, including information for the Agency for Toxic Substances and Disease Registry*
- *Discussing ethical implications of environmental health exposures such as right to know about community toxic spills*
- *Influencing regulatory controls such as community residential exposures in environmental health as appropriate*

Migrant Health

According to the National Center for Farmworker Health (1999), the migrant population is a diverse one, and its composition varies from region to region. However, it is estimated that 85% of all migrant workers are minorities, of whom most are Hispanic (including Mexican Americans as well as Mexicans, Puerto Ricans, Cubans, and workers from Central and South America). The migrant population also includes African Americans, Jamaicans, Haitians, Laotians, Thais, and other racial and ethnic minorities.

CASE STUDY

Polluted indoor air has become increasingly recognized as a potential public health problem. As an occupational health nurse, you have been asked to assess a small company with 75 workers who manufacture plant food. The workers have complained of headache, eye and throat irritations, and fatigue. Upon assessment, you find the company housed in a 30-year-old building with inconsistent maintenance. The ventilation system is old and has had cooling problems. The workers complain of incon-sistent heating and cooling and "stuffiness." You find a greater-than-expected incidence of asthma, worker sick days, and headaches requiring neurologist care.

1. What are some likely contributing factors to worker illness?

2. What should the nurse suggest that the owner do next in determining the contributing causes to the worker health problems?

3. What role could the occupational health nurse play in the prevention of future problems in this work environment?

Migrant and seasonal farmworkers hand-pick apples or peaches, harvest asparagus or chilies, stake up tomatoes, dig potatoes or beets, or work in a packing plant. Hand labor is especially vital to the production of the blemish-free fruits and vegetables, which American consumers demand. The fruit, vegetable, and horticultural industries in particular rely on the labor of migrant and seasonal farmworkers. Over the last decade, more than 85% of the fruits and vegetables produced in this country were hand harvested and/or cultivated. Although many people believe that fruit and vegetable production is declining in this country, in reality, domestic production has steadily increased over the last decade.

Farm labor is seasonal and intensive. Planting, thinning, and harvesting are not year-round activities. However, they are crucial to crop production, and the time frame in which they must occur is determined by the seasons and the weather. Failure to perform any of these activities at the appropriate time can result in a lost crop. The urgency to accomplish tasks according to nature's timetable compels farmworkers to work in the fields in all seasons and in all weather conditions, including extreme heat, extreme cold, rain, intense sun, and dampness.

Farmworkers' work hours accommodate the crops, not vice versa. Their work often requires stoop labor, working with the soil, climbing, carrying heavy loads, and having direct contact with plants. The plants and the soil are often treated with pesticides and chemical fertilizers. Some plants, such as tobacco and strawberries, exude chemicals that are toxic to humans or that can cause severe allergic reactions such as contact dermatitis. The Environmental Protection Agency estimates that 300,000 farmworkers experience acute pesticide poisoning each year. Anecdotal reports from clinicians indicate that many cases of pesticide poisoning are unreported because clients do not seek treatment or are misdiagnosed because the symptoms of pesticide poisoning can resemble those of viral infection.

Many of the health problems found in the general population, particularly among minorities and the poor, also affect migrant farmworkers. The hardships of life as a farmworker result in unique challenges to the health of these workers and their families.

Some health concerns are clearly attributable to the occupational hazards of farm work. Dermatitis and respiratory problems caused by natural fungi, dusts, and pesticides are common. Lack of safe drinking water contributes to dehydration and heat stroke. Other health conditions such as TB, diabetes, cancer, hypertension, depression, and HIV, which require careful monitoring and frequent treatment, pose a special problem for farmworkers who must move frequently.

Migrant and seasonal workers are a group of workers that could greatly benefit from occupational and environmental health nursing services. This can be done by providing direct care clinic services, educating workers about occupational health and safety hazards, and initiating workplace/community outreach. The occupational and environmental health nurse can have a major impact on health promotion and protection in this vulnerable population of workers.

CONCLUSION

Occupational health nursing is a specialty that provides nursing care to worker populations, creating and sustaining healthy and safe work environments. The specialty practice has grown enormously, encompassing expanded roles as independent practitioners, consultants, and policy makers. Expansion to focus on issues external to traditional workplace settings, including environmental health and migrant health, will be a significant and far-reaching opportunity. Prevention and health promotion are the cornerstones of care in occupational health nursing within an interdisciplinary framework. Research is critical in identifying work-related health issues and testing interventions to mitigate the risk. The specialty focus supports a healthy, productive workforce with not only a quality of work life but also a quality of life.

FYI

Labor Day Holiday—Why Do We Celebrate It?

Labor Day is usually celebrated with barbecues and picnics and is associated with the beginning of school. We rarely remember that Labor Day was created as a way for us to remember the tremendous labor struggles to improve worker conditions in the United States. In the 19th century, workers often worked 16-hour days, 6 and 7 days a week. Children were commonly used as a labor resource. Injuries were common, thousands of workers died, "caught in the grinding machinery of our growing industries" (p. 1319). In the labor market of today, despite improvements, workers continue to die in the workplace, while many more are injured, sometimes for life. We should remember all workers, past and present, on Labor Day. The authors encourage us to remember the "historical toll in lives and limbs that workers have paid to provide us with our modern prosperity . . . the continuing toil is far too high and that workers who died and continue to die in order to produce our wealth" (p. 1320). They deserve to be remembered and honored on Labor Day.

Source: Rosner & Markowitz, 1999.

CRITICAL THINKING ACTIVITIES

1. The next time you go to a fast-food restaurant, observe the potential for occupational hazards in the workers who serve your food. Are there prevention strategies that could prevent those hazards?

2. Ask one of the staff members at your nursing school about workplace hazards in the office. Ask him or her to describe what the most prevalent injury or illness associated with his or her work is. What could be done to prevent this risk?

3. Investigate your nurses association's position on workplace violence in health care. How can nurses protect themselves from this occupational hazard?

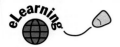 Explore Community Health Nursing on the web! To learn more about the topics in this chapter, use the passcode provided to access your exclusive web site: http://communitynursing.jbpub.com
If you do not have a passcode, you can obtain one at this site.

REFERENCES

American Association of Industrial Nurses (AAIN). (1976). *The nurse in industry.* New York: AAIN.

American Association of Occupational Health Nurses (AAOHN). (1996). *Code of ethics.* Atlanta: AAOHN.

American Association of Occupational Health Nurses (AAOHN). (1998). *Delivery of occupational and environmental health services.* Atlanta: AAOHN.

American Association of Occupational Health Nurses (AAOHN). (1999). *Standards of occupational health nursing practice.* Atlanta: AAOHN.

American Public Health Association. (1996). *The definition and role of public health nursing. A statement of the public health nursing section.* Washington, DC: American Public Health Association.

Brown, M. L. (1981). *Occupational health nursing.* Philadelphia: Springer.

Bureau of Labor Statistics. (1994). *Employment projections: 1994.* Washington, DC: U.S. Department of Labor.

Bureau of Labor Statistics. (1995). *Handbook of labor statistics.* Washington, DC: U.S. Department of Labor.

Bureau of Labor Statistics. (1999). *Employment projections: 1999.* Washington, DC: U.S. Department of Labor.

Burgel, B. (1993). *Innovations at the worksite: delivery of nurse-managed primary care services.* Washington, DC: American Nurses Association.

Centers for Disease Control and Prevention, U.S. Department of Health and Human Services. (1999). *National Institute for Occupational Safety and Health: National Occupational Research Agenda,* Publication Number 99-108. Atlanta: U.S. Government Printing Office.

Department of Health and Human Services (DHHS). (1996). *National Institute for Occupational Safety and Health: National Occupational Research Agenda.* Cincinnati, OH: U.S. Government Printing Office.

Department of Health and Human Services (DHHS). (2000). *Healthy People 2010: Conference edition.* Washington, DC: U.S. Government Printing Office.

Felton, J. (1985). The genesis of American occupational health nursing: Part I. *Occupational Health Nursing, 33,* 615–621.

Godfrey, H. (1978). One hundred years of industrial nursing. *Nursing Times,* Nov. 30, pp. 1966–1969.

Horstman, S. (1992). Industrial hygiene. In J. Last & R. Wallace (Eds.), *Public health and preventative medicine* (13th ed.) (pp. 547–550). Norwalk, CT: Appleton & Large.

Levy, B. & Wegman, D. (1995). *Occupational health: Recognizing and preventing work-related disease.* Boston: Little, Brown.

McGrath, B. J. (1945). Fifty years of industrial nursing. *Public Health Nurse, 37,* 119–124.

National Center for Farmworker Health. (1999). Who are America's farmworkers. Internet: www.NCFH.org.

Nightingale, F. (1869). *Notes on nursing. What it is and what it is not.* New York: Dover Press.

Rogers, B. (1994). *Occupational health nursing: Concepts and practice.* Philadelphia: W. B. Saunders.

Rogers, B., Agnew, J., & Pompeii, L. (2000). Occupational health nursing research priorities. *AAOHN Journal, 48*(1), 9–16.

Rogers, B., & Cox, A. (1998). Expanding horizons: Integrating environmental health in occupational health nursing, *AAOHN Journal, 46,* 9–13.

Rogers, B., Randolph, S., & Mastroianni, K. (1996). *Occupational health nursing guidelines for primary clinical conditions.* Beverly, MA: OEM Press.

Rosner, D., & Markowitz, W. (1999). Labor Day and the war on workers. *American Journal of Public Health,* September, 89(9), 1319–1321.

Slaney, B. (1984). *The development of occupational health nursing.* Philadelphia: W. B. Saunders.

Sluchak, TJ. (1992). Ergonomics: origins, focus, and implementation considerations. *AAOHN J, 40*(3), 105–112, 147–149.

Wright, F. S. (1919). *Industrial nursing.* New York: Macmillan.

Chapter 41

Advanced Nursing Practice in the Community

Mary H. Huch

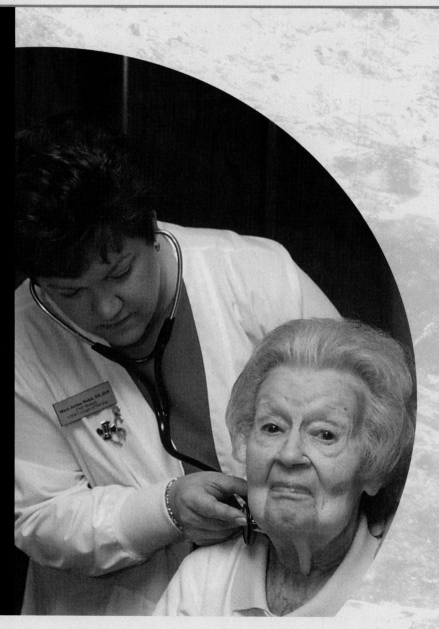

Life's picture is constantly undergoing change. The spirit beholds a new world every moment.

Rumi, Persian Sufi poet

QUESTIONS TO CONSIDER

After reading this chapter, answer the following questions:

1. What is advanced practice nursing?
2. What are the different roles for advanced practice nurses?
3. How have advanced practice roles developed?
4. What are the practice settings for advanced practice nurses?
5. How are advanced practice nurses reimbursed for their services?

KEY TERMS

Advanced practice nurse
Certification
Certified nurse midwives

Certified registered nurse
  anesthetists
Clinical nurse specialists

Nurse practitioners
Primary care

The specific role activities of advanced practice nurses are highly diverse, and role expansion is likely to continue well into the 21st century. New practice settings are emerging daily. These new practice arenas are continually being developed to meet health needs rather than just illness needs. Many people are looking for ways to stay healthy. People want to take control of their lives and health outcomes. The advanced practice nurse roles discussed in this chapter explore the ways these nurses contribute to the health and well-being of many individuals. The advanced practice nurses of the 21st century will be hindered only by their own reluctance to think in creative, innovative ways.

Advanced Practice Defined

The term *advanced practice* has been in the nursing literature for many years. In simplest terms, the **advanced practice nurse** is one whose preparation includes education and experience beyond the entry level for nursing practice.

The categories of providers included under the advanced practice umbrella have changed considerably since the term was first used. Originally, nurse anesthetists and nurse midwives were the only practitioners considered advanced practice nurses. Both specialties were well accepted and commonplace within the nursing profession in the early to mid 20th century. It was not until the 1960s that the roles of the clinical nurse specialist and nurse practitioner were described in the nursing literature.

Presently, four categories of nurse providers are considered advanced practice nurses: **certified registered nurse anesthetists, certified nurse midwives, clinical nurse specialists, and nurse practitioners.** Although all four of these groups are included as advanced practice nurses, the specific practice focus for each

group is quite different (Huch, 1995). See Box 41-1 for definitions of the four advanced practice nurse roles.

The following case studies provide good examples of the range of activities undertaken by advanced practice nurses.

BOX 41-1 DEFINITIONS OF ADVANCED PRACTICE NURSING ROLES

A nurse anesthetist is a registered nurse who completed a program of instruction for managing and sustaining life processes of a client while anesthetized during surgery.

A nurse midwife is a registered nurse who is educated to care for women during pregnancy, delivery, and afterward for issues related to women's health care. The newborn infant is also cared for by the nurse midwife.

A clinical nurse specialist is a registered nurse who has a minimum of a master's degree with study in a specialized area of clinical nursing.

A nurse practitioner is a registered nurse who has advanced educational preparation in the diagnosing, treating, and prescribing of medical therapies for disease processes.

CASE STUDY

Ms. Jones is a 51-year-old woman who comes to a primary care clinic for the first time because she has experienced "hot flashes" and "night sweats" for the past 2 weeks. As her primary care provider, the nurse practitioner elicits a detailed history of what has occurred. The symptoms are extensively explored, along with menstrual history, methods of birth control used, medications taken, and a complete health history. When comprehensive data are obtained, the nurse practitioner does a complete physical examination, including a pelvic examination. Various diagnostic tests are done, such as follicle-stimulating hormone (FSH) and luteinizing hormone (LH) levels, blood chemistries, a lipid profile, liver function studies, and a Pap smear.

Once the nurse practitioner has all of the necessary information, a return appointment with Ms. Jones is scheduled. During the next visit, the nurse practitioner explores what options are available to handle the annoying "hot flashes" and "night sweats" Ms. Jones is continuing to experience. The benefits and risks of hormone replacement therapy are thoroughly discussed with Ms. Jones to assist her in making a decision about beginning hormone replacement therapy. Other health-promotion measures such as a regular mammogram and monthly breast self-examination are also included in the discussion. Daily calcium carbonate supplementation along with regular exercise are prescribed for Ms. Jones. If Ms. Jones is a smoker, this is a good time for her to consider stopping. If Ms. Jones desires it, alternative therapies for dealing with the symptoms are also explored. If the FSH and LH levels are not indicative of the presence of menopause, counseling her on the use of birth control methods is important because pregnancy can occur if she is sexually active. A follow-up visit to the nurse practitioner in 1 to 2 months is scheduled to determine whether the planned therapies are effective in treating Ms. Jones's symptoms.

FYI

Community Clinical Nurse Specialist—A View from the Field

Mr. Smyth is a community clinical nurse specialist with an interest in geriatrics. He contracted with a retirement center to visit twice a week to address the health issues of the residents. Some of his activities include providing instructions on various medications the residents take, giving nutritional guidance to provide for an optimal diet, developing individualized exercise programs, and counseling clients about matters of concern. Besides the individualized information provided, he assesses the community to determine whether problems currently exist or whether there is the potential for the development of problems. The community health clinical nurse specialist's mission is to promote the health of the community. A proactive stance is taken rather than waiting for problems to occur.

The National Council of State Boards of Nursing (1992) established a definition of advanced practice nursing that includes the titles along with the level of learning and experience needed for each role:

> The advanced practice of nursing by nurse practitioners, nurse anesthetists, nurse midwives, and clinical nurse specialists is based on the following: a) knowledge and skills required in basic nursing education; b) licensure as a registered nurse; c) graduate degree and experience in the designated area of practice which includes advanced nursing theory; substantial knowledge of physical and psychosocial assessment; appropriate interventions and management of health care status (p. 22).

Historical Development of Advanced Practice Roles

The roles of advanced practice nurses are always changing. Examining each group of providers from a historical perspective provides a clearer understanding of the distinct roles and leads to an exploration of the usual work settings.

Certified Registered Nurse Anesthetists

The nurse anesthetist is one who, with advanced education, is responsible for keeping a client insensible to pain while maintaining vital functions during surgery. Nurses have long been involved in administering anesthesia in hospitals and outpatient surgery centers. As early as 1877, nurses administered anesthesia at St. Vincent's Hospital in Erie, Pennsylvania (Garde, 1996; Thatcher, 1984).

FYI

Nurse practitioners wrote 15 million prescriptions in 1998, up 66% from 1997. Nurse practitioners can write prescriptions in all 50 states and the District of Columbia, although in some states, a physician is required to co-sign the order.

The American Nurse, September/October 1999, 31(5), 8.

Certified Nurse Midwives

Mary Breckinridge, a British-trained nurse midwife, recognized the need for well-prepared midwives in rural Appalachia. She established the Frontier Nursing Service in 1925 and used British-trained nurse midwives because so few American nurse midwives were available. Traveling by horseback, these nurses helped with births and provided care for all women and babies in their assigned districts (Burkhardt, 1996; *Frontier Nursing Service*, 1997). From these humble beginnings, certified nurse midwives made a significant impact on reducing infant and maternal mortality.

In 1995, the American College of Nurse-Midwives (ACNM) was formed to meet the professional needs of nurse midwives. This group began to focus on the care of normal newborns and women (Burkhardt, 1996). Many contemporary nurse midwives practice in neighborhood health centers in urban and rural areas to provide total health care for women of all ages (Dorroh & Norton, 1996).

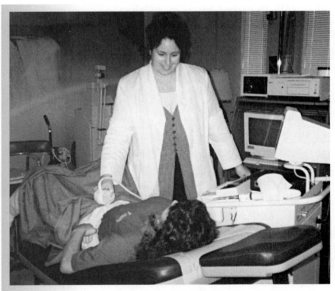

Family nurse practitioner conducting sonogram of a prenatal client.

Clinical Nurse Specialists

In the late 1960s, the nursing literature included many articles about clinical nurse specialists and nurse clinicians. About this time, nurses began to enroll in greater numbers in graduate programs of study and to focus on a particular area of practice (Georgopoulos & Christman, 1970; Reiter, 1966). It was shortly thereafter that the American Nurses Association provided a definition of the clinical nurse specialist, stating that the nurse possessed a master's degree and an area of clinical concentration (ANA, 1976).

For many years, acute care settings provided the primary area for employment of most clinical specialists. An exception to this acute care focus was the psychiatric clinical nurse specialist (Boyle, 1996). Within the acute care setting, the clinical specialist had a medical-surgical nursing focus, whereas the psychiatric clinical nurse specialist functioned in both inpatient and outpatient settings. Over time, the role of clinical nurse specialists has changed, and today they can be found in a wider variety of places: acute care settings (general units and intensive care units), rehabilitation centers, home health care, schools, and community settings (Daly & Mitchell, 1996; Good, 1992).

The community health clinical nurse specialist has a focus on the community as a whole rather than the individuals who constitute the community. This nurse tries to ascertain which individuals are in the high-risk populations. These activities are accomplished from the perspective of the entire community. The steps of the nursing process are used in promoting, maintaining, protecting, and restoring health of the populace. In addition, efforts are directed toward disease and disability prevention (Association of Community Health Nursing Educators, 1991).

Nurse Practitioners

In the 1960s, nurse faculty member, Loretta Ford, EdD, RN, from the University of Colorado School of Nursing, and Henry Silver, MD, from the University of Colorado School of Medicine, developed a postbaccalaureate pediatric nurse practitioner program at the University of Colorado. The faculty was intimately involved in evaluating nurses in this expanded role (Ford & Silver, 1967). These early nurse practitioners were taught new skills, such as using an otoscope and doing urinalysis, that today have become common activities for all nurses. A 20-month period of clinical training followed an intense 4-month period of classroom instruction. One important component of the nurse practitioner's education was the development of the ability to decide when the situation was beyond his or her scope of practice and to make the appropriate referral (see Conversation with box on p. 978).

From these origins, various other nurse practitioner programs have been instituted throughout the United States. Many early programs awarded a certificate at the completion of a course of study that varied from a few weeks to as long as 2 years. As the role of nurse practitioner gained greater acceptance, more programs were offered at the master's level. By the late 1990s, it was necessary to have a master's degree to take most nurse practitioners certification examinations. The following Research Brief shows how nurse practitioners are viewed by the recipients of their care.

RESEARCH BRIEF

Langner, S. R., & Hutelmyer, C. (1995). Patient satisfaction with outpatient human immunodeficiency virus care as delivered by nurse practitioners and physicians, Holistic Nursing Practice, 10, 54–60.

A survey was undertaken of 53 HIV-positive clients who visited an ambulatory care clinic. The questionnaire asked for ratings of satisfaction with the care providers—nurse practitioners, interns, residents, or internal medicine staff physicians. In general, nurse practitioners were rated considerably more favorably than the physicians by this group of clients. One reason that may account for the difference was that nurse practitioners cared for the clients on a consistent basis, whereas the house physicians rotated through the clinic and did not know the clients as well. It was more likely that a client would see the same nurse practitioner at each visit, but not very likely that the client would see the same physician each time. Concerning client education, nurse practitioners were seen more favorably (72% versus 58%) than physicians. Nurse practitioners have a strong focus on client teaching, and this could account for the difference in ratings. This study makes clear the importance of continuity of care and client education in client satisfaction with a caregiver.

Education Issues and Scope of Practice

Although there are some similarities in educational preparation, the scope of practice for each role is different. Each of these advanced practice nurses functions in a different way when providing care for clients.

Certified Registered Nurse Anesthetists

Although this group of providers is included under the title of advanced practice nurses, they do not ordinarily practice in a community setting. Information related to education and scope of practice can be obtained from the American Association of Nurse Anesthetists.

Certified Nurse Midwives

Pathways to becoming a midwife are quite varied today. Some programs are available for non-nurses who take the national examination and then become certified midwives. These individuals include physicians' assistants, family physicians, and other non-nurse learners (Burkhardt, 1996). Three types of programs are available to registered nurses who want to become certified nurse midwives. An education outcome can be precertification, a certificate (requires a bachelor's degree), or a graduate program.

Graduates of these nursing programs are eligible to sit for the certification examination of the ACNM, and the graduates are identified as certified nurse midwives.

The ACNM has been active in setting guidelines for directing the practice of all midwives. Midwives care for women during the antenatal, intrapartal, and postpartal periods and also care for their newborns after delivery. Midwives play a large part in family planning and gynecological care.

Whatever the educational background, certified nurse midwives are an essential force in providing better outcomes for pregnant women and their infants. Because of the focus on preventive care, nurse-midwifery practice has resulted in lower rates of infant mortality (ACNM, 1997; Dorroh & Norton, 1996).

Clinical Nurse Specialists

The clinical nurse specialist has had the most consistency in educational preparation of all the advanced practice nurses. This specialty evolved to provide a means for master's prepared nurses to remain clinically active and to decrease fragmented client care. Until the development of this role, masters'-prepared nurses generally became educators or administrators.

Nurse educators were responsive to this role and supported it from its inception. The strong focus on providing client care lent credibility to the usefulness of this role. The 1964 Nurse Training Act provided financial support for nurses wishing to become clinical nurse specialists. Receiving financial support made it easier for a nurse to return to school for a master's degree. The funding also provided tuition and a monthly stipend to assist with living expenses (Hamric, 1989).

No certificate programs exist that prepare for this role, although some agencies confer a similar title on nurses who work in a specialized area. Some of these titles are nurse clinician, nurse specialist, and clinical nurse. However, without a master's degree, these nurses should not call themselves clinical nurse specialists.

Beyond advanced study of a clinical practice area, the clinical nurse specialist curriculum focuses on specific competencies to be acquired for future practice. These competencies include being an expert practitioner, educator, consultant, and researcher. The clinical nurse specialist uses these competencies to improve the quality of life of the client or community (Hamric, Spross, & Hanson, 1996).

Clinical nurse specialists can be found in many practice arenas. As an expert practitioner, the clinical nurse specialist provides critical thinking, expert decision making, a high level of clinical judgment, and skill in determining care for selected clients or populations. Because of the preparation at the master's level, this nurse brings a wealth of advanced knowledge to the practice arena.

The community health clinical nurse specialist provides instruction for staff, consumers, and the community because education is at the forefront of clinical activities for this practitioner. Staff instruction can occur in planned or informal settings. When an unexpected teaching situation arises, the clinical nurse specialist acts to provide needed information for the staff or care recipient. The clinical nurse specialist may meet the learning needs of consumers by providing information on newly available therapies or means to improve the health of a community (Kupina, 1995).

As a consultant, the clinical nurse specialist is called on to share some expert knowledge with other professionals who are possibly from a complementary discipline. In this role, the clinical nurse specialist must not only provide information and possible recommendations for action, but should also help the other professionals develop their own problem-solving skills. It is always important that the consultant not promise more than can be delivered. To do so is a sure way of losing credibility (Menard, 1987).

The role of the researcher involves a range of activities. Research activities can range from something as simple as looking up treatment methods based on studies done by another person to something as complex as being fully responsible for all aspects of a research study. Although the clinical nurse specialist may be called on by other researchers to assist in data gathering, it is more likely that he or she would be the one developing and implementing the research study. Because of educational preparation at the master's level, the clinical nurse specialist should have the academic preparation to fully engage in research studies.

Clinical nurse specialists can be found in many practice sites. Health care settings employ clinical nurse specialists to provide the in-depth knowledge base needed for complex client care. Both children and adults are the recipients of this specialized knowledge base. As with other areas in nursing practice, the clinical nurse specialist is becoming even more specialized. The clinical nurse specialist is now an integral part of many critical care units. The role of the psychiatric specialist has moved beyond the traditional inpatient and outpatient settings into the home (Ward-Miller, 1996).

One of the most positive aspects of this movement is that the nurse can see clients in their own environment. Community health clinical specialists have the unique ability to merge nursing practice and public health to affect the health of the community. Another vital activity of the clinical nurse specialist in the community is functioning as a case manager (Daly & Mitchell, 1996; Good, 1992).

These advanced practice nurses can be found in some private and joint practices with physicians. The community health clinical specialist has much to offer in implementing a community-based model of care. Independent practice is an area in which the community health clinical specialist can be of value. The community health clinical nurse specialist will play a vital role in the public's health as we continue in the 21st century.

The role of the community health clinical nurse specialist is well explicated in the writings of Robinson, Mead, and Boswell (1995). These clinical specialists at the Portland Veterans Affairs Medical Center took part in the role evolution of the community health coordinators. Three areas were the target population for their services; namely, home health, extended care screening, and contracted community nursing home care. They provided for a smooth transition from the hospital to the community and helped overcome some barriers to comprehensive health care.

Nurse Practitioners

As with most of the other advanced practice nurses, educational pathways have been variable for nurse practitioners. The first educational programs occurred out of the mainstream of higher educational institutions. Rogers (1972) was an outspoken critic of nurse practitioner programs, insisting they were not nursing practice, but medical practice. Other nursing leaders at the time held a similar viewpoint. Often, in these early programs, graduates received a certificate upon completion of their studies even when instruction took place within a university setting (Huch, 1992).

It was during the 1970s that concerted efforts were made to establish standards for the education of nurse practitioners. The National League for Nursing took the lead and stated that a nurse practitioner should have a master's degree as the outcome of the educational program. The National Organization of Nurse Practitioner Faculties (NONPF) has established accreditation criteria for nurse practitioner educational programs (NONPF, 1997). By the late 1990s, almost all education programs for nurse practitioners were in higher education settings, with a master's degree awarded upon completion of the program. Only a few certificate programs remain in the United States today.

As with the first practitioners, the **primary care** setting is where the greatest abundance of practitioners can be found. Primary care is any setting that accords the first entry into the health care system. Practice sites include pediatric, adult health, geriatric, obstetrical/gynecological, and family care clinics (Hawkins & Thibodeau, 1996). According to a survey in *The Nurse Practitioner* (1997), ambulatory care settings employ approximately 91% of nurse practitioners.

A more recent trend (early to mid-1990s) is the development of acute care nurse practitioners. The number of medical residents available to provide care in the acute care setting was declining; thus, a need for another caregiver was created. To meet the need, many universities began acute care nurse practitioner programs. Approximately 7% of nurse practitioners (*The Nurse Practitioner,* 1997) are employed in inpatient settings. The goal for this practitioner, as with other nurse practitioners, is to provide high-quality, cost-effective care and to do so from a nursing perspective.

Within these various settings, nurse practitioners assist clients in managing illness through diagnosis and pharmacological and nonpharmacological means, providing health-promotion teaching, and counseling. Nurse practitioners in all states except Ohio have some measure of prescriptive authority, but the extent of that authority is quite variable (Lancaster & Lancaster, 1993). Some states allow the nurse practitioner to legally prescribe any drug without requiring a collaborative physician. Some states limit nurse practitioners to writing prescriptions only for noncontrolled drugs, but still without requiring a collaborating physician. Yet other states require a physician's signature along with the nurse's for both noncontrolled and controlled substances (Pearson, 1999).

Each state's nurse practice act regulates the specific scope of practice for this subgroup of advanced practice nurses. The rules and regulations of the state board of nursing further delineate the legal activities for the nurse. Nurse practitioners should consult the legal statutes for the states in which they plan to practice.

Healthy People 2010

The objectives of *Healthy People 2010* provide a blueprint for the practice of community health clinical specialists and primary care nurse practitioners into the 21st century and beyond. The following box lists a sample of *Healthy People 2010* objectives that community health clinical nurse specialists and nurse practitioners can use.

Credentials

Credentialing is the process of obtaining a certificate or diploma attesting to a predetermined fact. Most advanced practice nurses are required to have certification showing that a minimal competency level has been achieved. The **certification** process involves the submission of evidence of completion of a program of study, verification of a minimum number of clinical practice hours, the application for the certification examination, and documentation of a current registered nurse license. Six different certification boards offer certification examinations for the various categories of advanced practice nurses.

The American Association of Nurse Anesthetists Council on Certification of Nurse Anesthetists is the certifying body for nurse anesthetists. The Division of Accreditation that accredits educational programs of the ACNM oversees nurse midwifery educational programs. The ACNM Certification Council administers the national certification examination (Varney, 1987). The Certification Council also administers an examination to non-nurse midwives, although they are designated as clinical midwives rather than clinical nurse midwives.

The American Nurses Credentialing Center (ANCC) administers many certification examinations to clinical specialists and nurse practitioners. For a nurse to be eligible for one of these examinations, specific clinical preparation in the examination area is needed. Applicants can be certified in more than one area if they meet the educational and practice requirements of the examination. Many states require that nurse practitioners be certified before recognizing them as advanced practice nurses with prescribing privileges. Generally, clinical nurse specialists do not have to meet the same certification requirement for practice. The ANCC has certification examinations for community health clinical nurse specialists. The candidates for this examination must have a master's degree or higher and a stipulated number of practice hours. This examination is a cooperative effort with the American Public Health Association, Public Health Nursing Section (ANCC, 1999)

A nurse practitioner can be certified in more than one area through ANCC, but it is also possible to be certified by a different group. The American Academy of Nurse Practitioners administers a national certifying examination for adult and family nurse practitioners. Individual state boards of nursing make the determination of which certifying examination will be recognized.

The National Association of Pediatric Nurse Associates and Nurse Practitioners (NAPNAP) provides the certification mech-

HEALTHY PEOPLE 2010

SAMPLE OBJECTIVES TO BE USED BY NURSE PRACTITIONERS AND COMMUNITY HEALTH CLINICAL NURSE SPECIALISTS

Access to Quality Health Services
Primary Care

1.4   Increase the proportion of persons who have a specific source of ongoing care.

1.5   Increase the proportion of persons with a usual primary care provider.

Arthritis, Osteoporosis, and Chronic Back Conditions

2.7   Increase the proportion of adults who have seen a health care provider for their chronic joint symptoms.

Cancer

3.11   Increase the proportion of women who receive a Pap test.

3.12   Increase the proportion of adults who receive a colorectal cancer screening examination.

Diabetes

5.4   Increase the proportion of adults with diabetes whose condition has been diagnosed.

5.14   Increase the proportion of adults with diabetes who have at least an annual foot examination.

Immunization and Infectious Diseases
Infectious Diseases and Emerging Antimicrobial Resistance

14.12 Increase the proportion of all tuberculosis patients who complete curative therapy within 12 months.

14.18 Reduce the number of courses of antibiotics for ear infections for young children.

Maternal, Infant, and Child
Prenatal Care

16.6   Increase the proportion of pregnant women who receive early and adequate prenatal care.

Risk Factors

16.10 Reduce low birth weight (LBW) and very low birth weight (VLBW).

16.11 Reduce preterm births.

Mental Health and Mental Disorders
Treatment Expansion

18.6   Increase the number of persons seen in primary care who receive mental health screening and assessment.

Source: DHHS, 2000.

anism for pediatric nurse practitioners. Similar requirements described for the other groups hold for this application process.

The National Certification Corporation (NCC) offers certification in women's health (OB/GYN) and neonatal nursing. This group reviews course content, clinical experiences, and learning activities to decide whether a nurse is qualified to take the examination.

Reimbursement
Medicare
Medicare is the U.S. federally funded health insurance program for elders and persons with disabilities. Advanced practice nurses should be adequately compensated for the care they provide, but federal law regulates who can be compensated and in what amount (Lancaster & Lancaster, 1993). Safriet (1992) advanced the position that advanced practice nurses should be adequately compensated for their services, and until this is done, there will be a barrier to effective use of advanced practice nurses.

The Rural Nursing Incentive Act of 1991 provided funds for direct reimbursement of nurse practitioners and clinical nurse specialists practicing in rural areas. The Omnibus Budget Reconciliation Act (OBRA) made provision for indirect reimbursement to nurse practitioners and clinical nurse specialists. With indirect reimbursement, a physician must also been involved in the care of the client for payment of funds to occur. Legislative appropriation of these reimbursement funds led to an increase in the number of nurse practitioner positions.

The Balanced Budget Act of 1997 (Section 4511) brought about a major change in Medicare reimbursement practices. Nurse practitioners and clinical nurse specialists were eligible for direct reimbursement for services without regard for the setting of the practice. The intent of the law was to provide cost-effective, quality care to all U.S. citizens.

Medicaid

Medicaid programs are joint federal and state efforts to provide for the health care needs of low-income persons of an individual state. The federal government provides matching funds to each state, but the state is the body that sets specific guidelines for its program. Benefits offered through Medicaid are highly variable depending on the state. Advanced practice nurses are eligible to receive reimbursement based on individual state statutes.

Likewise, certified registered nurse anesthetists and certified nurse midwives can file applications for reimbursement to the appropriate funding source. It is important that all states enact legislation to provide for nondiscrimination of health care providers when performing services within their scope of practice (Safriet, 1992).

Private Insurance

Guidelines for reimbursement for advanced practice nurses are highly variable due to the many private insurance plans in existence in the United States. The plans sometimes include the nurse provider in the preferred provider network, but other times, the advanced practice nurse is viewed as outside the network; generally less coverage is then afforded for the nurse's services. This places an undue burden on those with minimal resources. More and more networks are seeking to include nurse practitioners among their credentialed providers (Kremer & Faut-Callahan, 1998).

Of particular concern when discussing reimbursement issues is the fact that advanced practice nurses often receive less payment than a physician when the same service is provided. Advanced practice nurses have been shown to provide high-quality care that is equivalent to that provided by physicians. Therefore, advanced practice nurses should be paid an equitable fee for services. Efforts of organized nursing must continue to be directed toward correcting these inequities (Safriet, 1992).

Role Differentiation

The specific role functions of clinical nurse specialists and nurse practitioners are somewhat blurred as these roles continue to evolve within the health care arena. Nurse practitioners originally practiced in primary care settings in the community, and clinical nurse specialists provided services within an acute care setting. An exception to this pattern was the community health clinical specialist who had a focus on individuals, families, and groups within the community. This health care provider was positioned to be a leader in meeting public health needs.

Because of declining revenues within the higher education setting, administrators are examining ways of consolidating programs for greater cost-effectiveness. Although advanced practice nurses are moving into a greater variety of practice settings, research is show-ing that there are many similarities between the roles of nurse practitioners and clinical specialists (Elder & Bullough, 1990; Fenton & Brykczynski, 1993; Forbes, Rafson, Spross, & Kozlowski, 1990; Hunsberger, Mitchell, Blatz, Paes, Pinelli, Southwell, French, & Soluk, 1992; Schroer, 1991; Sheehy & McCarthy, 1998).

There are some marked benefits and liabilities to the merger of these roles. By merging the titles, the number of advanced practice nurses under one title would increase considerably (Schroer, 1991). The clinical nurse specialists could potentially increase their scope of practice to include prescriptive privileges and thus benefit from direct reimbursement from third-party payers (Page & Arena, 1994). One liability of a combined role is the need to lengthen programs of study to provide enough time to truly develop the new role. Given that so many graduate students attend class part-time because of job and family commitments, it seems this would be a major burden on these students. Time will tell whether this role merging will continue or whether there will be a clearer delineation of the roles.

Practice Arenas
Acute Care Settings

All four types of advanced practice nurses can be found in acute care settings. In each instance, the nurse has specialized education and experience to fulfill the roles. As an expert practitioner, the clinical nurse specialist may be found on a general hospital unit such as neurology, oncology, or pediatrics. Often, the clinical nurse specialist will become even more specialized and practice only in a neonatal intensive care unit or a specialized adult critical care unit.

Nurse practitioners prepared for practice in acute care settings are working with groups of clients to manage care while the individuals are hospitalized. Some nurse practitioners have hospital admitting privileges and see clients in both the acute care and primary care settings. Often, the acute care practitioners are "on call" and respond to the unexpected events that can occur during hospitalization.

Hospitals or groups of emergency department physicians employ nurse practitioners to see persons who come to the emergency department when the situation does not warrant emergency treatment. This setting is known as a *fast track*. These practitioners may be prepared as acute care nurse practitioners, adult nurse practitioners, emergency nurse practitioners, or family nurse practitioners. Individuals with acute problems such as sore throats, earaches, low back pain, or diarrhea are seen by these practitioners. After a thorough examination, the problem is treated and usually resolves relatively quickly. The emergency department staff physicians see those persons with urgent problems. If the nurse practitioner finds a more complex situation than originally determined, the emergency physician may be consulted or the person may be transferred to the care of the physician.

Clinics

Primary care clinics (places of first entry into the health care system) have long been the sites of care of certified nurse midwives and nurse practitioners. For many people in rural or economi-

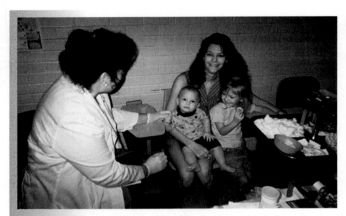

Family nurse practitioners (FNPs) see patients across the life span.

cally depressed areas, advanced practice nurses may be the only resource for health care. Any of the specialties of nurse practitioners focusing on primary care may be found in health care clinics. Funding for health clinics may be provided by state or federal governments and at times a combination of the two. Other clinics are funded through private sources. Private sources include foundations, groups of individuals, and single owners. It is common for a nurse practitioner or group of practitioners to open a health clinic to serve the general public (Sheehy & McCarthy, 1998). These clinics often have a strong focus on health teaching in addition to providing care for individuals with acute illnesses. For persons with stable chronic illnesses, the nurse practitioner can follow and treat according to accepted protocols.

A growing trend is for nurse practitioners to be hired by physicians who have a specialty practice. Orthopedic surgeons may have a collaborating nurse practitioner who may do the initial history and physical examination, make rounds at the hospital, do client teaching, and provide follow-up. Gastroenterologists have hired nurse practitioners to do sigmoidoscopies in addition to history and physical examinations, as well as follow-up with stable clients. These are just two examples of other areas where nurse practitioners may be found.

An important group of clinics that must be considered is those administered by the National Health Service Corps (NHSC), which is part of the U.S. Public Health Service. The NHSC is charged with providing primary health care to underserved areas. Those communities with the greatest need are targeted to receive services. Nurse practitioners and some other groups of health care providers can receive financial assistance for their education, while making a commitment to work in an underserved area.

The Indian Health Service (IHS) is another agency of the U.S. Public Health Service that provides health care to Native Americans. Various types of clinics are established as needs are identified. Nurse practitioners often serve as primary care providers for the Native American population. The nurse-managed clinics usually have a cost savings over the alternative of a physician-managed clinic or a visit to the emergency department (Berry, 1997).

Long-Term Care Facilities

Many residents of long-term care facilities are frail elders. Changes in health status can occur quickly because so many of them have more than one chronic disease. Regular, routine medical visits are mandated by federal regulations to provide cost-effective, quality care. The regulations allow for a nurse practitioner and physician to share a nursing home practice; thus, the residents receive an enhanced level of care. The knowledge base of advanced practitioners can be a means of securing needed care before complications occur. While practicing in long-term care facilities, the advanced practice nurse also serves as a role model and teacher to the nursing home staff (Snyder & Mirr, 1995).

Educational Institutions

Advanced practice nurses bring a wealth of information to the school health setting. At one time, the nurse was the person who applied a bandage and had students lie on a cot until they felt better. Nurses are now involved in many aspects of health promotion for students. (Chapter 39 furnishes a broader discussion of the school health nurse role.) In many states, school-based clinics that provide primary health care for the students and their families have been established. Services range from providing care for minor illnesses and injuries to family planning and pregnancy counseling. Most of these school-based clinics are managed by nurse practitioners.

Nurse practitioners are also commonly found in college health centers as first-line providers of care. Within these settings, the full gamut of nurse practitioner functioning is called into play. The college health center, like any other primary care clinic, offers a range of services from physical examinations, treatment for minor illnesses, x-ray examinations, and dispensing of pharmaceuticals, to counseling for problems.

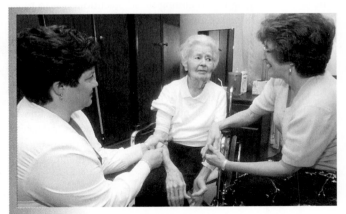

Dr. Mary Huch, chapter author (right), adult nurse practitioner, with elder client in long-term care facility.

Innovations in Health Care Delivery in the Community

Nursing Centers

The need for an alternative way of meeting the health care needs of underserved citizens throughout this country prompted nursing faculty in schools of nursing to open nursing centers. Both clinical nurse specialists and nurse practitioners are critical to the operation of these centers. Nursing centers have multiple purposes that include providing direct client care, functioning as a site for faculty clinical practice, and providing clinical experiences for both graduate and undergraduate students. Health teaching, routine physical examinations, maternal-infant care, primary care services, and counseling are some of the services provided by these centers. Funding for nursing centers is provided in many ways, including grant funds, private payment, Medicare, Medicaid, private insurance, and private donors. In some centers, there is no fee for services, but other centers do charge fees as either a flat fee or on a sliding scale. Nursing centers are often located in places that are more accessible to those who are uninsured or underinsured (Watson, 1996).

Case Management

The increased cost of care delivery and earlier discharge of clients from hospitals has opened the door for nurses to help clients through the maze known as health care delivery. Determining measurable, realistic outcomes takes a person with advanced knowledge. Advanced practice nurses are well positioned to serve as case managers, which may include interactions while clients are well, during hospitalization, and after discharge. Case managers strive to increase self-care abilities in the most cost-effective manner (Papenhausen, 1990). Community health clinical nurse specialists are often case managers. Home health agencies are an ideal work setting in which to implement this advanced practice nursing role (Zwanziger, Peterson, Lethlean, Hernke, Finley, DeGroot, & Busman, 1996).

Holistic Practice

One of the emerging trends among nurse practitioners is to function from a holistic perspective, moving beyond traditional medical therapies. What this means is that traditional care is provided along with what are known as *complementary approaches.* The complementary approaches include massage therapy, acupuncture, relaxation techniques, herbal therapy, meditation, and prayer. (Chapter 16 explores complementary health practices in great detail.) To use such therapies effectively, all nurses must have additional knowledge of the effects and hazards of selected approaches. Advanced education and the autonomy of independent practice make advanced practice nurses effective advocates for these therapies.

A CONVERSATION WITH . . .

Dr. Loretta Ford, who with Dr. Henry Silver started the first nurse practitioner program in 1965 at the University of Colorado Health Sciences Center, was asked to share some thoughts about advanced practice nurses.

"Have advanced nurse practitioners contributed to improved outcomes in health care?"

"Advanced practice nurses have contributed positively to improved outcomes in health care by putting "health" back into a medicalized system through the advanced practice nurses' orientation, preparation, commitment, and scholarship in professional nursing principles of prevention, patient education and empowerment, and political acumen in changing the systems of care."

"Advanced practice nurses have provided quality care while decreasing costs of service, and though some data have been collected on cost savings, more needs to be done. Longitudinal studies are especially needed to document behavioral changes in patients' lifestyles, use of health care services, and outcomes. Common sense would tell that the different costs of professional education, pay scales, role flexibility of advanced practice nurses as well as the growing recognition that many so-called health problems are not medical in nature and require different approaches."

"The practice arenas for advanced practice nurses increased very rapidly in recent years. Do you think this will affect the scope of practice in the future?"

"The scope of nursing practice has been expanding since the early 1900s and there's no reason to suspect it will diminish. Indeed, it will expand rather wildly. The expansions in knowledge and technology, communication, transportation, etc. will not only enlarge the scope of practice, but open many avenues of practice heretofore not imagined or even dreamed of. The challenge will be for professional nursing to envision the future in its broadest configuration and begin the preparation of those who will inherit the future. Advanced practice nurses who are creating the future will leave a legacy of knowledge, research, and philosophical thought upon which future generations can build. There's no time to lose, 'carpe diem.'"

—Loretta Ford, EdD, RN, FAAN
Personal communication, March 1998.

CONCLUSION

Although the nurse practitioner role is a relatively new one, dramatic progress has been made in the evolution and implementation of the advanced practice nurse. The historical development of the role has been shaped by consumer and system demands and has faced role challenges from within the nursing profession and with other health care professionals. Advanced practice nurses can now function in all 50 states.

The move to more standardized educational preparation has become a reality. Licensure and certification issues will remain concerns and challenges for the advance practice nurse in the community health setting. With full integration into the health care delivery system, the advance practice nurse provides quality health care to diverse populations in varied settings in the promotion of health.

CRITICAL THINKING ACTIVITIES

1. Mr. Johnson is an 85-year-old, widowed nursing home resident. He has lost 20 pounds over 4 months. He is very close to his ideal body weight. He is able to eat, but he often refuses to do so, even when the staff attempts to feed him. Occasionally, he drinks a nutritional supplement that is left at his bedside. Mr. Johnson is cognitively aware of his surroundings, although he often just closes his eyes when a care provider approaches. His family wants everything possible to be done for him, including insertion of a feeding tube. Mr. Johnson does not verbally express his wishes about the feeding tube placement. As the clinical nurse specialist in the nursing home you are called to work with Mr. Johnson and his family. What course of action would you take in this situation?

2. Explore the similarities and differences in the roles of advanced practice nurses.

3. Appraise the value of advanced practice nurses being reimbursed by third-party payers for client care visits.

4. Research how people decide who their primary care provider will be.

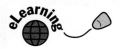

Explore Community Health Nursing on the web! To learn more about the topics in this chapter, use the passcode provided to access your exclusive web site: http://communitynursing.jbpub.com
If you do not have a passcode, you can obtain one at this site.

REFERENCES

American College of Nurse Midwives. (1997). Midwifery education. www.acmn.org/educ/doacnmpr.htm.

American Nurses Association, Congress on Nursing Practice. (1976). *Description of practice: Clinical nurse specialist.* Kansas City, MO: ANA.

American Nurses Credentialing Center (ANCC). (1999). Certification catalog. www.nursingworld.org/ancc/certify/catalogs/1999/cs99/cccscomm.htm.

Association of Community Health Nursing Educators. (1991). *Essentials of master's level nursing education for advanced community health nursing practice.* Louisville, KY: Author.

Berry, R. A. (1997). A nurse practitioner-managed after-hours clinic for a Native American reservation. *Journal of the American Academy of Nurse Practitioners, 9,* 165–170.

Boyle, D. M. (1996). The clinical nurse specialist. In A. B. Hamric, J. A. Spross, & C. M. Hanson (Eds.), *Advanced nursing practice: An integrative approach* (pp. 299–336). Philadelphia: W. B. Saunders.

Burkhardt, P. (1996). Nurse midwifery: Advanced practice nursing? *Nursing Clinics of North America, 31,* 439–448.

Daly, C. M., & Mitchell, R. D. (1996). Case management in the community setting. *Nursing Clinics of North America, 31,* 527–534.

Dorroh, M., & Norton, S. F. (1996). The certified nurse-midwife. In A. B. Hamric, J. A. Spross, & C. M. Hanson (Eds.), *Advanced nursing practice: An integrative approach* (pp. 395–420). Philadelphia: W. B. Saunders.

Elder, R. G., & Bullough, B. (1990). Nurse practitioners and clinical nurse specialists: Are the roles merging? *Clinical Nurse Specialist, 4,* 78–84.

Fenton, M. V., & Brykczynski, K. A. (1993). Qualitative distinctions and similarities in the practice of clinical nurse specialists and nurse practitioners. *Journal of Professional Nursing, 9,* 313–326.

Forbes, K. E., Rafson, J, Spross, J. A., & Kozlowski, D. (1990). The clinical nurse specialist and nurse practitioner: Core curriculum survey results. *Clinical Nurse Specialist, 4,* 63–66.

Ford, L. C. (1998). Personal communication. March, 1998.

Ford, L. C., & Silver, H. K. (1967). The expanded role of the nurse in child care. *Nursing Outlook, 15*(8), 43–5.

Frontier Nursing Service. (1997). Available via Internet: www.achiever.com/freehgmp/kynurses/fns.html.

Garde, J. F. (1996). The nurse anesthesia profession. A past, present, and future perspective. *Nursing Clinic of North America, 31,* 567–580.

Georgopoulos, B. S., & Christman, L. (1970). The clinical nurse specialist: A role model. *American Journal of Nursing, 70,* 1030–1039.

Good, M. E. (1992). The clinical nurse specialist in the school setting: Case management of migrant children with dental disease. *Clinical Nurse Specialist, 6,* 72–76.

Hamric, A. B. (1989). History and overview of the CNS role. In A. B. Hamric & J. A. Spross (Eds.), *The clinical nurse specialist in theory and practice* (2nd ed.) (pp. 3–18). Philadelphia: W. B. Saunders.

Hamric, A. B., Spross, J. A., & Hanson, C. M. (1996). *Advanced nursing practice: An integrative approach.* Philadelphia: W. B. Saunders.

Hawkins, J. W., & Thibodeau, J. A. (1996). *The advanced practice nurse* (4th ed.). New York: Tiresias Press.

Huch, M. H. (1992). Nurse practitioners and physician assistants: Are they the same? *Nursing Science Quarterly, 5,* 52–53.

Huch, M. H. (1995). Nursing sciences as a basis for advanced practice. *Nursing Science Quarterly, 8,* 6–7.

Hunsberger, M., Mitchell, A., Blatz, S., Paes, B., Pinelli, J., Southwell, D., French, S., & Soluk, R. (1992). Definition of an advanced nursing practice role in the NICU: The clinical nurse specialist/neonatal practitioner. *Clinical Nurse Specialist, 6,* 91–96.

Kremer, M. J., & Faut-Callahan, M. (1998). Reimbursement for expanded professional nursing practice services. In C. M. Sheehy & M. C. McCarthy (Eds.), *Advanced practice nursing: Emphasizing common roles.* Philadelphia: F. A. Davis.

Kupina, P. S. (1995). Community health CNSs and health care in the year 2000. *Clinical Nurse Specialist, 9,* 188–190, + 198.

Lancaster, J. & Lancaster, W. (1993). Nurse practitioners: Health care providers whose time has come. *Community Health, 16*(2), 1–8.

Langner, S. R., & Hutelmyer, C. (1995). Patient satisfaction with outpatient human immunodeficiency virus care as delivered by nurse practitioners and physicians. *Holistic Nursing Practice, 10,* 54–60.

Menard, S. W. (1987) The CNS as consultant. In S. W. Menard (Ed.). *The Clinical Nurse Specialist.* (pp. 127–143). New York: John Wiley and Sons.

National Center for Health Statistics (1999) *Healthy People 2000 Review, 1989-99.* Hyattsville, MD: Public Health Service.

National Council of State Boards of Nursing. (1992). *National council of state boards of nursing position paper on the licensure of advanced nursing practice.* Chicago: NCSBN.

National Organization of Nurse Practitioner Faculties. (1997). *Criteria for evaluation of nurse practitioner faculties.* Washington, DC: Author.

The Nurse Practitioner. (1997). A comparative analysis of primary care nurse practitioners and physician assistants. *The Nurse Practitioner, The American Journal of Primary Health Care, 22*(1), 14–17.

Page, N. E., & Arena, D. M. (1994). Rethinking the merger of the clinical nurse specialist and the nurse practitioner roles. *Image: Journal of Nursing Scholarship, 26,* 315–318.

Papenhausen, J. L. (1990). Case management: A model of advanced practice? *Clinical Nurse Specialist, 4,* 169–170.

Pearson, L. J. (1999). Annual update of how each state stands on legislative issues affecting advanced nursing practice. *The Nurse Practitioner, The American Journal of Primary Health Care, 24*(1), 16–24.

Reiter, F. (1966). The nurse-clinician. *American Journal of Nursing, 66,* 274–280.

Robinson, D. K., Mead, M. J., & Boswell, C. R. (1995). Inside looking out: Innovations in community health nursing. *Clinical Nurse Specialist, 9,* 227–229, + 235.

Rogers, M. E. (1972). Nursing: To be or not to be. *Nursing Outlook, 20,* 42–46.

Safriet, B. J. (1992). Health care dollars and regulatory sense: The role of advanced practice nursing. *Yale Journal on Regulation, 9,* 417–488.

Schroer, K. (1991). Case management: Clinical nurse specialist and nurse practitioner, converging roles. *Clinical Nurse Specialist, 5,* 189–194.

Sheehy, C. M., & McCarthy, M. (1998). *Advanced practice nursing: Emphasizing common roles.* Philadelphia: F. A. Davis.

Snyder, M., & Mirr, M. P. (Eds.). (1995). *Advanced practice nursing: A guide to professional development.* New York: Springer.

Thatcher, V. S. (1984). *History of anesthesia with emphasis on the nurse specialist.* New York: Garland Publishing.

Varney, H. (1987). *Nurse-midwifery* (2nd ed.). Boston: Blackwell Scientific.

Ward-Miller, S. (1996). The psychiatric clinical specialist in the home care setting. *Nursing Clinics of North America, 31,* 519–525.

Watson, L. J. (1996). A national profile of nursing centers. *The Nurse Practitioner, The American Journal of Primary Care, 21*(3), 72–81.

Zwanziger, P. J., Peterson, R. M., Lethlean, H. M., Hernke, D. A., Finley, J. L., DeGroot, L. S., & Busman, C. L. (1996). Expanding the CNS role to the community. *Clinical Nurse Specialist, 10,* 199–202.

Chapter 42

Health Ministries: Health and Faith Communities

Emily Chandler and Ruth D. Berry

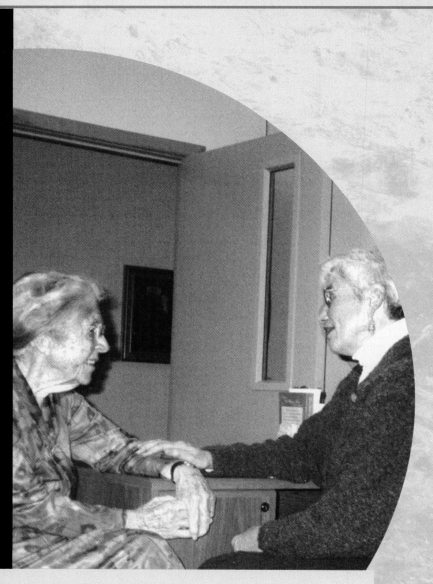

Wouldn't it be wonderful if faith groups adopted one small area and made sure that every single child was immunized . . . that every person had a basic medical exam . . . that every woman who became pregnant would get prenatal care?

Are these possible?

We believe the answer is yes.

CHAPTER FOCUS

Development of Health Ministries

History of Ministering: Hospitals, Hospitality, and Religious Communities

Nightingale's Legacy: The Relationship of Nursing to Early Models

Philosophical Underpinnings

Health Ministry in Action

The Faith Community

Models of Health Ministry

Structure of Health Ministries

Relationship Between Community Health Nursing and Faith Communities

Parish Nurse

Activities of Parish Nurses

QUESTIONS TO CONSIDER

After reading this chapter, answer the following questions:

1. What are health ministries?
2. How did health ministries begin?
3. How does spirituality relate to health?
4. How is the faith community an ideal setting for the role of the community health nurse?
5. What are examples of models of health ministries?
6. What is parish nursing?
7. How can nurses function to promote health in health ministry programs?

KEY TERMS

Assets mapping

Extrinsic religiosity

Faith community

Health ministries

Intrinsic religiosity

Parish nursing

Development of Health Ministries

History of Ministering: Hospitals, Hospitality, and Religious Communities

Health ministry, in its broadest sense, is a concept that encompasses spirituality, spiritual well-being, and activities that may be carried out by a specific faith community alone or in partnership with other organizations. **Health ministries** incorporate the spiritual foundations and practices of the faith community to promote mutual caring for the greatest potential of whole-person wellness. The notion of ministering to the sick has ancient beginnings that reach back beyond Florence Nightingale's time. The history of "ministering" comes from the earliest accounts of efforts to help and to care for the unfortunate, often those who were unable to afford private care in their homes. "Hospitality" was offered by religious communities who saw it as their responsibility to provide comfort and care. Hospitals originated as places where this ministering to (care of) the sick took place. Religious communities, both lay and formal, have a history of providing advocacy and access to care. Concern for the underserved focused on the disadvantaged, the elderly, women, children, persons with disabilities, and the chronically ill.

Health ministries have again become a viable option in community health care because of numerous trends in society. An aging population is not only increasing in numbers, but raising issues of values and quality of life, as well as caring for those who now are living longer. Vulnerable and frail persons continue to be underserved. Responsibility for self-care is promoted in a managed care environment. Patients are encouraged to remain out of the illness care system by staying healthy.

Individuals, families, and communities need to know how to make healthy choices about health options. Holistic health centers of the 1970s were instrumental in bringing individuals and families together with physicians, clergy, and nurses to determine strategies for achieving better health. The team approach emphasized preventive health practices and personal responsibility for health care. The World Council of Churches (1990) entered into dialog regarding wholeness, health, and healing as central to faith and the Creator. The Council endorsed the caring community as a means of restoring wholeness and healing. Building community could enhance mutual concern and overcome barriers of suffering and injustice with faith communities as the focus of interventions.

The Carter Center at Emory University and the Park Ridge Center for the Study of Health, Faith and Ethics addressed faith communities as an important public health resource and emphasized the advantages of churches having an active role in attaining *Healthy People 2000* and *2010* objectives (DHHS, 1990, 2000). Formed in 1995, the Faith and Health Caucus of the American Public Health Association has as a major objective encouraging partnerships between faith and health institutions to promote health.

Nightingale's Legacy: Relationship of Nursing to Early Models

Early models of health ministry can be traced to Florence Nightingale and her own preparation for nursing. Believing that her purpose was to care for the sick, the underserved, and the disadvantaged, Nightingale sought nursing training, but the only formal education in caring for the sick available to her was a 3-month experience at the Institution of Deaconesses at Kaiserworth, Dusseldorf, Germany. The Institution had 100 beds, where 116 deaconesses (so-called Protestant nurses) were in training to provide care. It has been argued that her primary purpose was not necessarily religious, but spiritual (Dossey, 1998). Historically, Nightingale followed a long line of healers—shamans, witches, midwives, and deaconesses. Nightingale wanted to answer what she believed to be her vocation—her call. Her primary commitment was to actualizing her spiritual convictions in acts of social justice.

Recent attention to Nightingale's philosophical leanings show how committed she was to the integration of spirituality in nursing, clearly differentiating between spirituality and religion, which she saw as only one possible expression of spiritual life. She distinctly articulated a concept of spirituality that was broader than religion. Spirituality was, for her, a connection between an inner self and a higher reality was by creative energy. Such energy was the most powerful resource for healing (Macrae, 1995).

Nightingale, it seems, was as ahead of her time in health ministry and spirituality in nursing as she was in epidemiology and community health nursing. Now the growing commitment to holistic care is pushing nursing and medicine, as well as other disciplines to reexamine the place of spirit in relationship to body and mind. Differences between spirituality and religion, and extrinsic and intrinsic religiosity are poorly understood and often badly articulated (Zinnbauer, Pargament, Cole, Rye, Butter, Belvich, Hipp, Scott, & Kadar 1997). The following provides examples of the ranges of competing categories:

- *Spirituality (Barnum, 1996; Dyson, Cobb, & Forman, 1997; Halstead & Mickley, 1997; McSherry & Draper, 1998)*
- *Spiritual well-being (Chandler, 1997; Fehring, Miller, & Shaw, 1997)*
- *Spirituality and healing (Burton, 1998; Cerrato, 1998)*
- *Patient's spiritual needs (Brown-Saltzman, 1997; Martsolf, 1997)*
- *The role of faith in health (Ellison & Levin, 1998; Matthews, McCollough, Larson, Koenig, & Swyers, 1998; Oman & Reed, 1998)*
- *The relationship of health ministries to community health (Chatters, Levin, & Ellison, 1998; Culp, 1997; Wallace & Forman, 1998).*

RESEARCH BRIEF

Oman, D. & Reed, D.(1998). Religion and mortality among the community-dwelling elderly. American Journal of Public Health, *88(10), 1469–1475.*

This study of 1,931 older residents of Marin County, California, analyzed the association between attending religious services and all cause mortality over a 5-year period, looking at six confounding factors: demographics, health status, physical functioning, health habits, social functioning, and support and psychological state. Persons who attended religious services had lower mortality rates than those who did not, and religious attendance tended to be slightly more protective coupled with high social support. This study lends support to the existence of a "protective effect" of religious attendance on health; a broad implication is the potential benefit of partnerships between religious organizations and health promotion efforts.

Philosophical Underpinnings

The philosophical underpinnings of faith communities remain essentially unchanged. At their best, communities of faith seek ways to continue a tradition of service, often to those who need it most.

The commitment is to health and wholeness for self and others. Participation in advocacy, health education, promotion, and illness prevention are intrinsically linked to spiritual health. Such a health ministry functions within a self-understanding of

RESEARCH BRIEF

Fehring, R. J., Miller, J. F., & Shaw, C. (1997). Spiritual well being, religiosity, hope, depression, and other mood states in elderly people coping with cancer. Oncology Nursing Forum, *24(4): 663–671.*

One hundred elderly people with a diagnosis of cancer were administered measures to determine the relationships between spiritual well-being, religiosity, hope, depression, and other mood states. Each person was administered an **intrinsic** and **extrinsic religiosity** index, a spiritual well-being scale, the Miller hope scale, and the Profile of Mood States scale. A consistent positive correlation was found among intrinsic religiosity, spiritual well-being, hope, and positive mood states. Significantly higher levels of hope and positive moods existed in elderly patients with high levels of intrinsic religiosity and spiritual well-being.

compassion and care that encompasses faith, lived out in their concept of care, and hope, actualized within a context of care, and love, which becomes the blueprint for the conduct of care.

Health Ministry in Action
The Faith Community

The **faith community** gives professional nursing a unique setting to practice with a diverse population. Members of the faith community represent the entire developmental age span. Families, as members of faith communities, comprise the entire array of "family-makeup" represented in the United States. Families of the elderly never-married, widow, or widower living alone; the single mom; the unmarried young adult, career male or female; the 'blended' families; and other one-parent families are all members of faith communities or congregations. The traditional two-parent family with one or more children participates in activities, ascribes to the religious dogma, and embraces the faith community rituals to add a spiritual dimension to their lives.

The members gain inner strength to cope with life situations; give meaning to life's existence, its joys, concerns, and challenges; and collectively find support from other members of the group. Congregations with predominately young families might concentrate on early childhood education efforts or activities of a more active and younger adult population.

Congregations that have predominately middle-aged and older adults might find that their focus will be primarily on life transitions of that age group, caregiving concerns, faith maturation issues, and life fulfillment later in one's life journey. On the other hand, congregations that encompass a broader age spectrum have the challenge and opportunity to deal with crossgenerational and intergenerational issues. They can learn from each other among the various age groupings, and they can find service opportunities within their congregation.

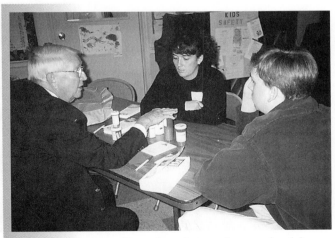

Pharmacist counseling church members at health fair about prescription drug therapy.

Another feature of the faith community is the cohesiveness inherent in the group. The term *connectedness* more adequately describes the cohesiveness and belongingness often found among members of a faith community. Connectedness with the Creator (identified as God, Higher Power, or the Supreme Being) of the faith community is a unique attribute of this community cohesiveness. The bond of connectedness with the Creator becomes the basis for the common bond of the faith community, which is evident in the interactions among families and various age groups. The strength of these relationships provides a protective effect for members of the faith community and often extends beyond the benefit of simple social support (Strawbridge, Shema, Cohen, Roberts, & Kaplan, 1998).

Connectedness is also evident in marking significant life passages. Members across the entire life span experience connectedness with family, friends, preceding generations, future generations, and the faith community around major transitions such as birth, marriage, and death. Events pivotal in the life of faith communities include baptism, christening, bris, confirmation, bar mitzvah, anniversaries, and funerals. In addition to the comfort that ritual provides at nodal events, attendance at religious services has been found to have a significant beneficial effect on health and longevity (Kark, Shemi, Friedlander, Martin, Manor, & Blondheim, 1996; Koenig, Cohen, George, Hays, Larson, & Blazer, 1997; Strawbridge, Cohen, Shema, & Kaplan, 1997).

Assisting families to make choices with their loved ones for a peaceful death and to deal with the associated grief is a major responsibility for nurses in faith communities (Chandler, 1999). The opportunity to intervene with people whose histories are known within a faith community is especially meaningful. Walking beside individuals and families in times of joy or sorrow, dur-

ing celebrations of beginnings and endings, fosters connectedness of members with one another, with the caregivers, and with the entire faith community.

Issues of health and wholeness, respect for the body, responsibility, and respect for life in its fullest and richest dimensions are important to congregations that take health ministry seriously. When individuals and congregations are themselves healthy, or whole, they are more likely to be responsive to needs in the wider community.

Models of Health Ministry

Within the local congregation (church, mosque, or temple), health ministries often interact with smaller groups on formal and informal bases, such as age-appropriate faith educational classes, women's and men's services, prayer groups, governing councils, and congregational staffs. Incorporating appropriate health concerns with these groups may be a consequence of identifying needs in a particular group, media or public policy concerns, or at the prompting of a health professional such as the community health nurse. For example, a group of women who have a women's prayer circle may have concerns about menopause changes.

There are as many examples of health ministry activities a congregation can initiate as there are creative ideas within the congregation. The vision is enhanced by the input of many different people, often bringing their personal and professional gifts to the enterprise. Starting a health ministry can have a galvanizing effect on a community; few people are politically opposed to health, and the resultant shared goals have the serendipitous effect of forging bonds in disparate groups within the community. Knowledge of how systems, subsystems, and interfaces operate is invaluable, as is expertise in group behavior and a sense of hu-

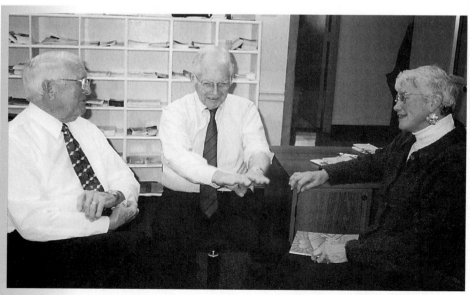

Chapter author, Ruth Berry (right), counseling church members between church services.

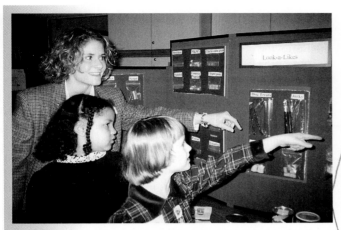

Health fair at church provides opportunities for the nurse to discuss drug use with children.

mor. Most of all, the effort is more likely to come to fruition if goals are mutually agreed upon in advance. For example, a group of ministers within a church district may be having stress-related health concerns. The nurse could meet with the group and assist them in identifying concerns and developing networks within the larger church community.

Health promotion at all levels is a good place to begin planning. What resources can be matched with what needs? What partnerships can be explored? There is good reason that many parish nurses have come from the ranks of community health nurses. They bring savvy, experience, and the ability to coalesce groups to the effort.

Health education in the church community takes the form of classes, literature, newsletters, and Internet-based information. Support groups, especially those that are age-focused, such as day care for preschool children or elderly community members, are real contributions to a community's well-being, as are issue-focused groups that an provide a forum for shared experiences such as separation, or bereavement.

Community service initiatives such as care teams, Habitat for Humanity (a housing volunteer group), and Operation Read and Stephen's Ministries (a literacy program) are all health ministries. Space and time for support groups—Alzheimer's Caregivers and self-help groups, such as AA—fills a larger community health need.

Structure of Health Ministries

Congregations respond to the mandate to care in a variety of ways. In formal or informal fellowship, they generate discussion of areas of interest or concern within the congregation. Other times, a single incident or experience in a faith community is an impetus for concerted dialog or action. At other times, one individual might be instrumental in stirring interest in a group that becomes a working committee. The faith community as an entity and groups that function within it are representative of

Lassiter's "established groups" (1996, p. 441). These groups have the advantage of existing bonds because they are members of the faith community. Members already know how groups function within the congregation, how to work together cooperatively, and who some of the effective leaders are. These ties and a common interest in health are helpful in the formation of a committee intentionally focusing on wellness.

A wellness committee gathers together persons with a common interest who are willing to further explore health and health-related issues. Wellness committees may be called *Faith and Health Cabinets, Wholeness in Health Teams, Parish Nurse Advisory Committees,* or *Congregational Health Councils.* Whatever the term, the group forms around the faith and health—physical, emotional, and spiritual—of the congregation.

The membership of a wellness committee includes both lay and professional members. Seven to twelve persons work well together. Membership should represent the lives and interests of the congregation as well as various health disciplines. The charge is to uncover the many dimensions of what it means to be a healthy and caring congregation. Nurses, social workers, physicians, dentists, hospice workers, caregivers, widows, youth, child-care staff, clergy, and representatives of church governing body are examples of potential volunteer professionals who can lead rich discussions for program planning. An initial assessment of the congregation needs to include any previous surveys or assessments of the congregation and the components within it. A simple walk by the nurse with members elicits comments that are invaluable in assessing the values and priorities of individuals:

> *"This room is a lively place when the young moms get together, watch their little ones play, and talk about the joys and challenges of parenting."*
>
> *"I recall when Alice began the first home delivered meals for our town in this church kitchen."*
>
> *"This mural of names painted by youth is so important to the Fellow and Senner families because the names of their deceased children are there."*
>
> *"This is where the Women's AA group meets."*

In addition to listening and recording, a visual survey of spiritually significant symbols and items is helpful. An environmental assessment should include indoor and outdoor signs, physical accessibility, reading materials, lighting, and emergency equipment.

Following the walk-through, an important next step is to acknowledge and catalog skills, gifts, talents, and possible capabilities of members and groups within the church. This approach, patterned after **"assets mapping"** described by Kretzmann and McKnight (1993) and Ammerman and Parks (1998), emphasizes the strengths and abilities of the congregation and will form the framework of subsequent possibilities and activities. The model also emphasizes strengths and competencies. The assets mapping model is particularly adaptable to faith communities because terms such as *gifts, talents, interests,* and *journeys* or *experiences* are common language in congregations. Members have opportunities to share their skills in church activities and may be able to redirect the skills to achieve new goals. Focusing on the capabilities, talents, and potentials of selected populations motivates the community or, in this case, the congregation and wellness committee to view healthy potential outcomes.

Traditionally, assessments result in the generation of a number of problems or needs. Community health nurses also engage in assessments and they include multiple sources of data, including demographics, health status indicators, group beliefs, and expressed needs. A concentrated effort to build on the identified strengths of the congregation is important. These interests and abilities, which represent positive assets endorsed by Kretzmann and McKnight, would also yield comprehensive involvement in health outcomes with traditional methods. Successful use of traditional community health nursing assessment processes with faith communities is described by Miskelly (1995). Such a program skillfully used the needs assessment process and incorporated *Healthy People 2010* objectives in an assessment for program planning within the church community. Intervention such as education, support groups, and counseling can be effectively constructed around strengths and needs identified in the assessment.

Additional assessment information is gained from the experiences of others who have embarked on health ministry services. The denominational or national faith community body can be contacted. Surveys of web sites, literature, and videos are helpful. The committee could also ask a nurse to attend one of the meetings to assess in what ways the congregation might benefit from this resource.

Health fairs are often a valuable first activity for the wellness committee. Not only do they engage in a large number of persons providing and receiving at one time, but they also serve to create awareness of a wide variety of issues. Health fairs serve to generate data that are helpful for further planning and evaluation. The scope of the activity can be very broad and comprehensive to involve multiple congregational members who have a personal interest in health and wholeness. The events can also include agencies represented in the community. Health fairs can also focus on narrower topics and thus respond to very intentional wishes and concerns that are identified. See Case Study on the following page.

Relationship Between Community Health Nursing and Faith Communities

Parish Nursing

An appropriate and challenging intervention for the community health nurse is putting the theological foundations of health ministries into action. Because the professional discipline of nursing incorporates the physical, emotional, cultural, and spiritual domains of practice and because professional nursing partners with professionals from a variety of disciplines and community members with varying life experiences, health ministry

activities are a natural arena for nurses working in community-based, population-focused practice. **Parish nursing** is one response to the societal trends and health care delivery system changes of the last decades of the 20th century. During the mid-1980s, professional nursing practice expanded into more independent practice arenas with the development of nursing centers, and parish nursing evolved out of holistic health centers. The movement's early beginnings included both the model of six congregations guided by Lutheran General Hospital, Chicago, and the collaborative efforts in rural Iowa with the Northwest Center on Aging. By the mid-1990s, more than 2,000 parish nurses were serving congregations in the United States as well as other countries; the nurses are in faith communities that include Christian, Muslim, and Jewish gatherings. Parish nurses are often key facilitators in health ministries of faith communities.

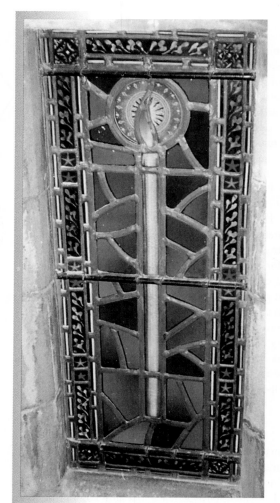

The stained glass of the candle depicts spiritual connectedness to the Creator, light, warmth, comfort, conscience, hope, and continuity.

Courtesy of Second Presbyterian Church, Lexington, Kentucky.

CASE STUDY

A Health Fair—Medicines and More

"Medicines and More" was the result of interest expressed on the part of members of the Wellness Committee of Second Presbyterian Church, Lexington, Kentucky. Comments from a retired health professional and from an older adult caregiver noted that they were concerned about numerous conversations and observations regarding confusion with medications. Quickly, the committee's discussion included stories of inquiries regarding multiple names for medicines, complex over-the-counter preparations, duplicate medicines for the same ailment, values and dangers of herbal preparations, problems eating or not eating food with medicines, medication errors indicating the need for reinforcement of emergency assistance, and others.

Members decided a fair would reach many people quickly. Although a major target was the older population, the committee believed that the information was valuable for members of all ages, for families as well as for individuals who were living alone. Because members already gathered on Sunday mornings for educational and worship services and because many elderly persons regularly participated in the monthly "Retirees Lunch," it was decided to plan the event to coincide with established habits. The committee further decided that because they wanted to provide information applicable for all ages and for the total congregation, they would schedule the fair during and following the Retirees Lunch in a room adjacent to the dining room. Families and those members not participating in the lunch were guided directly to the fair location following worship service. Retirees would be the special fair participants after lunch.

Upon agreeing on a number of objectives, the members listed tasks and eagerly offered to take responsibility for the many jobs. These jobs included marketing and publicity, obtaining resources, volunteering for hosting the various exhibits, taking blood pressure readings, greeting community presenters, and monitoring flow on the day of the fair.

The parish nurse contacted the local health department nutritionist and the university's college of pharmacy. A pharmacy brown-bag event was very popular, and the nutritionist provided helpful information regarding food-medicine interaction, supplements, and herbal preparations. Committee members contacted a local hospital's home care agency for information on Lifeline emergency calling. The senior nursing student contacted the local police department for 911 guidelines, supplied various phones for demonstration and practice, and obtained literature and posters at the State Pamphlet Library. In collaboration with the parish nurse, a County Cooperative Extension "Look-a-Likes" display was updated. Children and adults were able to view models and a brochure depicting potentially dangerous and confusing foods, medicines, and household products.

To encourage participation at all exhibits and to obtain evaluation data, members who completed surveys were eligible to win loaves of whole-wheat variety breads. The committee reviewed the evaluations within 2 weeks, reported the results and extended thanks to planners and attendees in the congregation's newsletter, and gained information for planning future programs regarding nutrition and exercise.

Effective and enjoyable health fairs can be simpler or more elaborate than the one described. The community presenters gained a new resource for their information. Both the pharmacists and the nutritionist expressed that they had never envisioned the benefits of providing health information in a faith community setting, and the county's extension agency appreciated help in renewing their display and obtaining feedback for additional outreach options. Collaborating with these professionals and their agencies created new partnerships with mutual benefits. Planning fairs to promote healthy behaviors is encouraged by Dillon and Sternas (1997).

The *Scope and Standards of Parish Nursing,* prepared by the Health Ministries Association, Inc. (HMA), was adopted by the American Nurses Association in 1998. The HMA is a professional interfaith organization that encourages faith communities to work with professionals, lay individuals, and agencies to promote health and wellness. Both nurses and others interested in health ministries comprise the membership. The 1998 document describes to the profession and to the public this evolving "specialty practice of nursing and of health ministry" (HMA/ANA, 1998, p. 3). Furthermore, the document clearly describes the independent practice of nursing, as defined by the jurisdiction's nursing practice act, in health promotion within the context of the client's values, beliefs, and faith practices. The client focus of a parish nurse is the faith community, including its family and individual members and the community it serves. (See Box 42-1.)

Basic preparation courses recommended for the parish nurse and endorsed by the International Parish Nurse Resource Center consists of at least 30 hours of course work in parish nursing. Information can be obtained from the Center,

---

BOX 42-1 THE CARTER CENTER'S INTERFAITH HEALTH PROGRAM: REALIGNING COMMUNITY ASSETS THROUGH COLLABORATION OF FAITH COMMUNITIES AND HEALTH ORGANIZATIONS

ALIGNING ASSETS OF FAITH AND HEALTH COMMUNITIES IN BUILDING HEALTHIER COMMUNITIES

The Carter Center's interest in the role of faith communities in improving community health began in the 1980s. A national symposium, "Closing the Gap," signaled the beginning of concerted efforts to bring together the most significant health science and the most relevant knowledge and experience from theology for both the faith community and health science and health service institutions. At that time, The Carter Center identified faith communities as the most underused resource group, with potential to help in closing the gap for improving America's health.

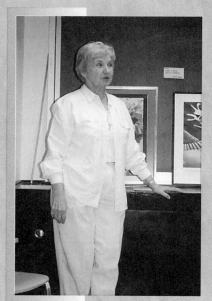

Anna Frances Wenger, PhD, RN, FAAN, The Carter Center.

In 1989, a conference on Striving for Fullness of Life: The Church's Challenge in Health *was sponsored by The Carter Center and Wheat Ridge Foundation. This conference focused on building healthy lives through public health measures such as preventing disease, disability, and premature death. This proved to be an important step forward, but it did not address the need for shifts in how congregations viewed their roles in the larger community and how health institutions and organizations perceived the assets of congregations.*

The Interfaith Health Program was formed in 1992 to respond to the challenge of helping to build healthier communities by engaging leaders from the health sciences and theology along with community representatives from health services and congregations to find ways to realign faith and health assets for the good of the community.

The Five Gap Model was used to ask the right questions when searching for strategies. The gaps include the following:

- *The gap between what is already known and what is applied*
- *The gap between what every faith group affirms as their concern for social justice and what they do*
- *The gap between successful working models and general application in other communities*
- *The gap perpetuated by faith groups working in isolation from each other and health agencies*
- *The gap between present wants and future needs*

Using the Five Gap Model, we focused on promotion of congregational health ministries, one of the key strategies of the Interfaith Health Program. The Atlanta Health Ministry Model was developed and then used in two African American communities and one multicultural community in Atlanta. This health ministry model was based on the participatory approach proposed by Paulo Freire, the Brazilian grassroots educator and author of Pedagogy of the Oppressed. *Some of the core*

BOX 42-1 THE CARTER CENTER'S INTERFAITH HEALTH PROGRAM: REALIGNING COMMUNITY ASSETS THROUGH COLLABORATION OF FAITH COMMUNITIES AND HEALTH ORGANIZATIONS—CONT'D

principles of the Atlanta Health Ministry Model (Droege & Wenger, 1997, p. 14) are as follows:

- Education is never neutral; it is either liberating or domesticating.
- People will act on issues that evoke strong feelings.
- People are creative and intelligent with the capacity for action.
- Genuine dialog is needed if communities are to share, listen, and learn.

Several key action steps characterized the approach used in Atlanta. First, a working group of 15 religious leaders participated in a 6-month planning process to determine the most effective way to enlist faith communities to increase engagement in health-promotion activities. This process served to nurture a network of potential collaborators.

Second, in each neighborhood, local pastors (or priests, rabbi, and imam) were invited to join a network of congregations, with each network governed by a Health Ministry Council. This council was formed by the participating congregations and staffed by a network coordinator. Third, the training of Congregational Health Promoters was at the heart of the program. The training program was coordinated by the Nell Hodgson Woodruff School of Nursing at Emory University, with nursing instructors who understood the participatory teaching-learning process, leading the training sessions.

The goal of this approach was to build on the capacities of the congregations and communities rather than to fix problems or to predetermine what needs to be learned.

Each participating congregation designated two natural leaders from within the congregation to join the training program which consisted of 20 to 24 hours of 2- to 3-hour sessions. Although the emphasis was on lay health leadership, some professionals such as nurses and social workers participated in the training. As the need was expressed by the participants, local health resource persons came to discuss specific health services in the community. When the trainees recognized the need to learn more about a resource, such as nutritional information or heart

health resources, the nursing instructor would make the connections for them, always emphasizing how they can assume that role in the future.

So, what has happened in these neighborhoods since the initial training period? In a largely African American community, Atlanta Health Ministries, a nonprofit organization with 501C3 status, was established. It has several active committees, with one of them being Congregational Health Promoters. In a very multiethnic community, there is a Congregational Health Ministry program as part of the Chamblee-Doraville Ministry Center. A Congregational Health Ministry Coordinator, who is a Parish Nurse employed by St. Joseph's Mercy Care System, conducts training sessions in Spanish and English and serves as a mentor for all of the congregational health promoters in the neighborhood, which includes Korean, Vietnamese, African American, Hispanic, and dominant culture American congregations.

A commitment to cultural openness is inherent for all of the initiatives of the Interfaith Health Program. As boundaries are spanned among disciplines and within communities, the persons engaged in faith and health ministries need to constantly renew their commitment to learn about the meaning of faith and health within the worldviews of the people. "Cultural openness refers to a life-long stance that promotes cultural self awareness and continuing development of transcultural skills" (Wenger, 1998, p. 164). Respect for differences, although important, is not enough (Wenger, 1998). Transcultural knowledge and skills are essential components when engaging in health ministries and building partnerships.

Two other initiatives of the Interfaith Health Program are directed toward moving the faith and health movement forward. Whole Communities Collaborative is a network of faith and health leaders from five specific communities within the United States where local working groups exchange ideas and develop local activities that bring faith-based communities and health organizations together for the good of the larger community or neighborhood. The other initiative is referred to as the Faith and Health Consortium. This network focuses on academic/community partnerships. There are five sites in the United States and one in South Africa where at least a school of theology or seminary and a

Continued

> ## BOX 42-1 THE CARTER CENTER'S INTERFAITH HEALTH PROGRAM: REALIGNING COMMUNITY ASSETS THROUGH COLLABORATION OF FAITH COMMUNITIES AND HEALTH ORGANIZATIONS—CONT'D
>
> *school of public health have formed an agreement to promote disciplinary and interdisciplinary courses, research studies, and service projects that involve the integration of faith and health concepts. Schools of nursing, medicine, social work, and allied health are included whenever possible. The Faith and Health Consortium working groups always include community partners because of the underlying premise that the education of professionals, in addition to research and service projects, needs ongoing involvement with representatives from the community to keep the academic endeavors grounded within sociocultural contexts. Both of these networks have developed collaborative relationships through regular monthly conference calls and periodic meetings attended by representatives from the local site working groups.*
>
> *Building partnerships between health institutions and faith communities requires an appreciation of assets or strengths that are already present within the community. Most of the work of the Interfaith Health Program focuses on alignment of assets for improvement of community health. Faith-based congregations are one of the most enduring assets within a community. Gary Gunderson (1997, 1998), director of the Interfaith Health Program, has outlined eight key strengths of congregations that highlight congregations as strategic partners in building healthier communities. These strengths are as follows:*
>
> 1. The power to accompany, to be physically present
> 2. The power to convene in small and large groups across interest lines
> 3. The power to connect, to form human networks across which resources flow
> 4. The power to frame, to story, to set events and data in a meaningful context
> 5. The power to give sanctuary to people, programs, ideas, and dialog
> 6. The power to bless, forgive, and nurture hope amid its opposite
> 7. The power to pray and to mark the boundary between holy and human
> 8. The power to endure and to maintain the sense of time and development
>
> *The challenge for health professionals and congregational leaders is to intentionally search for ways that the assets of both health and faith structures can be aligned for the benefit of the community at large. Our aspiration is that the most relevant health science and the most mature faith will guide the alignment of assets that will build strong partnerships for healthier communities.*
>
> *Anna Frances Z. Wenger, PhD, RN, FAAN*
> *Affiliate Faculty, Neil Hodgson Woodruff School of Nursing*
> *Faith and Health Consortium Coordinator*
> *Interfaith Health Program*
> *Rollins School of Public Health*
> *Emory University*
> *Atlanta, Georgia*

which advocates, develops, and promotes quality programs and current resources. The Center provides consultation and is on the cutting edge of research in parish nursing. The annual *Westberg Symposium* provides the valued benefits of education and networking. Spiritual maturity, professional practice experience, competent communication and negotiation skills, and a commitment to assessment of personal holistic health are necessary.

First, parish nursing's philosophy maintains that the spiritual dimension is central to the practice (Solari-Twadell & McDermott, 1999). The intentional and compassionate caring of nursing evolves from the spiritual dimension inherent in all humankind. Second, parish nurses affirm that their focus is the faith community and its ministry. Third, strengths of the congregation are paramount. The fourth component supports congregational and community partnerships that become vital aspects of programs. The fifth component addresses the continuous, dynamic process among health, spiritual health, and healing. From the philosophy, parish nurses have a basis for appropriate educational and experience preparation, for functions of the specialty, and for wide reaching health ministry activities.

Activities of Parish Nurses

In collaboration with the wellness committee, the parish nurse assists with and often initiates the effort for the congregational assessment. The appendix following this chapter shows an assessment compiled by a wellness committee. The committee reviewed survey forms and guidelines and decided that they wanted a manageable questionnaire that could be administered during a 10-minute period of the worship service. They also wanted to offer options that were nonthreatening and readily acceptable by persons with a wide experience of wellness and illness. Thus, nonthreatening educational literature was offered and followed by classes and support groups. Topics were intermingled; parenting, spiritual support practices, caregiving, and chronic illnesses were listed with concerns such as substance abuse, mental illness, communicable disease, and violence, which are more often inadequately addressed in communities. Their health questionnaire can be altered to meet the unique wishes or interests of any wellness committee and its congregation. The survey should be evaluated, results prioritized, and a report submitted with recommendations for action. The implementations and outcomes should be evaluated. This process would be repeated annually.

Overall, parish nurse services address health, wholeness, and healing within the context of the faith community served. With an emphasis on health promotion at all levels, the nurse considers individuals and families across the life span and partners with the congregation as community. At times, the parish nurse may serve several congregations that may form a cluster or alliance.

In addition to working closely with wellness committees, usual functions of the parish nurse include providing personal health counseling and health education, teaching personal lifestyle management skills, initiating and facilitating referrals to congregations and community resources, advocating and encouraging support resources, and integrating faith and health (Berry, 1994; Solari-Twadell & McDermott, 1999). Providing pastoral care is a major priority. Nursing activities corresponding to these functions are valued by members of the faith community. Responsibilities of parish nurses include establishing group programs; making visits to homes, hospitals, and nursing homes; meeting regularly with the pastoral staff; and participating in worship services of the community. The implementation of both the concept of the specialty as well as functions of the practice have resulted in creative, innovative, compassionate activities and nursing interventions (Berry, 1994; Culp, 1997; Magilvy & Brown, 1997; Solari-Twadell, Truty, & Ryan, 1994; Weis, Matheus, & Schank, 1997).

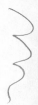

Parish nurses as community health nurses incorporate these community-based and population-focused roles in the practice with faith communities. Parish nurses may monitor care provided by other providers to ensure members the most seamless care possible. Parish nurses communicate with health care providers, discharge planners, family members, and others. They may also engage congregation members in posthospital supportive activities at home. To embrace the population-focus as well, the skills of partnering with community members and agencies, advocating for the most appropriate framework of care; facilitating health promotion at all three levels of prevention; and evaluating results are important components of parish nurse practice.

While assisting the congregation to strive for positive physical, spiritual, and emotional health outcomes, the parish nurse experienced in community health nursing can interpret and incorporate the goals of *Healthy People 2010* (DHHS, 2000; Magilvy & Brown, 1997; Marty, 1990; Miskelly, 1995; Weis, Matheus, & Schank, 1997). The numerous objectives that target schools, workplace, and communities with health issues that are also represented in the congregation are readily addressed in faith communities for reasons mentioned in the description of the structure of health ministries. In the 21st century, faith communities should become aware of the leading health indicators included in *Healthy People 2010*. Congregations will continue endeavors to achieve the *Healthy People 2010* goals because they are consistent with overall missions of justice and mercy in faith communities. The integration of responsibility for individual and collective health and wholeness is consistent with eliminating health disparities, increasing quality and years of healthy life, improving systems for personal and public health, and promoting healthful behaviors and communities.

. . . .

Say what is easily forgotten.
Do what is easily overlooked.
Think what is everlasting.
Hugh Prather, Spiritual Notes to Myself (1998),
Berkeley: Conari Press

. . . .

CONCLUSION

New and innovative endeavors are emanating out of the convergence of faith and health in health ministries. Growth of the partnerships between health and faith came about because of the increasing need to fill the ever-widening gaps brought about by economic and legislative constraints. The faith communities' history of caring and volunteerism were sought to be part of the solution to health care access, especially in health education, health promotion, and advocacy. Welfare reform legislation certainly demanded numerous community responses to care for those who could not speak for themselves.

Faith communities are also beginning to be seen as a neutral place to increase awareness of justice and social concern in relation to health care. The confusion and dilemmas brought about by the changes and complexity of the health care delivery system have left people at all economic levels poorly informed about how to navigate and use the system.

Community health nursing has emerged as a significant participant in these new developments. Nursing's traditional concern for the disadvantaged and underserved coincides with the mandate of the faith communities to care for those same populations. Creative forms of health ministries allow nurses to carve out innovative roles—bringing the best of community health nursing to the task. See Box 42-2 for a list of resources.

CRITICAL THINKING ACTIVITIES

1. Identify a health problem in your home community that could be addressed by building a potential partnership with a local faith community.

   - In what ways could a faith community address the problem to enhance public sector efforts?
   - What kind of partnerships could be forged with the faith community to enhance their contribution?
   - What are the steps that need to be taken to initiate a plan?
   - How will your own faith experience influence your participation?

BOX 42-2 RESOURCES

PRINT

Multifaith Information Manual
Kali Turner, B. (Ed.). Ontario Multifaith Council on
  Spiritual and Religious Care.
Multifaith Resource Center, 45 Windy Hill Ct.,
  Wofford Heights, CA 93285
Phone/fax: (619) 376-4691

*Partners in Healing: Healthcare Organizations and
  Parish Communities*
Describes why health care organizations and
  parishes should cooperate and do what each does
  best to create healthy living environments.
Catholic Health Association, 4455 Woodson Rd.,
  St. Louis, MO 63134-3797
Phone: (314) 427-2500; fax: (314) 427-0029; e-mail
  address: cha@healthonline.com

Beginning a Health Ministry: A How-to Manual
Health Ministries Association, PO Box 7853,
  Huntington Beach, CA 92646
Phone: (800) 852-5613, (714) 965-0085

*The Whole Church Catalogue for Congregational
  Health Ministries*
Division for Church & Society
Lutheran Church in America, 8765 W. Higgins Rd.,
  Chicago, IL 60173
Resource for people starting a health ministry in
  their congregation.

Multifaith Calendar
The purpose of the multifaith calendar is to facilitate
  understanding of other peoples' major religious hol-
  idays and festivals.
Multifaith Resource Center, 45 Windy Hill Ct.,
  Wofford Heights, CA 93285

The Jewish Healing Center
141 Alton Ave., San Francisco, CA 94116

VIDEOS

*Congregations who care: The ministry of health &
  wholeness*
Produced by the Office of Health Ministries
Presbyterian Church, 100 Witherspoon St.,
  Louisville, KY 40202-1396
Models of health ministries and parish nursing within
  congregations.

*Striving for fullness of life: The church's challenge in
  health*
Produced by Wheat Ridge Ministries.
Phone: (630) 766-9066
Conference on health ministries held at the Carter
  Center, Atlanta

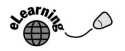

**Explore Community Health Nursing on the web! To learn more about the topics
in this chapter, use the passcode provided to access your exclusive web site:**
http://communitynursing.jbpub.com
If you do not have a passcode, you can obtain one at this site.

REFERENCES

Ammerman, A., & Parks, C. (1998). Preparing students for more effective community interventions: Assets assessment. *Family and Community Health, 21,* 32–45.

Barnum, B. S. (1996). *Spirituality in nursing: From traditional to new age.* New York: Springer.

Berry, R. (1994). A parish nurse. In Office of Resourcing Committee on Preparation for Ministry. *A day in the life of . . . . A kaleidoscope of specialized ministries.* Louisville, KY: Presbyterian Church (USA): Distribution Management Service.

Brown-Saltzman, K. (1997). Replenishing the spirit by meditative prayer and guided imagery. *Seminars in Oncology Nursing, 13*(4), 255–259.

Burton, L. A. (1998). The spiritual dimension of palliative care. *Seminars in Oncology Nursing, 14*(2), 121–128.

Cerrato, P. L. (1998). Spirituality and healing. *RN, 61*(2), 49–50.

Chandler, E. (1999). Care of dying patients and their families. In T. Buttaro, J. Trybulski, T. Bailey, & J. Kook. *Primary care: A collaborative approach*. St. Louis: Mosby

Chandler, E. (1997). *Spirituality and well-being in older adults*. Unpublished doctoral dissertation. Claremont, CA: Claremont School of Theology.

Chatters, L. M., Levin, J. S., & Ellison, C. G. (1998). Public health and health education in faith communities. *Health Education and Behavior, 25*, 689–699.

Culp, L. (1997). Health ministries: Caring for body and soul. *Registered Nurse Journal, 9*, 8.

Department of Health and Human Services (DHHS). (1990). *Healthy people 2000: national health objectives* (Publication number 91-50213). Washington, DC: U.S. Government Printing Office.

Department of Health and Human Services (DHHS). (2000). *Healthy people 2010: Conference edition*. Washington, DC: U.S. Government Printing Office.

Department of Health and Human Services, Public Health Services (DHHS, PHS). (June, 1998). *Healthy people in healthy communities: A guide for community leaders*. Washington, DC: US Government Printing Office.

Dillon, D. L., & Sternas, K. (1997). Designing a successful health fair to promote individual, family, and community health. *Journal of Community Health Nursing, 14*, 1–14.

Dossey, B. M. (1998). Florence Nightingale: A 19th century mystic. *Journal of Holistic Nursing, 16*(2), 111–165.

Droege, T., & Wenger, A. F. Z. (1997). *Starting point: Empowering communities to improve health—a manual for training health promoters in congregational coalitions*. Atlanta: The Carter Center.

Dyson, J., Cobb, M., & Forman, D. (1997). The meaning of spirituality: A literature review. *Journal of Advanced Nursing, 26*(6), 1183–1188.

Ellison, C. G., & Levin, J. S. (1998). The religion-health connection: Evidence, theory, and future directions. *Health Education and Behavior, 25*, 700–720.

Fehring, R. J., Miller, J. F., & Shaw C. (1997). Spiritual well being, religiosity, hope, depression, and other mood states in elderly people coping with cancer. *Oncology Nursing Forum, 24*(4), 663–671.

Gunderson, G. R. (1997). *Deeply woven roots: Improving the quality of life in your community*. Minneapolis: Fortress Press.

Gunderson, G. R. (1998). Aligning assets for community health improvement, *The Medical Journal of Allina,7*(4), 2–5.

Halstead, M. T., & Mickley, J. R. (1997). Attempting to fathom the unfathomable: descriptive views of spirituality. *Seminars in Oncology Nursing, 13*(4), 225–230.

Health Ministries Association/American Nurses Association. (1998). *Scope and standards of parish nursing practice*. Washington, DC: American Nurses Publishing.

Julkunen (Eds.), *The 23rd. Annual nursing research conference 1997, Transcultural Nursing—Global unifier of care, facing diversity with unity* (pp. 162–168). Kuopio, Finland: Kuopio University Publications E. Social sciences 59.

Kark, J. D., Shemi, G., Friedlander, Y., Martin, O., Manor, O., & Blondheim, S. H. (1996). Does religious observance promote health? Mortality in secular vs religious kibbutzim in Israel. *American Journal of Public Health, 86*, 341–346.

Koenig, H. G., Cohen, H. J., George, L. K., Hays, J. C., Larson, D. B., & Blazer, D. G. (1997). Attendance at religious services, interleukin-6, and other biological parameters of immune function in older adults. *International Journal of Psychiatry in Medicine, 27*(3), 233–250.

Kretzmann, J. P., & McKnight, J. L. (1993). *Building communities from the inside out: A path toward finding and mobilizing a community's assets*. Chicago: ACTA Publications.

Lassiter, P. G. (1996). Group approaches in community health. In M. Stanhope & J. Lancaster (Eds.), *Community health nursing: Promoting health of aggregates, families, and individuals*. (4th ed.). St. Louis: Mosby.

Macrae, J. (1995). Florence Nightingale's spiritual philosophy and its significance for modern nursing. *Image: Journal of Nursing Scholarship, 27*(1), 8–10.

Magilvy, J. K., & Brown, N. J. (1997). Parish nursing: Advanced practice nursing model for healthier communities. *Advanced Practice Nursing Quarterly, 2*, 67–72.

Martsolf, D. S. (1997). Cultural aspects of spirituality in cancer care. *Seminars in Oncology Nursing, 13*(4), 231–236

Marty, M. (Ed.). (1990). *Healthy people 2000: A role for America's religious communities*. Chicago: Park Ridge Center.

Matthews, D. A., McCullough, M. E., Larson, D. B., Koenig, H. G., & Swyers, J. P. (1998). Religious commitment and health status: A review of the research and implications for family medicine. *Archives of Family Medicine, 7*(2), 118–124.

McSherry, W., & Draper, P. (1998). The debates emerging from the literature surrounding the concept of spirituality as applied to nursing. *Journal of Advanced Nursing, 27*, 683–691.

Miskelly, S. (1995). A parish nursing model: Applying the community health nursing process in a church community. *Journal of Community Health Nursing, 12*, 1–14.

Oman, D., & Reed, D. (1998). Religion and mortality among the community-dwelling elderly. *American Journal of Public Health, 88*(10), 1469–1475.

Solari-Twadell, P. A., Truty, L., & Ryan, J. A. (1994). *Congregational health services.* Park Ridge, IL: Lutheran General Hospital.

Solari-Twadell, P. A., & McDermott, M. A. (Ed.). (1999). *Parish nursing: Promoting whole person health within faith communities.* Thousand Oaks, CA: Sage Publications.

Strawbridge, W. J., Shema, S. J., Cohen, R. D., Roberts, R. E., & Kaplan, G. A. (1998). Religiosity buffers effects of some stressors on depression but exacerbates others. *Journal of Gerontology, 53B*(3), S118–S126.

Strawbridge, W. J., Cohen, R. D., Shema, S. J., & Kaplan, G. A. (1997). Frequent attendance at religious services and mortality over 28 years. *American Journal of Public Health, 87*(6), 957–961.

Wallace, J. M., & Forman, T. A. (1998). Religion's role in promoting health and reducing risk among American youth. *Health Education and Behavior, 25,* 721–741.

Weis, D., Matheus, R, & Schank, M. J (1997). Health care delivery in faith communities: The parish nurse model. *Public Health Nursing, 14,* 368–372.

Wenger, A. F. Z. (1998). Cultural openness, social justice, global awareness: Promoting transcultural nursing with unity in a diverse world. In P. Merilainen & K. Vehvilainen-Wenger, A. F. Z. (1999). Cultural openness: Intrinsic to human care, *Journal of Transcultural Nursing, 10*(1), 10.

World Council of Churches. (1990). *Healing and wholeness: The churches' role in health.* Geneva: World Council of Churches.

Zinnbauer, B., Pargament, K., Cole, B., Rye, M., Butter, E., Belvich, T., Hipp, K., Scott, A., & Kadar, J. (1997). Religion and spirituality: Unfuzzying the fuzzy. *Journal for the Scientific Study of Religion, 36*(4), 546–564.

APPENDIX

PARISH NURSE SERVICE HEALTH QUESTIONNAIRE

Dear Friends,

In order to plan for the ongoing wellness program parish nurse service, it is important to know what the congregation's needs are in regard to health issues. This questionnaire was designed to gather that information primarily from adults. Another survey will address the young people more specifically. We would appreciate your assistance in answering the following questions. ALL INFORMATION will be anonymous and will be used for planning services for this congregation.

PLEASE return your questionnaire today if at all possible. If you have any health related concerns that you would like to discuss with the parish nurse, or if you would like to receive literature we might have, please call the church (254-7768), or leave a message at 323-5684, so that the parish nurse will be able to contact you.

THANK YOU for your time and help.
Wellness Committee—Second Presbyterian Church
Ruth D. Berry, Parish Nurse

1. Classes, support groups, or information packets may be developed to meet interests and needs of people at Second to enhance physical, emotional and spiritual health. Please indicate if you would be interested in any of the following. You may mark as many as you like.

   _____ Living with chronic illness
   _____ Adolescent health issues
   _____ Coping with cancer
   _____ Caring for elderly parents
   _____ Parenting
   _____ Single parenting
   _____ Step parenting
   _____ Humor
   _____ Substance abuse
   _____ Alcoholics Anonymous
   _____ Smoking cessation
   _____ Interpersonal relationships
   _____ Safe baby-sitting
   _____ Spiritual direction
   _____ Women's health issues
   _____ Men's health issues
   _____ Childbirth preparation
   _____ Pre-retirement planning
   _____ CPR instruction
   _____ Human sexuality
   _____ Psalm study
   _____ Coping with AIDS
   _____ First aid
   _____ Weight control
   _____ Divorce recovery
   _____ Exercise groups
   _____ Normal aging process
   _____ Values clarification
   _____ Healthy eating
   _____ Adult children of alcoholics
   _____ Living wills/advance directives
   _____ Loss and grief
   _____ Marriage enrichment
   _____ Prayer
   _____ Bible study
   _____ Health care access
   _____ Childbirth preparation
   _____ Values clarification
   _____ Memory disorders
   _____ Alzheimer's disease
   _____ Conflict resolution
   _____ Hormone replacement therapy
   _____ Attention deficit disorders
   _____ Other

2. Which of the health-promotion classes or groups do you think that Second needs most? Place a star to the RIGHT of the item.

3. How would you rate your health?
   Excellent   Good   Fair   Poor

4. Do you engage in regular exercise?   Yes   No
   If yes, how often _____

5. Do you have a regular physical exam?   Yes   No
   If yes, how often _____

6. Do you have regular dental exams?   Yes   No
   If yes, how often _____

7. Do you regularly wear a car seat belt?   Yes   No

8. CHECK ANY of the following conditions that you have or have had in the past:
   _____ Heart disease
   _____ High blood pressure
   _____ Arthritis
   _____ Diabetes
   _____ Cancer
   _____ Emotional problems
   _____ Allergies
   _____ Depression
   _____ Lung disease
   _____ Physical disability
   _____ Substance abuse
   _____ Other

   Please provide the following information about yourself:

9. Sex: Male _____   Female _____

10. Age _____

11. Marital status: Single _____, Married _____,
    Separated _____, Divorced _____,
    Widow(er) _____

12. Education:
    _____ Elementary
    _____ High school
    _____ Technical school
    _____ Two years college
    _____ Four years college
    _____ Beyond college

13. Number of children at home:
    _____ Under 1 year
    _____ 1-4 years
    _____ 5-6 years
    _____ 6-10 years
    _____ 11-14 years
    _____ 15-18 years
    _____ Over 18 years

14. Employment:
    _____ Not working
    _____ Work at home
    _____ Work part-time
    _____ Work full time
    _____ Plan to retire in 5 years
    _____ Retired

15. Which worship service do you usually attend?
    _____ 8:30 a.m.
    _____ 11:00 a.m.
    _____ neither

16. What day of the week would you be interested in attending classes or a group?
    Sun ___, M ___, TU ___, W ___, TH ___, F ___, SAT ___

17. Would you need child care?   Yes   No

18. Need transportation?   Yes   No

19. What health concern is most important to you?
    _____ Chronic illness
    _____ Catastrophic illness
    _____ Substance abuse
    _____ Related financial issues
    _____ Stress
    _____ Fitness
    _____ Aging
    _____ Grief
    _____ Other

20. Any other topics that you would like the Wellness Committee to consider?

Scope and Standards of Public Health Nursing Practice

Scope of Public Health Nursing Practice

- *Public health nursing is the practice of promoting and protecting the health of populations using knowledge from nursing, social, and public health sciences.*

- *Public health nursing is population-focused and community-oriented.*

- *The goal is the prevention of disease and disability for all people.*

- *Public health nurses most often partner with nations, states, communities, organizations, and groups, as well as individuals, in completing health assessment, policy development, and assurance activities.*

- *Public health nurses assess the needs and strengths of the population, design interventions to mobilize resources for action, and promote equal opportunity for health.*

Tenets of Public Health Nursing

1. *Population-based assessment, policy development, and assurance processes are systematic and comprehensive.*

2. *All processes must include partnering with representatives of the people.*

3. *Primary prevention is given priority.*

4. *Intervention strategies are selected to create healthy environmental, social, and economic conditions in which people can thrive.*

5. *Public health nursing practice includes an obligation to actively reach out to all who might benefit from an intervention or service.*

6. *The dominant concern and obligation is for the greater good of all of the people or the population as a whole.*

7. *Stewardship and allocation of available resources supports the maximum population health benefit gain.*

8. *The health of the people is most effectively promoted and protected through collaboration with members of other professions and organizations.*

Standards of Care

Standard I: Assessment
The public health nurse assesses the health status of populations using data, community resources identification, input from the population, and professional judgment.

Standard II: Diagnosis
The public health nurse analyzes collected assessment data and partners with the people to attach meaning to those data and determine opportunities and needs.

Standard III: Outcomes Identification
The public health nurse participates with other community partners to identify expected outcomes in the populations and their health status.

Standard IV: Planning
The public health nurse promotes and supports the development of programs, policies, and services that provide interventions that improve the health status of populations.

Standard V: Assurance—Action Component of the Nursing Process for Public Health Nursing
The public health nurse ensures access and availability of programs, policies, resources, and services to the population.

Standard VI: Evaluation
The public health nurse evaluates the health status of the population.

Standards of Professional Performance

Standard I: Quality of Care
The public health nurse systematically evaluates the availability, accessibility, quality, and effectiveness of nursing practice for the population.

Standard II: Performance Appraisal

The public health nurse evaluates his or her own nursing practice in relation to professional practice standards and relevant statutes and regulations.

Standard III: Education

The public health nurse acquires and maintains current knowledge and competency in public health nursing practice.

Standard IV: Collegiality

The public health nurse establishes collegial partnerships while interacting with health care practitioners and others, and contributes to the professional development of peers, colleagues, and others.

Standard V: Ethics

The public health nurse applies ethical standards in advocating for health and social policy, and delivery of public health programs to promote and preserve the health of the population.

Standard VI: Collaboration

The public health nurse collaborates with the representatives of the population and other health and human service professionals and organizations in providing for and promoting the health of the population.

Standard VII: Research

The public health nurse uses research findings in practice.

Standard VIII: Resource Utilization

The public health nurse considers safety, effectiveness, and cost in the planning and delivery of public health services when using available resources to ensure the maximum possible health benefit to the population.

Note: These standards are to be used in conjunction with other American Nurses Association documents, such as *Nursing's Social Policy Statement* (1995), the *Code for Nurses with Interpretive Statements* (1995), standards of nursing practice for a specific population, and the public health nursing statement of the American Public Health Association (1996).

Source: Quad Council of Public Health Nursing Organizations. (1999).Scope and Standards of Public Health Nursing Practice. Washington, DC: American Nurses Association, American Nurses Publishing.

Index

A

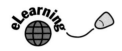

CRITICAL THINKING ACTIVITIES

1. What are the advantages of public health nurses working in the private health sector?

2. Compare the role of the public health nurse of today with that of public health nurses at the turn of the 20th century. What are the challenges common to both roles?

3. Using the three priorities of prevention, protection, and health promotion identified by Dr. Salmon in her model "Construct for Public Health Nursing," give examples from your own practice in community health nursing that illustrate these three priorities.

Explore Community Health Nursing on the web! To learn more about the topics in this chapter, use the passcode provided to access your exclusive web site: http://communitynursing.jbpub.com
If you do not have a passcode, you can obtain one at this site.

REFERENCES

American Nurses Association (ANA). (1991, June). *Nursing's agenda for health care reform: Executive summary*. Washington, DC: Author.

American Nurses Association (ANA). (1980). *ANA social policy statement*. Washington, DC: Author

American Public Health Association (APHA). (1996, March). *The definition and role of public health nursing. A statement of the Public Health Nursing Section*. Washington, DC: American Public Health Association.

Anderson, E. T., & McFarlane, J. M. (1966). *Community as a partner: Theory and practice in nursing*. Philadelphia: JB Lippincott.

Association of Community Health Nursing Educators (ACHNE). (1995). *Essential of baccalaureate education for community health nursing*. Louisville, KY: University of Kentucky.

Association of State and Territorial Directors of Nursing. (1998). *Partners for progress*. Unpublished work.

Bender, K. (1995). Staphylococcus food poisoning in a university cafeteria. In Soule, B., Larson, E. L., & Preston, G. A. (Eds.), *Infections and nursing practice*. St. Louis: Mosby.

Centers for Disease Control and Prevention (CDC). (1989, June 23). Multiple outbreaks of staphylococcal food poisoning caused by canned mushrooms. *Morbidity and Mortality Weekly Report, 38*(24), 1–2.

Hanlon, J. J., & Pickett, G. E. (1974a). Historical perspectives. In *Public health administration and practice* (pp. 22–44). St. Louis: Mosby.

Hanlon, J. J., & Pickett, G. E. (1974b). Community nursing services. In *Public health administration and practice*. St. Louis: Mosby.

Heinrich, J. (1983). Historical perspectives on public health nursing. *Nursing Outlook, 32*(6), 317–320.

Institute of Medicine (IOM). (1988). *The future of public health*. Washington, DC: National Academy Press.

Milbank Memorial Fund Commission. (1976). *Higher education for public health: A report*. New York: Prodist.

Mississippi Department of Archives. (1920–1980).*Correspondence, memoranda, and reports*. Mississippi Department of Health, Record Group 51, Public Health Nursing Division, Vol. 36. Jackson, MS: Author.

Mississippi Department of Archives. (1922–1982). *Historical files*. Mississippi Department of Health, Record Group 51, Public Health Nursing Division, Vol. 317. Jackson, MS: Author.

Salmon, M. E. (1993). Public health nursing: The opportunity of a lifetime. *American Journal of Public Health, 83*(1), 674–675.

Soros, G. (1997). The capitalist threat. *The Atlantic Monthly, 279*(2), 45–58.

White, M. S. (1982, November-December). Construct for public health nursing. *Nursing Outlook, 30*, 527.

Chapter 38

Home Visiting, Home Health, and Hospice Nursing

Karen Saucier Lundy, Karen B. Utterback,
Debra K. Lance, and Mary E. Stainton

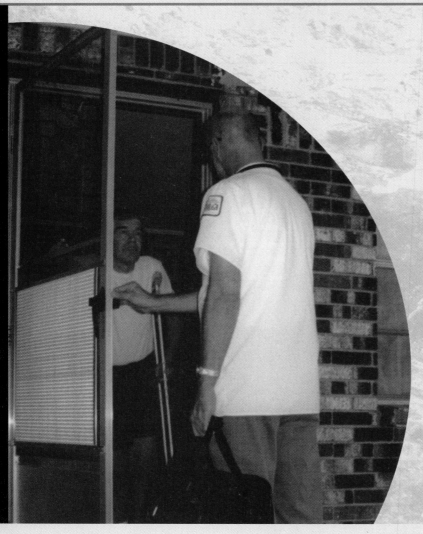

Historically, homes were the earliest practice settings for community health nurses. Clients were seldom in hospitals, but recovered from illness at home and learned about disease prevention and treatment at home; as always, nurses reached out to them. Home health care was established in the latter part of the 19th century, as nursing schools began graduating more and better trained professional nurses. Influencing this movement to home care was the explosion of scientific knowledge about microorganism transmission and communicable disease and the accompanying advancement in technology.